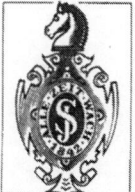

Jiro Suzuki (Ed.)

Advances in Surgery for Cerebral Stroke

Proceedings of the International Symposium on
Surgery for Cerebral Stroke, Sendai 1987

With 318 Figures

Springer Japan KK

Prof. JIRO SUZUKI, M.D.
Division of Neurosurgery
Institute of Brain Diseases
Tohoku University
School of Medicine
Sendai, 980 Japan

ISBN 978-4-431-68316-2   ISBN 978-4-431-68314-8 (eBook)
DOI 10.1007/978-4-431-68314-8

Typesetting: Asco Trade Typesetting Ltd., Hong Kong

Preface

Cerebral stroke is an extremely common disease which strikes suddenly and leaves its victims in a seriously disabled state; its prevention remains a medical problem of the highest priority. Though the techniques for neurosurgical treatment following onset were already considered at the beginning of this century when the first surgical attempts were made, there is still room for significant developments in this area.

Radiography of the cerebral vessels developed by Moniz in 1927 and the subsequent widespread use of angiography have gradually led to neurosurgical treatment of cerebral aneurysms, arteriovenous malformations, and other vascular abnormalities, but many unresolved problems remain.

Computed tomography and microsurgical techniques have become major weapons in the surgeon's armory and notable advances have been made in the surgical therapy of cerebral infarction and hypertensive intracerebral hemorrhage. However, the surgical treatment of cerebral stroke—whether due to aneurysm, AVM, or other mechanisms—has been limited to therapy during the chronic stage following onset; even today, surgical therapy for stroke is not universally accepted as appropriate.

Nonetheless, toward the possibility of acute-stage treatment of cerebral stroke, further progress has been made possible by the emergence of magnetic resonance imaging, positron-emission tomography, and digital subtraction angiography, as well as advances in intravascular neurosurgery and the development of brain-protective agents. It has now become possible to save the lives of stroke victims in the acute stage following onset and to obtain favorable functional recovery.

In the light of these recent developments, in May 1987 a symposium was held in Sendai, Japan, devoted to the surgical treatment of stroke, in which some 1000 neurosurgeons from 45 countries around the world participated. The scale and success of that symposium testify to the extent of the interest and expectations of neurosurgeons throughout the world concerning developments in this direction.

With the help of the many participants, we have also been able to produce this volume of the symposium proceedings. It goes without saying that the speed with which the proceedings have been completed has been due to the enthusiasm of the speakers and discussants; however, special thanks must also be expressed to the staff of Springer-Verlag, who have encouraged and promoted this undertaking from the outset, and to the two Sendai neurosurgeons, Dr. Motonobu Kameyama and Prof. Takashi Yoshimoto, whose tireless efforts have made this volume possible. This project has been executed with a grant from the Commemorative Association for the Japan World Exposition.

Following the considerable achievements of surgery for stroke as of 1987, it is our sincere hope that neurosurgeons will be able to make still further contributions to the treatment of this disease, which threatens the lives of so many people throughout the world.

Sendai, Japan, March 1988   JIRO SUZUKI

Table of Contents

RTD 3. Bypass Surgery

RTD 4. Nonsurgical Treatment for AVMs

RTD 5. Scientific Basis for Cerebral Infarction

Part 3. Selected Papers

Part 1. Special Lectures

New Brain Protective Agents and Clinical Use

Jiro Suzuki[1]

It has long been held that if the cerebral blood flow is stopped for only 3–5 min, the recovery of brain cells in the region of the occlusion is already impossible.

Hypothermic anesthesia was effective in prolonging the permissible time for occlusion of cerebral vessels in my experiences in aneurysmal surgery.

However, hypothermic anesthesia is being attacked due to many difficulties, including the danger of cardiac arrest and the fact that a lengthy period is required both in cooling and rewarming the patient's body temperature. Thus, I had in the back of my mind the thought that there must be some other way to prolong the period for safe vascular occlusion. One day during 1969, a 54-year-old woman was admitted to our clinic suffering from a ruptured MCA aneurysm with severe heart disorders. The anesthetist refused to use hypothermic anesthesia to avoid cardiac complications.

I was mistakenly confident that surgery could be successfully completed on this patient without hypothermic anesthesia. A severe premature rupture occurred during surgery and, in order to treat the neck of the aneurysm, temporary occlusion of the feeding M1 and draining M2 arteries was required for a full 50 min. There was no reason to be optimistic about the recovery of normal brain functions in this patient after 50 min of occlusion. I found her to have normal consciousness and complete control over her arms and legs. I was surprised to see this.

The only possibility was that the 1000 cm³ 20% mannitol, which had been administered immediately before craniotomy to reduce the brain volume, had somehow been effective in prolonging the period of safe vascular occlusion.

This incident was the starting point for what has been more than 15 years of research by trial and error to demonstrate the pharmacological effects of mannitol and to develop new cerebral protective agents.

Using various kinds of animals, we started to attempt to develop the ideal animal models of cerebral infarction which would allow us to demonstrate clearly the effects of mannitol.

It proved, however, to be an extremely difficult task to regularly produce a focus of infarction at the same location, same size, and same grade which, moreover, could be controlled in an animal which would survive for many days following production of the infarction. At last, using a unilateral temporal approach at the base of the brain of the dog, all four vessels, namely the internal carotid artery, the anterior and middle cerebral arteries, and the posterior communicating artery, were occluded under a surgical microscope. Then, a focus of infarction confined to the anterior portion of the thalamus was developed on the side of the vascular occlusion (Fig. 1). Soon we found that, if an EEG electrode were inserted into the focus in the anterior thalamus, it was possible to identify only those animals which showed extreme EEG changes. In this way, 100% of the animals used

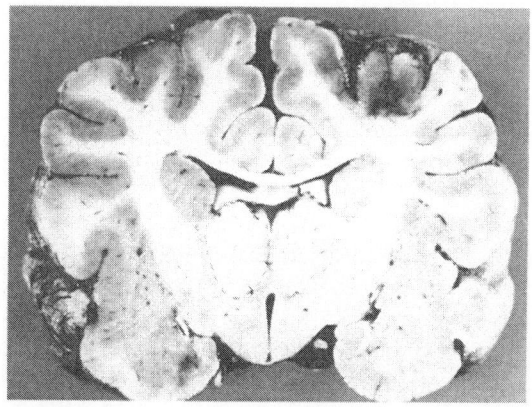

Fig. 1. Focus of infarction confined to anterior portion of thalamus

[1] Division of Neurosurgery, Institute of Brain Diseases, Tohoku University School of Medicine, Sendai, Japan

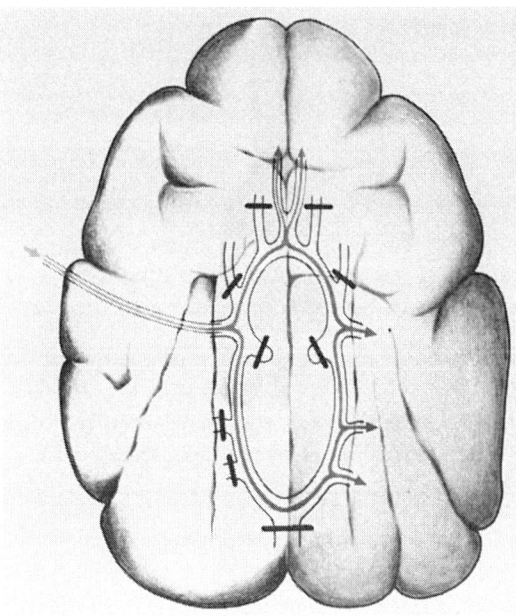

Fig. 2. Separation of circulation to the brain from the systemic circulation by occlusion

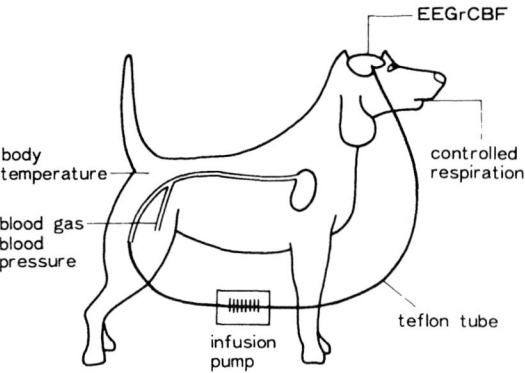

Fig. 3. Schema of infusion pump

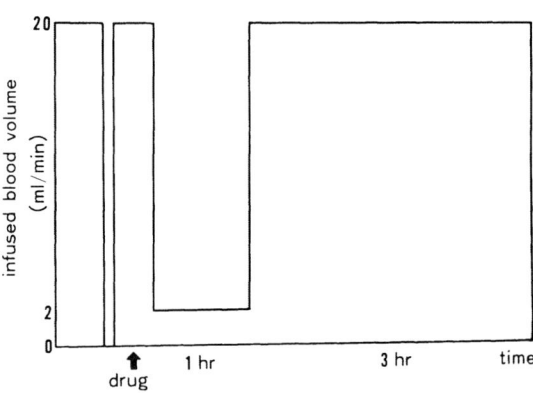

Fig. 4. Program of the experiment

in any given experiment could be prepared with infarctic foci confined to that region of the brain.

We, the many neurosurgeons in Sendai, have done many animal experiments and clinical data about the capability of brain protection of 20% mannitol and have reported our results in numerous papers [1]. However, it was still totally unclear what mechanisms were involved in mannitol's ability to suppress cerebral infarction. It worked, but the effective mechanism was not known. Since I was already aware that mannitol is a known free radical scavenger of OH radicals, it was apparent that, if mannitol's free radical scavenger action were the cause of the suppression of cerebral infarction, then similar effects should be obtainable from many other known free radical scavengers.

The animal model to test the protective effects on the brain of many available drugs was one using the dog, where, using a unilateral temporal approach, all of the trunk arteries at the base of the brain are identified under a surgical microscope and no damage to the brain itself is brought about.

As shown in Fig. 2, by means of occlusion of a combination of these vessels at the base of the brain, circulation to the brain can be entirely separated from the systemic circulation.

Using a narrow cannula inserted into a unilateral middle cerebral artery (MCA) and connected to the femoral artery through a perfusion pump, it is possible to gain full control over the flow of blood to an entire cerebral hemisphere. In other words, when the pump is switched off, blood flow falls to zero, and, when the pump is accelerated, the blood flow increases (Fig. 3).

The first step in the experiments was, therefore, to turn the pump off, observe the rapid attenuation of all electrical activity of the brain, and thereby confirm that cerebral blood flow is occurring through the pump. Circulation to the brain was of course then restored to its original level and the drugs under study were administered systemically.

Thereafter, cerebral blood flow was reduced to 10% its normal value and a state of extreme cerebral ischemia was maintained for 1 h. After 1 h had elapsed, blood flow was returned to normal for 3 h and the changes in electrical activity were monitored (Fig. 4). The effectiveness of the drugs was then evaluated from the level of electrical activity after the completion of 3 h of

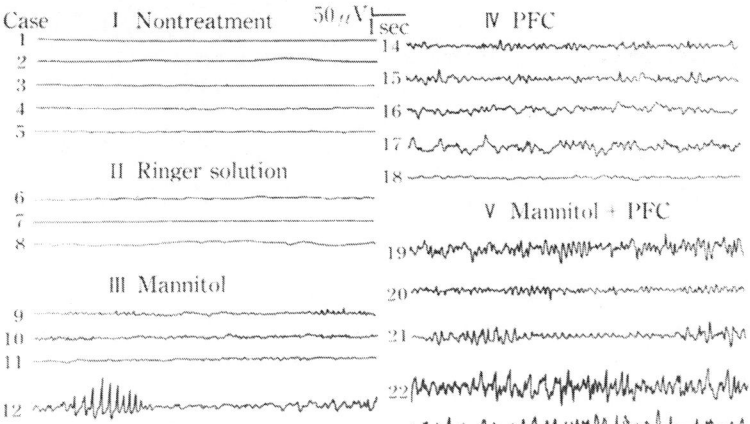

Fig. 5. Summary of results with EEG

Table 1. Summary of results

	Grade 0	Grade 1	Grade 2	Grade 3	Grade 4
Nontreatment	6	1	—	—	—
Mannitol	—	—	2	1	2
Vitamin E					
100 mg/kg p.o.	1	—	2	2	1
30 mg/kg i.r.	—	—	—	1	2
10 mg/kg i.r.	1	2	1	—	1
DMSO	—	—	—	1	1
Vitamin C	1	3	1	—	—
Glycerol	—	3	—	—	—
Dexa	—	2	2	1	—
Y-9179	2	1	1	1	—
MY-103	—	2	—	2	1
Vitamin E + Dexa + Mannitol	—	—	—	—	3
PFC + Vitamin E + Dexa + Mannitol	—	—	—	—	5

Numbers are the numbers of experimental dogs

recirculation.

It was found that the electrical activity was completely flat in all animals which had been administered Ringer's solution or nothing at all (Fig. 5). In contrast, some EEG activity remained following 20% mannitol administration and the electrical activity was shown more actively in animals administered mannitol and perfluorochemicals (PFC). Little positive effect was brought about by glycerol, but dexamethasone had some effect. We have thus far studied a variety of drugs said to be free radical scavengers and have found that not only mannitol, but several drugs have protective effects on the brain. Particularly noteworthy have been the surprisingly good effects of combined therapy with mannitol, vitamin E, and dexamethasone (Table 1). These results have led to the hypothesis that mannitol's effects are due specifically to its action as a free radical scavenger.

We were first obliged to demonstrate whether or not the free radical reaction actually occurs during infarction. For this purpose we used a chemiluminescence method in which the emission of relevant photons was shown ($^1O_2 \rightarrow {}^3O_2$ with the emission of $h\nu$ photon). We then investigated whether or not these free radical scavengers—mannitol, vitamin E, and the steroids—can suppress photon emission.

We developed a rat infarction model in which severe, global ischemia was produced for these experiments in a chemiluminescence method. This rat model involved the occlusion of basilar artery at the base of the brain and the application of an aneurysm clip to the bilateral common carotid arteries. By controlling the duration of the temporary clipping on bilateral common carotid arteries, it was possible to freely produce many kinds of conditions of cerebral ischemia.

In comparison with the four-vessel occlusion

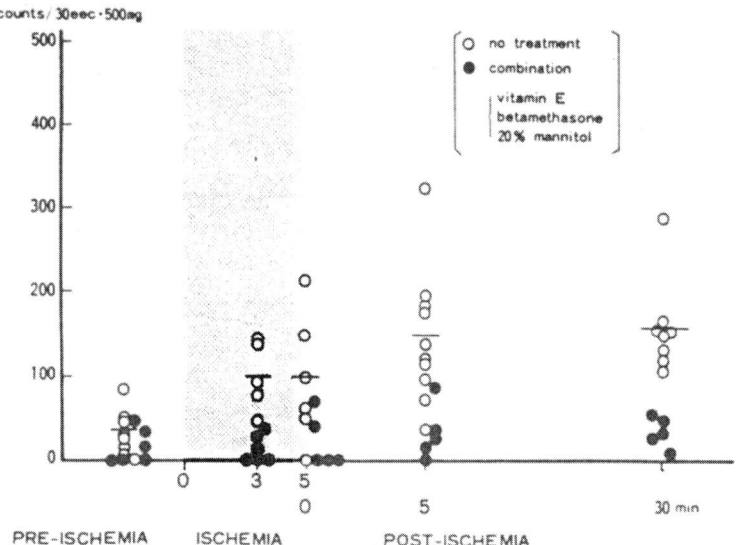

model developed by Pulsinelli and used widely throughout the world, we have found our rat infarction model to be vastly superior [1].

Using our model, photon emissions due to the free radical reaction were already apparent after 5 min of vascular occlusion. Following recirculation, the photon count increased further. These findings indicate that the free radical reaction occurs in the early period of ischemia and shows a marked, transient increase due to the increased supply of oxygen following recirculation (Fig. 6).

When the above three drugs—which we nicknamed the Sendai Cocktail—were administered prior to ischemia, the number of photons were suppressed throughout the entire course of the experiment. In this way, the scavenger effects of these drugs were clearly demonstrated.

We have also performed experiments in which mice were placed in a hypoxic chamber with 4% oxygen and 96% nitrogen. In the untreated control animals and ones treated by some drugs, all died within 3 min of the start of the hypoxia. But I was particularly impressed by the fact that all animals, showed convulsions prior to death (Fig. 7).

We then tried pretreatment with the anticonvulsant, Aleviatin, namely phenytoin, before placing the mice in the hypoxic chamber and, sure enough, they survived for 60 min or more. I was truly surprised at this finding.

We then performed ischemia experiments using the perfusion pump model in dogs, identical to that which I have already introduced. Surprisingly, phenytoin was found to be more

effective, due to dose-dependency, than any of the drugs we had previously tried. Also, we could prove by the chemiluminescence method that phenytoin is not a free radical scavenger and it will be effective as a stabilizer of cell membranes. Administering what we have called Sendai Cocktail, that is, mannitol, vitamin E, and phenytoin, the protective effects of this cocktail on the ischemic brain have been remarkably good, with nearly complete suppression of brain edema in all dogs. We currently use the Sendai Cocktail—which contains 10 ml 20% mannitol, 10 mg vitamin E, and 10 mg phenytoin per kg—which we believe to be the most effective combination of drugs at the present time in protecting the brain from the cerebral ischemia (Fig. 8).

I would like to explain in more detail about the pharmacological effects of Sendai Cocktail. If cerebral blood flow is reduced to 30% of the normal level with recirculation at 5.5 h from the starting of ischemia, already brain electrical activity is permanently affected (Fig. 9).

In contrast, if this Cocktail is given 30 min from the start of 30% ischemia, there is some electrical activity even during 30% ischemia. Then, if cerebral blood flow is returned to full capacity again at 5.5 h from the start of the ischemia and Cocktail is given every 2 h, there is a remarkable recovery of electrical activity which is sustained for at least 10 h (Fig. 10).

If blood flow is reduced to 30% and the Cocktail is given within 1 h following the start of the ischemia, there is recovery of the EEG, but there is not recovery if 2 h of ischemia have elapsed

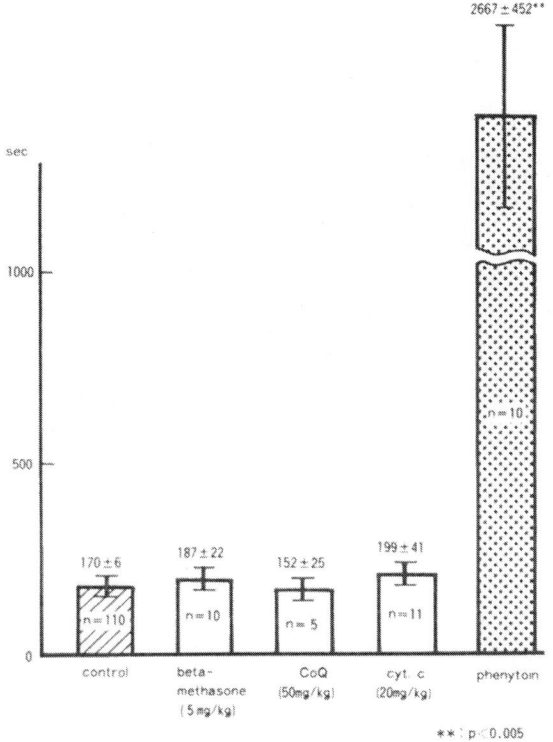

Fig. 7. Effect of phenytoin on survival time

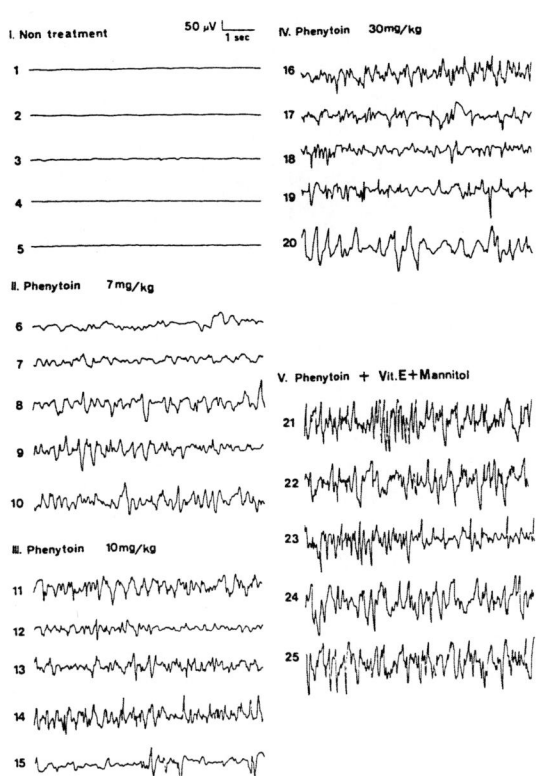

Fig. 8. Effect of different concentrations of phenytoin and Sendai Cocktail

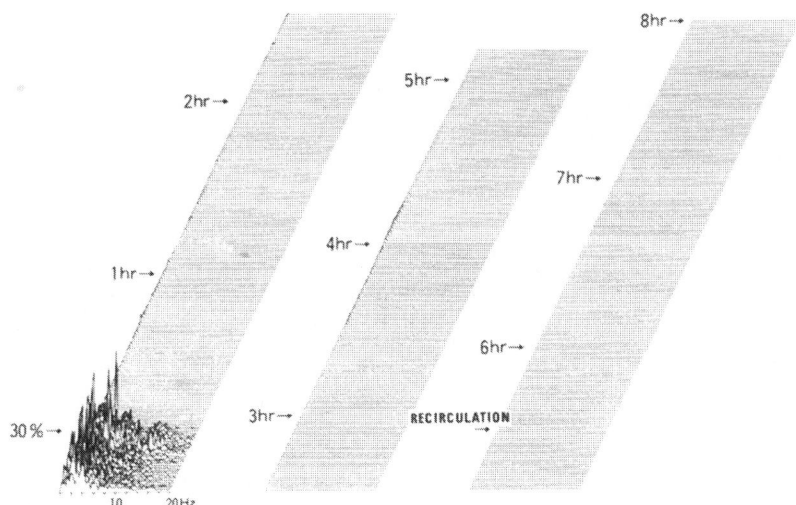

Fig. 9. Effect of recirculation in untreated controls (30% ischemia)

without Cocktail. I believe if the start of the administration of Cocktail is delayed, the brain will not be able to recover.

Using our infarction model controlled by a perfusion pump at will, the relationship between the level of cerebral blood flow and the duration of the ischemia can be demonstrated.

In the case of 10% of the normal level of CBF, the critical irreversible point of EEG from the start of ischemia is at 20 min in the untreated cases and at 60 min in Cocktail cases. Namely, the critical time is, prolonged to 60 min from 20 min by Cocktail in the cases of 10% of the normal CBF (Fig. 11).

In the case of 20% ischemia, this critical period is at 30 min in the control group and 120 min

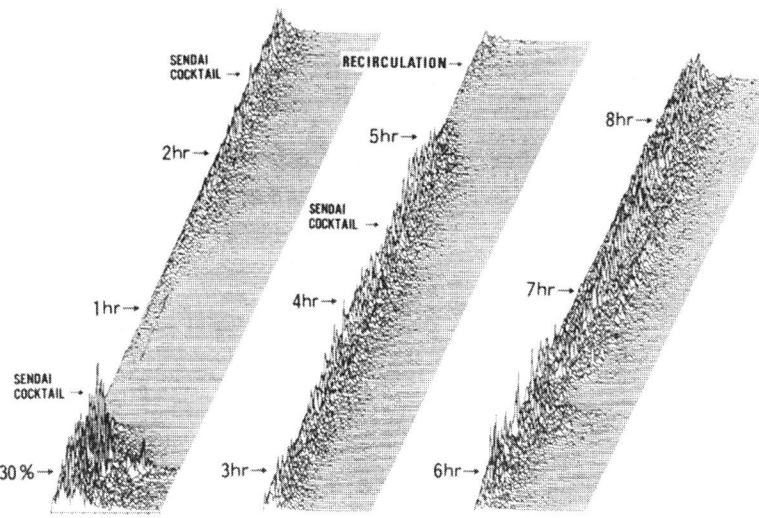

Fig. 10. Effect of recirculation in treated group (30% ischemia)

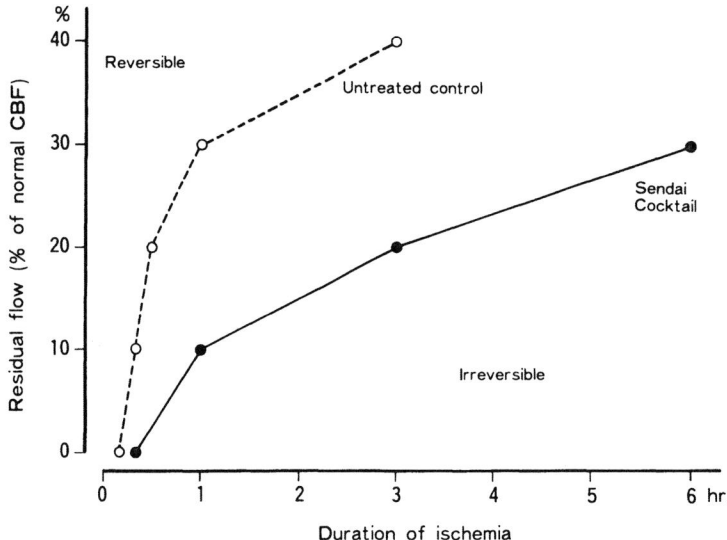

Fig. 11. Functional recovery of ischemic brain as related to degree and duration of ischemia

in the Cocktail group; at 30% ischemia, 60 min in the control group and 360 min in the Cocktail group. I believe you can see the effectiveness of this Cocktail in the respective ischemia grades.

How long after the administration of the Sendai Cocktail will it still have protective effects? Within its effective period, how long a period of vascular occlusion can the brain withstand? That is, when one dose of Sendai Cocktail is administered to a 50-kg patient over a period of 30 min, the drug will be effective for a period of about 100 min: during that 100-min period, any combination of intracerebral vessels can be temporarily occluded for a period of up to 40 min. When still longer vascular occlusion is required to complete the surgical operation, 5 min of re-

circulation is necessary following 40 min of occlusion; then up to 40 min of vascular occlusion can be allowed again. If this period of vascular occlusion exceeds the 100-min effective period, a further dose of Cocktail must be given. I have performed radical surgery on more than 2000 cases of ruptured cerebral aneurysm by my own hands, many of which were in the acute period following onset. More than 1500 cases of them were operated upon using mannitol and Cocktails which were developed by us (Table 2).

The clinical technique using the Cocktail which I currently use is as follows (Fig. 12): Immediately prior to making a direct approach to the aneurysm, the Cocktail is administered. The feeding and draining arteries of the aneurysm are then identified and temporarily

Table 2. Aneurysm site and surgical results

Site	No. of cases	Excellent	Good	Fair	Poor	Dead
AcomA	651	406	109	64	39	33 (5.1%)
ICA	455	286	78	35	32	24 (5.3%)
MCA	368	225	63	42	26	12 (3.3%)
ACA	86	61	7	6	8	4 (4.7%)
V-BA	68	32	13	7	10	6 (8.8%)
Multiple	372	188	83	43	24	34 (9.1%)
Total	2000	1198	353	197	139	113 (5.7%)

AcomA anterior communicating artery, *ICA* internal carotid artery, *MCA* middle cerebral artery, *ACA* anterior cerebral artery, *V-BA* vertebro-basilar artery

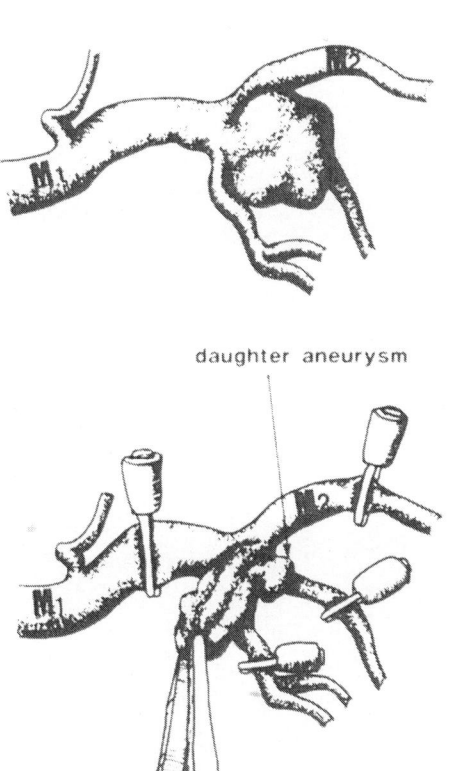

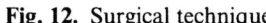

daughter aneurysm

Fig. 12. Surgical technique

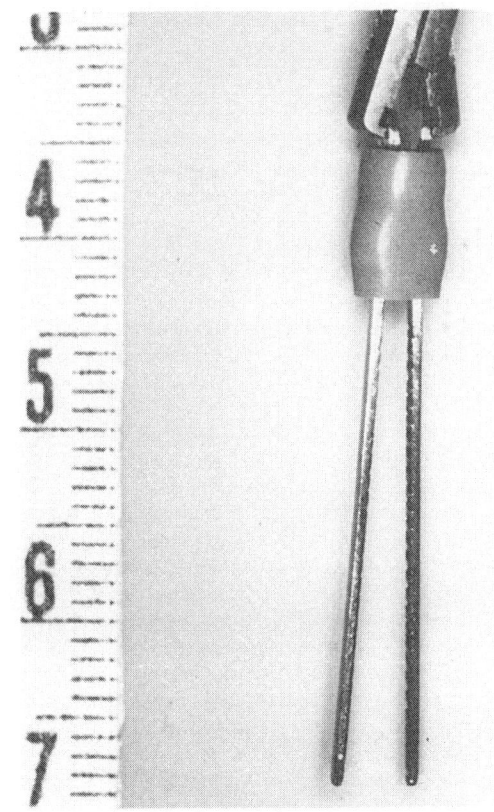

Fig. 13. Jiro's temporary clip

occluded to bring the pressure within the aneurysm to zero, applying temporary clips to all feeding and draining arteries of the aneurysm. Dissection of the aneurysm itself can then be done quickly and safely.

The temporary clip must have a weak blade pressure of about 40 g. A long, Jiro's temporary clip is 24 mm in length and 40 g (Fig. 13). This temporary clip is very convenient to put on and take off from the deeply seated artery. Because this clip is long the tip of the clip can be picked up

from any direction easily during the surgery, it is well-suited for this procedure. As the intra-aneurysmal pressure will decrease to zero by temporal clipping on both feeders and drainers of the aneurysm, the aneurysm itself can be grasped with a pincet and the area behind the aneurysm neck can be observed with certainty without overlooking the presence of a daughter aneurysm, or another important artery lying immediately behind the aneurysm. With this technique, treatment of the aneurysm can be

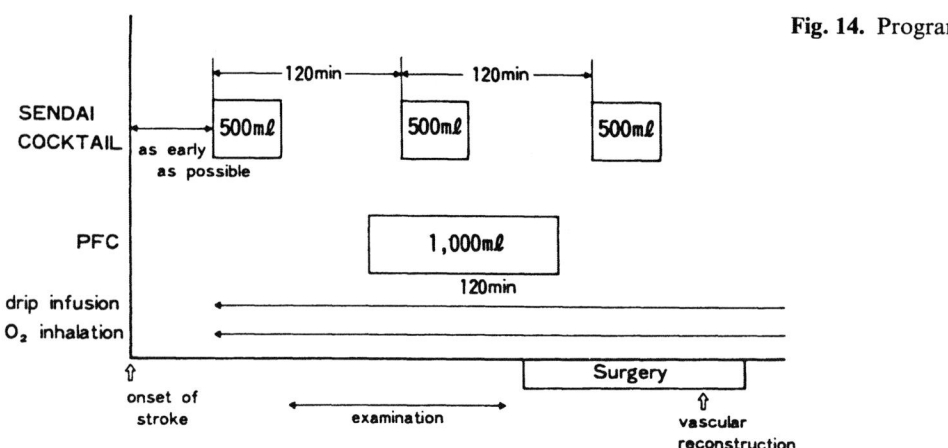

Fig. 14. Program of treatment

Table 3. EC-IC bypass for progressing stroke under administration of Sendai Cocktail

Case no.	Age (years)	Sex	Angiographic finding	Preoperative most severe paresis		Speech disturbance	Onset to refbw (days)	Result
				Arm	Leg			
1	29	F	rt. IC occl	3	4	−	4	Ex
2	51	M	rt. IC sten	3	4	−	5	Ex
3	50	M	lt. IC sten	2	3	+	5	Ex
4	58	M	lt. IC occl	4	2	+	2	Ex
5	64	M	Lt. M_3 steb	4	4	+	4	Ex
6	54	M	rt. M_1 occl	3	4	−	2	Ex
7	52	M	rt. M_1 occl	4	4	−	1	Ex
8	58	M	lt. M_1 occl	2	2	−	2	G
9	61	M	lt. M_1 sten	4	4	+	6	G
10	57	M	rt. M_{1-2} sten	1	4	−	3	G
11	61	M	lt. M_1 occl	2	3	+	1	G
12	62	M	lt. M_2 occl	3	3	+	9	G
13	57	M	rt. IC occl	3	4	−	5	G
14	41	M	lt. M_1 sten	2	2	−	5	G
15	69	F	rt. M_2 occl	2	3	−	2	F
16	51	M	lt. M_1 occl	2	2	+	2	F
17	71	M	rt. M_1 sten	4	4	+	6	F
18	59	M	lt. IC occl	2	3	+	8	D

Ex excellent, *G* good, *F* fair, *D* dead

done more quickly and more safely.

Recently, we have wedged a balloon catheter into various small cerebral arteries via the femoral artery and then inflated the balloon to occlude the arteries temporarily using the Cocktail. Thus, I could perform upon the successful excision of a partially thrombosed giant aneurysm on the basilar artery. At first, this aneurysm shadow disappeared in angiography by occlusion using a balloon at the top of the basilar artery. Though I could not see any feeders to the aneurysm behind the giant aneurysm in the operative field, I could resect the aneurysm without bleeding due to the balloon, then could perform the successful neck clipping. Occlusion time of the basilar artery was 40 min. The patient's course was uneventful after the operation.

I have also succeeded in the total excision of a large, subtentorial arteriovenous (AV) malformation by using two balloon catheters to occlude blood flow of the feeders from the basilar artery. Occlusion time of the arteries was 40 min.

We have also used the Cocktail to suppress the progress of cerebral infarction in the very early period following the onset of the infarction. We then identify in cerebral angiograms those vessels which have occluded and proceed immediately to bypass surgery and/or embolectomy. Of course, if the patient had no indication for the surgery, we chose some conservative treatment (Fig. 14).

Good results have been obtained in this way compared with cases without such treatment. Yoshimoto's paper in the round table discussion of this problem shows the details of our results.

When, however, the administration of the Cocktail has been delayed and there has already appeared a low density area in CT scans, there is the fear of hemorrhagic infarction and severe brain edema after the recanalization by both surgery and medication, and we believe that already the opportunity for embolectomy or bypass surgery has been lost.

Therefore, I believe that the cases suffering from cerebral infarction have to be managed as first class emergency cases in their very acute stage.

In the case of slow progressive cerebral infarction, when symptoms are taking a slow, down-hill course, effective therapy can be obtained by using Sendai Cocktails and then performing bypass surgery or thromboendarterectomy.

I can therefore confidently recommend this therapeutic method in cases of slow progressive stroke. Only one patient of 18 cases treated by our method was lost by cardiac complication after the surgery (Table 3).

As I have outlined here, my colleagues and I have spent some 18 years in the development of new cerebral protective agents and have used them clinically with good results in many cases of cerebral aneurysm, AV malformation and recently in the acute stage of cerebral infarction.

By means of further study and clinical application, it will undoubtedly be possible to establish even better therapeutic techniques for those cases of acute stage cerebral infarction which have not previously been suitable for both medical and surgical treatment. By so doing, we will be able to not only make genuine advances in the treatment of acute stage cerebral infarction, but also further expand the indication of effective neurosurgical treatment for other cerebral diseases.

Reference

1. Suzuki J (1987) Treatment of cerebral infarction. Springer Vienna New York

Ischemic Neural Lesions in Cerebral Stroke

Keiji Sano[1]

Ischemic Lesions in Subarachnoid Hemorrhage (SAH)

When hemorrhage occurs in the subarachnoid space, intracranial pressure (ICP) inevitably rises, dependent upon the amount and distribution of the subarachnoid blood [30, 31].

The ICP changes associated with aneurysmal rupture have been incidentally recorded at the time of rebleeding in SAH patients under continuous ICP monitoring [31]. Two different pressure patterns were found in patients who had verified recurrent hemorrhages. One was associated with massive hematoma while the other occurred with edema but only minimal hematoma; the terms "hemorrhagic-compressive lesion: SAH type II" and "ischemic-edematous lesion: SAH type I" have been used for these two conditions.

In SAH type I, a majority of rebleedings were arrested at epidural pressure (EDP) levels of approximately the diastolic blood pressure. The EDP then returned to considerably lower levels within minutes. In SAH type II, the ICP approached the systolic blood pressure and both aneurysm leakage and cerebral blood flow (CBF) were arrested, usually leading to death within hours. It was suggested that those pressure patterns were determined by factors such as the volume of extravasated blood, the vasomotor reaction, and the intracranial spatial buffering capacity [30].

The ICP elevation following aneurysmal rupture was shown to be of such an extent as to temporarily exceed the diastolic blood pressure [30, 31].

CBF is determined by the formula:

$$CBF = k \times PP/CVR = k \times (SAP - ICP)/CVR$$

in which PP is perfusion pressure, CVR is cerebrovascular resistance, k is constant, and SAP is systemic arterial pressure [27].

This formula indicates that the brain is exposed to severe global ischemia when the ICP is extremely elevated following aneurysmal rupture. Although this global ischemia appears to play an important role in the occurrence of acute ischemic neurological deficits, its exact evaluation as to the severity and duration has been difficult to perform in clinical situations. For the purpose of investigating the initial ischemic event following SAH, we undertook an experiment using an animal SAH model [4].

SAH was induced by extraction of a needle (4-0 atraumatic needle with thread) previously inserted into the intracranial portion of the internal carotid artery; cerebrospinal fluid (CSF) leakage during the experiment was strictly avoided. The animal (adult mongrel dog) was initially anesthetized with halothane inhalation during the operative procedure. Then the dog was immobilized with gallamine infusion and mechanical ventilation was instituted. The regional cortical blood flow (rCBF) measured by the use of a thermocouple, epidural pressure (EDP), cisterna magna pressure (CMP), systemic arterial pressure (SAP), and electroencephalogram (EEG) were continuously monitored during the experiment. Three hours after induction of SAH, the brain was perfused with a mixed solution of formalin and carbon black solution to examine the state of cerebral microcirculation.

With this SAH model, ICP patterns very similar to those in human SAH were reproduced. Further, the concomitant changes in other parameters, such as rCBF, SAP, and EEG, were recorded. The ICP patterns obtained could be divided into two types. In pattern I, ICP rose abruptly near the arterial diastolic pressure, stayed there for several minutes, and then gradually fell to a level slightly higher than normal. The time course of rCBF was almost a mirror image of that of ICP, except that there was an

[1] Department of Neurosurgery, Teikyo University School of Medicine, Tokyo, Japan

overshoot before returning to the original level. The magnitude and duration of this rCBF overshoot tended to be more pronounced as the ICP elevation was greater. EEG activity was invariably suppressed while ICP was elevated, but it gradually improved as rCBF showed an overshoot and then came back to a normal level. However, at 3 h after SAH, EEG still showed some slowing. In pattern II, ICP elevation was so severe and prolonged that rCBF remained depressed during the experiment and there was no recovery of EEG activity. In most cases, a marked elevation of SAP (Cushing reflex) occurred. This caused a further elevation of ICP, but did not help to improve the depressed rCBF.

Three hours after induction of SAH, the brain was perfused with carbon black solution and perfusion defects were examined in coronally cut brain slices. To our surprise, perfusion defects of variable extent were found in a high percentage of SAH type I animals (20 of 26). Their distribution was always symmetrical and showed a predilection for localization in the thalamus, basal ganglia, and cortical arterial boundary zones, conforming to the pattern of no-reflow phenomenon (NRP) originally reported by Ames et al. [1]. In the majority of the SAH type II animals, the area of nonfilling in the cerebral hemispheres was quite extensive, sparing a small area in the region of the hypothalamus. The infratentorial structures showed good filling even in this condition. These results suggest that, compared to other types of transient global ischemia, SAH is particularly liable to develop NRP. However, since the ischemia observed in SAH type I was not extended much (within 10 min), being followed by an immediate reactive hyperemia in the cortical area, it seems possible that what we observed was not real NRP but delayed hypoperfusion. The ICP patterns I and II of our SAH model corresponded quite well to SAH type I and II as described by Nornes [30], respectively. It may be emphasized that moment to moment alterations of ICP and CBF corresponded well with each other. CBF changes occurred as predicted by the above formula, except for the overshoot in pattern I. This overshoot of rCBF represents reactive hyperemia, which is known to occur following a temporary increase of the CSF pressure. The results of our experiment support Nornes's view that the pressure patterns following aneurysmal rupture show the whole range from full spatial compensation (SAH type I) to total decompensation (SAH type II) [30]. This

Table 1. SAH due to aneurysm rupture (acute stage)

Amount and Distribution of Blood
  Increased ICP
  AIND (acute ischemic neurological deficit)
    →Patient's Conditions (Grades)
    Transient global ischemia, impaired autoregulation, decrease in CBF, systemic hypertensive (Cushing) response, vascular engorgement, brain swelling, microcirculatory disturbance, selective vulnerability of the brain, etc.
  Delayed Cerebral Vasospasm
    →DIND (delayed ischemic neurological deficit)
Sites of hemorrhage ⎤
Acute hydrocephalus ⎬ →Grades
Intracerebral hematoma ⎦
Rebleeding
Patient's other pathological conditions
Age

ICP intracranial pressure

increased ICP heralds a series of symptoms which may be termed direct effects of SAH or acute ischemic neurological deficits (AINDs) (Table 1). AINDs include transient global ischemia, impaired autoregulation, decrease in cerebral blood flow (CBF), systemic hypertensive response or Cushing response, vascular engorgement of the brain, brain swelling, microcirculatory disturbance, excessive release of excitatory neurotransmitters to cause neuronal hypermetabolism in decreased CBF resulting in selective vulnerability of the brain. AINDs also affect the vascular reactivity which may contribute to the development of delayed vasospasm. AINDs influence the neurological conditions of the patient which can be expressed as grades. If the status of a patient with SAH is in a good grade, such as grade I of Hunt, it means the patient has minimal AIND. Grades III, IV, or V imply that AINDs are of a considerable or severe degree. Recent evidence suggests that oxygen-derived free radicals may be abundantly produced in ischemic tissues, accounting for at least part of the damage that results [12, 28].

When the subarachnoid clot is of a considerable amount, delayed cerebral vasospasm or arterial spasm will occur around a week or so after SAH, accompanied by neurological symptoms or delayed ischemic neurological deficits (DINDs).

This vasospasm and DIND, the so-called direct effect of SAH or AIND, and, thirdly, rebleeding of aneurysms are the three greatest causes of mortality and morbidity in SAH patients. According to Kassell and Torner [18], among the causes of disability and death in 1272 patients with SAH, vasospasm comprises 33.5%, direct effect 25.5%, and rebleeding 17.3%.

Since the most influential factors on the outcome of SAH patients are rebleeding, cerebral vasospasm, and direct effects of subarachnoid blood, the most essential therapies of SAH patients are prevention of rebleeding of aneurysms, prevention or treatment of cerebral vasospasm, and, if possible, lessening the direct effects of SAH.

Theoretically, rebleeding can be prevented by clipping of aneurysms in the very early stage [46]. Concurrent intracerebral hematomas can also be removed by early surgery. Acute hydrocephalus, if present, can be treated by ventricular drainage or shunting. Thus, there may be a possibility of decreasing the direct effects of SAH, at least to some extent. Then cerebral vasospasm comes to stand in our way as the toughest problem to struggle with in the treatment of aneurysmal SAH.

Late or chronic cerebral vasospasm or more exactly, the arterial spasm which appears in 40%–80% of SAH cases, or in about 45% of the cases remaining through the 2nd week of SAH of our series [41], exerts a crucial influence on the mortality and morbidity of the patients.

This arterial spasm has several characteristics. First, it usually appears after some time lag from the onset of subarachnoid hemorrhage (SAH) [41, 42]. In our studies, it appeared first on day 4 (the day of SAH being day 0) and, on the average, on day 7.6 ± 2.5 in the natural course. Even postoperative vasospasm appeared with nearly the same interval from the onset of SAH, namely, on the average, on day 6.7 ± 1.6. Second, there is a close correlation between the development of vasospasm and subarachnoid clots, as pointed out by many investigators [40]. One may say, "without subarachnoid clots, no vasospasm." Third, in arteries of the other parts of the body which have bled, there is no sustained arterial contraction comparable to chronic cerebral vasospasm.

Vasospasm As a Deficiency Syndrome

Any theory concerning the pathogenesis of the vasospasm should be able to explain these characteristics. In the late 1970s, Asano, Tanishima, Sasaki, and their co-workers in my department fostered an idea that cerebral vasospasm might be caused by free radical reactions and subse-

quent lipid peroxidation initiated by clot lysis [6, 44, 48, 61].

All parts of the body are provided with manifold defense mechanisms against free radicals, especially active oxygen species (hydrogen peroxide H_2O_2, hydroxyl radical $\cdot OH$, superoxide anion $O_2 \cdot^-$, singlet oxygen $^1O_2$) which are generated in the reduction process of oxygen molecules. These defense mechanisms, however, are very poor in the brain tissue [9] or almost undetectable in the CSF of the higher mammals, including man.

For instance, the glutathione peroxidase level in the human serum is 0.126 ± 0.014 unit/ml, whereas that in the human CSF is 0.003 ± 0.001 unit/ml. Vitamin E is measured as 0.77 mg/dl in the human serum and is undetectable in the human CSF; catalase is 0.054 unit/min per ml in the human serum and undetectable in the CSF. These substances are known as potent free radical scavengers, or antioxidants, found in most tissues. We believe one of the adverse phenomena caused by this lack of free radical scavengers in the CSF is chronic or delayed cerebral vasospasm discussed here [43, 44, 47]. Therefore, cerebral vasospasm can be regarded as a sort of deficiency syndrome—due to deficient defense mechanisms in the CSF. This view has recently been shared also by other authors [51].

When bleeding occurs in the subarachnoid space, hemolysis soon occurs and oxyhemoglobin (oxyHb) is liberated. Upon conversion of oxyHb to methemoglobin, superoxide anion is released [29], which, in turn, directly or indirectly through hydroxyl radical, singlet oxygen, or alkoxyl radical, initiates free radical reactions such as peroxidation of polyunsaturated fatty acids (PUFAs) in the biomembrane. PUFAs are known to be most susceptible to free radical attacks. It is also known that some degradation products of hemoglobin, such as hematin, iron ions, and methemoglobin, possess a powerful catalytic action in the conversion of PUFAs to their peroxidized forms, namely, hydro- and endoperoxides. Besides, leukocytes, which usually are found in and around subarachnoid clots, may also produce activated oxygen species such as superoxide. Therefore, it seems reasonable to assume that hemolysis triggers free radical reactions leading to lipid peroxidation.

As is well known, superoxide is converted by superoxide dismutase (SOD) to hydrogen peroxide in normal conditions. Hydrogen peroxide is finally inactivated by catalase or glutathione peroxidase. However, if these enzymatic activities are lowered or if iron (Fe^{2+}, Fe^{3+}) complexes are present, superoxide and hydrogen peroxide produce very active singlet oxygen and hydroxyl radicals by the so-called Haber-Weiss reaction. Superoxide may also react with PUFA hydroperoxides, which are present as impurities in PUFAs, to produce alkoxyl radical. These active free radicals, such as hydroxyl radical, singlet oxygen, and alkoxyl radical, are known to react with PUFAs in the biomembrane and produce fatty acid free radicals, which easily combine with oxygen to become lipid peroxide. This step of the reaction produces more free radicals which propagate new reactions. Thus, a chain reaction of lipid peroxidation is initiated.

Unlike other parts of the body, CSF is almost lacking in defense mechanisms (vitamin E, glutathione peroxidase, etc.) against free radicals. During SAH, these defense mechanisms are at first supplied by the extravasated blood itself, but rapidly decrease and, after 3 days, become insufficient to prevent the free radical chain reactions from propagating.

In the CSF of patients with SAH ($n = 32$), it was found that TBA (thiobarbituric acid)-reactive substances had increased, especially in cases which developed vasospasm [6, 48]. The presence of TBA-reactive substances (TRS) has been regarded as representing the presence of lipid peroxides.

The TRS value is, however, an indirect index of lipid peroxides. In order to directly prove lipid peroxidation in SAH, the CSF of a patient with SAH was periodically collected and fractionated using an octadecylsilyl silica column. The fraction eluted with 15% ethanol-water was analyzed by high-performance liquid chromatography (HPLC) detecting at 238 nm (conjugated diene). Several peaks were recognized in accordance with the occurrence of angiographic and symptomatic vasospasm. One of the peaks, which appeared on day 7 after SAH, was identified as 5-hydroxy eicosatetraenoic acid (5-HETE) with the aid of HPLC and gas chromatography-chemical ionization mass spectrometry (GC-MS) by our collaborators. No peak was observed with HPLC corresponding to hydroxy eicosatetraenoic acids (HETEs) or hydroperoxy eicosatetraenoic acids (HPETEs) in the CSF obtained from normal controls (patients with cervical spondylosis).

In ten patients with SAH, semi-quantitative analysis of 5-HETE in the CSF was performed by measuring the peak identified as 5-HETE on HPLC. A close correlation was observed be-

tween the occurrence of cerebral vasospasm (angiographical and symptomatic) and the appearance of 5-HETE in the CSF (in lumbar CSF obtained by lumbar puncture and cisternal CSF obtained by cisternal drainage, especially in the latter) [43]. 5-HETE appeared in the CSF with some time lag after SAH. Identification of 5-HETE indicates formation of its precursor, 5-hydroperoxy eicosatetraenoic acids (5-HPETE), and proves the occurrence of lipid peroxidation in the CSF of SAH patients. This, however, does not exclude the possibility of the formation of H(P)ETEs other than 5-HETE or of prostaglandin endoperoxides and their derivatives, since, in the above examination, analysis of these substances was not technically feasible.

Asano et al. persistently found a large amount of 12-HETE in subarachnoid clots in experimental SAH in dogs. This is understandable because 12-HETE is known to be produced by platelets (human). The precursor of 12-HETE, 12-HPETE, is known to exert stimulatory actions on 5-lipoxygenase which is present in leukocytes (human) or in the arterial wall. This may explain the fact that 5-HETE (5-HPETE) was found in the CSF of SAH patients. 12-HPETE (12-HETE) or 5-HPETE (5-HETE) activates lipoxygenases, constricts arterial smooth muscles, inhibits prostacyclin (PGI_2) synthesis and EDRF (endothelium-derived relaxing factor), and is a chemoattractant for leukocytes and smooth muscle cells. Leukotrienes (LT) which derive from 5-HPETE also have various actions. LTC_4 increases the vascular permeability and LTB_4 stimulates the chemotaxis and the release of superoxide from leukocytes, which is shown to inactivate EDRF. Therefore, almost all features of vasospastic arteries described below are within the spectrum of the known activities of these lipoxygenase products.

Rapid decreases of glutathione peroxidase and vitamin E in the CSF of SAH patients after day 3, and a decrease of PGI_2 in the artery after day 2, as shown by Sasaki et al. [52] in dogs, may well explain the time lag in the appearance of cerebral vasospasm.

We have observed histological changes in patients who died of vasospasm following rupture of intracranial aneurysms, namely subendothelial thickening (the endothelium must have also been damaged, but this was difficult to confirm because of a dropping out of the endothelium) and myonecrotic changes in parts of the media. In experimental models of vasospasm, the most striking changes seen by electron microscopy were also intimal or endothelial changes and some myonecrotic changes in the tunica media. As a matter of fact, the earliest morphological change in experimental SAH was the endothelial damage (granules and vesicles) which appeared from one to several hours after injection of blood into the cistern.

In the experimental evaluation of the "free radical reactions-lipid peroxidation" hypothesis, the link between the generated lipid peroxides and the occurrence of vasospasm has yet to be proved. In this regard, Sasaki et al. [54] showed that cisternal injection of 15-hydroperoxy eicosatetraenoic acid (15-HPETE or 15-HPAA) caused prolonged vasospasm in dogs, which resembled vasospasm following SAH. Electron micrography of those arterial samples revealed disappearance of myofibrils, pyknotic changes of nuclei, and the appearance of vacuoles as well as of electron-dense granules in scattered parts of the tunica media, and, above all, a remarkable destruction of the endothelial cells with thickening of the subendothelial layer and corrugation of the elastic lamina.

These histological changes, especially the endothelial damage, can be regarded as the toxic effects of lipid peroxides, free radical injury, or free radical vasointoxication, because the endothelial changes appear before arterial constriction becomes manifest, and free oxygen radicals, especially hydroxyl radicals, are known to cause endothelial lesions [25].

PGI_2 synthesis in the endothelium must be impaired by this endothelial damage. In addition, lipid hydroperoxides, e.g., 15-HPETE, are well known as inhibitors of the synthesis of PGI_2 from endoperoxides [10]. As stated earlier, peroxidation of PUFAs is increased in SAH. This means an increase in the endoperoxides and hydroperoxides of PUFAs. Endoperoxides become sources of prostaglandin synthesis and, from these, vasoconstrictive thromboxane A_2 (TXA_2), $PGF_{2\alpha}$, D_2, E_2, etc., will be produced. Hydroperoxides inhibit PGI_2 synthesis, resulting in a decrease of PGI_2 in the vessel wall. If there is endothelial damage, platelets in the bloodstream come there to adhere and aggregate, producing TXA_2 and other vasoconstrictive substances. Sasaki et al. [50] found an increase of endothelial permeability or disruption of the blood-arterial wall barrier in the major cerebral arteries following experimental SAH in dogs, allowing infiltration of plasma constituents into the arterial wall.

In the presence of endothelial damage or blood-arterial wall barrier disruption, the artery, being devoid of or deficient in PGI_2 or EDRF, would be exposed to the unopposed vasocontractile action of TXA_2 and of other vasocontractile substances released from the aggregated platelets or other blood elements. The sustained elevation of TXA_2 and other vasoconstrictive substances in the face of decreased PGI_2 and EDRF will inevitably result in a prolonged contraction of cerebral arteries [14].

The CSF, which is a good protector of the brain against mechanical forces, has one defect or fault in its chemical structure; deficiency of free radical scavengers. Cerebral vasospasm is most probably caused by this defect. This fact may remind the readers of Hamlet's words about "men carrying the stamp of one defect whose virtues shall in the general censure take corruption from that particular fault" (*Hamlet*, act I, scene 4).

Vasoconstrictor Agents in the CSF of SAH Patients

It is well documented that the CSF from patients with aneurysmal SAH may induce smooth muscle contraction [7]. However, development of symptomatic vasospasm is not paralleled by an increase in vasoconstrictive activity in the CSF: such activity was shown to be highest in the early stage of SAH when vasospasm had not yet developed. This finding led Brandt et al. [7] to hypothesize that cerebral vasospasm may be due to a disturbance of the protective mechanisms in the arterial wall maintaining normal vessel tone (PGI_2 or its metabolite), even in the presence of vasocontractile substances in the perivascular space. In their experiments using human cerebral artery strips, indomethacin, which inhibits cyclooxygenase and consequently inhibits PGI_2 synthesis, increased the CSF-induced contraction. On the other hand, PGI_2 and its metabolite, 6-keto-PGE_1, reversed the contractions induced by CSF, as well as by norepinephrine, serotonin, and $PGF_{2\alpha}$. These findings are in accordance with our view.

Sasaki tried to identify the vasoconstrictor agents in CSF from patients with SAH [49]. When the CSF of patients with or without vasospasm was applied to isolated canine basilar artery strips, the artery segments showed contraction. In order to identify the vasoconstrictor agents, experiments were done to reverse the

CSF-induced contraction with specific pharmacological antagonists. The contraction was not reversed by methysergide (serotonin blocker), mepyramine (histamine blocker), phenoxybenzamine (blocker of alpha action of norepinephrine), proparanol (blocker of beta action of nerepinephrine), or atropine (acetylcholine blocker). Therefore, serotonin, histamine, norepinephrine, and acetylcholine were eliminated as the prime vasoconstrictor agents in the CSF.

Since vasocontractile activity of lipid peroxides or prostaglandins has been said to be related to the disulfide form of the sulfhydril structure of the biomembrane [3], Sasaki investigated the action of two disulfide-reducing agents; dithiothreitol (DTT) and dithioerythritol (DTE). Both of these chemicals inhibited the CSF-induced contraction. Furthermore, N,N'-propylenebisnicotinamide (AVS), which is a hydroxyl radical scavenger and an inhibitor of the contractions induced by lipid hydroperoxides, also showed an inhibitory effect on the CSF-induced contraction [49].

These results strongly speak for lipid peroxides or prostaglandins as the prime vasoconstrictor agents in the CSF of SAH patients. Contraction induced by potassium application was not inhibited by DTT or by DTE, both of which had inhibited the CSF-induced contraction. Therefore, potassium has little to do with the vasocontractile activity of CSF.

Liszczak et al. [26] and Zervas et al. [64] described a rete vasorum in the adventia which was permeable even to large proteins and was in continuity with the subarachnoid space in dogs and cats. Therefore, it is reasonable to assume that vasoactive substances in the subarachnoid space can easily penetrate the cerebral arteries, in which case the cerebral artery will incur the effects of vasoconstrictive substances from the lumen side as well as from the side of the subarachnoid space. Furthermore, PGI_2 or EDRF, which inhibit these vasoconstrictive effects, are decreased in the arterial wall. It is no wonder that the artery becomes spastic.

Thus, the pathogenesis of cerebral vasospasm in SAH may be summarized as follows: Free radical reactions, especially lipid peroxidation, are initiated by clot lysis because of insufficient defense mechanisms in the CSF against free radicals. These defense mechanisms are especially insufficient after day 3. Each constituent of these free radical reactions (such as lipid hydroperoxides) has vasocontractile capacity [6, 61]. Furthermore, the endothelium and the media of the

artery incur free radical injury (toxic effects of free radicals). Because of the endothelial damage and the inhibitory effects of the lipid hydroperoxides on PGI_2 synthesis, the arterial wall PGI_2 level drops to a very low value. Vasoconstricitive substances act on the arterial wall not only from the side of the subarachnoid space, but from the lumen side as well, because there is constant adhesion and aggregation of platelets to the damaged endothelium and these platelets produce TXA_2 and other vasoconstrictive substances which are unopposed by PGI_2 or EDRF. Furthermore, because of the increase of endothelial permeability or disruption of the blood-arterial wall barrier [50], plasma constituents penetrate into the arterial wall to cause intimal thickening and to release vasocontractile substances. Thus, the artery falls into a state of chronic vasospasm with characteristic histological changes. Figure 1 schematically summarizes the above-mentioned changes leading to delayed ischemic neurological deficit (DIND). Changes or findings referred to in the review by Kassell et al. [17] are also added.

Treatment of Cerebral Vasospasm

Various treatments are summarized in Table 2. Presently, there is no optimal treatment as to the prevention or reversal of the arterial narrowing and prevention or reversal of DINDs. Development of such agents is badly needed. In relation to the "free radical reactions-lipid peroxidation" hypothesis, the results of recent three double blind clinical trials will be reported below.

Double blind clinical trial using a free radical scavenger AVS. If lipid peroxides generated from free radical reactions are the cause of vasospasm, it must be shown that administration of an antioxidant or a free radical scavenger is effective, at least to a considerable extent, in the prevention or amelioration of vasospasm. To test this, Asano et al. [5] used AVS (N,N'-proplylenebisnicotinamide), a potent hydroxyl radical scavenger, soluble in both oil and water, which has an inhibitory action on activation of lipoxygenase by lipid peroxides, in experimental vasospasm.

SAH was induced in dogs by intracisternal injection of blood and subsequent changes in the basilar artery diameter were evaluated by angiography. First, intrathecal administration of AVS 3 days after SAH caused prompt resolution of preexisting chronic vasospasm for 3–4 h.

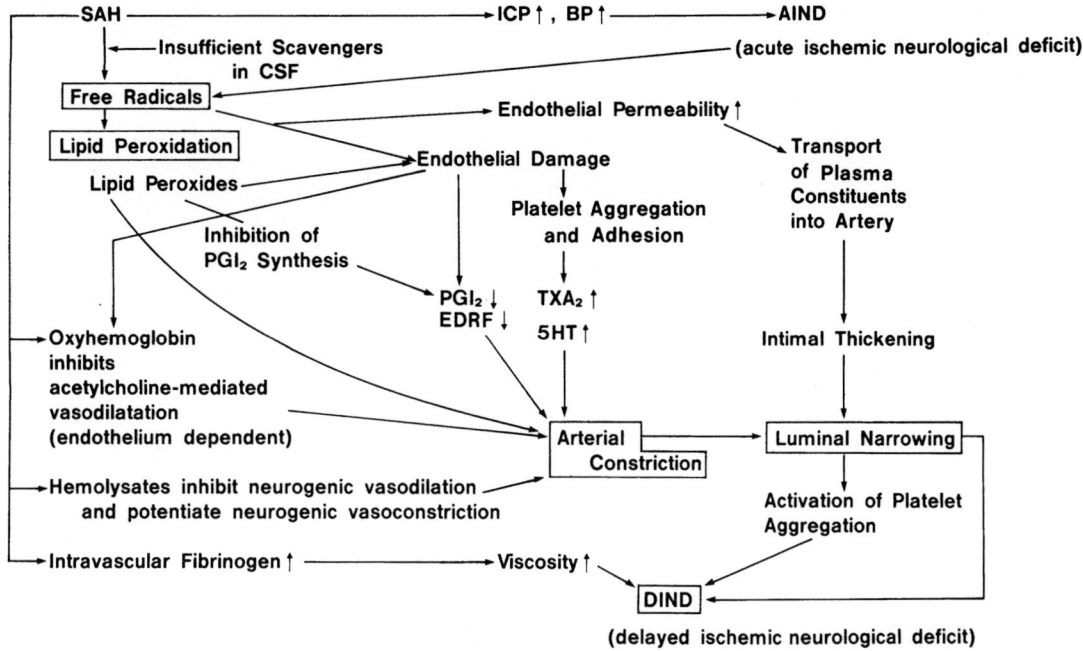

Fig. 1. Changes leading to delayed ischemic neurological deficit (*DIND*). *SAH* subarachnoid hemmorhage, *ICP* intracranial pressure, *BP* blood pressure, *AIND* acute ischemic neurological deficit, *PGI*$_2$ prostacyclin, *EDRF* endothelium-derived relaxing factor, *TXA*$_2$ thromboxane A$_2$

Next, continuous intravenous administration of saline (control) or AVS was performed for 4 days. In the control group, early and chronic spasm was observed on daily angiograms. In the AVS-treated group, early spasm was only moderately inhibited, but the occurrence of chronic spasm was remarkably suppressed in a dose-dependent fashion. Because of these encouraging results, a double blind clinical trial was planned involving 17 institutes. A total of 211 cases of SAH with grades I-IV of Hunt (without modification) received intravenous drip infusion for 8 h of 4 g/day of AVS (H group), 2 g/day of AVS (L group), or placebo (P group) for 14 days starting before day 4 of SAH, usually on day 2 or day 3. Clipping of the aneurysm was usually performed before or during administration of the drug. However, in ten cases among 71 cases of H group and in three cases among 73 cases of P group, clipping of the aneurysm was not performed because of poor general conditions. Neurological evaluation of the patients was done just after completion of the therapy, and at 1 month and 3 months after the onset of SAH. Angiography and computed tomography (CT) were also performed.

Occurrence of paralysis of the arm or the leg or both was significantly reduced in the L and H groups as compared with the P group at 1 month and 3 months after the onset of SAH ($P < 0.01$). The same is true with cases that had no paralysis before the therapy and later developed paralysis.

Occurrence of symptomatic spasm, as evaluated from changes of consciousness and neurological conditions just after completion of the therapy, was the lowest in the H group (35.8%), then in the L group (43.6%), and then in the P group (50.8%). In accordance with this, occurrence of low-density areas on CT was significantly low in the L group (40%) as compared with the P group (57.7%) ($P < 0.05$) just after completion of the therapy. Occurrence of angiographic spasm was also low in the H and L groups as compared with the P group. No serious side effects were noted in the H and L groups.

Double blind clinical trial using a TXA$_2$ synthetase inhibitor OKY-046. The decreased synthesis of PGI$_2$ would shift the reciprocal relationship between TXA$_2$ and PGI$_2$ toward a disproportionate synthesis of TXA$_2$, which further leads to the release of ADP and serotonin from the platelets, to platelet aggregation, and, finally, to local vasoconstriction. Therefore, it may well be expected that correction of the imbalance between TXA$_2$ and PGI$_2$ would be useful in therapy for

Table 2. Possible modes of therapy against vasospasm

1. Removal of perivascular clot by early surgery and cisternal drainage and/or irrigation
2. Hemodynamic improvement of impaired cerebral circulation
    Elevation of systemic arterial pressure (dopamine, etc.)
    Hypervolemia
    Albumin, dextran, mannitol, etc.
3. Cerebral protection against ischemia by drugs
    Barbiturates
    Y-9179 (nizofenone)
4. Use of free radical scavengers
    Vitamin E
    Barbiturates
    Y-9179 (nizofenone)
    1,2-bis(nicotinamido)-propane (AVS)
    Mannitol, etc.
5. Suppression of platelet aggregation and pharmacological modification of prostaglandin synthesis
    Ticlopidine
    Phosphodiesterase inhibitors (papaverine, phthalazinol, etc.) (see 9)
    Cyclooxygenase inhibitors (indomethacin, aspirin, etc.)
    Lipoxygenase inhibitors
    Phospholipase A_2 suppression (steroids)
6. Inhibition of thromboxane A_2 synthesis and/or stimulation of prostacyclin synthesis
    OKY-046 (Sodium (E)-3-[4-(1-imidazolylmethyl)phenyl]-2-propenoate)
    Y-9179 (nizofenone)
    Trapidil
    Prostacyclin and its analogues
7. Calcium antagonists
    Nimodipine
    Nifedipine
    Nicardipine
    Diltiazem
    Cinnarizine
    Verapamil
8. Adenyl cyclase stimulation
    $Beta_2$-adrenergic drugs
        Isoproterenol ($beta_1$ + $beta_2$) (+ lidocaine)
        Salbutamol (mainly $beta_2$)
9. Phosphodiesterase inhibition
    Papaverine, methylxanthines, ascorbic acid, aminophylline, diazoxide, chlorpromazine, reserpine, Hydralazine
10. Combination of 8 and 9
    Salbutamol + amionphylline
11. Use of exogenous cyclic AMP or one of its congeners
    Dibutyryl cyclic AMP
12. Guanyl cyclase inhibition
    Phenoxybenzamine (blocking serotonin, alpha-adrenergic drugs and cholinergic drugs)
    Phentolamine (alpha blocker)
    Methysergide, reserpine, kanamycin (serotonin blocker)
    Atropine (cholinergic blocker)
    Prostaglandin-$F_{2\alpha}$ blocker (?)
    Sodium nitroprusside (alpha blocker) +
    Phenylephrine (alpha stimulator with little effect on the cerebral vessels)
13. Combination of 9 and 12
    Aminophylline + nitroprusside + dopamine
14. Angiotensin-converting enzyme inhibition
    Teprotide
15. Topical application of drugs
    Lidocaine
    Nicardipine
    Papaverine
    Prostacyclin and its analogues

cerebral vasospasm.

Sasaki et al. [53] tested a thromboxane synthetase inhibitor, OKY-1581, in experimental SAH in dogs. The drug was proved to be effective for amelioration of angiographical vasospasm. A similar but chemically more stable thromboxane synthetase inhibitor, OKY-046, was also found to be effective for the treatment of experimental vasospasm.

A total of 256 cases of SAH, in which aneurysm clipping was completed by day 3, received OKY-046, 400 mg/day (H group), 80 mg/day (L group), or placebo (P group) by intravenous continuous drip infusion for 10–14 days following surgery. The occurrence of angiographical vasospasm or of low-density areas on CT (on day 21 or later) was significantly reduced in the L group, if the preoperative Glasgow Coma Score was 14 or less (which corresponded to grade III or worse). Analysis of activities of daily life (ADL) at 1 month after the onset of SAH showed that the L group showed better ADL than the other groups if the preoperative Glasgow Coma Score was 14 or less. There was no significant difference in the occurrence of angiographical spasm, or of low density on CT or in ADL among H, L, and P groups if the preoperative Glasgow Coma Score was 15.

Double blind clinical trial using nizofenone. Protection of the brain against ischemia using barbiturates or nizofenone (Y-9179) is important. Nizofenone, a cerebral protector and a free radical scavenger, has less side effects than barbiturates. A recent cooperative double blind clinical trial [32, 39] showed that the group treated with this drug was superior to the placebo group ($P < 0.05$) in the "disability status scale" 1 month after development of vasospasm, although development of vasospasm was not prevented. (Administration of the drug was initiated before vasospasm developed and continued for 5 days and, if vasospasm developed, for an additional 5 days.)

One of the main reasons why many neurosurgeons hesitate to perform early surgery (which is the best means to prevent rebleeding of aneurysms) even on grades I or II patients, is fear of postoperative vasospasm, which is actually only remotely related to surgery itself. Therefore, if future investigations yield effective drugs for prevention or cure of chronic cerebral vasospasm (DIND) as well as for the treatment of acute ischemic neurological deficit (AIND), the treatment of ruptured intracranial aneurysms will be so changed that very early surgery to prevent rebleeding of aneurysms combined with removal of as much subarachnoid clot as possible and fashioning of cisternal drainage will be performed, accompanied by ample administration (systemic or topical) of such drugs. Then the results of treatment of ruptured intracranial aneurysms will be greatly ameliorated.

Ischemic Lesions in Vascular Occlusion

Neurons are susceptible to ischemia more than any other cells in the body. If ischemia lasts for a considerable time, neurons quickly die because of energy failure due to lack of oxygen and glucose. This is called "acute ischemic neuronal death." If ischemia is relatively brief, some neurons may die in several hours, or, at most, within 24 h, a phenomenon called "maturational neuronal death [15]. Some neurons may recover their metabolic and functional activities and then die several days later. The last phenomenon was first described in the gerbil hippocampus by Kirino and his co-workers [19-24] and was termed "delayed neuronal death." The delayed neuronal death has been attracting the interest of not only basic scientists but of clinicians because elucidation of the underlying mechanism of this phenomenon points toward the development of treatments for ischemia-evoked pathological processes [24, 38].

The hippocampal change, selective damage of CA_1 neurons or neurons in Sommer's sector [57], has been known to occur in epileptic seizures, ischemia-anoxia insults, and also in cases of hypoglycemia. This has been called the Ammon's horn sclerosis and its pathogenetic mechanism has long been the target of hot debate, e.g., the Pathoklise theory of Vogt versus the vascular theory of Spielmeyer [45].

The clinical importance of this phenomenon was revived by Sano and Malamud [45], who stated this hippocampal change might become an epileptogenic focus for temporal lobe seizures. This idea was enlarged by Falconer [11] and led him to perform temporal lobectomies including the hippocampus for the treatment of intractable epilepsy.

Recently, a new concept on the pathogenesis of hippocampal injury has emerged [38]. The new concept has been proposed through approaches to the problem from three different directions. The first one is experimental studies on epileptic neuronal damage. The second is experimental works on ischemic neuronal injury in selectively vulnerable regions in the brain. The third approach, which played a special role in combining the two preceding approaches and in prompting us to unify hypotheses of pathogenesis, involves researches on neuronal damage caused by various neurotoxins. Among these toxins, certain putative neurotransmitters and their agonists have come to attention. There is a significant body of evidence that these substances exert their noxious effect by causing excessive excitation of neurons. The patterns of the "excitotoxic" damage in the hippocampus were proved to be almost identical to those seen in epileptic patients or in postanoxic/ischemic brain. Therefore, it may be justified to call this new concept on the pathogenesis of delayed neuronal death of the hippocampus the "excitotoxicity" theory. The most probable candidate of intrinsic excitotoxins is an excitatory putative neurotransmitter, glutamate.

The Mongolian gerbil (*Meriones unguiculatus*) was introduced as an experimental animal for stroke. It was revealed that ischemia in the gerbil is due to a lack of an interconnection in the circle of Willis at the base of the skull. Almost all gerbils have no connection between the carotid and the vertebrobasilar circulation. At the beginning, the gerbil was used as a focal ischemia model by occluding the unilateral carotid artery [15, 16]. Later, it was realized that bilateral occlusion of the carotid arteries brings about uniform forebrain ischemia, during which blood flow is close to zero [58, 59]. In most of gerbils subjected to 5 min of ischemia by bilateral carotid occlusion, hippocampal damage is seen throughout the dorsal hippocampus [19-21]. The CA4 (the end-plate) pyramidal cells show a fast change. They become darkly stained with shrunken cell bodies and empty spaces surrounding them. This change becomes obvious within 3-6 h following ischemia. The rapid cell change in CA4 corresponds to the previously known ischemic cell change. The change in the CA1 sector (Sommer's sector) develops slowly. On day 1 following brief ischemia, no definite alteration is seen except that the cell nucleus occasionally looks more inhomogeneous than normal. On day 2, the pyramidal cells show a slight clumping of the nuclear chromatin and slits develop in the basal side of the cytoplasm. These initial signs of alteration are followed by extensive destruction of most of the pyramidal cells when observed on the 4th day. The change in the majority of the CA1 neurons is slow but progressive. The full-

blown pathological state is only seen after the 4th day by light microscopy, but an insidious process starts to take place by 24 h following brief ischemia. This slow change is clearly detected by electron microscopy [21]. The main findings are an accumulation of increased endoplasmic reticulum (ER) cisterns, an increase of dark granules unbound by a membrane, and a disaggregation of polyribosomes into monoribosomes. These changes are never seen in the normal CA1 neurons. The delayed neuronal death in the hippocampal CA1 subfield is a novel type of cell change after ischemia. The changes which follow brief ischemic insult have been studied in the rat as well [22, 34, 36, 56].

Except for several differences in minor detail, pathological alteration in the hippocampus following ischemia are quite similar in both gerbils and rats. In view of the resemblances in pathological findings and structural similarity of the normal hippocampus among various species, the alteration in the hippocampus following ischemia exhibited by various species including man may be fundamentally identical to the changes seen in the rodents.

Delayed neuronal death in the CA1 neurons observed following brief ischemia in the rodent is a slow alteration and is not similar to acute ischemic cell death, which is well known as developing shortly after relatively prolonged, severe ischemia. It takes almost 2 days to detect definite morphological changes in the CA1 neurons, which herald delayed extensive neuronal death. During this period following recirculation, there is no selective decrease in cerebral blood flow in the hippocampus which can account for the selective neuronal damage [58, 59]. There is no impairment of energy metabolism which is compatible with extensive neuronal damage in the hippocampus. Arai et al. [2] examined the CA1 subfield in the gerbil ischemia model biochemically and confirmed that there is no decrease of ATP that can account for cell deterioration. Pulsinelli and Duffy [35] also noticed a similar change in the energy metabolism in their rat model. They found that the imbalance of regional blood flow and glucose metabolism does not correlate with the pattern of neuronal injury [36]. All of these experimental results indicate that neurons in the hippocampus die following brief ischemia without any definite "classic" reason to die.

Suzuki et al. [59] studied the gerbil CA1 neurons electrophysiologically following brief ischemia. They found that the CA1 neurons are electrically active for 1 day after ischemia. This means, at least electrophysiologically, the neurons in the CA1 sector are alive for a certain period following brief ischemic insult. If this hypothesis is valid, neurons, following ischemia, are left in an unstable state between death and survival. As a consequence, there is the possibility of salvaging dying neurons following ischemia. To examine this hypothesis, experiments on drug effects were performed. When pentobarbital was given immediately following ischemic insult, it showed a definite, reproducible, favorable effect on the survival of CA1 neurons following brief ischemia [24]. The effective dosage was 20–40 mg/kg. The favorable effect of baributurates was not seen if injection was done 1 h after ischemic insult. Other chemical agents such as nizofenone (Y-9179) [60] (12.5–25 mg/kg) or diazepam (10–20 mg/kg) could also ameliorate the ischemic hippocampal lesion ($P < 0.01$). The same is probably true with phenytoin. All of these drugs are known to have a sedative activity on neurons. This result may suggest that CA1 neurons are not only electrically active, but they are "hyperactive" during the recirculation period following brief ischemia. The reason for this hyperactivity may be explained by literal hyperexcitation of neurons or by a lack in inhibition, which could lead to excessive firing. The lack in inhibition hypothesis is not likely since Francis and Pulsinelli [13] did not detect any selective decrease in the activity of glutamic acid decarboxylase (GAD), an enzyme related to gamma-aminobutyric acid (GABA), in the CA1 sector following ischemia. On the contrary, a certain type of interneuron, presumably GABAergic, in the CA1 sector is rather tolerant to ischemia [16]. There is increasing evidence that a putative amino acid neurotransmitter, glutamate, is involved in the pathogenesis of ischemic hippocampal cell damage. In the CA1 subfield, it is well known that most of the neurons have abundant glutamate receptors. Given a sufficient concentration of glutamate, these neurons show sustained burst discharges which trigger excessive Ca^{2+} influx. To protect the hippocampal neurons from noxious hyperexcitation, provoked, most likely, by glutamate, Simon et al. [55] blocked N-methyl-D-aspartate (NMDA) receptors using aminophosphonoheptonoic acid (AP-7), and showed that AP-7, injected into the hippocampus, dramatically reduced the neuronal damage. Recently, Wieloch et al. [63] and Pulsinelli [33] independently found that removing the glutamergic excitatory input into the

hippocampus protects the hippocampus from ischemic damage. This means that ischemic injury is dependent on the presence of excitatory afferents. The phenomenon of "deafferentation protection" is also known in the pathogenesis of kainate (glutamate agonist) lesions. All of these experimental results on ischemic hippocampal damage are compatible with the hypothesis of hyperexcitation induced by glutamate.

The detrimental effects of glutamate are not restricted to the hippocampal neurons. Choi [8] recently found that neocortical neurons were sensitive to brief applications of glutamate, but it took up to a day to show cell damage if glutamate was washed out quickly. Futhermore, glutamate is believed to be involved in the pathogenesis of hypoglycemic brain injury [62].

It has gradually been realized that vulnerability of neurons to certain noxious insults such as hypoxia/anoxia, hypoglycemia, or sustained seizure activities, is inevitably related to the properties of neurons. Although any biological organisms which live in an aerobic condition are destined to die when oxygen and metabolic substrates are withdrawn, cell death seen in neurons occurs far earlier than such general cell destruction. Rothman [37] cultured the rat hippocampal neurons obtained from an embryo and tested their vulnerability to anoxia. He found that, before the establishment of synapses between cultured neurons, they were less susceptible to anoxia. However, as soon as neurons started to communicate by synapses, they became vulnerable to oxygen deprivation. At this state, he added $MgCl_2$ to block synaptic activity and noticed that neurons could survive an anoxic insult. This result may suggest that synaptic activity is closely related to the neuronal vulnerability to anoxia or ischemia. The neurotransmitter mediating synaptic communication in these cultured neurons is, presumably, glutamate. This evidence indicates that glutamate neurotoxicity and synaptic transmission are the key phenomena linked in the pathogenesis of neuronal injury in many, if not all, cerebral ischemia/anoxia, hypoglycemia cases, or epileptic seizures.

Recent advances in this field have proposed the optimistic view that the brain can be protected from various detrimental insults by reducing the release of a certain neurotransmitter or by blocking receptors which combine with the transmitter. This approach seems to dramatically improve our capability in managing cerebral ischemia/anoxia or hypoglycemia patients. The problem, however, may not be that simple. There are at least several barriers to break through in order to put this mode of therapy to practical use. Amino acid antagonists currently available work at a relatively higher concentration and poorly cross the blood-brain barrier. Even if more potent and more diffusible chemicals are developed, we must circumvent the possible side effects of the substances. Since amino acid transmitters are found all through the neuraxis, there is no guarantee that such an agent is safely used without unexpected adverse effects on the vital neural functions.

Most of the information accumulated on the glutamate toxicity is related to a relatively brief insult, which may not induce widespread destruction of the brain. We have to realize that, in clinical ischemic insults, neurons could be already at an irreversible state when the detrimental insults are resolved. It is hard to believe that such cell death is also mediated by neurotransmitters. Neurons are salvable when suitable therapy is instituted following a brief period of ischemia/anoxia or hypoglycemia. However, this seems to be the case only when treatment is initiated early enough. There are so many difficulties we must overcome in the treatment of ischemic neural lesions.

References

1. Ames A III, Wright RL, Kowada M, et al. (1968) Cerebral ischemia: II. The no-reflow phenomenon. Am J Pathol 52:437–447
2. Arai H, Lust WD, Passonneau JV (1982) Delayed metabolic changes induced by 5 min of ischemia in gerbil brain. Trans Amer Soc Neurochem 13:177
3. Asano M, Hidaka H (1979) Contractile response of isolated rabbit aortic strips to unsaturated fatty acid peroxides. J Pharmacol Exp Ther 208:347–353
4. Asano T, Sano K (1977) Pathogenetic role of no-reflow phenomenon in experimental subarachnoid hemorrhage in dogs. J Neurosurg 46:454–466
5. Asano T, Sasaki T, Koide T, Takakura K, Sano K (1984) Experimental evaluation of the beneficial effect of an antioxidant on cerebral vasospasm. Neurol Research 6:49–53
6. Asano T, Tanishima T, Sasaki T, Sano K (1980) Possible participation of free radical reactions initiated by clot lysis in the pathogenesis of vasospasm after subarachnoid hemorrage. In: Wilkins RH (ed) Cerebral arterial spasm. Williams and Wilkins, Baltimore, pp 190–201
7. Brandt L, Ljunggren B, Anderson KE, Hindfelt B, Teasdale G (1981) Vasoconstrictive effects of human post-hemorrhagic cerebrospinal fluid on cat pial arterioles in situ. J Neurosurg 54:351–356
8. Choi DW (1985) Glutamate neurotoxicity in cortical cell culture is calcium-dependant. Neurosci. Lett. 58:293–297
9. Cohen G (1983) Catalase, glutathione peroxidase, superoxide dismutase, and cytochrome P-450. In: Lajtha A (ed) Handbook of neurochemistry, vol. 4. Plenum Press, New York, 2nd edn., pp 315–330
10. Dusting GJ, Moncada S, Vane JR (1977) Prostacyclin (PGX) is the endogenous metabolite responsible for relaxation of coronary arteries induced by arachidonic acid. Prostaglandins 13:3–15
11. Falconer MA (1974) Mesial temporal (Ammon's horn) sclerosis as a common cause of epilepsy. Aetiology, treatment, and prevention. Lancet Sept 28:767–770
12. Flamm ES, Demopoulos HB, Seligman ML, Poser RG, Ransohoff J (1978) Free radicals in cerebral ischemia. Stroke 9:445–447
13. Francis A, Pulsinelli W (1982) The response of GABAergic and cholinergic neurons to transient cerebral ischemia. Brain Res 243:271–278
14. Gorman RR (1978) Prostaglandins, thromboxanes, and prostacyclin. Biochemistry and mode of action of hormones. Int Rev Biochem 20:81–107
15. Ito U, Spatz M, Walker JT, Klatzo I (1975) Experimental cerebral ischemia in Mongolian gerbils. Part I. Light microscopic observations. Acta Neuropathol (Berl) 32:209–223
16. Kahn K (1972) The natural course of experimental cerebral infarction in the gerbil. Neurology (Minneap) 22:510–515
17. Kassell NF, Sasaki T, Colohan ART, Nazar G (1985) Cerebral vasospasm following aneurysmal subarachnoid hemorrhage. Stroke 16:562–572
18. Kassell NF, Torner JC (1984) The International Cooperative Study on timing of aneurysm surgery: An update. Stroke 15:566–570
19. Kirino T (1982) Delayed neuronal death in the gerbil hippocampus following ischemia. Brain Res 239:57–69
20. Kirino T, Sano K (1984) Selective vulnerability in the gerbil hippocampus following transient ischemia. Acta Neuropathol (Berl) 62:201–208
21. Kirino T, Sano K (1984) Fine structural nature of delayed neuronal death following ischemia in the gerbil hippocampus. Acta Neuropathol (Berl) 62:209–218
22. Kirino T, Tamura A, Sano K (1984) Delayed neuronal death in the rat hippocampus following transient forebrain ischemia. Acta Neuropathol 64:139–147
23. Kirino T, Tamura A, Sano K (1984) Delayed neuronal death in the hippocampus following brief ischemia. In: Bes A, Braquet P, Paoletti R, Siesjö BK (eds) Cerebral ischemia. Elsevier, Amsterdam, pp 25–34
24. Kirino T, Tamura A, Sano K (1986) A reversible type of neuronal injury following ischemia in the gerbil hippocampus. Stroke 17:455–459
25. Kontos HA, Wei EP, Povlishock JT, Dietrich

WD, Magiera CJ, Euis EF (1980) Cerebral arteriolar damage by arachidonic acid and prostaglandin G_2. Science 209:1242–1245

26. Liszczak TM, Varsos VG, Black P, Kistler JP, Zervas NT (1983) Cerebral arterial constriction after experimental subarachnoid hemorrhage is associated with blood components within the arterial wall. J Neurosurg 58:18–26

27. Lundberg N, KjälLquist A, Kullberg G, et al. (1974) In: Krayenbühl H (ed) Advances and technical standards in neurosurgery, vol. 1. Springer, Vienna, pp 3–59

28. McCord JM (1985) Oxygen-derived free radicals in postischemic tissue injury. N Eng J Med 312: 159–163

29. Misra HP, Fridovich I (1972) The generation of superoxide radical during the autoxidation of hemoglobin. J Biol Chem 247:6960–6962

30. Nornes H (1973) The role of intracranial pressure in the arrest of hemorrhage in patients with ruptured intracranial aneurysm. J Neurosurg 39: 226–234

31. Nornes H, Magnaes B (1972) Intracranial pressure in patients with ruptured saccular aneurysm. J Neurosurg 36:537–547

32. Ohta T, Kikuchi H, Hashi K, et al. (1986) Nizofenone administration in the acute stage following subarachnoid hemorrhage. Results of a multicenter controlled double-blind clinical study. J Neurosurg 64:420–426

33. Pulsinelli WA (1985) Deafferentation of the hippocampus protects CA1 pyramidal neurons against ischemic injury. Stroke 16:144

34. Pulsinelli WA, Brierley JB, Plum F (1982) Temporal profile of neuronal damage in a model of transient forebrain ischemia. Ann Neurol 11: 491–498

35. Pulsinelli WA, Duffy TE (1983) Regional energy balance in rat brain after transient forebrain ischemia. J Neurochem 40:1500–1503

36. Pulsinelli WA, Levy DE, Duffy TE (1982) Regional cerebral blood flow and glucose metabolism following transient forebrain ischemia. Ann Neurol 11:499–509

37. Rothman SM (1983) Synaptic activity mediates death of hypoxic neurons. Science 220:536–537

38. Rothman SM, Olney JW (1986) Glutamate and the pathophysiology of hypoxic-ischemic brain damage. Ann Neurol 19:105–111

39. Saito I, Asano T, Ochiai C, et al. (1983) A double-blind clinical evaluation of the effect of nizofenone (Y-9197) on delayed ischemic neurological deficits following aneurysmal rupture. Neurol Res 5:29–47

40. Saito I, Sano K (1979) Vasospasm following rupture of cerebral aneurysms. Neurol Med Chir (Tokyo) 19:103–107

41. Saito I, Sano K (1980) vasospasm after aneurysm rupture: Incidence, onset, and course. In: Wilkins, RH (ed) Cerebral arterial spasm. Williams and Wilkins, Baltimore, pp 294–301

42. Saito I, Ueda Y, Sano K (1977) Significance of vasospasm in the treatment of ruptured intracranial aneurysms. J Neurosurg 47:412–429

43. Sano K (1983) Cerebral vasospasm and aneurysm surgery. Clin Neurosurg 30:13–58

44. Sano K, Asano T, Tanishima T, Sasaki T (1980) Lipid peroxidation as a cause of cerebral vasospasm. Neurol Res 2:253–272

45. Sano K, Malamud N (1953) Clinical significance of sclerosis of the cornuammonis: Ictal "psychic phenomena". Arch Neurol Psychiatry 70:40–53

46. Sano K, Saito I (1980) Early operation and washout of blood clots for prevention of cerebral vasospasm. In: Wilkins RH (ed) Cerebral arterial spasm. Williams and Wilkins, Baltimore, pp 510–513

47. Sano K, Sasaki T, Watanabe T, Asano T (1981) Cerebral vasospasm: The result of lipid peroxidation leading to inhibition of prostacyclin biosynthesis in the cerebral artery. Neurosurgeons (Tokyo) 1:105–111

48. Sasaki T, Asano T, Sano K (1980) Cerebral vasospasm and free radical reactions. Neurol Med Chir (Tokyo) 20:145–153

49. Sasaki T, Asano T, Takakura K, Sano K, Kassell NF (1984) Nature of the vasoactive substance in CSF from patients with subarachnoid hemorrhage. J Neurosurg 60:1186–1191

50. Sasaki T, Kassell NF, Yamashita M, Fujiwara S, Zuccarello M (1985) Barrier disruption in the major cerebral arteries following experimental subarachnoid hemorrhage. J Neurosurg 63:433–440

51. Sasaki S, Kuwabara H, Ohta S (1986) Biological defence mechanism in the pathogensis of prolonged cerebral vasospasm in the patients with ruptured intracranial aneurysms. Stroke 17:196–202

52. Sasaki T, Murota S, Wakai S, Asano T, Sano K (1981) Evaluation of prostaglandin biosynthetic activity in canine basilar artery following subarachnoid injection of blood. J Neurosurg 55:771–778

53. Sasaki T, Wakai S, Asano T, Takakura K, Sano K (1982) Prevention of cerebral vasospasm after SAH with a thromboxane synthetase inhibitor OKY-1581. J Neurosurg 57:74–82

54. Sasaki T, Wakai S, Asano T, Watanabe T, Kirino T, Sano K (1981) The effect of a lipid hydroperoxide of arachidonic acid on the canine basilar artery. An experimental study on cerebral vasospasm. J Neurosurg 54:357–365

55. Simon RP, Swan JH, Griffiths T, Meldrum BS (1984) Blockade of N-methyl-D-aspartate receptors may protect against ischemic damage in the brain. Science 226:850–852

56. Smith M-L, Auer RN, Siesjö BK (1984) The density and distribution of ischemic brain injury in the rat following 2-10 min of forebrain ischemia. Acta Neuropathol (Berl) 64:319–332

57. Sommer W (1880) Erkrankungen des Ammonshorns als aetiologisches Moment der Epilepsie. Arch Psychiat Nervenkr 10:631–675

58. Suzuki R, Yamaguchi T, Kirino T, Orzi F, Klatzo I (1983) The effects of 5-minute ischemia in Mon-

golian gerbils: I. Blood-brain barrier, cerebral blood flow, and local cerebral glucose utilization changes. Acta Neuropathol (Berl) 60:207–216

59. Suzuki R, Yamaguchi T, Li CL, Klatzo I (1983) The effects of 5-minute ischemia in Mongolian gerbils: II. Changes of spontaneous neuronal activity in cerebral cortex and CA1 sector of hippocampus. Acta Neuropathol (Berl) 60:217–3222

60. Tamura A, Asano T, Sano K, Tsumagari T, Nakajima A (1979) Protection from cerebral ischemia by a new imidazole derivative (Y-9179) and pentobarbital. A comparative study in chronic middle cerebral artery occlusion in cats. Stroke 10:126–134

61. Tanishima T, Asano T, Sasaki T, Sano K (1979)

Role of peroxidation in the genesis of cerebral arterial spasm. Acta Neurol Scand (Suppl) 60:484–485

62. Wieloch T (1985) Hypoglycemia-induced neuronal damage prevented by an N-methly-D-aspartate antogonist. Science 230:681–683

63. Wieloch T, Lindvall O, Blomqvist P, Gage FH (1985) Evidence for amelioration of ischaemic neuronal damage in the hippocampal formation by lesions of the perforant path. Neurol Res 7:24–26

64. Zervas NT, Liszcak TM, Mayberg MR, Brack PM (1982) Cerebrospinal fluid may nourish cerebral vessels through pathways in the adventitia that may be analogous to systemic vasa vasorum. J Neurosurg 56:475–481

Future Aspects of Surgery for Cerebral Stroke

Mahmut G. Yaşargil[1]

The sense of presence is related to the distinctive attributes of our information from the past and the quality of concepts we have conceived for the future. We realize that the human being is distinctly unique. In a sense, man possesses a "neuronal compass" which can guide him to his intellectual destiny. He has evolved from a purely instinctual creature to a rational, reflective, and self-steering being.

The architectural arrangement of the brain is of an old construction. A billion-year-old brain stem, with a 500-million-year-old diencephalon and cerebrum, is coupled to a telencephalon which is 30 million years old. The holistic imagination is postulated to be a function of the cortex. It potentiates and modifies the drives of the limbic system. In many instances, perhaps it is the limbic and lower archaic systems which control the cortex. These reciprocal abilities must always be delicately balanced. Therefore, it is necessary to exercise caution and careful judgement in order to avoid the rigidities and inflexibilities of archaic instincts, learned dogmas, and computerized analysis.

Since the very beginning, human beings were apparently aware of the enigmatic brain and its importance in life. During ancient times, Pythia in Delphi spoke in oracles, answering many delicate questions. Here we see her receiving advice from Apollo, who is the holy guardian of medicine in Greek mythology. The calcarine bones of the goat were a popular way of predicting the future in Asia and the Near East. Do we believe nowadays to have better methods of predicting the outcome of an insult in a patient with neurovascular disease?

Four billion-year-old earth and two million-year-old human brain; two dynamic, hitherto insufficiently explored creations of nature with similarities in both their morphology and function (Fig. 1).

[1] Neurosurgical Department, University Hospital, Zurich, Switzerland

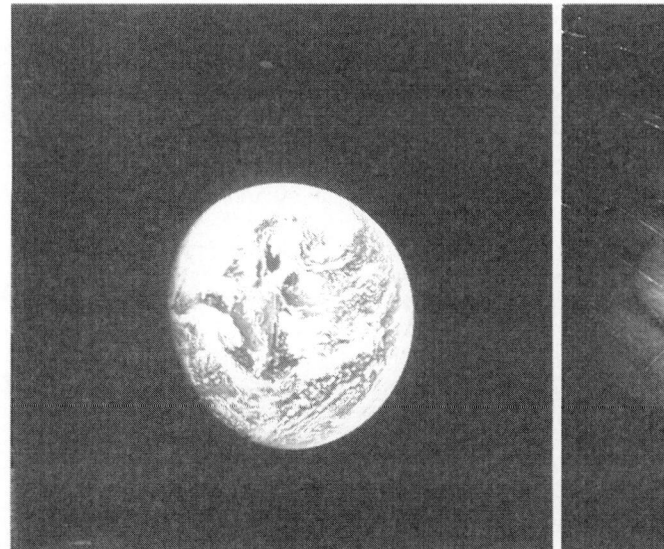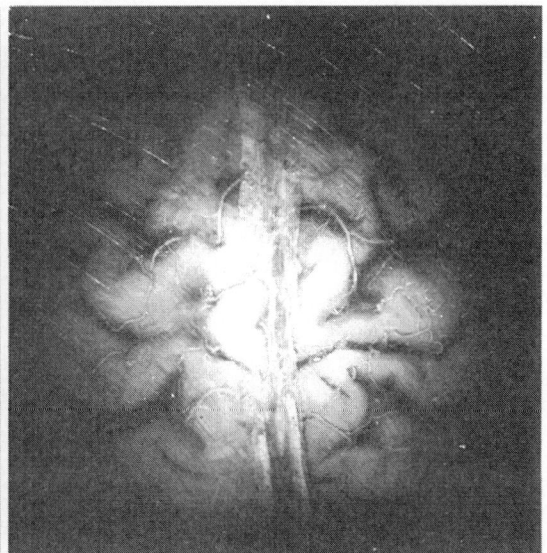

Fig. 1a, b. Two dynamic creations of nature. **a** Earth. **b** Human brain

What incessant urge drives our brain to explore and investigate not only our environment, from the particles of the atom up to the clusters of galaxies in the cosmos, but also to examine and understand its own construction and function? Intensive research work is in progress to decipher the function of the complicated network of the neuronal system. Vascular research is concentrated on puzzling out the network of the capillary system. The great Dutch anatomist Frederik Ruysch (1638–1731), who performed the most perfect injection preparations of the vascular system, expressed enthusiastically, "The whole of life emanates from capillaries."

Papyrus Smith, the oldest manuscript (2700–4000 years old), translated and published by Breasted [3] in 1930, contains descriptions of injured brains in 27 cases and the term "brain" written for the first time in hieroglyphs. Breasted remarked that the author of this papyrus "knew of the cardiac system and was surprisingly near recognition of the circulation of the blood."

The written word "brain" as a Chinese character means, as a pictogram, "animal, skull, hairs, and mind." When was this character written for the first time?

The abbreviations of terms used for diagnosis and therapy in cases of neurovascular disease, taken from the recent monograph of Barnett et al. [1], and the newest monograph of Suzuki [17], look like modern hieroglyphs.

A monumental, allegoric fresco of Diego Rivera, at the entrance to the National Institute of Cardiology in Mexico City, demonstrates dramatically the history of research work concerning blood circulation. The study of the historical aspects connected with the research of blood circulation results in the discovery of fascinating and discerning views. On the one hand, there are precise observations and descriptions of the morphology and physiology of the general and cerebral blood circulation and, on the other hand, there are many speculative conclusions.

Two prophetical remarks faced us at the beginning of the new age: Roger Bacon (1214-1294), who set the stage for modern scientific thinking in the 13th century, gave us this extraordinary and worthy aphorism: "Truth can emerge sooner from error than from confusion." The aphorism of Francis Bacon (1561-1625), made 382 years later, runs as follows: "*Tantum possumus quantum scimus*" (The more we know the more we can).

On April 17, 1616, Harvey presented his discovery of the circulation of the blood. His book was published in 1628. This was a real breakthrough in understanding the blood circulation. Vascular anatomy was transformed into physiology. Thomas Willis published his book 30 years later, containing the first functional explanation of the circle arteriosus cerebralis. Malpighi, in 1661, described for the first time the capillaries, thus supplying the missing link in the investigations and conclusions of Harvey.

Two English pioneers of medicine should be mentioned: It was William Hunter, at the beginning of the 18th century, who first suggested the term "anastomosis" to denote the union of two vessels, whereas the term "collateral" was introduced by his younger brother, John Hunter. It was John Hunter who ligated the femoral artery in a case of popliteal aneurysm and thus proved the efficiency of the collateral arterial circulation. Before this, he had performed studies on the collateral system of the external carotid artery in deer.

During the past 200 years, there has been an overwhelming increase and acceleration in research activities concerning cerebral blood vessels and cerebral blood circulation. Each decade in our century has brought us great scientific and technical advances (Table 1). Within the last 40 years, we have been witness to the unique development of sophisticated techniques which measure the rCBF and cerebral metabolism (Table 2).

Table 1. Development in neurodiagnostic techniques

Year	Development
1900–1920	X-ray, LP
1920–1970	PG, MG
1930s	Cer. angiography, EEG
1940s	Kety-Schmidt, radionuclides
1950s	rCBF, catheter angiography
1960s	Doppler-sonography, rheology, spinal angiography
1970s	CT, Xe-CT, SPECT, PET
1980s	MRI, NMR-spectroscopy, EEG-EP-brain mapping, MRI-projection-angiography, MEG, superselective staging angiography

LP, PG pneumography, *MG* myelography, *rCBF* regional cerebral blood flow, *CT* computd tomography, *SPECT* single photon emission CT, *PET* positron emission tomography, *MRI* magnetic resonance imaging

Table 2. Literature of the measurement of blood flow and metabolism of the brain

Author	Year	Author	Year	Author	Year
Fick	1870	Obrist et al.	1967	Fieschi et al.	1980
Kety-Schmidt	1945	Oeconomos et al.	1969	Siesjö	1981
Gibbs et al.	1947	Kogure et al.	1969	Olsen et al.	1981
Shenkin et al.	1948	Hossmann et al.	1973	Sokoloff et al.	1981
Schneider	1950	Branston et al.	1974	Jones	1982
Lassen and Munck	1955	Sundt et al.	1974	Phelps et al.	1982
Greitz	1956	Symon et al.	1974	Herscowitch et al.	1983
Hirsch	1957	Michenfelder et al.	1975	Reivich et al.	1983
Brockman and Jude	1960	Heiss	1976	Raichle et al.	1983
Lassen and Ingvar	1961	Ter-Pogossian et al.	1978	Mazziotta and Phelps	1986
Gottstein et al.	1961	Yoshimoto et al.	1978	Barnett et al.	1986
Meyer et al.	1963	Ogawa et al.	1979	Suzuki et al.	1987
Plum et al.	1963	Astrup	1980		
Nemoto et al.	1965	Seki et al.	1980		

The fact is that abundant data have been described which cover the manifold thresholds of brain energy systems such as blood flow, circulation time, temperature, oxygen, CO_2, glucose, and lactate thresholds. Also, ionic equilibrium, as well as thresholds of functional and morphological needs, have been described. Definitions have been created, such as "ischemic penumbra" or "luxury perfusion." Despite all this information and knowledge, we are still not fully equipped for our duties at the patient's bedside. In a given case with cerebrovascular disease, there is, even now, insufficient knowledge available concerning the metabolic requirements and the blood supply of affected and nonaffected brain tissue.

Medieval doctors tried their best to decipher a differential diagnosis by observing the yellow color of a urine sample. Are we not somehow in the same situation as our medieval colleagues? We are studying the different gray colors and tones of computerized tomography (CT) scans and magnetic resonance imaging (MRI) to find at least some indirect answers concerning the actual pathophysiological condition of the brain of our patient. We realize, however, that we are at the very beginning.

We have still to develop a system which will be of most benefit to everyday neurodiagnostic practice: for instance, a repeatable, noninvasive, three-dimensional imaging of regional cerebral blood flow; as well as biochemical and metabolic activities, and an instant mapping of the brain, including general and local cerebral functions and their needs.

Special Features of Brain Vessels

We are fully aware that vessels are not just tubes. They are organs with a special architecture and special biochemical activities. In all organs, the arteries are accompanied by two veins, lymphatic vessels, vasa vasorum, and a rich network of nerves. This is not the case in the central nervous system (Fig. 2).

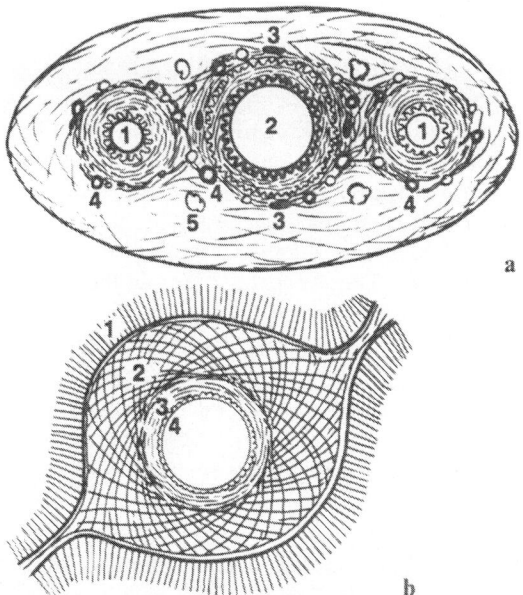

Fig. 2. a Organization of the peripheral vessels. *1* concomitant veins, *2* artery, *3* nerves, *4* vasa vasorum, *5* lymphatic vessels. **b** Organization of a brain artery *1* cortex, *2* arachnoidal fibers, *3* media of a cerebral artery, *4* endothelium of a cerebral artery

The cerebral vessels are not only entirely different from the vessels of other organs, they have, in addition, significant architectural and biochemical differences which vary in the many regions of the brain. Bell [2] stated in his paper concerning the history of the study of the cerebral circulation and the measurement of cerebral blood flow:

Charles Roy and Sir Charles Sherrington, working in Cambridge in 1890, measured the diameter of the brain in the open skull and were the first to suggest an intrinsic local control of the CBF (cerebral blood flow), corresponding with local variation in functional activity: the chemical products of cerebral metabolism contained in the lymph which bathes the walls of the arterioles of the brain can cause variations of the calibre of the cerebral vessels: that in this reaction the brain possesses an intrinsic mechanism by which its vascular supply can be varied locally in correspondence with local variations of functional activity. Unfortunately, their foresight was refuted by Leonard Hill who, in his Hunterian Lectures in 1896, stated that the cerebral circulation followed passively the changes in systemic blood pressure.

The newest investigations have shown that the endothelial cells of the capillaries are capable of producing 10% of the CSF.

Collateral System of the Arteries of the Brain

With the institution of serial cerebral angiography in the 1950s, the importance and significance of angiography for the visualization of the collateral circulation and its complex annular formations was demonstrated. We were forced to realize and accept that the extra- and intracranial collateral systems escaped visualization of a selective type. They appeared here and there only by chance. Even in cases of vascular occlusion, their appearance on the X-ray remained in doubt. Using superselective angiography techniques routinely, the collateral system can now be visualized more regularly. There is reasonable hope that in the near future the cerebral collateral system will be visualized properly and adequately with the help of microcatheters. More detailed information about the actual condition and function of the cerebral collateral system and its standards will be greatly appreciated. It will not only assist in making conclusive decisions concerning the treatment of occlusive vascular disease, but will also be useful when deciding the treatment of aneurysms, arteriovenous malformations (AVMs) and tumors.

Vascularization Patterns of the Brain in Convex and Central Areas

We are accustomed to accept that the vascularization of the central nervous system is divided into two main compartments—supra- and infratentorial, or carotid- and vertebro-basilar systems—and the two separated compartments of the hemispheres. In reality, there is a further valid separation: convex (pallial) and central areas, which have separate and different arterial and venous patterns of vascularization. During the development of the cerebral and cerebellar hemispheres, the leptomeningeal arteries receive a rich collateral network, whereas the arteries of the central areas seem to have a very poor collateral network. Is perhaps this information an outdated dogma? Daily experience with the surgery of deep central AVMs demonstrates clearly a rich paraventricular network of perforating arteries.

The lenticulostriate arteries especially seem to be "terminal arteries," but the origins of these arteries exhibit many variations in their alteration, reciprocity, and mutuality. Sophisticated research (infarct models) on the study of regional cerebral blood flow and metabolism is frequently related to the selective ligature of the middle cerebral artery in animals, particularly in cats, dogs, and monkeys. There are no remarks in these publications as to whether the ligature was made proximal or distal to the origin of the lenticulostriate arteries. Does there exist any precise anatomical study concerning the variation of lenticulostriate arteries in any of these animals that were investigated? It seems to me that further precise anatomical studies of the perforators are absolutely essential to clarify the diagnostic and therapeutic parameters concerning vascular disease of the central nervous system. Serial angiography studies in cases of stroke show us that the relation of the site of occlusion to the lenticulostriate arteries can be an essential factor in determining the natural history and course of the disease.

Vascular Surgery

The exciting history of vascular surgery within the last 2000 years can be mentioned only punctually (Tables 3, 4).

Susruta, a great surgeon of India, used large ants ("deo"-in Bengali) for the purpose of clamping arteries and preventing the discharge of blood. If the ants, after they had bitten, were divided in the middle, their mouths continued biting. This was the first biotechnical ligature.

The pioneer work in vascular surgery was accomplished 80 years ago by Carrel [4, 5]. His technique was adopted and modified for microvascular surgery by Jacobson and Suarez [10].

The evolutionary development of new neurodiagnostic modalities is integrated into the development of surgical treatment. Both advance simultaneously and perpetuate each other.

The surgery of carotid arteries was pioneered by Eastcott, Pickering, and Rob in 1954 [7]. Prophetic remarks of the great American neurologist Miller-Fisher were published in 1951 [14]:

It is even conceivable that some day vascular surgery will find a way to by-pass the occluded portion of the artery during the period of ominous fleeting symptoms. Anastomosis of the external carotid artery or one of its branches with the internal carotid artery above the area of narrowing should be feasible.

Woringer and Kunlin [20] succeeded in performing for the first time an extra-intracranial bypass graft on a 62-year-old patient.

The development of microvascular surgery in the 1960s made it technically possible to reconstruct intracranial arteries. This operation for patients with occlusive intracranial vascular disease has been approached with great apprehension and hesitation, because the indications for surgery in such cases have not been delineated. Clinical experience has shown that neither the

extent nor the number of occlusions solely determine the symptoms and their evolution. In each individual case, there is no precise method to determine whether spontaneous recovery or repeated attacks with progression of the disease will occur.

Interestingly, the routine use of serial angiography has shown spontaneous extra-intracranial collaterals not only in cases of AVMs and fistulas, but also in cases with occlusion of the internal carotid artery (ICA). Nature has shown us that in some cases such an extracranial-intracranial collaterals (EIA) is indicated. But which clinical parameter should we follow?

Even 20 years later, the indications for reconstructive cerebrovascular surgery cannot be set down as a definite or general rule, not even with the help of CT, MRI, SPECT, and PET. The decision for surgery should be made at the bedside of each patient. It is totally and absolutely individual and mainly related to the status of the collateral system. Any judgement relating to the collateral system requires a profound knowledge of anatomy, and is dependent on high-quality serial angiography and wide clinical experience.

There is a broad scale of possible primary and secondary insufficiencies of the arterial collateral system of the brain (Table 5). However, not all patients present with the expected related symp-

Table 3. Important figures in vascular surgery

Surgeon	Time
Susruta of India	600 B.C.
Rufus of Ephesus	1st century A.D.
Antyllus	2nd–3rd century
Abulcasis of Cerdoba	10th century
Ambroise Paré	16th century
John Hunter	18th century

Table 4. Important figures in modern vascular surgery

Name	Year
Alexis Carrel	1902
C.C. Guthrie	1912
Dos Santos	1946
Kunlin	1948
Eastcott, Pickering, and Rob	1954
Jacobson and Suarez	1960

Table 5. Primary and secondary insufficiency of the arterial collateral system of the brain

1. Congenital anomalies of the circle of Willis
   Aplasia, hypoplasia
   Persistent prim. arteries
2. Occlusive diseases of the vessels
   Cardiac origin
   Atherosclerosis
   Primary arteritis, secondary arteritis
   Moyamoya
   Fibromuscular dysplasia
   Hematological disorders
3. Spasm (mainly after subarachnoidal bleeding by rupture of aneurysms)
4. Brain edema
5. Steal syndrome
   Occlusion
   Fistula
   AVM
6. Compression (tumor, aneurysm, AVM)
7. Trauma: head and neck
   Direct lesion
   Indirect lesion (fat, air) } of the vessels
8. Iatrogenic
   Angiography
   Neurosurgery

toms and even these occur in different degrees of intensity.

Until now our decisions in this field have been nothing more than mere, vague guesses. This has compelled us to place more weight on the "art of medicine" than on the "science and technique of medicine."

We should be grateful for the Cooperative Study, an immense task completed by Barnett et al. [1]. This study was necessary to stop the wide, uncritical use of bypass surgery as a therapy for stroke. The "warning shot" provoked by the study should not, however, hinder further diagnostic and therapeutic action, for this will ultimately result in accomplishing a better understanding of occlusive brain vessel disease and its surgical therapy.

At present, we find ourselves in a very dynamic phase of scientific and technical development which will open new perspectives concerning the cerebral hemodynamics, CSF, and metabolic, biochemical, and biophysical activities of the brain. For the present and for the future, we need more knowledge concerning the anatomy, physiology, biochemistry, and biophysics of the brain. We need more possibilities for the instant measurement of the functions and needs of the brain. We need better instruments and apparatus for brain surgery. We should also be more competent in performing microsurgical techniques and this can only be achieved by patient and consistent exercise and practise in the laboratory.

The remarks of the British philosopher, Whitehead, in his book *Adventures of Ideas*, seem to me the best advice for us [19]:

Systems, scientific and philosophic, come and go. Each method of limited understanding is at length exhausted. In its prime each system is a triumphant success: in its decay it is an obstructive nuisance. The transitions to new fruitfulness of understanding are achieved by recurrence to the utmost depths of institution for the refreshment of imagination.

References

1. Barnett HJ, Mohr JP, Stein BM, Yatsu FM (1986) Stroke, vols. 1-2. Churchill Livingstone, Edinburgh

2. Bell BA (1984) A history of the study of the cerebral circulation and the measurement of cerebral blood flow. Neurosurgery 14:238–246
3. Breasted JH (1930) Edwin Smith surgical papyrus. University of Chicago Press, Chicago, pp 164–174
4. Carrel A (1908) Results of the transplantation of the blood vessels, organs and limbs. J Am Med Ass 51:1662–1667
5. Carrel A (1907) The surgery of blood vessels. Johns Hopkins Hosp Bull 20:18–28
6. Donaghy RMP, Yaşargil MG (1967) Microvascular surgery. Thieme, Stuttgart
7. Eastcott HHC, Pickering GW Rob, CG (1954) Reconstruction of internal carotid artery. Lancet II:994–996
8. Gänshirt H (1972) Der Hirnkreislauf. Thieme, Stuttgart
9. Greitz T, Invar, DH, Widén L (1985) Positron emission tomography. Raven, New York
10. Jacobson JH, Suarez EL (1960) Microsurgery in anastomosis of small vessels. Surg Forum 11:243–245
11. Lougheed WR, Gunton RW, Barnett HJM (1965) Embolectomy of internal carotid, middle and anterior cerebral arteries. J Neurosurg 22:607–609
12. Major RH (1954) A history of medicine, vol. 1 Charles C. Thomas, Springfield
13. Meyer JS (1975) Modern concepts of cerebrovascular disease. Spectrum Publication, Holliswood
14. Miller-Fisher C (1951) cited by Toole [18]
15. Phelps ME, Mazziotta JC, Schelbert HR (1986) Positron emission tomography and autoradiography. Raven, New York
16. Roy CS Sherrington CS (1890) On the regulation of the blood supply of the brain. J Physiol 11:85–108
17. Suzuki J (1987) Treatment of cerebral infarction. Springer, Vienna
18. Toole JF (1984) Cerebrovascular disorders, 3rd edn. Raven, New York, p 125
19. Whitehead AN (1933) Adventures of ideas. Cambridge, New York, p 163
20. Woringer E, Kunlin J (1963) Anastomose entre la carotide primitive et la carotide intra-crânienne ou la sylvienne par greffon selon la technique de la suture suspendue. Neurochirurgie 9:181–188
21. Yaşargil MG (1969) Microsurgery. Thieme, Stuttgart, pp 95–119
22. Yaşargil MG, Krayenbühl H, Jacobson JH (1970) Microneurosurgical arterial reconstruction. Surgery 67:221–233

Ischemia Secondary to Atherosclerosis
Protection and Treatment

HENRY J.M. BARNETT[1]

It is a distinct pleasure to pay tribute to Prof. Jiro Suzuki. In the wide world of our profession, he ranks as a great man. Longfellow, the distinguished American poet, described the tireless energy, determination, tenacity, and dedication of Jiro Suzuki when he wrote this poem:

The heights by great men reached and kept
Were not attained by sudden flight,
But they, while their companions slept,
Were toiling upward in the night.

(The Ladder of St. Augustine)

Under our leader and source of inspiration, Jiro Suzuki, we are all working for a common purpose during this symposium. I am reminded in a way of Alexander the Great. He had three units in his army. First were the Companions. They were elite and were noblemen. They may be thought of as the counterpart of the neurosurgeons. Second were the Cavalry. They too were elite, skilled, and innovative and might be regarded as the counterpart of the neuroradiologists or, in another context, the statisticians. Finally, there were the Foot Soldiers. They were reliable, disciplined, necessary, and poorly paid. They may be seen as the counterpart of the neurologists. No group alone was effective except in small skirmishes. Together they employed a common purpose and conquered the known world. Our common purpose today and in the years ahead of us is to wage many battles and in time to win the war against stroke.

The Progress of the War to Date

Battles are being won. There has been a 5% decline per year for several years in stroke mortality and an overall decline of 50% over 25

years. This has coincided with our ability to control blood pressure, to treat and prevent heart disease (one stroke in four is heart-related), and sweeping dietary changes. We also recognize now, without equivocation, that cigarette smoking causes stroke and there is some evidence that patients on low potassium diets are more prone to stroke [13]. All these factors have played a role in the realm of primary prevention.

Secondary prevention has been the preoccupation of most of us but in the background, based on lower-profile research and good medical practice, our enemy has already sounded this major retreat. This sharp change in the background requires that all potential therapeutic evaluation strategies come into clear focus. Compared with the major standard of the randomized trial, all the other yardsticks are of limited value in the search for unequivocal and definitive answers regarding therapy. Recently, on two occasions, a distinguished professor of surgery told a group of us that without a clinical trial an experienced surgeon knows when he is likely to benefit a patient. I wish I had such faith and could accept such an unscientific viewpoint. It is not being anti-surgery to oppose this thinking; it might be antitraditional. It is not antipharmaceutical to deny claimed benefit for a poorly evaluated drug. Both in medicine and in surgery, there are many examples of the widespread misuse of drugs and procedures which persisted for years and even for decades unit a critical analysis was achieved.

In evaluating therapy, historical controls overlook the dramatic decline going on in the background. Nonrandomized comparisons introduce selection bias and the presence of unexpected population differences skew the results. Indeed, they may be skewed in favor of the treatment that is allegedly useful and thus be blatantly contrived. To continue my analogy, experience and prognostic studies are useful

[1] Department of Clinical Neurological Sciences, The University of Western Ontario, London, Ontario, Canada

guides to the identification of the strength of the enemy but are not in themselves acceptable weapons for critical evaluation.

In the light of modern scientific methodology and biostatistics, and with the firm conviction that disregard for these techniques may lead to very misleading conclusions, I would like to examine briefly the four major strategies used by neurologists and neurosurgeons in secondary stroke prevention.

Anticoagulants

In heart-related thromboembolism, which is outside the framework of this talk, the value of anticoagulants is being established and some carefully designed clinical trials are in progress, which it is hoped will remove some of the lingering uncertainties here.

In noncardiac conditions, a few of which are germane to my topic, their use is strictly empirical. They have never properly been evaluated in atherothrombotic TIA. In progressing stroke, which in the Stroke Data Bank Registry currently being compiled in the United States occurs in 16.3% of ischemic strokes, their use was evaluated in one controlled study and the benefit was doubtful [7].

A series of case studies has been conducted in our institution into the visualization of thrombi in arteries, a condition regarded by some as a reason for emergency surgery. Antithrombotic agents in this pilot study, which was neither controlled nor randomized, yielded a better outlook than did prompt surgery [3].

Platelet Inhibitors

Since we launched the first controlled trial of aspirin in 1970, eight studies have now been completed. In the Canadian study, there was an overall 30% reduction in stroke and death [4]. In the French study, there was a 50% reduction in stroke and stroke death [2]. In the British study of 2435 patients, there was a 20% reduction in the risk of stroke and vascular death [18]. In the European study of 2500 patients, there was a 33% reduction in stroke and death [9]. No trials of persantine alone have been carried out in sufficient numbers to be of any consequence. When combined with aspirin, persantine confers no additional benefit from stroke reduction. A trial on ticlopidine therapy

will be concluded in 1988. In the trial, 3000 patients are being examined and it will give definitive answers as to the benefit of this potential treatment. In the meantime, it can be claimed that aspirin is of moderate benefit in stroke prevention, probably in both males and females, and a dose of one to four tablets per day has been shown to be useful.

Carotid Endarterectomy

In the light of four particular factors, there is a growing concern about this very common procedure: (a) It was not shown to prevent stroke in the two randomized trials that were conducted. (b) Stroke is declining and in this light all therapies with risk must be reexamined. (c) The procedure is proliferating and is probably done twice as often as it should be. (d) It is not done without real risk to the patient. With these observations in mind, we must ask ourselves what we know about the use of this procedure in a variety of circumstances. The evidence for its usefulness in asymptomatic disease is weak. In my opinion, such patients should not be operated on except in rare circumstances until the randomized clinical trials recently launched in asymptomatic patients are concluded. It is my prediction that indications for endarterectomy in asymptomatic patients will then virtually disappear.

There are those who regard some clinical and radiological conditions as indicative of the need for emergency endarterectomy. This includes the patient with thrombus in the artery. This is a high-risk circumstance and anticoagulants appear to be safer than surgery during the time that it requires for the dissipation of the thrombus [3].

Claims are made that the procedure is being done better with greater experience. Data from large surveys do not support this claim although there is no doubt that in some units it is a reasonable postulate [10]. The important question to be asked is: Is it a clearly beneficial procedure? Quite possibly, it will be shown to be so and in the most expert hands it will almost certainly be shown to be so. It has to be admitted, however, that it has never been proven. Hundreds of thousands of uncontrolled anecdotes obstruct the view and cast shadow rather than light. Its popularity is not a useful guide to its value. As the Nobel laureate Pauling noted: "Scientific truth is rarely obtained by a majority vote."

There are perceived high-risk groups. These perceptions are reasonable, albeit, unproven hypotheses and for the time being stand as little more than speculation. Claims commonly made about the "hemodynamic lesion" all tend to overlook the compelling importance of collateral variability. Sweeping claims about the significance of the degree of obstruction without considering the collaterals are misleading. An important paper appeared from St. Louis early this year [15]. In 19 patients, the PET scanner was used to identify the degree of hemodynamic compromise in TIA subjects. There was an even split between normality and major compromise despite varying degrees of obstruction and the conclusion was that the degree of stenosis meant less than the existence of the detectable collaterals in determining the hemodynamic compromise. The 158 London, Ontario subjects in the Canadian aspirin study were followed for 10 years [14]. Eighty of them had a so-called surgically significant lesion in the carotid artery. The likelihood of an ipsilateral stroke was the same as that of a stroke in another vascular territory (2.9% and 2.6% per year, respectively). The likelihood of death equalled the sum of both these stroke risks (5.5% per year). The degree of ulceration in the milder stenotic cases was of more consequence than the degree of narrowing. In all of the subgroups which have been perceived to be at higher risk, we are woefully short of adequate data.

The short- and the long-term benefit of carotid endarterectomy has been the subject of careful enquiry by a committee appointed by the American Neurological Association and chaired by Whisnant [6]. Utilizing the best currently available data, it appears that the nonoperated TIA patient has a 5% risk for the first 3 years and 3% risk of morbidity and mortality thereafter. If patients face a 10% operative risk, there is no hope of benefitting and conferring significant years of stroke-free survival upon them. With a 4% operative risk, benefit begins to appear at approximately 18 months. All these calculations are based on the best published nonsurgical data bases and are gleaned from observations made in the past, not the present. Contemporary randomized trials are urgently needed and in my opinion are an ethical demand upon neurosurgeons, vascular surgeons, and neurologists. One such study is underway and already has enrolled more than 1000 patients in Britain and Europe. One will commence in late 1987 in North America and the full backing of the North American neurosurgeons in this audience is requested. It would be reckless of us to pretend that

we have sufficient data in existence today. The profession and the public are looking with skepticism on such statements.

EC/IC Bypass for Stroke Prevention in Arteriosclerosis

The results here are disappointing. Some workers became and remain angry because of the results of the International Cooperative Study. I grieve especially for my closer neurosurgical friends and for nobody more than Peerless. He randomized more of his patients into the study than any another surgeon in the worldwide effort. His perioperative morbidity and mortality were the best in the study and his patency rate was 100%. Neither of these figures came from his own review; such a data source would be regarded as scientifically unacceptable in methodological circles; the results were assessed by outside independent evaluation.

The following summary covers the main points relative to the analyses performed in this trial:

The overall negative results have been published, are well known, and include the primary analyses as well as the major subgroups [8]. All the primary analyses and those of the major subgroups were negative including the 74 patients with continuing events in the presence of bilateral carotid occlusion. There were distressingly negative results in patients with continuing symptoms despite carotid occlusion and in middle cerebral artery stenosis.

The functional status of all patients was assessed at 3-monthly intervals [11]. There was a measurable overall improvement in the surgical patients. Unfortunately, it was not quite as much as in the control group, but it clarifies and explains the impression held by many surgeons that the operation is satisfactory to the patient.

A luxuriant anastomosis was not as good in terms of prediction of stroke-free survival as was a lesser one.

Patients with so-called vulnerable preoperative collaterals did less well than those with good preoperative collaterals. Nature has superior capabilities in this regard than we do [1].

Patients with recent events, as occurred in 600 of those entered, proved to be less rather than more likely to benefit [1]. It must be recalled that all patients were required to have had at least one event within 3 months of entry.

There was a trend to benefit in the Japanese

and Taiwanese centers compared with the overall figures, as there was in Memphis and in a scattering of small and large centers worldwide. If a treatment is only slightly worse than a control in a trial which is large enough to meet the demands of a proper sample-size requirement, there will be centers just above and just below the benefit line, as in this study. None reached anything close to significance and the confidence limits were wide due to the small numbers in individual centers.

An abstract at this meeting states that the bypass study was flawed. I urge all of you to read very carefully the hard data as well as the soft retrospective data, speculation, and surmise contained in the March 1987 issue of the New England Journal of Medicine [1, 16, 17].

Nonrandomized patients are a source of distortion in a trial if it is recognized that there are a number of patients of a certain type not submitted to the randomization process. No data have been produced to indicate that such a unique subgroup was diverted from the trial by the collaborators. If there are such data, we urge its publication. We kept track of the patients who were not randomized. The neurologists' forms unfortunately were frequently not submitted. They gave only a guide as to the reasons why patients were not submitted to randomization. We did not stress their use. A more important form was filled out by the participating surgeons. At the time of submission of the results paper, the week after the discussions at the final workshop of all collaborators and the presentation of results to the World Congress of Neurosurgery, these data had not been computed. We have now conducted and published a careful review of these data. The findings are as follows:

Three variations of center cooperation are disclosed [1]. Firstly, a small number of centers lost interest early. The surgeon moved or died and these compose group I in Table 1. In group II, strict adherence to the contractual agreement was pursued. In these 52 centers, which entered 87% of the patients into the trial, only 1.3 patients every 5 years were deviated per center from the study and operated upon outside the study. Patients were not eligible but could be operated on outside the study if there were medical exclusions or if they refused to sign a legally required consent. In these cooperative centers, the ratio of those randomized to all those who were operated upon outside the study was 1:1. Compared with other large surgical trials this is a unique record. In the big CASS trial, the ratio was 24 not randomized to 1 randomized and yet the positive

Table 1. NonRandomized surgical patients

	Group I (9 centers)	Group II (52 centers)	Group III (10 centers)
Randomized patients	34	1191	152
Medical exclusions	20	925	494
Refused consent	10	258	207
Deliberate diversions	5	66	24

Centers in group I dropped out of the study early; centers in group II submitted the large majority of their eligible patients for randomization; centers in group III failed to randomize the majority of their patients

conclusions from that study are acceptable [5]. In contrast to the cooperative 52, we had ten centers (Group III) who did not adhere to the spirit of the collaborative effort nor to the written agreement. The ratio of nonrandomized to randomized patients was 5:1. Fortunately these ten centers entered a disproportionately small total number of patients. The claim is now being made that these deviated patients contained the "real candidates" for this operation. The challenge for these centers, and they know who they are, is to disclose and publish these data. This disclosure alone, and no amount of rhetoric, will substantiate the accusation that this study was flawed. An analysis of the results repeated after eliminating the data from centers in group III gives identical results to the analyses which included their data.

The Rand Corporation was commissioned by the NIH to make a study of clinical research [12]. Their report, which included the bypass trial, identified five reasons why clinicians choose to quarrel with the results of clinical studies which go against their views: (a) Reverence for authority; (b) respect for tradition; (c) the "Olympian" view that practice is superior to "mere research" (d) doing something is better than doing nothing; (e) the effect of acceptance on financial and educational investments.

Julius Caesar in De Bello Gallico stated "Men nearly always believe what they wish." Francis Bacon, 1600 years later, said much the same thing: "For what a man had rather were true, he more readily believes." We all wanted to believe that Yaşargil had introduced a golden era in stroke reduction by surgery. We were disappointed. I suggest that we stop looking over the EC/IC battlefield for any signs of survivors. We cannot muster from this survey a viable, let alone an impregnable, army in the war against stroke. Conceivably, a few platoons may be lingering somewhere. It behoves us to recall what happened when Alexander the Great died at the age of 32. Fierce jealousies bred of arrogance and greed ripped apart his three-tiered and previously invincible army. They quarrelled, fought, poisoned, and murdered each other and in a few years were incapable of fighting a battle let alone a war. As one of the very few neurologists privileged to attend the meeting in Sendai, I would urge vascular neurosurgeons to continue to move ahead arm-in-arm with neurological and biostatistical colleagues to make further inroads into stroke prevention.

I close by reminding you of what was said 200 years ago by David Hume, a man who did not believe in all of the miracles claimed by the Christian church: "The onus of proof for unusual claims rests with the claimant."

References

1. Barnett HJM, Sackett D, Taylor W, et al. (1987) Are the results of the extracranial-intracranial bypass trial generalizable? NEJM 316:820–824
2. Bousser MG, Eschwege E, Haguenon M, et al. (1983) "AICLA": controlled trial of aspirin and dipyridamole in the secondary prevention of atherothrombotic cerebral ischemia. Stroke 14: 5–14
3. Buchan A, Gates P, Pelz D, Barnett HJM. Intraluminal thrombus in the cerebral circulation. Stroke
4. Canadian Cooperative Study Group (1978) A randomized trial of aspirin and sulfinpyrazone in treated stroke. NEJM 299:53–59
5. CASS Principal Investigators and Their Associates (1983) Coronary artery surgery study (CASS): a randomized trial of coronary artery bypass surgery. Circulation 68:939–950
6. Committee on Health Care Issues, American Neurological Association (1987) Does carotid endarterectomy decrease stroke and death in patients with transient ischemic attacks? Annals of Neurology 22:72–76
7. Duke RJ, Bloch R, et al. (1986) Intravenous heparin for the prevention of stroke progression in acute partial stable stroke: a randomized controlled trial. Ann Int Med 105:825–828
8. EC/IC Bypass Study Group (1985) Failure of extracranial-intracranial arterial bypass to reduce the risk of ischemic stroke. NEJM 313:1191–1200
9. ESPS Group (1987) The European stroke prevention study. Lancet 1351–1354
10. Fode NC, Sundt TM, Robertson JT, et al. (1986) Multicenter retrospective review of results and complications of carotid endarterectomy in 1981. Stroke 17:370–376
11. Haynes B et al. (1987) Functional status changes following medical or surgical treatment for cerebral ischemia. JAMA 257:2043–2046
12. Kahan JP, Neu CR, Hammons GT, Hillman BJ (1987) The decision to initiate clinical trials of current medical practices. Rand, Santa Monica
13. Khaw K-T, Barrett-Connor E (1987) Dietary potassium and stroke-associated mortality. NEJM (1986) 316:235–240
14. Lauzier S, Cote R, Ogunyemi A, Hopkins M, Vandervoort M, Barnett HJM (1986) Predictive value of cerebral atheroma in 158 patients—a 10 year follow-up. Stroke 17:127 (abstract)
15. Powers WJ, Press GA, Grubb RL Jr, Gado M, Raichle ME (1987) The effect of hemodynamically significant carotid artery disease on the hemodynamic status of the cerebral circulation. Ann Int Med 106:27–35
16. Relman AS (1987) The extracranial-intracranial arterial bypass study: What have we learned? NEJM 316:809–810.
17. Sundt TM (1987) Was the international randomized trial of extracranial-intracranial arterial bypass representative of the population at risk? NEJM 316:814–816
18. UK-TIA Study Group. The UK-TIA aspirin trial: the interim results. Br Med J

Future Aspects of Surgery for Cerebral Stroke

CHARLES G. DRAKE[1]

Predictions of future events, particularly in surgery and its technology, are at best conjecture, but I believe they are best surmised from reflections on the past and review of the current states of the art.

Surgery for Ischemic Stroke

The vast majority of strokes have an ischemic origin from thromboembolism related to atherosclerosis of extracranial and intracranial arteries and heart disease. Because of the time factor from complete ischemia to cerebral cell death—a matter of minutes—most surgery has been preventive in nature, to restore flow and remove sources of thromboembolism by removing upstream atheromatous stenosis and ulceration, extracranial to intracranial (EC-IC) bypass of inaccessible lesions, and heart valve replacement.

Cerebral revascularization early after acute ischemic stroke has been of little avail and complicated by conversion of bland to hemorrhagic infarctions. Logistically, because of the time interval leading to cell death, it may well be impossible to use any brain cell protective measure before infarction occurs, unless the event occurs in hospital. The very early removal of a carotid or middle cerebral embolus occurring in hospital rarely seems to have been of value. Whether the deep barbiturate coma that was induced within 20 or 30 min, as in our cases, was protective is speculative.

To date, revascularization to improve flow to the marginally ischemic penumbra to reduce infarct size has also been disappointing except for a few anecdotal experiences. Stroma-free hemoglobin and fluorocarbons will undoubtedly have their trial when approved.

Although as much as 25% of strokes result from thromboembolism from diseased hearts, the only significant surgical role has been replacement of diseased valves. Rarely, a ventricular aneurysm with mural thrombosis has been excised when the first embolus has been to a systemic vessel. Perhaps in the future, plication of the bag-like fibrillating auricle may reduce the risk of mural thrombosis in that disorder.

Occasionally, large or giant aneurysms present with transient ischemic attacks (TIAs) or even a completed small infarct. Surgical obliteration of the aneurysm not only removes the risk of bleeding, but of repeated embolic stroke as well.

Carotid endarterectomy is the most common brain revascularization procedure. Ordinarily, it is used only after TIAs, but now asymptomatic lesions are being removed. There is mounting concern amongst neurologists and neurosurgeons about its overall efficacy.

There have been only two randomized clinical trials of carotid endarterectomy, but neither adequately addressed the benefit or lack of benefit of the procedure. Whisnant's careful review of the literature concluded that carotid endarterectomy may be of value provided the procedures are performed with a sufficiently low complication rate [4]. The postoperative mortality/stroke morbidity would probably have to be less than 1% to effect a 50% reduction in stroke after 5 years of follow-up. Even the best published surgical results probably have produced only about a 33% reduction in stroke after 5 years. If, as he suggests, the overall combined mortality and stroke morbidity is probably between 6% and 10%, then it is possible that the net effect of carotid endarterectomy is unfavorable. In that about 150 000 carotid endarterectomies were done last year in the United States, at great expense, it seems therefore that a carefully controlled clinical trial is warranted to determine the subgroups most likely to benefit.

It seemed inconceivable that EC-IC bypass revascularization of the middle cerebral artery

[1] Division of Neurosurgery, The University of Western Ontario, London, Ontario, Canada

territory would not be efficacious in preventing stroke after TIA from surgically inaccessible lesions. Yet, in a recent trial, it was not shown to be of benefit over the best medical management in general or in any of the many subgroups examined, regardless of the abundance of the new perfusion. This was true even for severe middle cerebral artery disease and even in the prevention of a subsequent infarction in the same hemisphere.

There could be no doubt that this bypass could support the middle cerebral circulation in view of our experience with giant aneurysm surgery. In ten patients, where the M1 could be deliberately occluded by tourniquet after EC-IC bypass for giant middle cerebral aneurysm, none had other than transient hemispheric ischemia and all had excellent outcomes. Remarkably, in three patients aged 9, 11, and 18 years, respectively, where M1 occlusion was done even though the bypass had failed, the M2 circulation was perfused by immediately available and luxurious leptomeningeal collaterals from the A2 and P2 without deficit. That bypass would supply the M2 branch distribution is not surprising, but in nine patients, the whole of the M1, as well as the M2, was isolated for giant carotid bifurcation aneurysms. This was done either by proximal A1 clipping and tourniquet occlusion of the terminal carotid (seven cases) or detached balloon occlusion of the petrous carotid where crossflow from A1 was scant or absent (two cases). All had excellent results, for the bypass filled the M1 retrogradely as well as its lenticulostriate branches.

That bypass did not hold its promise for stroke prevention was startling to the neurosurgical world. Why additional blood flow was not important in the face of apparent hemodynamic insufficiency beyond atheromatous stenosis is still not understood. It may be that thromboembolism, rather than reduced flow, or the gradual over development of the circle of Willis and leptomeningeal collaterals in the medically treated patients is the more important factor.

Even so, some neurosurgeons have not accepted the results of the study completely, feeling that there must be some groups of patients that should benefit, either in the prevention of stroke or in improvement of brain function from increased perfusion of marginally ischemic regions. As Yaşargil said, the results of the Bypass Study must be accepted under the parameters of that study. The study was done impeccably, with complete integrity and 100% follow-up by the principal investigators. If other atheromatous situations exist which are unknown to most and might benefit, then they must be subjected to a similar controlled study. The burden of proof looms large, for the numbers are likely to be small if existent. If the transiently ischemic brain had an incapacitating headache as a part of its syndrome, akin to the heart's angina, then the intracranial bypass procedure might still flourish.

Bypass for vertebrobasilar occlusive disease may provide benefits in a few cases where posterior communicating or other collaterals are insufficient, providing the morbidity of these procedures can be reduced.

While balloon angioplasty seems to have earned a place in the treatment of systemic and coronary atherosclerosis, there has been concern about its use in cervical and intracranial arteries because of downstream embolic effects from the detritus and the negligible time of safe ischemia for surgical repair of arterial tears or thrombotic occlusion. Although the few intracranial angioplasties reported have carried high morbidity, there is a considerable radiological literature building for balloon angioplasty for cervical carotid disease, apparently with minimal morbidity.

The use of thrombolytics for acute infarctive stroke is already under trial by the intravenous route. The elapsed time factor will be critical and surely will need to be under an hour, unless a cytoprotective agent becomes available for early protection. There have been tentative selective cerebral artery perfusions for lysis of local thrombosis, although these were performed several hours or more after the event.

Surely the largest future for neurosurgery in the prevention of stroke is the carotid endarterectomy, for about half of ischemic strokes result from ulcero-occlusive disease of this vessel in the neck. There must be subgroups of this disease which will benefit providing very low operative morbidity is maintained. It is too early to know whether balloon angioplasty in the carotid will be safe and effective, but certainly there will be more trials by the radiologists in North America.

Intracranial endarterectomy must have a marginal future because of the necessity to preserve the orifices of the vital perforating vessels. All novel surgical management of atherosclerotic disease must be compared with the current natural history as modified by the best medical therapy. Already the incidence of stroke has been reduced by nearly 50% in only 25 years, largely through the reduction of risk factors. Now on the horizon, as I have learned from Dudrick [1] and now Mullan, is a means not only to prevent atherosclerosis but actually to reduce the atheromatous plaque by avoiding certain amino acids and the use of cholesterol transferase inhibitors.

Surgery of Hemorrhagic Stroke

Cerebral hemorrhage in all its forms is responsible for about 10% of all strokes. Its origins can be divided into hypertensive and nonhypertensive etiologies.

Hypertensive cerebrovascular disease has been the most frequent cause, accountable for about 75% of hemorrhagic strokes. These hemorrhages occur in particular locations, mostly the basal ganglia, brain stem, and cerebellum, and are readily recognized by CT scanning. However, its incidence is declining coincident with a similar decline in the frequency and severity of hypertension, because of its widening therapeutic control. Surely the future for this disorder will be the early recognition and control of hypertension. In compliant patients, life expectancy is not dissimilar to those not so afflicted. The prospect of surgical relief of essential hypertension by decompression of the left medulla oblongata seems remote even in concept.

I am not convinced that intracerebral clot removal from this or other causes leads to a significant improvement in brain function over that which would occur with natural lysis and absorption. I suspect the surgical benefits from the open removal of clots or the stereotactic use of lytic agents and aspiration is marginal for hemorrhages which are not life threatening. Clot should be removed when life threatening and when a reasonable quality of life can be expected. Cerebellar hematomas and infarctions must be monitored very carefully.

Nonhypertensive causes of intracranial hemorrhage, from a surgical viewpoint, are divisible into blood dyscrasia, including chronic oral anticoagulation and angiopathies (e.g., amyloid), and vascular anomalies.

Aside from the removal of life-threatening hematomas, the avoidance of bleeding from dyscrasia is a matter for medical control.

Aneurysms and arteriovenous malformations (AVMs) constitute the largest challenge to neurosurgery for the future of intracranial bleeding. Although less common than others forms, hemorrhage from these anomalies are unique in occurring in a younger population, and their catastrophic bleeding can be prevented now only by surgical means, with the reward of long and useful lives. Aneurysms probably account for 6% of hemorrhagic stroke and AVMs for 1%.

Intracranial Aneurysms

It is just 50 years since an intracranial aneurysm was first clipped by Dandy, on 22 March 1937. In that half century, much has been learned about the natural history of aneurysms, the morbid consequences of their rupture, and their surgical treatment.

Currently, the technical problems for obliteration of virtually all small saccular aneurysms anywhere on the brain circulation are solved, with overall surgical success rates bettering 90% for most sites in patients in reasonable condition, even after early surgery and the risks of vasospasm.

For large aneurysms, up to 2.5 cm in diameter, some problems remain, particularly in certain sites of complex branching with many perforating vessels. Still, success rates, even for the upper basilar artery, are approaching 90%, particularly with the use of the temporary clip.

Operations for giant aneurysms in any numbers have been reported only in recent years. Even though our experience includes nearly 600 cases, there are still some problems to be overcome, although the tandem or parallel fenestrated clip technique has been very rewarding (Tables 1, 2).

Cavitron evacuation of tough, adherent thrombus is spectacularly easier and safer, although the instrument needs to be miniaturized and have several angles.

For the anterior circulation, the success rate is 86% and two of three can be clipped (Table 1).

For the posterior circulation, the results are poorest for those on the basilar artery—only 68% success overall, partly because only one in three can be clipped. However, if the brain stem involvement is minor, the success rate rises to about 75%. With severe brain stem disorder, little more than a third have good outcome (Table 2).

Giant posterior cerebral and vertebral aneurysms have good results, equivalent to those on the anterior circulation.

The tragedy in the midst of all this technical success is that just over half of those who rupture

Table 1. Giant aneurysms: anterior

n	Excellent	Good	Poor	Dead
257	190 (74%)	31 (12%)	22 (8.5%)	14 (5.5%)

Table 2. Giant aneurysms: posterior

n	Excellent	Good	Poor	Dead
323	144 (44.5%)	77 (24%)	68 (21%)	34 (10.5%)

an aneurysm and reach hospital have a satisfactory outcome. About 30% who die never reach a hospital. This awful morbidity is due principally to devastating rebleeding or ischemia with vasospasm, but also, in smaller numbers, to communicating hydrocephalus and medical and surgical complications. The future, therefore, rests primarily with the prevention of rebleeding and ischemia and improvement in the management of certain large and giant aneurysms.

Rebleeding, the most common complication, is the most tragic and devastating. Three factors will be important in its prevention. First is recognition that an initial bleeding has occurred, particularly by physicians but also by the patients and their families. This aspect of the tragedy is not in surgical hands, although we must promote a continuing education campaign, not only to our students and physicians, but to the public as well. It is the largest problem. In Ontario, with a population of 9 million, only 40% of patients who rupture an aneurysm receive surgical treatment. The second important factor is to completely prevent rebleeding by operation as early as is practical and safe. Third, rebleeding can be retarded by about 50% with antifibrinolysins; there is no good evidence that these drugs are the cause of any increase in ischemic deficit. Factor 13 may be an even more potent antifibrinolysin and may even retard the release of the vasoactive agents.

The best deterrent to rebleeding in hospital is early operation. The return to early operation which began in Japan and in Europe in the late 1970s can be expected to continue, even though a study on the timing of surgery showed that it was little better than delayed surgery, except in patients who were in very good condition. In the analysis of all the factors for this disappointment, only two seemed important. It has been newly discovered that the peak of rebleeding was in the first 24 h, before which few patients could be operated upon. This period accounted for at least 5% of early rebleeding, which dropped about 1% per day thereafter, but down to 0.5% per day if antifibrinolysins were

used. Also, because early surgery and antifibrinolysins prevented rebleeding, many of these patients survived only to become victims of vasospasm. The incidence of infarction was doubled, so that the final outcome was little changed, whether the surgery was early or delayed.

Ischemia with vasospasm has therefore emerged as the most important complication of SAH to be overcome. In spite of over 25 years of research and trials of every conceivable vasoactive agent, no drug has emerged that reliably and credibly alters either the caliber of the arteries or the ischemia. Even the exact cause of the phenomenon is unknown, although it is likely to be multifactorial. Only volume expansion with improved rheology and artificial hypertension have proved fairly reliable. In our clinic, about 60% of patients who develop an ischemic deficit are relieved completely or to a satisfactory degree.

The endovascular balloon dilatation of spastic, large basal arteries, introduced in Leningrad, is interesting. However, whether perfusion beyond the large arteries, in the smaller vessels, will be improved remains to be seen.

Hope prevailed that early and complete removal of clot from the cisterns would prevent vasospasm. It proved not to be easy or complete, not without injury to pial banks, and only marginally effective, except perhaps after very early operations. Whether catheter irrigation for clot lysis with plasminogen activators will be safer and more effective remains to be seen.

Calcium channel-blocking agents, more specific for cerebral arteries, are now under intense study. There is promise that ischemia may be lessened significantly, but whether it will be from decline in the intensity of vasospasm or to one or more of the other actions of the drug must yet be determined. The results of the Canadian study on nimodipine suggest the latter is more likely, for, in spite of a significant decline in ischemic deficit, there was no alteration of the incidence or severity of the vasospasm [2]. Perhaps the next attack will be on the free radicals in the arachidonic acid cascade.

Historically, the surgical obliteration of

aneurysms has been centered around four basic methods:

1. Hunterian proximal ligation, occasionally with trapping
2. Neck clipping or ligation
3. Wrapping with gauze and/or plastic
4. Intraluminal thrombosis, now using thrombogenic wire
5. Endoaneurysmal balloon detachment, a recent innovation

Since the state of the art of neck clipping and parent arterial reconstruction for giant aneurysms with fenestrated clips has reached such levels of success, I view the technical future for neurosurgeons as centered on these techniques. They could be expanded to most giant saccular aneurysms, now unclippable, if safer means for prolonged circulatory arrest can be developed, such as with new cytoprotective agents or cardiopulmonary bypass without heparin, which is under development. With enough time, an otherwise impossible aneurysm could be opened, the thrombus evacuated with the cavitron, and a neck fashioned for repair. There is a need for clip miniaturization, including the appliers, and the potential for applying a clip at virtually any angle.

Hunterian proximal arterial occlusion, which has been so successful when tolerated, with and without bypass, will remain on standby for those whose necks cannot be repaired and for certain giant fusiform aneurysms.

EC-IC bypass for unclippable giant carotid bifurcation and middle cerebral aneurysms with tourniquet occlusion of M1 is a proven method. Whether bypass will play a role in giant anterior or posterior cerebral artery aneurysms is doubtful. The leptomeningeal collateral to these circulations has been so vigorous that no deficit has resulted from proximal ligation of the four isolated anterior cerebral arteries and only in two of 16 P2 arteries. Where bilateral A1 or A2 occlusion is contemplated, one A2 bypass with a side-to-side A2 anastomosis would probably be essential. Bypass to protect a few basilar or bilateral vertebral artery ligations may prove helpful where the posterior communicating collaterals are marginal. However, a vigorous P2 or superior cerebellar bypass is likely to cause failure of the upper basilar artery occlusion as its retrograde flow will maintain aneurysm filling and prevent thrombosis as occurs so often in the presence of a large posterior communicating artery.

For internal carotid occlusion, detached balloon occlusion in the petrous segment has largely replaced clamp occlusion in the neck in our unit, because initial temporary balloon occlusion is also predictable for collaterals and the dead space from which thromboembolism may arise is lessened. However, detached balloon occlusion of intracranial arteries has not been used for fear of blocking the orifices of vital perforating vessels.

Coating with mesh or plastic probably has a limited future for only certain cases such as small fusiform aneurysms with branches arising from the sac. If a saccular aneurysm can be dissected and completely freed, as it must be for coating, then usually more definitive measures can be applied. A few giant fusiform middle cerebral aneurysms can be encased, but the more common fusiform S-shaped atherosclerotic aneurysm of the basilar artery and its perforators cannot be separated from the brain stem.

Induced intraluminal thrombosis of the sac by transcranial methods, such as iron filings or thrombogenic wire, has not received wide acceptance. The neck is seldom occluded and the base of the sac simply "blows out" to form another dangerous aneurysm, as occurred in all three cases attempted in our unit.

Only occasionally is a ligature used now, although in some respects it is best of all for a complete neck occlusion which doesn't produce "dog ears." However, ligatures tend to kink the branches at large necks and there is more risk in their application. They may be useful for narrowing a large neck for clipping.

Giant fusiform aneurysms pose special problems in that the whole wall of the artery is diseased and collateral arterial supply is essential for two circulations: that of the terminal branches feeding the territory of the diseased artery and that of the many vital perforating branches arising from the sac. The former may be supplied with bypass if necessary, but for all but the middle cerebral, the existing circle of Willis or leptomeningeal collateral usually suffices. However, to occlude the interior of a fusiform aneurysm with thrombus beyond a proximal occlusion, or with any other material, one runs the risk of infarction in the perforating territories. Rarely can a peripheral fusiform sac be excised with reconstruction of the parent artery.

We now have experience with over 80 cases, only a few of which were atherosclerotic in origin. Most have occurred in a younger age group, mostly in the first four decades of life, and remain of undetermined etiology. Nearly all have been treated by proximal occlusion, occasionally trapping, with reasonable success rates, especially on the anterior circulation (86%): however, only 60% on the posterior circulation had good outcomes. The results were better when the patient was in good condition or only a short segment of the basilar artery was involved. That terminal branch collateral was available was not surprising in view of the experience with other giant aneurysms. What was remarkable was the frequency with which perforator collaterals were naturally available to the basal ganglionic region and brain stem in this age group. Unfortunately, this availability is not predictable or testable, even with the tourniquet, for it awaits occlusion of the perforators by thrombosis within the aneurysm. To provide collaterals here by surgical means is almost beyond my imagination. Perhaps ultramicrosurgery, about which some speculate, may allow reanastomosis of lenticulostriates, etc.

It is difficult to see a therapeutic future for the large, fusiform, S-shaped atherosclerotic aneurysm involving most of the basilar artery. If bilateral vertebral occlusion could be done under continuous anticoagulation, its growth might be curtailed. Balloons could be detached in both vertebral arteries, but even the short time off heparin to remove the catheter might well result in thrombosis of the sac with massive brain stem infarction. Severely stenosing vertebral clips might halt progression.

Well remembered is the reaction of the neurosurgical world when, in 1974, Serbinenko published his paper first describing his endovascular detachment of occluding balloons in the large arterial feeders to cerebral arteriovenous malformations (AVMs) and two aneurysms [3].

Although AVMs were pursued by this technique, especially after Kerber's modification of Dotter's calibrated leak balloon, little more was heard about intracranial aneurysms in the next decade, except for detached balloon occlusion of parent carotid or vertebral arteries. A few large extracranial aneurysms, mostly cavernous, were treated by intraluminal detached balloons, but there were problems with deflation of the balloons, balloon embolism, thromboembolism, and infection. Recently, surgeons from Moscow, Kiev, and Leningrad have rekindled interest with reports of their gradually increasing experience over 15 years with detached balloon occlusion of selected cerebral aneurysms. In Kiev, there was preservation of the parent arteries in 406 of 451 cases attempted, with good results in 80%. Remarkably, it is said that there is complete obliteration of the neck in nearly all cases in recent years.

Experience with this technique in Japan and North America is growing. In San Francisco, parent artery preservation was possible in 42 of 126 cases, with good results in 88%. The detached balloons are now filled with HEMA, which polymerizes slowly and, like silicone, prevents deflation. However, being water soluble, it will not cause massive embolization if still liquid when the balloon bursts. Yet, the risks of balloon detachment and rupture and thromboembolism remain.

It is difficult to understand why the neck of the aneurysms obliterated with detached balloons are said not to "blow out" to form another dangerous aneurysm underneath, as occurs with other methods of endoaneurysmal thrombosis such as wire or a small residual neck after clipping. It may be due to some hemodynamic difference, the unyielding nature of the balloon, or, perhaps, longer follow-up is needed.

The other probable future for SAH is the recognition of those who unknowingly harbor intact aneurysms. More are being discovered with CT scanning for other reasons. However, three-dimensional magnetic resonance (MR) imaging is imminent with computer reconstruction of the circle of Willis and its major branches down to a few millimeters. If the risk factors for aneurysm could be identifed, then a screening program might be possible. Yet the risk factors remain unknown except perhaps for cystic disease, coactation, and the rare family history. It has been suggested that collagen III may be deficient in patients with aneurysms. A study using noninvasive screening of aortic compliance is underway in London to look for any relationship.

The time to operate on an aneurysm is before it ruptures to avoid the morbidity of SAH and have an extremely low operative risk. As it is possible that, by middle age, 2% of the population harbor aneurysms of dangerous size, prophylactic aneurysm surgery might assume enormous proportions. In that only about 60% of aneurysms over 6 mm ultimately rupture, upwards of 40% of these operations would be unnecessary, as it is unlikely that predictability of those that will rupture will ever occur.

Arteriovenous Malformations

While other vascular malformations afflict the brain, cavernous, venous, and telangiectasis, the arteriovenous malformation (AVM) remains of most concern to neurosurgeons. For many years, after the pioneering efforts of Olivecrona in resection of AVMs in the 1930s, physicians looked upon them as much more benign than aneurysms, managing them with control of epilepsy and headache. Surgeons operated on the smaller lesions, mostly in noneloquent brain or those which had ruptured with a clot which usually had dissected part of the malformation from its bed. Of course, those early operations were done only with Bovie coagulation, ligatures, and silver clips. It was soon learned that clipping of feeding vessels was of no use in preventing bleeding, so there was little surgical enthusiasm for blind embolization with beads when it was introduced.

In contrast to aneurysms, the hemorrhage is intracerebral or intraventricular in two-thirds of all cases. Prevention of bleeding or rebleeding is the major reason for neurosurgical intervention, but it must be with a very low mortality and morbidity rate to better the natural history of the disorder, which only recently is coming to light. Once discovered, the annual bleed rate is between 1% and 2.5%, but the morbidity is less than that for ruptured aneurysm: death results in 10%-20% of the cases, but 60% of the survivors are normal or not seriously impaired. There is some inverse relationship between bleeding and the size of the malformation.

The current and future options for the management of AVMs are likely to remain surgical excision, embolization, radiation, or combinations of the above.

Site and size of AVMs are the major considerations for all managements. Our experience with over 500 cases suggests that surgical excision remains the treatment of choice and, with bipolar coagulation and the microscope, we have reached the state where most small AVMs (nidus of 2.5 cm) can be removed with minimal morbidity from most brain regions, including some on the surface but not deep in the brain stem. In the basal ganglia, this includes the caudate striatum, putamen insula, and anterior and dorsolateral thalamus. Although an involved anterior limb of the internal capsule can be taken, the genu and posterior limb must be preserved.

More discretion is needed for medium AVMs (nidus of 2.5–5 cm), particularly in basal ganglionic regions, but most others, even in eloquent brain regions, can be removed, although the dissection must be directly on the coils of the mass in the yellow glial plane.

Large AVMs (nidus of 5 cm) remain the largest surgical problem for the future. Their surgical morbidity has been the highest while their natural history is probably the most benign, at least for bleeding. It has been calculated that, to significantly improve the natural history of intact AVMs, surgical mortality must be in the order of 1% and the morbidity 10%. Because of their size, large hemispheric AVMs commonly encroach on or are in eloquent brain regions, the Rolandic, left Sylvian fissure, and cerebellar peduncles. Large AVMs are unlikely to be removed from deep ganglionic or brain stem regions except when only the tail of the lesion is invading.

The major surgical problem with removal of large AVMs is the fear of injury to motor, speech, and brain stem regions, the safe control of every deep, fragile, feeding vessel, and diminishing the afterload effect to prevent intra- and postoperative bleeding.

For those felt to be in or deep to functional cortical areas, craniotomy under local anesthesia is emerging as a valuable adjunct. It is remarkable how often the motor or speech areas are narrowly displaced from their presumed location with electrocorticographic mapping so that dissection down that side of the lesion can be carried out safely while constantly monitoring the patients ability to speak or move.

In our experience, it was not the removal of the AVM from its bed of eloquent brain that caused neurological catastrophe, but the intra- and particularly postoperative bleeding, especially in the posterior fossa. The incidence was related directly to the size of the AVM. It was the pursuit of deep spurting feeders that had been ruptured by the old bipolar forceps into or under eloquent brain that caused injury to deep pathways. The new thermal-diffusing nonsticking bipolar forceps have vastly improved the safety of removing large AVMs by averting tearing and popping of the small fragile feeding arteries that must be coagulated and divided safely on the first attempt. Since their introduction 2 years ago, there has not been a major problem with bleeding, intra- or postoperative, in our unit, although most large lesions have been staged with preoperative embolization.

Occasionally, during or after the removal of huge AVMs, sudden brain swelling with a cascade of bleeding from the deeper walls of the cavity has occurred and has been difficult to control. This has been described as "break through" bleeding based on diversion of the large flow into dysautoregulated vessels surrounding the AVM. To my knowledge, such dysautoregulation has not been shown to exist. While some of this bleeding may be shown in a few instances to be due to residual AVM, our belief is that most of it is the result of the arterial afterload from removal of the sump of the surrounding hypoperfused vascular bed and of fragile bipolar hemostasis. The diversion of this high flow, now under normal pressure, ruptures some of these abnormal fragile vessels which were poorly secured by coagulation. When it occurs, finger occlusion of the carotid in the neck usually dramatically reduces the brain swelling and the bleeding then is controllable. For large cerebral AVMs, the neck should be draped into the field so that a Selverstone clamp can be nearly closed on the internal carotid. The clamp can be removed later without the risk of thromboembolism. Delayed closure of the craniotomy for an hour or so is also wise with tests of hypertension and the Valsalva maneuver. Operative or preoperative embolization staging seems to have reduced this problem.

Embolization alone by radiologists or even more vigorously and extensively through craniotomy has failed to obliterate all but a few AVMs, and the nidus seems to recannulate in a few months or years. There is no evidence that partial obliteration alters rebleeding. We have abandoned embolization, transfemoral or intraoperative, except for preoperative staging to reduce arterial afterload and rarely for headache or steal. I am not yet convinced that preembolization assists the technical dissection, for the radiologists seldom can embolize the troublesome deep fragile feeders. Exceptions are when the embolization occludes the "nose" of the AVM, such as large lesions in the corpus callosum, the occipital lobe, and cerebellum.

It was little known until 1975 that radiation had an effect on AVMs. Since then, many have been treated with X-ray, focussed gamma, the proton Bragg peak, and, recently, electrons. However, there has been little discernible effect except on small lesions less than 2.5 cm, where the wipe-out rate with focussed gamma is spectacular—better than 90% with only a 3% morbidity from radiation necrosis. It seems not possible to irradiate large AVMs with effective doses and protect surrounding brain. The 8 or 10 Gy now used for them seem not enough.

Two futures for the treatment of AVMs seem probable; one surgical and the other embolization and radiation, probably in combination. The surgical future for medium and large AVMs will center on complete control of the fragile feeding arteries and the avoidance of afterload by staging which are the only real barriers to removal of all but huge lesions involving much of one or both hemispheres.

Staging, surgically, by embolization, or both, will probably be routine. Intraoperatively, the AVM could be collapsed by some form of profound regional hypotension such as temporary occlusion of all available major feeding arteries by clip or tourniquet, and even by transfemoral temporary balloon occlusion of deeper inaccessible feeding vessels. Such prolonged occlusions may become very safe if new cytoprotective agents are discovered. If cardiopulmonary bypass pump runs without heparin become a reality, then a soft shrunken AVM could easily be dissected from its bed after temporary exsanguination with arrest under deep hypothermia after the easier surface dissection had been done. Preliminary cortical mapping under local anesthesia will be very helpful where the lesion is in or near eloquent brain regions.

However, radiation and embolization will have their days of trial, although the risk of bleeding in the interval must be faced. The use of focussed gamma radiosurgery will increase for small AVMs, even in noncritical regions. While embolization and radiation are now ineffective for large AVMs, they can be combined. The search has begun for new perfusates for embolization which may suffuse more completely into AVMs. During the injection, some form of temporary circulatory arrest should be helpful, which could be total or local with temporary occluding balloons.

It is even conceivable that neurosurgeons might see little of AVMs in the future. The small ones could be irradiated. For the large ones, interventional and therapeutic radiologists could combine their methods, embolizing them to the extent possible and submitting the remaining smaller nidus to irradiation to complete the obliteration.

A year ago a journalist for the New York Times asked me what effect would occur in the craft of neurosurgery because of diagnostic radiologists' use of endovascular balloon techniques. He had been told that, within a decade, neurosurgeons would no longer be operating on intracranial aneurysms. There was no question that the diagnostic radiologists who had moved into interventional radiology were exerting a profound influence in many of surgery's anatomic fields. It was also equally true that their skills had been advancing steadily in the decade or so after the introduction of balloon techniques. Yet there are many problems that seem unlikely to be overcome easily; the various geometries of aneurysms and their origins, their fragility, and the lack of direct control of either the vehicle or the embolic material or aneurysmal rupture. In addition, radiologists have to face a neurosurgical success rate well over 90% for ruptured aneurysms in patients in reasonable condition.

Even so, balloon technology is in its infancy and I predict again that there will be a concerted effort in the next decade by interventional radiologists in North America and surgeons elsewhere to offer a less invasive and safer alternative to craniotomy to obliterate intracranial aneurysms by detached balloons, even with plastic. Balloon technology was introduced by surgeons and has remained in their hands in Russia and Japan. However, in Europe and North America, it has been taken over by neuroradiologists, probably because it was looked upon and misjudged by surgeons as minor in scope and technical demand, time consuming, and it was not "cutting" surgery. Also, there was the barrier to the use of appropriate X-ray machines which require professional radiological guidance and are so costly to reduplicate. Not to be denied is the radiologists manipulative skills using modern imaging navigation of all arterial streams with catheters. Yet I suspect most know aneurysms and AVMs only as shadows on an X-ray plate or a TV screen and have not seen their infinite variety, complexity, and fragility as seen at craniotomy, or know the breadth of their morbidity.

Before it is too late, my belief, recently acquired, is that some young neurosurgeons in North America and Europe should become involved with the new imaging and the escalating endovascular techniques. At least in the beginning, it should be done in partnership with their radiological colleagues, for considerable learning and skills must be acquired. In this way, development would be complementary rather than competetive. These are very new and different surgical adventures and it seems important that surgeons, with their ingenuity and wider knowledge of the intimate pathology, should be involved in their development and final placement in neurovascular therapeutics.

This paper began with the question of predictions for the future and mine may well have but a short temporal span. When I look back on my surgical life, now over 35 years, the changes in surgery, its art and science, have been remarkable and profound. The next generation of neurosurgeons will be faced with technology and science not yet born and some still not dreamed. Advances are often unanticipated and come often not from intraspecialty expertise but from other fields of endeavor. The enquiring investigative surgeon must remain alert for developments in fundamental science and new technology and become involved with their application to surgical disease.

References

1. Dudrick SJ (1987) Regression of atherosclerosis by the intravenous infusion of specific biochemical nutrient substrates in animals and humans. Ann Surg 206:296–315
2. Petruk K, West M, Mohr G, Weir B et al. (1988) Nimodipine treatment in poor grade aneurysm patients. Results of a multicentre double-blind, placebo controlled trial. J Neurosurg
3. Serbinenko FA (1974) Balloon catheterization and occlusion of cerebral vessels. J Neurosurg 41:125–145
4. Whisnant JP (1987) Does carotid endarterectomy decrease stroke and death in patients with transient ischemic attacks? Chairman, Committee on Health Care Issues. American Neurological Association. Ann Neurol 22:72–76

Part 2. Round Table Discussions (RTD)

RTD 1. Posterior Circulation Aneurysm

Posterior Circulation Aneurysms

Sydney J. Peerless and Charles G. Drake[1]

Introduction

More than 1400 patients with aneurysms arising
from the vertebral and basilar arteries have been
operated upon in the neurosurgical unit at the
University of Western Ontario in the past 35
years. The majority (1100) underwent surgical
treatment since 1970 and, therefore, enjoyed the
benefits of contemporary neuroradiology, anesthesiology, and the use of the operating microscope and microtechniques. Throughout this
period, a system of pre- and postoperative management, anesthetic technique, and operative
approach has evolved.

Despite the relatively inaccessible location of
these aneurysms in the confining space in front of
the brain stem, the majority of patients with
small aneurysms can be operated upon successfully and with a morbidity and mortality not
dissimilar to aneurysms of the anterior circulation. Beside excellent neuroanesthesia and technical and psychological preparedness to work in
this confined space, a detailed appreciation of the
anatomy is necessary. The most important pre-
dictors of outcome, however, are the grade of
patients going into the operating room and
the size of the aneurysm. Whereas a combined
morbidity and mortality of 8% has been experienced in small aneurysms, the risk of operation rises progressively as the aneurysm enlarges
to 32% with giant aneurysms of the posterior
circulation. Similarly, grade 1 and 2 patients have
a significantly more favorable outcome, with
most of the postoperative disability being accounted for by effects of the original bleed,
vasospasm, and possibly the added insult of
operation on an already injured brain.

[1] Division of Neurosurgery, The University of Western Ontario, London, Ontario, Canada

Approach to the Upper Basilar Artery

A minor controversy exists over the optimal approach to the upper basilar artery. The subtemporal, transsylvian, and combined approaches
each have strong advocates. We have favored the
subtemporal approach in the vast majority
of aneurysms originating on the basilar artery
above the anterior inferior cerebellar artery
(AICA) for the following reasons: The distance
from the scalp to the aneurysm is the shortest
from this approach; most of the aneurysms have
a neck that is narrowest in the anterior/posterior
direction and, therefore, accept the clip in the
lateral approach most easily; the critical perforators arising off the origin of the P1 bilaterally
and off the terminal basilar artery are posterior
and can be seen and separated from the neck and
protected before clipping; and, finally, the subtemporal approach is faster and allows more
efficient use of limited operating room time. The
transsylvian approach is also valuable in that the
fundamentals of the exposure are more familiar
to most neurosurgeons and it is particularly useful for high-lying aneurysms arising from the
elongated basilar arteries, where the neck of the
aneurysm is more than 1 cm above the posterior
clinoid. Although initially the amount of brain
retraction to reach the basilar bifurcation from
the transsylvian approach is less, the exposure
can be confining with access limited by perforating vessels arising off the posterior communicating artery and may require temporary retraction
of the carotid and middle cerebral arteries. As
well, the transsylvian approach gives the
surgeon only limited exposure of the posterior
cerebral and basilar perforators. A combined
transsylvian-subtemporal approach provides the
advantages and disadvantages of both expo-
sures, but can be extremely useful for large
broad-necked aneurysms, extending the visibility
and providing the opportunity for safe clipping
from either access. Familiarity with the anatomy,
complete confidence in the approach, and pre-

vious experience are all important determinants as to how the surgeon should approach these aneurysms but, in our opinion, one should be familiar with all these methods and, in any one case, the patient should be positioned, fixed in the pin headrest, and draped in such a way that any or all of the approaches can be utilized.

Temporary and Permanent Clips

Most of these aneurysms have been operated upon under moderate to deep generalized hypotension. In the early years, we used Arfonad, then subsequently sodium nitroprusside, and in the past 6 years increased inhaled concentration of isoflurane to produce the lowering of blood pressure. However, in recent years, we have been more frequently using a temporary clip on the basilar artery, with the patient normotensive, with excellent success. Our rediscovery of the temporary clip technique, stimulated by Suzuki and the Sendai school, has proved to be successful, both because of the apparent measure of protection provided by mannitol and the introduction of temporary clips with gentle closing pressures by Suzuki, Sugita, and others. The temporary clip not only dramatically reduces the risk of intraoperative rupture but, more importantly, will most often make the aneurysmal sac soft enough to be gently but deliberately deformed by the dissector, permitting precise definition of the neck and separation of surrounding important structures. For the upper basilar artery, we commonly use intermittent temporary basilar artery occlusion for periods averaging 3.5 min. However, as many as 20 intermittent clippings of the basilar artery have been utilized and some for as long as 20 min with no untoward effects. We have utilized the temporary clip for intermittent upper basilar artery occlusion in more than 100 cases with no recognized permanent complications.

All of the small aneurysms, that is less than 1.25 cm in diameter, have been clipped. Of the large aneurysms, 92% have also been secured directly with clips. However, of the 353 giant aneurysms with diameters greater than 2.5 cm, only 42% could be treated with neck clipping. In the past several years, we have come to use the Sugita clip almost exclusively. Drake's aperture modification of the Sugita clip is particularly useful for aneurysms of the upper basilar artery to permit clipping of the neck while the fenestration encircles and protects the P1 and its perforators, the perforators alone, and the oculo-

motor nerve. For those aneurysms with large bulky necks, the aperture clip permits clipping the neck in sections by using the tandem principle. This tandem technique makes use of the stronger closing pressures over a short length of blade to secure a portion of the neck so that one, two, or more aperture clips are placed across the neck with portions of the aneurysm still filling within the aperture, which is finally closed with a straight clip. Once again, the subtemporal approach makes multiple clip occlusion of an aneurysm neck possible that may be impossible in the narrow space of the pterional-transsylvian approach.

We have rarely attempted to wrap or coat aneurysms of the posterior circulation. More often, we have been impressed with the futility of coating, having spent many anxious hours patiently removing muscle, scar, gauze, and glue when redoing aneurysms that seemed at the first exposure by another surgeon to have been too dangerous or too difficult to clip. Wrapping and coating, in our opinion, is a far inferior treatment unless the sac is completely encased, and gives little protection against further enlargement or rupture. Usually a posterior circulation aneurysm that can be completely wrapped or encased in a reinforcing material can almost always be clipped.

Approach to Aneurysms of the Lower Basilar and Vertebral Arteries

Aneurysms below the AICA, that is vertebral–PICA, vertebral junction, basilar fenestration, and those few aneurysms arising off the lower basilar artery not adjacent to a named branch, can most often be exposed via the suboccipital approach. The side of the exposure is determined by consideration of two factors—the side of the neck and distance. Normally, we prefer to approach the neck side of these aneurysms rather than the fundus side. This practice has three advantages. The first, and most important, is that the surgeon can expose the aneurysm from its least hazardous side while gaining the opportunity to have proximal and distal control of the parent artery and to see with greater clarity the associated branches at the neck. Moreover, because these aneurysms tend to balloon out asymmetrically within the narrow space at the base, causing the basilar artery to be displaced away from the fundus, the exposure distance is somewhat smaller on the neck side than on the fundus side. Obviously, for aneurysms of the vertebral artery, the approach is made most often on the side from which the vertebral artery enters the skull but even then, with large sacs or with marked tortuosity and displacement of the vertebral artery, we have occasionally found it useful to clip finally the neck of the aneurysm across the front of the brain stem. Rarely, lower basilar artery aneurysms have been clipped through the subtemporal-transtentorial approach, again in circumstances where the aneurysm was large and ballooning downward, making exposure of the neck more straight-forward from above. For those aneurysms at the AICA, below the AICA, or at the vertebro-basilar (V-B) junction, particularly when large, multilobed, with a broad neck, or when the surgeon is uncertain of the anatomical detail, a combined transtentorial-suboccipital approach can be ideal.

The combined transtentorial-suboccipital approach provides a wide access to the whole length of the basilar artery. This exposure is gained by extending the normal suboccipital craniectomy upward and laterally to unroof the confluence of the transverse and lateral sinus and to join the bony removal afforded by a low middle and posterior temporal craniotomy. The bone at the base, including the mastoid, is removed away until flush with the floor of the temporal fossa and posterior slope of the petrous bone. After gently elevating the temporal lobe and identifying the vein of Labbé, the tentorium is divided behind the trochlear nerve and continued posteriorly and laterally to the petrous base. The dura of the posterior fossa is divided anterior to the lateral sinus so that the two dural incisions can be linked after dividing, between ligatures, the petrosal sinus. The isolated dural leaflet continuing the vein of Labbé and the intact transverse and lateral sinus system can then be retracted gently backward with the temporal lobe and cerebellum to view the whole brain stem and the vessels from the distal vertebrals to the distal basilar artery. One needs free mobility of the microscope to be able to see both above and below the trigeminal and seventh and eighth cranial nerves. One must also be cautious to avoid excessive retraction so as not to stretch and injure the tender cochlear nerve. This exposure usually permits a detailed evaluation of the anatomy, temporary proximal occlusion or trapping of the basilar or vertebral arteries, and sufficient room to place and align clips in a fashion to obliterate the neck of an otherwise complex aneurysm. It also provides sufficient room to decompress the sac once the neck is

clipped by removing the clot and formed thrombus causing deforming pressure on the brain stem.

Results

The overall results by grade for surgical patients harboring small and large aneurysms, excluding those patients with giant aneurysms, are summarized in Table 1. Patients judged to have excellent results are neurologically normal. Those listed as good have detectable neurological signs, but have returned to full activity including work and are not restricted in their day-to-day life. Patients have been classified as having a poor result if they are unable to return to work or are dependent on others for their activities of daily living. Overall, we have achieved an 89% excellent or good result in these patients. These numbers, of course, are a composite of more than 30 years' experience, beginning with the first attempts to deal with these aneurysms by the senior author, which resulted in a 50% mortality. In the past 5 years, we have been able to achieve an average of 95% excellent or good results overall, with the most troublesome aneurysms still being those sacs arising from the terminal basilar artery. Theoretically, preventable complications such as inadvertent perforator injury or major branch vessel occlusion from imperfectly placed clips, postoperative unrecognized extradural or subdural hematoma, and cardiopulmonary complications continue to take their toll. As well, vasospasm with secondary resulting cerebral ischemia and rebleeding among unsecured and incompletely secured aneurysms remain the most feared complication and the most important factor causing the patient's ultimate poor outcome.

Table 1. Posterior circulation aneurysms results by grade (1080 patients)

Grade	E	G	P	D
0	108	12	4	1
1	559	65	23	25
2	119	46	21	9
3	22	23	23	9
4		2	7	2
Total	808	148	78	46
	89%		11%	

E excellent, *G* good, *P* poor, *D* dead

Table 2. Basilar bifurcation aneurysms (small and large)

Grade	E	G	P	D
0	55	8	3	
1	274	43	16	15
2	76	29	18	4
3	13	14	16	3
4		1	4	
Total	418	95	57	22
	87%		13%	

Table 3. Basilar-SCA aneurysms

Grade	E	G	P	D
0	28	2		
1	84	5	3	2
2	16	9	3	1
3	3	4	3	
Total	131	20	9	3
	93%		7%	

Table 4. Basilar aneurysms between the SCA and AICA

Grade	E	G	P	D
0	4	2		
1	29	3	3	3
2	5	2		2
3	1	1	2	1
Total	39	8	5	6
	81%		19%	

Table 5. Vertebral-basilar junction aneurysms

Grade	E	G	P	D
0		1		
1	38	3		1
2	6	4		2
3	1	2		
4		1	1	1
Total	45	10	2	4
	90%		10%	

Table 6. Vertebral-PICA aneurysms

Grade	E	G	P	D
0	11			
1	109	7	1	4
2	15	2		
3	2	2	1	1
4			2	1
Total	137	11	4	7
	93%		7%	

Table 7. Posterior cerebral aneurysms

Grade	E	G	P	D
0	10			1
1	25	4		
2	1			
3	2		1	3
Total	38	4	1	4
	89%		11%	

Tables 2–7 summarize the operative results on patients harboring aneurysms up to 2.4 cm in diameter by site and grade. Our largest experience by far has been with those aneurysms arising at the basilar bifurcation. Our results at this site and for those relatively few patients whose aneurysms arose at the origin of the anterior inferior cerebellar artery and up to, but not including, the superior cerebellar artery remain patients with aneurysms in whom we have had the least success. These aneurysms remain perhaps the greatest technical challenge to the neurosurgeon because of the narrow, difficult access and the close proximity to vital and vulnerable structures.

Today, for small and large aneurysms, the combined risk for morbidity and mortality of small and large (but not giant) aneurysms of the posterior circulation is 5%. It is similar in our unit whether the aneurysm is operated upon early (within the first 96 h) or late. The most important single factor to predict outcome is the condition (grade) of the patient going into the operation.

References

1. Drake CG (1979) The treatment of aneurysms of the posterior circulation. In: Carmel PW (ed) Clinical neurosurgery, vol. 26. Williams and Wilkins, Baltimore pp 96–144
2. Peerless SJ, Drake CG (1985) Posterior circulation aneurysms. In: Wilkins RH Rengachary SS (eds) Neurosurgery. McGraw-Hill, New York, pp 1422–1437

Surgical Management of Posterior Inferior Cerebellar Artery Aneurysms

James I. Ausman, Balaji Sadasivan, Fernando G. Diaz, Ghaus M. Malik, and Manuel Dujovny[1]

Introduction

Posterior inferior cerebellar artery (PICA) aneurysms are rare and make up 0.65%–3% of all intracranial aneurysms [11, 21]. In 1953, Rizzoli and Hayes first reported successful surgical treatment of a PICA aneurysm operated in 1947 [25]. Since then, there have been several reports on the surgical management of PICA aneurysms [6, 7, 11, 13, 15, 21]. However, as these aneurysms are rare, surgical experience with them has generally been limited. We present our experience over the past 9 years with 11 patients who underwent clipping of PICA aneurysms.

Summary of Cases

The records of the Henry Ford Hospital were reviewed for the period 1 January 1979 to 30 June 1987. There were over 500 cases of cerebral aneurysms treated surgically, of which 11 were of PICA aneurysm.

The age of these patients ranged from 24 to 78 years (Table 1). There were seven females and four males in this study. Three of the patients did not have subarachnoid hemorrhange (grade 0) [12]; three patients were gradeI; one patient was grade II; four patients were grade III.

All the patients underwent four-vessel cerebral angiography to demonstrate the aneurysm and its relationship to the vertebral artery (VA) and PICA. Six of the aneurysms were on the left and five on the right. There were two giant aneurysms (> 2.5 cm) [27]. All the aneurysms were on the proximal segment of the PICA at or near the VA-PICA junction. There were no distal PICA aneurysms in this study.

We treated all the patients with dexamethasone

and phenytoin preoperatively. After induction, a Swan-Ganz catheter, a Foley catheter, an arterial line, and a spinal drain were inserted. The patients were operated in the lateral decubitus position, with the head flexed and in a headholder.

A paramedian straight or retromastoid incision was made and the suboccipital muscles divided. If necessary, the occipital artery can be preserved as it could be needed for a bypass procedure to the PICA if clipping of the aneurysm occluded the proximal PICA. The muscle dissection was carried caudally up to the C2 level. A suboccipital craniectomy extended to the foramen magnum. In some of the earlier cases, part of the posterior arch of the C1 vertebra was also removed. During the craniectomy, the patients were given intravenous furosemide and mannitol. The dura was then opened so that flaps of dura were reflected on the sigmoid sinus, transverse sinus, and the midline. At this stage, the spinal drain was opened and cerebrospinal fluid (CSF) drained continuously. The microscope was then utilized. The cerebellum was retracted and the cisterna magna opened to drain additional CSF.

Our technique usually involved identifying the intracranial vertebral artery to obtain proximal control. The dissection was then carried out on the PICA distal to the aneurysm. The VA distal to PICA was then identified to obtain distal control. The base and neck of the aneurysm were then dissected free and clipped. In five of the cases, temporary clipping was used. When temporary clipping was used, 250 mg thiopental, 100 mg lidocaine, and 12.5 g mannitol were given several minutes before the temporary clips were placed. The blood pressure was maintained at normal or slightly elevated levels. The clips were usually placed on the proximal and distal VA, and on the PICA. Sugita or Yasargil temporary clips with 40–80 g closing force were used on the VA. Kleinert-Kutz clips were used for the PICA. In the five patients in whom temporary clipping

---

[1] Department of Neurological Surgery, Henry Ford Hospital, Detroit, Michigan, USA

Table 1. Summary of cases

Age(yrs)	Sex	Grade	Surgical procedures	Temporary clipping	Result
51	F	I	Clipping of left PICA aneurysm	None	Excellent
48	F	0	Clipping of left PICA aneurysm	None	Excellent
37	M	I	Clipping of left PICA aneurysm	None	Excellent
59	F	II	Clipping of right PICA aneurysm	None	Excellent
78	F	III	Clipping of right PICA aneurysm	30 min	Died
50	M	III	Clipping of right PICA aneurysm	35 min	Fair
73	F	III	Clipping of left PICA aneurysm	None	Fair
55	F	III	Clipping of giant left PICA aneurysm	9 min	Good
38	M	0	Clipping of giant right PICA aneurysm	90 min	Good
24	M	0	Clipping of right PICA aneurysm	None	Excellent
69	F	I	Clipping of left PICA aneurysm	8 min	Excellent

PICA posterior inferior cerebellar artery

was used, the clamp time was 8 min, 9 min, 30 min, 35 min, and 90 min. After the aneurysms were clipped and the temporary clips removed, blood flow into the VA and PICA was checked. In the later cases, a microdoppler was used to check for blood flow in these vessels.

In all 11 patients, the aneurysm was identified and clipped. In one patient, the PICA was found to arise from the dome of the aneurysm. In this patient, after the aneurysm was clipped, there was no blood flow in the PICA distal to the aneurysm. The PICA was divided distal to the aneurysm and an end-to-side anastomosis to the opposite PICA was performed. This patient required 90 min of temporary clipping to do both the clipping of the aneurysm as well as the reconstruction of the posterior circulation. No deficit occurred as a result.

Our results were divided into the five categories described by Dujovny et al. [8]. We had excellent or good results in grade 0, grade I, and grade II patients (seven patients). Among the four grade III patients, we had one good result and two fair results.

There is one mortality in this study. The patient was a 78-year-old female with grade III subarachnoid hemorrhage. Angiograms showed a 5-mm right PICA aneurysm. On the 2nd postbleed day, a retromastoid craniectomy was performed and the dura opened. The cerebellum was retracted and the aneurysm identified. The brain was swollen and the exposure was limited. As the neck was being dissected, bleeding developed from the superior aspect of the neck. The VA was clamped proximal and distal to the PICA and a 10–0 Nurolon stitch was placed at the point. The

aneurysm was dissected and a Sugita clip placed across the neck. In order to get a better view of the area, the dome of the aneurysm was excised and an aneurysmorrhaphy was done. After 30 min of clamp time, the temporary clips on the VA were removed. Initially, there was no blood flow in the VA. The Sugita clip was removed and there was no back-flow from the PICA. After a few minutes, blood flow returned to the VA. The Sugita clip was replaced over the neck of the aneurysm. There was no flow in that PICA vessel. A right cerebellar tonsillectomy was done. In the immediate postoperative period, the patient was awake and alert. However, she developed multiple complications and deteriorated neurologically. A CT scan showed a right cerebellar infarction. Angiography showed occlusion or severe stenosis of the right VA and proximal basilar artery. She died 2 months after her surgery.

Discussion

The natural history of aneurysms of the vertebrobasilar system is associated with a high mortality. Richardson's study showed that the mortality of untreated posterior circulation aneurysms was higher than untreated anterior circulation aneurysms [24]. Eight of fourteen untreated posterior fossa aneurysms died of aneurysm rupture during follow-up in Uihlein and Hughes's report [33]. Gillingham found that all 26 of his patients with posterior circulation aneurysm who were treated without operation died within 3 years [9].

In the past two decades, improvements in angiography, such as transfemoral catheterization, subtraction, and magnification, have improved the preoperative assessment of these aneurysms. The use of the operating microscope for the delicate dissection of posterior circulation aneurysms has improved the results of surgical treatment.

Clinical Characteristics

The average age in our study (55 years) was similar to that found in other studies [4, 11, 13, 18, 25]. Our study showed an approximate 2:1 preponderance of females, again similar to other studies [4, 11, 13, 25]. All 11 aneurysms in this study were located at or near the PICA-VA junction. There were no cases of distal PICA aneurysm. Most other series and literature reviews report a 10%–20% incidence of distal PICA aneurysm [11, 21, 34]. Two of the eleven aneurysms were giant aneurysms (18%) [27]. This was a lower percentage than that reported by Kempe (31%) [15] but higher than that reported by Drake and Peerless (3%) [7] or Hudgins et al. (0%) [11].

Surgical Management

The PICA, the largest and most distal branch of the VA, is intimately related to the medulla, the inferior portion of the fourth ventricle, the inferior vermis, the tonsils, and the inferior aspect of the cerebellar hemisphere [19, 28]. The PICA has the most variable course of all the cerebellar arteries and this is the primary determinant of the location of the aneurysm [16]. The aneurysms usually occur at the branching points and at curves and point in the direction that blood flow would have taken if the curve or branching had not been present. The PICA-VA aneurysm usually arises at a curve where the VA turns medially to join the contralateral VA. The sac of the aneurysm commonly points superiorly and slightly posteriorly to be against the medulla. In the normal course of the PICA, this point usually lies 10 mm above the foramen magnum in the anterolateral subarachnoid space between the medulla, skull base, and lower cranial nerves. The PICA usually arises posterior or lateral to the aneurysm neck. In the lateral approach to the aneurysm, this facilitates preservation of the PICA [34]. The PICA takes a variable course through the rootlets of cranial nerves IX through XII. Frequently, it may even touch cranial nerves

VII and VIII [16]. Damage to the cranial nerves is a major cause of morbidity in PICA aneurysm surgery [11].

Aneurysms at the proximal PICA may be approached with the patient in the sitting, prone, supine, or lateral positions. We have approached these aneurysms with the patient in the lateral position for the following reasons:
1. Decreased risk of air embolism or hypotension as compared to the sitting position
2. Less retraction on the cerebellum as gravity causes it to fall away, as compared to the prone position
3. Less risk of meningitis or CSF leak as compared to the transclival approach in the supine position
4. Better visualization of the PICA [34]

In the earlier cases, we removed part of the posterior arch of the Cl vertebra. In the later cases, we found that we could do the operation without removing the arch.

We have used temporary clipping of vessels since 1981 and found it useful [2]. This procedure is based on Suzuki's method which involves the use of low gram force aneurysm clips for the shortest possible occlusion time [32]. Temporary clipping does not generally appear to have any deleterious effect and has been found to be useful by other neurosurgeons [17, 20, 35]. During temporary clipping, we use mannitol to improve cerebral blood flow [14], lidocaine to stabilize the sodium-potassium pump in the membrane, and barbiturates as cerebral protective agents [3, 20]. We feel this regimen allows a safe temporary occlusion time of at least 30–40 min [2].

In one patient in this study, after the aneurysm was clipped, an end-to-side PICA-to-PICA anastomosis was done. Our experience with reconstruction of the intracranial circulation as part of the surgical treatment of aneurysms began in 1981 [1, 2]. So far, we have performed reconstructive surgery after clipping of the aneurysm in eight cases of giant aneurysms. There procedures are technically difficult and only a few other cases have been reported [5, 10, 30, 31, 36].

The results in our study are similar to other reports in the literature. Of our patients, 73% did well. We had one mortality (9%). Yamaura et al. have reported on 21 PICA aneurysms [34]. Two patients died preoperatively. They had no postoperative deaths. Hudgins et al. have reported on 21 surgically treated cases [11]. There was a 10% mortality and a 20% occurrence of serious morbidity. Drake and Peerless have reported their experience with 146 cases [7]. Of those patients, 84% did well and there was a 6% mortality.

References

1. Artero JC, Ausman JI, Dujovny M, et al. (1985) Middle cerebral artery reconstruction. Surg Neurol 24:5–11
2. Ausman JI, Diaz FG, Dujovny M (1986) Reconstruction of the intracranial circulation. In: Kikuchi H, Fukushima T, Watanabe K (eds) Intracranial aneurysms. Nishimura, Niigata, pp 284–291
3. Bruce DA (1978) The pathophysiology of increased intracranial pressure. Upjohn Kalamazoo
4. Chou SN, Ortiz-Suarez HJ (1974) Surgical treatment of aterial aneurysms of the vertebrobasilar circulation. J Neurosurg 41:671–680
5. Dolenc V (1922) End-to-end suture of the posterior inferior cerebellar artery after the excision of a large aneurysm: Case report. Neurosurg 11:690–693
6. Drake CG (1978) Treatment of aneurysms of the posterior cranial fossa. Prog Neurol Surg 9:122–192
7. Drake CG, Peerless SJ (1986) Posterior circulation aneurysms. In: Kikuchi H, Fukushima T, Watanake K (eds) Intracranial aneurysms. Nishimura, Niigata, pp 336–348
8. Dujovny M, Charbel F, Berman SK, Diaz FG, Malik G, Ausman JI (1987) Geriatric neurosurgery. Surg Neurol 28:10–6
9. Gillingham FJ (1982) In: Youmans JR (ed) Neurological surgery: A comprehensive reference guide to the diagnosis and management of neurosurgical problems. WB Saunders, Philadelphia, vol. 3, pp 1715–1717
10. Hopkins LN, Budny JL, Castellani D (1983) Extracranial-intracranial arterial bypass and basilar artery ligation in the treatment of giant basilar artery aneurysms. Neurosurg 13:189–194
11. Hudgins RJ, Day AL, Quisling RG, et al. (1983) Aneurysms of the posterior inferior cerebellar artery: A clinical and anatomical analysis. J Neurosurg 58:381–387
12. Hunt WE, Kosnik EJ (1974) Timing and perioperative care in intracranial aneurysm surgery. Clin Neurosurg 21:79–89
13. Jamieson KG (1964) Aneurysms of the vertebrobasilar system. Surgical intervention in 19 cases. J Neurosurg 21:781–797
14. Kassell NF, Baumann KW, Hitchon PW, et al. (1981) Influence of a continuous high dose infusion of mannitol on cerebral blood flow in normal dogs. Neurosurg 9:283–286
15. Kempe LG (1979) Aneurysms of the vertebral artery. In: Pia HW, Langmaid C, Zierski J (eds) Cerebral aneurysms: Advances in diagnosis and therapy. Springer, Berlin, pp 119–120
16. Lister JR, Rhoton AL Jr, Matsushima T, et al. (1982) Microsurgical anatomy of the posterior inferior cerebellar artery. Neurosurg 10:170–199
17. Lyunggren B, Saveland H, Brandt L, et al. (1983) Temporary clipping during early operation for ruptured aneurysm. Preliminary report. Neurosurg 12:525–530
18. Locksley HB (1966) Report on the Cooperative Study of Intracranial Aneurysms and Subarachnoid Hemorrhage. Section V, Part I. Natural history of subarachnoid hemorrhage, intracranial aneurysms, and arteriovenous malformations. Based on 6368 cases in the cooperative study. J Neurosurg 25:219–239
19. Margolis MT, Newton TH (1974) The posterior inferior cerebellar artery. In: Newton TH, Potts DG (eds) Radiology of the skull and brain, vol. 2 Mosby, St. Louis, pp 1710–1774
20. Marshall LF, U HS (1983) Treatment of massive intraoperative brain swelling. Neurosurg 13:412–414
21. Pasqualin A, DaPian R, Scienza R, et al. (1981) Posterior inferior cerebellar artery aneurysm in the fourth ventricle. Acute surgical treatment. Surg Neurol 16:448–451
22. Rand RW, Jannetta PJ (1967) Micro-neurosurgery for aneurysms of the vertebral-basilar artery system. J Neurosurg 27:330–335
23. Rhoton AL Jr, Jackson FE, Gleave J, et al. (1977) Congenital and traumatic intracranial aneurysms. CIBA Clin Symp 29(4):2–40
24. Richardson AE (1968) The natural history of patients with intracranial aneurysms after rupture. Prog Brain Res 30:269–273
25. Rizzoli HV, Hayes GJ (1953) Congenital berry aneurysm of the posterior fossa. Case report with successful operative excision. J Neurosurg 10:550–551
26. Rothman SLG, Azarhia B, Kier EL, et al. (1973) The angiography of posterior inferior cerebellar artery aneurysms. Neurorad 6:1–7
27. Sahs AL, Perret GE, Locksley HB, et al. (1969) Intracranial aneurysms and subarachnoid hemorrhage: A cooperative study. Lippincott, Philadelphia
28. Shrontz CE, Dujovny MD, Diaz FG, et al. (1987) Arterial anatomy and revascularization of vertebrobasilar circulation. In: Woods HF (ed) Cerebral blood flow: Physiologic and clinical aspects. McGraw-Hill, New York, pp 716–719
29. Sekhar LN, Nelson PB (1983) A technique of clipping giant intracranial aneurysms with the preservation of the parent artery. Surg Neurol 20:361–368
30. Smith RR, Parent AD (1982) End-to-end anastomosis of the anterior cerebral artery after excision of a giant aneurysm. Case report. J Neurosurg 56:577–580
31. Sundt TM Jr, Piepgras DG, Honser OW, et al. (1982) Interposition saphenous vein grafts for advanced occlusive disease and large aneurysms in the posterior circulation. J Neurosurg 56:205–215
32. Suzuki J, Kwak R, Okudairo Y (1979) The safe

time limit of temporary clamping of cerebral arteries in the direct surgical treatment of intracranial aneurysm under moderate hypothermia. Tohoku J Exp Med 127:1–7

33. Uihlein A, Hughes RA (1955) The surgical treatment of intracranial vestigial aneurysms. Surg Clin North Amer 35:1071–1083

34. Yamaura A, Ise H, Makino H (1981) Radiometric study on posterior inferior cerebellar aneurysms with special reference to accessibility by the lateral suboccipital approach. Neurol Med Chir 21:721–733

35. Yaşargil MG (1969) Reconstructive and constructive surgery of the cerebral arteries in man. In: Yaşargil MG (ed) Microsurgery applied to neurosurgery. Academic Press, New York, pp 82–119

36. Yaşargil MG (1984) Microneurosurgery, vol. 2 Thieme, Stuttgart

Posterior Circulation Aneurysms

Lindsay Symon[1]

Discussion of posterior circulation aneurysms is inevitably influenced by the work of Drake and his colleagues. Over the past 20 years, Drake has accumulated vast experience of posterior circulation aneurysms which is unparalleled in any other clinic in the world. In our own clinic, posterior circulation aneurysms represent just less than 10% of proven aneurysmal origin of subarachnoid haemorrhage and as a result my own personal experience in operating on nearly a thousand aneurysms is of the direct operative obliteration of just 72 posterior circulation aneurysms. Of these, 50 have been at the top of the basilar artery, ten at the posterior inferior cerebellar origin, and the others scattered throughout the basilar distribution. Twelve giant posterior circulation aneurysms have been operated on remote from subarachnoid haemorrhage.

This paper, therefore, addresses the techniques of approach to an aneurysm in which an experienced aneurysm surgeon may find himself faced with a situation less than familiar. Where a clinic has operated on over a thousand basilar aneurysms familiarity of approach will necessarily change the view of the surgeons.

Basilar Tip and Proximal Posterior Cerebral Aneurysms

The standard subtemporal approach here recommended by Drake is widely used but has considerable disadvantages if attempts are being made to undertake early aneurysm surgery. It requires deep retraction and even with division of the tentorium or tying it down by a stitch to the floor of the middle fossa it is a difficult approach in the presence of appreciably raised tension.

Though Drake and Peerless now use a linear incision as for the standard Frazier approach to the trigeminal ganglion, most less experienced surgeons will prefer a straightforward mid-temporal flap turned down above the ear followed by the development of a straightforward four-burr hole flap carried right down to the floor of the temporal fossa. It is essential in this approach that no ridge of bone is left above the floor of the temporal fossa, and if necessary any residual shelf of bone above the floor must be removed flush with an air drill. The position of Labbé's vein should be identified in the preoperative work-up and a number of veins crossing the area from the temporal lobe to the floor of the fossa must often be divided although strenuous effort should be made to preserve Labbé's vein itself. The depth of retraction particularly in the acute brain swelling associated with recent subarachnoid haemorrhage means that the brain must be carefully protected with Lintine, which must be removed very carefully by lavage at the end of the operation rather than simply lifted off the underlying brain. The self-retaining Yasargil retractor is essential and as the tentorial hiatus is approached, Drake's manoeuvre of placing a suture through the free edge of the tentorium, avoiding the fourth nerve and anchoring the edge of the tentorium to the floor of the temporal fossa, may be of some help. This counteracts the upward slope of the medial part of the tentorium and provides access to the hiatus. In the approach to the hiatus, the posterior communicating artery and terminal carotid artery may provide a guide towards the upper basilar. Under the microscope the arachnoid may be opened over these structures, they can be visualised fairly easily even in the presence of subarachnoid haemorrhage through the intact arachnoid and avoided. The third nerve is almost directly in the field, should be protected with a cotton patty, but nevertheless is frequently injured in the course of such procedures. The partial or complete third nerve palsy which ensues invariably

[1] Gough-Cooper Department of Neurological Surgery, Institute of Neurology, Queen Square, London, England

shows recovery provided the nerve is not severed. As I have noted above, this approach carries the authority of the world's most experienced posterior circulation surgeon and must, therefore, be regarded as adequate for the majority of aneurysms at the upper end of the basilar artery. However, in my own experience and that of others it is a difficult and constricted exposure in the presence of brain swelling and although Drake himself has indicated that resection of the temporal lobe has never been necessary in his series of basilar tip aneurysms, my own personal preference in approach to these lesions remains the extended sylvian approach, as recommended by Yaşargil, together with, if necessary, partial resection of the medial part of the temporal lobe.

There remain, however, certain aneurysms at the top of the basilar artery which must be approached by a mid-temporal route. These are the aneurysms which drop backwards from the top of the basilar artery, indenting the upper stem. Dissection of these anteriorly, while possible, can be extremely difficult, and the classic Drake approach carries the enormous advantage of rendering the position of the sheaf of posterior perforators coming from the top of the basilar more immediately accessible. It may be difficult to identify these and difficult to dissect them from a more anterior approach. As Drake has pointed out these may be swept off the posterior aspect of an aneurysm of the upper basilar when they have been confidently identified, the author's preference being to use some blunt but not narrow instrument, a MacDonald dissector for example, to carry these gently back from the posterior aspect of the aneurysm before applying a clip. The salient disadvantage of the mid-temporal approach lies in the identification of the opposite posterior cerebral artery, the first segment of which may be quite closely applied to the contralateral aspect of the aneurysm neck.

While most surgeons will employ the mid-temporal or Drake approach from the right side, it may be occasionally essential to perform the approach from the left side; although this will apply particularly to proximal posterior cerebral artery aneurysms on the left.

The sub-temporal zone remains one of the most epileptogenic of areas and following extensive retraction of this region it is essential to maintan the patient on anti-convulsants for at least a year following surgery.

Extended Anterior Temporal Approach with Anterior Temporal Lobectomy

This approach from the right side is the author's usual technique of approach to upper basilar aneurysms with rare exceptions. The flap used is essentially the small fronto-temporal flap for anterior circulation aneurysms with its posterior limb carried a little further back but the incision still lying in front of the ear coming down to the tragus. The dissection essentially follows the posterior communicating artery and third nerve backwards from the terminal carotid artery picked up in the inner end of the sylvian fissure, and a degree of retraction or resection of the temporal lobe conditioned by the amount of room available in the individual case. It is the author's invariable practice to divide the bridging veins from the sylvian fissure to the sphenoparietal sinus to enable lateral retraction of the tip of the temporal lobe; should there appear any potential difficulty in obtaining sufficient access, the anterior 1 in. of the temporal lobe is resected into the tentorial hiatus and twin retraction is placed posteriorly, one on the stem of the resected lobe, and a superior one gently on the upper part of the lobe behind the line of the middle cerebral artery. Retractor pressure on the middle cerebral should be carefully avoided, particularly if hypotension is employed, as considerable ischaemia of the evocative cortex may be induced. I was drawn to this approach as suitable for the upper basilar artery as a result of my experience in the radical excision of craniopharyngioma. The tentorial hiatus is a limited structure and its anterior compartment anterior to the brainstem is in fact quite close to the posterior curve of the internal carotid artery, separated by no more than three-quarters of an inch. In addition to this, an approach from the posterior clinoid backwards has a merit of starting at approximately the same level as the terminal basilar and overcomes the problem of the necessary extensive upward retraction of the mid-temporal lobe, which is inherent in the mid-temporal approach. The greater advantage, however, is the access to both posterior cerebral arteries. Visualisation of both is more readily available from this approach and provided the position of the posterior perforators can be verified and these can be swept off by a curved dissector passed round the posterior part of the neck of the aneurysm then the application of a clip is in the author's experience considerably easier by this route than by the lateral approach. No one can deny that the broad neck of a basilar aneurysm encroaching upon one or both posterior cerebral arteries represents a considerable technical problem. I have not found it necessary to employ fenestrated clips and the present considerable variety of curved clips has proved on the whole adequate. Very rarely, a low basilar bifurcation has necessitated removal of one posterior clinoid process for access using an air drill.

Combined Supra- and Infratentorial Approach to the Lateral Aspect of the Tentorial Hiatus

This approach gives incomparable access to the clivus from the posterior clinoid to the foramen magnum and this author has used it for clivus meningiomas, for larger difficult aneurysms of the basilar artery anywhere over its entire length and for tumours that have extensive spread in the middle and posterior fossas, such as apical petrous meningiomas or cholesteatomas of the tentorial hiatus. The use of this approach in aneurysms of the upper basilar artery carries the advantage that following division of the lateral sinus anterior to the insertion of Labbé's vein, upward retraction of the mid-temporal region with the posterior leaf of the tentorium completely protects the venous drainage of the temporal lobe and simultaneous downward retraction of the upper part of the cerebellum together with the division of the petrosal venous system if necessary gives an incomparable view of the tentorial hiatus with much less brain retraction than is necessary by the purely supratentorial approach.

An essential preliminary in the planning of this approach is a detailed analysis of the venous drainage of the hemispheres. The position of Labbé's vein should be carefully charted. As a rule it enters the lateral sinus sufficiently posteriorly to enable division of the lateral sinus anterior to the insertion of Labbé's vein as described. Very occasionally if Labbé's vein enters the sinus exactly at the junction of the lateral and sigmoid, it may be necessary to divide the lateral sinus behind Labbé's vein. This is a distinct disadvantage, however, since its limits the upward retraction of the temporal lobe. Possibly preferable is a more extensive dissection of the base of the petrous pyramid to enable division of the upper sigmoid rather than the transverse sinus, with

a consequent facility for upward retraction of Labbé's vein with the temporal lobe as before. The situation of the sinus communication at the torcular Herophili must be assessed. One transverse sinus, that receiving the blood from the superior sagittal sinus, is usually dominant and it is often the right, but provided there is good communication at the torcular and a substantial contra-lateral sinus, then division of either may be safely accomplished. It was the experience of ENT surgeons who regularly divided the sigmoid sinus on either side without problem that brought this to the author's attention, but there is no doubt that if inadequate or no communication at the torcular exists or if one lateral sinus is absent then the division of the single lateral sinus is unsafe and should not be performed.

Where this approach has been performed for tumours of the tentorial hiatus then of course the site chosen will depend upon the one giving the greatest access, but where the approach is to the basilar artery then it is the author's view that the ease of approach from the right side for a right-handed surgeon renders this the side of choice. It may seem strange that such an extended low approach should be considered for aneurysm of the top of the basilar, but in effect the capacity to follow the basilar artery up from the mid-pons and to look up into the tentorial hiatus is of enormous advantage where one is dealing with a very large basilar aneurysm, as will be discussed in the management of giant aneurysms. Temporary occlusion of the major afferent artery considerably reduces the tension of a giant sac and this approach renders the anatomy of the basilar artery itself, the posterior communicating artery and proximal posterior cerebral vessels easily displayed in the field. The fourth nerve is at risk in the dissection and must be carefully avoided.

Approach to the Lower Part of the Basilar Artery and Posterior Inferior Cerebellar Artery

Anterior inferior cerebellar artery aneurysms constitute the commonest lower aneurysm in the posterior circulation and these and aneurysms up to the middle third of the basilar may be readily approached by a lateral posterior fossa exposure. Where one is dealing with posterior inferior cerebellar artery aneurysm, the choice of side, of course, is dictated by the laterality of the posterior inferior cerebellar. Where the aneurysm is from the lower part of the basilar trunk then the surgeon has the choice either of approaching across the fundus from the side to which the aneurysm is pointing, or from the contra-lateral side in the hope that he will reach the neck. The anatomy of each individual aneurysm will determine this, but the author has almost invariably approached from the side of the fundus largely because the fundus will dissect space between the brainstem and the clivus and provided the surgeon is prepared to undertake temporary proximal occlusion of the basilar and, if necessary, temporary distal occlusion also, control of the circulation is possible should the aneurysm rupture.

In fashioning the lateral sub-occipital approach, choice of position is important. In the author's view, the lateral or "park bench" position is essential, the seated position carries the enormous disadvantage that induced hypotension is extremely dangerous and the surgeon is working upwards with extended arms, an extremely uncomfortable situation should emergencies arise. In the positioning of the patient appropriate protection of downward prominences is well described elsewhere (Drake, Symon) and the incision, starting above the asterion and running down the posterior face of the mastoid sloping towards the foramen magnum, is a standard incision used for many lateral posterior fossa lesions such as acoustic neuroma. For the posterior inferior cerebellar artery aneurysms it is essential that the incision provide an adequate exposure of the foramen magnum and the foramen magnum rim itself must be removed well laterally to avoid any lip of bone getting in the surgeon's way as he passes round into the lateral part of the foramen. The actual position of the posterior inferior cerebellar in the foramen varies; in some instances it may be quite low, almost in the foramen itself, in others quite high depending on the curvature of the vertebral artery and posterior inferior cerebellar artery. In one of the author's cases, the PICA was so far medially carried, that the aneurysm was almost in the foramen of Magendie. The twelfth nerve may be at risk since it may hook round the vertebral close to the origin of posterior inferior cerebellar artery.

Aneurysms higher on the basilar artery require extreme care in dissection above or between the posterior cranial nerves. For this reason, since there is a great deal more room between the two fifth nerves or between the fifth and the seventh and eighth than there is between seven and eight, and nine, ten, eleven, careful consideration should be given in a mid-third basilar aneurysm as to whether it may not be easier to approach this either as Drake has described by a sub-temporal approach, or as I would prefer by a combined supra- and infratentorial approach, rather than from a purely posterior fossa route. The combined supra- and infratentorial approach has a great deal more capacity for access than either of the other two and has been used for the rare giant central third basilar aneurysms attacked by the author (two cases).

Conclusions

Posterior circulation aneurysms will continue to constitute a major challenge to the majority of aneurysm surgeons simply because they are not common. Anterior circulation aneurysms represent part of the stock-in-trade of the majority of neurosurgical clinics and the small fronto-temporal flap with the basal approach through the cisterns provides excellent access to anterior cerebral, middle cerebral or posterior communicating and terminal carotid aneurysms for most surgeons. Familiarity breeds ease of handling. The posterior circulation aneurysm on the other hand turns up several times a year in most clinics, it is a less than familiar entity and even with the accumulated experience of the approach to the tentorial hiatus implicit in the handling of central tumours it still represents a difficult lesion. A giant aneurysm of the top of the basilar artery is possibly one of the most demanding operations in surgery. Silverberg in the United States and Rice-Edwards in the United Kingdom have used cardiac arrest and hypothermia but it remains in this author's view somewhat doubtful that in the management of a severely ill patient with recent subarachnoid haemorrhage, the added complications of such an extensive procedure can be justified. However, extended experience will be necessary to demonstrate whether techniques of temporary vascular occlusion associated with peri-operative monitoring will so increase the ease of routine vascular surgery that results even for the larger aneurysms of the top of the basilar will approach the acceptability which anterior circulation aneurysms have now obtained.

Posterior Circulation Aneurysms

W. Richard Marsh and Thoralf M. Sundt, Jr.[1]

Since 1969, 218 aneurysms of the posterior circulation have been operated upon in our department. Of this group, 131 were saccular (size less than 15 mm), 47 were globular (15–25 mm), and 40 were giant aneurysms (greater than 25 mm). Aneurysms were seen at all the usual sites. Timing of operation was determined by the patient's clinical condition and there was a trend toward operation after the 1st week following subarachnoid hemorrhage. All saccular and globular aneurysms were treated by direct clipping. Most of the giant aneurysms could be directly clipped, often only with the use of a "booster" clip. Those giant aneurysms which could not be directly clipped were treated by proximal ligation of the parent artery with or without bypass. The overall results show 165 of 218 patients (75.6%) having an excellent or good outcome; 20 patients (9.2%) had a poor outcome from their illness and/or treatment; 33 patients (15.2%) died. The results are discussed with respect to aneurysm location, aneurysm size, patient preoperative grade, and timing of surgery.

Successful operative treatment of aneurysms of the posterior circulation has evolved more slowly than that of aneurysms of the anterior circulation. Schwartz in 1948 was the first surgeon to obliterate successfully an aneurysmal sac embedded in the pons [4]. All case reports of such aneurysms prior to 1950 followed inadvertent encounters during an operation for a presumed tumor. Drake reported the first series in 1961 [1]. Reviewing the literature at the point, a total of only 47 cases had been reported and the results of operative treatment were discouraging. In 1965, Drake updated his own series to 14 patients and clarified the critical importance of the perforating vessels in the region of the basilar caput [2]. The advances in neuroradiology leading to successful imaging of both vertebral arteries and,

finally, routine safe cerebral angiography via the transfemoral route in the early 1970s has allowed visualization of these lesions. But it was only with the application of the operating microscope to neurosurgery and the development of microinstrumentation and progress in the engineering of clips that successful operative treatment became possible.

Subarachnoid hemorrhage (SAH) remains the most common indication for operation. The natural history of untreated but ruptured posterior circulation aneurysms is extremely poor: 60% of such patients die within 6 months and of these deaths, 60% are due to recurrent hemorrhage [6]. One year following recovery from the initial hemorrhage, the annual rebleed rate remains 2%–4%.

Globular (15–25 mm) and giant (>25 mm) aneurysms may produce local symptoms from mass effect or obstructive hydrocephalus. It is our belief that these unruptured but symptomatic lesions require operative treatment because the risk of subsequent rupture is quite high. Indeed, recent data suggest a worrisomely high rate of rupture for any aneurysm more than 10 mm in size [5].

Indications for operation for the smaller, unruptured saccular aneuryms are less clear and must be individualized. The decision will rest on an honest appraisal by the surgeon of the pathological anatomy and the results of his own operating experience. Generally, we have not clipped such a small incidental aneurysm which was unruptured unless it could be safely exposed during the operation for a ruptured anterior circulation aneurysm. There is a worldwide trend toward early aneurysm surgery after SAH. In our department, the timing of operation is determined primarily by the condition of the patient and the location of the aneurysm. Consideration for early surgery is given to all patients who are grade I. If a patient has experienced only a "mild" bleed and shows little subarachnoid blood on CT scanning, then early operation is

---

[1] Department of Neurological Surgery, Mayo Clinic, Rochester, Minnesota, USA

Table 1. Location and results in 218 cases of posterior circulation aneurysms

Location	Results				
	Excellent	Good	Poor	Death	Total
PICA	39	6	2	4	51
Basilar caput	73	20	14	21	128
Basilar trunk	18	9	4	8	39
Total	130	35	20	33	218

undertaken. However, we feel that in many patients harboring aneurysms in the region of the basilar caput it is wise to delay operation until the effects of the acute hemorrhage subside. Elevation of the temporal lobe and satisfactory exposure of the vasculature in the region of the aneurysm seems more dangerous early after SAH. Our only indication for early operation in grade III or IV patients is a localized mass.

Operative management involves lumbar spinal drainage, 20% mannitol with or without furosemide if the temporal lobe is to be elevated, and intraoperative hypotension during the critical dissection of the aneurysm neck. Mean systemic arterial pressures in the range of 50–60 mmHg are maintained primarily by the volatile anesthetic (isoflurone), supplemented with nitroprusside. If temporary occlusion of a parent vessel is necessary, then the blood pressure is maintained in the patient's normotensive range and the neural tissue rendered ischemic is protected by a preocclusion administration of barbiturate.

The surgical approaches have been adequately described elsewhere by many authors and will not be described here in detail. Aneurysms in the region of the basilar caput are approached either in the manner of Yaşargil et al. from the pterion [7] or in the manner of Drake beneath the temporal lobe [3]. The decision regarding approach is made based upon the relation of the aneurysmal neck to the dorsum sellae and the projection of the fundus. All other posterior circulation aneurysms occurring at or above the anterior inferior cerebellar arteries are approached in a subtemporal manner; those superior cerebellar basilar artery aneurysms projecting to the left are approached from the left whereas the others are approached from the right. The aneurysms occurring at the vertebro-basilar junction and along the intracranial vertebral artery are best approached through a retromastoid craniectomy with the patient in a modified park bench pos-

ture. Distal posterior inferior cerebellar artery (PICA) aneurysms are approached by a midline suboccipital craniectomy with the patient either sitting or prone.

A total of 218 aneurysms of the posterior circulation have been treated in such fashion by our department since May 1969. Of the total group, 128 aneurysms were in the region of the basilar caput, 51 were PICA aneurysms arising either at the vertebral junction or more distal in the vessel's course, and 39 occurred along the basilar trunk. Four categories were used for judging the results of surgery: (a) excellent, normal employment, with normal mentation and little or no neurological deficit; (b) good, neurological deficit but with normal mentation and employment; (c) poor, anything less than full activity; and (d) death. Any death within 6 months is reflected in the mortality figure. The overall results are given in Table 1: 130 with excellent outcome, 35 with good outcome, 20 with poor outcome, and 33 deaths. The site-specific result for the three categories of aneurysm is given in the same table.

When the results are correlated with size of aneurysm (Table 2), it is appreciated that many of the poorer results were in patients with larger aneurysms. Thus, there were 47 globular aneurysms (15–25 mm), among which there were eight poor results and six deaths for a combined major morbidity/mortality rate of 30%. Similarly, there were 40 giant aneurysms (>25 mm), among which there were six poor results and ten deaths for a combined major morbidity/mortality rate of 40%. These are to be compared with the smaller saccular aneurysm subgroup (<15 mm), in which the combined major morbidity/mortality rate was 15%.

Table 3 presents the outcome data with respect to preoperative grade of the patient by the Botterell classification. All grade 0 patients harbored globular or giant aneurysms which were symptomatic by virtue of mass effect. Table 3 confirms

Table 2. Size and results in posterior circulation aneurysms

Size (mm)	Results				
	Excellent	Good	Poor	Death	Total
<2	0	0	0	0	0
2–3.9	6	0	0	0	6
4–5.9	19	4	1	2	26
6–7.9	20	4	3	5	32
8–9.9	16	5	0	0	21
10–14.9	26	7	2	6	41
15–19.9	18	4	4	3	29
20–24.9	9	2	4	3	18
25 or >	15	9	6	10	40
Total	129	35	20	29	213[a]

[a] Size not registered in five cases

Table 3. Results and preoperation grade in posterior circulation aneurysms

Botterell preop grade	Results				
	Excellent	Good	Poor	Death	Total
0	35	6	4	9	54
1	63	12	4	10	89
2	25	9	6	3	43
3	7	5	4	5	21
4	0	3	2	6	11
Total	130	35	20	33	218

the intuitive belief that poorer results are to be expected in patients injured neurologically by the effects of their hemorrhage. If one looks only at the patients in grades 1 and 2, the group for whom early operation is often considered, a major morbity of 7.5% and mortality of 10% are noted.

Aneurysms of the posterior circulation continue to remain a challenge. Our overall results indicated a 76% excellent or good result. If one considers only saccular aneurysms (<15 mm), then 85% of patients enjoyed an excellent or good outcome. Further advances in the surgical treatment of this condition rest on earlier diagnosis and treatment as well as the development of effective therapy for cerebral vasospasm.

References

1. Drake CG (1961) Bleeding aneurysms of the basilar artery: direct surgical management in four cases. J Neurosurg 18:230–238
2. Drake CG (1965) Surgical treatment of ruptured aneurysms of the basilar artery: experience with 14 cases. J Neurosurg 23:457–473
3. Drake CG (1979) The treatment of aneurysms of the posterior circulation. Clin Neurosurg 26:96–144
4. Schwartz HG (1948) Arterial aneurysm of the posterior fossa. J Neurosurg 5:312–316
5. Wiebers DO, Whisnant JP, Sundt TM Jr, O'Hallon WM (1987) The significance of unruptured intracranial saccular aneurysms. J Neurosurg 66:23–30
6. Winn HR, et al. (1980) The natural history of vertebral basilar aneurysms. Presented at the AANS, April 1980
7. Yaşargil MG, et al. (1976) Microsurgical pterional approach to aneurysms of the basilar bifurcation. Surg Neurol 6:83–91

Surgical Treatment of Posterior Circulating Aneurysms

Akira Yamaura[1]

Probably the first successful operation for a posterior circulation aneurysms was performed by Olivercrona in 1932 for a right peripheral posterior inferior cerebellar artery (PICA) aneurysms, which was trapped and excised [4]. A basilar aneurysm was surgically treated by Gillingham in 1958. Drake (1961), Logue (1964), and Jamieson (1964) pioneered utilization of a subtemporal approach in the treatment of basilar aneurysms. In 1975, Yaşargil et al. reported a frontolateral route to basilar bifurcation (BA-BIF) aneurysms [10]. A technical note of the transsylvian approach to aneurysms of the terminal portion of the basilar artery and of the lateral suboccipital approach to vertebral aneurysms will be discussed from our experience.

The incidence of posterior circulation aneurysms is generally believed to be 5%–10% of all intracranial aneurysms. The most common site is the BA-BIF (33%), followed by the basilar (BA) trunk (24%) and vertebral (VA)-PICA junction (31%) in our series of a total of 216 cases [9].

Neuroradiological Study

Radiometric Study for Transsylvian Approach

In the anterior-posterior view of carotid arteriography, a triangular space, defined by the internal carotid artery (ICA) and middle cerebral artery (MCA) above and the base of the skull below, is an entrance for the transsylvian approach to BA. Therefore, important factors in determining the difficulty of the operation are the height of the ICA arch and the height of the aneurysm neck. The distances to such key points from the base line between the anterior and the posterior clinoid

processes were measured. When the ICA arch was high, complications of the operation were not often seen; when the aneurysm neck was located very high, much heavier retraction on the ICA and proximal MCA was required to gain access to the aneurysm. In our series, oculomotor paresis or hemiparesis were less often seen when the ICA bifurcation was located between 5 and 10 mm above the base line. The incidence of postoperative complications did not seem to be related to the depth of the surgical field, defined as the distance between the ICA bifurcation and aneurysm neck [6]. The feasibility of an approach through the carotid-optic space is determined by the length of the Al segment of the anterior cerebral artery (ACA) and length of the intracranial ICA and its curve (Fig. 1). Information as to the length and caliber of the posterior communicating artery (P COMM A) is also important for selection of the route (Fig. 2). When P COMM A is small in caliber and long, the route should be lateral to P COMM A, which is early displaced medially by a retractor. With a well-developed but short P COMM A, a space between perforators from P COMM A should be utilized.

Radiometric Study for Lateral Suboccipital Approach

A simple radiometric study was very useful in management of VA aneurysms. The following distances to the aneurysm neck were measured: (a) From the midline on an AP view; (b) from the posterior wall of the clivus on lateral views; and (c) from the foramen magnum on lateral views. In the initial 14 cases of VA-PICA aneurysms, there was a greater chance of postoperative complications when the aneurysm was located within 10 mm of the midline and posteriorly more than 13 mm from the clivus [8]. On AP views, most VA-PICA aneurysms arose at the knee-shaped corner of the VA. The location of the aneurysms was classified into the following three categories

[1] Department of Neurosurgery, Chiba University School of Medicine, Chiba, Japan

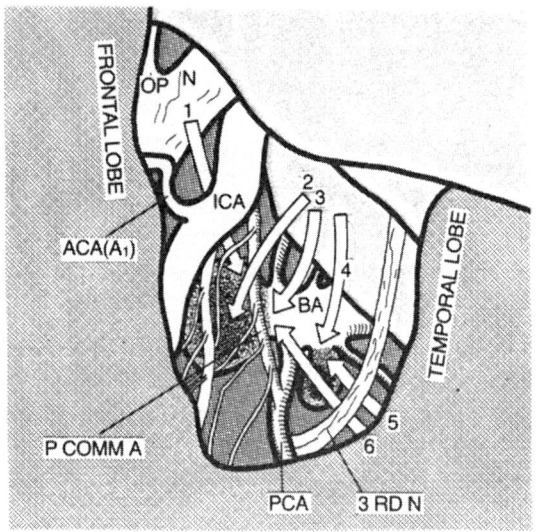

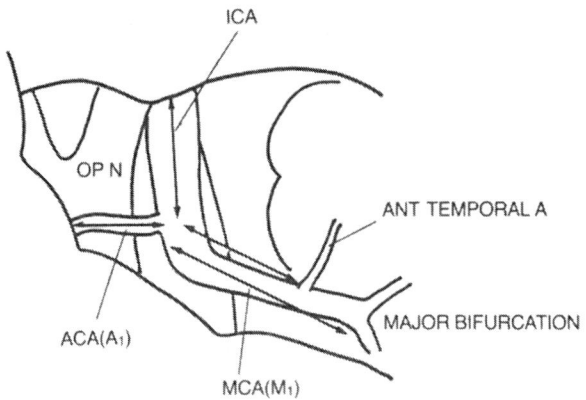

Fig. 1. Variety of approaches to aneurysms of the terminal portion of basilar artery. Route *1* between optic nerve (*OP N*) and internal carotid artery (*ICA*). Route *2* between *ICA* and posterior communicating artery (*P COMM A*). Route *3* lateral to *ICA* and *P COMM A*. Route *6* subtemporal approach to basilar bifurcation. Routes *4, 5* approaches to basilar artery (BA)-superior cerebellar artery (SCA) aneurysm

Fig. 2. Radiometry for selection of routes for basilar bifurcation aneurysms. *OP N* optic nerve, *ICA* internal carotid artery, *ACA* anterior cerebral artery, *MCA* middle cerebral artery, *ANT TEMPORAL A* anterior temporal artery

(Fig. 6): Type A, the aneurysm was located just above the knee of the VA; type B, just below the knee; type C, at some distance below the knee of the markedly elongated VA. Care should be taken not to include the distal portion of the VA in an aneurysm clip with type A aneurysms because the distal portion of the VA is hidden behind the aneurysm. Appreciation of the size of each VA is required when a proximal clip occlusion is the choice of treatment for a fusiform aneurysm or a dissecting aneurysm of the VA.

Fusiform aneurysm and dissecting aneurysm entirely differ in their pathology, natural history, and indication of surgery. From a practical standpoint, however, it is very difficult to differentiate these two conditions on vertebral arteriography. During investigation of a subarachnoid hemorrhage, vertebral arteriography shows a fusiform dilatation associated with some narrowing of the parent artery. This situation occurred in 30% of the VA aneurysms in our series. Such a lesion could be: (a) a ruptured dissecting aneurysm of the VA; (b) an unruptured arteriosclerotic fusiform aneurysm; or (c) a ruptured saccular aneurysm with a thrombus in the aneurysmal lumen and with spasm of its parent artery. The pathognomonic sign of a dissecting aneurysm is the presence of contrast media in an intramural dissecting space, pearl and string sign, pearl reaction, rosette sign, tapering, occlusion, intimal flap, and indicative pouch in arteriography. Unfortunately, such well-known signs have not been helpful in diagnosis in our experience. Dissecting aneurysms in the MCA, ICA, and VA are encountered more commonly in young male patients. There is no significant atherosclerosis, and in the acute stage, a typical "dark red or brown" intramural hematoma is observed during surgery. Dissecting aneurysms usually present as ischemia due to obstruction of the parent artery. When dissection involves the VA, however, dissecting aneurysms may present as subarachnoid hemorrhage. Friedman et al. reported that 20 of 25 cases of dissecting aneurysms of the posterior circulation presented as subarachnoid hemorrhage [3].

Indication and Contraindication for Surgery

The indication for surgery on posterior circulation aneurysms does not differ significantly from those of anterior circulation aneurysms. In grade III, surgery is indicated only when the patient can be aroused and the verbal response is reasonably correct. The age of patients per se is not a con-

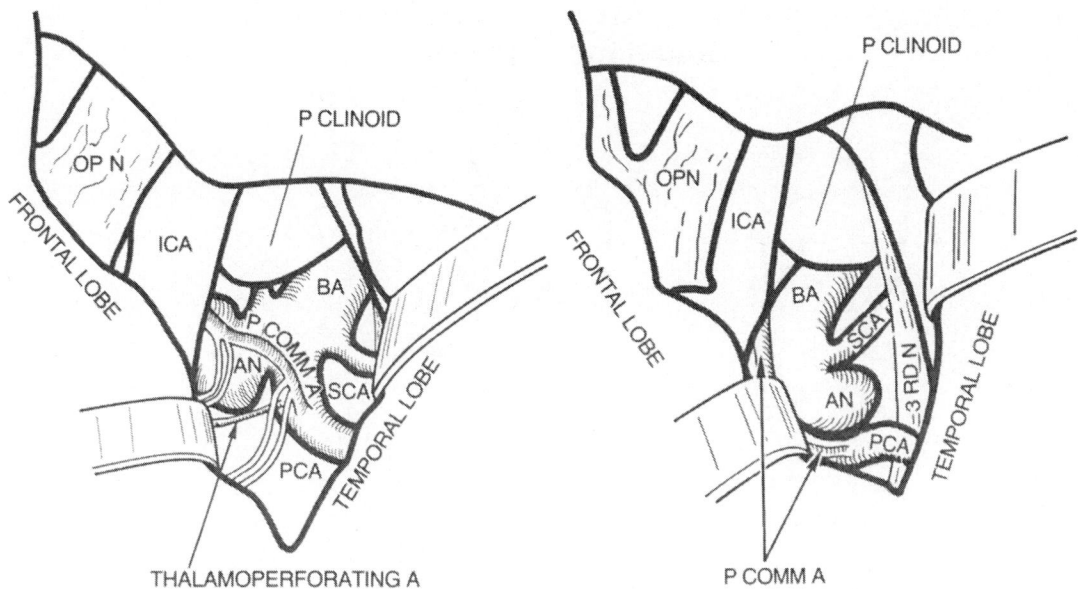

Fig. 3. Schema of transsylvian approach to basilar bifurcation aneurysm. *OP N* optic nerve, *ICA* internal corotid artery, *P CLINOID* posterior clinoid, *BA* basilar artery, *P COMM A* posterior communicating artery, *AN* aneurysm, *SCA* superior cerebellar artery, *PCA* posterior cerebral artery

Fig. 4. Schema of transsylvian approach to basilar artery-superior cerebellar artery aneurysm. *OP N* optic nerve, *ICA* internal corotid artery, *P CLINOID* posterior clinoid, *BA* bosilar artery, *P COMM A* posterior communicating artery, *AN* aneurysm, *SCA* superior cerebellar artery, *PCA* posterior cerebral artery

traindication to surgery. Six of eight patients over 70 years of age underwent surgery and achieved full recovery. Among these six patients, there were four BA-BIF aneurysms, one distal posterior cerebral artery (PCA) aneurysm, and one VA-PICA aneurysm.

Technical Note of Transsylvian Approach to Aneurysms at Terminal Portion of Basilar Artery

Craniotomy

A free bone flap of 3 × 4 cm is turned to perform an ordinary frontolateral craniotomy. The pterion is rongeured sufficiently.

Opening the Sylvian Fissure

The most important part of this approach is opening the sylvian fissure "widely"—at least over 3–4 cm length. Then deeper dissection is carried out to expose the main trunk of the MCA and the entire length of the ICA. A bridging vein from the anterior temporal lobe is usually preserved. An anterior temporal artery sometimes

restricts the mobilization of the MCA-ICA arch, but none of these arteries was severed in our series. Wide dissection of the sylvian fissure is essentially harmless and will actually serve to protect the brain, the artery, and the cranial nerves from heavy retraction when a critical point is reached. For a high-position or low-position BA-BIF aneurysm, which is the most difficult type to treat, a wide opening of the sylvian fissure is essential.

Approach to Terminal Portion of Basilar Artery

The ICA and proximal portion of the MCA are gently retracted medially with a 3- to 5-mm-wide retractor (medial retractor) (Figs. 3, 4). The temporal lobe is retracted laterally with the use of a second retractor (lateral retractor). Liliequist's membrane is then opened, and a wide view of the interpeduncular and prepontine cisterns is obtained. A BA-superior cerebellar artery (SCA) aneurysm is most safely managed at this stage.

P COMM A

P COMM A and its branches often hide a BA-BIF aneurysm, particularly when the latter is

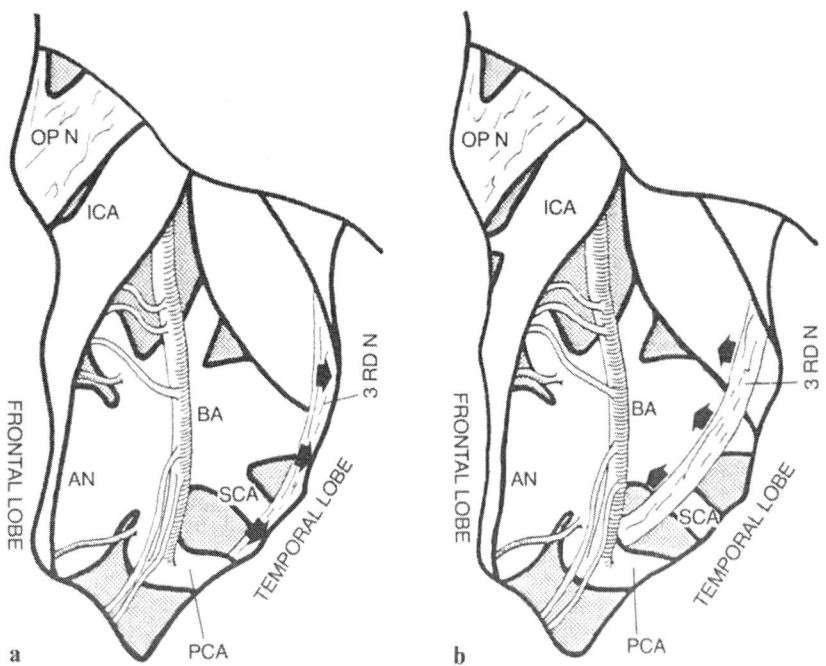

Fig. 5a, b. Protection of oculomotor nerve (*3RD N*). **a** *3RD N* is away from the surgical field when the arachnoid is dissected only medial to the nerve. **b** *3RD N* may be injured when the nerve is entirely dissected. *OP N* optic nerve, *ICA* internal carotid artery, *AN* aneurysm, *BA* basilar artery, *SCA* superior cerebellar artery, *PCA* posterior cerebral artery

located at a high position or, is large, when P COMM A is short and well developed, or when P COMM A originates at the very proximal portion of the ICA. In these situations, developing a space between the perforators of P COMM A would offer a better chance for perfect clipping of the more difficult BA-BIF aneurysm (Fig. 1). The author has utilized this space in approximately 50% of operations on BA-BIF aneurysms.

Thalamoperforating Artery

Every effort should be made to preserve these perforators from the P1 segment of the PCA [2, 5]. A severely disabled condition may result from involvement of these arteries. A large BA-BIF aneurysm with a broad neck often has a very close relationship with such perforators. Surgeons should always be aware of the presence of these important perforators on the contra-lateral side. If these perforators are well developed and cannot be separated from the aneurysm, a fenestrated clip should be tried.

Oculomotor Nerve

In order to minimize postoperative oculomotor nerve palsy, dissection of the arachnoid should

be limited only to the medial aspect of the nerve (Fig. 5). The nerve is gently displaced from the surgical field because of shrinking of the intact arachnoid lateral to the oculomotor nerve. Postoperative oculomotor paresis occurred in less than 30% of our patients.

Technical Note of Lateral Suboccipital Approach to Vertebral Aneurysms

For a right-handed surgeon, the patient is best positioned prone for a left-sided lesion and lateral for a right-sided lesion. This is true when the aneurysm is located very high in the posterior fossa and close to or beyond the midline.

Suboccipital Craniectomy

For most VA aneurysms, a suboccipital craniectomy (3 × 4 cm) is made as lateral as possible (lateral suboccipital approach).

Intradural Procedure

Retractors are so arranged that the cerebellar hemisphere is displaced posteriorly. One of the first landmarks to look for is the eleventh cranial

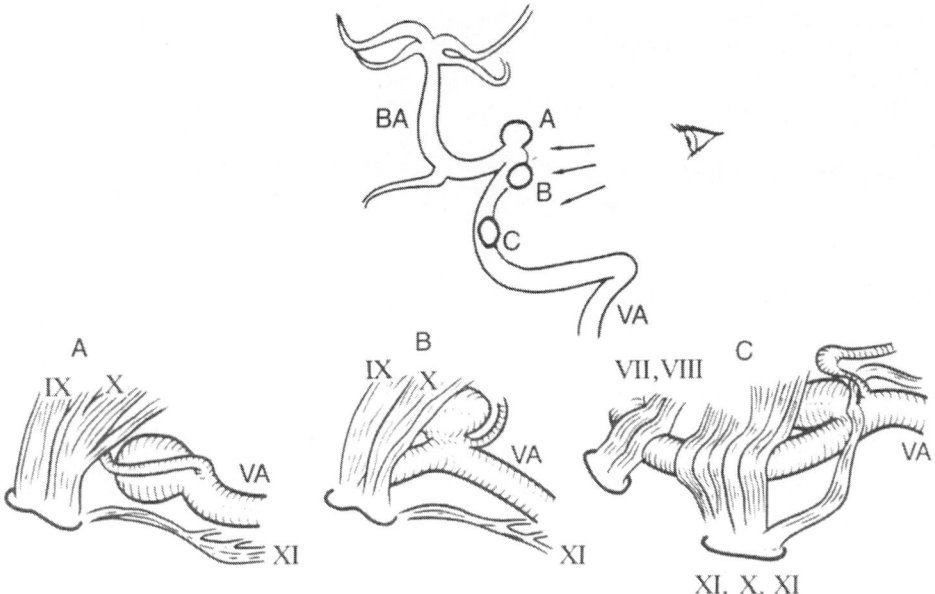

Fig. 6. Classification of VA-PICA aneurysm—types A–C. Care should be taken in type *A* not to involve the distal vertebral artery, where the distal portion of the vertebral artery is hidden behind an aneurysm. *BA* basilar artery, *VA* vertebral artery

nerve, which is then followed to the jugular foramen; the ninth and tenth cranial nerves are identified. The VA-PICA aneurysm is approached via a space between the ninth and tenth cranial nerves on the one hand and the eleventh cranial nerve on the other. The twelfth cranial nerve can be seen coursing across the VA at the origin of the PICA.

Clipping of VA-PICA Aneurysm

From a surgical point of view, VA-PICA aneurysm are classified into three types as described above (Fig. 6). In type A, the aneurysm is located just above the knee of the VA, and the distal portion of the VA is hidden behind the aneurysm. Thus, care should be exercised so as not to include the distal VA in a clip.

Proximal Clip Occlusion of VA

This technique is used for a dissecting aneurysm of the VA only when the opposite VA is dominant or at least equivalent to the involved VA. In our experience, this technique has been effective in protecting against recurrent hemorrhage. It may be unsafe to place a clip distal to the PICA, which is the classic maneuver, in the presence of a long distal VA. This should be done only in a patient in whom the VA distal to the origin of the PICA

is short and the surgeon can confirm that there are no perforators from this segment of the VA.

Results of Treatment

Short-Term Follow-Up Studies

The incidence of oculomotor paresis following surgery on BA-BIF and BA-SCA aneurysms is a matter of concern. In our series, the incidence was 24% in 34 patients with BA-BIF aneurysms and 25% in 22 patients with BA-SCA aneurysms treated via the transsylvian approach. Most of the oculomotor paresis was minimal. These results are much better than those reported in the literature [7]. Cruciger et al. [1] found postoperative oculomotor palsy in 21 (68%) of 31 patients who were operated on for BA-BIF aneurysm via the subtemporal approach. Both the literature and our own experience would indicate that use of the transsylvian approach is less traumatic to the oculomotor nerve.

In our series of 37 patients with BA-BIF aneurysms treated via the transsylvian approach and subtemporal approach, there were seven patients (19%) with postoperative hemiparesis. Two were associated with anterior circulation aneurysms, which were responsible for bleeding.

Within 3 months of surgery for BA-BIF and

BA-SCA aneurysms in our series, there were three deaths. A severely disabled postoperative condition occurred in three and two patients with BA-BIF and BA-SCA aneurysms, respectively. Major bleeding during surgery was the most important cause of a poor outcome. All of the initial seven patients who were operated on via a subtemporal approach showed some complications, and one patient died.

Among 46 patients operated on for aneurysms of the VA and its branches, seven (15%) had ninth and tenth cranial nerve palsy, including one patient whose recovery was prolonged and three patients with abducens paresis, none of whom had permanent deficits. Otherwise, the postoperative course in VA aneurysms was benign. There were no postoperative deaths and no patient had a severely disabling condition.

Long-Term Follow-Up Studies

A long-term follow-up study was carried out on 123 postoperative patients over a period of more than 12 months. There was only one additional death in BA-SCA aneurysm and another death due to meningitis 4 months after transoral transclival surgery for mid-BA aneurysm. In summary, in the author's series, five deaths among 123 patients operated on for posterior circulation aneurysms of all sites and followed up for more than 12 months were related to surgery. Approximately 80% of the survivors returned to lead a normal life.

References

1. Cruciger MP, Hoyt WF, Wilson CB (1981) Peripheral and midbrain oculomotor palsies from operations for basilar bifurcation aneurysms in a series of 31 cases. Surg Neurol 15:215–219
2. Drake CG (1978) Treatment of aneurysms of the posterior cranial fossa. Prog Neurol Surg 9:122–194
3. Friedman AH, Drake CG (1984) Subarachnoid hemorrhage from intracranial dissecting aneurysm. J Neurosurg 60:325–334
4. Höök O, Norlen G, Guzman J (1963) Saccular aneurysms of the vertebral basilar arterial system. A report of 28 cases. Acta Neurol Scand 19:271
5. Peerless SJ Management of aneurysms of posterior circulation. In: Youmans JR (ed) Neurological surgery, vol. 3. Saunders, Philadelphia, pp 1715–1763
6. Saeki N, Rhoton AL Jr (1977) Microsurgical anatomy of the upper basilar artery and the posterior circle of Willis. J Neurosurg 46:563–578
7. Yamaura A (1985) Surgical treatment of posterior circulation aneurysms: I, II. Contemporary Neurosurgery 7(12):1–8, 7(13):1–8
8. Yamaura A, Ise H, Makino H (1981) Radiometric study on posterior inferior cerebellar aneurysms with special reference to accessibility by the lateral suboccipital approach. Neurol Med Chir 21:721–734
9. Yamaura A, Ise H, Makino H (1982) Treatment of aneurysms arising from the terminal portion of the basilar artery. With special reference to the radiometric study and accessibility of trans-sylvian approach. Neurol Med Chir 22:521–532
10. Yaşargil MG, Antic J, Laciga R, et al. (1975) Microsurgical pterional approach to aneurysms of the basilar bifurcation. Surg Neurol 6:83–91

Surgical Treatment of Basilar Aneurysms

Takamasa Kayama[1] and Jiro Suzuki[2]

Introduction

Surgical management of basilar artery aneurysms is still difficult despite the introduction of microneurosurgical techniques. Since 1961, we have developed various safety surgical techniques to deal with ruptured cerebral aneurysms and have reported on aneurysms of the anterior circle of Willis [7, 8, 11]. In the present study, we evaluate our direct operations on basilar aneurysms over the past 25 years, directing particular attention to the surgical methods employed. We discuss these cases and describe special surgical techniques which involve temporary vascular occlusion with the administration of the "Sendai Cocktail."

Subjects

Fifty-three patients with single basilar aneurysms underwent direct operation in the 25 years 3 months from June 1961 to October 1986. The sites of the aneurysms included the bifurcation of the basilar artery ($n = 33$), the P1 region of the left posterior cerebral artery ($n = 2$), the left side of the bifurcation of the basilar and superior cerebellar artery ($n = 6$), the right side of the same site ($n = 10$), and the proximal portion of the right ($n = 1$) and left ($n = 1$) superior cerebellar arteries (Fig. 1).

Surgery was performed within 7 days after onset in four cases, within 8–14 days in eight cases, and after 15 or more days in 41 cases. The preoperative condition, according to the grading system of Hunt and Kosnik, was grade I in 19 cases, grade I a in 14, grade II in 12, grade III in seven, and grade IV in one case. No patients were assessed as grade V.

The surgical approach was subtemporal in 37 cases, frontotemporal in 13, and bifrontal in three.

Operating Techniques

The patients were placed in the supine position and a pillow was inserted under the shoulder. The head was tilted about 90° to the left or right. The side of approach to the aneurysm we employed depended on which side was nearest to the aneurysm; in the case of midline aneurysms, the approach was under the nondominant temporal lobe. When the sagittal surface of the head was inclined 10°–15° relative to the bed, it was possible to allow the temporal lobe to fall forward and thus provide a sufficient field of vision. Slight retraction was applied to the temporal lobe. The dura mater was opened if the brain was judged to be protruding, the sphenoidal ridge was re-

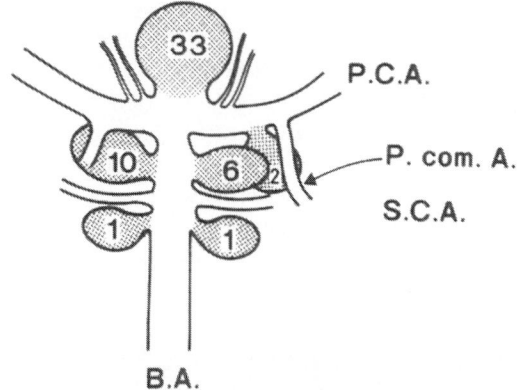

Fig. 1. Site distribution of 53 cases of basilar artery aneurysm, which were operated upon from June 1961 to October 1986. *PCA* posterior cerebellar artery, *P com A* posterior communicating artery, *SCA* superior cerebellar artery, *BA* basilar artery. *Figures* refer to the number of cases

[1] Department of Neurosurgery, Sendai National Hospital, Sendai, Japan
[2] Division of Neurosurgery, Institute of Brain Diseases, Tohoku University School of Medicine, Sendai, Japan

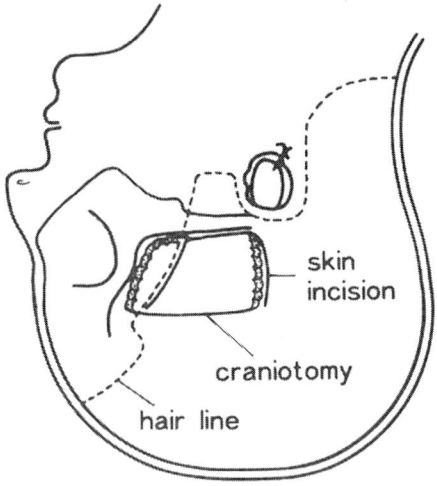

Fig. 2. Skin incision and craniotomy for the sub-temporal approach we use. Skin incision is recommended in the so-called keel form, which has the advantage of exposure as close to the base of the skull as possible

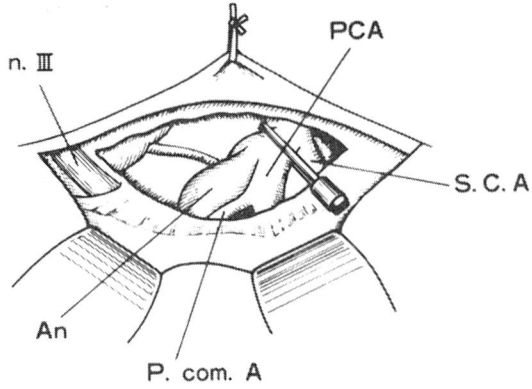

Fig. 3. Schema of operation. Note that a temporary clip should be placed on the basilar artery prior to dissect aneurysm under administration of the Sendai cocktail *PCA* posterior cerebral artery, *SCA* superior cerebellar artery, *P com A* posterior communicating artery, *An* aneurysm, *n III* third cranial nerve

moved, and cerebrospinal fluid was aspirated from the suprachiasmal cistern, whereby the brain became less taut (Fig. 2).

A thin cotton pledget was used to cover the surface of the temporal lobe and protect the brain. Labbé's vein was carefully preserved and every effort was made to avoid damaging any structures. Next, the temporal lobe was elevated so that the notch of the tent was discernible. The course of the third cranial nerve or posterior communicating artery would make the basilar artery invisible; therefore, before dissection of the aneurysm, a temporary clip was placed on the basilar artery, avoiding sites of severe arteriosclerosis (Fig. 3). It is important before temporary interruption of blood flow to administer intravenously, a mixture of 500 ml 20% mannitol, 500 mg vitamin E, and 500 mg phenytoin (known as the "Sendai Cocktail") for 30 min to protect the brain against ischemic insult. Thus, the dissection of the aneurysm was performed under bloodless conditions. After complete dissection of the aneurysm, the aneurysmal neck was ligated with thread, and then a permanent clip was applied. When clipping is performed, it is essential to identify the routes of the superior cerebellar and posterior cerebral arteries on the opposite site and be certain that the tip of the clip is placed only on the aneurysm. Since in many cases the opposite superior cerebellar artery is hidden from view by the aneurysm, it is important to reconfirm the position of the clip after

it is in place. When the neck of the aneurysm has to remain after ligation and clipping because it is broad or hard due to arteriosclerosis, the remaining neck should be covered with pieces of muscle and Aron alpha-adhesive after release of the temporary occlusion clip and restoration of normal blood flow. This procedure should begin from the opposite side to the visible site in the operation field.

In some cases, these procedures require considerable time. If blood flow has to be interrupted for more than 40 min, it is possible to restore the circulation for 5–10 min and then again use temporary occlusion, providing an additional Sendai Cocktail is administered immediately. In this way, even lengthy procedures can be completed under bloodless conditions.

It is also important to preserve the third cranial nerve during these procedures, although there have been cases in which the third cranial nerve was damaged at the rupture of the aneurysm. In such instances, the nerve is fused to the aneurysm sac and the two must be separated with great care. With our method, the fourth cranial nerve is rarely visible, but when the operative field is enlarged by cutting open the edges of the tent there is no damage to the fourth cranial nerve.

When large aneurysms cover the entire operative field, it may be difficult to secure the basilar artery. In such cases, a ballon is inserted into the basilar artery or the body of the aneurysm. This useful method for temporarily stopping the blood flow has been applied successfully in recent years.

Results

In these 53 cases, the operative results were excellent in 20 (37.7%), good in 13 (24.5%), fair in seven (13.2%), and poor in eight (15.1%). There were five deaths (9.4%); all the deaths occurred in the early part of the series. In two cases, the temporal lobe was injured by damaging Labbé's vein and by too much retraction on the temporal lobe. In another, there was a massive intraoperative hemorrhage from the aneurysm before the basilar artery could be secured. One patient had a contusional intracerebral hemorrhage in the frontal lobe with the bifrontal approach. Finally, in one case of moyamoya disease, the basilar artery blood flow was occluded for 21 min (Tables 1, 2)

For the 48 surviving patients, the findings of examinations performed at discharge were compared with the results of follow-up evaluations obtained up to 6 months after discharge. Patients whose condition was good or fair at the time of discharge subsequently improved and showed good or excellent states. There were no cases of recurrent hemorrhages. The long-term morbidity in 48 cases, excluding those who had died by discharge, was 8.4% (Table 3).

Discussion

There have been many reports concerning various approaches to basilar aneurysms, but the most frequently used approach are the transsylvian [3, 9], in which the sylvian fissure is divided, and the temporopolar [2], which is basically the same as the transsylvian approach except that the temporal lobe is pulled back and a large division is made in the sylvian fissure. The subtemporal approach for basilar artery aneurysm surgery was described by Drake [1], but there have been few other reports on this method. The lack of its wide application is attributable to the fact that the retraction on the brain is greater than with the other approaches: Early in our series, there were some cases of contusions of the temporal lobe because of this much retraction, but we found that brain damage can be minimized through aspiration of cerebrospinal fluid from the suprachiasmal cistern, allowing access to the base of the temporal lobe during craniotomy. With such an approach, preservation of Labbé's vein is important, and it is freed up to the entry of the transverse sinus. It should be noted that the course of Labbé's vein differs among individuals, and in cases where it passed through the middle of the operative field and had to be cut, venous congestion occurred postoperatively. This resulted in cerebral edema or the formation of an intracerebral hematoma, which adversely influenced the outcome. This method provides a larger operating field than with the transsylvian approach, and the field can be created at the site of the basilar aneurysm, regardless of its height.

Using the technique of temporary vascular occlusion, one can safely and successfully treat the cerebral aneurysm. Before 1971, moderate

Table 1. Surgical results on discharge ($n = 53$ patients)

	Excellent	Good	Fair	Poor	Dead
Number	20	13	7	8	5
Percentage	37.7	24.5	13.2	15.1	9.4

Excellent capable of working; *Good* capable of working, with minimum neurological or psychic impairment; *Fair* capable of walking with help, and/or psychic impairment and/or aphasia; *Poor* incapable of walking, with or without consciousness disturbance

Table 2. Causes of deterioration in mortality

Age	Sex	Site	Craniotomy	Temporary occlusion time (min.)	Cause
63	F	Lt. BA.-SCA	Lt. keel form	45	Labbe's vein cut temporary lobe damage
40	M	Lt. BA.-SCA	Lt. keel form	63	rebleeding during surgery
48	F	Basilar bif.	Bifrontal	25	Rt. frontal lobe ICH
43	M	Rt. BA.-SCA	Rt. keel form	32	Lt. temporal lobe damage
46	M	Basilar bif.	Lt. Front-temporal	21	Moyamoya Disease

Table 3. Comparison of operative results on discharge and in follow-up study

Results on discharge	No. of cases	Results at follow-up					
		Excellent	Good	Fair	Poor	Dead	Unknown
Excellent	20	17	0	0	0	0	3
Good	13	3	8	0	0	0	2
Fair	7	2	3	2	0	0	0
Poor	8	1	0	1	3	1*	2
Total	48	23 (47.9%)	11 (22.9%)	3 (6.3%)	3 (6.3%)	1 (2.1%)	7 (14.6%)

(8.4%)

* Died due to pneumonia
 Follow up rate: 85.4%,
 Follow-up duration average 3Y7M (6M to 8Y1M)

hypothermia of approximately 27 °C was used during surgery to protect the brain from the ischemia that might result from temporary stoppage of cerebral blood circulation. Now, however, the brain can be protected from the effects of ischemia for up to 40 min of blood flow stoppage by intravenous administration of the Sendai Cocktail [5, 6, 10]. As Fig. 4 shows, there was no clear relationship between the results of surgery and the duration of blood flow interruption. In some cases, the outcome was poor when the stoppage was brief and in others good results were achieved when it was lengthy. Results of our animal experiments [4–6, 10], which were performed over a period of more than 15 years in our institute, indicate that blood flow can be safely halted for up to 40 min; it can be briefly restored and then stopped again if another Sendai Cocktail is administered. While the blood flow is interrupted, placement of the clip at a severely arteriosclerotic site might result in injury to the inner membrane of the vessel. Another contraindication to this technique is moyamoya disease; one of our patients with this condition lost consciousness after 21 min of blood flow stoppage and died. Also, we do not apply the clip used to interrupt the blood flow with great force; weak pressure is sufficient. We use a clip with a pressure of 30–50 g when it is open [7, 8].

The clip temporarily stops the blood flow in the basilar aneurysm before its dissection; if dissection precedes the temporary clipping, a massive hemorrhage often occurs during the dissection procedure. Applying the clip to the basilar artery and dissecting and treating the aneurysm after the blood pressure in the aneurysm has dropped is considered a safe and complete

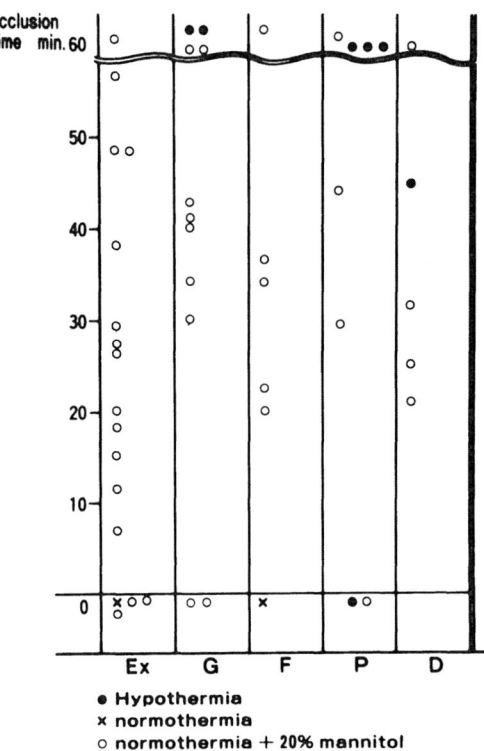

Fig. 4. Correlation between operative results and occlusion time of basilar artery

approach to treatment, including treatment of the neck of the aneurysm. In treating the aneurysmal neck, it is important to ligate the neck with thread, which makes complete clipping of the neck possible. If the neck has hardened due to arteriosclerosis and this persists even after ligation and clipping, pieces of muscle are put on sequentially, starting at the opposite side facing the operating field. Based on the fact that there were no cases of recurrent hemorrhage in the long-term follow-up study [11], it appears that these procedures are better than clipping alone.

Conclusion

In this paper, we present surgical management of basilar artery aneurysms with special reference to the temporary cerebrovascular occlusion method under the administration of cerebral protective agents in the Sendai Cocktail.

We usually use a subtemporal approach, which provides a large operating field; the field can be created at the site of the basilar aneurysm, regardless of its height. In the surgery, care should be taken to preserve the vein of Labbé and to avoid injury to the third and fourth cranial nerves. It is necessary to use a temporary cerebrovascular occlusion method utilizing administration of the Sendai Cocktail. This method does not adversely affect the outcome and makes for safe and complete surgery. To treat the aneurysm neck, it is also necessary to ligate the neck with thread, which ensures complete clipping.

References

1. Drake CG (1978) Treatment of aneurysms of the posterior cranial fossa. Prog Neurol Surg 9:122–194
2. Sano K (1980) Temporopolar approach to aneurysms of the basilar artery at and around the distal bifurcation: Technical note. Neurol Res 2: 361–367
3. Sugita K, Kobayashi S, Shintani A, Mutsuga N (1979) Microneurosurgery for aneurysms of the basilar artery. J Neurosurg 51:612–615
4. Suzuki J (1974) A method of prolongation of temporary stopping of the cerebral blood flow. 33rd Annual meeting of the Japan Neurosurgical Society, Sendai, Japan, Oct. 22, 1974 (in Japanese)
5. Suzuki J, Fujimoto S. Mizoi K, Oba M (1984) The protective effect of combined administration of anti-oxidants and perfluoro-chemicals on cerebral iachemia. Stroke 15:672–679
6. Suzuki J, Imaizumi S, Kayama T, Yoshimoto T (1985) Chemiluminescence in hypoxic brain: II. Cerebral protective effect of mannitol, vitamin E and glucocorticoid. Stroke 16:695–700
7. Suzuki J, Mizoi K, Yoshimoto T (1986) Bifrontal interhemispheric approach to aneurysms of the anterior communicatng artery. J Neurosurg 64: 183–190
8. Suzuki J, Yoshimoto T, Kayama T (1984) Surgical treatment of middle cerebral artery aneurysms. J Neurosurg 61:17–23
9. Yaşargil MG, Antic J, Laciga R, Jain KK, Hodosh RM, Simth RD (1976) Microsurgical pterional approach to aneurysms of the basilar bifurcation. Surg Neurol 6:83–91
10. Yoshimoto T, Sakamoto T, Watanabe T, J Suzuki (1978) Experimental cerebral infarction: III. Protective effect of mannitol in thalamic infarction in dogs. Stroke 9:217–218
11. Yoshimoto T, Uchida K, Kaneko U, Kayama T, Suzuki J (1979) An analysis of follow-up results of 1000 intracranial sarcular aneurysms with definitive surgical treatment. J Neurosurg 50:152–157

Discussion

Vanderwerf (Amsterdam): What do the panel think about operating on posterior basilar aneurysms in the acute stage. Do they think there is a difference if the operation is carried out early or late? Second, why are grades III and IV grouped together? In our experience, there is always a big difference in the outcome of grade III and IV patients. Third, when do you decide to clip or section the posterior communicating artery (PCoA) when it is not certain whether a temporary clip is required? Are you sure that the opposite PCoA is patent and when do you resite?

Peerless (Ontario): In answer to your second question, we grouped patients of grades III and IV simply to obtain balanced groups numerically. I agree that grade IV patients are very different. With such small numbers of patients, the divisions are quite artificial.

Symon (London): With regard to the first question, I think whether posterior circulation aneurysms can be managed acutely depends entirely on the experience of the surgeon: If the surgeon has performed a large number of basilar aneurysms the operation becomes a matter of routine. However, under conditions of raised intracranial pressure, particularly if there is some evidence of cerebral edema, the options will be reduced. The assessment of the difficulty of the procedure is important: If the operation looks straightforward I will perform it as soon as possible, just as for an anterior circulation aneurysm. But if I think it will be a very difficult cap basilar dissection I prefer to wait until the patient has recovered from the acute effects of the hemorrhage. Then, however, the situation may arise of a patient in grade I with a large subarachnoid clot who is not operated upon and whose condition deteriorates over a period of a few days and vasospasm develops. The surgeon then regrets not having operated earlier. I feel there is no clear answer here; I would like to operate early, but I still have my reservations.

Marsh (Rochester): I would concur with what Dr. Symon has said. Elevating the temporal lobe in the acute stage in patients with little blood incurs great risks. While it is difficult not operating on a well patient through fear of renewed hemorrhage we feel this is better than operating on a potentially curable patient and then encountering difficulties in surgery.

Kayama (Sendai): Our experience in the acute stage is rather limited. While awaiting operation, rerupture sometimes occurs in the patient. Given an easy case, it may be better to operate.

Ausman (Detroit): We would agree with Dr. Symon. Theoretically, the arguments in favor of early surgery are quite strong. The best way to prevent rebleeding is to clip the aneurysm and it would seem reasonable when treating the arterial narrowing in cerebral ischemia (vasospasm) to secure the aneurysm before volume loading the patient and using hypertension. Definite data on management morbidity and mortality with respect to early versus late surgery would be helpful here. We do not have enough experience to arrive at a conclusion.

Yamaura (Chiba): We have carried out surgery at the acute stage in some cases but were not too happy with the results. At present, we prefer to operate in the 2nd week, particulary in basilar bifurcation or midbasilar aneurysm, which may require heavy retraction of the brain. However, if the patient has PICA aneurysm or distal PCA aneurysm, which are straightforward type we may operate at any time. In answering the third question of Prof. Vanderwerf, we have experience of about 70 cases of basilar bifurcation, but I have never severed the PCoA though in some cases I had to include it in the clip. I have never divided PCoA to approach basilar bifurcation aneurysms.

Marsh: I do not have the precise figures, but we

have often divided the PCoA provided that the vessel was small, the opposite PCA large, and the P1 segment on the operating side of good size so as to provide satisfactory exposure.

Peerless: We have divided the PCoA probably less than about ten times. We are very concerned with the collateral circulation in aneurysm surgery and so are reluctant to divide one of the most important collaterals in the posterior circulation. We feel it is rarely necessary and potentially hazardous.

Symon: I have only divided the PCoA when I thought the dissection was stretching the two main perfusing branches to the hypothalamus. It should only be done if the PCoA is small and it is believed to be really necessary.

Yamaura: If the PCoA is obtrusive in the surgical operation I think it is a good idea to create space between the perforating arteries so as to approach the basilar bifurcation aneurysm, particularly if the latter is very high.

Suzuki (Osaka): I think the incidence of vasospasm in ruptured aneurysms of the posterior circulation is the same as ruptured aneurysms of the anterior circulation. How does the panel feel about this?

Peerless: That has certainly been our impression. The incidence is identical in the two groups; it is related to the amount of blood spilled into the subarachnoid space not to the actual source of the blood.

Samii (Hanover): My first question is in how many cases have you been unable to clip the aneurysm, unable to identify the surrounding arteries, occluded these arteries, and only realized this postoperatively on angiography? Second, in two cases, we have carried out reconstruction of the posterior cerebral artery and PICA in a fusiform aneurysm. Is this necessary? Have you carried out this procedure with fusiform aneurysms?

Peerless: All our small aneurysms were clipped. Of the large aneurysms, about 85%–90% were clipped. In giant aneurysms, less than 50% were clipped. About 10% of the aneurysms operated upon need immediate reoperation usually because some portion of the neck of the aneurysm is still open, some portion of the dome is still

filling, or occasionally because of dangerous narrowing of the origin of the posterior cerebral artery or narrowing of the terminal basilar artery. Unfortunately, when the clip was imperfectly placed so as to damage the perforating vessels or major branch vessels, damage to the brain had already occurred before the clip could be removed. We did not then reoperate to obtain a better angiographic result. A point to be stressed here is that all of these patients should have a postoperative angiogram even if the aneurysm was punctured at the time of surgery and collapsed. We are often surprised to find an aneurysm still filling in the postoperative angiogram. These patients need to undergo reoperation. We have not resected a fusiform aneurysm and tried to anastomose it. We have generally had poor results with this fusiform giant atherosclerotic aneurysm despite trying different approaches, such as proximal occlusion or direct partial clipping or wrapping.

What is the time limit for temporary occlusion in posterior aneurysm and what is the incidence of vascular spasm during and after operation?

Peerless: We use intermittent temporary clipping: We attach the clip, perform some of the dissection, and then remove the clip so as to allow reperfusion. The average clip time is 3.5 min, with six or seven applications in any one case. We had one patient in whom a temporary clip was kept on the basilar artery continuously for the 100 min because the aneurysm had ruptured. The patient, a 69-year-old woman, recovered from the procedure with no deficit. We have not found with any certainty that the basilar temporary clipping safety time can be monitored with a somatosensory-evoked potential. Sometimes, a patient recovers consciousness with a neurological deficit, though we cannot be certain that this was due to the temporary clip. With regard to vasospasm, the incidence in our unit is now about 30% angiographic vasospasm and 15% symptomatic vasospasm, with about half of the latter being sick with the vasospasm and requiring treatment.

Handa (Hamamatsu): You frequently use bypass in giant aneurysms in the anterior circulation. What about the posterior circulation?

Peerless: We have done this less than a dozen times since we can deal with these aneurysms with proximal occlusion without a bypass using the collateral circulation. The collateral circulation close to giant aneurysms is more expedient than the anterior circulation.

Kayama: What do you think of the use of a ligature to make a neck on a large-based aneurysm?

Peerless: We have performed this on occasions but less often in recent years.

Commentator, *Yaşargil* (Zurich): Remarkable progress has been made in recent years. Not so long ago, basilar aneurysms were regarded as inoperable. Now, in 1400 operated cases the morbidity and mortality are 10% in London, Ontario. We now have to try and reduce this figure to the 1%–2% of anterior circulation aneurysms. From Dr. Peerless' presentation, there seems to be a tendency to operate as soon as possible on the basis of the patient's consciousness. Patients with grades I and II of consciousness do much better than those in grades III and IV. I also believe that conscious patients should be operated upon. Perhaps with the advent of new technologies, such as PET and MRI, the decision as to the which patients require operation will be facilitated. In London, Ontario over the past 20 years, 1400 patients with vertebrobasilar aneurysm have been operated upon, which was 50% or fewer of the whole aneurysms. Normally, 5%–10% of cases are vertebrobasilar aneurysms; 7% of my 1600 cases were vertebrobasilar aneurysm. The size of the aneurysm is very important as is the condition of the patient, but the direction of the aneurysm also plays a big role. Superior posteriorly directed aneurysms are easily operated in basilar aneurysms, even in middle to large cases. Superior anteriorly directed aneurysms are similar. However, posteriorly and inferior posteriorly directed aneurysms cause problems if they become large because then the perforators become incorporated in the wall. In such cases, I do not know how to proceed. It is important that we learn more about the perforators. According to the anatomical study of Minkovic, there is only one perforator from P1 in 5%–10% of cases and there are natural anastomoses between the perforators in the ventrobasilar system.

Drake: I have great faith in temporary clips if they are light—about 30–50 g. We have performed hundreds of operations and did angiography in every one, but there was no evidence of injury to the artery except in one case. The introduction of temporary clips has altered the whole position. Since their introduction, we have achieved about a 95% rate of good outcomes in patients who were in good condition and had small basilar bifurcation aneurysms; the result has been favorable in over 90% of large aneurysms. The most difficult basilar aneurysm I find is when it is low and hidden behind the clivus; the perforators run up behind the aneurysm and the P1s go up on either side. A transsinus approach may be attempted here if the confluence is not good or if a large sigmoid or lateral sinus is present that is not suitable for division. It is very easy to take a temporal flap, remove the mastoid, drill off the petrosal apex, and divide the superior petrosal sinus; the sigmoid and lateral sinus can then be retracted with anterior cerebellum. The vein of Labbé must, however, be behind the confluence; if it is in front this approach cannot be used.

RTD 2. Moyamoya Disease

Statistical Study of Japanese Cases of Moyamoya Disease

Akira Nishimoto, Hideyuki Kuyama, and Hitohisa Niimi[1]

A statistical study of Japanese cases of moyamoya disease was begun in 1974, when the Research Committee for Vascular Disorders of the Central Nervous System was first organized by the Ministry of Health and Welfare of the Japanese government. Before the investigation by this committee, individual studies had been published with 96 cases in 1966 [8] and 1968 [9] by Nishimoto et al. 363 cases in 1971 [4] and 463 cases in 1984 [1] by Kudo, and with 518 cases in 1974 [7] and 1975 [6] by Nishimoto et al.

In this study, a total of 1370 cases of true or definite moyamoya disease are evaluated, consisting of the authors' accumulated 518 cases before the committee, 667 definite cases used in the committee study between 1974 and 1981 [10], and 185 definite cases of the same study between 1983 and 1985 [2] (Tables 1, 2). True or definite cases were diagnosed and selected from the study by the bilaterality of the typical cerebral angiographic findings [5]. Among 1370 cases, 544 were male and 826 were female, showing a female preponderance. There were 633 cases of children under the age of 15 years and 737 cases of adults above 16 years. Two peaks of frequent occurrence were observed at the ages between 0–5 years and 30–39 years (Fig. 1).

The committee divided the cases into four clinical types: transient ischemic attack (TIA) type, infarction type, epilepsy type, and hemorrhagic type. A total of 649 cases with follow-up study were evaluated statistically in relation to each clinical type (Table 2b). Among the 649 cases, seven cases showed two clinical types: therefore, a total of 656 incidents of the different types were studied.

Frequency of each clinical type at onset showed no differences between male and female (Table 3). However, TIA and infarction types were more common in children (50% and 32%, respectively), while the hemorrhagic type was seen in 65% of the adults (Table 4). Clinical types in relation to age are shown by percentage of each type in Fig. 2 and by percentage of each age period in Fig. 3. Main clinical types which had a preceding attack of a different type are listed in Table 5. TIA and epilepsy attacks were often seen as preceding attacks in patients of infarction type.

Treatment was divided into medical and the surgical groups (Table 6) and the numbers and the percentages of both treatment in each clinical type are listed in Table 7. The TIA type was more often treated surgically while the hemorrhagic type was treated more conservatively. The methods of surgical treatment and the technics of cerebrovascular reconstructive surgery, with

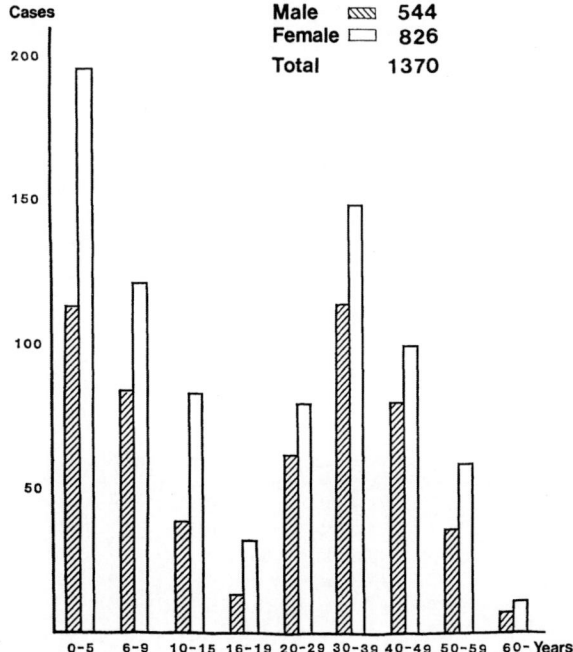

Fig. 1. Age and sex distribution

[1] Department of Neurological Surgery, Okayama University Medical School, Okayama, Japan

Table 1. Reported statistical studies of moyamoya disease

Period	Group	Author	Probable	Definite	Total
–1971	Keio University	Kudo	/	/	463
1973–1974	Okayama University	Nishimoto	/	/	518
1974–1975	Research Committee for Vascular Disorders of Central Nervous System	Nishimoto	69	120	189
1976–1978	Committee; National Cardiovascular Center	Yamaguchi	/	/	590
1976–1978	Committee; Okayama University	Nishimoto	201	389	590
1974–1981	Committee; Okayama University	Nishimoto	0	464	464*
1977–1982	Committee; National Cardiovascular Center	Yamaguchi	238	591	829
1983–1985	Committee; National Cardiovascular Center	Kikuchi	26	185	211
–1985	Committee + Keio University; Kudo, Kitamura, Gotoh, Handa	Handa	301 Undifferentiated cases 417	845	1563

* 464 responses to 667 surveys of definite moyamoya disease for long term follow-up

Table 2a. Statistics of definite 1370 moyamoya cases

Period	Group	Author	No. of cases
1973–1974	Okayama University	Nishimoto	518
1974–1981	Committee, Okayama University	Nishimoto	667
1983–1985	Committee, National Cardiovascular Center	Kikuchi	185
Total			1370

Table 2b. Study according to clinical types

Period	Group	Author	No. of cases
1974–1981	Committee, Okayama University	Nishimoto	464[a]
1983–1985	Committee, National Cardiovascular Center	Kikuchi	185
Total			649

[a] 464 responses to 667 surveys

Table 3. Clinical types at onset

	Male	Female	Total
TIA	71 (30%)	125 (30%)	196 (30%)
Infarction	74 (31%)	107 (26%)	181 (28%)
Hemorrhage	70 (29%)	144 (35%)	214 (33%)
Epilepsy	15 (6%)	34 (8%)	49 (7%)
Asymptomatic	5	3	8
Others	3	2	5
Unknown	2	1	3
Total	240 (100%)	416 (100%)	656 (100%)

Seven cases had two clinical types (overlapped)

Table 4. Clinical types at onset

	Child	Adult	Total
TIA	177 (50%)	19 (6%)	196 (30%)
Infarction	113 (32%)	68 (22%)	181 (28%)
Hemorrhage	16 (5%)	198 (65%)	214 (33%)
Epilepsy	44 (13%)	5 (2%)	49 (7%)
Asymptomatic	0	8	8
Others	2	3	5
Unknown	0	3	0
Total	352 (100%)	304 (100%)	656 (100%)

Seven cases had two clinical types (overlapped)

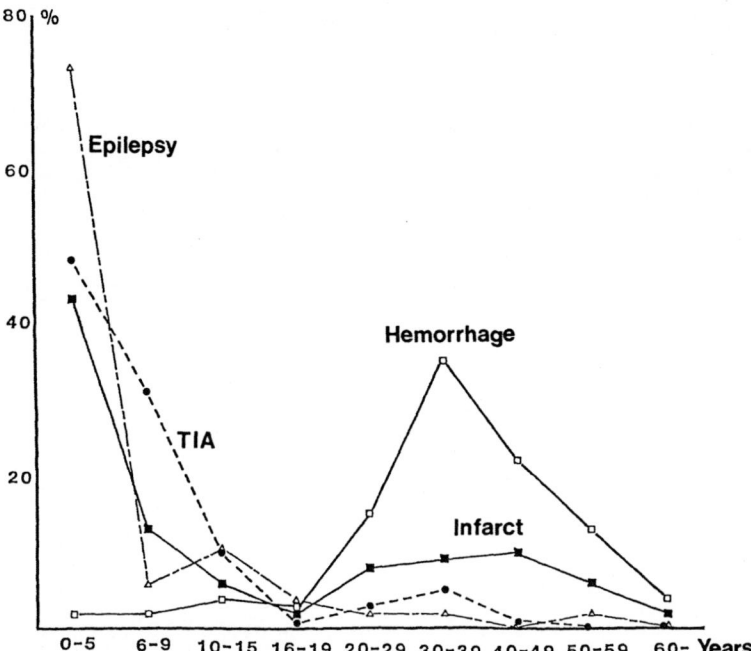

Fig. 2. Clinical type and age distribution. *TIA* transient ischemic attack

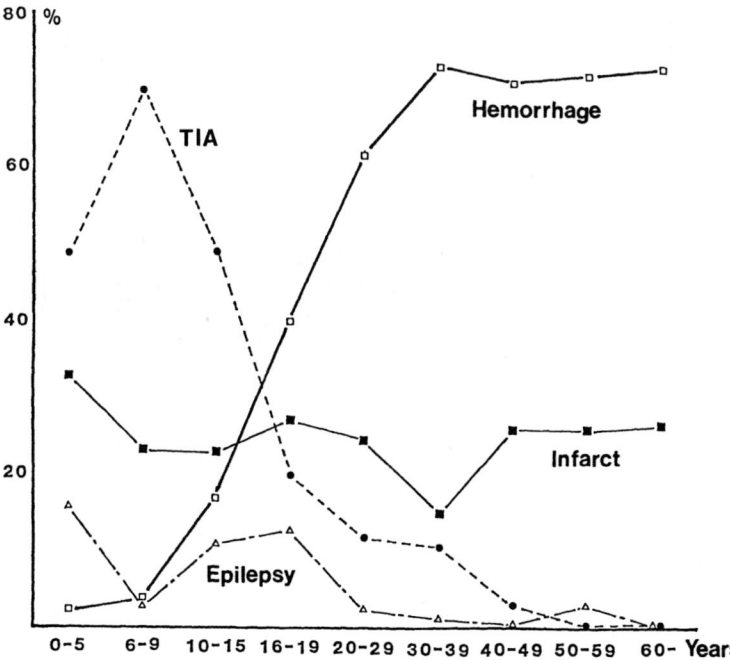

Fig. 3. Relationship between type of moyamoya disease and age at onset. *TIA* transient ischemic attack

their numbers and percentages, are listed in Tables 8 and 9. STA-MCA (superficial temporal artery—cortical branch of middle cerebral artery) anastomosis was previously a common technique, but EDAS (encephalo-duro-arterio-synangiosis) has become more common recently. EDAMS is the authors' technique [3], and is a combination of EMS (encephalo-myo-synangiosis) and EDAS with a dural strip infolding technique.

The results of medical and surgical treatment (Table 10) and those related to each clinical type (Tables 11, 12) are demonstrated. Medical and surgical cases are almost equal in number and their results are almost the same. In TIA and infarction cases, the outcome of surgical treatment seems to be a little bit more favorable compared with those of medical treatment, but not significantly so.

Table 5. Main clinical types and their preceding attacks

	Preceding attack				
	TIA	Infarction	Hemorrhage	Epilepsy	Unknown
TIA	/	6	2	8	1
Infarction	56	/	2	20	1
Hemorrhage	13	5	/	2	1
Epilepsy	7	3	2	/	0

TIA transient ischemic attack

Table 6. Treatment

	Medical	Surgical	Unknown	No treatment	Total
Child	133 (40%)	192 (58%)	3 (1%)	2 (1%)	330 (100%)
Adult	192 (60%)	119 (37%)	1 (1%)	7 (2%)	319 (100%)
Total	325 (50%)	311 (48%)	4 (1%)	9 (1%)	649 (100%)

Table 7. Treatment and clinical types

	Medical	Surgical	No treatment	Unknown	Total
TIA	62 (19%)	127 (40%)	3	4	196 (30%)
Infarction	92 (28%)	88 (28%)	1	0	181 (28%)
Hemorrhage	131 (40%)	78 (25%)	5	0	214 (33%)
Epilepsy	30 (9%)	19 (6%)	0	0	49 (7%)
Asymptomatic	8	0	0	0	8
Others	4	1	0	0	5
Unknown	1	2	0	0	3
Total	328 (100%)	315 (100%)	9	4	656 (100%)

Seven cases had two clinical types
TIA transient ischemic attack

Table 8. Method of surgical treatment

Method	No.	Percent
Reconstructive surgery	286	79
Removal of hematoma	33	9
Cervical sympathectomy	24	7
Others	36	10
Total	361	100

The outcome in all of the cases of moyamoya disease is shown in Tables 13 and 14. Childhood cases were more favorable, with an 80% good outcome, while adult cases had a 62% good outcome. In addition, adult cases had a 16% mortality rate, mostly due to intracranial hemorrhage. TIA and epilepsy types showed good clinical outcome in most of the cases, with a more unfavorable outcome in the infarction and hemorrhagic types. This study was made by letter inquiry with the authors' (1973–1974) and the committee's (1974–1985) forms to neurosurgical, neurological, and pediatric clinics in Japan. The authors also made efforts to select the true moyamoya cases from the answered forms according to the committee's criteria, i.e., the typical bilateral angiographic findings. The authors believe this statistical study may give an update outline of moyamoya disease in Japan.

Table 9. Reconstructive surgery and operative side

	Unilateral surgery	Bilateral surgery		Total
		One side	Other	
STA-MCA	38	56	40	144 (35%)
EMS	18	20	17	55 (13%)
EDAS	26	48	52	126 (30%)
EMAS	3	1	1	5 (1%)
EDAMS	0	3	3	6 (1%)
STA-MCA&EMS	16	30	41	87 (21%)
Others	2	0	0	2
Total	103	158	154*	415 (100%)

* Type of surgical procedure was not described in four cases. *EMS* encephalo-myo-synangiosis, *EDAS* encephalo-duro-arterio-synangiosis, *EMAS* encephalo-myo-arterio-synangiosis, *EDAMS* encephalo-duro-arterio-myo-synangiosis, *STA-MCA* superficial temporal artery—middle cerebral artery anastomosis

Table 10. Results of treatment

	Good	Fair	Poor	Dead	Unknown	Total
Medical	223 (69%)	30 (9%)	13 (4%)	31 (9%)	28 (9%)	325 (100%)
Surgical	231 (74%)	24 (8%)	12 (4%)	23 (7%)	21 (7%)	311 (100%)
No treatment	8	0	1	0	0	9
Unknown	2	0	0	0	2	4
Total	464	54	26	54	51	649

Good active to self-sustaining, *Fair* partially assisted, *Poor* totally assisted to bedridden

Table 11. Outcome of medical treatment

	Good	Fair	Poor	Dead	Unknown	Total
TIA	51 (82%)	3 (5%)	0 (0%)	1 (2%)	7 (11%)	62 (100%)
Infarction	47 (51%)	23 (25%)	8 (9%)	6 (6%)	8 (9%)	92 (100%)
Hemorrhage	92 (70%)	3 (2%)	4 (3%)	22 (17%)	10 (8%)	131 (100%)

Good fully active to self-sustaining, *Fair* partially assisted, *Poor* totally assisted to bedridden, *TIA* transient ischemic attack

Table 12. Outcome of surgical treatment

	Good	Fair	Poor	Dead	Unknown	Total
TIA	116 (93%)	1 (1%)	2 (2%)	0 (0%)	5 (4%)	124 (100%)
Infarction	54 (70%)	12 (16%)	5 (6%)	2 (3%)	4 (5%)	77 (100%)
Hemorrhage	25 (65%)	8 (21%)	1 (3%)	3 (8%)	1 (3%)	38 (100%)

Ratings and abbreviations as in Table 11

Table 13. Outcome

	Good	Fair	Poor	Dead	Unknown	Total
Child	279 (80%)	30 (9%)	13 (4%)	5 (1%)	20 (6%)	347 (100%)
Adult	185 (62%)	24 (8%)	13 (4%)	49 (16%)	31 (10%)	302 (100%)
Total	464 (72%)	54 (8%)	26 (4%)	54 (8%)	51 (8%)	649 (100%)

Ratings as in Table 11

Table 14. Outcome and clinical types of moyamoya disease

	Good	Fair	Poor	Dead	Unknown	Total
TIA	174 (89%)	4 (2%)	2 (1%)	1 (0%)	15 (8%)	196 (100%)
Infarction	107 (59%)	36 (20%)	13 (7%)	9 (5%)	16 (9%)	181 (100%)
Hemorrhage	134 (63%)	13 (6%)	10 (5%)	41 (19%)	16 (7%)	214 (100%)
Epilepsy	41 (84%)	2 (4%)	1 (2%)	1 (2%)	4 (8%)	49 (100%)
Asymptomatic	7	0	0	1	0	8
Others	4	0	0	0	1	5
Unknown	2	0	0	1	0	3

Ratings and abbreviation as in Table 11

References

1. Handa H, Yonekawa Y, Gotoh Y, et al. (1984) Filing of 1500 cases of spontaneous occlusion of the circle of Willis. Report of Research Committee for the Spontaneous Occlusion of the Circle of Willis, pp 14–20 (in Japanese)
2. Kikuchi H, Karasawa J, Negata I, et al. (1985). All Japan statistical study of the cases of spontaneous occlusion of the circle of Willis. Report of Research Committee for the Spontaneous Occlusion of the Circle of Willis, pp 19–25 (in Japanese)
3. Kinugasa K, Honma Y, Kuyama H, et al. (1985). Surgical treatment of moyamoya disease: Encephaloduroarteriomyosynangiosis (EDAMS). 14th Japanese Conference on Surgery of Cerebral Stroke, p 76 (in Japanese)
4. Kudo T (1971) Abnormal cerebrovascular network. 18th Nihon-Igakkai-Soukaikaishi, pp 1253–1273 (in Japanese)
5. Nishimoto A (1979) Moyamoya disease. Neurol Med Chir 19:221–228 (in Japanese)
6. Nishimoto A, Mizukawa N (1975) So-called moyamoya disease. Neurolog Med 3:37–45 (in Japanese)
7. Nishimoto A, Mizukawa N, Ohashi T, et al. (1974) Moyamoya disease. Report of Research Committee for Vascular Disorders of the Central Nervous System, pp 51–57 (in Japanese)
8. Nishimoto A, Sugiu S, Takeuchi S (1966) Cerebrovascular malformation of the circle of Willis. Brain Nerve 18:508–513 (in Japanese)
9. Nishimoto A, Takeuchi S (1968) Abnormal cerebrovascular network related to the internal carotid arteries. J Neurosurg 29:255–260
10. Nishimoto A, Ueda K, Honma Y (1982) Long-term follow up study of spontaneous occlusion of the circle of Willis. Report of Research Committee for the Spontaneous Occlusion of the Circle of Willis, pp 60–73 (in Japanese)

Clinical Manifestation and Pathology of Moyamoya Disease in Northeast China

An Analysis of 54 Cases

Jing-xian Suo[1]

Moyamoya disease was reported and named by Suzuki in 1969 [5] for the first time. From 1980 through 1985, 54 cases have been reported in Northeast China [1–4]. Forty-two of them were diagnosed by cerebral angiography and 12 patients were confirmed by autopsy.

Clinical Material

Of the 54 cases, 36 were male; 18 were female. Among these cases, 14 were children and the other 40 were adults.

Clinical Manifestation

Thirty-seven adult patients were of the intracranial hemorrhagic type and suffered headache, vomiting, convulsions, aphasia, and motor disturbance. Seventeen patients were of the ischemic type and were considered to have transient ischemic attack (TIA), hemiparesis, hemiplegia and mind disorder. Among these 17 cases, three were adults and 14 were teenagers and children. Eighteen patients in the intracranial hemorrhagic group became unconscious, 15 of them were complicated by tentorial herniation, and, among these 15 cases, four had decerebrate rigidity.

Angiographic Findings

Cerebroangiography was performed on 42 patients. Thirty-two of them had undergone bilateral carotid percutaneous punctures and ten had had only unilateral examination.

The main findings in the angiograms were stenosis of the upper portion of the internal carotid siphon and nonfilling of the anterior and middle cerebral arteries. The aberrant vascular networks appeared as "a puff of smoke" at the base of the brain (Figs. 1, 2).

CT Scan

Eleven patients received CT scanning. Multiple local low density areas were found in five patients with brain ischemia (Fig. 3). However, high-density areas appeared in six patients with intracerebral hemorrhage, particularly in patients with bleeding of less than 20 ml. These patients were not easily confirmed by cerebroangiogram, because the arrangement of brain arteries was abnormal. The CT scan is more significant in the diagnosis of hemorrhagic moyamoya disease as it is able to locate the origin and quantity of bleeding.

Treatment and Results

Craniotomy and evacuation of hematoma were performed immediately after admission for six patients with intracerebral hemorrhages: All of them survived. Ten were ischemic patients. Three of them were treated with STA-MCA anastomosis, and seven were treated with temporal muscle covering the cerebral surface. All of the ten cases had good results as their hemiparesis improved in varying degrees.

Twenty-six patients received conservative treatment. Among them, 12 patients improved in varying degrees and ten patients recovered. Unfortunately, no improvement was shown in four patients.

Pathological Examination

Twelve patients died within 24 h after admission. Postmortem examinations showed intracerebral

[1] Department of Neurosurgery, Norman Bethune University of Medical Sciences, Chang-chun, Jilin, People's Republic of China

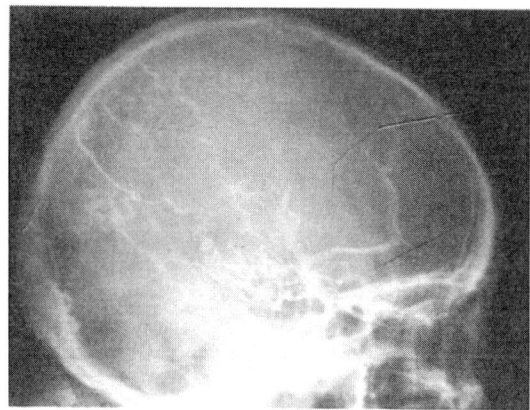

Fig. 1. Carotid arteriograph demonstrating the narrowing of the upper portion of the carotid siphon and nonfilling of the anterior and middle cerebral arteries. The aberrant smokelike vascular networks are visible

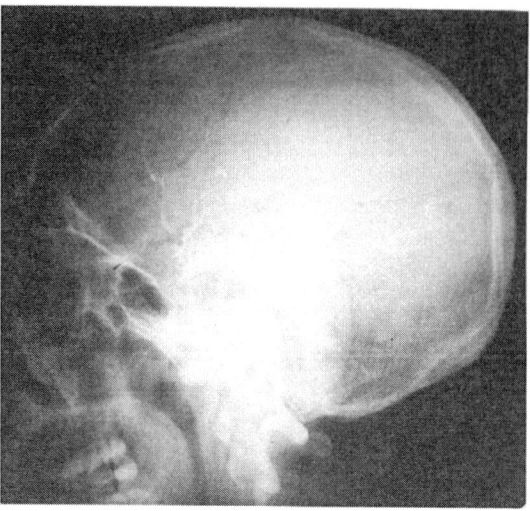

Fig. 2. Vertebral angiograph showing basal moyamoya

hemorrhage and cerebral herniation in seven of these patients. Five patients died of primary intraventricular hemorrhage: In these patients, the tortuous vascular networks and their ruptures were seen on the lateral wall of the lateral ventricle after removing the clot, and the origin of bleeding was discovered.

Agenesia of the circle of Willis was found in all of the deceased patients. The main arteries of the circle of Willis had narrowed, with the diameters of some vessels were less than 1.0 mm.

Double right anterior cerebral arteries were found in one patient. One of them had derived from the anterior communicating artery and the left anterior cerebral artery had become threadlike. These findings indicate congenital agenesia of the vessels (Fig. 4). The pathological examination showed that the retiform vessels came from the deep perforating branches derived from the anterior and middle cerebral arteries and posterior communicating artery (Fig. 5). A light-microscopic study of the specimens of the middle cerebral arteries showed nearly total obliteration of the lumen, degeneration, tortuousity and discontinuity of the elastic fiber layer, and infiltration of the adventitia with leukocytes (Fig. 6).

Discussion

From 1980 through 1985, there were 54 cases of moyamoya disease reported in Northeast China. Among them, 37 cases had suffered from intracranial hemorrhage and 17 cases from cerebral ischemia, in the hemorrhagic group. Five patients with primary intraventricular hemor-

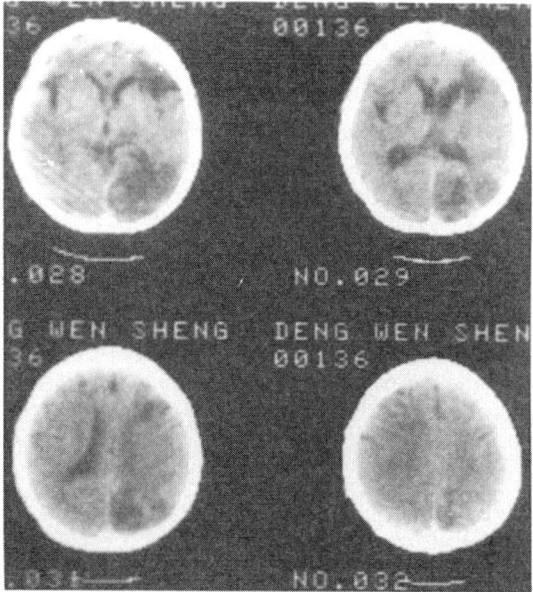

Fig. 3. CT scan of a case of ischemic type moyamoya disease demonstrating multifocal low density areas and no displacement of the lateral ventricle

rhage had been postmortally examined: They were found to have tortuous vascular networks on the wall of the dilated lateral ventricle. This might have been the origin of the bleeding. It was also shown that the subarachnoid bleeding and come from lateral ventricular hemorrhage, which was often misdiagnosed as primary subarachnoid bleeing.

Cerebroangiography seems essential for the diagnosis of moyamoya disease, but sometimes,

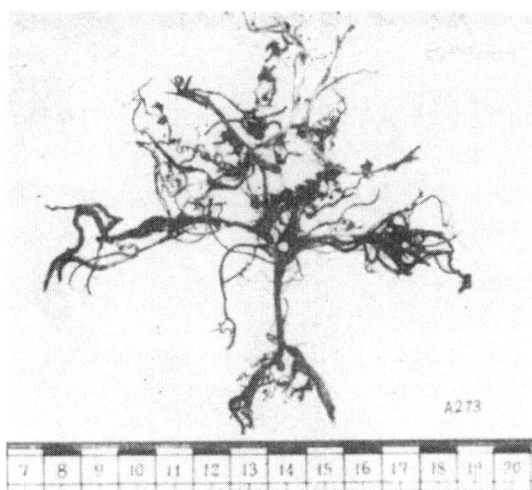

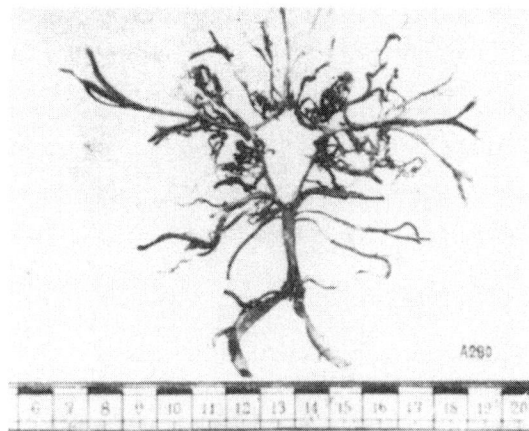

Fig. 4. A dissected Willis circle showing thin bilateral carotid arteries, middle cerebral arteries and many accumulated tortuous vessels; posterior cerebral artery, basal artery and vertebral artery are dilated and thick

Fig. 5. A dissected Willis circle showing the basal moyamoya and three anterior cerebral arteries, two on the right and one of them derived from the anteior communicating artery; the left anterior cerebral artery is very thin

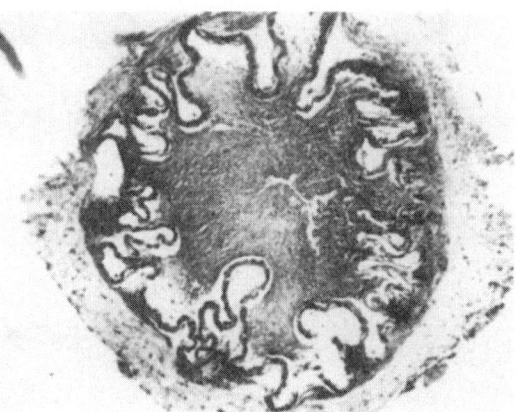

Fig. 6. Light microscopic study of a specimen of a middle cerebral artery showing nearly total obliteration of the lumen as well as degeneration, tortuousity and discontinuity of the elastic fiber layer. The media is atrophied and the adventitia is infiltrated by leukocytes

when the hematoma is not large enough, a CT scan is needed. In such cases, anterior and middle cerebral arteries appear unfilled and an aberrant arrangement of vessels is often present on the cerebroangiogram. In this series, four cases of intracerebral hematoma, which were confirmed by CT scan afterwards, could not be seen on the cerebroangiogram. It's recognized that moyamoya vessels were collaterals of cerebral vessels. During operations on patients with intracerebral hematoma, these vessels should not be destroyed. Satisfactory results were obtained in six cases with intracerebral hematoma in this report.

The pathogenesis of moyamoya disease may be a congenital abnormality of cerebral vessels, and we have found by pathological examinations the circle of Willis to be agenetic or markedly thin. All the cases, including the case with three anterior cerebral arteries mentioned above, supported the congenital agenesis theory. However, congenital deformity of cerebral vessels can not explain the proliferation of vascular intima, infiltration of intima and adventitia of vessels with monocytes. It's reasonable to accept the explanation by Liu Duosan [4] that chronic intravascular inflammation may result in the narrowing or occlusion of the vessels on the basis of congenital abnormality of the circle of Willis. Eventually, aberrant vascular networks grow in order to form collaterals. The exact nature of vascular inflammation is not known yet. Therefore, further investigation is necessary.

References

1. Dai C et al (1985) Moyamoya disease. Hei-Long-Zan Med 5:22
2. Fan H (1985) "Foggy" disease complicated with intracerebral hemorrhage. Cerebr Stroke Neurol Dis 2:211
3. Liu T, Lee C (1984) Intraventricular hemorrhage resulting from "Foggy" disease. Cerebr Stroke Neurol Dis 1:22
4. Liu T et al (1980) Abnormal net like vessels at the base of the brain: their pathology and clinical manifestation. Chin Neuropsychol 13:129
5. Suzuki J (1969) Cerebrovascular "Moyamoya" disease. Arch Neurol 20:288

Table 1. Age distribution and clinical presentations

Group	Sex		Age (yrs)					
	Male	Female	5–15	16–25	26–35	36–45	46–55	55–
Hemorrhagic	30	15	13	10	10	11	1	0
Ischemic	15	16	10	8	4	5	3	1
Total	45	31	23	18	14	16	4	1

Table 2. Past history in 76 cases with moyamoya disease

	Children	Adults
Pulmonary tuberculosis		3
Frequent cold	2	3
Mumps	1	
Cholecystitis		1
Rheumatism		1
Nasal furuncle		1
Epilepsy	2	
Epistaxis	2	3

Table 3. Symptoms and signs in 76 cases with moyamoya disease

Symptoms and signs	Children	Adults
Hemorrhagic group	13	32
Sudden coma	10	16
Hemiplegia	6	9
Sensory disturbances	2	1
Aphasia	2	8
Unsteady gait	2	
Divergence of eyes		1
Decerebrate rigidity		2
Cerebral herniation	3	3
Headache	12	23
Vomiting	7	19
Intracranial hematoma	5	14
Ischemic group	10	21
Sensory disturbances	3	8
Aphasia	5	14
Coma	1	2
Mental disturbances		1
Headache	1	4

angiogram and CT scan are presented in Tables 4 and 5.

Surgical Treatment

Surgical treatment was performed in 31 cases (Table 6).

Among the nine cases with hematoma removal, three hemorrhages were in the basal ganglion or further into the third ventricle. All of the three patients died after operation.

In six cases who underwent STA-MCA bypass, only two showed obvious improvement in neurological features postoperatively.

Angiography was performed between 1 month and $1\frac{1}{2}$ years after operation in six cases who had received encephaloduralarteriosynangiosis. Three of them demonstrated newly formed fine vessels between the superficial temporal artery and the underlying cortex, and three other cases did not. Surgical treatment seemed to be beneficial to half the number of cases with improved neurological deficits but they were not coincident with the new vessel formation.

Forty-five cases were not treated surgically and two patients died of ischemic coma.

It seems that the prognosis of both surgical and nonsurgical treatment from these few cases are similar, except for those who had large intracranial hematoma in need of emergent surgery.

Follow-Up

Only 20 cases were available for follow-up study in a period of 6 months to 6 years after discharge from the hospital. Among them, 13 were hemorrhagic and seven ischemic. Surgical treatment had been performed in four cases for evacuation of hematoma and in six cases for synangiosis. The other ten patients were treated conservatively. All the patients mentioned above without reference to surgical or conservative treatment showed some clinical improvement, but one, who had been in the late stages of cerebral herniation when admitted to the hospital, remained unconsciousness 6 months after evacuation of his intracranial hematoma. The number is too small to indicate whether surgical treatment is beneficial for ischemic moyamoya patients.

Moyamoya Disease in Beijing

CHUNG-CHENG WANG and JI-ZONG ZHAO[1]

Seventy-six cases of moyamoya disease were encountered between 1977 to 1985 in our institute. Forty-five of them were males and 31 females. They were 4–57 years of age with an average of 22.9 years. Their clinical presentations showed evidence of intracranial hemorrhage in 45 cases (59.2%) and cerebral ischemia in 31 (40.8%) (Table 1).

Past History

Twelve patients had a history of infection prior to the onset of the present illness (Table 2).

One case had two transfusions at a month interval. The second transfusion was followed by the onset of moyamoya disease.

Clinical Manifestation

Clinical presentation can be divided into two classes: hemorrhagic and ischemic (Table 3).

All the hemorrhagic cases were documented with bloody CSF or CT-scanning. Two cases presenting hemorrhage had also had a history of hemihypoesthesia and hemiparesis 1 month and 6 months earlier. In the 19 cases with intrahematoma, eight were in the cerebral parenchyma, seven in the lateral ventricle, and two in the third ventricle and fourth ventricle each.

Cerebral Angiography

In 39 cases, a complete serial angiography was performed (Table 4). It seems that in some moyamoya patients one internal carotid artery may become diseased first and then another, but they soon reach a similar magnitude. Their stenosed changes first appear in C1, 2 (Fig. 1) and then spread to their proximal and distal parts, even to M1 and C3-5. Along with the stenosed change of the internal carotid artery, collateral circulation is gradually established, mainly from the basovertebral system (Fig. 2) and the middle meningeal and ophthalmic arteries (Fig. 3). The basovertebral system supplies the branches of the anterior artery by retrograde filling and supplies the middle cerebral artery through the enlarged posterior communicating artery. The middle meningeal artery becomes enlarged and tortuous, providing blood to the branches of the anterior cerebral artery, as does the ophthalmic artery. The amount and magnitude of the collaterals established are basically parellel to the development of carotid stenosis. The moyamoya vessels at the base of the brain are usually like puffs of smoke, but in a few cases the vessels may be thick and tortuous even in a shape of something like AVM. Two cases also had one saccular aneurysm each on the distal branches of the posterior cerebral arteries. The findings from serial

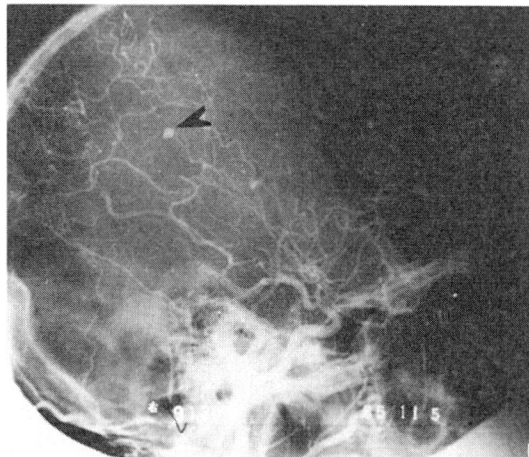

Fig. 1. Lateral view of carotid angiogram, showing the C1, narrowing of C2, and a saccular aneurysm on the branch of the PCA. *Arrow* aneurysm

[1] Beijing Neurosurgical Institute, Beijing. People's Republic of China

Table 4. Serial angiogram findings

	No. of cases
Internal carotid artery	
Bilateral occlusion	7
Bilateral stenosis	16
One occlusion and one stenosis	9
One stenosis and one normal	7
Moyamoya network	
Fine vessels	30
Thick and tortuous vessels	9
Collateral circulation	
From external carotid to internal carotid artery	
From meningeal arteries to cerebral arteries	21
From ophthalmic artery through ethmoid arteries to cerebral arteries	17
From occipital artery to cerebral artery	3
From posterior circulation to anterior circulation	
From branches of PCA to branches of ACA	37
From posterior communicating artery to MCA	25

PCA posterior cerebral artery, *ACA* anterior cerebral artery, *MCA* middle cerebral artery

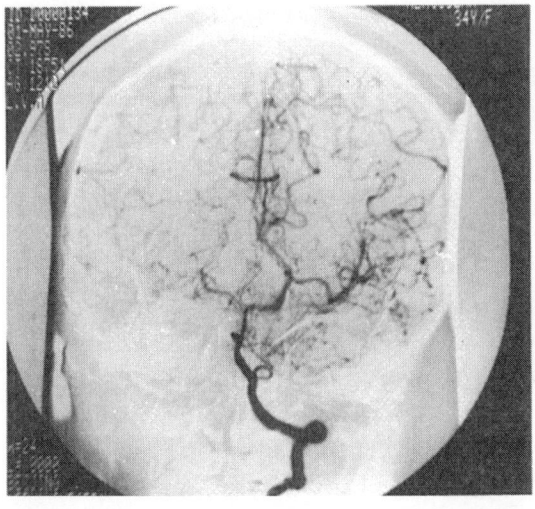

Fig. 2. Vertebral angiogram in a case of moyamoya disease. The middle cerebral artery is well filled from the posterior communicating artery and the branches of the anterior cerebral artery are filled from the cortical branches of the posterior cerebral artery

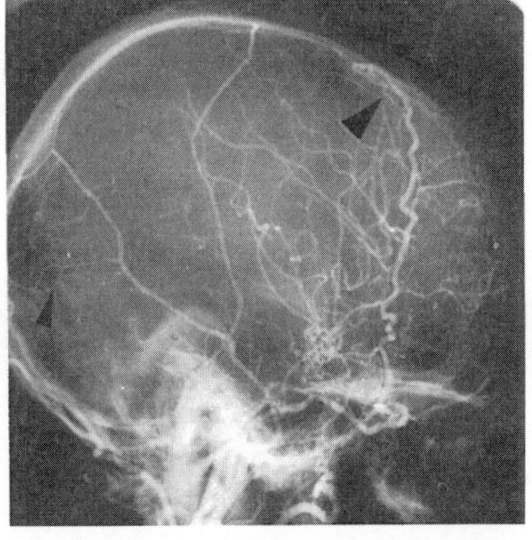

Fig. 3. Lateral view of carotid angiogram in moyamoya disease. The middle meningeal and ophthalmic arteries are dilated and tortuous, providing blood to the anterior cerebral artery system. *Large arrow* collected circulation via superficial tenporal artery; *Small arrow* collected circulation via middle meningeal artery

Pathology

The cerebral arteries of seven cases of moyamoya disease demonstrated by angiography and operation were observed by light, transmission and scanning electron microscopy (Figs. 1–4). In two cases, the lumen of the terminal portion of the internal carotid artery was completely occluded by proliferating connective tissue. The characteristic pathological change was extensive destruction of myocytes and of the internal elastic lamina. Degeneration and necrosis of myocytes was obvious in the media. A great number of condensed organelles and other elements of cellular destruction were dispersed throughout the interstitium. The media was thinned. The proliferated

Table 5. CT Scan in 32 cases

	Children	Adults
Cerebral infarction		
Low density in frontal lobe	1	5[a]
Low density in temporal lobe		1
Low density in fronto- temporal lobe	1	1
Low density in occipital lobe		1
Cerebral hemorrhage		
High density in basal ganglion		5
High density in white matter	1	2
Generalized atrophy of brain		
Large ventricles and subarachnoid spaces	2	9
Normal	1	2

[a] Low density on both sides in one case

Table 6. Surgical treatment in 31 cases

Operative procedure	No. of cases
Removal of hematoma	9
Encephaloduralarteriosynangiosis	16
STA-MCA bypass	5
Omentum transplantation to brain surface	1

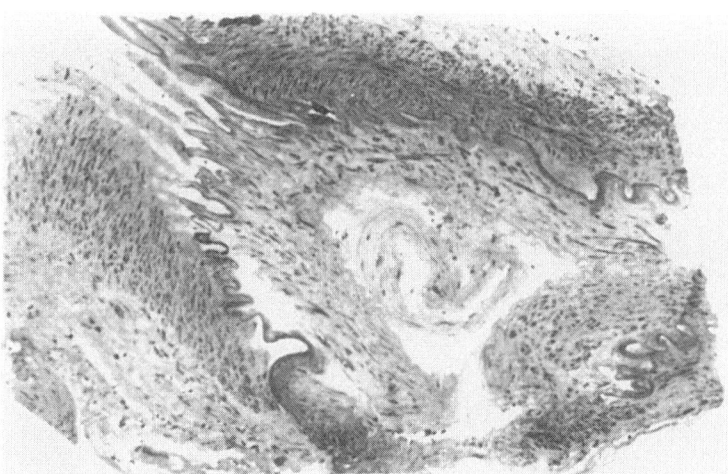

Fig. 4. Terminal portion of internal carotid artery. The lumen is occluded by connective tissues, the intima thickened, and media thinned. Epoxy section, basic fuchsin-methylene blue stain (× 110)

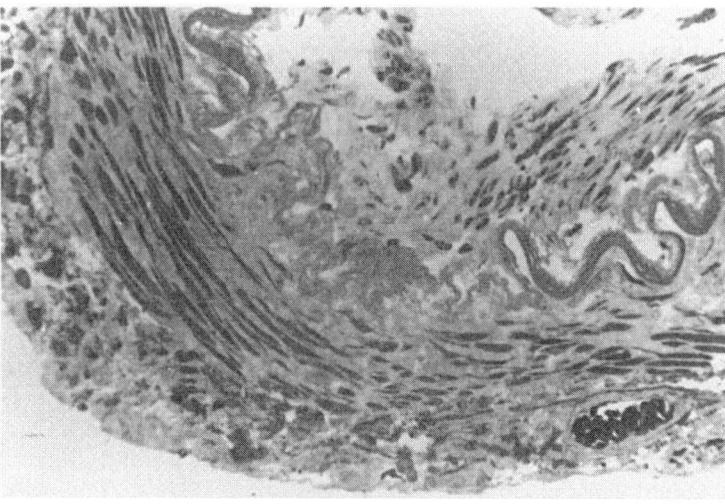

Fig. 5. Terminal portion of internal carotid artery. The internal elastic lamina is in-folded, thickened or thinned, and disintegrated. Epoxy section, basic fuchsin-methylene blue stain (× 420)

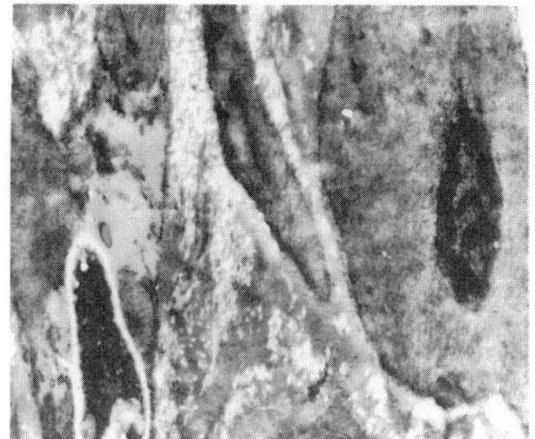

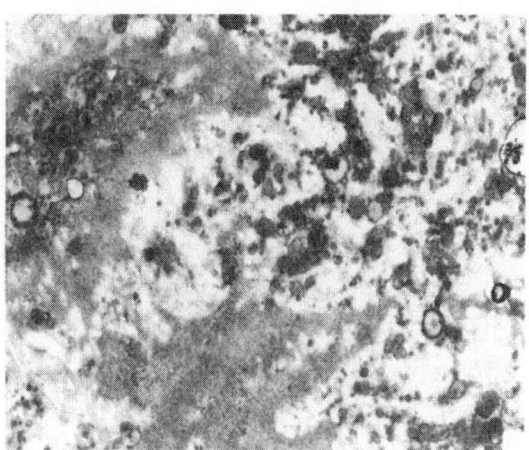

Fig. 6. The smooth muscle cell in the media of internal carotid artery is necrosed with interruption of plasma membrane, pyknosis of nucleus, and intracellular edema. Uranyl acetate and lead citrate ($\times 7\,200$)

Fig. 7. The smooth muscle cell of the intima of internal carotid artery is necrosed, its plasm membrane has disappeared. Many condensed organelles are dispersed throughout the interstitium. Uranyl acetate and lead citrate ($\times 13\,700$)

myocytes in the intima showed the same destructive changes as in the media. The internal elastic lamina was excessively infolded and was thickened or thinned, disrupted or disintegrated in the same areas. Identical but less severe and more localized changes were seen in three middle cerebral arteries (M2 and M5) and two collateral arteries at the base of brain. These changes suggest that moyamoya disease is a progressive disorder characterized by repeated myocyte destruction occurring over a long period.

Discussion

The etiology of moyamoya disease is not clear yet. Suzuki et al. [4] were impressed by the frequency of a past history of chronic inflammation in the cervical region in patients with moyamoya disease. They injected foreign protein into mongrel dogs and found that the internal carotid bifurcation showed many of the pathological changes seen in moyamoya disease. Suzuki et al. suggested that there may be some relations between infection and moyamoya disease. Twelve of our patients had a distinct infection history prior to the onset of moyamoya disease, such as tuberculosis, rheumatoid, and influenza. Moyamoya in another case seemed to be related to a second blood transfusion. When 10 ml blood had been infused intravenously, the patient became allergic and developed a hemiplegia the following day. Some authors reported lepto-

spirus as a causing factor of moyamoya disease in central China.

The diagnosis of moyamoya disease depends on cerebral angiography which is characterized by the following: (a) stenosis or occlusion of the terminal internal carotid artery, mostly bilateral but not necessarily symmetrical; (b) abnormal vascular networks formed at the base of the brain, which are usually like puffs of smoke, but in some cases their vessels are thick and tortuous; and (c) collateral circulation established between anterior and posterior cerebral circulations, between extra- and intracranial vessels.

Vascular networks at the base of brain in ischemic patients are usually like puffs of smoke. In the contrast, in hemorrhagic patients, they may be thick, tortuous and irregular, even in the shape of AVM. The ischemic anterior cerebral circulation is mainly supplied by the vertebro-basilar system, meningeal and ophthalmic arteries. The supplied anterior and middle cerebral arteries are of normal caliber in most ischemic cases but of large caliber in one-third of the hemorrhagic ones.

Many surgical procedures have been developed to improve the neurological deficit or prevent its deterioration in moyamoya patients. Perivascular cervical sympathectom, superior cervical ganglionectomy [4], and STA-MCA anastomosis [2] have been reported as beneficial. As the arteries of some children may be of inadequate size to perform anastomosis, other surgical techniques have been developed successfully, such as encephalomyosynangiosis [5], encephaloduralarteriosynangiosis [3], and cerebroarteriosynangiosis [1]. However, we can not draw an affirmative conclusion from the few cases we treated surgically.

References

1. Bulagura S, Farris WA (1985) Treatment of moyamoya disease by cerebroarteriosynangiosis. Surg Neurol 23:270–274
2. Karasawa J, Kikuchi H, Furuse S, Kawamura J, Sakaki T (1978) Treatment of moyamoya disease with STA-MCA anastomosis. J Neurosurg 49:679–688
3. Matsushima Y, Fukai N, Tanaka K, Tsueuoka S, Inaba Y, Aoyagi M, Ohno K (1981) A new surgical treatment of moyamoya disease in children: A preliminary report. Surg Neurol 15:313–320
4. Suzuki J, Takaku A, Komada N, Sato S (1975) An attempt to treat cerebral moyamoya disease in children. Child Brain 1:193–206
5. Takenchi S, Tsuchida T, Kobayashi K, Fukuda M, Ishii T, Tanaka R, Ito J (1983) Treatment of moyamoya disease by temporal muscle graft: encephalomyosynangiosis. Child Brain 10:1–15

Moyamoya Disease in Shanghai

Yu-quan Shi[1]

Moyamoya disease is infrequent in Shanghai. Upon review of all the cerebral angiographies performed in Hua Shan Hospital since 1961, only 42 cases which showed the characteristic radiological features of moyamoya disease were found. In comparision with the higher prevalence rates in other parts of our country such as Wupei province, Northern Jiangsu, and Guangxi province, where hundreds of cases have been reported in Chinese medical literature, the incidence of moyamoya disease in the Shanghai district is much lower. Among the 42 cases, 27 had their clinical data available for retrospective study, which was done by Wang and Tan in 1983. Their thesis, entitled "*Brain base abnormal vascular network; Clinical and radiological analysis of 27 cases*" was published in the Chinese Medical Journal 98(8): 583–590, 1983. Since then, another four cases have been seen in our hospital, making the sum total 31 cases upon which my discussion was based.

Among the 31 cases of moyamoya disease, there were 21 males and 10 females. Their age ranged between 4 to 48 years. There were six cases in the juvenile group (aged under 19) and 25 cases in the adult group (aged over 20). Three cases had been treated surgically. There were three patients who died in the hospital; autopsies were performed on two of them.

The clinical manisfestations differed between the juvenile and adult groups. Five of the six juvenile moyamoya cases showed motor paralysis of extremities together with some speech disturbances and headaches. The onset of the disease was gradual in five cases and abrupt in one case. There were two cases of intracerebral hemorrhage associated with mental retardation. The main clinical characteristics of the adult group are those of SAH or intracerebral hemorrhage. Acute SAH occurred in 20 of the 25 cases and was associated with vomiting, impairment of consciousness in different degrees, motor paralysis in some cases and choked discs in five cases. Transient ischemic attack of the carotid system occurred in four of the 25 cases. The attack usually lasted for a few hours and the patient recovered spontaneously without any residual neurological deficits. In one of the 25 cases, there were seizure attacks with sudden falling and unconsciousness which disappeared completely in a few minutes without any discomfort to the patient.

Radiological Findings

CT scanning of the brain had been done in only three cases, one of which showed an entirely normal picture. In one case, a large area of low density in the left cerebral hemisphere was seen, suggesting a cerebral ischemic infarction. In another case, an irregular area of increased density with slight displacement of the lateral ventricles to the right was shown in the depth of the left hemisphere indicating there was an intracerebral hemorrhage. The cerebral angiographic pictures of these cases are quite self-explanatory. Altogether, 46 carotid angiographies and one vertebral angiography had been done in these 31 cases. In all cases, narrowing of varying degrees was observed in the distal part of the carotid siphon (i.e., C1 and C2 segments of the internal carotid artery with irregularity of the inner lining of the lumen. In some cases, the middle part of the carotid siphon (i.e., C3 and C4) were also involved but rarely were the proximal part (i.e., C5) or the extracranial part of the internal carotid artery (ICA) involved. Both the anterior cerebral artery (ACA) and middle cerebral artery (MCA) were faintly or incompletely filled, with their initial part (i.e., A1, A2 and M1, M2) very much narrowed. The ophthalmic artery and

---

[1] Department of Neurosurgery, Hua Shan Hospital, Shanghai Medical University, Shanghai, People's Republic of China

the PCA were usually dilated and their distal branches communicated with the terminal branches of ACA and MCA and showed retrograde flow within the latter in some cases. There were fine abnormal, vascular networks (moyamoya vessels) of variable sizes seen at the base of the brain. From these vessels, some branches of the ACA or MCA may have initiated. Collateral circulation was also seen in some cases between the branches of the external carotid artery (ECA) and the dural and subpial vessels of the brain in the temporal, occipital, and frontal facial regions.

Of the two autopsies on the three patients who died in the hospital, one was done on a child of 4 years. He had a history of irregular fever, chronic productive cough, abdominal distention, emaciation for 7 months, right-sided hemiplegia dysphasia, and headaches for 2 months. A CSF examination showed an increase in lymphocytes, elevated protein and a reduction of sugar and chlorides. A left carotid angiography revealed a narrowing of the C1 and C2 segments of the ICA, A1 and A2 of the ACA, and M1 of the MCA. There was a fine, abnormal vascular network in the basal ganglia region. The distal branches of the ECA were dilated and anastomosed with the cortical branches of the left cerebral hemisphere. The clinical diagnosis was disseminated pulmonary tuberculosis, tuberculous meningitis, tuberculous peritonitis and moyamoya disease. Postmortem examination revealed miliary tuberculosis in the lungs, liver, peritoneum, and meninges with tuberculous endarteritis of the major cerebral arteries and a fresh thrombosis.

The second autopsy was of an adult man of 49 years. He had had repeated attacks of SAH in his last year with progressive visual impairment. The left carotid angiogram showed a marked narrowing of the C1 segment of the ICA and the proximal segments of the ACA and MCA. There were moyamoya vessels at the base of the brain. Postmortem examination confirmed the pathological changes in the cerebral vessels. There were a marked thickening and bending of the internal elastic membrane and fibrous proliferation of the media of the arteries. Since the cerebral vascular reconstructive surgery was started late in China, a majority of these cases were treated conservatively by our neurological colleagues, by means of antibiotics, steroids, vasodilators, low molecular dextrane, vitamins, etc., with fairly good results. However, there were three cases treated by surgery; one case by evacuation of an intracranial hematoma, one case by intracranial transposition of free omental graft, and one case by STA-MCA bypass. All these cases were discharged in improved condition. At present, we are not in the position to conclude which treatment is better, but we intend to operate on all those patients who show progressive symptoms of cerebral ischemia. As to the etiology of moyamoya disease, I think that both the congenital and the acquired forms may exist, but in our country, the majority of the cases seems to be of the acquired form. Any pathological conditions which may effect the cerebral arteries in early life may also give rise to the characteristic features of moyamoya disease. The abnormal vascular network seen at the base of the brain represents the collaterals as the result of the stenosis of major cerebral arteries. It has been mentioned that many pathological conditions, such as basal meningitis, cerebral tumors, intracranial trauma, leptospirosis, syphilis, tuberculosis, post irradiation, etc., are able to effect cerebral vessels. In our country, leptospiral arteritis seemed to be more prevalent, since many such cases showed positive histories of exposure, and the leptospiral coagulation resolution tests and serum complement fixation tests for leptospirosis were positive. These cases usually respond well to penicillin treatment. This probably explains the favorable results achieved following conservative treatment in our series.

Moyamoya Disease in Korea

A Cooperative Study

Kil Soo Choi[1]

Introduction

This study is based upon the collected data investigated by written inquiry from 33 institutions with neurosurgery residency programs in Korea. The first typical moyamoya disease in Korea was reported by Kim and Cho under the title of *Hemangiomatous Malformation of the Brain* at the Korean Neurosurgical Society meeting in 1969.

Incidence

The total number of patients with moyamoya disease in Korea from 1969 through 1986 was 289. There were 130 males and 159 females.

Age

Study of patients' ages show no distinct ages of high prevalence. The ages are evenly distributed in each decade (Table 1).

Symptoms and Signs

Among our 289 cases, headache was the most common symptom, followed by intracranial hemorrhage, motor disturbance, speech disturbance, and seizure, in that order of frequency (Table 2).

Familial Occurrence

We have experienced two cases of moyamoya disease in parent-sibling and two cases in siblings, as well as one case in identical twins (Table 3).

Angiography

According to the characteristic angiographic findings, moyamoya disease has been categorized into two types in our studies: typical moyamoya disease and atypical, or moyamoya-like, disease. By considering true moyamoya disease to be a lesion in which there is progressive stenosis and occlusion of the distal portion of the internal carotid artery (ICA) bilaterally, patients with unilateral abnormalities should not be considered to have true moyamoya disease. Therefore, we refer to these cases as atypical moyamoya, or moyamoya-like, disease in order to distinguish them from true moyamoya disease.

Table 1. Age distribution

Age (years)	No. of cases
0–10	52
11–20	45
21–30	44
31–40	55
41–50	56
51–60	34
61–70	2
71–80	1
Total	289

Table 2. Symptoms and signs

	No. of cases	%
Headache	150	52
Intracranial hemorrhage	103	36
Motor disturbance	61	21
Speech disturbance	58	20
Seizure	55	19
Mental disturbance	33	11
Visual disturbance	20	7
Fever	13	5
Sensory disturbance	12	4
Involuntary movement	12	4

[1] Department of Neurosurgery, College of Medicine, Seoul National University, Seoul, Korea

Table 3. Familial occurrence

	No. of cases
Father—son	1
Father—daughter	1
Sibling	2
Identical twins	1
Total	5

Table 4. Moyamoya-like disease

	No. of cases
One-sided moyamoya disease	
With contralateral normal vessels	40
With contralateral MCA obstruction	8
With contralateral ACA obstruction	1
With contralateral ICA stenosis	1
Moyamoya vessels	
With bilateral MCA obstruction	10
Total	60

MCA middle cerebral artery, *ACA* anterior cerebral artery, *ICA* internal carotid artery

Table 5. Angiography

	No. of cases
Typical moyamoya disease	224
Atypical, or moyamoya-like, disease	60
Incomplete angiographic study	5
Total	289

Table 6. EEG and CBF findings

Findings	No. of cases
EEG	
Normal	10
Abnormal	35
Total	45
CBF	
Normal	2
Abnormal	6
Total	8

CBF cerebral blood flow

Table 7. CT scan findings

Findings	No. of cases
Normal	16
Ischemia/infarction	150
Hemorrhage	74
ICH	32
IVH	29
ICH + IVH	11
SAH	2
Total	240

Typical moyamoya disease was found in 224 cases, whereas moyamoya-like disease was found in 60 cases (Table 4). In five cases, the angiographic study was incomplete and unsatisfactory to meet the criteria of moyamoya disease. Of 60 patients with atypical moyamoya disease 40 are reported to have normal angiographic picture on the contralateral hemisphere (Table 5).

Associated Lesions

Nine patients are associated with aneurysms, one patient with arteriovenous malformations (AVM), and one patient with a persistent primitive trigeminal artery (PPTA).

EEG and CBF

EEG study showed normal findings in ten cases and abnormal findings in 35 cases. Regional cerebral blood flow (CBF) was measured by the ^{133}xenon inhalation technique in eight patients. Six of eight patients showed low values of mean hemispheric blood flow in both hemispheres (Table 6).

Computed Tomography

Among 240 CT scans, 16 patients were reported to have normal findings. Cerebral ischemia or infarction was diagnosed in 150 patients, whereas hemorrhage was diagnosed in 74 patients. Among these 74 cases with hemorrhage, IVH was found in 29 patients. Subarachnoid hemorrhage (SAH) was seen in only two patients (Table 7).

Pathology

The first autopsy case in Korea was reported by Cho in 1973. It was a 47-year-old-Korean

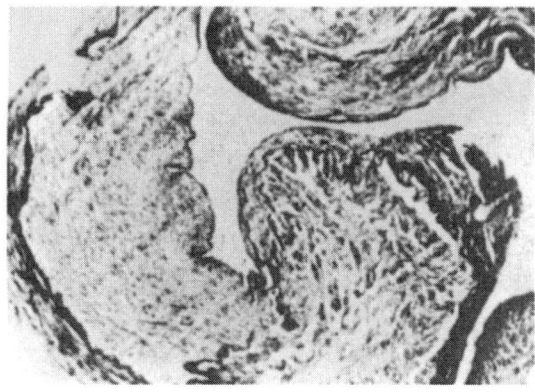

Fig. 1. The nodular pattern of intimal thickening of right proximal anterior cerebral artery was characteristic in our autopsy case

Table 8. Surgical treatment

	Type of procedure	No. of cases
Ischemic group	STA-MCA anastomosis	12
	EMS	19
	STA-MCA anastomosis + EMS	3
	EDAS	2
	Total	36
Hemorrhagic group	CVD for IVH	11
	Hematoma evacuation for ICH	18
	Total	29

STA-MCA superficial temporal artery-middle cerebral artery, *EMS* encephalomyosynangiosis, *EDAS* encephaloduroarterisynangiosis, *IVH* intraventricular hemorrhage, *ICH* intracerebral hemorrhage, *CVD* continuous ventricular drainage

woman with moyamoya disease who died of SAH. In the postmortem study, the major blood vessel of the base of the brain showed irregular thickening and tortuosity of the elastic membrane of the intima. No inflammatory reaction was found. The nodular pattern of intimal thickening was characteristic (Fig. 1).

Surgical Treatment

Over the last 10 years, two types of surgical procedures—STA-MCA anastomosis and encephalomyosynangiosis (EMS)—are thought to be the most frequently used therapeutic techniques for the treatment of the ischemic group of moyamoya disease. We have performed 13 STA-MCA anastomoses and 22 EMS procedures over the last 10 years. A newly developed surgical procedure, (EDAS), was recently performed in only two pediatric patients. The outcome of each surgical procedure is generally accepted as favorable in our study (Table 8).

Acknowledgments. The author is grateful to the Directors of Neurosurgery of the following hospitals for their generous support and cooperation in providing the collected data about moyamoya disease in Korea: Capital Armed Forces Hospital; Chonbuk National University Hospital; Chonnam National University Hospital; Chosun University Hospital; Chung-Ang University Hospital; Chungnam National University Hospital; Daegu Catholic Hospital; Ewha Womans University Hospital; Fatima Hospital; Hae-Wha Hospital Korea University; Hangang Sacred Heart Hospital; Hanyang University Hospital; Kangnam Sacred Heart Hospital; Kangnam St. Mary's Hospital; Keimyung University Dong San Medical Center; Koryo General Hospital; Kosin Medical College & Gospel Hospital; Kyung Hee University Medical Center; Kyungpook University Hospital; Maryknoll Hospital; Masan Koryo General Hospital; National Medical Center; Paik Hospital Busan Inje College; Presbyterian Medical Center; Pusan National University Hospital; Seoul Paik Hospital; Seoul National University Hospital; Soonchunhyang University Hospital; Wallace Memorial Baptist Hospital; Wonkang University Hospital; Wonju Christian Hospital; Yeungnam University Hospital; Yonsei University Severance Hospital

Moyamoya Disease in Taiwan

Chun-Jen Shih[1] and Chain-Fa Su[2]

Introduction

"Moyamoya", a word indicating a puff of smoke, names a disease showing stenosis or occlusion of the intracranial arteries at the base of skull and abnormal vascular networks (intraparenchymatous anastomosis) in the region of the basal ganglia. It was first described, on angiography, by Nomura [5] and Takeuchi [8]. A variety of synonyms have been suggested, including "cerebral juxtabasilar telengiectasis," "cerebral arterial rete," "rete mirabile," and "cerebral arterial rete mirabile." Previously considered to be confined to Japan, moyamoya disease has recently been reported sporadically all over the world [2–4, 6]. In Taiwan, this rare disease is occasionally uncovered at large neurological centers. However, the epidermiology of the disease is, as yet, unclear. In the present joint study, 26 cases were retrospectively assesed in order to delineate the general aspects of this disease in Taiwan.

Materials and Methods

Twenty-six records collected from five large neurological centers (Tri-Service General Hospital, Veterans General Hospital, National Taiwan University Hospital, Kaohsiung Medical School Hospital, and Chang-Gung Memorial Hospital) during the period from January 1978 to October 1986 were assessed. These hospitals usually perform cerebral angiography upon evidence of a cerebral vascular accident, ischemia or hemorrhage, provided patients have no obvious history of hypertension. One patient showing moyamoya-like vessels and stenosis of arteries at the base of the skull was excluded from this study because of an eventual diagnosis of optic glioma. We adopted the characteristic angiographic findings proposed by the reseach committee of the Ministry of Welfare and Health of Japan (MHWJ) [1]. The diagnostic criteria used are as follows: (a) stenosis or occlusion beginning at the termination of the intracranial internal carotid artery and also at the origin of the anterior and middle cerebral arteries; (b) abnormal vascular network in the region of the basal ganglia; (c) above-mentioned findings symmetrical on both sides, and (d) transdural anastomosis (rete mirabile).

Results

Table 1 summarizes the age, sex, type, CT findings, location, clinical symptoms, and angiograhpic characteristics of the patients. There were 18 males and eight females with a male dominance (1:0.44). Incidence is about 0.018 patients per 100 000 persons a year in Taiwan. Age ranged from 4 to 62 years with an average of 32.8 years. Our sample comprises five children (below age 14) and 21 adults with a peak incidence occurring between 30 and 50 years (Fig. 1). The clinical symptoms were the same as those caused by cerebrovascular accident, ischemia, or hemorrhage. Headache, motor paresis, vomiting, unconsciousness, or transient ischemic attacks were frequently observed when the patients were admitted to the hospital. One case having infarctions over both frontal lobes showed symptoms of psychoorganic syndrome and mental retardation.

CT scans showed 18 patients with either intracerebral, subarachinoidal or intraventricular hemorrhages while cerebral infraction was demonstrated in only eight cases. In addition, cerebral infarction was more frequently found in children and teenage patients (below age 20) than in those above age 20. Cerebral infraction

[1] Department of Health, The Executive Yuan, Republic of China
[2] Department of Surgery, National Defense Medical Center and Tri-Service General Hospital, Taipei, Republic of China

Table 1. Summary of 26 cases of moyamoya disease

Case	Age	Sex	Type	CT	Location	Symptoms	Angiogram
1.	4	M	Complete stroke	CI	Lt. PO	Motor paresis, TIA	A1,A2,A3
2.	6	M	Complete stroke	CI	Rt. FP	Motor paresis	A1,A2
3.	6	F	Complete stroke	CI	Lt. FT	Motor paresis, TIA, speech disturbance	A1,A2,A3,A4
4.	9	F	Hemorrhage	ICH	Lt. FT	Headache, unconsciousness	A1,A2
5.	11	M	Hemorrhage	IVH, SAH	Lt. V	Headache, vomiting, motor paresis	A1,A2,A3
6.	16	M	Complete stroke	CI	Rt. T	Headache, motor paresis, unconsciousness	A1
7.	18	M	Complete stroke	CI	Rt. B	Headache, vomiting, motor paresis	A1,A2
8.	19	F	Hemorrhage	ICH	Rt. FT	Headache, vomiting, motor paresis	A1,A2,A3
9.	27	M	Complete stroke	CI	Rt. P	Motor paresis	A1,A2
10.	31	M	Hemorrhage	ICH	Rt. FTP	Headache	A1,A2
11.	33	F	Hemorrhage	IVH	Bil. V	Headache, vomiting, unconsciousness	A1,A2
12.	35	M	Hemorrhage seizure	IVH	Bil. V	Headache, vomiting, motor paresis	A1,A2,A3
13.	37	F	Hemorrhage	IVH, SAH	Bil. V	Headache, vomiting	A1,A2,A3
14.	37	M	Hemorrhage	SAH	Bil.	Headache	A1,A2,A3
15.	37	M	Hemorrhage	IVH, SAH	Bil. V	Headache, vomiting, unconsciousness	A1,A2,A3
16.	38	F	Hemorrhage	IVH	Bil. V	Headache, vomiting, unconsciousness	A1,A2,A3
17.	40	M	Hemorrhage	ICH, IVH	Rt. FTP	Headache, vomiting	A1,A2,A3
18.	42	F	Hemorrhage	IVH, SAH	Rt. F	Headache, vomiting, unconsciousness	A1,A2
19.	44	M	Hemorrhage	IVH, SAH	Rt. T	Headache, vomiting, unconsciousness	A1,A2,A3
20.	45	M	Hemorrhage	IVH	Rt. V	Headache, motor paresis	A1,A2,A3
21.	45	M	Complete stroke	CI	Bil. F	Psycho-organic syndrome, mental retardation	A1,A2,A3
22.	49	M	Complete stroke	CI	Lt. O	Visual disturbance, motor paresis	A1,A2,A3,A4
23.	49	M	Hemorrhage	IVH, SAH	Bil. V	Headache, vomiting	A1,A2,A3
24.	51	F	Hemorrhage	ICH	Rt. TP	Headache, visual disturbance, unconsciousness	A1,A2,A3
25.	62	M	Hemorrhage	CI, SAH	Lt. T	Headache, vomiting	A1
26.	62	M	Hemorrhage	ICH, CI	Bil. TP	Visual disturbance, unconsciousness	A1,A2,A3

CI cerebral infarction, *IVH* Intraventricular hemorrhage, *SAH* Subarachnoid hemorrhage, *ICH* Intracerebral hemorrhage *A1* stenosis or occlusion beginning at the termination of the intracranial internal carotid arteries or at the origin of the anterior and middle cerebral arteries; *A2* Intraparenchymatous anastomosis in the region of the basal ganglia; *A3* Above mentioned findings symmetrical on both sides; *A4* Transdural anastomosis (rete mirabile); *F* frontal, *T* temporal, *P* parietal, *O* occipital, *V* ventricle

Table 2. Comparison of epidermiology in moyamoya disease between Japan and Taiwan

	Japan	Reference no.	Taiwan
Case no.	829 (1955–1982)	7	26 (1978–1986)
Incidence	0.1 patients/100 000 per yr	10	0.018 patients/100 000 per yr
Incidence of juvenile and adult cases	Child: 65.2% Adult: 34.8%	8	Child: 19.2% Adult: 80.8%
Peak age incidence	0–5 years and 30–40 years	8	30–40 and 40–50 years
Male:female	1:1.4	7	1:0.4
Family history	13/147 cases	7	None

occurred in five of eight patients (62.5%) below age 20, but in only 3 of 18 patients (16.7%) above age 20.

Cerebral angiography was indispensable in the diagnosis of moyamoya disease. CT scan and angiography were performed on all patients in this series. Fifteen patients showed all of the following angiographic findings: (a) stenosis or occlusion beginning at the termination of the intracranial internal carotid artery or the origin of the anterior and middle cerebral arteries; (b) intraparenchymatous anastomosis in the region of the basal ganglia; and (c) the above-mentioned findings symmetrical on both sides. However, while seven patients demonstrated (a) and (b) of the above findings, two patients had (a) only. In addition, two patients showing the above three findings developed transdural anastomosis (rete mirabile). Aneurysms in combination with moyamoya disease were not found in this series.

Discussion

Comparison of the epidemiology in moyamoya disease between Japan and Taiwan is shown in Table 2. Moyamoya disease is as rare in Taiwan as it is in Europe and North America. Only 0.018 patients per 100 000 persons per year were diagnosed as having the disease. In addition, our data did not show a peak age incidence in juvenile cases. In our study, peak incidences can be found at 30–40 and 40–50 years (Fig. 1). The incidence of juvenile cases reported by Suzuki (65.2%) were much higher than that of Taiwan (19.2%). The Japanese juvenile cases showed a peak age incidence at 0–5 years with an average age of 4.5 years [7]. However, it is worth emphasizing that different incidence rates may have been the result of the more common use of cerebral angiograms in Japan in patients less than 5 years old with the symptoms of cerebral vascular accident.

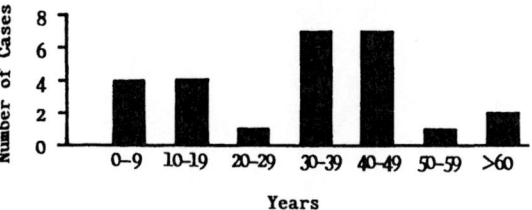

Fig. 1. Age distribution at onset

It is interesting to note that the sex incidence showed a male predominance in our study while a female predominence is evident in all Japanese series [1, 9, 10]. Moreover, the family tendency was not found in our cases.

Judging from the CT scans, we can divide the clinical manifestations of these cases into ischemic and hemorrhagic types. It has been estimated by the research committee of the MHWJ that the ischemic type is predominent in juvenile cases (81%). However, the hemorrhagic type is more common in adult cases (60%) [10]. Our results showed five of eight cases (62.5%) below age 20, but only three of 18 cases (16.7%) above age 20, were cerebral infarctions and, therefore, conform with Japanese findings.

Summary

Incidence of moyamoya disease in Taiwan is about one sixth of that of Japan. Age peak incidence is at 30–40 and 40–50 years and no family tendency could be traced. An interesting predominance of males was shown in the present series while a female predominence is evident among all of the Japanese series. Judging from the CT scans, the ischemic type was more frequently found in juvenile or teenage cases. Adult cases usually showed a hemorrhagic pattern.

References

1. Gotch F (ed.) (1983) Annual report (1982) of the research committee on spontaneous occlusion of the circle of Willis ("moyamoya" disease). Ministry of Health and Welfare, Japan
2. Krayenbuhl HA (1975) The moyamoya syndrome and the neurosurgeon. Surg Neurol 4:353–360
3. Lee MLK, Cheung EMT (1973) Moyamoya disease as a cause of subarachnoid hemorrhage in Chinese. Brain 96:623–628
4. Meriwether RP, Barnett HG, and Echols DH (1976) Moyamoya disease as a cause of subarachnoid hemorrhage in a negro patient. J Neurosurg 44:620–622
5. Nomura T (1961) Atlas of cerebral angiography. Tokyo, Igaku-shoin pp 192–195
6. Quest DO, Correl JW (1985) Basal arterial occlusive disease. Neurosurgery 17:937–941
7. Suzuki J (1986) Moyamoya disease: Epidermiology and symptomatology, cerebral angiography. Springer, Berlin Heidelberg, pp 7–52
8. Takeuchi K (1961) Occlusive disease of the carotid artery. Shiukei Keukyu no Shimpo 5:511–543
9. Yamaguchi T, Tashiro M, Minematsu K, Kitamura K (1980) Summary of Japanese survey of occlusion of the circle of Willis. In: Reports by the research committee on spontaneous occlusion of the circle of Willis. Japanese Ministry of Health and Welfare, Tokyo, pp 13–22
10. Yonekawa, Y, Handa H, Okuno T (1986), Moyamoya disease: diagnosis, treatment, and recent achievement. In: Barnett HJM, Stein BM, Mohr JP, Yatsu FM (eds) Stroke. Churchill Livingstone, pp 805–829

Moyamoya Disease in Hong Kong

H.L. Wen[1], Z.D. Mehal[1], John C.K. Kwok[1], Y.W. Chan[2], and C.S. Kay[2]

Introduction

Moyamoya disease is a rare chronic occlusive cerebrovascular disease which was first described as a type of occlusive disease of the internal carotid artery [15, 24]. The clinical pictures of the disease are variable, presenting as hemiplegia, paraplegia, convulsive seizures, headaches, speech disturbances, involuntary movements of the extremities, and mental retardation. The peak age incidence cycle appeared between one to five years and another at 30 years of age. However, the clinical pictures are different between these two groups. The patients under 15 years old often showed recurrent episodes of ischemic cerebrovascular accidents which produced permanent speech or mental defect. In the adult the mode of presentation is signs and symptoms of subarachnoid hemorrhage with poor prognosis.

The angiographic appearance of moyamoya disease is typical and is characterized by marked stenosis or complete occlusion of the distal internal carotid arteries with poor visualization of the anterior and middle cerebral arteries at their proximal ends. The fine vascular network which develops at the base of the brain [12–14, 20, 22, 23] is termed moyamoya, which means something hazy, like a puff of cigarette smoke drifting in the air [20–23].

It has been reported that this disease is confined to the Japanese [7]. Since then, reports have been appearing in the literatures from other parts of the world, with reports of small numbers of cases or even a single cases [1–6, 8–11, 16–19, 25]. In this paper we review the papers that have been reported in the literature on moyamoya disease in Hong Kong, and add two of our cases.

_____
Departments of Neurosurgery[1] and Neurology[2], Kwong Wah Hospital, Kowloon, Hong Kong

Case Reports

Case I

A 44-year-old Chinese female was first admitted to the Caritas Medical Center (CMC), Kowloon, on 16 December 1985. She had been in perfect health. The night prior to admission to the CMC, she woke up from her sleep and went to the toilet. On her way back to her room she collapsed and passed out for about 10 min. Due to the noise produced by the fall, her husband woke up and found her on the floor. There were no convulsions. After regaining consciousness, she found out that she could not move the left side of her body and accordingly she was admitted to the CMC. After preliminary investigation, including lumbar puncture which showed blood-stained CSF and a CT scan taken on 25 December 1985, which showed a right intracerebral hematoma, she was treated conservatively at CMC and was improving. Later whe was transferred to our hospital on 8 January 1986.

There was no history of high blood pressure or cardiovascular disease nor was there diabetes mellitus. The family history showed no neurological or vascular diseases.

Physical examination. The patient was fully conscious, able to speak but was not able to move the extremities of the left side on command but able to do so on painful stimulation. There was left facial weakness of central type. The pupils were equal and reacting to light. The reflexes were hypoactive on the left and normal on the right. Hypoesthesia was noted on the left side of the face and body. Babinski's sign was negative. The body temperature was 37 °C, respiration was 20/min, pulse was 85/min and blood pressure was 120/80.

Laboratory tests. Routine blood, urine, and blood chemistry tests revealed to be within normal ranges. The leptospira agglutination test proved negative.

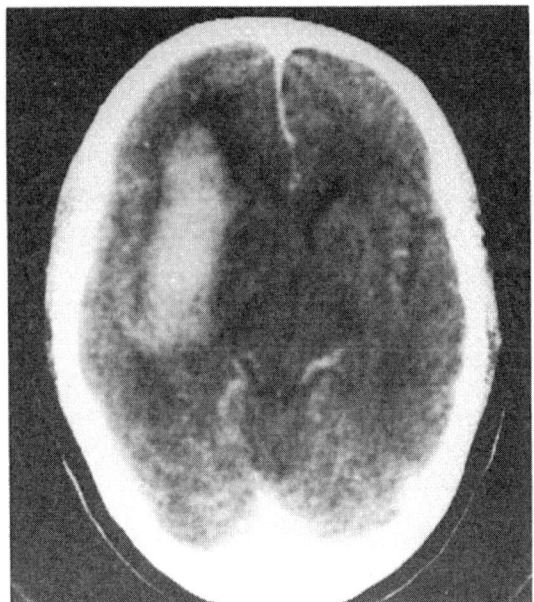

Fig. 1. Initial CT scan taken on 25 December 1985, showing a large right intracerebral hematoma

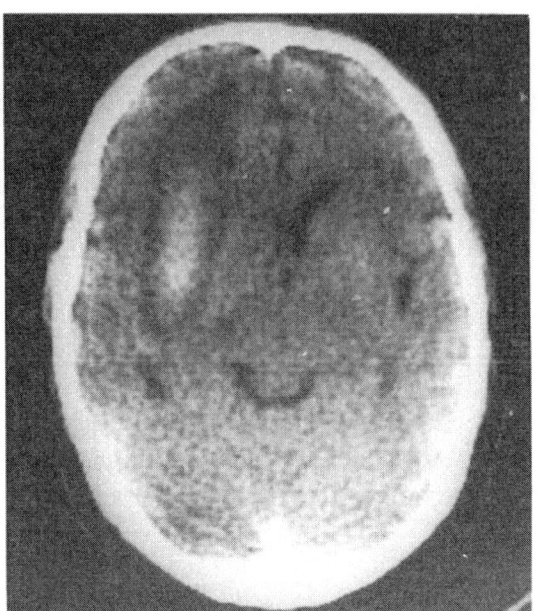

Fig. 2. Repeated scan taken on 13 January 1986, showing the right intracerebral hematoma resolved

Computed tomography. The CT scan showed a large hematoma present on the right side, extending from the anterior parietal to the mid-parietal lobe. It was associated with a small edema causing marked distortion of the ventricle and a shift of the midline structure to the left. The posterior fossa was normal (Fig. 1). A repeated CT scan on 13 January 1986 showed the right intracerebral hematoma was resolving (Fig. 2) and on 14 November 1986 an area of hypodensity was noted (Fig. 3). The diagnosis was right intracerebral hematoma.

Carotid angiography. Right carotid angiogram was performed on 23 January 1986. The anterior communicating artery and right middle cerebral artery were not visualized. The posterior communicating artery was prominent and anastomotic vessels were demonstrated. Numerous small anastomotic vessels at the basal region were shown to be typical of moyamoya disease. Left carotid angiography showed the internal carotid artery was stenotic, sparing some middle cerebral artery branches. Basal anastomotic vessels were seen (Figs. 4, 5).

Clinical course. After admission to CMC, the patient's condition improved. She was given physiotherapy from which she gradually regained some of her strength on the left side. At the time of transfer to our hospital, she still had the left hemiplegia. Upon discharge, she was

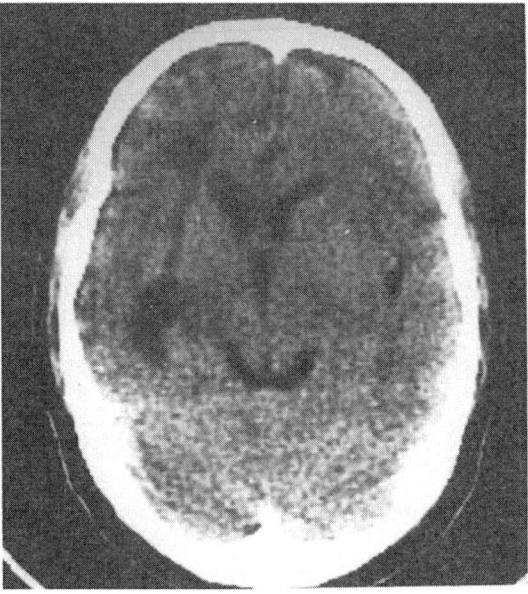

Fig. 3. CT scan taken on 14 November 1986, showing hypodense area at previous site of hemorrhage on the right

walking with the help of a tripod stick. When seen on 13 October 1986, she was still limping. The left extremities were much weaker than the right. Hypoesthesia of the left side of the face and the whole of the left side of the body was noted. The reflexes were hyperactive on the left. There

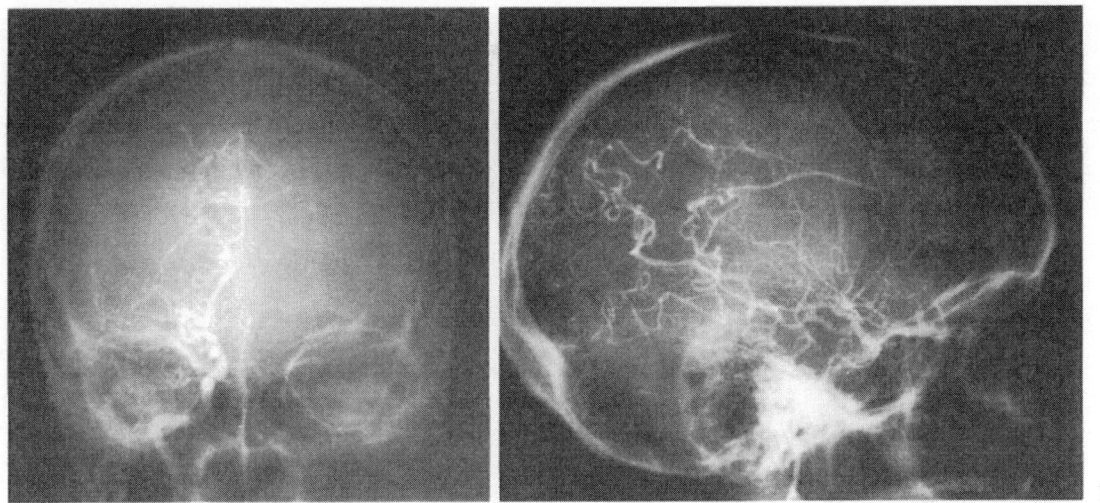

Fig. 4a, b. Right carotid angiogram. **a** Anteroposterior and **b** lateral views demonstrate the anterior and right middle cerebral arteries were not visualized. Posterior communicating artery and anastomotic vessels were prominent. Numerous anastomotic vessels at the basal region were shown to be typical of moyamoya disease

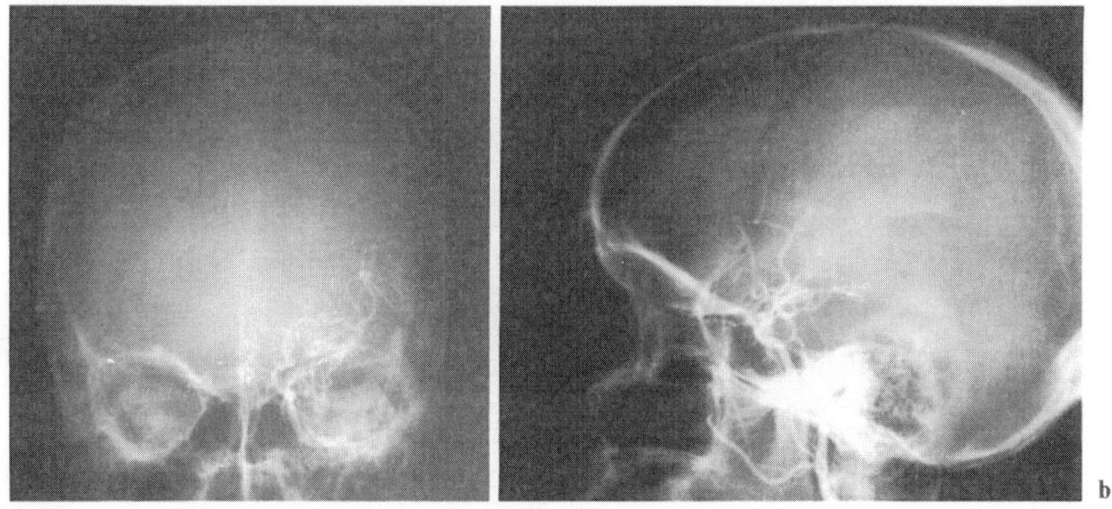

Fig. 5. Left carotid angiogram. **a** Anteroposterior and **b** lateral views. The internal carotid artery was stenotic sparing some middle cerebral artery branches. Basal anastomotic vessels were seen

was a left homonymous hemianopia and a left astereognosis. There was no positive Babinski's sign. There was left facial weakness. The fundi were normal. The pupils were equal and reacted to light.

Case II

A 65-year-old Chinese female was admitted to Kwong Wah Hospital (KWH), Kowloon, because of generalized convulsion. She was apparently in good health until 26 June 1986 at about 10 a.m., when she developed headache mainly in the front of her head. She then went to the Buddhist temple to pray, which was about $1\frac{1}{2}$ from her home. While praying, she noted slurred speech, which lasted 3 min, with dizziness. The headache had persisted but not too severely. Following this, she was found with twitching of the face, jerky movements of the body and limbs, and unconscious. The ambulance was called and she was admitted to KWH.

There was no history of high blood pressure or cardiovascular disease. There was no diabetes mellitus. There was no family history of neurological or vascular disease.

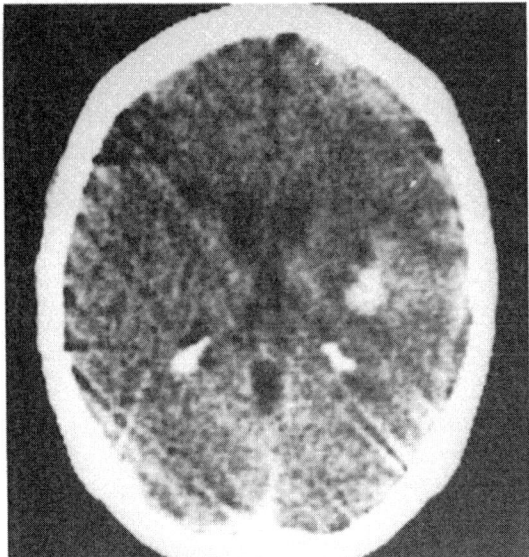

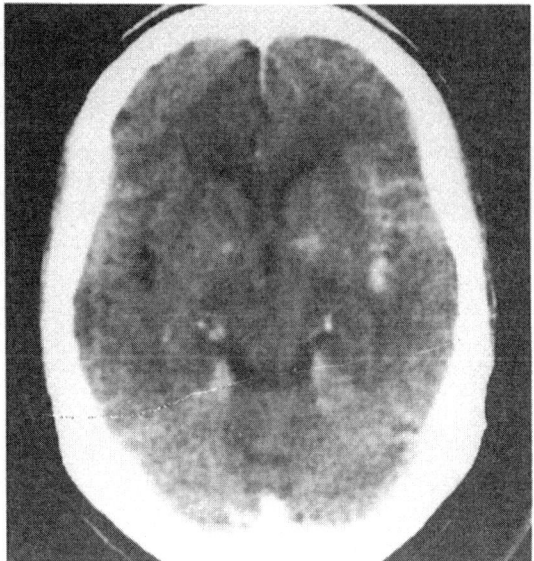

Fig. 6. CT scan taken on 2 July 1986 showing a small blood clot in the left internal capsule and the ventricles

Fig. 7. Repeated CT scan showing resolution of the hemorrhage. Following contrast injection, mottle or tortuous, and serpiginous type of enhancement were observed at the site of the previous hemorrhage, suggestive of AV malformation

Physical examination. The patient was in a comatose state with grimaces of the face and twitching of the whole body. The pupils were small but equal in size. The mouth was foaming with saliva. The neck was supple. The chest demonstrated coarse breathing sound but was otherwise within normal. The abdomen revealed a right upper quadrant old scar due to a previous operation for gall stones 10 years before. The extremities could be moved, with the deep reflexes greatly exaggerated on both sides but equal. There was no positive response of the Babinski's sign. The body temperature was 38.8 °C, respiration was 20/min and regular, pulse was 83/min, and blood pressure was 130/80.

Laboratory tests. Routine blood, urine, and blood chemistry tests were all within normal ranges.

Computed tomography. A CT scan taken without dye on 2 July 1986 showed a small blood clot in the left internal capsule and in the ventricles without a shift of the midline structure to the right. A repeated CT scan on 11 July 1986 showed resolution of the hemorrhage which was demonstrated on the previous scan of 2 July 1986 with minimal edema noted. The ventricular system was normal. There was no midline shift (Fig. 6). Following injection of contrast media, mottle, or tortuous, and serpiginous types of enhancement were observed at the site of the previous hemorrhage. The findings were consis-

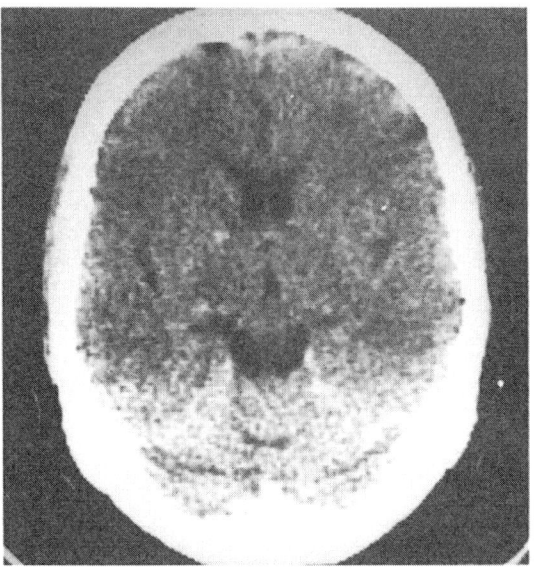

Fig. 8. Repeated CT scan on 13 October 1986 showing hypodensity in the previously bleeding area

tent with arteriovenous malformation. No abnormally enhanced vessels were seen in the right cerebral hemisphere or posterior fossa. The basal cisterns were not remarkable (Fig. 7). A repeated CT scan on 13 October 1986 showed hypodensity in the previously bleeding area

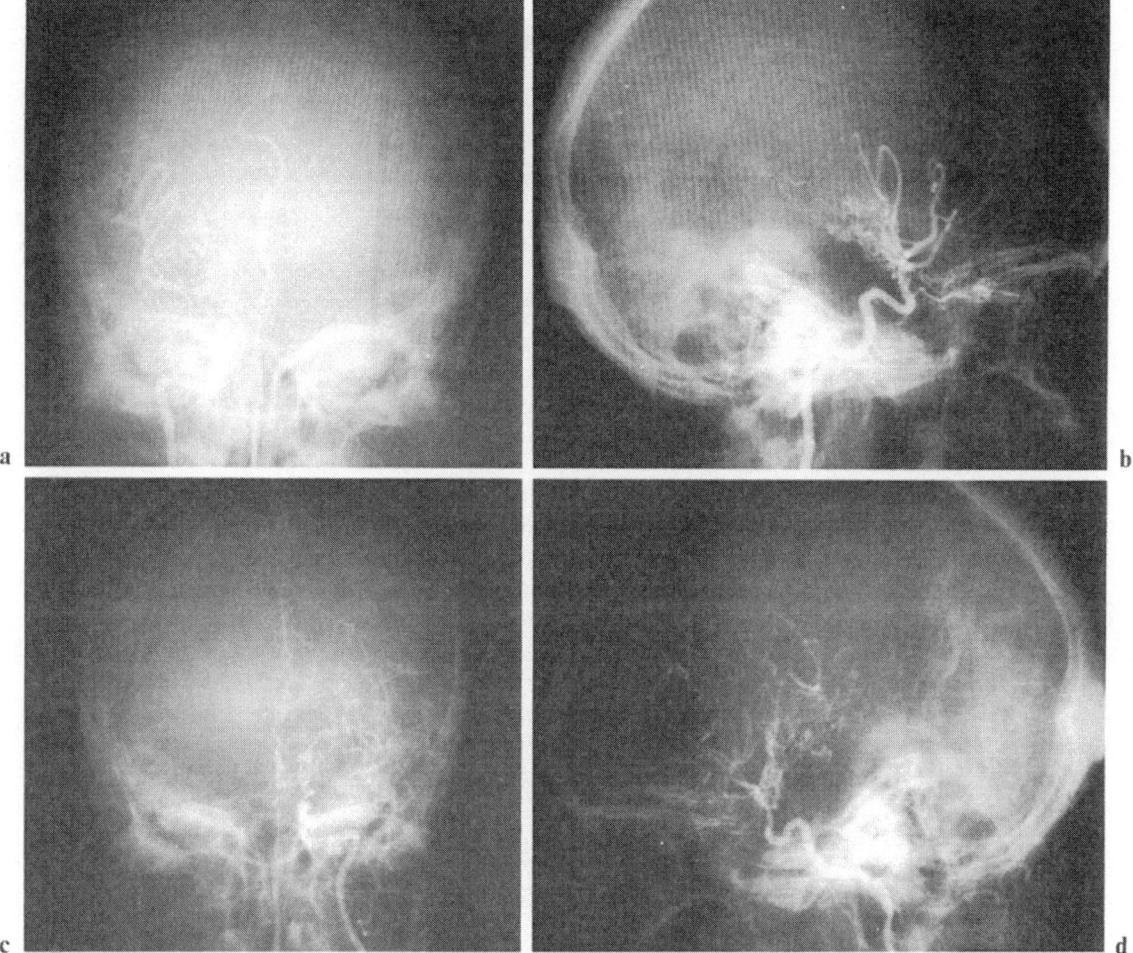

Fig. 9a–d. Bilateral carotid angiogram. **a, c** Anteroposterior and **b, d** lateral views taken 20 days after onset of symptoms, showing bilateral occlusion of the internal carotid artery. Distal to the ophthalmic artery, a fine leash or netlike vessels arising at the base of the brain were noted, resembling moyamoya disease

(Fig. 8). The diagnosis was small intracerebral hemorrhage on the left.

Carotid angiography. It was carried out bilaterally 20 days after the onset of the symptoms, and showed bilateral occlusion of the internal carotid artery. Distal to the ophthalmic artery, a fine leash or netlike vessels arising at the base of the brain were seen, resembling those of moyamoya disease (Fig. 9).

Clinical course. After admission to the hospital the patient was treated conservatively for her convulsions which subsided 5 h later. She was noted to be stuporous but opened her eyes and followed orders. There was spontaneous movement of the extremities. The next day she was fully conscious and complaining of severe head-

ache, which was bursting in nature and gradually subsided. Upon neurological examination prior to discharge from the hospital, she was found to be neurologically, within normal range and was discharged from the hospital on 26 July 1986. She was last seen on 13 November 1986 and was in good health with no neurological deficit.

Discussion

In reviewing the papers that were published on moyamoya disease in Hong Kong, we could only collect four papers [2, 5, 8] (Table 1). One by Lee and Cheung [8] reported 11 cases of moyamoya disease in the Chinese population of Hong Kong between 1970 and 1972. Nine of them (82%)

Table 1. Moyamoya disease in Hong Kong

Authors	Years data collected	No. of cases	Female to male ratio		Age(yrs)	Source
			F	M		
Lee et al.	1970–1972	11	6	5	29–59	Brain (1973)
Chan et al.	1977–1980	20	9	11	21–66	Proc. Roy. Australasian Coll. Radiol. (1980)
Huang et al.	1980–1982	16	8	8	22–70	Neurol. (1983)
Huang	1980–1985	24	8	16	7–59	Personal communication
Wen et al.	1985–1986	2	2	0	44 and 65	Present paper

were of subarachnoid hemorrhage—one because of speech defect and hemiparesis and another because of aphasia alone. The ages varied from 29 to 59 years with a female to male ratio of 6:5. Compared with the published cases, they were older with fewer females. All these cases were diagnosed by cerebral angiography.

Chan and Lau [2] reported 20 cases. The ages varied from 21 to 66 years with a female to male ratio of 9:11. In this group, the presenting symptoms of subarachnoid hemorrhage occurred in 80% of the cases. Other presenting symptoms included paralysis, visual disturbance, speech disturbance and neurofibromatosis. All were diagnosed by cerebral angiography. Six cases had associated aneurysms—four from moyamoya vessels, one from the posterior cerebral artery and one from the opposite anterior cerebral artery—and two presented with intracerebral hematoma. STA–MCA anastomosis was performed in one patient.

Huang et al. [5] in an unpublished paper, presented 16 cases of moyamoya disease in adults with the ages varied from 22 to 70 years. The cases were collected from 1980 to 1982. The female to male ratio was 8:8. The authors noted that the predominant cases were of subarachnoid hemorrhage or infarction occurring in the young, nonhypertensive subject and the paper emphasized microbiological study. They found the sensitized erythrocytes lysis test for leptospirosis showed a total absence of reaction in 60% of blood donors, while six cases of confirmed moyamoya disease patients tested showed titers of 1/10 to 1/60, suggesting the possibility of past leptospiral infection. This result was found to be compatible with the results reported from China [10].

Through personal communication, we found that Huang collected 24 cases from 1980 to 1986, from different hospitals in Hong Kong. There were eight females and 16 males, the youngest being 7 years old and the oldest 59. All were diagnosed by cerebral angiography, of which 16 cases had prior CT scan. There were nine cases of subarachnoid hemorrhage and ten cases of infarcts. The infarct cases occurred in the younger age group. The other five cases presented themselves because of headache, syncope, aphasia and hemiparesis.

A total of 73 cases of moyamoya disease, including the two cases presented in this paper, moyamoya were found in Hong Kong from 1970 to 1986. However, this does not represent the true figures for Hong Kong as no report on the incidence of this disease was made from 1973 to 1976. On the average, one would expect to see five to six cases per year of moyamoya disease in Hong Kong. Again, this data may not be correct as many cases with symptoms and signs of infarct or subarachnoid hemorrhage may not be referred to the regional hospital for cerebral angiography, especially those that were seen by private practitioners. In Hong Kong, the patients were mainly adult and their presenting symptoms were that of hemorrhage. Our two cases presented themselves because of intracerebral hemorrhage and in case I, a CT scan revealed a huge intracerebral hematoma on the right, which gradually resolved. As there was no progression of symptoms and signs, she was treated conservatively. The same was true with case II, though the hematoma noted by the CT scan was not large. Both patients were seen again on 13 October 1986 and CT scans done on both of them showed the intracerebral hematomas had been resolved, leaving an area of hypodensity at the original sites of the hematomas. This would confirm the reported cases in the literatures that adults presented themselves commonly with symptoms and signs of cerebral hemorrhage, be it subarachnoid, ventricular, or intracerebral. Infarction is said to occur more commonly in younger patients but it also can be seen in adults.

Summary

Seventy-three cases of moyamoya disease were collected in Chinese patients who have been living in Hong Kong from 1970 to 1986. The majority of the cases was comprised mainly of adult males. The mode of presentation of the disease was cerebral hemorrhage.

Acknowledgments. We wish to thank Mr. BL Wong of the B.L. Wong & Co., Hong Kong for his keen interest in and funding of our work. We also wish to thank Mr. H.T. Lo of KWH, Kowloon for his clerical assistance.

References

1. Busch HFU (1969) Unusual collateral circulation in a child with cerebral occlusion. Psychiat Neurol Neurochirurg 72:23–28
2. Chan FL, Lau Roy SF (1980) Moyamoya disease in Chinese. Proc. 31st Ann. Meet. Royal Australasian Coll. of Radiologists, Oct. 4, 1980 p D25
3. Galligioni F, Andrioli GC, Martin G, Briani S, Iraci G (1971) Hypoplasia of the internal carotid artery associated with cerebral pseudoangiomatosis. Am Roentgen 112:251–262
4. Hoare AM, Keogh AJ, (1974) Cerebrovascular moyamoya disease. Br Med J 1:430–432
5. Huang CY, Chan FL, Seto WH (1983) Moyamoya disease: A clinical, radiological and microbiological study. Neurol (Suppl. 2) 33:165
6. Krayenbuhl HA (1975) The moyamoya syndrome and the neurosurgeon. Surg Neurol 4:353–360
7. Kudo T (1968) Spontaneous occlusion of circle of Willis: disease apparently confined to Japanese. Neurology 18:485–496
8. Lee MLK, Cheung EMT (1973) Moyamoya disease as a cause of subarachnoid hemorrhage in Chinese. Brain 96:623–628
9. Lepoire J, Tridon P, Montaut J, Hepner H, Renard M, Picard L (1969) Malformations angiomateuses arterio-arterielles du systeme carotidien. Neurochirurg 15:5–18
10. Liu XM, Ruan XZ, Cai Z, Yu BR, He SP, Gong, YH (1980) Moyamoya disease caused by leptospiral cerebral arterities. Chin Med J 93:599–604
11. Meriwether RP, Barnett HG, Echols DH (1976) Moyamoya disease as a cause of subarachnoid hemorrhage in a negro patient. J Neurosurg 44:620–622
12. Nishimoto A, Sugiu R, Mannami T, (1964) Hemangiomatous malformation of bilateral internal carotid artery at the base of brain. Preliminary Report Proc. Ann. Meet. Neuro-Radiol. Ass., Tokyo, Jap. 5:2–9
13. Nishimoto A, Sugiu R, Mannami T (1965) Hemangiomatous malformation of bilateral internal carotid artery at the base of brain. Brain Nerve 17:750–756
14. Nishimoto A, Sugiu R, Takeuchi S (1966) Malformations of the circle of Willis, presenting a peculiar cerebral angiographic picture: Cases encountered in Japan. Brain Nerve 18:508–513
15. Nomura T (1961) Atlas of cerebral angiography, 1st edn. Igaku-shoin, Tokyo, pp 192–195
16. O'Sullivan DJ (1973) Cerebrovascular moyamoya disease. Proc Austral Neurol Ass 9:73–79
17. Poór G, Gács G (1974) The so-called moyamoya disease. J Neur Neurosurg Psychiat 37:370–377
18. Simon J, Sabouraud O, Guy G, Turpin J (1968) Un cas de maladie de Nishimoto; A propose d'une maladie rare et belaterale de la carotide interne. Rev Neurol 119:376–383
19. Sogaard I, Jorgensen J (1975) Familial occurence of bilateral intracranial occlusion of the internal carotid arteries (moyamoya). Acta Neurochirurg 31:245–252
20. Suzuki J, Kowada M, Asahi M, Takaku A (1963) A study on disease showing singular cerebral angiographical findings which seem to be new collateral circulation. Proc. 22nd Meet. Jap. Neurosurg. Soc.
21. Suzuki J, Takaku A (1969) Cerebrovascular 'moyamoya' disease: disease showing abnormal netlike vessels in base of brain. Arch Neurol 20:288–299
22. Suzuki J, Takaku A, Asahi M, Kowada M (1965) Diseases showing the "fibrille"—like vessels at the base of brain. Brain Nerve 17:767–776
23. Suzuki J, Takaku A, Fukusawa H (1966) Cerebrovascular 'moyamoya' disease among the Japanese on study of autopsy case. Neurol Med Chir 8:269–270
24. Takeuchi K (1961) Occlusive disease of the carotid artery. 5:511–543 (in Japanese)
25. Taveras JM (1969) Multiple progressive intracranial occlusions: A syndrome of children and young adults. Am J Roentgen 106:235–268

Moyamoya Disease in Thailand

Charas Suwanwela[1]

It is well known that the attention of neurosurgeons around the world was drawn to the existence of moyamoya disease by Suzuki of Sendai, who also gave it its present name. It was indeed very appropriate to discuss this disease at the meeting in Sendai. One of the most puzzling aspects is the apparently high prevalence among Japanese. An inquiry into the geographical distribution of this strange disease of unknown etiology would therefore be interesting.

Thailand is in Southeast Asia. Geographically it is a tropical region, 7°–20° north of the equator, while Japan is 31°–40° north. Bangkok is about 4600 km from Tokyo and about 5000 km from Sendai. Even though both Thais and Japanese are Asian and Mongolian, they are of different ethnic stock. Certain other diseases also show different patterns of occurrence: For instance, the fronto-ethmoidal encephalomeningocele is much more common in Thailand.

Inquiries to Neurosurgical Services

An inquiry was made to neurosurgeons actively practicing at neurosurgical centers in Thailand, both in Bangkok and the provinces. There have been only a few cases of moyamoya disease diagnosed at each neurosurgical service. Thailand has a population of 50 million, which is served by about 60 neurosurgeons. Most major neurosurgical centers are in Bangkok, which has a population of over 5 million. All neurosurgical services have facilities for cerebral angiography and are able to diagnose moyamoya disease from the angiographic findings. Most would subject patients with spontaneous intracranial hemorrhage to angiography. One can therefore be fairly certain that moyamoya disease is a rare entity in Thailand.

Prevalence at Chulalongkorn Hospital

The Chulalongkorn Hospital is the teaching hospital of the Faculty of Medicine, Chulalongkorn University. It has about 1200 inpatient beds, including a neurosurgical unit with 42 beds. The close proximity and collaboration with the neurology unit in the care of patients with stroke syndromes and the special interest in the syndrome of acute and progressive neurological deficits in infancy and childhood would certainly assure the diagnosis of moyamoya disease whenever one is admitted to the hospital. It has been a policy that adults with spontaneous intracranial hemorrhage and children with cerebral vascular disease syndrome are subjected to cerebral angiography. It would therefore be unlikely that cases of moyamoya disease are missed.

In the past 24 years, from 1963 to 1986, we have performed 6458 cerebral angiographies. Only four cases which fit Suzuki's definition of moyamoya disease, e.g., bilateral carotid artery stenosis or occlusion with fine neovasculatures at the base of the brain and no apparent cause for arterial disease were encountered. In addition, there were cases with cortical telangiectasia seen in cerebral angiography, representing collateral circulation in response to carotid artery occlusion from various diseases such as purulent meningitis and disseminated lupus erythrematosus. Cases of tuberculous meningitis were seen with carotid artery narrowing and occlusion but no moyamoya was found.

Among the four patients diagnosed as having moyamoya disease, three were adults, aged 24, 30, and 40 years. Intracranial hemorrhage, mainly intraventricular and intracerebral was present in these three cases. No apparent cause was discernable.

Computed tomography was done in the 30-year-old male who had a small intraventricular hemorrhage and, in the enhanced study, abnormal vessels were seen around the left lateral ventricle. It was thought to be an angioma. Cerebral

---

[1] Section on Neurological Surgery, Faculty of Medicine, Chulalongkorn University, Bangkok, Thailand

angiography, however, revealed occlusion of the internal carotid arteries and moyamoya vessels.

One 5-year-old child had a progressive left hemiparesis over a 1-week period. The computed tomogram revealed an increased density of the brain in the temporal region which showed further enhancement of the lesion, similar to a hemorrhagic infarct. Angiography revealed occlusion of the carotid arteries and moyamoya vessels. It must be noted also that this child had had a beta-thalassemia and had required repeated blood transfusions since his early childhood.

Conclusion

Moyamoya disease is rare in Thailand. The prevalence is much lower than in Japan. Occlusion of internal carotid arteries from various causes such as meningitis and arteritis may also give rise to collateral vessels which show moyamoya appearance in the angiogram.

Moyamoya Disease in the Philippines

Romeo H. Gustilo[1]

Moyamoya disease, a very challenging and attractive medical entity, has been the subject of numerous scientific investigations and dissertations. Neurosurgical and neurological societies, both nationally and locally, especially in Japan, have focused attention on it by dedicating portions of conferences to the discussions of its pathology, etiology, and varied clinical manifestations. The advent of angiography in the early 1940s and its perfection soon after offered a great advance in the understanding of the anatomical characteristics of this syndrome as it was thought then. The main characteristic and important trait of moyamoya disease is the fact that its pathology is centered in the cerebrovascular area [7], mainly in the basal region of the brain. The basal blood vessels show an abnormal, hazy netlike pattern and fine beaded appearance secondary to abnormally develop collaterals and transdural anastomosis in this region. There is narrowing or even occlusion of the carotids in the region of the siphon [5] resulting in symptoms affecting consciousness, motor disturbances such as plegia and palsies, and other neurological manifestations. Children and adults have been known to have suffered with this affliction which is predominant in females.

The disease in its early phase was thought to be a syndrome and various authors and researchers have given it different names. In 1968, Kudo called it the spontaneous occlusion of the circle of Willis [5]. In 1970, Urbanek [9] called it the Nishimoto-Takeuchi-Kodo disease. Kudo, at that point, thought this disease to be limited to the Japanese race. However, more cases with similar angiographic findings were later reported from other countries. In 1969, Taveras [8] reported cases in children and young adults with multiple progressive intracranial arterial occlusions. Similar reports [2, 3, 6] from other countries followed.

Incidence of this disease seem to show predominance in the female sex. Gadoth [1] suggests two clinical groups: one of children with a primary form of moyamoya with the classical symptomatology, benign in character and with no demonstrable angiographic worsening. The second group consists of children and adults who develop an "acquired" the progressive form of moyamoya, with various underlying diseases such as tuberculosis, meningitis, atherosclerosis, neurofibromatosis, and vascular stenosis of the major extracranial vessels.

The etiology of moyamoya disease is unknown. Congenital factors are highly considered. The disease is seen more in Japanese females and the high familial occurence suggests the possibility of it being a hereditary vessel malformation. Kitahara [4] supports the theory that genetic and immunologic disturbances may underly the pathogenesis of moyamoya.

Anastomosis of the superficial temporal artery and cortical branches of the middle cerebral artery has offered encouraging results.

Philippine medical literature and direct inquiry from foremost and senior neurologists, neuroradiologist and neurosurgeons have failed to establish the presence of a fully documented and classical case of moyamoya (G. Gamez, M. Perez, and B. Adapon, personal communication) in the Philippines.

[1] Department of Neurological Sciences, Makati Medical Center, and Neurologica Surgery, Faculty of Medicine and Surgery, University of Santo Tomas, Manila, The Philippines

References

1. Gadoth N, Hirsch M (1980) Primary and acquired forms of moyamoya syndrome: Review and three cases reports. Isr J Med 16:370–377
2. Hardwood-Nash DC, McDonald P, Argent W (1971) Cerebral arterial disease in children: angiographic study of 40 cases. Am J Roentgenol Rad Therapy Nucl Med 111:672–686
3. Hila SK, Solomon, GE, Gold AP, Carter S (1971)

Primary cerebral arterial occlusive disease in children: I. Acute acquired hemiplegia. Radiology 99: 71–86

4. Kitahara T, Okomura K, Semba A, Yamamuza A, Makino H (1982) Genetic and immunologic analysis on moyamoya. J Neurol Neurosurg Psychiat 45:1048–1052

5. Kudo T (1968) Spontaneous occlusion of circle of Willis: Disease apparently confined to Japanese. Neurology 18:485–496

6. Simon J, Sabourgaund O, Guy G, Turpin J (1968) Un cas de maladie de Nishimoto: A propos d'une maladie rare et bilaterale de la carotide interne. Rev Neurol 119:376–383

7. Suzuki J, Takeku A (1969) Cerebrovascular moyamoya disease. A.M.A. Arch. Neurol Psychiat 20: 288–299

8. Taveras JM (1969) Multiple progressive intracranial arterial occlusions: Syndrome of children and young adults: Caldwell Lecture. Am J Roentgenol Rad Therapy Nucl Med 106:235–268

9. Urbanek K, Farkova KE (1970) Nishimoto-Taekuchi-Kudo disease: Case report. F. Neurol Neurosurg Psychiat. 33:671–673

Moyamoya Disease: The Australian Experience

GEOFFREY TOAKLEY[1]

Since the original arteriogram and description of this disease in 1955 by Shimizu and Takeuchi, and Suzuki's reporting of cases in 1963, it has been thought that this disorder is a rare one chiefly involving Japanese for whom: it would appear cerebral vascular disorders are a great deal more common than for Western people.

Slowly but surely it has been realised that the disease is one which occurs worldwide. In Australia, a large country in area, approximately the size of the continental USA, with 16 million people chiefly scattered in the capital cities of the southeast corner, one has had to obtain statistics by writing to neurosurgical units. This was done, and all were kind enough to send me notes of patients they had had with this disease over the last ten years.

Some 18 cases have now been found. Five were under 20 years of age.

The presentation took two forms:
a) Ischemic attacks, rather like transient ischemic attacks with carotid stenosis, but often with sustained hemiparesis
b) Cases presented with hemorrhage

Of the 18 cases, ten were female and eight were male. Arteriograms were done in all cases. These showed varying degrees of the classic picture of bilateral carotid stenosis with a spreading blockage on the internal carotid artery upward into the A1 or M1 (Fig. 1). Types of collateral circulation such as ethmoidal, striate, and vault anastomoses were found (Fig. 2). Where CT scans were done, local infarcts were seen differing in size from patient to patient.

In the latest Australian Year Book, one Australian of 32 is an Asian, but there were no Asian patients in this series. One patient, a female aged 7 years of French extraction coming from New Caledonia, presented recurrent episodes of hemiparesis. She was found to have coarctation of the aorta and this was repaired at the age of 9 years.

Stenosis of the distal internal carotid artery (IAC) and posterior communicating arteries as well as stenosis on the left side IAC were found (Figs. 3–5). It is interesting to note that, though almost complete obstruction of the distal IAC occurred, the child, when last seen, had no residual defects. Only one case had progressive dementia. This was a 27-year-old female, who, 10 months prior to the onset of mental deterioration, had had a motor vehicle accident. It was stated that she was knocked out but on the way to the hospital in an ambulance she had a fit. CT scans showed multiple infarcts which were obviously a great deal worse than one would have expected from a head injury as described. Arteriography gave the diagnosis of moyamoya.

So far as treatment is concerned in these cases, no sympathectomies were performed. Eight cases had external carotid middle cerebral artery anastomoses: One case had only encephalodural-

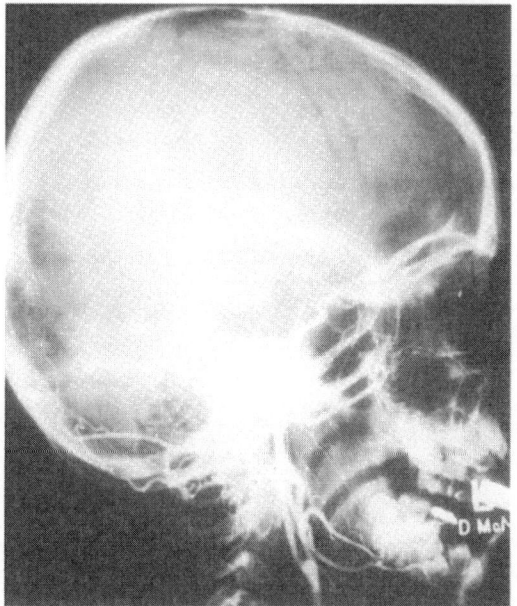

Fig. 1. Carotid stenosis, old infarct

[1] Alexandra, Wickham Terrace, Brisbane, Australia

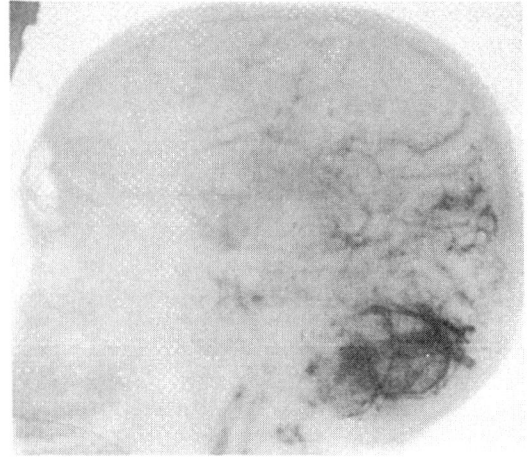

Fig. 2. Ophthalamic and deep collaterals, old infarct

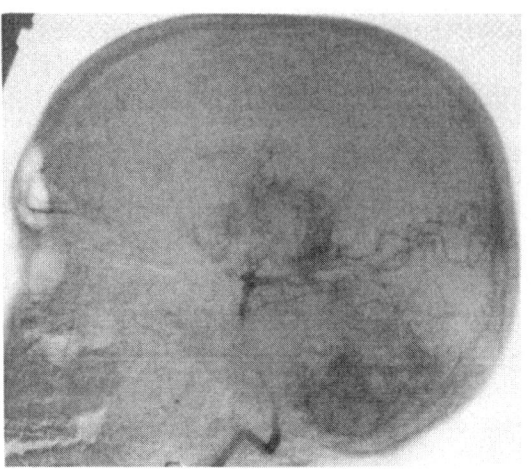

Fig. 3. L-CA and collaterals

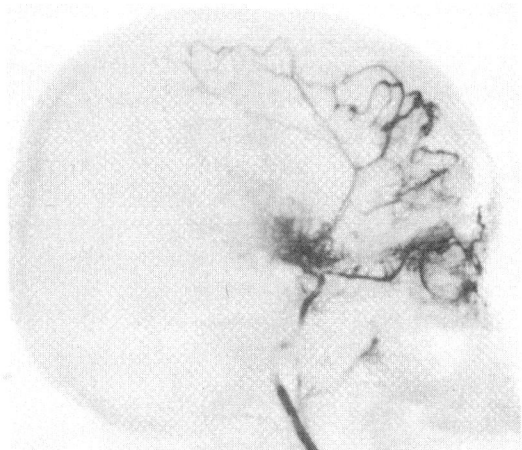

Fig. 4. Right vertebral

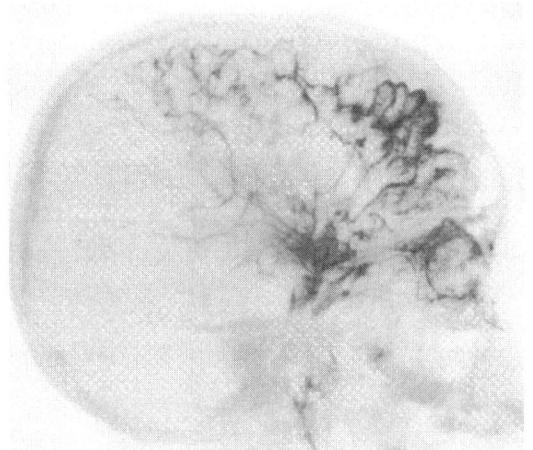

Fig. 5. Collaterals middle cerebralartery and PC

synangiosis. My own personal experience is of three cases in the above series. None of these were operated upon.

All appear to be in stable condition with minimal symptoms and no signs. In summary, in the past ten years there have been 18 cases of proven moyamoya disease in Australia. It is possible that there have been more cases investigated by neurologists or general physicians and that the series here presented is an underestimate of the total occurrence in Australia. Recently two papers of a couple of cases have been presented in the Australian Medical Journal. Figures indicating the progression of the girl are presented with coarctation and the progressive disorder of the female patient with multiple infarcts and dementia is shown.

Moyamoya Disease in South America

Reinaldo Poblete[1]

Introduction and Method

For many years, Japanese neurosurgeons have insistently postulated that moyamoya disease only pertains to Japan and, when occurring in other places, it only affects people of Japanese ancestry. It is clear that the disease exists in other continents and races as well.

To prepare this manuscript on moyamoya in South America, an inquiry was sent to each of the neurosurgical societies, to their FLANC representatives and to the more prominent neurosurgeons of the region. The inquiry asked for the following data—age, sex, and clinical description exams, angiography, operation, and evolution.

Almeyda (Brazil), Franco (Ecuador), and Krivoy (Venezuela) answered the inquiry. The data were compiled in Chile with a case presented by Schijman (Argentina) at the 28th Annual Meeting of the Argentinian Association of Neurosurgery held in Santa Fe in August 1986.

No answer was received from other countries, with the exception of Benedeck who informed us that no moyamoya patients had been diagnosed in Uruguay.

Inquest Results

The illness manifests itself through the two classic clinical forms described by Suzuki and Takaku [9], either as transient ischemic crisis (more frequent in children) or as the ictal form with subarachnoidal hemorrhage (more frequent in young adults) with the typical angiographic representation and CT findings of moyamoya.

The occurrence of the collateral circulation of the moyamoya type depends upon the following factors—a bilateral obstructive lesion of the carotids, at least two lesions at the circle of Willis, the age of the patient and the stage of the disease [1, 2, 8, 9].

Analysis of Information Received

Argentina. At the 28th Annual Meeting of the Argentinian Association of Neurosurgery, Schijman presented an abstract of a classic case of moyamoya disease in a 4–year–old male child with a very good response to bilateral encephalo-myosynangiosis. Angiographic control showed collateral circulation of moyamoya–type irrigating medial cerebral and anterior cerebral arteries.

Brazil. Almeyda from Sao Paulo sent us reports of ten cases at the 9 du Julio Hospital. They are all classic cases of moyamoya disease, with no sex bias but with a preponderance of young adults over children.

In cases 7 and 8, he performed bilateral arteriodurasynangiosis, in 1982 and 1983, respectively, without obtaining collateral circulation.

Cases 1 and 10 should be noted because the first was an association of moyamoya with a left parasagittal meningotelial meningioma and the other showed the association of moyamoya with an arterial aneurism of the anterior communicating artery. In these cases, the tumor was excised and the aneurism clipped.

Ecuador. Franco sent a report of a case of a $1\frac{1}{2}$ year old girl with epilepsy and transient ischemic crisis. A slide of the angiographic study showed the typical lesion of moyamoya disease.

Venezuela. Krivoy reported four cases of classic moyamoya disease, both clinically and angiographically. These were not published or presented by the physicians in charge.

Chile. Castro, Head of Neuroradiology at the Instituto de Neurocirugia, presented our experi-

[1] Instituto de Neurocirugia, Santiago, Chile

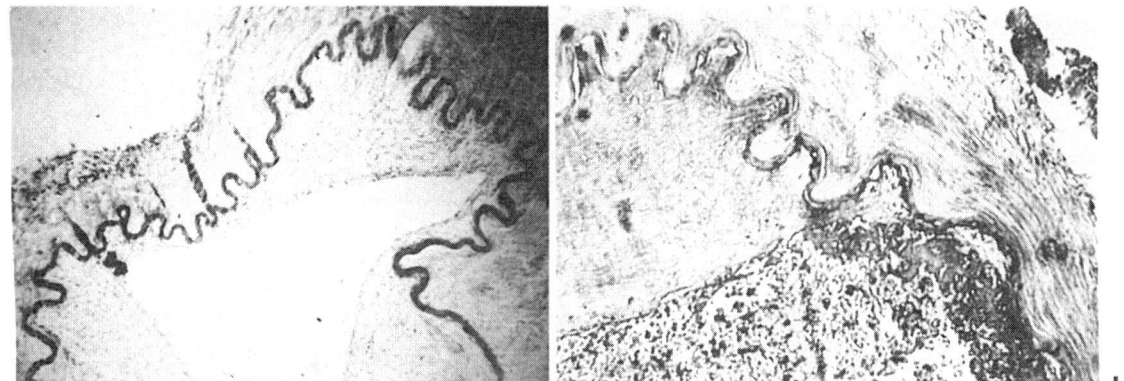

Fig. 1a, b. Case 1 MLC. Eccentric reduction of the lumen due to proliferation of tunica media and connective tissue, mucoid degeneration of the intima; thromboangiitis obliterans

ence at the 10th Symposium of Neuroradiology held at Punta del Este, Uruguay in 1974. It consisted of 26 patients, with the classic features of moyamoya which were reported the same year in Nevrocirucia (Chile) [1].

The most relevant findings of this series are the following:

a) Incidence was predominant among females (17 women; 9 men)
b) 80% of the patients were less than 30 years old
c) There was frequent association with focal sepsis of the head and neck (30.8%)
d) There was a clear seasonal prevalence (21 of the 26 patients admitted during autumn and summer)
e) The disease is rarely fatal
f) In these cases, the angiographic study either contributed to or hastened death

Findings of Autopsy Studies

Case 1 (MLC—Obs: 27869). Intracranial thromboangiitis obliterans involving both sylvian arteries; eccentric reduction of the lumen due to proliferation of tunica media and connective tissue; indemnity of elastic and muscular layers; mild inflammatory mononuclear infiltration of the adventitia (Fig. 1).

Case 2 (MMO—Obs: 1747–9776). A type of lesion resembling a poliarteritis involving *exclusively* brain arteries; mono- and polymorphonuclear infiltration of all artery coating structures, especially the adventitia; lamination of the elastica and thickening of the middle coat at the intrapetrosal segment of both carotid arteries;

thrombus developing at the bifurcation of the right carotid siphon; recent anemic infarct, left cerebral atrophy due to old vascular occlusion (Fig. 2).

Case 3 (CRP—Obs: 32382). Thromboangiitis obliterans confined to brain vessel involving both middle cerebral arteries and anterior communicating artery; lesion similar to case 1 but more accentuated, especially the hyperplasia of the intima; organized and canalized thrombus with two secondary lumens are visible (Fig. 3).

In these three cases, the arterial pathology was only in the brain arteries with absolute indemnity of extracranial arterial branches. The embolic source was not recognized in any of the three cases.

The finding of histological lesions of different ages in a single patient (case 2) suggests the existence of subclinical and cronically evolving arteritis with episodes of accutization [1].

In 1984, at Hospital Van Buren, Valparaiso, Chile, Quintana operated on an 18–year–old patient with transient ischemic crisis. He performed a bilateral encephaloduraarteriosynangiosis with a 5–month interval between both operations. He obtained good results.

In 1986, Zuleta and Candia, of the Instituto the Neurocirugia, operated on a 14–year–old boy (IEA—Obs: 56239) with a clinical presentation, CT and angiographic studies typical of moyamoya. Postoperative course was good.

Thus, although only Brazil, Venezuela, and Chile answered the inquest, moyamoya disease exists in South America: Additional support for this conclusion are the cases reported by Schijman of Argentina and Franco of Ecuador.

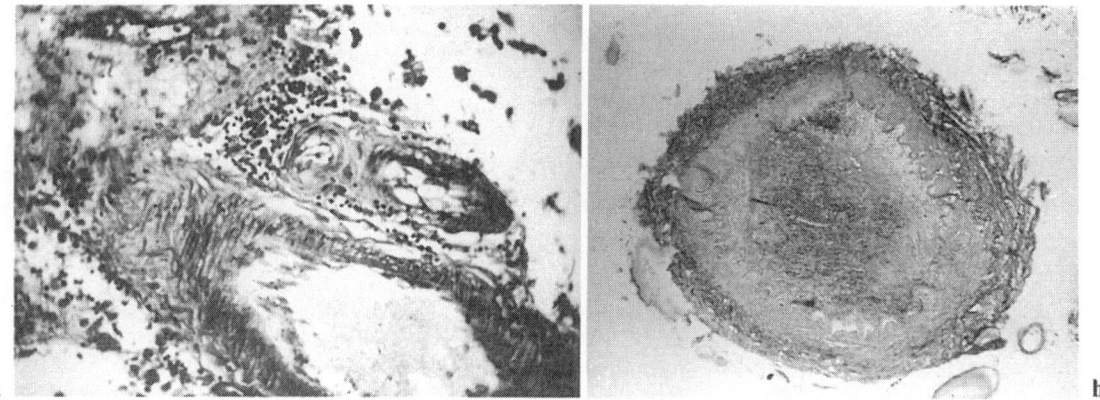

a   b

Fig. 2a, b. Case 2 MMO. Mono- and polymorphonuclear infiltration of all artery structures, specially the adventitia; organized thrombus; periarteritis nodosa type

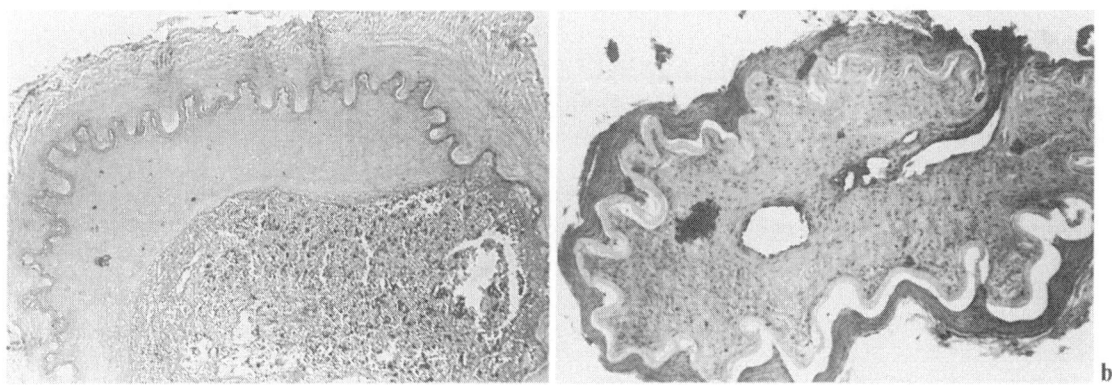

a   b

Fig. 3a, b. Case 3 CRP. Hyperplasia of the intima and organized and canalized thrombus (two secondary lumens); thromboangiitis obliterans

Pathogenesis. Reviewing the literature, the scarcity of anatomopathological data is confirmed, since the disease in general is not fatal. Moreover, only seldom is the lesion explored for surgical purposes, allowing only the biopsy of the thrombus or embolus and not the resection of the vessel wall for histology.

The diagnosis of arteritis is based on clinical findings and angiographic and CT alterations.

Angiographic studies are performed in patients with ictal clinical onset due to hemorrhage, in patients with recurrent transient ischemic crisis with worsening of the disease and in those for whom the CT shows a typical image of moyamoya.

In general, angiography is not done on patients with a compensated ischemic vascular presentation that does not recur, either because it is though that surgical and/or medical treatment will not be of help or because of the inherent risks of the procedure.

Bickerstaff [2], Shillito [8], Taveras [10], and Harwood-Nash et al. [3] point out the frequency of infections of the pharynx, tonsils, head, cervical region, and exanthemas preceding arteritis and the importance of this in the pathogenesis of moyamoya. Upon this, they agree with Malamud [6], Pouyanne [7], Kudo [5], and Basauri et al. [1].

Malamud [6] reports a typical case of periarteritis nodosa of the small meningeal arteries of the surface of cerebral hemispheres, of the heart and some more chronic lesions of the trachea, esophagus, gastrointestinal tract, and kidneys. These extracranial lesions are not present in case 2.

Pouyanne [7], when referring to the primary carotid arteritis as a leading factor for arterial obliteration, states that arteritis may be due to the accumulation or inflammation of the Buerger, periarteritis nodosa, etc.

The more recent concept that periarteritis nodosa and thromboangiitis obliterans (Leo

Buerger) are due to an allergic/hyperergic reaction offers a more satisfactory pathogenic explanation for moyamoya disease.

For Malamud [6], pathogenesis may be attributed to anaphylactic hypersensibility to different antigens, some of which could be bacteria.

In Malamud's case, the beginnings of the disease follow an infection of the upper respiratory tract, continued by the general compromise of several organs and an intense process of cerebral necrosis clearly not in proportion with the extension and localization of the arteritis. This facts suggests an allergic reaction [6].

This same reaction could explain the three patients of our 1974 series who died following angiography, in which the autopsy findings in two of them showed a thromboangiitis obliterans and in the other a type of lesion similar to periarteritis nodosa.

Could the deaths be attributed to another allergic reaction, this time to the contrast media, not in proportion to and superimposed on the one that caused the moyamoya?

Let us remember that Shillito [8] and Hilal et al. [4] remark upon the lack of complications in the angiographic studies of their patients, this being in agreement with the innocuous character of the exam in the other 23 patients of our 1974 series.

In 1974, Basauri et al. [1] advised us to pay attention to the number of contrast media injections and to the needless repetition of angiographic studies.

In light of these remarks, it is essential to perform angiographies in these patients with the previous medication of glucocorticoides or H1 blockers.

Acknowledgments. The author wishes to thank Dr. Ariel Gómez (Biochemiotry Lab), Drs. Renato Chiorino, Arturo Zuleta, and Guillermo Candia (Dept of Pathology), and Mr. Oscar Castro (Photography Lab) and Ms. Raquel González for their valuable contributions to the preparation of this manuscript.

References

1. Basauri L, Castro M, Langhi R, Rojas G, Ibañez H (1974) Occlusive arterial disease in children and young adults: Analysis of 26 cases: I. Clin Asp Neurocir (Chile) 32:40–49
2. Bickerstaff ER (1964) Aetiology of acute hemiplegia in childhood. Br Med J 2:82–87
3. Harwood-Nash DC McDonald MB, Argent W (1971) Cerebral arterial disease in children: An angiographic study of 40 cases. Am J Roentg 3:672–686
4. Hilal SK, Solomon GE, Gold AP, Carter S (1971) Primary cerebral arterial occlusive disease in children I. Acute acquired hemiplegia. Neuroradiology 99:71–86
5. Kudo T (1968) Spontaneous occlusion of the circle of Willis: A disease apparently confined to Japanese. Neurology 18:485–496
6. Malamud N (1945) A case of periarteritis nodosa with decerebrate rigidity and extensive encephalomalacia in a five–year–old child. J Neuropathol Exp Neurol 4:82–92
7. Pouyanne H, Arné L, Loiseau P, Mouton L (1957) Considerations sur deux cas de thrombose de la carotide interne. Rev Neurol 97:525–530
8. Shillito J (1964) Carotid arteritis: A cause of hemiplegia in childhood. J Neurosurg 21:540–551
9. Suzuki J, Takaku A (1969) Cerebrovascular moyamoya disease. Arch Neurol 20:288–299
10. Taveras JM (1969) Multiple progressive intracranial arterial occlusion: A syndrome of children and young adults. Am J Roentg Rad Ther Nucl Med 106:235–268

Long-Term Follow-up Study of STA-MCA Anastomosis and EMS in Moyamoya Disease

Jun Karasawa[1], Haruhiko Kikuchi[2], Izumi Nagata[2], Susumu Miyamoto[2], Hisashi Shishido[1], Toshiaki Tazawa[1], and Hajime Touho[1]

Summary

The condition of 62 children with moyamoya disease was followed after cerebral revascularization. The mean follow-up period was 87 months. For revascularization, 42 cases were treated with superficial temporal artery—middle cerebral artery (STA-MCA) anastomosis and encephalomyosynangiosis (EMS) on both sides, nine with only EMS on both sides, and the remaining 11 with STA-MCA anastomosis on one side and with EMS on the other side. Clinical improvement was obtained in 61 among 62 cases. Complete remission without any neurological deficits was obtained in 27 cases. Speech disturbance worsened in the remaining one. Though postoperative improvement in the motor and speech function was satisfactory in most of the cases, these surgical procedures could not restore the visual field defect caused by completed stroke. Minor deficits in the intellectual function persisted in 14 cases.

Introduction

For moyamoya disease, a progressive cerebrovascular occlusive disease associated with the development of several collateral pathways, effectiveness of cerebral revascularization has been reported [1–14].

However, a confusing variety of surgical procedures were proposed, and any long-term follow-up study has been rarely published [1–14]. The authors have treated 152 children with this disease with STA-MCA anastomosis and/or EMS. In this study, we clinically evaluated 62 cases which were followed for more than 56 months.

[1] Department of Neurosurgery, Osaka Neurological Institute. Toyonaka, Osaka, Japan
[2] Department of Neurosurgery, Faculty of Medicine, Kyoto University, Kyoto, Japan

Cases

Sixty-two consecutive cases of moyamoya disease were studied for their postoperative course. Follow-up duration varied from 56 to 146 months. The mean follow-up period was 87 months. Each case was under 15 years old (upon) first admission. For surgical revascularization, STA-MCA anastomosis and EMS were performed on 95 sides in 53 cases and EMS was performed on 29 sides in 20 cases. Clinical manifestations, motor and sensory disturbance, speech disturbance, mental retardation, involuntary movement, visual field defect, etc., were evaluated. Operative results were classified into three groups: improved, unchanged, and worsened. Improvement was divided into complete remission, moderate improvement, and slight improvement. Complete remission was defined as complete disappearance of neurological deficits without transient ischemic attack (TIA). Moderate improvement indicates remarkable improvement in neurological symptoms with or without sporadic TIA of mild degree.

Results

Table 1 indicates activity of daily life (ADL) after surgical revascularization. Postoperative improvement in clinical manifestations are summarized in Table 2. Table 3 demonstrates the operative results found in this long-term follow-up study. Clinical improvement was obtained in 61 cases among 62 children. The remaining one showed an aggravation of speech disturbance, though motor function improved remarkably. Complete remission of the clinical symptoms except for visual field defect was noted in 27 cases, moderate improvement in 26 cases, and slight improvement in eight cases. Mental retardation and minor intellectual deficits were seen in 30 cases before operation. They persisted postoperatively in 14 cases. Visual field defect was newly

Table 1. Postoperative daily activity after long-term follow-up

Surgical procedure	No. of cases	Excellent	Good	Fair	Poor	Dead
STA-MCA anast. + EMS on both sides	42	20	17	3	2	0
EMS on both sides	9	3	6	0	0	0
STA-MCA anast. + EMS on one side + EMS on the other side	11	4	3	3	1	0
Total	62	27	26	6	3	0

(Mean follow up period = 56 months, 1986 July)

Table 2. Postoperative improvement of clinical manifestations after revascularization

Symptoms and signs	No. of cases (preop.)	Complete remission	Moderate improvement	Slight improvement	Unchanged	Worsened
Motor weakness	46	16	21	9	0	0
Sensory disturbance	15	10	1	4	0	0
Speech disturbance	23	9	2	3	8	1
Mental retardation or intellectual deficits	30	4	4	8	14	0
Involuntary movements	4	4	0	0	0	0
Visual field defect	3	0	0	0	3	2
Swallowing disturbance	5	0	0	2	3	0

(Mean follow up period = 56 months, 1986 July)

developed postoperatively in two children. STA-MCA anastomosis and EMS could not restore the visual field defect from completed stroke in three cases. In 53 cases among 62, social life has been possible with or without slight limitation. Only three cases depend on aid for daily life. Figure 1, a typical postoperative external carotid angiography, shows extensive irrigation from STA-MCA anastomosis and EMS.

Discussion

Progressed cerebrovascular occlusive lesions with the development of several peculiar collaterals has been mentioned as the pathological feature of moyamoya disease. In children, most cases showed cerebral ischemic symptoms, which may have been induced by the motions linked with hyperventilation such as crying, running, or inflating a balloon. In order to prevent cerebral ischemic attacks, several procedures have been proposed [1–14]. Because of the confusing variety of surgical procedures, operative indication,

operative methods, and their results are controversial [1–14]. Since 1973, the authors have treated moyamoya disease with STA-MCA anastomosis and with EMS. We make it a principle to perform both STA-MCA anastomosis and EMS in children with moyamoya disease. Only EMS is done when postoperative hemorrhagic infarct may be anticipated in cases with impending stroke, or when an appropriate recipient cortical artery could not be found during operation in our initial cases. In recent cases, the STA is anastomosed to the intrasylvian portion of the MCA. Thus, anastomosis was possible in every recent case. EMS is an associated surgical procedure rather than an independent one. This long-term follow-up study is to show the clinical effectiveness of STA-MCA anastomosis and EMS for moyamoya disease.

Clinical manifestations, motor weakness, and sensory disturbance improved in each case without exception (Table 2). Postoperative improvement in motor symptoms was satisfactory in 37 among 46 cases. In contrast, mental retardation or minor intellectual deficits persisted in about

Table 3. Long-term operative results

Surgical procedure	No. of cases	Complete remission	Moderate improvement	Slight improvement	Unchanged	Worsened
STA-MCA anast. + EMS on both sides	42	20	16	6	0	0
EMS on both sides	9	3	5	1	0	0
STA-MCA anast. + EMS on one side + EMS on the other side	11	4	5	1	0	1
Total	62	27	26	8	0	1

(Mean follow up period = 56 months, 1986 July)

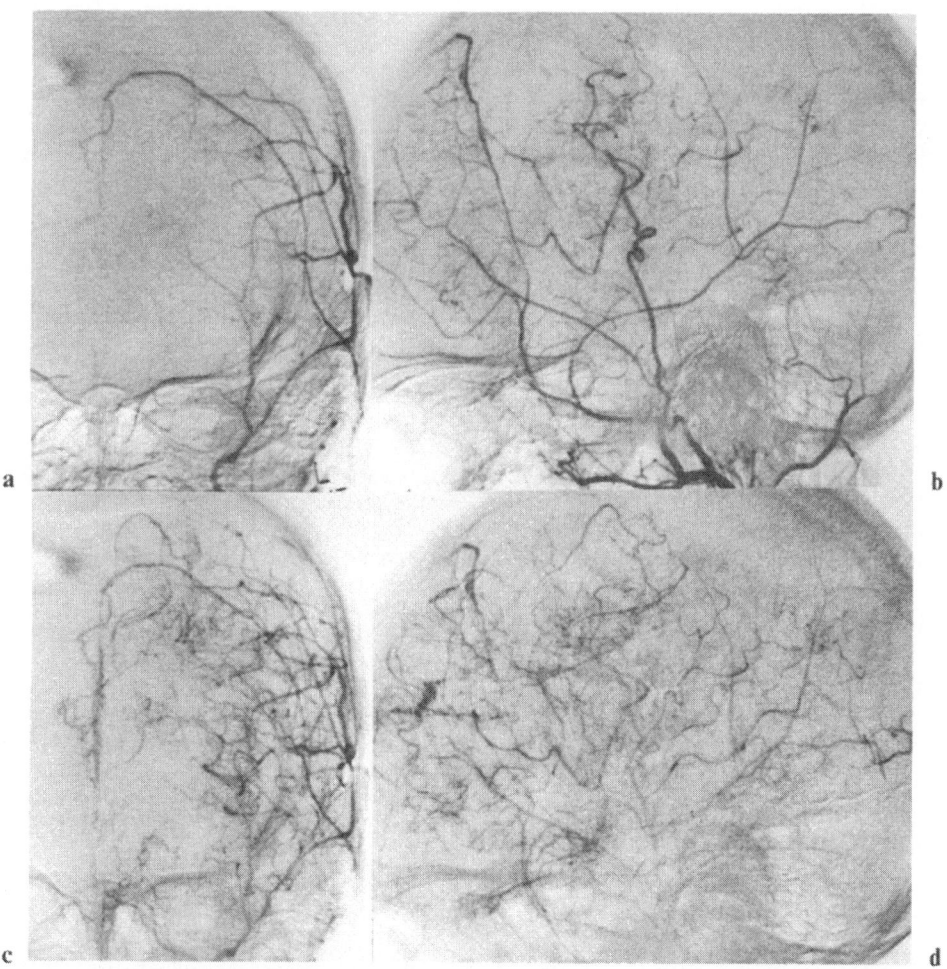

Fig. 1a–d. Typical postoperative external carotid arteriogram **a** Early arterial phase (A-P view). **b** Early arterial phase (lateral view). **c** Late arterial phase (A-P view). **d** Late arterial phase (lateral view). Extensive irrigation from external carotid system via STA-MCA anastomosis and EMS is demonstrated

half of the cases (14 of 30). Visual field defect from completed stroke could not be restored by STA-MCA anastomosis or EMS. In addition, newly developed visual field defect was noted during long-term follow-up in two cases. In moyamoya disease, cerebrovascular occlusive lesions do exist also in the posterior circulation [12]. Although STA-MCA anastomosis and EMS can exert indirect benefits to the posterior cerebral artery (PCA), distribution by redistribution of cerebral blood flow, persistent occlusive lesions may progress in the PCA in some cases [12]. In such cases, these surgical procedures cannot prevent stroke in the visual cortex. For revascularization of the PCA distribution, especially of the visual cortex, other procedures, such as omentum transplantation, may be needed.

For revascularization of the MCA distribution in moyamoya disease, several surgical procedures have been introduced [1–14]. These can be divided into two groups. One is a direct anastomotic bypass operation such as an STA-MCA anastomosis. The other is a nonanastomotic indirect procedure such as EMS or encephaloduroarteriosynangiosis (EDAS). The procedures of the latter group present few technical difficulties. However, due to the use of a nonanastomotic procedure, it is not certain that the operative result will be satisfactory and postoperative irrigation from the external carotid system may be poor in certain cases. Since the recipient artery has a thin wall and small caliber, some technical training is necessary for STA-MCA anastomosis in this disease. This direct anastomotic procedure, however, has a certain operative result. As described before, we make it a rule to perform STA-MCA anastomosis in each case: EMS is rather an associated procedure. In 53 cases among 62 (85.5%), complete remission or moderate improvement followed STA-MCA anastomosis and/or EMS. In these cases, social life was possible. These satisfactory results indicate the effectiveness of STA-MCA anastomosis and EMS as a surgical treatment in moyamoya disease.

References

1. Amine ARC, Moody RA, Meeks W (1977) Bilateral temporal-middle cerebral artery anastomosis for moyamoya syndrome. Surg Neurol 8:3–6
2. Balagura S, Farris WA (1985) Treatment of moyamoya disease by cerebroarteriosynangiosis. Surg Neurol 23:270–274
3. Boone SC, Sampson DS (1978) Observations on moyamoya disease: A case treated with superficial temporal-middle cerebral artery anastomosis. Surg Neurol 9:189–193
4. Cahan LD (1985–1986) Failure of encephaloduro-arterio-synangiosis procedure in moyamoya disease. Ped Neurosci 12:58–62
5. Ishii R, Koike T, Takeuchi S, et al. (1983) Anastomosis of the superficial temporal artery to the distal anterior cerebral artery eith interposed cephalic vein graft. J Neurosurg 58:425–429
6. Karasawa J, Kikuchi H, Furuse S, et al. (1977) A surgical treatment of moyamoya disease: Encephalomyosynangiosis. Neurol Med Chir 17:29–37
7. Karasawa J, Kikuchi H, Furuse S, et al. (1978) Treament of moyamoya disease with STA-MCA anastomosis. J Neurosurg 49:679–688
8. Karasawa J, Kikuchi H, Kawamura J, et al. (1980) Intracranial transplantation of the omentum for cerebrovascular moyamoya disease: A two-year follow-up study. Surg Neurol 14:444–449
9. Karasawa J, Kikuchi H, Kuriyama Y, et al. (1985) Determination of local cerebral blood flow by use of stable xenon and CT in moyamoya disease: Clinical, angiographic and blood flow assessments of the effects of bypass surgery. In: Handa H, Kikuchi H, Yonekawa Y (eds) Microsurgical anastomoses for cerebral ischemia. Igakushoin, New York, pp 247–255
10. Matsushima Y, Fukai N, Tanaka T, et al. (1981) A new surgical treatment of moyamoya disease in children: A preliminary report. Surg Neurol 15:313–320
11. Matsushima Y, Inaba Y (1984) Moyamoya disease in children and its surgical treatment. Child Brain 11:155–170
12. Miyamoto S, Kikuchi H, Karasawa J, et al. (1986) Study of the posterior circulation in moyamoya disease: II. Visual disturbances and surgical treatments. J Neurosurg 65:454–460
13. Nakagawa Y, Tsuru M, Mabuchi S, et al. (1985) Reconstructive surgery in 28 cases of moyamoya disease: Operative methods outcome, and postoperative angiography. In: Spetzler RF, et al. (eds) Cerebral revascularization for stroke. Thieme-Stratton, New York, pp 308–317
14. Takeuchi S, Tsuchida T, Kobayashi K, et al. (1983) Treatment of moyamoya disease by temporal muscle graft: Encephalomyosynangiosis. Child Brain 10:1–15

Encephaloduroarteriosynangiosis

A New Operation to Treat Moyamoya Disease

Yoshiharu Matsushima[1]

Moyamoya disease is an unusual form of chronic cerebrovascular disease in which the bilateral distal internal carotid arteries (IC) and circle of Willis become progressively narrower [3, 6]. To compensate for a decrease in blood supply to the brain due to this arterial narrowing, the collateral systems for the brain are activated and the blood flow per these collaterals progressively increases in inverse proportion to the progress of IC narrowing, by gradually replacing the collaterals of the internal carotid system with the collaterals of the external carotid system which has more capacity in blood flow. [4, 6].

Figure 1 show our scheme of collaterals to the brain in which the brain is surrounded by seven systems of collaterals which we have named as A to G systems [4].

The A system is the intracerebral anastomosis and is the anastomoses between the perforating arterial branches entering into the brain from the base of the brain (basal perforators) and from the surface of the brain (medullar branches of the cortical arteries). They are anastomosed with each other mostly at the external angle of the lateral ventricle as demonstrated in the angiograms of moyamoya patients (Fig. 2). The B system is the basal communicans and stands mainly for the circle of Willis. Moyamoya disease is caused by an insufficiency of this system.

The C system is the cortical leptomeningeal anastomoses. These are end-to-end anastomoses among each principal cerebral artery on the surface of the brain, as are well demonstrated in the angiograms of moyamoya patients (Fig. 3).

The D system is the dural network. The dural arteries are anastomosed with each other as if the brain were covered with a mesh hat (Fig. 4).

The E system is the extracranial network. As is well known in cases of bleeding from scalp injuries, the blood flow to the scalp and its accessory

tissues is extremely abundant, and the arteries also connect with each other and form networks (Fig. 4).

The F system is the functional anastomosis and represents the blood flow increase by non-anatomical causes, such as the elevation of $PaCO_2$, cervical sympathectomy, and superior cervical ganglionectomy.

The G system is the ground communications system. The principal blood vessels to the brain are connected in the neck. We call this the ground communications system as it is the system of collaterals beneath the skull. The brain is surrounded by these seven more or less concentric layers of collateral systems. The D and E systems, which are fed by the external carotid system, are difficult to be utilized as collaterals to the brain, as the brain is too much isolated from these systems by the cranium and the subarachnoid fluid space (Fig. 5).

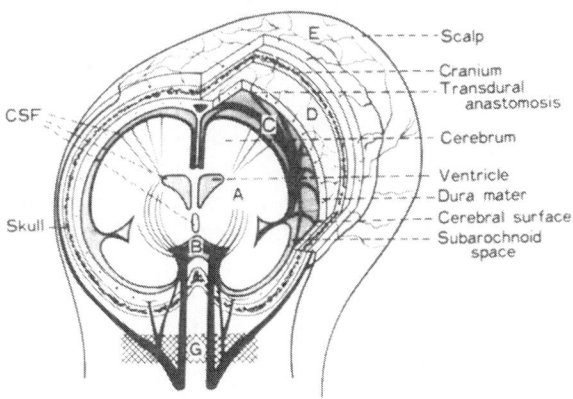

Fig. 1. Collateral systems to the brain. There is a subarachnoid fluid layer between the C and D systems and the cranium between the D and E systems. Both prevent the D and E systems (external carotid circulation) from being easily utilized as collaterals. *A* anastomosis intracerebralis, *B* basal communications, *C* cortical leptomeningeal anastomosis, *D* dural networks, *E* extracranial networks, *F* functional collaterals, *G* ground communications

[1] Department of Neurosurgery, Tokyo Medical and Dental University, Tokyo, Japan

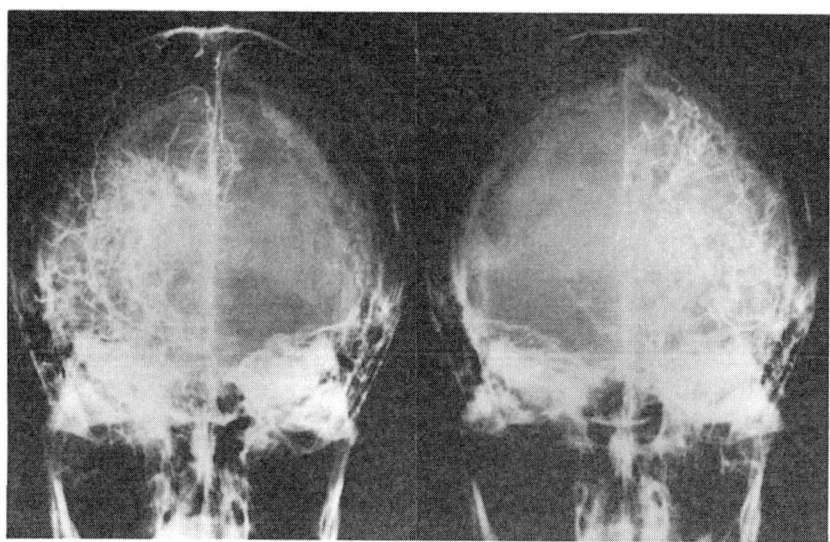

Fig. 2. Moyamoya vessels of a typical moyamoya patient seen equally prominent on both sides

In moyamoya disease, the B system becomes progressively insufficient, and the A and C systems operate first to compensate for the blood flow decrease caused by the B system insufficiency. The A system becomes prominent and develops so-called moyamoya vessels which are obvious on the angiograms of moyamoya patients (Fig. 2).

The C system also becomes prominent at the same time, but this change is not so obvious as these cortical arteries can normally be seen in the cerebral angiograms of patients without moyamoya. The D and E systems, which usually do not suffer in moyamoya disease and have an abundant blood supply, are still not well utilized as collaterals to the brain during the early stages of brain oligemia due to such obstacles as the cranium and the subarachnoid fluid layer.

In the course of time, however, the D and E systems form anastomoses with the C system called transdural anastomoses (Fig. 4) [6], possibly through the enlargement of the minimal arterioles. The latter are present in such tissues as pacchionian granulations, bridging veins, arteries, and cranial nerves which physically connect or bridge the dura mater and the brain.

The increase in blood flow via the external carotid system thus developed results in virtually natural healing in unnoticed moyamoya disease. In normal moyamoya disease, however, reversible or irreversible cerebrovascular ischemia sometimes occurs before an adequate increase in blood flow through the external carotid system is obtained.

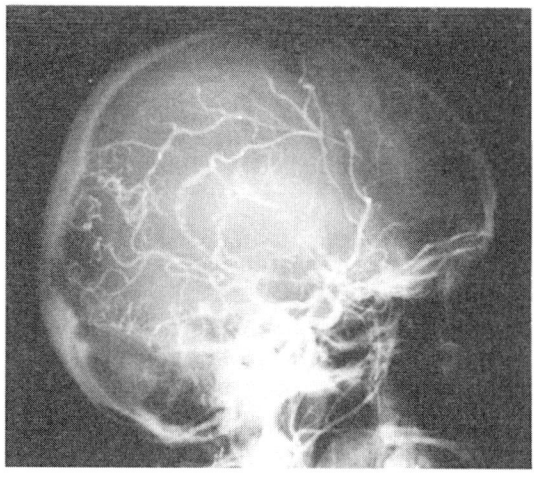

Fig. 3. Typical cortical leptomeningeal anastomoses seen in a moyamoya patient

According to this concept, it is necessary to surmount the two obstacles, the cranium and the water layer, if we are to treat the moyamoya patient before ischemic or infarctive episodes occur.

To surmount the two obstacles surgically, it is necessary to fenestrate the cranium and to bridge the subarachnoid space by inserting granulation tissue through a dural wound.

Our new operative method, encephaloduro-arteriosynangiosis (EDAS) is an operative procedure which has been developed to help the formation of collaterals to supply a sufficient blood

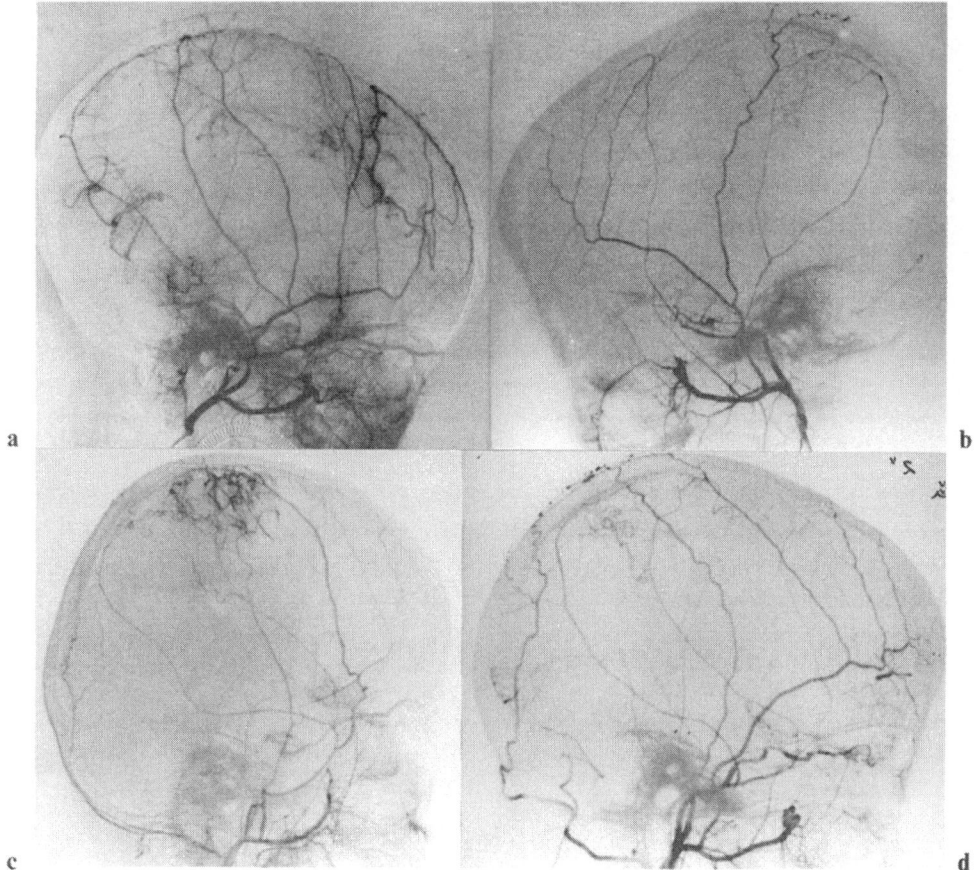

Fig. 4a–d. Prominent D and E systems seen in moyamoya patients. These systems are anastomosed with the C systems through transdural anastomoses in a later phase of moyamoya disease

Fig. 5. There are two obstacles for the collaterals to the brain to be developed between the external carotid and internal carotid systems—the cranium and the subarchnoid fluid layer. In cerebrovascular moyamoya disease, only moyamoya vessels feed the brain

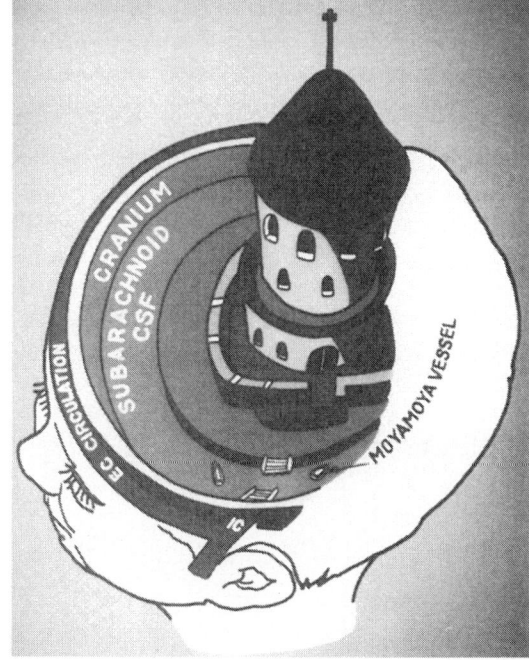

flow to the brain from the external carotid system, and promote the natural healing of moyamoya disease.

The operative procedure (Fig. 6) is to push the scalp artery, which is the principal artery of the E system, down to the surface of the brain with a strip of galea. The D and E systems are anastomosed by suture attaching the scalp artery to the dura mater, and the D system is connected with the C system, bridging the subarachnoid fluid layer by spontaneous anastomoses growing

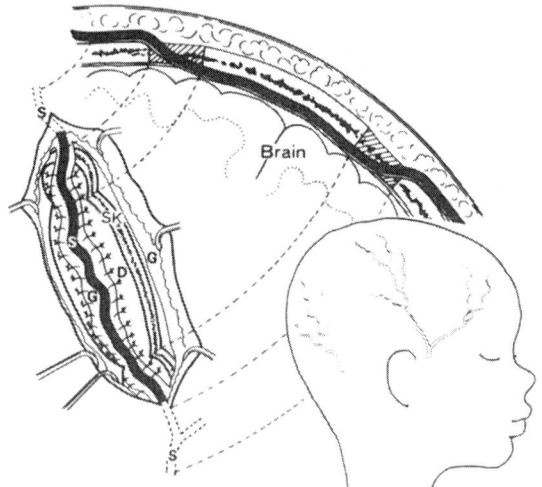

Fig. 6. Encephaloduroarteriosynangiosis and the scalp arteries (*S*) usually used as donors. *D* dura mater, *G* galea, *SK* skull

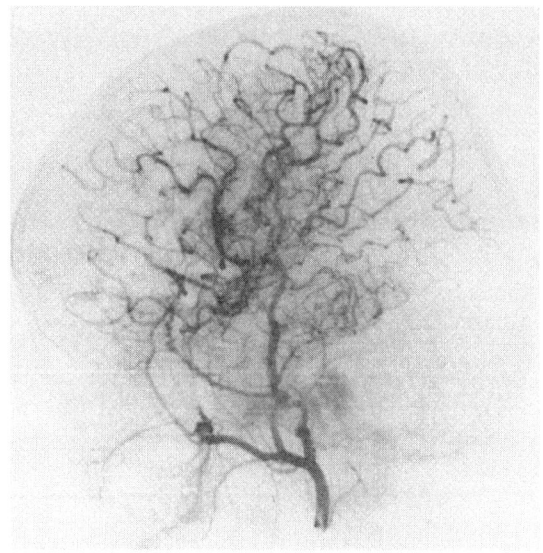

Fig. 7. A selective external carotid angiogram of a moyamoya patient who underwent encephaloduroarteriosynangiosis 9 months earlier. Note the total hemisphere is visualized by selective external carotid angiography which normally shows no cerebral vessels

in the granulation tissue developing between the dura mater and the brain. The most important point of this operation is that it does not sacrifice the preexisting collaterals, as seen in Figs. 4 and 5, as opposed to STA-MCA anastomosis or EMS, which we used in the past. Figure 7 shows an external carotid angiogram of a moyamoya patient who underwent EDAS 9 months earlier. The whole hemisphere is visualized through the parietal branch of the STA, which is the donor artery.

The revascularization of the brain usually occurs proportional to its requirement [1], and symptoms of the patient decrease accordingly [5].

We performed this operation on 96 sides in 51 pediatric moyamoya patients and obtained excellent results in all of them, possibly proving justification of the above-mentioned approach, which we introduced in the development of our new operative method to treat this interesting chronic cerebrovascular insufficiency.

References

1. Matsushima Y, Aoyagi M, Fukai N, Tanaka K, Tsuruoka S, Inaba Y (1982) Angiographic demonstration of cerebral revascularization after encephaloduroarteriosynansiosis (EDAS) performed on pediatric moyamoya patients. Bull Tokyo Med Dent Univ 29:7–17
2. Matsushima Y, Fukai N, Tanaka K, Tsuruoka S, Inaba Y, Aoyagi M, Ohno K (1981) A new surgical treatment of moyamoya disease in children: A preliminary report. Surg Neurol 15:313–320
3. Matsushima Y, Inaba Y (1984) Moyamoya disease in children and its surgical treatment: An introduction of a new surgical procedure and its follow-up angiograms. Child Brain 11:155–170
4. Matsushima Y, Inaba Y (1986) The specificity of the collaterals to the brain through the study and surgical treatment of moyamoya disease. Stroke 17:117–122
5. Matsushima Y, Tomita H, Takei H, Yamaguchi T, Takasato Y, Tsuruoka S, Fukumoto T, Kuroiwa T, Takada Y, Niimi Y, Inaba Y (1985) Changes in symptoms after encephaloduroarteriosynangiosis (EDAS) in pediatric moyamoya disease. In: Spetzler RF, Carter LP, Selman WR, Martin NA (eds) Cerebral revascularization for stroke. Thieme, New York, pp 578–583
6. Suzuki J, Kodama N (1983) Moyamoya disease: A review. Stroke 14:104–109

Revascularization Surgery for 50 Patients with Moyamoya Disease

Yoku Nakagawa[1], Hiroshi Abe[2], Hiroyasu Kamiyama[2], Yutaka Sawamura[2], Satoshi Gotoh[3], and Takeshi Kashiwaba[4]

Moyamoya disease is a disease characterized by chronic occlusion of the circle of Willis with subsequent development of fine vascular networks in the ganglionic region and is common in Japanese people. The term "moyamoya" means puff of smoke in Japanese and represents the characteristic angiographic findings of these fine vascular networks. Although reconstructive surgery for moyamoya disease is widely accepted now [1, 2, 5–8], there is still no definite consensus as to surgical indication for patients with hemorrhagic attack [6] and as to selection of operative method for each patient [5–8].

This article offers the overall surgical results of our experiences, introduces new operations devised by the senior author and also refers to surgical intervention for patients with hemorrhagic attack.

Overall Surgical Results

Subjects

Fifty patients who underwent various revascularization surgery were subjected to this evaluation. Ages at operation were under 16 years in 17 patients and over 16 years in 33 patients. Clinical patterns at operation were ischemic in 27 patients, hemorrhagic in 19 patients and mixed (ischemic and hemorrhagic) in four patients. Of 50 patients, 22 presented with neurological signs at the time of operation, as shown in Tables 1 and 2.

[1] Department of Neurosurgery, Kushiro Rohsai Hospital, Kushiro, Japan
[2] Department of Neurosurgery, Hokkaido University Hospital, Sapporo, Japan
[3] Department of Neurosurgery, Asahikawa Red Cross Hospital, Asahikawa, Japan
[4] Kashiwaba Neurosurgical Hospital, Sapporo, Japan

Operative Methods

Encephalomyosynangiosis is an operation to place temporal muscle on the surface of the brain and suture it with the free edge of the dura mater, in expectation of a development of anastomosis between the arteries in the muscle and the pial arteries of the middle cerebral artery territory (Table 3). Schematic drawings of each stage of operative procedures of encephalomyosynangiosis are shown in Fig. 1. Encephaloduroarteriosynangiosis was devised by Matsushima et al. [4]. Initially, a superficial temporal artery (usually parietal branch) is dissected and bone and dura mater are opened. The dissected superficial temporal artery is placed on the surface of the brain and dura mater is closed by suturing with the surrounding tissues of the dissected superficial temporal artery. Finally, the bone flap is replaced. Encephalomyoarteriosynangiosis is described in detail below.

Outcome

The average follow-up periods after reconstructive surgery were 40 months. Thirty-four patients (68%) were assessed to be in excellent condition, since there was no episode of ischemic and/or hemorrhagic attack in all cases after operation except for two cases indicated with an asterisk (Table 1) who developed transient ischemic attacks 14 months and 20 months following surgery. The neurological deficits present in eight patients at the time of operation subsided in three patients and were markedly improved in five patients following surgery (Table 1). Fifteen patients (30%) were assessed to be in good condition (Table 2). Of the 15 patients in this group, 13 presented neurological deficits of moderate to marked degree at the time of operation. Two patients (cases 35, 37) showed another minor hemorrhagic attack 30 months and 31 months, respectively, following STA-MCA anastomoses.

Table 1. Patients with excellent postoperative outcomes

Case no.	Age at operation (yrs)	Clinical type	Postoperative follow-up		Postoperative changes in neurological signs
			Years	Months	
1	34	H	7	6	Asymptomatic at operation
2	41	H	7	2	Calculation and recent memory disturbance markedly improved
3	9	H	6	8	Asymptomatic at operation
4	33	I	6	8	Right hemiparesis subsided
5	40	M	6		Asymptomatic at operation
6	13	I	5	11	Left hemiparesis subsided; intellectual disturbance markedly improved
7	18	I	5	11	Right hemiparesis subsided
8	43	I	5	11	Calculation and recent memory disturbance markedly improved
9	28	M	4	11	Asymptomatic at operation
10	26	I	4	2	Asymptomatic at operation
11	29	I	4	1	Asymptomatic at operation
12	19	H	3	10	Right hemiparesis subsided
13	36	H	3	9	Asymptomatic at operation
14	43	H	3	8	Asymptomatic at operation
15	28	I	3	8	Gerstmann's syndrome markedly improved
16	6	I	3	8	Asymptomatic at operation
17	47	H	3	7	Asymptomatic at operation
18	17	I	3	5	Asymptomatic at operation
19	10	I	3	4	Asymptomatic at operation
20	33	I	2	10	Asymptomatic at operation
21	54	H	2	10	Asymptomatic at operation
22	7	I	2	2	Asymptomatic at operation[a]
23	12	I	2	1	Asymptomatic at operation
24	5	I	1	10	Asymptomatic at operation
25	51	H	1	9	Asymptomatic at operation
26	28	H	1	8	Asymptomatic at operation
27	6	I	1	6	Asymptomatic at operation[a]
28	38	H	1	6	Asymptomatic at operation
29	11	I	1	1	Asymptomatic at operation
30	38	I	1		Asymptomatic at operation
31	36	M		11	Asymptomatic at operation
32	46	I		9	Slight dementia markedly improved
33	41	M		3	Asymptomatic at operation
34	9	I		1	Asymptomatic at operation

[a] There was no ischemic attack and/or hemorrhagic episodes in all cases after operation except for these two cases indicated who developed transient ischemic attack 14 months and 18 months following surgery

There was no definite diminution of basal moyamoya vessels on the angiogram of case 35 taken 26 months following surgery, regardless of rich collaterals via the anastomosed superficial temporal artery. A 5-year-old boy unfortunately died of subdural hematoma on the unoperated side 7 months following STA-MCA anastomosis with encephalomyosynangiosis (Table 2). His postoperative course before the appearance of the hematoma was satisfactory with good recovery of motor function. The occurrence of sub-dural hematoma may have been related to the intake of 300 mg of aspirin per day for 3 months.

Case Presentation

Case 18. A 17-year-old senior high-school girl was admitted to our hospital with frequent episodes of right or left hemiparesis lasting for 5–10 min, which began at the age of 13 years (Table 1). These episodes were frequently noted during

Table 2. Patients with good and poor postoperative outcomes

Case no.	Age at operation (yrs)	Clinical type	Postoperative follow-up		Postoperative changes in neurological signs	Ischemic attack	Hemorrhagic episode
			Years	Months			
Good							
35	35	H	8		Right hemiparesis subsided; intellectual disturbance markedly improved	−	+ (minor)
36	48	H	7	9	Right hemiparesis and aphasia improved	−	−
37	37	H	7	6	Asymptomatic at operation	−	+ (minor)
38	42	H	4	6	Right hemiparesis and aphasia moderately improved	−	−
39	4	I	3	9	Asymptomatic at operation	+ (decreased)	−
40	4	I	3	5	Right upper limb paresis and aphasia improved	−	−
41	31	H	3		Intellectual disturbance improved	−	−
42	5	I	1	11	Right hemiparesis and aphasia improved	−	−
43	35	H	1	10	Right hemiparesis and aphasia improved	−	−
44	49	I	1		Right lower quadrantanopsia slightly improved	−	−
45	8	I		11	Mental retardation and right hemiparesis slightly improved	−	−
46	8	I		9	Involuntary movement improved	−	−
47	6	I		6	Mental retardation slightly improved	+ (decreased)	−
48	38	H		2	Left hemiparesis moderately improved	−	−
49	48	H		1	Right hemiparesis and aphasia slightly improved	−	−
Poor							
50	5	I	7 (dead)		Right hemiparesis and aphasia improved → dead	−	+ (subdural hematoma of right side)

exercise or with Valsalva's maneuver. She was asymptomatic at admission and a CT scan revealed the presence of a small, low-density area in the right parietal region. She underwent STA-MCA bypass with encephalomyosynangiosis on both sides. The episode of hemiparesis gradually decreased and subsided 3 months following surgery.

Right carotid angiograms before (Fig. 2a) and 7 months after the operation (Fig. 2b–d) are demonstrated. Following surgery, the basal moyamoya networks (indicated by the asterisk in Fig. 2b) were definitely decreased in size

and surgically created collaterals were visualized via the branches of the external carotid artery (Fig. 2c, d).

New Operation: EMAS

Change of Operative Method from 1978 to 30 September 1986

Table 4 shows various operative methods performed by the authors from 1978 to 30 Septem-

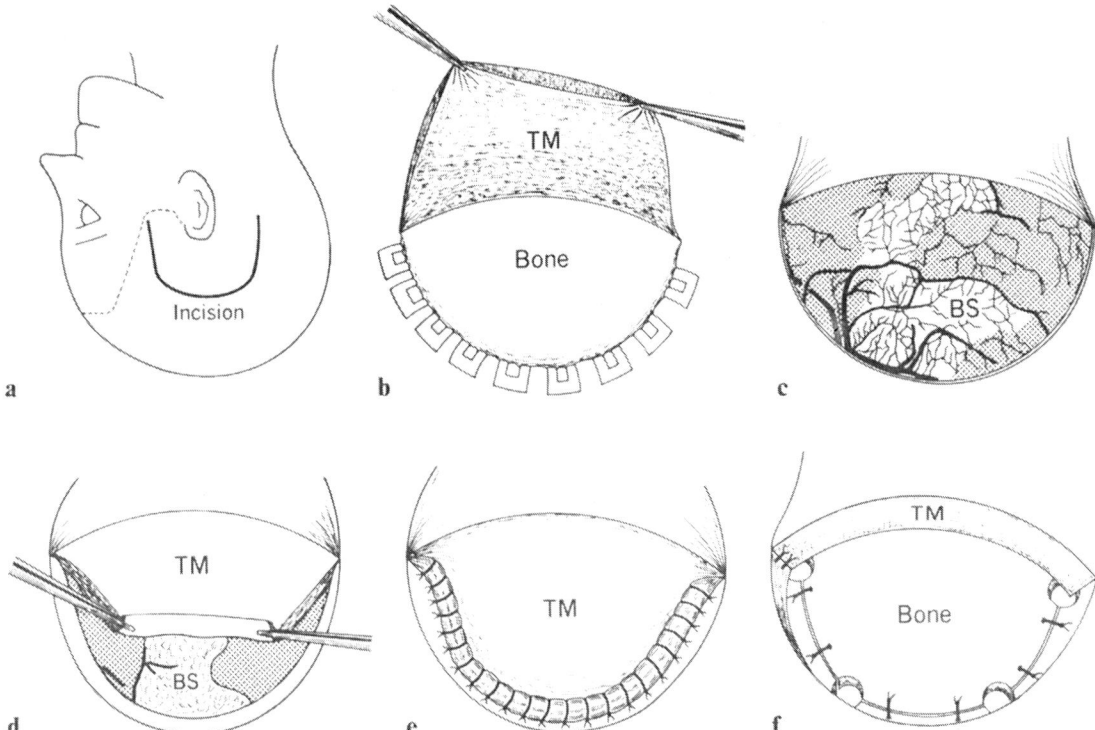

Fig. 1a–f. Schematic drawings of each stage of operative procedures of encephalomyosynangiosis **a** Marking of skin incision. **b** Dissection of temporal muscle (*TM*). **c** Exposure of brain surface (*BS*). It is important that relatively thick branches of the middle meningeal artery are kept uninterrupted, since the branches possess the future possibility of supplying blood into the intradural vessels. **d** Temporal muscle (*TM*) is about to be placed on the brain surface (*BS*). **e** Completion of covering the brain surface with temporal muscle (*TM*). **f** Replacement of bone flap (*TM* temporal muscle); 2–3 mm of the edge of the bone flap on the temporal muscle side is removed to enable smooth insertion of the muscle under the bone flap. Care is needed not to cut out too much of the bone edge since its removal of a wider piece causes depression of the scalp

Table 3. Various operative methods performed for 50 patients

Operations	No. of cases	Sides
Bilateral	40	
Unilateral	10	
Total	50	
STA-MCA bypass		11
Encephalomyosynangiosis		21
Encephalomyosynangiosis with STA-MCA bypass		17
Encephalomyoarteriosynangiosis		36
Encephalomyoarteriosynangiosis with STA-MCA bypass		3
Encephaloduroarteriosynangiosis		2
Total		90

ber 1986. Initially, the authors did an STA-MCA bypass. However, follow-up postoperative angiograms in some cases showed that bypassed superficial temporal arteries became smaller as time passed, possibly due to a progression of the occlusive process on the cortical arteries of the middle cerebral artery. Therefore, we performed encephalomyosynangiosis or encephalomyosynangiosis combined with STA-MCA bypass. Recently the authors started to do encephalomyoarteriosynangiosis (EMAS).

EMAS

EMAS is an operative procedure, newly devised by the senior author, in which a dissected branch of superficial temporal artery, with its distal end

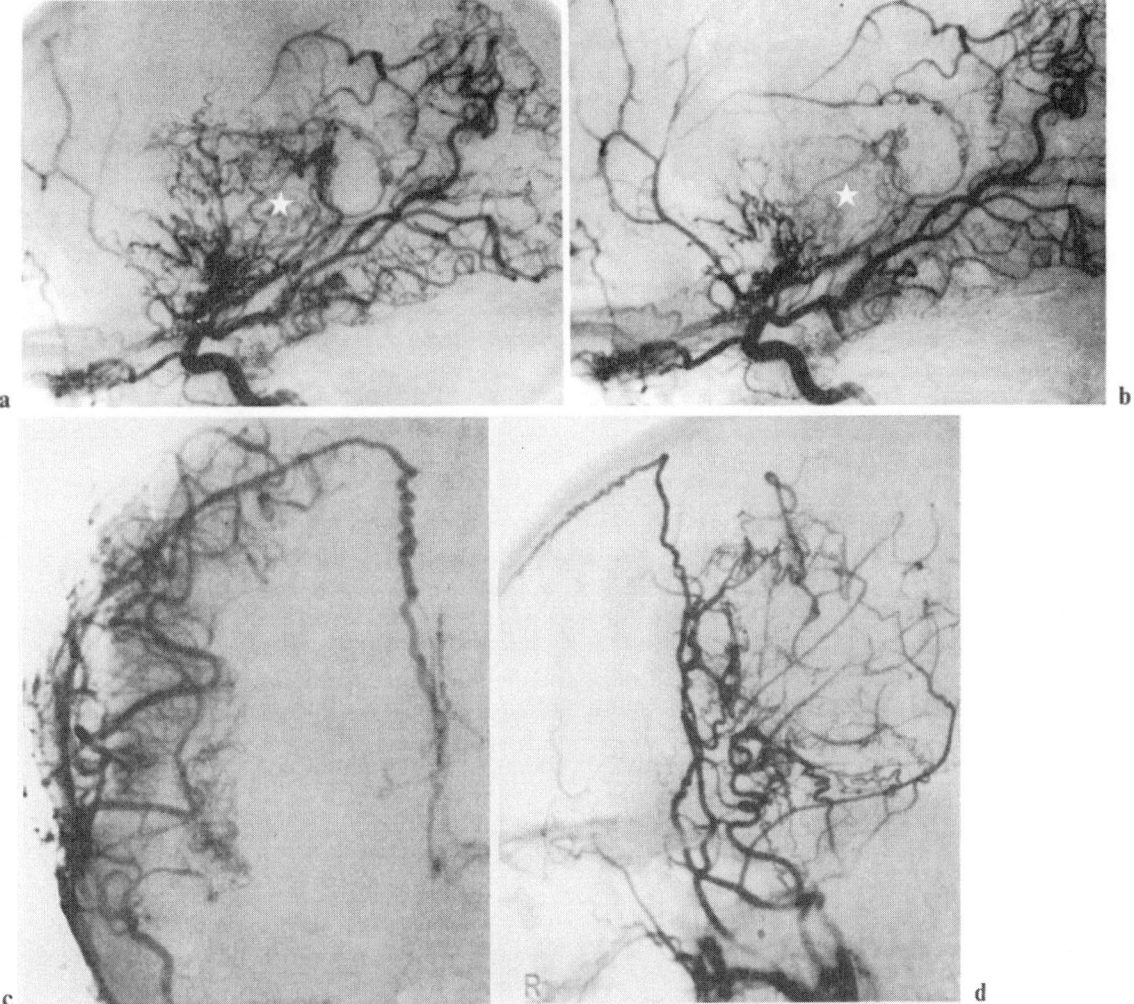

Fig. 2a–d. Right carotid angiogram of case 18 who underwent STA-MCA bypass with encephalo-myosynangiosis on this side. Shown are the right internal carotid angiograms taken **a** before and **b** right internal and **c, d** external, carotid angiograms taken 7 months after operation. Following the surgery, basal moyamoya networks were definitely decreased in size (*asterisk* **b**) and surgically created collaterals are well visualized via branches of the external carotid artery (**c, d**)

ligated, is placed on the surface of the brain. EMAS was attempted in the absence of a suitable recipient artery for anastomosis. The authors named this procedure encephalomyoarteriosynangiosis (EMAS) since encephalomyosynangiosis is simultaneously performed. Recently, we intentionally tried to place a superficial temporal artery on the surface of the brain with its lumen patent since the patent superficial temporal artery is more likely to promote neovascularization rather than the ligated one.

Schematic drawings of each stage of operative procedures of EMAS are given in detail in Fig. 3.

Outcome of Patients Who Underwent EMAS

EMAS alone was performed on 36 sides in 24 patients. A superficial temporal artery was placed on the surface of the brain with its distal end ligated in 15 sides and with its lumen patent in 21 sides. Ages at operation were under 16 years in 11 patients and over 16 years in 13 patients. Clinical patterns at the time of these operations was ischemic in 16 patients, hemorrhagic in six patients and mixed in two patients. The mean follow-up period was 24 months following surgery.

Table 4. Change in operative methods from 1978 through September, 1986

Operative methods	1978	1979	1980	1981	1982	1983	1984	1985	1986 until Sept. 31	Total
STA-MCA bypass	4	5	2							11
Encephalomyosynangiosis		2	3	2	3	2	4	2	3	21
Encephalomyosynangiosis with STA-MCA bypass	1	2	2	1	4	4		3		17
Encephalomyoarteriosynangiosis (EMAS)										
STA with distal end ligated			1		6	5	2	1		15 } 36
STA with lumen patent						2	3	9	7	21
Encephalomyoarteriosynangiosis (EMAS) with STA-MCA bypass							2	1		3
Encephalduroarteriosynangiosis					1	1				2
Total	5	9	8	3	14	14	9	17	11	90 sides

Of 13 patients who were asymptomatic at the time of operation, no ischemic and/or hemorrhagic attack was noted in 12 patients and ischemic attack was reduced in frequency and severity in one patient. Of 11 patients who were symptomatic at the time of operation, there was marked improvement or disappearance of symptoms in four patients and improvement of symptoms in seven.

Postoperative Angiography

Operative Methods and Postoperative Angiographic Findings

Postoperative angiography was performed on 40 sides in 27 patients (Table 5). The mean interval between operation and postoperative angiography was 7 months. Development of collaterals via branches of the external carotid artery were graded excellent, good and fair. "Excellent" means that all or nearly all main branches of the middle cerebral artery were well visualized from branches of the external carotid artery. "Fair" means that filling into the middle cerebral artery branches remained faint and "good" is between "excellent" and "fair".

Development of neovascularization was excellent in 23 sides, good in 11 sides, and fair in eight sides. The incidence of decrease of basal moyamoya networks was 55% in all. Of various operative methods, excellent development of neovascularization was obtained in encephalomyosynangiosis with STA-MCA bypass and

EMAS. STA-MCA bypass alone produced no long-lasting sufficient filling of the branches of the middle cerebral artery through the anastomosed superficial temporal artery, possibly due to the progression of the occlusive process including the anastomosed recipient artery.

Operative Methods and Arteries Contributing to Neovascularization

Table 6 summarizes operative methods and arteries contributing to neovascularization. Among the various procedures, encephalomyosynangiosis combined with STA-MCA bypass, EMAS, and EMAS with STA-MCA bypass have advantages in that the three main branches of the external carotid artery—the superficial temporal artery, the deep temporal arteries, and the middle meningeal arteries—are capable of contributing to future neovascularization into intradural vessels. In addition, no interruption of the cortical branches of the middle cerebral artery is required, which indicates that EMAS is very safe procedure.

Surgery for Patients with Hemorrhagic Attack

A survery of Japan by Kudo and Fukuda [3] in 1976 showed that 10 of 58 patients (17%) whose age at onset was over 16 years had repeated hemorrhagic attack, and six of these ten patients died. Follow-up periods ranged from a few years

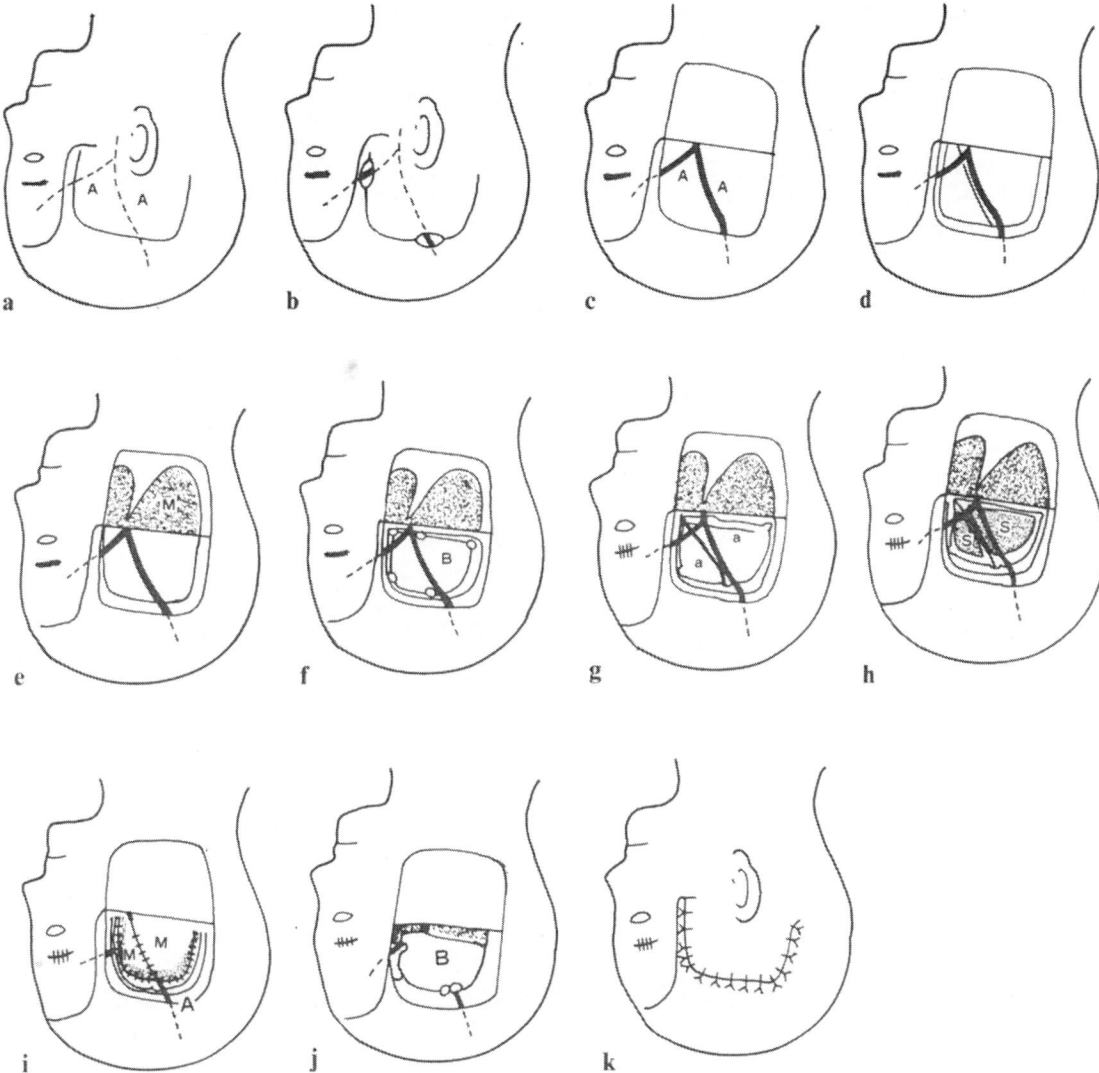

Fig. 3a–k. Stages of operative procedure of encephalomyoarteriosynangiosis (EMAS) **a** Markings of skin incision and of superficial temporal artery (STA, dotted line, indicated with *A*). **b** Dissection of two branches of STA. It is important to dissect STA branches under the marking of the skin incision before injection of local anesthetic drugs to avoid constriction of the STA with the anesthetic drugs. **c** Completion of dissection of the STA and reflection of skin flap. **d** Incision of temporal muscles indicated with continous line. **e** The temporal muscle (*m*) is reflected split to keep the stream of the STA. **f** Site of burr holes and extent of bone flap (*B*). Completion of craniotomy without interruption of STA is essential. **g** Exposure of dura mater. *a* represents branches of middle meningeal artery. **h** Opening of dura mater. *S* indicates surface of brain. It is important that relatively thick branches of middle meningeal artery are kept uninterrupted, since the branches possess the future possibility of supplying blood into the intradural vessels. **i** Completion of covering of brain surface and two branches of STA with temporal muscles (*M*). Temporal muscles are sutured with dura mater. *A* indicates STA. **j** Replacement of bone flap (*B*). **k** Completion of skin suture

to 10 years. A recent survey [9] has also revealed that 33% of the 175 patients having moyamoya disease with hemorrhagic attack seek medical attention because of repeated bleeding. The mortality from repeated bleeding was 30% in this survey. In our series, 2 of 19 patients (11%) showed

minor repeated bleeding and the mortality from repeated bleeding was 0%. Follow-up periods were 49 months on the average. The results highly indicate that surgical treatment should be applied to patients with hemorrhagic attack. However, longer follow-up periods and more precise post-

Table 5. Operative methods and postoperative angiographical findings*

Operative methods		Development of neovascularization (sides)			Incidence of decrease of basal moyamoya networks (%)
		Excellent	Good	Fair	
STA·MCA bypass	8	1	1	6	0
Encephalomyosynangiosis	8	6	3	1	50
Encephalomyosynangiosis with STA·MCA bypass	12	8	4	0	83
Encephalomyoarterosynangiosis (EMAS)	12	8	3	1	67
Total	40 sides in 27 patients	23	11	8	55

* The mean interval between operation and postoperative angiography was 7 months

Table 6. Operative methods and arteries contributing to neovascularization

Operative methods	Arteries contributing to neovascularization			
	Superficial temporal artery		Deep temporal arteries (temporal muscle)	Middle meningeal arteries
	Interruption needed during bypass	No interruption		
STA-MCA bypass	●			
Encepahlomyosynangiosis			●	●
Encephalomyosynangiosis with STA-MCA bypass	●		●	●
Encephalomyoarteriosynangiosis (EMAS)		●	●	●
Encephalomyoarteriosynangiosis (EMAS) with STA-MCA bypass	● (one branch of STA)	● (one branch of STA)	●	●
Encephaloduroarteriosynangiosis		●		

operative evaluations are needed before the superiority of surgery can be determined.

Conclusion

Revascularization surgery for moyamoya disease was beneficial for reducing or arresting ischemic attack.

Encephalomyosynangiosis with STA-MCA bypass or EMAS, as devised by the senior author, were found to be the most preferable operative methods in terms of promotion of neovascularization.

Revascularization surgery seemed to decrease the chance of repeated bleeding by reducing the number of moyamoya vessels that function as collateral pathways.

References

1. Karasawa J, Kikuchi H, Furuse S, Sakaki T, Yoshida Y, Ohnishi H, Taki W (1977) A surgical treatment of moyamoya disease: Encephalomyosynangiosis. Neurol Med Chir (Part 1), 29–37 (in Japanese)
2. Karasawa J, Kikuchi H, Furuse S, Kawamura J, Sasaki T (1978) Treatment of moyamoya disease with STA-MCA anastomosis. J Neurosurg 49: 679–688
3. Kudo T, Fukuda S (1976) Spontaneous occlusion of the circle of Willis: A disease entity, its pathology and clinical features. Adv Neurol Sci 20:750–757 (in Japanese)
4. Matsushima Y, Fukai N, Tanaka K, Tsuruoka S, Inaba Y, Aoyagi M, Ohno K (1981) A new surgical treatment of moyamoya disease in children: A preliminary report. Surg Neurol 15:313–320
5. Nakagawa Y, Gotoh S, Shimoyama M, Ohtsuka

K, Mabuchi S, Sawamura Y, Abe H, Tsuru M (1983) Reconstructive operation for moyamoya disease: Surgical indication for the hemorrhagic type and preferable operative methods. Neurol Med Chir 23:464–470 (in Japanese)

6. Nakagawa Y, Tsuru M, Gotoh S, Shimoyama H (1984) Reconstructive operation for moyamoya disease with hemorrhagic attack: Does surgical intervention reduce the chance of repeated bleeding? In: Handa H, Kikuchi H, Yonekawa Y (eds) Microsurgical anastomoses for cerebral ischemia. Igakushoin, New York, 233–239

7. Nakagawa Y, Tsuru M, Mabuchi S, Sawamura Y, Houkin K, Gotoh S, Kashiwaba T (1984) Reconstructive surgery in 28 cases of moyamoya disease, operative methods, outcome and postoperative angiography. In: Spetzler RF, Carter LP, Selmon WR, Martin NA (eds) Cerebral revascularization for Stroke. Thieme-Stratton, New York, pp 308–317

8. Nakagawa Y, Abe H, Sawamura Y, Kamiyama H, Gotoh S, Kashiwaba T (1988) Revascularization surgery for moyamoya disease. Neurol Res 10 (to appear)

9. Nishimoto A, Ueda K, Honma Y (1983) Follow-up study on outcome of occlusion of the circle of Willis (in Japanese). In: Gotoh F (ed) Proceedings of the Research Committee on Spontaneous Occlusion of the circle of Willis ("Moyamoya Disease") of the Ministry of Health and Welfare, Japan, pp 66–74

CBF and Metabolism in Moyamoya Disease Following Cervical Sympathectomy

Motonobu Kameyama, Satoru Fujiwara, Akira Takahashi, Akira Ogawa, Hiroo Sato, and Jiro Suzuki[1]

Due to the fact that there are still many uncertainties concerning the pathogenesis of moyamoya disease, no effective and reliable methods for prevention and treatment of this disease have become firmly established so far. In childhood moyamoya disease, the onset usually presents as symptoms of cerebral ischemia due to repeated transient ischemic attacks (TIAs). The disease gradually progresses and, at a certain stage the symptoms of brain ischemia disappear. At the next stage, many adult cases manifest symptoms of intracranial hemorrhage, particularly intraventricular hemorrhage [9]. For treatment of such pathology, various methods for increasing blood flow to the brain have been attempted.

On the basis of various research findings, we suspect that the cervical sympathetic nerves are critically involved in the development of moyamoya disease. We are currently performing superior cervical ganglionectomy (SCG) and perivascular sympathectomy (PVS) at the cervical portion of the internal carotid artery, the results of which are relatively favorable therapeutically [8, 10]. In this paper, the surgical procedure of PVS and SCG for moyamoya disease and its clinical results are described.

Theoretical Background

We have previously reported that there are sympathetic nerve fibers reaching the walls of the arteries of the human brain down to the size of arterioles, and that they are particularly abundant in the arteries around the circle of Willis [6]. Moreover, in animal experiments, we have shown that the sympathetic nerve endings within the arterioles of the intracranial internal carotid arterial system originate in the superior cervical ganglion [7]. Since these sympathetic fibers which are distributed to such vascular walls have vasoconstrictive effects, we surmised that PVS and SCG at the cervical region would resulted in the dilatation of the vessels of the internal and external carotid arterial systems, increase blood flow along collateral pathways, and therefore constitute a therapeutic technique for cerebral circulatory insufficiency.

Surgical Procedure

With the patient's head tilted slightly contralaterally (Fig. 1), the cervical region is somewhat extended and a skin incision is made from slightly above the height of the mandibular angle after tracing the anteromedial edge of the sternocleidomastoid muscle, which is then pushed externally.

The common carotid artery and the bifurcation of the internal carotid artery and external carotid artery are then exposed. Perivascular denervation is easily accomplished, provided a wheel is made between the adventitia and media by saline injection. The PVS is performed in the entire region, approximately 10 mm below the carotid bifurcation and over a length of approximately 10 mm along the internal carotid artery. It is known that a superior cervical ganglion is present at a site somewhat rostromedioposterior from the bifurcation of the internal and external carotid arteries and on the longus capitus muscle, but it can sometimes be difficult to find. However, the sympathetic trunk nerves can always be discovered by searching in this vicinity, provided that one has a good conception of the topographic anatomy. By following the trunk nerves rostrally, the superior cervical ganglion will be discovered.

The communicating branches of this ganglion are served as far as possible and the entire ganglion is removed. During this procedure, some pressure is inevitably put on the internal carotid

[1] Division of Neurosurgery, Institute of Brain Diseases, Tohoku University School of Medicine, Sendai, Japan

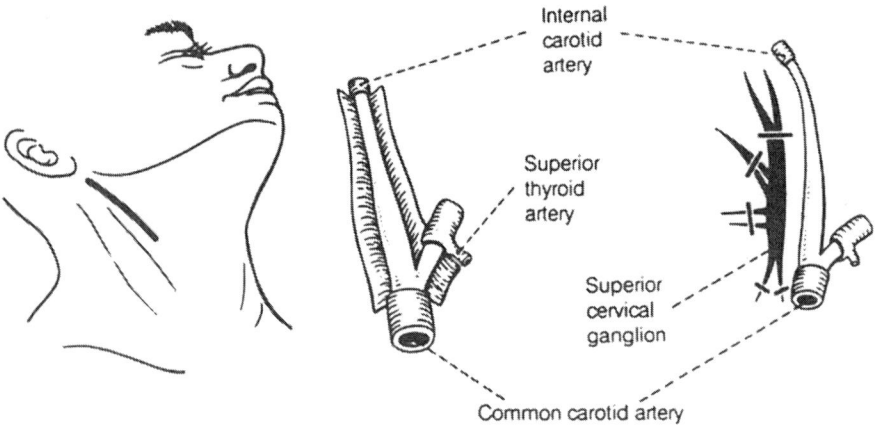

Fig. 1. Schemes of the right superior cervical ganglionectomy and the cervical perivascular sympathectomy. Skin incision (*left*), cervical perivascular sympathectomy (*center*), and superior cervical ganglionectomy (*right*)

artery in the medial direction, but pressure which would cause occlusion should be avoided. Moreover, care must be taken not to bring about damage to the vagus or the hypoglossal nerves.

Such perivascular denervation cannot be performed bilaterally in a single operation; at least 2 weeks recovery time should be allowed following unilateral denervation before the contralateral operation is attempted.

Clinical Results

In our more than 100 cases of moyamoya disease, these therapeutic surgical procedures have been used in 40 child cases (less than 15 years of age) and 20 adult cases, all with symptoms of cerebral ischemia. In the early days, there were cases in which only unilateral PVS was performed: however, in recent cases, bilateral PVS and SCG have been routinely carried out.

Among the 40 child cases in which PVS and SCG were performed, 28 cases (70%) showed improvement of symptoms during the follow-up period of up to 14 years (Table 1). With regard to the change in the symptoms, the following results were obtained. Of the 35 cases who had shown TIA-like symptoms, 24 had complete disappearance of such attacks. All of the eight cases who had shown involuntary movements showed disappearance of such symptoms. Among the 17 patients who had shown deficits of intelligence, one of the 11 mild cases showed a return of IQ to a normal range and eight showed some improvement. Among the cases with IQs below 50, there

were no improvements (Table 2). In the 20 adult cases, improvements were seen in six of the eleven cases with motor disturbances, in three of the four with speech disturbances, in two of the four with visual acuity abnormalities, and in four of the nine with psychic symptoms (Table 3). The EEG findings also supported the effectiveness of this surgical treatment (Table 4). In other words, in nearly all of the patients there were some improvements in the symptoms of moyamoya disease. Moreover, such improvements were seen in the early postoperative period and continued thereafter. The majority of the cases showing improvements were those which had had bilateral PVS and SCG, and most of those not showing improvements had had incomplete or unilateral surgical treatment.

Changes in CBF and Metabolism Following PVS and SCG

Since we have experienced many cases in which frequent episodes of TIA had ceased just after the PVS and SCG, we currently believe that these surgical procedures have immediate effects. However, recently we have added encephaloduroarteriosynangiosis (EDAS), developed by Matsushima et al. [5], with the expectation that it will increase cerebral blood flow through collateral circulation into the vessels of the brain surface from the superficial temporal artery.

During the operation, sequential changes in CBF and cerebral tissue O_2 and CO_2 were measured, using electrodes placed on the surface of

Table 1. Surgical treatment and results for child cases

Operation	Results			
	Improved	Unchanged	Aggravated	Total
Bilateral PVS	1	2	1	4
Unilateral PVS, contralateral PVS + SCG	3	3	0	6
Bilateral PVS + SCG	24	4	2	30
Total	28 (70.0%)	9 (22.5%)	3 (7.5%)	40

PVS perivascular sympathectomy, *SCG* superior cervical ganglionectomy

Table 2. Results of surgical treatment in child cases

Symptom	Presurgery (cases)	Follow-up	
Episode of TIA	35	No episode	24
		Improved	8
		Worsened	3
Involuntary movement	8	Cured	8
Mental handicap	17		
Educationable (50 < IQ < 80)	11	Normal range	1
		Improved	8
		Stationary	2
Uneducationable (IQ < 50)	6	Stationary	6

TIA transient ischemic attack

Table 3. Results of surgical treatment in adult cases

Symptom	Presurgery (cases)	Follow-up	
Motor disturbance	11	Improved	6
		Stationary	5
Sensory disturbance	4	Improved	1
		Stationary	3
Speech disturbance	4	Improved	3
		Stationary	1
Visual disturbance	4	Improved	2
		Stationary	2
Mental handicap	9	Improved	4
		Stationary	5

the brain via craniotomy for EDAS, together with the measurement of common carotid flow and blood pressure. Throughout the operation, blood gases were kept constant. In the 12 cases investigated, common carotid flow, cerebral tissue O_2 and CO_2, and systemic blood pressure did not show significant change: however, CBF increased 18.8% at 30 min after SCG with statistical significance (Fig. 2).

Table 4. EEG findings following surgical treatment

	Improved	Unchanged	Aggravated	Total
Children	31 sides	15	5	51
Adults	9	2	0	11
	40 (64.5%)	17 (27.4%)	5 (8.1%)	62

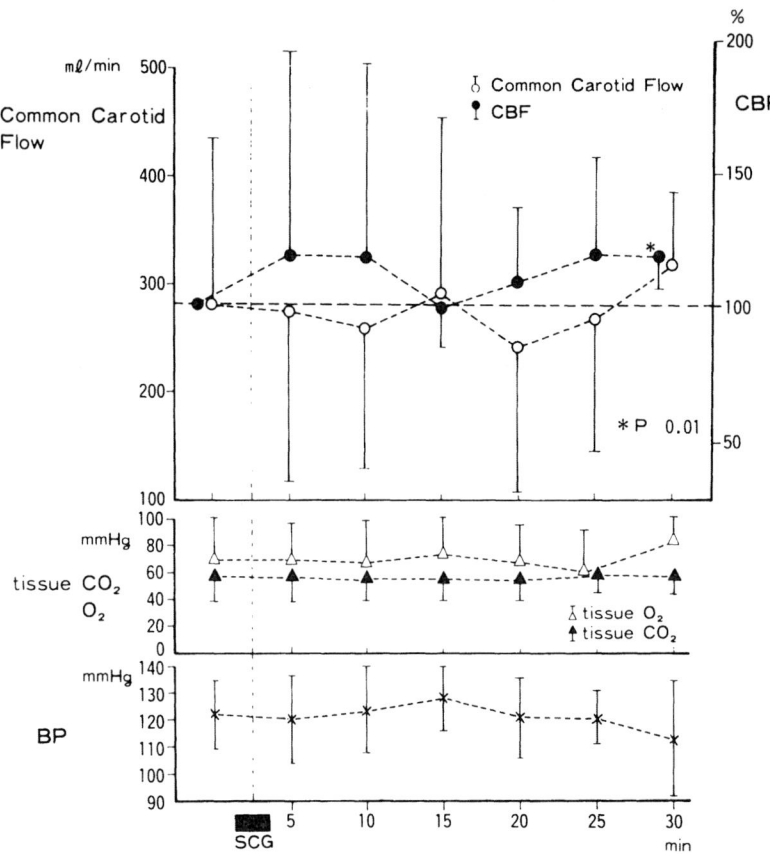

Fig. 2. Sequential changes in the cerebral blood flow (*CBF*) and metabolism after superior cervical ganglionectomy (*SCG*)

Discussion

The natural course of moyamoya disease results in recurring mild deficits in most cases. Particularly in juvenile cases, progressive aggravation occurs in some 30% and mild deficits in 30%, so that more than one-half of juvenile cases of moyamoya disease have lasting neurological deficits. A relatively small number of children are capable of returning to fully normal social lives. The facts again emphasize the need for successful treatment for this disease.

In recent years, various intracranial techniques, such as superficial temporal artery to middel cerebral artery (STA-MCA) anastomosis [2–4], encephalomyosynangiosis (EMS) [1], and EDAS have been proposed for the treatment of moyamoya disease, and there are many reports of favorable surgical results using these techniques. It cannot be said, however, that STA-MCA anastomosis is always a safe technique. Additionally, the recipient arteries at the surface of the brain are small and narrow in moyamoya

disease. Also, although the EMS technique was developed because of the problems of finding an appropriate recipient artery, it requires adhesion between a portion of temporal muscle, fascia, or dura mater, and the surface of the brain to allow for the development of collateral pathways. This region of adhesion is widespread and, consequently, there is the remaining concern that this could become an epileptic focus subsequently or that adhesion could be torn due to slight trauma and the damage to the brain tissue could be the source of intracranial hemorrhage. Furthermore, the superficial temporal artery or middle meningeal artery, which will be the feeding artery of the vault moyamoya, must be cut, and this could actually lead to a decrease in CBF.

We have found that quite effective results were obtained when PVS and SCG were performed on both sides, with each side treated several weeks apart. Also, the effectiveness of these procedures was proven by the significant increase of CBF during the operation. The advantages of these techniques are the simplicity of the surgical method, the lack of intracranial invasion, and uncommon side effects. Since these techniques have immediate effects, we believe that PVS and SCG should be the first choice for surgical treatment. Along with the EDAS procedure, which allows for the accelerated development of collateral pathways but does not require invasion of the brain tissue, these procedures would constitute a safer and more effective means of treating moyamoya disease.

References

1. Karasawa J, Kikuchi H, Furuse S (1977) A surgical treatment of moyamoya disease: Encephalo-myosynangiosis. Neurol Med Chir (Tokyo) 17: 30–37
2. Karasawa J, Kikuchi H, Furuse S, Kawamura J, Sasaki T (1978) Treatment of moyamoya disease with STA-MCA anastomosis. J Neurosurg 49: 679–688
3. Kikuchi H, Karasawa J (1976) Extra-intracranial arterial anastomosis in ten patients with moyamoya syndrome. In: Schmiedek P (ed) Microsurgery for stroke. Springer, Berlin, pp 260–263
4. Krayenbühl HA (1975) The moyamoya syndrome and the neurosurgeon. Surg Neurol 4: 353–360
5. Matsushima Y, Fukai N, Tanaka K, Tsuruoka S, Inaba Y, Aoyagi M, Ohno K (1981) A new surgical treatment of moyamoya disease in children: a preliminary report. Surg Neurol 15: 313–320
6. Sato S, Suzuki J (1975) Anatomical mapping of the cerebral nervi vasorum in the human brain. J Neurosurg 13: 559–568
7. Sato T, Sato S, Suzuki J (1979) Correlation with superior cervical sympathetic ganglion and sympathetic nerve innervation of intracranial artery: Electron microscopical studies. Brain Nerve (Tokyo) 31: 375–384
8. Suzuki J (1986) Treatment. In: Suzuki J (ed) Moyamoya disease. Springer, Tokyo, pp 105–117
9. Suzuki J, Kodama N (1983) Moyamoya disease–a review. Stroke 14: 104–109
10. Suzuki J, Takaku A, Kodama N, Satoh S (1975) An attempt to treat cerebrovascular moyamoya disease in children. Child Brain 1: 193–206

Discussion

Kitamura (Fukuoka): Dr. Shih, Dr. Suo, and Dr. Gustilo pointed out a lower incidence in Southern Asia than in Japan. Dr. Choi you have collected a great many data; could you comment on the differences in incidence between South Korea and Japan.

Choi (Seoul): Thus far, no national survey of the incidence of moyamoya disease has been conducted in South Korea, so it is difficult to answer your question. Recently, about 30 new patients have been reported each year; this is for a population of about 40 million. The Japanese incidence is about 100/year for a population of about 120 million. So the Korean figure is comparable with that for Japan given the difference in population. Why is the incidence so high in Korea? I think it is because of the ethnic similarities and similarities in climate and diet to Japan.

Kitamura (Fukuoka): Does Dr. Toakley think there is a difference in the incidence between Asians and Caucasians from your experience in Australia?

Toakley (Brisbane): I don't think there is. We have had 18 cases over a period of 10 years, which for a population of about 16 million works out at about the same incidence as that reported for Japan. The series only included Caucasians; there are no dietary similarities between Japan and Australia. This figure of 18 may in fact be an underestimate since it only includes patients who went to neurosurgical units or university departments of radiology.

Commentator, *Suzuki* (Sendai): In Thailand, Australia, Hong Kong, and the Philippines, there is a very low incidence of moyamoya disease, in Shanghai, Beijing and Changchun the incidence is higher, and in Korea and Japan the incidence is higher still. We need to know more about this interesting disease in various countries, especially in child cases.

Barnett (Ontario): A multicenter randomized therapeutic trial should now be carried out to evaluate the various anastamotic procedures, the remarkable ideas of Prof. Suzuki, and, because of the possibility of immune system breakdown, the use of new immunosuppressants, including cyclosporine. No evaluation of a rare disease with such a chronic course and variable form can be definitive without random assignment and long-term follow-up. This is the big challenge to Japanese neurosurgeons and neurologists to carry out this study with convincing control populations.

RTD 3. Bypass Surgery

Extracranial-Intracranial Bypass Surgery

James I. Ausman, Fernando G. Diaz, and Balaji Sadasivan[1]

Ischemic cerebrovascular disease may be due to embolism, hemodynamic compromise, or small vessel occlusive disease. The extracranial-intracranial (EC-IC) bypass surgery was introduced as a treatment for the hemodynamic causes of cerebral ischemia in 1967. It was based on the logical assumption that the brain is like other organs in the body and that symptoms caused by hypoperfusion to a region can be prevented by increasing the blood flow to that region. In the EC-IC bypass operation, blood flow is improved distal to the occluded or stenotic artery, thereby increasing the perfusion of the ischemic areas.

It has been shown experimentally that focal brain ischemia occurs as a result of imbalance between regional cerebral blood flow (CBF) and regional metabolic demands [8]. There are consistent regional CBF threshholds for functional impairment and for structural integrity. Sustained regional CBF below these threshholds results in neurological dysfunction and tissue damage, respectively. The EC-IC bypass has been shown to improve CBF ipsilateral to the bypass or in both hemispheres by xenon blood flow techniques, xenon computerized tomography (CT), and positron emission tomography (PET) scanning detection methods. In addition, the donor vessel has been found to enlarge after EC-IC bypass [9] and a large volume of flow through the superficial temporal artery has been documented. The EC-IC bypass has also been shown to improve oxygenation and cortical metabolism. Several clinical series support the usefulness of the bypass operation.

The results of the EC-IC Bypass Study [5], which was presented in Toronto in July 1985 and published in *The New England Journal of Medicine* in November 1985, concluded that in the 1377 patients studied, bypass surgery was no more effective than the best medical care in reducing stroke or stroke-related deaths. The large number of centers involved (71), the many patients in the study (1377), the enormous effort involved (8 years of work), the high cost of the study (more than $9 million), and the apparent scientific design have made the study appear definitive. Based on the findings of the study, it has been suggested that the bypass operation be completely discarded as a form of treatment for stroke patients. The results of the EC-IC Bypass Study contradict a large body of clinical and experimental research that preceded the study.

If the conclusions of the Bypass Study are unequivocally accepted as being correct, many basic questions will be raised and be required to be answered. Why does the brain not act like other organs and show benefit when hypoperfusion is corrected? Why does the improvement in CBF and cerebral metabolism documented in patients after EC-IC bypass have no value in the clinical management of stroke patients? We hope those who embrace the conclusions of the EC-IC Bypass Study will direct their research efforts towards answering these questions.

On the other hand, the results of the Bypass Study, although apparently valid for the 1377 patients studied, may not be applicable to the general population of stroke patients or to the group of patients currently being treated with the bypass operation. The conduct of the study was initially praised and the study was held up as a model. It was assumed that the data collection was meticulous and its evaluation exhaustive. The principal investigators did not report any discrepancies or problems in data collection.

Ausman and Diaz [1], in their critique of the EC-IC Bypass Study, noted that, in at least 2 of the 71 centers, there was evidence that eligible patients were not entered into the study. Sundt's survey [11] of 57 of the 71 participating centers revealed that 2572 patients who should have been in the study were operated outside the study. Information provided by the principal investigators to the committee appointed by the

[1] Department of Neurosurgery, Henry Ford Hospital, Detroit, Michigan, USA

American Association of Neurological Surgeons (AANS) has produced even more discrepancies (Table 1) which do not correlate with the information provided by the participating centers [3]. The AANS committee has been unable to resolve these discrepancies despite an on-site visit. We do not know why the principal investigators were unaware of the discrepancies in the data, or, if they were aware of it, why it was not disclosed at the time the results were published.

The discrepancies raise two serious questions. The first pertains to collection of all data. Were they collected in the same, inadequate manner? Unlike the data from which Sundt and the AANS discovered the discrepancies, the rest of the data have not been subjected to similar independent review. Will an investigation into the data collection method reveal similar large discrepancies, in say the actual number of fatal strokes in the medical and surgical group? We do not know.

The second question is whether any prerandomization bias existed. We now know that only a fraction of the patients who should have entered the study were actually included in the study. Is this fraction representative of the whole group?

Dudley has suggested two approaches to try to overcome this problems [4]. First, randomization may be undertaken before consent is sought, and the subgroup that is excluded by failure to obtain consent can then be analyzed not only for its standard characteristics but also for the proportions that would have entered each treatment arm. Second, even if this is not done, excluded patients must have their treatment recorded and be followed up with the same rigorous standards that pertain to those who have been included. The study failed to take any of those precautions and, therefore, selection bias by doctors, patients, or both cannot be excluded. Bias must therefore be assumed.

Relman has discussed some of the factors in prerandomization bias [10]. One factor involved is the surgeon's understandable reluctance to randomize patients referred for what the surgeon believes to be beneficial treatment. The surgeon would more likely enter into the study patients in whom the benefit was uncertain (low benefit group) or patients not in danger of suffering a stroke as a result of randomization and possible nonsurgical treatment (low risk group). This may explain why the natural history of stroke in the patients entered into the study was less ominous than predicted.

In the largest participating center in the United States coming closest to full randomization of cases and with the least prerandomization bias, a trend favoring surgical patients was found by the principal investigators [11].

The population of stroke patients who will benefit most from a bypass operation will be those with a hemodynamic problem. There is no attempt to identify this population in the study. The study does not appear to have many patients who fall into this category.

In 22% of the patients, there were no CT scan evaluations at the time of entry into the study. In this group, we cannot rule out intracerebral hemorrhage as the cause of the stroke. In the remaining 78% of the patients, we do not know what proportion had a hemodynamic problem. More than a third (38%) of the patients in the study had internal carotid occlusion with no further ischemic symptoms since their initial ischemic event. This group of patients is unlikely to have a hemodynamic problem and most neurosurgeons today do not treat this group with bypass surgery.

In the evaluation of patients, to identify the group of patients with a possible hemodynamic problem, we feel four-vessel angiography with a careful study of the natural collateral circulation is important. Almost half (44%) of the patients in the study did not have a selective four-vessel study. Barnett and his colleagues dismiss the importance of natural collaterals and refer to a 1982 study [7] in which there was no correlation between natural collaterals and the ability to predict the amount of angiographic flow that will develop and be imaged through the surgical collaterals (bypass) [2]. This study, conducted by Fox et al. [7], involved 431 patients who were included in the surgical group of the Bypass Study. Of these, 249 patients had angiographic evidence of occlusion of the internal carotid artery. In the study, the authors found that "the angiography done preoperatively is adequate in all cases to show the lesions, but the degree of completeness is variable." They were, therefore, unable to draw any correlation between the collaterals (for which the data was inadequate) and outcome. The inadequacy of the angiography in the study also resulted in their concluding that the time at which the postoperative angiography was done is not important. This is a conclusion that conflicts with data from a study of serial angiograms which showed that the superficial temporal artery (STA) increases in diameter with time [9]. Thus, Barnett and his colleagues have

Table 1. Discrepancies in the data provided by the principal investigators on the number of patients operated outside the study

Source of information	Total no. of patients operated outside the study	Breakdown of patients operated outside the study			
		Ineligible	Clinician refused to enter patient	Patient refused entry	Eligible but not randomized, no reason given
NEJM, Nov. 7, 1985, p 1192, opening sentence in Results section	118	—	—	—	—
NEJM, Nov. 7, 1985, p 1192, subsequent discussion in Results section	178	—	52	115	11
NEJM, March 26, 1987, p 818, information in list of "Procedures Performed by Centers" provided by S.J. Peerless in July 1986	1906	1604	109	—	193
NEJM, March 26, 1987, p 819, Table 2. Data Provided to the committee at the site visit, Sept. 17, 1986	1900	—	104	—	—
NEJM, March 26, 1987, p 819, additional total given to the committee during site visit, Sept. 17, 1986	1646	1542	104	—	—
NEJM, March 26, 1987, p 819, Table 3. Data sent to the committee after the site visit, Oct. 28, 1986	2009	1439	95	475	—
Sundt's survey of 57 of 71 centers	2572	—	—	—	—

made sweeping conclusions about angiography based on inadequate data.

In the decade since the Bypass Study began, there have been advances in the evaluation of CBF in patients. Xenon blood flow, xenon CT, and PET are being used to identify patients with hemodynamic problems. Even if the conclusions of the EC-IC bypass study could be extrapolated to the general population of patients undergoing the operation, it would apply to a population of patients selected based on criteria existing in 1977, in whom CT scans were not routinely done, cerebral angiography was often incomplete, and CBF studies were not considered necessary. The selection criteria for surgery in 1987 is certainly very different.

Meaningful analysis of the group of patients with middle cerebral stenosis (MCS) or middle cerebral occlusion (MCO) is not possible because of the postrandomization bias introduced by the redistribution of tandem lesions into other groups. The tandem lesion group represented 17%–19% of those entered while those with pure MCS and MCO represented 4% of the total in each medical and surgical subgroup [6]. Between March 1985 and the publication of the results in November 1985, the principal investigators redistributed the tandem lesion group and this increased the MCS and MCO group to 13%–14% and 11%–12%, respectively. The predominance of tandem lesions in the MCS and MCO groups makes conclusions about pure MCS and pure MCO of questionable value.

The EC-IC Bypass Study has shown that the bypass operation has an extremely low mortality (0.6%) and morbidity (2.3%) and a very high technical success rate (96% patency by angiography). Despite the operative mortality and morbidity, the outcome in the surgical and medical groups were the same in the study. This was because although the patients in the surgical group had a higher fatality in the 1st year, this was balanced by a lower fatality rate at the 5-year follow-up period. This aspect of the study needs to be evaluated further.

The AANS committee believes that the conclusions of the EC-IC Bypass Study was too sweeping. Dudley [4] believes that "this [Bypass Study] conclusion cannot be supported from the trial, and the organizers are *being uncompromising and rigid* in continuing to claim on their evidence that the operation must be laid to rest."

We agree with both the AANS committee and Dudley. We believe the study should be seen in proper perspective and its conclusions should be more modest. The data collection process of the study should be reviewed to discover what went wrong so that these mistakes will not be repeated in any future clinical trial.

The clinician still has the problem of how to deal with patients who present in the clinic with a history of transient cerebral ischemia (TIA) or minor stroke. We advocate complete evaluation of these patients before deciding which patient would likely benefit from the operation. A cardiac work-up, CT scan, complete cerebral angiography, and CBF studies form a part of our evaluation. We perform the bypass operation for patients who have a surgically inaccessible stenosis or occlusion and who have presumed hypoperfusion of the corresponding hemisphere or who continue to have TIAs despite a trial of best medical therapy.

References

1. Ausman JI, Diaz FG (1986) Critique of the EC-IC bypass study. Surg Neurol 26:218–221
2. Barnett HJM, Fox A, Hachinski V, et al (1986) Further conclusions from the extracranial-intracranial bypass trial. Surg Neurol 26:227–235
3. Committee of the American Association of Neurological Surgeons (1987) The extracranial-intracranial bypass study. NEJM 316:817–820
4. Dudley HAF (1987) Extracranial-intracranial bypass, one; clinical trials, nil. Br Med J 294:1501–1502
5. EC-IC Bypass Study Group (1985) Failure of extracranial-intracranial bypass to reduce the risk of ischemic stroke. Results of an international randomized study. NEJM 313:1191–1200
6. EC-IC Bypass Study Group (1985) The International Cooperative Study of extracranial-intracranial arterial anastomoses (EC/IC bypass study): Methodology and entry characteristics. Stroke 16:397–406
7. Fox AJ, Taylor DW, Peerless SJ (1985) Pre-existing collateral pathways: A factor determining success in EC-IC bypass surgery? In: Handa H, Kikuchi H, Yonekawa Y (eds) Anastomoses for cerebral ischemia. Igaku-Shoin, New York, pp 153–157
8. Jones TH, Morawetz RB, Crowell RM, et al. (1981) Threshholds of focal cerebral ischemia in awake monkeys. J Neurosurg 54:773–782
9. Latchaw RE, Ausman JI, Lee MC (1979) Superficial temporal-middle cerebral artery bypass: A detailed analysis of multiple pre- and postoperative angiograms in 40 consecutive patients. J Neurosurg 51:455–465
10. Relman A (1987) The extracranial-intracranial arterial bypass study—what have we learned? NEJM 316:809–810
11. Sundt T (1987) Was the international randomized trial of extracranial-intracranial arterial bypass representative of the population at risk? NEJM 316:816–816

Extracranial-Intracranial Bypass for Cerebral Revascularization

Robert F. Spetzler and Mark N. Hadley[1]

Introduction

Cerebral revascularization for ischemia remains a viable treatment option in the armamentarium of the neurovascular surgeon. The International Cooperative Study of Extracranial to Intracranial Arterial Anastomoses has helped to redefine the indications for these procedures and has improved our understanding of the pathophysiology of cerebrovascular ischemia. In this monograph we will outline our approach to cerebral revascularization, discuss patient selection criteria, and review our surgical techniques and results.

Theoretical Considerations

Revascularization of the brain and brainstem in the treatment of ischemia has great theoretical merit. A vascular conduit from the extracranial circulation to the intracranial circulation circumventing vessel occlusion or stenosis should be expected to provide a significant additional nutrient blood supply and ameliorate symptoms of ischemia secondary to hypoperfusion. Several individual investigator series have documented improved neurological function following extracranial-intracranial (EC-IC) bypass with long-term resolution of symptoms [2, 3, 7, 9]. Cerebral blood flow studies employing several measurement techniques have demonstrated a marked increase in regional cerebral blood flow in previously ischemic regions following bypass surgery [7].

This rationale and these observations appeared to be invalidated by the findings from the recent International Cooperative Study of EC-IC Arterial Anastomosis [10]. Patients in that study who underwent bypass surgery had a worse outcome and more ischemic symptoms and strokes than did patients randomized to medical treatment. At first glance, it appeared that the EC-IC bypass was an excellent surgical procedure but was *without specific indications* and of *no proven benefit*.

Since the initiation of the EC-IC bypass study, much has been learned about the pathophysiology of cerebrovascular ischemia. The results of the Cooperative Study have been analyzed in detail, and the indications for cerebral revascularization have been redefined [1, 10]. Anterior and posterior EC-IC revascularization procedures are now being utilized in a much more rational and judicious manner and, as a result, are performed much less frequently than prior to the announcement of the Cooperative Study results. The EC-IC bypass procedure does have merit; however, patients must be carefully selected. Only those individuals who have recurrent transient ischemia *due to hypoperfusion* which is *refractory* to optimal medical management and who are acceptable surgical candidates with respect to anesthetic risk should be considered for EC-IC revascularization.

The most heralded and frequently performed EC-IC anastomosis has been the superficial temporal artery to middle cerebral artery (STA-MCA) bypass for anterior circulation disease. Several variations of this procedure have been performed including STA to middle meningeal artery bypass, a "bonnet" bypass to the contralateral MCA, and the use of various interposition grafts (vein, artery, prosthetic grafts) in attempts to augment cerebral blood flow [2–4, 7]. Several bypass options exist in the treatment of posterior circulation ischemia including STA to posterior cerebral artery (STA-PCA), STA to superior cerebellar artery (STA-SCA), STA to anterior inferior cerebellar artery (STA-AICA), and STA to posterior inferior cerebellar artery (STA-PICA) anastomoses [3, 7]. Frequently the occipital artery, rather than the STA, will be used as the extracranial vascular conduit when attempt-

[1] Division of Neurological Surgery, Barrow Neurological Institute, Phoenix, Arizona, USA

ing revascularization of the AICA or PICA vascular distributions.

Patient Selection

The majority of patients with cerebral ischemia have symptoms due to thromboembolism [1, 7]. Patients with TIAs or stroke from hemodynamic vascular insufficiency nonetheless represent a significant minority. Often, multiple factors are operating simultaneously to produce symptoms in an individual patient. Great care must be taken to correctly diagnose cerebrovascular insufficiency. Vague complaints, such as light-headedness, dizziness, or headache, must be accompanied by more concrete signs and symptoms of hemodynamic compromise and must correlate with demonstrable pathology on the radiological studies. All patients with symptomatic cerebrovascular disease are evaluated with angiography, computerized tomography (CT), stable xenon cerebral blood flow CT, and, recently, magnetic resonance imaging (MRI).

Compulsive four-vessel head and neck angiography (including aortic arch views) is essential to document vascular occlusion or stenosis, the presence or absence of collateral blood supply (or a steal phenomenon), and the location and caliber of extracranial vascular channels. CT studies help identify regions of infarction and provide critical information about ventricular size and the presence of other mass lesions (e.g., cyst, tumor, hematoma, AVM) which might mimic ischemic disease. The stable xenon CT documents regions of relative hypoperfusion, and the MRI studies provide information regarding acute ischemic events and multiple infarctions and give precise views of the brainstem and posterior fossa structures, which are poorly visualized on CT scans.

All patients undergo detailed medical evaluations, including a cardiological work-up for a potential cardiac embolic source. Attendant medical problems are brought under optimal control. If patients remain symptomatic despite trials of aspirin or anticoagulants and they are reasonable candidates for surgery (from an anesthetic risk perspective), then they are considered for a cerebral revascularization procedure. The procedure to be performed is based on individual pathology-anatomy with the bypass directed at the ischemic region of greatest need.

Technical Considerations

Several aspects of the general operative anesthetic management of patients treated with cerebral revascularization procedures are the same irrespective of the specific anastomosis to be performed. All operations are performed under general anesthesia with maintenance of normotension, normocapnia, and adequate oxygenation ($PO_2 > 100$ torr). All patients receive intraoperative monitoring of EEG by compressed spectral analysis and somatosensory and brainstem auditory evoked potentials [3, 6, 7]. Heparin (100 units/kg) is administered intravenously before intraoperative occlusion of the recipient vessel and is not reversed at the conclusion of the procedure. Aspirin (5 grains t.i.d.) is administered preoperatively and continued postoperatively.

Before vascular clamping of the recipient vessel, barbiturates (thiopental, 1–3mg/kg loading dose) are administered to achieve EEG burst suppression. During the period of vessel occlusion, barbiturates are continued at a dose adequate to maintain burst suppression. If hypotension occurs before burst suppression, pressors (usually dopamine) are administered to maintain normotension [3, 6, 7]. Shunts are not used.

The Shaw hemostatic scalpel (Oximetrix Inc., Mountain View, CA) is employed to make the skin incision and to perform the initial dissection. This instrument provides excellent hemostasis and allows a rapid, bloodless approach to both the donor and recipient vessels. A portable Doppler unit is often employed early in the procedure to map the course of the donor vessel when it is otherwise not apparent by inspection. When performing the intracranial anastomosis, a small plastic dam is placed beneath the recipient artery and a Microvac suction (Microvac, PMT Inc., Hopkins, MN) is placed beneath or near the dam to constantly clear cerebrospinal fluid from the operative field [3, 6]. When using a vein interposition graft, great care must be taken to avoid damage to the vessel during harvest. All side branches must be tied securely, and the orientation of the interposition graft once in place must be rechecked to avoid kinking or twisting and compromise of the lumen.

All procedures are performed utilizing the operating microscope with its superb optics, lighting, and magnification. Following surgery, patients are monitored in the intensive care unit for management of postoperative hypo- or hypertension. Patients usually receive follow-up angiography within the first postoperative week and follow-up stable xenon CT studies prior to discharge from the hospital.

Anterior Circulation

STA-MCA anastomoses are performed with the patient in the supine position with the patient's head rotated to one side, exposing the temporoparietal region of the ischemic side. The parietal branch of the superficial temporal artery is most frequently used as the donor vessel. In our experience, the frontal branch is frequently already participating in the collateral supply to the region of ischemia. The donor vessel is dissected free from the scalp first and then a small temporoparietal craniotomy is performed through the same scalp incision.

Posterior Circulation

The patients who undergo a posterior circulation revascularization procedure are placed in the modified park bench or prone position, depending on the specific vascular anastomosis to be performed. The Midas Rex drill (Midas Rex, Ft. Worth, TX) is used to create the bony exposure and is particularly efficacious for a posterior fossa craniectomy. All bone flaps are replaced at the completion of the surgery. These patients (posterior circulation procedures) have a modest incidence of postoperative aseptic meningitis and/or communicating hydrocephalus (5 of 32 patients [16%]) and must be treated appropriately [3, 7].

Table 1. Procedures (1987–1986)

Procedure	No.
Anterior circulation	
STA-MCA bypass	115
Vein interposition	43
Posterior circulation	
OCCIP-PICA	19
STA-SCA	8
STA-PCA	3
Vein interposition	2
Total	190

Table 2. Variations of autogenous venous interposition anastomoses

Procedure	No.
Anterior circulation ($n = 43$)	
SCA-MCA	23
CCA-MCA	4
SCA-ECA/STA-MCA	4
CCA-ICA	3
"Bonnet" (STA-contralateral MCA)	2
CCA-ECA/STA-MCA	1
ICA-MCA	1
ECA-MCA	1
SCA-CCA	1
ICA-ICA	3
Posterior circulation ($n = 2$)	
ECA-PCA	1
SCA-PCA	1
Total	45

SCA subclavian artery

Surgical Results

To date, 190 revascularization procedures have been performed (RFS) (Tables 1, 2). A total of 158 procedures have been directed at the treatment of anterior circulation disease, 43 of which were vein interposition grafts (Fig. 1). Thirty-two EC-IC bypasses have been performed in the treatment of vertebrobasilar insufficiency, two of which were vein interposition grafts (Figs. 2, 3).

Follow-up was achieved in 170 patients (90%). Eighteen of these patients died, mostly as a result of severe cardiopulmonary disease. The patency rate of the STA-MCA anastomoses was 95%, the patency rate of the posterior circulation anastomoses (excluding the vein grafts) was 96%, and the patency rate of the vein interposition grafts was 82% (median follow-up = 16

months). Eighty-two percent of patients were relieved of their symptoms, 12% had a reduction in symptoms, and 6% had no improvement in their preoperative status. There was zero operative mortality and less than 5% morbidity for the series as a whole.

Discussion

Extracranial to intracranial vascular anastomosis procedures are efficacious in the treatment of selected patients with brain ischemia. The number of patients who are candidates for these procedures represents a small percentage of the total population of patients with symptomatic cerebrovascular disease. Prior to the Cooperative EC-IC bypass study, we treated a wide variety of patients with cerebral ischemia with bypass (a maximum of 70 in 1 year). We now restrict the use of EC-IC revascularization to a limited, select group of patients who have nonembolic cerebrovascular insufficiency, which is unstable despite optimal nonsurgical therapy. We have averaged four procedures per year since the results of the study were made available.

The revascularization procedures are technically straightforward and high patency rates have been documented, albeit lower with vein interposition grafts [2, 3, 7, 9, 10]. Several series have documented improvement in acute ischemic symptoms and imply a reduction of stroke risk in treated patients [2, 3, 7, 9]. The serial examination of patients and the neuroradiological diagnostic battery which we have outlined facilitates the selection of patients who may most benefit from these procedures.

The use of microneurosurgical techniques and the operating microscope are essential to keep perioperative morbidity and mortality rates at an absolute minimum. We believe the practices of intraoperative heparinization, barbiturate-induced suppression of cerebral electrical activity, and perioperative blood pressure control are important adjuncts for successful EC-IC bypass surgery [3]. Antithrombotic therapy prevents thrombosis at the anastomotic site. Several studies have documented the beneficial effects of heparin on platelet aggregation (inhibition) and fibrin formation (inhibition) during vascular surgery [3, 6, 7]. Avoiding pharmacological heparin reversal and the use of pre- and postoperative aspirin contributes to the protection from perioperative thromboembolic events [6].

Barbiturates reduce the metabolic requirements of cerebral tissue and may be responsible for extending the tolerance of the brain for the reduction of substrate supply that occurs with ischemia [3, 5–8]. Several investigators have reported that barbiturates, in particular thiopental and pentobarbital, have the capacity to modify or prevent cerebral injury due to focal ischemia [5, 7, 8]. Barbiturate therapy is most efficacious when the agent is administered before a period of temporary focal ischemia which makes them a logical choice as a cerebro-protective agent during elective neurovascular surgery [5, 6]. We use barbiturate protection to the point of EEG burst suppression in all major neurovascular procedures and have had no untoward reactions or complications [3, 6]. Most importantly, in our experience, barbiturate therapy has been effective in protecting the brain during surgery. No

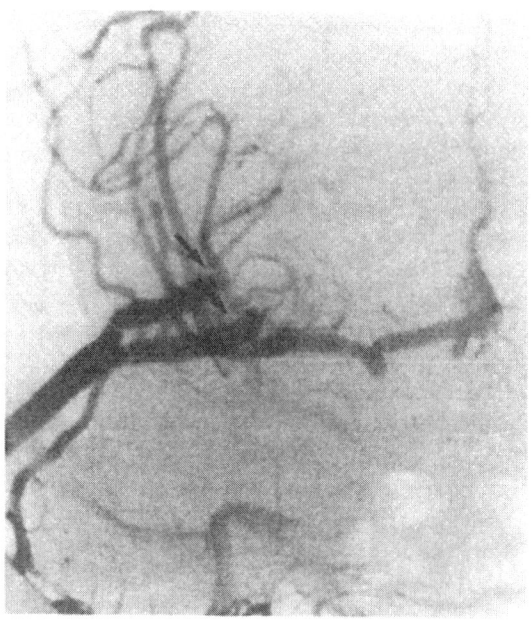

Fig. 1. Vein interposition graft from right ECA to the MCA. The "double barrel" anastomoses represent a high flow bypass alternative, indicated by *arrows*

patient in this series had a postoperative neurological deficit from ischemia as a result of clamping the recipient vessel to perform the anastomosis. Our experience in the use of barbiturate cerebral protection during carotid endarterectomy has been similar [6].

Strict blood pressure control in the operative and postoperative periods helps reduce the incidence of hypotensive ischemia (hypoperfusion) and hypertensive intracerebral hemorrhage [3, 6, 7]. In our experience, postoperative hypotension has been due to hypovolemia and close attention to the patients intraoperative fluids and cardiac parameters will avoid this potential complication. Postoperative hypertension has been common in the immediate postoperative period and is effectively treated by a constant infusion of sodium nitroprusside. As noted, patients who undergo posterior fossa revascularization procedures, particularly occipital artery-PICA, had an increased incidence of postoperative aseptic meningitis and/or communicating hydrocephalus [3]. Clinicians must be aware of these potential complications and treat them appropriately.

The decision to use a vein interposition graft is made when other anatomical collateral channels are either unavailable, too small, or already involved in the collateral circulation process [3, 4, 7]. We commonly use the saphenous vein as the interposition graft, which affords a wide variety

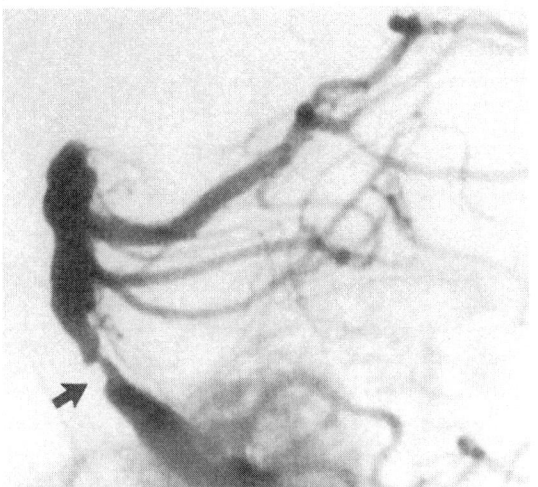

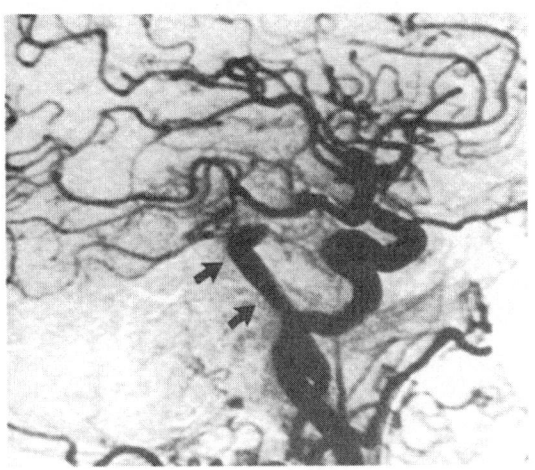

Fig. 2. Preoperative angiogram documenting severe basilar artery atherosclerotic disease, indicated by the *arrow*, in a patient with frequent drop attacks, dysphagia, dysarthria, and alternating hemiparesis

Fig. 3. Postoperative DSAA examination illustrating a high flow ECA to PCA vein interposition graft, indicated by *arrows*

of potential anastomoses employing either long or short segments (Figs. 1–3). The advantages of using a vein graft include its luminal diameter (much larger than an STA), the lack of atherosclerotic changes within the vein which are commonly found in the donor artery, the ability to provide immediate high flow rates to the recipient vascular bed, and the length of the vein (essentially unrestricted). The disadvantages of using a vein as a donor vessel include the necessity of harvesting an additional vessel, the performance of two anastomoses, the luminal size discrepancy between the vein and the recipient vessel, and reduced long-term patency rates [3, 4, 7]. All of these factors must be considered in the treatment of an individual patient.

In summary, the EC-IC bypass remains an important therapeutic option in the treatment of patients with cerebrovascular disease. Carefully selected patients will benefit from these procedures. Conscientious perioperative patient management and meticulous microneurosurgical techniques can minimize perioperative morbidity and mortality and improve long-term survival.

References

1. Awad IA, Spetzler RF (1986) Extracranial-intracranial bypass surgery: A critical analysis in light of the International Cooperative Study. Neurosurgery 19(4):655–664
2. Diaz FG, Umansky F, Mehta B, et al. (1985) Cerebral revascularization to a main limb of the middle cerebral artery in the sylvian fissure. J Neurosurg 63:21–29
3. Hopkins LN, Martin NA, Hadley MH, et al. (1987) Vertebrobasilar insufficiency: II. Microsurgical treatment of intracranial disease. J Neurosurg 66:662–674
4. Marano SR, Spetzler RF, Carter LP (1985) Autogenous saphenous vein interposition grafts for high flow augmentation of cerebral blood flow. BNI Quarterly 1(4):29–33
5. Selman WR, Spetzler RF, Roski RA, et al. (1982) Barbiturate coma in focal cerebral ischemia: Relationship of protection to timing of therapy. J Neurosurg 56:685–690
6. Spetzler RF, Martin N, Hadley MN, et al. (1986) Microsurgical endarterectomy under barbiturate protection: A prospective study. J Neurosurg 65:63–73
7. Spetzler RF, Selman WR, Carter LP, et al (1985) Cerebral revascularization for stroke. Thieme-Stratton, New York
8. Spetzler RF, Selman WR, Roski RA, et al. (1982) Cerebral revascularization during barbiturate coma in primates and humans. Surg Neurol 17:111–115
9. Sundt TM Jr, Whisnant JP, Fode NC, et al. (1985) Results, complications, and follow-up of 415 bypass operations for occlusive disease of the carotid system. Mayo Clin Proc 60:230–240
10. The EC-IC Bypass Study Group (1985) Failure of extracranial-intracranial arterial bypass to reduce the risk of ischemic stroke: Results of an international randomized trial. N Engl J Med 313:1191–1200

Investigation of the Cerebrovascular Reserve Capacity to Identify Patients with Chronic Brain Ischemia Who May Benefit from Bypass Surgery

P. Schmiedek, T. Kreisig, E. Moser, G. Leinsinger, and K. Einhäupl[1]

In response to the result of the EC-IC bypass study [8], which failed to show any benefit for the prevention of cerebral ischemia in the surgical group, it has been argued that surgery has been overused. Accordingly, it has been suggested that only so-called hemodynamic cases, with a decreased cerebral perfusion pressure due to insufficient collateral blood supply, should be candidates for cerebral revascularization. The identification of these hemodynamic cases, however, is not possible when using clinical criteria and is still difficult on the basis of diagnostic studies such as angiography or CT scanning of the brain. Positron emission tomography (PET), on the other hand, which undoubtedly provides superior information on cerebral circulation and metabolism is not readily available. Therefore, we have used regional cerebral blood flow (rCBF) studies, under stimulated conditions with the Diamox test, in order to investigate the regulatory capacity of the cerebral circulation [7]. These studies were performed before and after bypass surgery in order to find out whether there was any improvement of the cerebrovascular reserve capacity following surgery which could then be regarded as evidence in support of the beneficial effect of the operation in these patients.

Material and Methods

Thirteen patients were included in this study. According to their clinical and angiographic findings, all patients were thought to be candidates for extra-intracranial (EC-IC) bypass surgery and all were subsequently operated on. RCBF measurements were performed preoperatively and then repeated during the early and later postoperative period. In addition to flow studies under resting conditions, measurements were repeated 20 min following the intravenous injection of 1 g Diamox. The difference between the Diamox-induced rCBF increase and the resting rCBF was used to determine the cerebrovascular reserve capacity (CRC) and was calculated in ml/100 g/min. For measurement of rCBF, the xenon-133 inhalation technique with a rapidly rotating detector system with 64 seperate NaI crystals was used. Details of this single photon emission tomography (SPECT) technique have been previously published [1, 4]. With this method, rCBF can be measured simultaneously from three separate brain slices which are parallel to the orbitomeatal line and centered 1.5 and 9 cm above it. Each study lasted 4 min with 1 min for Xe-133 inhalation and 3 min for monitoring of isotope washout. The rCBF is then calculated from the sequence of four 1-min tomographic images, using a conventional algorithm. In this study, only flow measurements of the middle slice were taken into consideration, thus reflecting primarily blood flow within the area of the middle cerebral artery. At the conclusion of each study, the arterial pCO_2 was measured as well.

Results

According to the results of rCBF studies (Figs. 1, 2), the 13 patients could be divided into two groups. In the first group of seven patients, rCBF under resting conditions increased slightly postoperatively. Values of cerebrovascular reserve capacity (CRC), however, increased from 6.3 ± 5.0 ml/100 g/min to 10.2 ± 9.4 ml/100 g/min (early postoperative), to 14.7 ± 7.2 ml/100 g/min (late postoperative). In the second group of five patients, resting flow values again did not reveal any significant change postoperatively. However, in contrast to the first group, these patients had a comparatively higher CRC preoperatively with a mean of 12.0 ± 7.9 ml/100 g/min. Following surgery, a slight decrease of CRC was noted from

[1] Departments of Neurosurgery, Radiology and Neurology, Klinikum Grosshadern, University of Munich, Munich, Federal Republic of Germany

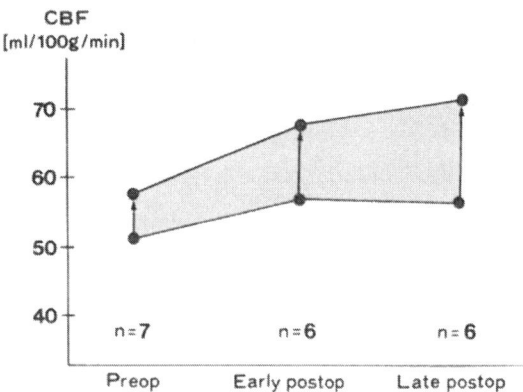

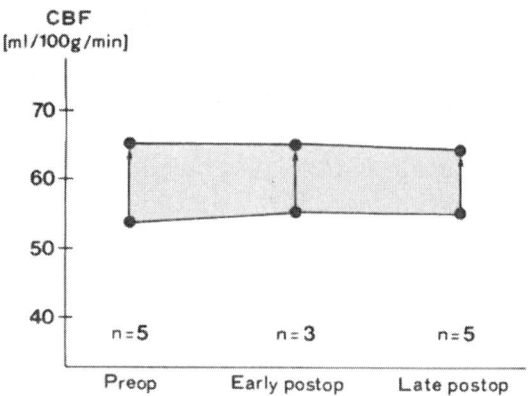

Fig. 1. Preoperative and postoperative CFB of group I. *CBF* cerebral blood flow

Fig. 2. Preoperative and postoperative CBF of group II. *CBF* cerebral blood flow

10.0 ± 9.6 ml/100 g/min (early postoperative) to 8.0 ± 6.4 ml/100 g/min (late postoperative). Except of preoperative CRC values, both groups were comparable with regard to clinical data, graft patency (evaluated by transcranial Doppler technique) and also with regard to the postoperative course.

Comments

Although the results of this study were derived from only a limited series of patients and from a retrospective analysis of data, they may be of some significance for the ongoing controversy concerning the value of EC-IC bypass surgery. RCBF studies under resting conditions, which have been reported repeatedly from patients with EC-IC bypass surgery, have been generally disappointing, because either no or only small and transient changes of rCBF were seen following surgery [3, 5]. The preliminary results of this study, however, suggest that, in a selected group of patients, a measurable effect of bypass surgery on cerebral hemodynamics can be shown, namely an increase of the CRC. Whether this finding is in accordance with recent PET studies, where a decrease of cerebral blood volume was found following bypass surgery, remains at present speculative [2, 7]. If, in this setting, an increase of the CRC would be associated with a decrease of the cerebral blood volume, then this would mean that similar or even identical information could be obtained with both techniques. This then might be of practical importance, because access to rCBF studies is certainly easier as compared with PET. Moreover, our results indicate that the CRC will increase more in those patients with a low preoperative CRC. There-

fore, the Diamox test may turn out to be useful in identifying patients according to their CRC who may be appropriate candidates for cerebral revascularization. This predictive value of the Diamox test for successful bypass surgery needs further confirmation, possibly by PET studies in addition to rCBF studies, under stimulated conditions.

References

1. Büll U, Moser EA, Schmiedek P, Leinsinger G, Kreisig T, et al. (1984) Dynamic SPECT with 133 xenon: Regional cerebral blood flow in patients with unilateral cerebrovascular disease: Concise communication. J Nucl Med 25:441–446
2. Gibbs JM, Wise RJS, Thomas DJ, et al. (1987) Cerebral hemodynamic changes after extracranial-intracranial bypass surgery. J Neurol Neurosurg Psychiatr 2:140
3. Halsey JH, Morawetz RB, Blauenstein UW (1982) The hemodynamic effect of STA-MCA bypass. Stroke 13:163–167
4. Henriksen L, Lassen NA, Paulson OB, Rommer P (1980) Evaluation of a new multi-crystal ECT system. Nucl Med 22–24
5. Meining G, Ulrich P, Köster E, Schürmann K (1983) Ergebnisse der atraumatischen Hirndurchblutungsmessung mittels Xenon-Inhalation nach EC/IC-Anastomose. Akt Neurol 10:208–211
6. Leblanc R, Tyler JL, Mohr G, et al. (1987) Hemodynamic and metabolic effects of cerebral revascularization. J Neurosurg 66:529–535
7. Vorstrup S, Henriksen L, Paulson OB (1984) Effect of acetazolamid on cerebral blood flow and cerebral metabolic rate for oxygen. J Clin Invest 74:1634–1639
8. The EC/IC Bypass Study Group (1985) Failure of extracranial-intracranial arterial bypass to reduce the risk of ischemic stroke: Results of an international randomized trial. N Engl J Med 313:1191–1200

Bypass Surgery: Indication, Timing, and Effectiveness

W. Richard Marsh and Thoralf M. Sundt, Jr.[1]

While the value of extracranial to intracranial (EC-IC) bypass operations in conjunction with planned major cerebral vessel occlusions for the treatment of aneurysms and tumors remains well-recognized, the usefulness of such surgery for any atherosclerotic cerebrovascular disease is controversial. Results of the EC-IC bypass trial have led to categorical statements by the principal investigators that there is no indication for EC-IC bypass for any atherosclerotic disease of the anterior circulation. Revelations regarding large numbers of patients operated outside the trial by participating centers cast some doubt on these conclusions. It is necessary to get clinical and follow up data on the patients undergoing superficial temporal to middle cerebral artery (STA-MCA) bypass at participating centers but who were withheld from the study to assess the meaning of the cooperative study. Our own experience with bypass includes 415 STA-MCA anastomoses for atherosclerotic cerebrovascular disease in 403 patients, seven superficial temporal to superior cerebellar artery anastomoses, 41 occipital artery to posterior inferior cerebellar anastomoses, and 146 saphenous vein grafts, atherosclerotic disease, and aneurysms of the anterior and posterior circulations. Current indications, operative technique, and analysis of results are to be presented.

In the two decades since Yaşargil developed and then successfully applied an anastomosis of the superficial temporal artery to the middle cerebral artery (STA-MCA bypass), we have seen a flowering of the technique and indications for operation. After the feasibility of the STA-MCA bypass was shown, many corollary procedures were demonstrated to be technically feasible: occipital to MCA bypass, occipital to PICA bypass, saphenous vein grafts to the MCA either on the cortical surface or in the Sylvian fissure, saphenous vein grafts to the posterior circulation, and short vein grafts interposed between scalp arteries and cerebral vessels. Applications were quickly seen for conditions other than occlusive cerebrovascular disease. Base of skull tumors involving the carotid artery and giant aneurysms requiring indirect treatment were *and are* important applications of the technique.

Occlusive cerebrovascular disease, however, remained the condition where the greatest hope was seen for application. Series of large numbers of operated patients were published by Yaşargil and Yonekawa, Samson, Lee, Chater, Sundt, and others, attesting both to the low morbidity and mortality from the operation and demonstrating a high rate of graft patency. A series of 403 such patients who underwent a total of 415 STA-MCA bypass operations was published from our institution several years ago [6]. The patients harbored the usual gamut of stenotic or occlusive anterior circulation lesions and had experienced a variety of cerebral or retinal ischemic symptoms. The neurological morbidity and mortality observed was low and consistent with that achieved by other surgeons. A retrospective analysis of this surgical series was undertaken to assist in judging the worth of the operation for anterior circulation occlusive disease [9]. A subgroup of 239 patients, 187 of whom experienced focal transient cerebral ischemia, 24 experiencing mild but nondisabling ischemic stroke, and 28 experiencing transient or persistent unilateral visual impairment due to ischemia, were studied. These patients had a variety of occlusive lesions of the anterior circulation. The control group for our analysis consisted of a series of patients who had experienced cerebral ischemic symptoms and who had undergone angiography for consideration of carotid endarterectomy. The two groups were not entirely comparable, therefore, but we were unable to show any benefit of the STA-MCA bypass with regard to survival in patients who had tran-

[1] Department of Neurologic Surgery, Mayo Clinic, Rochester, Minnesota, USA

sient ischemic attack (TIA), mild stroke, or transient monocular visual symptoms. Nor was there any benefit of the operation with respect to survival free of stroke. These observations reinforced our experience and led us to conclude in 1985 that a patient with a single TIA from an internal carotid artery occlusion was not at a great enough risk of stroke to justify a bypass operation. Others had arrived at similar conclusions if we interpret correctly the decline in frequency of STA-MCA bypass operations at various centers by the early 1980s.

Later that same year, the International Bypass Study was completed and presented [2]. Seventy-one institutions from North America, Europe, and Japan participated in a study, from 1977 to 1982, in which patients with occlusive disease of the anterior circulation, meeting certain medical entry criteria, were randomly assigned to medical or operative treatment. The results were published on 7 November 1985 in the New England Journal of Medicine. The study is heralded as a model of the way to evaluate effectiveness of a surgical treatment. Its design was impeccable and the internal validity of its results are unchallenged. The investigators concluded that the EC-IC bypass procedure, using a temporal artery pedicle anastomosed to a cortical middle cerebral artery branch, could not be shown to be of value in any of the subgroups analyzed and, in fact, was detrimental in two of the subgroups studied: those with severe middle cerebral artery stenosis and those with persistence of ischemic symptoms after an internal carotid artery occlusion.

Effective early criticism of the study was largely muted by the powerful design of the study. However, a recent series of three articles in the New England Journal of Medicine suggests that the external validity, or general applicability, of the study is at least open to question [1, 3, 4, 8]. This doubt has arisen because of the acknowledgement by all participants in this dialogue of a large number of patients treated at participating institutions contemporaneously with the study who were excluded from analysis. The exact number of patients involved was unclear but may be more than 3000 according to Sundt [8]. Recall that only 663 patients were operated upon in the randomized study. Some of the patients were ineligible for medical reasons, but a substantial number were eligible by medical criteria. Advocates of the operation contend that this revelation may fatally flaw the study while the investigators state forceful arguments in

defense of the analysis. At the very least, this exchange highlights the need in any future randomized study to document patients treated contemporaneously by participants but outside a design protocol in order to assess the role of any decision bias prior to randomization.

What is the state of the EC-IC bypass now? Is there no place for the operation? Can the results of the International Bypass Study by used to increase our understanding and more effectively treat out patients? We think so.

It is clear that the indications for bypass in occlusive cerebrovascular disease are more restrictive than 10 years ago. Most patients with stenotic or occlusive lesions experiencing a single TIA or a few TIA's affecting the anterior or posterior circulation are best treated with antiplatelet therapy and control of risk factors—particularly hypertension, cigarette smoking, diabetes, and exogenous cholesterol and saturated fat. However, patients not responding to the best medical therapy and experiencing frequent hemodynamic TIA's resulting from a high-grade stenotic or occlusive lesion of the anterior or posterior circulation without significant intervening medical illness, should be considered for operation. The type of operation is unclear as the bypass study shows that the standard STA-MCA bypass is likely ineffective. Other operations have been proposed, particularly grafts which immediately provide higher flow to the anterior or posterior circulation systems [5, 7]. The technique of anastomosis of the STA to the proximal MCA discussed by Ausman is one such example. The use of short vein grafts from the temporal artery as described by Little, or long vein grafts from the carotid artery to an intracranial vessels, are other such examples.

Our own experience is with 146 long vein grafts from the extracranial carotid artery to an intracranial vessel. Seventy-nine of the patients had advanced occlusive disease of the posterior circulation, nine patients were deteriorating because of unclippable giant aneurysms of the posterior circulation, 32 patients were experiencing progressive ischemia of the anterior circulation, and 26 patients had giant aneurysms of the anterior circulation. Graft patency in the first 65 cases was 75% (Table 1). However, after significant technical changes in graft preparation—including use of a Garrett line to prevent twisting of the graft, careful attention to not overdistend the vein with heparinized saline to avoid intimal rupture, patch grafting the proximal anastomosis, and use of a running suture at the distal

Table 1. Preparation of vein vs graft patency in 146 cases from December 1979 to March 1987

	Patency (%)	Twist or kink	Poor flow through proximal vessel	Distal athero- schlerosis	Pressure from subdural	Turbulance at distal suture line	Undertermined cause	Total
Before use of Garrett line and Shiley catheter (65 cases)	74	4	5	3	1	0	4	17
After use of Garrett line and Shiley catheter (81 cases)	93	0	4	0	0	1	1	6

Table 2. Vein graft patency: anterior and posterior circulation

	No.
Patent[a]	123
Acute occlusions	19
Late occlusions (after 30 days)	4
Total	146 (patency 84%)

[a] Includes three acute occlusions which required re-operation

Table 3. Bypass vein grafts: posterior circulation

Result	Occlusive disease	Aneurysms
Excellent	51	2
Good	11	2
Poor	5	2
Death	12	4
Total	79	9

Table 4. Bypass vein grafts: anterior circulation

Result	Occlusive disease	Aneurysms
Excellent	18	17
Good	3	4
Poor	4	3
Death	7	2
Total	32	26

anastomosis—patency in the overall group is now 84% (Table 2) and is 93% in the last 81 cases. Graft flows at operation were very high, averaging 100 ml/min for posterior circulation grafts and 110 ml/min for anterior circulation grafts. Excellent or good results, including relief of deficits existing prior to operation, were achieved in more than 70% of patients with occlusive disease of the posterior circulation and 45% of those with giant aneurysms of the posterior circulation (Table 3). The four deaths and one poor result were in patients with atherosclerotic fusiform giant aneurysms, for which we have found no satisfactory treatment. Sixty-five percent of those with progressing anterior circulation ischemia and 75% of those with giant aneurysms in the anterior circulation experienced excellent or good results (Table 4). Unquestionably, the operation carries substantially more risk than the standard STA-MCA bypass, but the patients on whom the operation has been performed were neurologically unstable and progressing over hours to days, not weeks or months, prior to operation.

Another operation which may prove to have applicability in patients with middle cerebral artery stenosis and persistent symptoms on medical treatment—a group faring worse in the surgical arm than the comparable medical group in the EC-IC bypass study—is that of an on-lay patch graft to the middle cerebral artery. We have had limited experience with several patients so treated in our department, with satisfactory results to date.

In summary, in the 20 years since its development and first application, we have seen an expansion in the techniques and indications for EC-IC bypass. The International EC-IC Bypass Study has shown that the often-used indications 10 years ago are too expansive. We still feel that indication for bypass operation is present in certain cases of skull base tumor and unclippable giant aneurysm. With respect to occlusive cerebrovascular disease, we will consider operation for patients who have a highly stenotic or occlusive lesion of the anterior or posterior circulation, have frequent TIAs, progressive stroke, or "slow stroke" which likely seem hemodynamic in origin, have poor angiographic collateral, and fail to respond to the best medical therapy.

A vein graft or anastomosis of temporal artery to proximal middle cerebral artery is the procedure used. In the instance of middle cerebral artery stenosis with a patient experiencing persistent symptoms and failing to respond to anticoagulation, an on-lay patch graft of the stenotic segment may be performed. We hope that new techniques such as patch grafting of the middle cerebral artery, other intracranial microvascular reconstructive techniques, or better medical therapy will eventually emerge from the critical analysis which the International EC-IC bypass study has given us.

References

1. Barnett HJM, et al. (1987) Are the results of the extracranial-intracranial bypass trial generalizable? N Eng J Med 316:820–824
2. EC/IC Bypass Study Group (1985) Failure of extracranial-intracranial arterial bypass to reduce the risk of ischemic stroke: Results of an international randomized trial. N Eng J Med 313:1191–1200
3. Goldring S, et al. (1987) The extracranial intracranial bypass study. N Eng J Med 316:817–820
4. Relman AS (1987) The extracranial-intracranial bypass study. N Eng J Med 316:809–810
5. Sundt TM, et al. (1982) Interposition saphenous vein grafts for advanced occlusive disease and large aneurysms in the posterior circulation. J Neurosurg 56:205–215
6. Sundt TM, et al. (1985) Results, complications, and follow-up of 415 bypass operations for occlusive disease of the carotid system. Mayo Clin Proc 60:230–240
7. Sundt TM, et al. (1986) Saphenous vein bypass grafts for giant aneurysms and intracranial occlusive disease. J Neurosurg 65:439:450
8. Sundt TM, et al. (1987) Was the international ramdomized trial of extracranial-intracranial arterial bypass representative of the population at risk? N Eng J Med 316:814–816
9. Whisnant JP, et al. (1985) Long-term mortality and stroke morbidity after superficial temporal artery-middle cerebral artery bypass operation. Mayo Clin Proc 60:241–246

Follow-up Xenon Enhanced CT-CBF Measurements in Patients Treated with STA-MCA Bypass

M. Samii, E. Kohmura, K. Holl, and N. Nemati[1]

STA-MCA bypass operation has been widely performed on patients with cerebrovascular occlusive disease since its introduction. It is intended to improve cerebral hemodynamics and consequently to reduce the incidence of further strokes. In 1985, however, the EC-IC Bypass Study Group published negative results about its clinical effectiveness in patients with arteriosclerotic arterial disease in the carotid and middle cerebral arteries [1]. This result urged the reconsideration of the hemodynamic efficacy of this operation.

From November 1984 to September 1985 follow-up cerebral blood flow (CBF) measurements were performed using xenon-CT method on 13 patients who were treated with STA-MCA bypass operation. The patients' age ranged from 44 to 75 years (mean = 58.9 years). The preoperative clinical picture was mild to moderate, with completed stroke in nine cases, reversible ischemic neurological deficit (RIND) in one case, transient ischemic attack (TIA) in two cases, and in one case, cavernous sinus syndrome due to a meningioma in the cavernous sinus. Unilateral internal carotid artery (ICA) occlusion with contralateral ICA stenosis was the main angiographic finding (Table 1). The surgical indication was decided on the basis of clinical and angiographic findings.

CBF study was performed using a prototype General Electric Xe CT Imaging System combined with GE CT 9800 Scanner. The details have been described in the literature [3, 5, 6]. After two baseline scans, six enhanced scans were performed in the same level during inhalation of a 33% xenon-0_2 mixture.

For follow-up purposes, the level cutting the basal ganglia was always selected. CBF data were analysed in a precise anatomical structure by placing a region of interest on the flow image.

CBF studies were performed preoperatively (mean = 9 days before the operation), directly postoperatively (mean = 9 days after the operation), and in the follow-up period (mean = 4.8 months postoperatively). Patency of the bypass was confirmed in all cases in the follow-up study by Doppler sonography.

Changes of CBF in the follow-up period are listed in Table 2. PCO_2 was not significantly different at the follow-up study. No significant CBF change could be observed at the follow-up study ($P > 0.05$). In some individual cases, however, improvement of CBF was observed.

Case 1. This 59-year-old male who had a history of transient right hemiparesis (RIND) 3 years ago, presented to us complaining of newly developed left hemiparesis. Angiography revealed occlusion of the right ICA and high-grade stenosis of the left ICA. CT scan (Fig. 1a) showed brain atrophy and a small infarct in the left frontal white matter. A flow map (Fig. 1b) revealed severely reduced CBF throughout the right hemisphere (R: 25 ml/100 cm^3/min, L: 40 ml/100 cc/min). STA-MCA bypass was performed on

Table 1. Angiographic findings of the operated patients

	No. of patients
ICA occlusion	
With contralateral ICA stenosis	7
Without contralateral ICA stenosis	2
ICA stenosis	
Bilateral	1
Unilateral	1
MCA occlusion	1
MCA stenosis	
Bilateral	0
Unilateral	1
VA occlusion	0
No stenotic lesion	0

[1] Neurosurgical Clinic, Nordstadt Hospital, Hannover, Federal Republic of Germany

Table 2. CBF change of operated patients

CBF	Operated side		Contralateral side	
	Preop	Postop (4.8 months)	Preop	Postop
Hemisphere	44 ± 8	45 ± 7	49 ± 7	49 ± 5
ACA	42 ± 8	43 ± 10	45 ± 9	46 ± 7
MCA	44 ± 10	44 ± 7	50 ± 6	52 ± 7
PCA	45 ± 13	45 ± 10	48 ± 10	42 ± 8

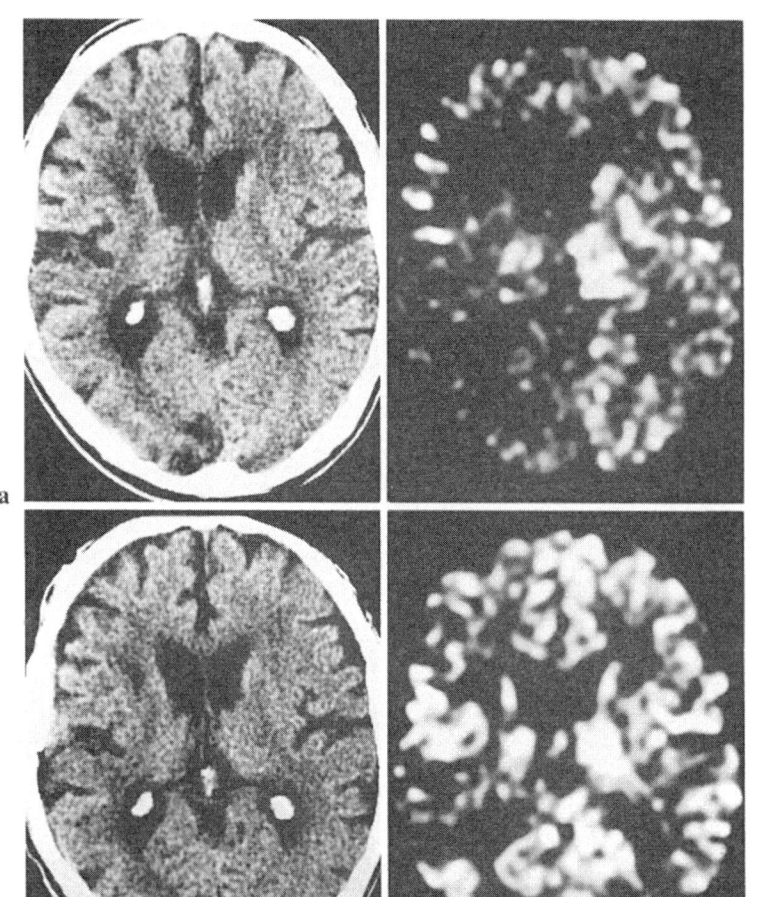

Fig. 1a–d. Case 1. **a** Preoperative CT. **b** CBF. **c** Postoperative CT. **d** CBF

the right side. Postoperative study (Fig. 1c, d) showed improved CBF (R: 39 ml/100 cm³/min, L: 51 ml/100 cm³/min).

Figure 2 shows the change of CBF ratio (symptomatic side/contralateral side) of each patient. No significant change could be observed as a whole. However, patients with preoperatively lowered CBF ratio tended to improve after the operation, and vice versa.

CBF improvement might be achieved postoperatively, if we would selectively operate on patients who have lowered CBF but relatively preserved anatomy. These results are in agreement with those of some others [4, 6]. Is there still room for the STA-MCA bypass operation in patients with cerebrovascular occlusive disease?

In the same period CBF was followed up also in 13 patients with cerebrovascular ischemic

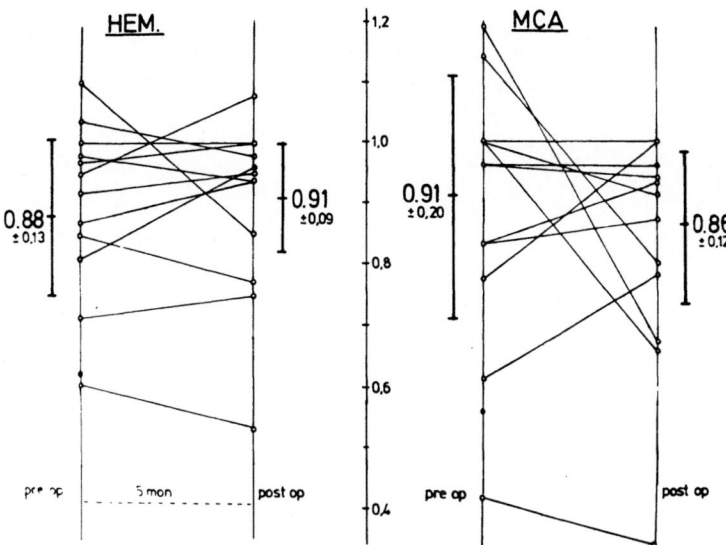

Fig. 2. Change of CBF ratio in the operated group. (symptomatic/contralateral side). No significant change was observed (paired Student's *t*-test)

symptoms, who were diagnosed as not suitable candidates for STA-MCA bypass operation. The age of patients ranged from 19 to 71 years (mean = 48 ± 14 years). Main symptoms were completed stroke in eight cases, RIND in two cases, and TIA in three cases. In this group no patient had ICA occlusion and the main angiograhical finding was ICA stenosis in six patients (Table 3). The follow-up period was almost the same as in the operated group (mean = 4.7 months). In this group as well, no significant CBF change was observed (Table 4).

In the individual case of non-operated group, however, the same tendency as the operated patients could be observed (Fig. 3). Was CBF increase after the operation achieved by the bypass?

An additionally interesting case should therefore be presented.

Case 2. This 60-year-old male, who had bilateral occlusions of the internal carotid arteries, had presented one month earlier with RIND composed of aphasia and weakness of the right arm.

CT scan showed relatively well preserved anatomical structures. A xenon CT study (Fig. 4a) showed remarkably reduced CBF in both hemispheres (R: 37 ml/100 cm³/min, L: 33 ml/100 cm³/min). STA-MCA bypass was performed on

Table 3. Angiographic findings of patients not operated

	No. of patients
ICA occlusion	
With contralateral ICA stenosis	0
Without contralateral ICA stenosis	0
ICA stenosis	
Bilateral	3
Unilateral	3
MCA occlusion	2
MCA stenosis	
Bilateral	1
Unilateral	1
VA occlusion	1
No stenotic lesion	2

Table 4. CBF change of the patients not operated

CBF	Symptomatic side		Contralateral side	
	Preop	Postop (4.7 months)	Preop	Postop
Hemisphere	51 ± 8	49 ± 6	56 ± 9	55 ± 6
ACA	49 ± 11	49 ± 9	53 ± 11	52 ± 8
MCA	54 ± 11	47 ± 10	58 ± 13	54 ± 8
PCA	47 ± 10	48 ± 10	56 ± 14	53 ± 7

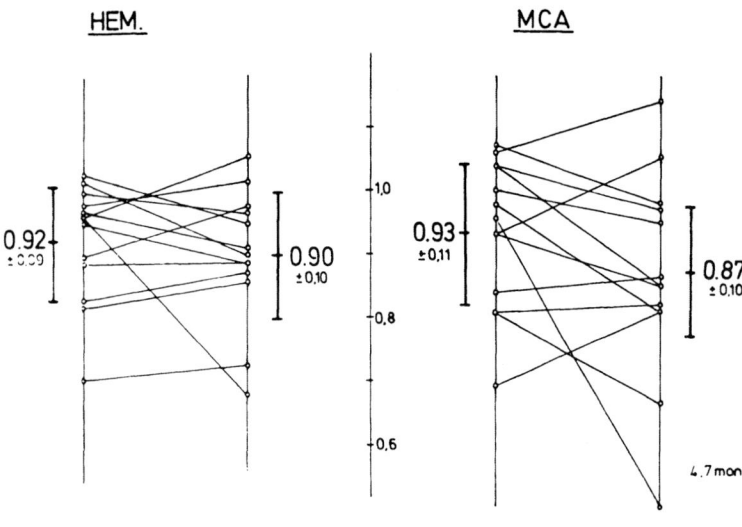

Fig. 3. Change of CBF ratio in the group not operated on (symptomatic/contralateral side). No significant change was observed (paired Student's *t*-test)

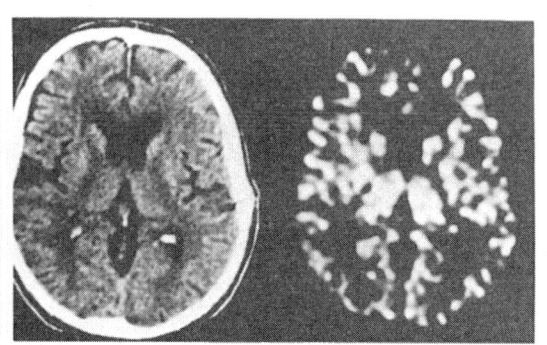

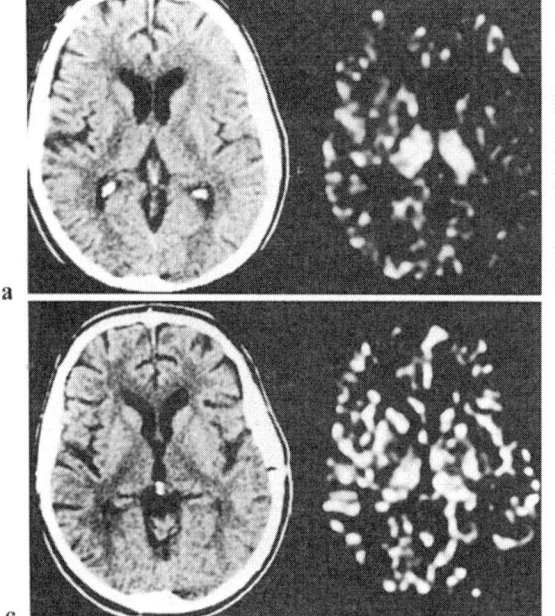

Fig. 4a–c. Case 2. **a** Preoperative study. **b** CBF study 3 months after the surgery. **c** The study under left STA compression

the left side based on his clinical symptom. CBF study 3 months later (Fig. 4b) showed a marked improvement in both hemispheres (R: 52 ml/100 cm³/min, L: 49 ml/100 cm³/min). Subsequently, we repeated CBF measurement under compression of the left STA. The patient presented no clinical change and the flow map (Fig. 4c) revealed only a small reduction (R: 45 ml/100 cm³/min, L: 45 ml/100 cm³/min).

What would happen if we had not operated on this patient?

In conclusion, our CBF study suggested that STA-MCA bypass operation cannot remarkably affect CBF at the resting state in patients with classical surgical indication, although improvement could be seen in some individual cases. The natural collateral circulation system plays a great role even after surgery, though STA-MCA bypass may improve the collateral reserve [2].

Neurosurgeons are actively engaged in selecting more suitable candidates in trying to improve results. However, we must carefully consider and evaluate the end results. A natural maturation of a collateral system might be responsible for the results, and the operation could play a moderate role in the natural history.

References

1. EC-IC Bypass Study Group (1985) Failure of extracranial-intracranial arterial bypass to reduce the risk of ischemic stroke. N Engl J Med 313: 1191–1200
2. Halsey JH Jr, Morawetz RB, Blauenstein UW (1982) The hemodynamic effect of STA-MCA bypass. Stroke 13:163–167
3. Kohmura E, Gürtner P, Holl H, et al. (1986) Erfahrungen mit der inhalation eines 33% igen xenon-(stable)-Sauerstoff-gemisches im Zusammenhang mit einer neuen methode zur lokalen Hirndurchblutungsmessung. Fortschr Röntgenstr 144:531–536
4. Schmiedek P, Gratzl O, Spetzler R, et al. (1976) Selection of patients for extra-intracranial arterial bypass surgery based on rCBF measurements. J Neurosurg 44:303–312
5. Yonas H, Wolfson SK Jr, Gur D, et al. (1984) Clinical experience with the use of xenon-enhanced CT blood flow mapping in cerebral vascular disease. Stroke 15:443–450
6. Yonas H, Gur D, Good BC, et al. (1985) Stable xenon CT blood flow mapping for evaluation of patients with extracranial-intracranial bypass surgery. J Neurosurg 62:324–333

EC-IC Bypass As a Potent Functional Collateral Circulation

Yasuhiro Yonekawa[1] and Yasunobu Gotoh[2]

Introduction

Effectiveness of extracranial-intracranial bypass (EC-IC bypass) has been hitherto reported from various points of view such as increase of regional cerebral blood flow (rCBF), improvement of cerebral metabolism and of neurophysiological function, although its effectiveness in stroke prevention could not be proven by the International Cooperative Study [5–7, 9]. This paper is to present our experience with and the importance of the EC-IC bypass as a new source of collateral circulation by analyzing the degree of postoperative hemodynamic changes over time; dilatation of the superficial temporal artery (STA) after construction of an EC-IC bypass, its feeding territory in the middle cerebral artery (MCA), and rCBF.

Materials and Methods

Around 250 bypasses have been performed for various cerebrovascular disease in the Department of Neurosurgery, Kyoto University Hospital, from 1977 through 1986. Among these patients, 60 recent patients over 30 years of age were selected for this analysis. All of these patients had atherosclerotic lesions confirmed by cerebral angiography, underwent EC-IC bypass surgery according to the criteria of case selection described elsewhere [7], and had follow-up angiography.

The diameter of the STA was measured on the angiogram and the rate of its postoperative dilatation was calculated as compared with its preoperative diameter (Fig. 1). The following branches of the postoperative feeding territory of the MCA through the STA was labelled on

[1] Department of Neurosurgery, National Cardiovascular Center, Osaka, Japan
[2] Department of Neurosurgery, Kyoto University Hospital, Kyoto, Japan

the angiogram according to a modified Ring's method [4]: (a) the orbitofrontal artery; (b) the anterior frontal artery; (c) the central sulcus artery; (d) the posterior parietal artery; (e) the angular artery; (f) the posterior temporal artery; (g) the anterior temporal artery; (h) the lenticulostriate artery.

Regional cerebral blood flow was measured with the inhalation method using ^{133}Xe. Three closely located regions of interest (ROI) were selected in the pre- and postoperative maps of rCBF and the ratio of their average values was calculated.

Results

Patients consisted of the following groups; MCA occlusion (16 cases), MCA stenosis (15 cases), internal carotid artery (ICA) occlusion (16 cases), and ICA stenosis (13 cases). All the bypasses constructed in these patients were patent as confirmed by follow-up angiography.

Dilatation of the STA over Time

Postoperative diameter of the STA increased in all but three cases during the whole postoperative course as compared with the preoperative one, amounting to 3.94 times maximally. The STA diameter decreased for a while during postoperative weeks 2 and 3 and became maximally dilated during weeks 21–30, amounting to 1.73 times on the average as compared with preoperative, diameter. Later on, the diameter tended to decrease and subsequently maintained its diameter of 1.55 times (Fig. 2).

The degree of dilatation was more remarkable in cases with stenotic lesions rather than in cases with occlusive lesions (Fig. 3): MCA occlusion 1.52 ± 0.14, MCA stenosis 1.84 ± 0.16, ICA occlusion 1.27 ± 0.05, ICA stenosis 1.63 ± 0.15, all occlusive lesions 1.39 ± 0.11, all stenotic lesions 1.74 ± 0.11

On reviewing CT scans, this tendency of STA

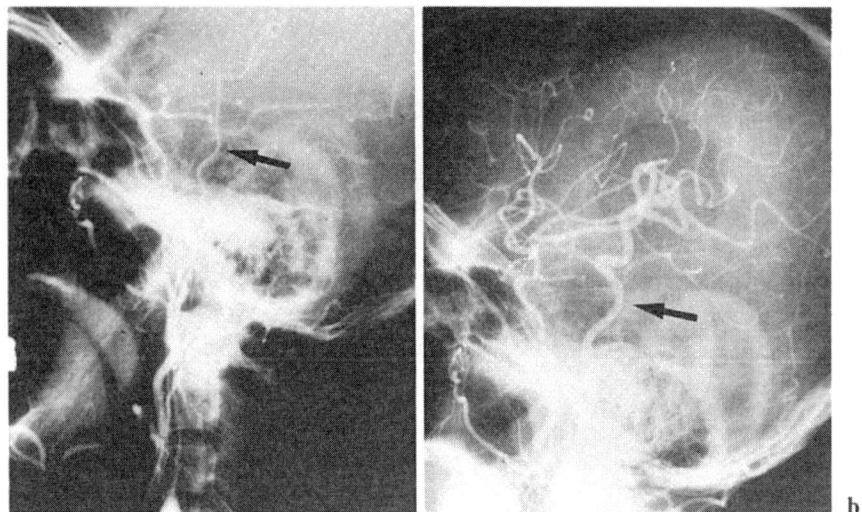

Fig. 1a, b. Postoperative dilatation of the STA. **a** Preoperative angiography. **b** Postoperative angiography. *Arrow* indicates dilatation of the STA

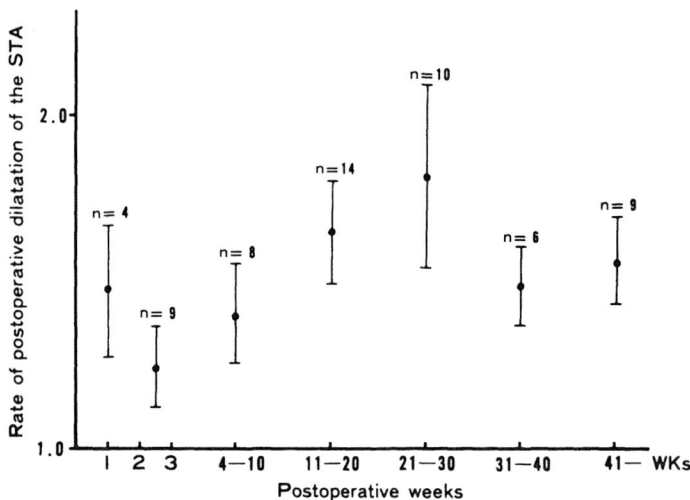

Fig. 2. Postoperative dilatation of the STA over time. Values are means $\pm$ SEM ($n = 60$)

dilatation was more marked in cases without cortical low density area (LDA) (1.72 ± 0.12) than in cases having it (1.48 ± 0.12) (Fig. 3).

Dilatation of the STA and Its Feeding Territory

The feeding territory, classified according to the method mentioned above, was labelled and its relationship to STA dilatation was plotted. A positive correlation was observed (Fig. 4).

CBF Findings and STA Dilatation

Absolute values of rCBF varied between a 25% increase or decrease postoperatively. A large proportion of patients tended to have increased rCBF during weeks 21 to 30 and later on had gradually decreased rCBF or regained preoperative values of rCBF. A positive correlation between postoperative changes of rCBF and the rate of STA dilation could not be found (Fig. 5).

Discussion

Postoperative dilatation of the STA up to three times, as compared with preoperative diameter, has been already reported at the early stage of EC-IC bypass surgery [3] and has been considered to reflect the need of the ischemic brain

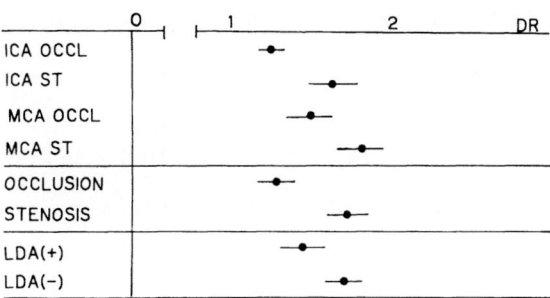

Fig. 3. Dilatation of the STA in various lesions. *DR* dilatation rate

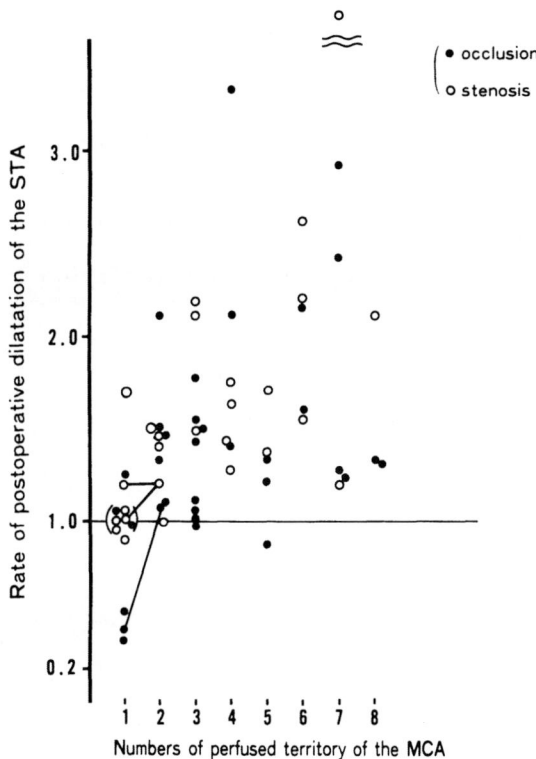

Fig. 4. Perfused territory of the MCA through the STA and STA dilatation

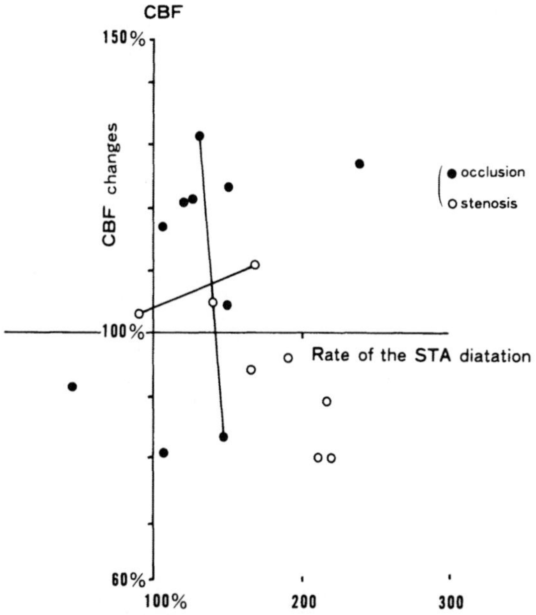

Fig. 5. CBF changes and STA dilatation

and/or is related to the pressure gradient between the STA and the MCA [2]. Our observation is considered to add a new aspect and to give some contrast to these interpretations. The degree of dilatation was rather less in cases with occlusive lesions and with cortical LDA on the CT scan than in cases with stenotic lesions and without cortical LDA. We know also from our experience that the STA does not dilate well in cases with moyamoya disease in the active phase in which cortical arterial pressure has been reported to be very low and inherent collateral circulation scarce [8].

Postoperative increase of rCBF (around 10%)

has been also reported with the peak described variously either at the 2nd week or 3rd month postoperatively [6, 9]. The degree of dilatation of the STA varied over time with its peak between the 11th and 30th weeks and stabilized later on. It correlated well with the width of the perfusion territory of the MCA through the STA but did not correlate well with postoperative increase of rCBF. Hence, the dilatation did not necessarily contribute to the increase of rCBF. This might have been caused by the fact the rCBF reflects the product of inherent collateral circulation and newly constructed bypass through the STA. Postoperative dilatation of the STA is considered rather to contribute to increasing the reserve of total collateral circulation.

The peculiarities of the behavior of the STA dilation was beyond our expectations. Dilatation of the STA is considered to result partly from the fact that blood flowing through the STA must overcome the inherent blood flow. The width of the vascular bed to be perfused and metabolic demands are considered also to play important roles in the dilatation. At any rate, a newly constructed bypass offers secure collateral circulation with an ample reserve capacity. Also, from this point of view, EC-IC bypass can not be discarded only from the results of the International Cooperative Study in which hemodynamic and metabolic study was not and could not be performed [7].

References

1. Iwata Y, Nakamura T, Hayakawa T, et al. (1985) Postoperative distribution of blood flow via the superficial temporal artery-middle cerebral artery anastomosis. Neurol Med Chir (Tokyo) 25:981–988

2. Kawase T, Tazawa T (1985) The pressure gradient and flow distribution of STA-MCA bypass. In: Spetzler RF, Carter LP, Selman WR, Martin NA (eds) Cerebral revascularization for stroke. Thieme-Stratton, New York, pp 143–147

3. Lachaw RE, Ausman JI, Lee MC (1979) Superficial temporal-middle cerebral artery bypass: A detailed analysis of multiple pre- and postoperative angiogram in 40 consecutive patients. J Neurosurg 51:455–465

4. Ring BA (1962) Middle cerebral artery: Anatomical and radiographic study. Acta Radiol (Stockholm) 57:289–300

5. Samson Y, Baron JC, Bousser MG, et al. (1985) Effects of extra-intracranial aterial bypass on cerebral blood flow and oxygen metabolism in humans. Stroke 16:609–616

6. Tanahashi N, Meyer JS, Rogers RL, et al. (1985) Long-term assessment of cerebral perfusion following STA-MCA bypass in patients. Stroke 16:85–91

7. The EC-IC Bypass Study Group (1985) Failure of extracranial-intracranial arterial bypass to reduce the risk of ischemic stroke: Results of an international randomized trial. N Eng J Med 313:1191–1200

8. Yonekawa Y, Handa H, Okuno T (1986) Moyamoya disease: Diagnosis, treatment and recent achievement. In: Barnett HJM, Stein BM, Mohr JP, Yatsu FM (eds) Stroke, vol. 2, Churchill Livingstone, New York, pp 865–829

9. Youkin D, Hungerbuhler JP, O'Conner M, et al. (1985) Superficial temporal-middle cerebral artery anastomosis: Effects on vascular neurologic and neuropsychologic function. Neurology 35:462–469

Bypass Surgery for Ischemic Cerebrovascular Disease

Akira Ogawa[1], Yoshiharu Sakurai[1], Takashi Yoshimoto[2], Motonobu Kameyama[2],
Jiro Suzuki[2], and Masatoshi Itoh[3]

Introduction

There continues to be debate about the effectiveness of and indication for extracranial to intracranial arterial bypass surgery (EIAB) as therapy for ischemic cerebrovascular disease. Particularly noteworthy are the negative conclusions drawn from the International Cooperative Study [8], which was undertaken to determine the effectiveness of such surgery in preventing the recurrence of transient ischemic attacks (TIAs) or reversible ischemic neurological deficits (RINDs). It has also been reported, however, that EIAB normalizes disturbances of cerebral hemodynamics [6, 9] and, indeed, the results of the International Cooperative Study itself did not indicate that EIAB surgery was ineffective in all varieties of ischemic cerebrovascular disease. Moreover, in light of the fact that, at an early stage following EIAB for slow progressing stroke, there is marked improvement in symptoms [7], effective results following vascular reconstruction can be expected in many patients in which ischemic symptoms have arisen due to hemodynamic mechanisms.

In the present report, we discuss the effects of EIAB, in our 18 cases of slow progressing stroke. We have also studied the cerebral blood flow (CBF) and metabolism of cases, in which bypass operations were performed for the purpose of preventing the recurrence of strokes, and we discuss the effectiveness of such surgery from the perspective of cerebral hemodynamics.

[1] Department of Neurosurgery, Stroke Center, Sendai National Hospital, Sendai, Japan
[2] Division of Neurosurgery, Institute of Brain Diseases, Tohoku University, School of Medicine, Sendai, Japan
[3] Division of Nuclear Medicine, Cyclotron RI Center, Tohoku University, Sendai, Japan

EIAB for Slow Progressing Stroke

Clinical Materials

We have performed EIAB in 18 cases of slow progressing stroke of the anterior circulation. The ages of the patients ranged from 29 to 71 years, and the responsible vascular lesions were as follows: four cases of occlusion of the internal carotid artery (ICA), two cases of ICA stenosis, seven cases of occlusion of the middle cerebral artery (MCA), and five cases of MCA stenosis (Table 1).

Indication for surgical therapy is determined as follows. On admission, patients are administered the Sendai cocktail (10 ml/kg 20% mannitol, 10 mg/kg vitamin E, and 10 mg/kg phenytoin), followed by anticoagulant therapy, administration of low molecular weight dextran, and induced hypertension therapy. If there are no improvements in neurological symptoms following such therapies, the responsible vascular lesion is identified in cerebral angiograms and, if there are no fresh low-density areas (LDAs) in CT scans which can account for the symptoms, vascular reconstruction is undertaken. The vascular reconstruction entailed anastomosis of the superficial temporal artery (STA) to the MCA in 13 cases, anastomosis of the occipital artery to the MCA in one case, anastomosis of the common carotid artery (CCA) to the MCA (using a vein graft) in two cases, and embolectomy plus STA-MCA anastomosis in two cases.

In order to study the indication for and effectiveness of the vascular reconstruction, comparisons were made of the preoperative neurological symptoms and the outcome at discharge. The Japan Coma Scale (III-3 Scale) was used to evaluate the level of consciousness, and the severity of the preoperative paresis was evaluated using DeJong's classification.

The patient's condition at discharge was classified into one of five groups: excellent (normal), good (mild neurological deficits, but normal

Table 1. EC-IC bypass for progressing stroke under administration of Sendai cocktail

Case no.	Age (yrs)	Sex	Angiographical findings	Preoperative Most severe paresis		Speech disturbance	Onset to reflow (days)	Result
				Arm	Leg			
1	29	F	Rt. IC occl	3	4	−	4	Ex
2	51	M	Rt. IC sten	3	4	−	5	Ex
3	50	M	Lt. IC sten	2	3	+	5	Ex
4	58	M	Lt. IC occl	4	2	+	2	Ex
5	64	M	Lt. M_3 sten	4	4	+	4	Ex
6	54	M	Rt. M_1 occl	3	4	−	2	Ex
7	52	M	Rt. M_1 occl	4	4	−	1	Ex
8	58	M	Lt. M_1 occl	2	2	−	2	G
9	61	M	Lt. M_1 sten	4	4	+	6	G
10	57	M	Rt. M_{1-2} sten	1	4	−	3	G
11	61	M	Lt. M_1 occl	2	3	+	1	G
12	62	M	Lt. M_2 occl	3	3	+	9	G
13	57	M	Rt. IC occl	3	4	−	5	G
14	41	M	Lt. M_1 sten	2	2	−	5	G
15	69	F	Rt. M_2 occl	2	3	−	2	F
16	51	M	Lt. M_1 occl	2	2	+	2	F
17	71	M	Rt. M_1 sten	4	4	+	6	F
18	59	M	Lt. IC occl	2	3	+	8	D

IC internal carotid artery, *M* middle cerebral artery, *Ex* excellent, *G* good, *F* fair, *D* dead

social life still possible), fair (moderate neurological deficits, normal social life not possible), poor (unable to walk even with assistance), and dead.

Results

On discharge, seven patients were in excellent condition, seven in good condition, three in fair condition, and one was dead (Table 1). Fourteen of the eighteen patients showed improvements postoperatively in the neurological symptoms which had been present preoperatively, and were capable of returning to normal social lives, a rate of improvement in neurological symptoms of 77.8%. The one fatality was due to pneumonia, giving a mortality of 5.6%. The morbidity rate was 16.7% (three of 18 cases). Among the morbid cases, one 71-year-old man underwent a CCA-MCA bypass operation using a vein graft, but suffered hemorrhagic infarction 3 weeks postoperatively and, consequently, had a fair outcome. The remaining two fair patients were cases of MCA occlusion which developed fresh emboli distally from the atheromatous occlusion. Low-density areas (LDAs) were seen in the territory of the perforating branches of the MCA, and no improvement in the symptoms was obtained. With regard to the relationship between the preoperative symptoms and prognosis, a tendency was found for severe paresis of extended duration not to improve following surgery.

CBF and Metabolism before and after EIAB

Among the cases in which EIAB was performed for ischemic cerebrovascular disease, measurements were made of the CBF and metabolism during the operation in 41 cases. Seven were cases of progressing stroke, in which vascular reconstruction was performed in the early period while symptoms were deteriorating (hereafter referred to as acute stage cases). The remaining 34 cases were patients with TIA or RIND, for which the EIAB was performed to prevent against further strokes (hereafter referred to as the chronic stage cases).

The vascular lesions in the acute stage cases were two cases of MCA stenosis and five cases of MCA occlusion. Among the chronic stage cases, there were 15 MCA stenosis cases, three MCA occlusion cases, ten ICA stenosis, and six ICA occlusion cases. These cases included 16 patients

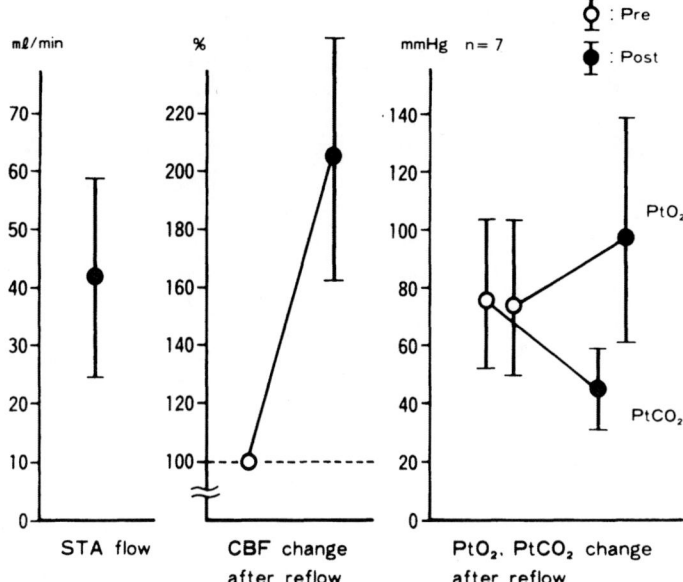

Fig. 1. Cerebral blood flow (*CBF*) and metabolism following EC-IC bypass for progressing stroke. *PtCO₂* tissue CO_2 tension, *PtO₂* tissue O_2 tension, *STA* superficial temporal artery

with TIAs, three with RIND, and 15 with minor completed strokes.

After completion of the anastomosis, a laser Doppler blood flow meter (Medpacific LD-5000) and probes (Tissue 0_2 sensor, Roche; FET tissue CO_2 sensor, Kurare) for measuring the tissue O_2 and CO_2 tension (PtO_2 and $PtCO_2$, respectively) were placed on the surface of the brain. Moreover, an electromagnetic blood flow meter (Nihon Kohden) was placed on the STA. After waiting for the stabilization of the electrode, recirculation was established, and the CBF and metabolism, before and after recirculation, was continuously recorded. Finally, by placing a pressure transducer on a branch of the STA, the STA-MCA pressure gradient was recorded.

Results

In the acute stage cases, a mean blood flow of 41.6 ± 17.5 ml/min was recorded at the STA, and the regional cerebral blood flow (rCBF) was found to increase approximately twofold. The PtO_2 was found to increase from 75 ± 30 mmHg prior to recirculation to 100 ± 39 mmHg afterwards. The $PtCO_2$ was at a high level prior to recirculation (76 ± 28 mmHg), but became normalized following recirculation (45 ± 18 mmHg) (Fig. 1). The STA-MCA pressure gradient was 84 ± 35 mmHg.

In contrast, in the chronic stage cases, the blood flow in the STA was 18 ± 16 ml/min after recirculation, and rCBF increased about 20%.

Only a small increase in PtO_2 was found (from 78 ± 20 mmHg to 80 ± 22 mmHg), and only a small decrease in $PtCO_2$ was seen (from 42 ± 12 mmHg to 40 ± 13 mmHg) (Fig. 2). The STA-MCA pressure gradient in the chronic stage cases was 44 ± 27 mmHg.

Discussion

The concept of "progressing stroke" has been advocated for neurological symptoms which progress stepwise or continuously. Although there have been reports of progressing stroke due to cardiac embolism, the vast majority are said to be due to hemodynamic mechanisms following thrombosis caused by arteriosclerosis. In fact, in our cases as well, the CBF and metabolism prior to vascular reconstruction showed high $PtCO_2$ and low PtO_2. Moreover, following recirculation and an increase in cerebral blood flow, there occurred normalization of both $PtCO_2$ and PtO_2 together with rapid improvements in neurological symptoms. The fact that the improvements in cerebral hemodynamics were accompanied by improvements in neurological symptoms clearly indicates that EIAB can be effective in cases of progressing stroke.

With regard to changes in clinical symptoms, we found that notable improvements occurred in 14 of the 18 cases (77.8%). Since it is reported that the natural course of this disorder leads to severe neurological sequelae in 64%–69% and

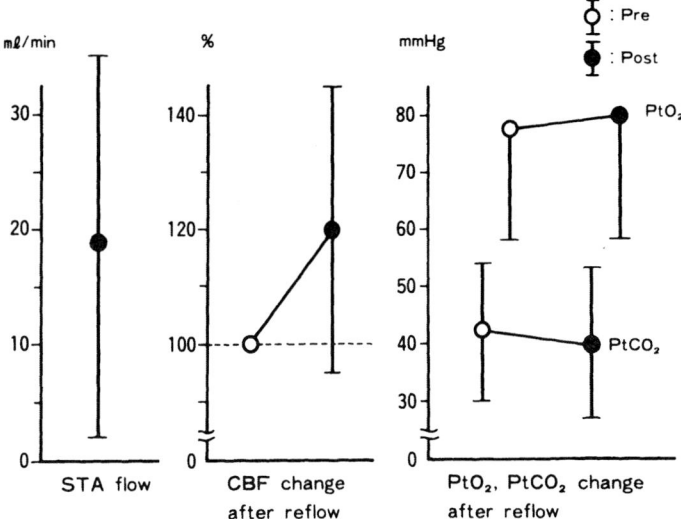

Fig. 2. Cerebral blood flow and metabolism following EC-IC bypass for prevention against further strokes. *Abbreviations* as in Fig. 1

death in 14% [5], the prognosis in surgically treated cases is clearly superior. Improvements in symptoms following EIAB in progressing stroke have previously been reported by several groups as being in the region of 50%–60% [4] and, together with our own results, we conclude that vascular reconstruction is indicated for progressing stroke.

In comparison with the reports of others on the surgical treatment of progressing stroke, our results have been favorable. One reason for this is our policy of administering brain protective substances, specifically the Sendai Cocktail, to such patients at the early stage of onset. These drugs have previously been shown to suppress ischemic changes in the brain, thus minimizing neurological sequelae.

Among those cases in which no improvements in symptoms were obtained, there was one case in which a vein graft was used for CCA-MCA anastomosis, and neurological sequelae remained postoperatively following hemorrhagic infarction. It is now thought that, in the vascular reconstruction of the already damaged ischemic brain in the acute stage of the disease, recirculation, using a high-flow bypass, should not be done. There were two other MCA occlusion cases in which improvements were not found in symptoms which had arisen postoperatively due to infarction in the region of the perforating branches. More recently, in cases with MCA occlusion, we determine the surgical method to be used once we have confirmed the condition of the occluded region. In cases where there is occlusion due to a fresh embolus located distally from the

occlusion, due to an M_1 atheroma, embolectomy is performed together with the bypass operation.

In cases where hemodynamic mechanisms are involved in the appearance of symptoms, such as progressing stroke or crescendo TIAs, the effectiveness of EIAB is evident both from the effects on cerebral hemodynamics and the improvement in clinical symptoms. It should be said, however, that the International Cooperative Study [8] was skeptical about the clinical effectiveness of EIAB undertaken to prevent recurrence in cases of TIA or RIND. There were, however, several shortcomings in that study, among which the following five points are noteworthy: (a) four-vessel study was not undertaken to determine the indication for surgery; (b) CBF and metabolism were not measured; (c) there remain uncertainties about the differential diagnosis of thrombosis and embolism; (d) the condition and selection of the recipient artery was not considered; and (e) there was no consideration of the severity of the arteriosclerosis of the donor artery, the STA, when deciding on the indication for surgery [1, 3].

In contrast, there have been many studies reporting on the effectiveness of intracranial vascular reconstruction from the perspective of cerebral hemodynamics. Cerebral blood flow, as measured by positron emission CT, has been shown to increase markedly at both cortical and subcortical sites following EIAB [9], and there has also been a report showing significant recovery of both CBF and cerebral metabolism [6]. In the present study, despite the fact that cerebral hemodynamic measurements were made during surgery immediately following the anastomosis,

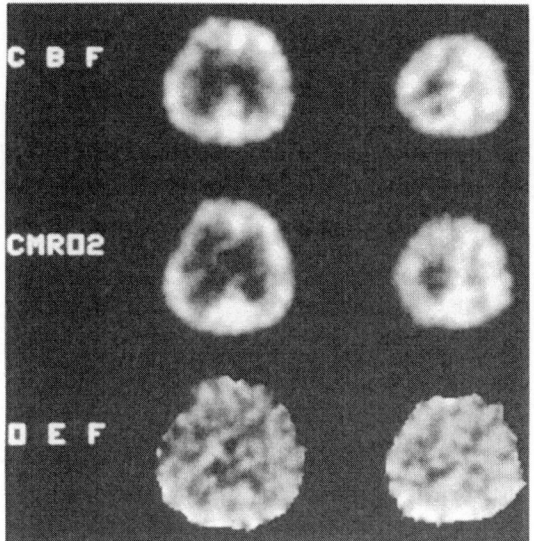 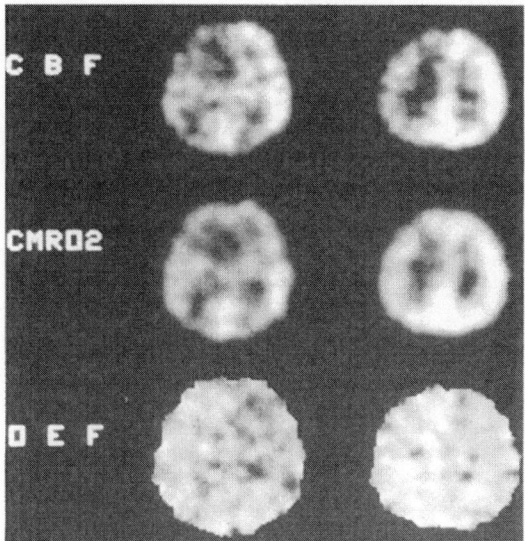

Fig. 3. Preoperative positron emission CT study on a patient with left internal carotid occlusion. Misery perfusion syndrome was observed *CBF* cerebral blood flow, *CMRO₂* cerebral metabolic rate of oxygen, *OEF* oxygen extraction fraction

Fig. 4. Postoperative positron emission CT study. Misery perfusion syndrome has disappeared. *Abbreviations* as in Fig. 3.

there was a significant 20% increase in CBF. In contrast, although the tissue oxygen and tissue carbon dioxide levels were within a normal range prior to the anastomosis, only minor changes were found following the surgery. When studied individually, it was found that, in approximately one-third of the cases, the blood flow in the STA exceeded 20 ml/min, and the increase in CBF exceeded 40%. Moreover, the STA-MCA pressure gradient averaged about 40 mmHg, and there was a considerable number of cases which showed notable effects in the cerebral metabolism. It is evident that these included a good number of cases in which the mechanism of onset of the ischemic symptoms was due to hemodynamic crisis. In the postoperative angiograms of such cases, extensive regions of the MCA were perfused from the STA. The present study was confined to the effects during surgery immediately following anastomosis. In the studies which have included sequential follow-up angiography following anastomosis, the STA has been found to become thicker and its area of perfusion to enlarge. Moreover, there have been reports indicating that there are continued improvements in oxygen consumption, glucose metabolism, and cerebral hemodynamics following surgery. Such findings suggest that vascular reconstruction in the chronic stage is effective in bringing about improvements in cerebral hemodynamics.

Finally, in positron emission CT studies, despite the fact that oxygen consumption is maintained, severe decreases in CBF have been observed. As a result, there emerges pathology indicative of high levels of oxygen extraction fraction—a syndrome which has been called the misery perfusion syndrome [2] (Fig. 3). In light of the fact that, by means of EIAB, improvements in cerebral ischemia occur and the uncoupling of cerebral metabolism and CBF disappears, we believe that there is indication for the bypass operation in such cases. In fact, in one case of this kind which we have experienced (left ICA occlusion), postoperatively, there occurred the normalization of the oxygen extraction fraction (Fig. 4). For determination of indication for surgery, study of the mechanisms of onset of the ischemic symptoms is required,using measures of cerebral hemodynamics, and it will be essential to establish a diagnostic method based on such techniques.

Conclusion

Therapeutic effectiveness following EIAB can be expected in cases of ischemic cerebrovascular disorders when the symptoms are due to hemodynamic mechanisms. Particularly for cases of progressing stroke, good results can be obtained using EIAB, both from the perspective of cerebral hemodynamics the improvement in clinical symptoms.

In contrast, in cases with TIA and/or RIND, where EIAB has been performed to prevent the further stroke, the increases in CBF following vascular reconstruction are small and the changes in tissue oxygen and tissue carbon dioxide of the cortex are also small. Nevertheless, despite the fact that measurements were made immediately following the anastomosis, approximately one-third of our cases showed marked increases in CBF and normalization of cerebral tissue oxygen and tissue carbon dioxide. In such cases, as well, good therapeutic results of the EIAB operation can be anticipated.

With regard to the indication for surgery, further study of the mechanisms of onset of ischemic symptoms is required, using techniques for measuring cerebral hemodynamics, and will be essential for the establishment of a certain diagnostic technique.

References

1. Ausman JI, Diaz FG (1986) Critique of the extra-cranial-intracranial bypass study. Surg Neurol 26:218–221

2. Baron JC, Bousser MG, Rey A, Guillard A, Comar D, Castaigne P (1981) Reversal of focal "misery-perfusion syndrome" by extra-intracranial arterial bypass in hemodynamic cerebral ischemia. A case study with ^{15}O positron emission tomography. Stroke 12:454–459

3. Day AL, Rhoton AL Jr, Little JR (1986) The extra-cranial-intracranial bypass study. Surg Neurol 26:222–226

4. Diaz FG, Ausman JI, Mehta B, Dujovny M, Reyes RA, Pearce J, Patel S (1985) Acute cerebral revascularization. J Neurosurg 63:200–209

5. Gentou E, Barnett HJM, Feields WS (1977) Cerebral ischemia: The role of thrombosis and anti-thrombotic therapy. Study group on antithrombotic therapy. Stroke 8:150–175

6. Samson Y, Baron JC, Bousser MG, Dderlon JM, David P, Comoy J (1985) Effects of extra-intracranial arterial bypass on cerebral blood flow and oxygen metabolism in humans. Stroke 16:609–616

7. Suzuki J (1987) Treatment of cerebral infarction: Experimental and clinical study. Springer, Vienna

8. The EC/IC Bypass Study Group (1985) Failure of extracranial-intracranial arterial bypass to reduce the risk of ischemic stroke. Results of an international randomized trial. N Engl J Med, 19:1191–1200

9. Yamamoto YL, Little J, Thompson C, Meyer E, Feindel W (1979) Positron tomography with krypton-77 for evaluation of topographical rCBF changes following EC-IC bypass surgery. In: Gotoh F, et al. (eds) 9th International Symposium of Cerebral Blood Flow and Metabolism, pp 522–523

Discussion

Commentator, *Gagliardi* (Florence): At the 8th International Symposium on Microsurgery for cerebral Ischemia in Florence, the following indications for EC-IC bypass were proposed: (a) The patients should have clear symptoms of anterior circulation ischemia, have failed conventional medical therapy (including antiplatelet therapy and control of risk factors), and have not suffered a major permanent neurological deficit. Other nonvascular causes for the symptoms should have been evaluated and excluded. (b) The patients should have no evidence of extensive tissue destruction on computed tomography of the brain. (c) Four-vessel cerebral angiography should demonstrate a lesion appropriate to the clinical picture and a compromised physiological collateral circulation. (d) Clinical and instrumental investigations should be strongly suggestive of hemodynamic compromise. All available diagnostic modalities (CBF, SPECT, transcranial doppler, PET, etc.) should be used to confirm the presence of hemodynamic compromise and to document the physiological response to surgical therapy. On the basis of these guidelines, since 1986 we have selected four or five patients for surgery who were suffering from recurrent TIA in spite of invasional medical therapy, antifibrinolytic, and heparin. All the patients were in a normal condition after bypass surgery and were no longer in need of medical aid. Of course, this is a small group and there has not been enough time to follow these patients up and make a conclusive evaluation. I think it is necessary to organize and develop an international registry where all cases can be gathered, followed up, and studied. Such an international registry would be the only way to evaluate the efficiency of anastamosis in selected patients.

Nakagawa (Kushiro): As mentioned by Dr. Yonekawa, I have investigated the current status of EC/IC bypass in Japan for the Japanese Neurosurgical Congress. About 900 cases of bypass surgery were performed in Japan last year; this represents 60% of the number in 1984. Dr. Ausman or Dr. Spetzler, how many cases of bypass surgery were performed in the USA last year? Has there been a decrease?

Spetzler (Phoenix): I think our decrease is much greater because the number of neurosurgeons in private practice doing bypass surgery is very small. Many of the major centers have stopped performing bypass entirely and others, like my center, have reduced the frequency a great deal. I do not know for sure, but I would say that the number is less than 10% of what was done prior to the announcement of the Cooperative Study.

Ausman (Detroit): In our center, the number went down by at least half to two-thirds.

Marsh (Rochester): I do not have the exact number for our institution, however, I would agree that it has gone down quite dramatically.

Brock (Berlin): It appears that the conclusions of the study apply to the patients included in the study. What should an institution do that has not selected its patients according to the criteria of the study? Should the institution continue as before? The conclusions of the study would not apply to this institution. I ask this question because we have always selected our patients according to different criteria and we have always performed neck surgery plus bypass in a single session when the external carotid artery required endarterectomy. We based our decision on the stump pressure following desobliteration at the neck.

Schmiedek (Munich): I think that is a difficult question because your patients still belong to the chronic cerebrovascular disease group and this group has been incorporated in the Bypass Study. You also have to consider the indications in the light of the results of the Bypass Study.

Spetzler: How does the stump pressure in the neck reflect the need for bypass?

Brock: We measure the pressure in the superficial temporal artery following endarterectomy of the neck and we see how much the increase in perfusion pressure is. We first dissect the superficial temporal artery, cannulate it, record the pressure, and then we go to the neck and we see what happens. The increase is remarkable. We do it in one session. The patients are sometimes old, and in these anesthesia presents a greater risk than the actual surgical procedure.

Samii: Is your strategy still the same after the International Study?

Brock: This is a big problem because I think that the major impact of this study was not on the neurosurgeons; it is the neurologists who no longer send us the patients. For example, in patients with discs the chances of being cured are about 95%–97%, however in the cases that are not successful the result may be a patient who after the operation is unable to speak whereas he was able to speak before surgery. This makes me reluctant to perform the operation.

Samii: I do not agree completely. Each of us has had this experience after bypass. However, we are not evaluating the immediate results of bypass surgery, we are looking at the developments after several years. In the cases I presented with bilateral carotid occlusion, there was strong reduction of CBF on both sides and the patient had aphasia and paresis on the right side. This was after the International Study. As a result of the CBF measurements, I decided to operate on this patient and I perfomed a left-sided cerebral bypass. Three months later, the patient had normal cerebral circulation; CBF was normal on both sides. I compressed the superficial temporal artery and I saw no change. Of course I do not attempt to operate on the other side when the patient already has good collateral circulation. So, personally, I am still confused.

Brock: It could be that with this bypass you gave the patient time to develop the collateral circulation. This being the case, it would make surgery a valid step.

Almefty (Jackson): What would the panel do if they had a patient who fulfilled the criteria of the study; they do not do EC/IC, put the patient on medical treatment, but the patient continues to be symptomatic? Would the panel then consider doing EC/IC?

Yonekawa (Osaka): We would do bypass surgery. Before that we would obtain CBF findings to confirm the hemodynamics.

Marsh: Unquestionably, bypass surgery would be considered. We would not conduct any other ancillary tests at the point.

Spetzler: I do not think that there is a quick answer here. We would look at the angiogram and see if there is anything in the common carotid artery. If after administering aspirin and stumpectomy the patient is still symptomatic, we carry out the Xenon- CT scan with the diamox test. About 10% of those patients have shown a decrease in flow that has been aggravated by the dimox and such patients we would consider candidates for bypass surgery.

Ogawa (Sendai): In our series, progressing stroke showed good recovery of the neurological deficits. In other words, progressing stroke caused by hemodynamic factors is considered to be a good indication for bypass surgery. However, in cases of TIA or RIND, it is important to determine whether the symptoms are related to the hemodynamics. We have to be very careful in differentiating whether the symptoms are due to hemodynamic mechanisms, small-vessel disease, perforating artery lesions, thrombolism, or embolism.

Samii: I do not think that our clinical and neurological techniques are sufficient to provide us with a secure answer to the main question. But I believe that with a superselective functional angiography, which will probably be developed soon, in combination with cerebral blood flow we will perhaps be able to select patients much better for bypass surgery than at present. I personally am still a little confused as to the indications for bypass.

Schmiedek: At our institute, we would seriously consider this patient for bypass surgery.

Brock: I think this is like operating on aneurysms in grade V: There is nothing to be gained by waiting; the surgeon must do something.

Ausman: I think the crux of the matter is that we are dealing with a disease of unknown etiology: We do not know in any individual patient if the cause is embolic or hemodynamic. We do not know the natural history and yet we must treat the patient. We are looking for the appropriate indications.

Raja (Maltan): Since Dr. Barnett's important paper of 1985, there has been a great deal of discussion and Dr. Ausman has succinctly described the present position. We are now trying to establish the true indications for operating on patients with cerebral stroke. I think that prior to release of the results of the International Studies presently examining this problem, those results should be reexamined by a second or third body. These studies will have a tremendous impact on clinical practice and I believe, therefore, it is in the interests of the patients that such checking of the results be carried out.

Sengupta (Newcastle): Before the recent paper was published in the New England Journal of Medicine, there were some criticisms about the validity of the trial. The journal suggests that the trial taken by itself with the population of patients and methods used is valid, but that it is now necessary to investigate those patients who did not appear in the study. What does the panel think about this?

Spetzler: I am not sure that what was written in the New England Journal of Medicine has made a great deal of difference to me. We tried to enter all our patients at Case Western Research into the study. One of our neurologists described a patient as having crescendo TIA with middle cerebral artery distribution. I was out of town at the time. The neurologist determined that the patient was in too critical a condition to be entered into the study and so the patient was managed outside the study. This well illustrates my belief that the same criteria were not always applied as to which patients should be included in the study and which should be left out: However, the great majority of patients we operated upon in what I may term our "enthusiastic" stage were the same ones we randomized in the study. We all had patients who showed tremendous progress. I think perhaps that there are some patients who we should not have put into the trial in the first place; they represent a very small minority of patients, but in these revascularization is appropriate hemodynamically, physiologically, and in terms of patient care. Caution has to be exercised here not to perform bypass on every patient with an angiographic lesion unless operative morbidity and mortality are to be reduced to zero.

Almefty: In bypass for a tumor or giant ameurysm to prevent occlusion of a major vessel, how many times was the operation successful and how often did patients suffer infarction despite a functioning bypass?

Yonekawa: Dr. Debrun reported recently that he performed EC-IC bypass in cases with intolerable balloon Matas test but that half became tolerable after the procedure. We have the same experience.

Spetzler: I think it depends on whether the case is a tumor where there are other possible causes of the various problems—middle cerebral artery occlusion, internal caotid artery occlusion, etc. I think the best results are with middle cerebral artery occlusion because the amount of dead space from where the artery is occluded is very small until the next branch. This is in contrast to the internal carotid artery occlusion, which despite a good bypass can have a delayed ischemic event occurring 3–4 days afterward; the latter is I believe an extension of the embolus. However, I think there is no doubt on the basis of experiments and clinical studies that the patient with middle cerebral artery distribution benefits from having had an occlusion before the bypass.

RTD 4. Nonsurgical Treatment for AVMs

Stereotactic Heavy-Particle Irradiation of Intracranial Arteriovenous Malformations

Yoshio Hosobuchi[1]

Introduction

Microsurgical techniques have made more feasible the total excision of arteriovenous malformations (AVMs) located in previously inaccessible areas of the brain, and with acceptable rates of morbidity and mortality. Nonetheless, there are still many AVMs that cannot be treated surgically, either because they are located deep within the brain or because of their enormous size or relatively benign clinical presentation. From September 1980 to December 1984, we treated 75 patients who had AVMs of this particular group with combined methods of intraluminal embolization, surgical occlusion of the arterial feeding vessels, and/or partial excision of the AVM, followed by stereotactic heavy-particle irradiation.

Materials and methods

Of 75 patients, 44 were female. The age range was 4–72 years, with a median of 32 years. The various locations of the AVMs are shown in Table 1. The majority of the patients had one or more hemorrhages as a presenting symptom (Table 2), although they generally showed minimal neurological deficit. Over 30% of the patients suffered from a chronic intractable headache of long duration requiring a significant quantity of opiate medication. The primary goal of embolization and surgery was to reduce the size of the AVM and the flow through it. A stereotactic irradiation treatment plan was developed based on a modified Leksell system [1]. A beamline configuration with the Bragg ionization peak of the 230 MeV/u helium-ion beam was generated using Lawrence Berkeley Laboratories' 184-in. synchrocyclotron (Berkeley, CA-USA) [1]. Total doses of 45 Gy equivalent are delivered to treat an area about 12 mm^3 to 35000 mm^3; average volumes in most patients treated ranged from 5000 mm^3 to 15000 mm^3. Total treatment was delivered within 1–3 days using one to six entry portals.

Results

The effects of treatment in this group of patients were reviewed in February 1987. Follow-up ranged from 26 to 78 months after radiation treatment. Every effort was made in all patients

Table 1. Location of AVM

Location	No. of patients
Frontal	8
Parietal	15
Temporal	3
Occipital	3
Thalamus	12
Basal ganglia	12
Hypothalamus	2
Vein of Galen	4
Cerebellum	11
Brain stem	1
Spinal cord	1
Carotid-cavernous fistula	3
Total	75

Table 2. Presenting history

Symptoms and signs	No. of patients	Percent
Hemorrhage without neuro-logical deficit	47	62
With neurological deficit	20	26.7
Chronic headache	27	36
Seizure	14	18.7
Progressive neurological deficit	6	8.0

[1] Department of Neurological Surgery, School of Medicine, University of California, San Francisco, California, USA

Table 3. Results of heavy particle irradiation of AVM: Review of 76 patients treated September 1980–December 1984 (February 1987)

Year	No. of Patients	Degree of thrombosis		
		Total (%)	>50% (%)	<50% (%)
1980	2	1 (50)	1 (50)	0
1981	5	3 (60)	1 (20)	1 (20)
1982	16	13 (81.25)	3 (18.75)	0
1983	30	16 (53.3)	9 (30)	4 (16.7)
1984	22	9 (40.9)	8 (36.4)	5 (22.7)
Total	75	42 (56)	22 (29.3)	11 (14.7)

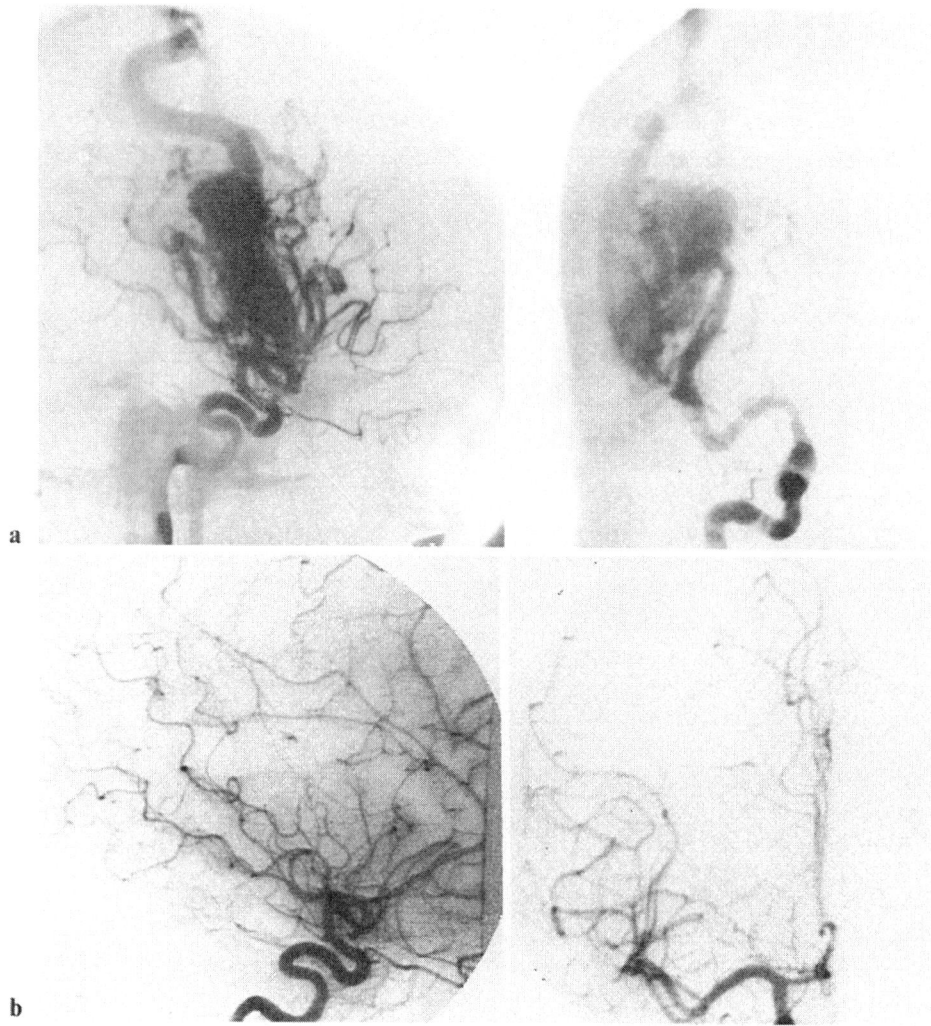

Fig. 1. a Lateral view of the right internal carotid arteriogram showing a large AVM in a 34-year-old female. She experienced two hemorrhages without any neurological deficit. **b** Lateral view of the right internal carotid arteriogram from the same patient 24 months following heavy-particle irradiation treatment

to obtain follow-up arteriograms and CT scans every 12 months for evaluation, until total thrombosis occurred. All 75 patients have been followed. The majority of AVMs began to decrease in size and flow after 12 months; in some patients total thrombosis occurred by the end of the second year after radiation therapy, although in other patients total thrombosis has not occurred even after 3 years (Table 3). At the end of February 1987, 54% of patients showed total thrombosis of their AVMs, 33% with over 50% thrombosis; 13% had less than 50% of their AVM thrombosed. It has been especially gratifying that patients who presented with relatively benign clinical history responded well to this mode of therapy (Fig. 1).

The complications of treatment are listed in Table 4. There was one death due to recurrent hemorrhage occurring within 12 months of treatment.

Conclusion

Stereotactic irradiation appears to be effective in causing partial or complete thrombosis of AVMs that are not surgically resectable. Use of heavy particles generated in cyclotron allows better spatial definition and dose-distribution than do other methods, allowing larger AVMs to be treated [1–3]. From these preliminary results, it is evident that heavy-particle irradiation therapy, like proton-beam therapy, does not offer protection from recurrent hemorrhage for at least 12 months, nor is it devoid of major complications.

Table 4. Complications

	No. of patients
Recurrent hemorrhage (3 occurred within 12 months of treatment, 1 occurred 34 months after treatment)	4 (1 death)
Worsening of neurological deficit (all occurred 12–23 months after treatment)	4
Sudden massive thrombosis of large AVM (2 with temporary obstructive hydrocephalus, 1 with diencephalic coma)	3

However, it does offer a noninvasive mode of therapy for AVMs that are difficult to treat surgically.

References

1. Fabricant JI, Lyman JT, Hosobuchi Y (1984) Stereotactic heavy-ion Bragg peak radiosurgery: Method for treatment of deep arteriovenous malformations. Br J Radiol 57:479–490
2. Kjellberg RN, Hanamura T, Davis KR, Lyons SL, Adams RD (1983) Bragg-peak proton beam therapy for arteriovenous malformations of the brain. N Engl J Med 309:269–274
3. Steiner LS (1984) Treatment of arteriovenous malformations by radiosurgery. In: Wilson CB, Stein BM (eds) Intracranial arteriovenous malformations. Williams and Wilkins, Baltimore, pp 295–313

Nonsurgical Treatment for AVMs

Van V. Halbach, Randall T. Higashida, and Grant B. Hieshima[1]

The treatment of choice of small symptomatic cerebral arteriovenous malformations (AVMs) in noneloquent regions is neurosurgical resection. In selected regions (deep structures, eloquent areas), the morbidity and mortality associated with surgical resection may exceed the risk from the disease itself. In selected patients, transvascular embolization may be of benefit in alleviating the symptoms or reducing the risks of the disease. Decisions as to the timing and type of treatment are complex and should by made by a team of neurologists, neurosurgeons, radiologists, and radiotherapists. Relatively few patients at our institution are treated by embolization alone; rather a combination of preoperative, intraoperative, and preradiation embolizations are far more common. A few of the more common indications for embolization are delineated below.

Headache

While there is an increased incidence of migraine headaches associated with cerebral AVMs, especially located in the occipital lobes, nonmigranous headaches are common. Patients with AVMs who have severe unilateral, pulsatile headaches often demonstrate significant dural supply to the AVM or have venous outflow obstruction, which places the draining veins and nidus under increased pressure. Embolization of the dural supply is safe and often alleviates the headaches. In patients with venous outflow restriction, diminishing the size of the nidus with embolization often relieves the headaches.

---

[1] Department of Radiology and Neurological Surgery, University of California Hospitals, San Francisco, California, USA

Progressive Neurological Deficits

In patients with cerebral AVMs and progressive neurological deficits unrelated to prior hemorrhage, there are many etiologies. Large AVMs in close proximity to eloquent regions may develop deficits or seizures secondary to cerebral ischemia in adjacent normal parenchyma. These patients are at high risk of developing normal perfusion pressure breakthrough following surgical resection or aggressive embolization. Staged embolization can often recover the associated deficits. Other potentially treatable sources of progressive deficits include mechanical compression from arterial aneurysms, venous varices, or draining veins. Venous hypertension transmitted to normal draining veins can result in neurological dysfunction. Increased venous pressure in the lateral sinuses can lead to decreased CSF absorption and cause elevated intracranial pressure. This can often be improved by embolization to reduce the flow to the nidus.

Hemorrhage

Complete obliteration of cerebral AVM by embolization is rare. It is unknown whether subtotal obliteration of cerebral AVMs by transvascular embolization lowers the risk of hemorrhage, and some preliminary reports with both particulate and liquid adhesives suggest an increased risk of hemorrhage following embolization. Therefore, our current goal is to try to identify the source of the hemorrhage and direct our treatment to the specific cause. Of the patients referred to our institution with a history of hemorrhage secondary to cerebral AVM, approximately 33% demonstrate an aneurysm within the nidus. These structures are small, seen on early arterial-phase angiograms, and may represent pseudoaneurysms which are actually the point of rupture of the

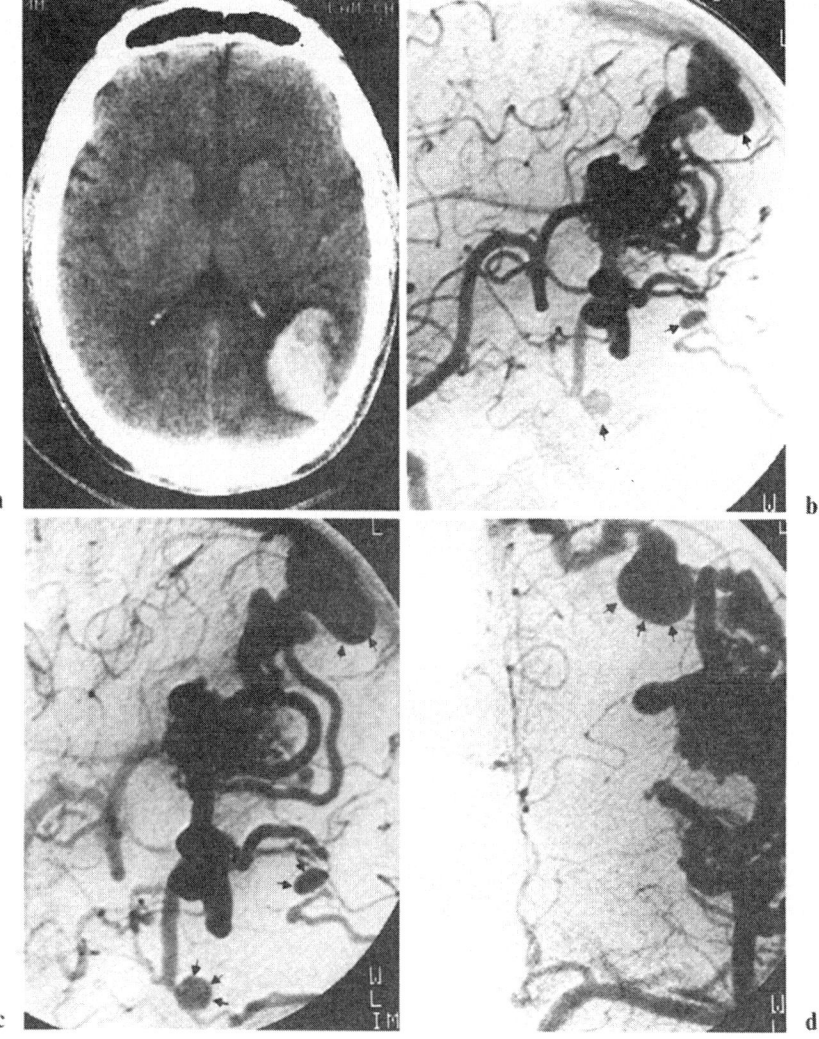

Fig. 1. a Non-contrast CT shows a parietal lobe hematoma. **b, c** Early and late arterial phase, internal carotid angiogram demonstrates a small AVM with venous occlusion and venous varices in draining veins. Note the late washout of contrast material. **d** AP view shows the varix in the draining vein to the superior sagital sinus. *Arrows* indicate the varices

nidus. Obliteration of these structures decreases the risk of subsequent bleeding. A large percentage of patients who hemorrhage demonstrate venous outflow obstruction. Figure 1 is from a 60-year-old man who presented with intraparenchymal hematoma. The angiogram demonstrates venous occlusions. Possible etiologies include mechanical kinking of the veins, or thrombosis or vascular damage to the drainage veins. This acquired venous occlusion places the draining vein and nidus under high pressure and increases the risk of hemorrhage. Severe venous occlusive disease is often associated with venous varices, aneurysms, or pseudoaneurysms. Diminishing the flow by embolization of the nidus may decrease the risk of hemorrhage; however it may also promote further thrombosis within the venous drainage and aggravate symptoms. Arte-

rial aneurysms in both common and uncommon locations in feeding arteries can cause hemorrhage. If neurosurgical procedures fail to alleviate the aneurysm, ballon occlusion of the aneurysm can be performed. Figure 2 is from a patient with repeated episodes of posterior temporal hemorrhages. The angiogram demonstrates a lobulated aneurysm. A ballon was positioned across the aneurysm and detached without deficits. The patient had no further episodes of hemorrhage.

Diminishing Nidus Size

The effectiveness of radiation therapy in diminishing nidus size is inversely proportional to the size and flow rate in cerebral AVMs. Transvas-

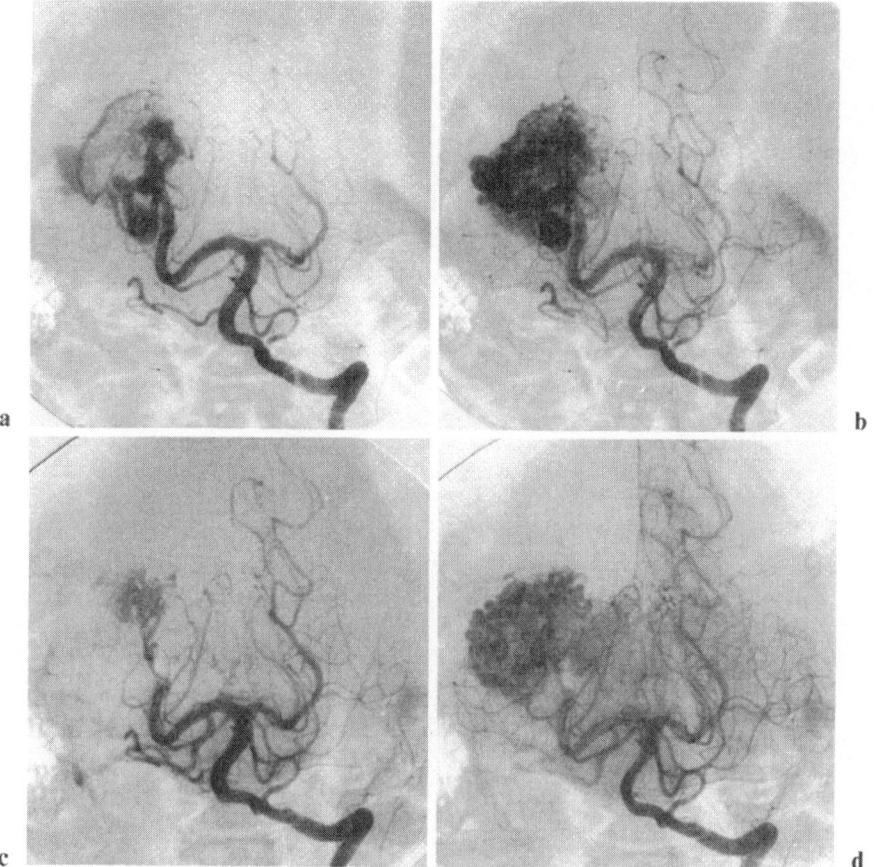

Fig. 2. a Vertebral artery injection, early arterial phase, shows a lobulated aneurysm located in the posterior temporal AVM. **b** Later phase shows the nidus of AVM. **c, d** Early and late phase angiogram shows obliteration of the aneurysm

cular and intraoperative embolization can decrease the size and flow to an AVM and improve both surgical and radiation therapy.

Surgical Adjunct

Preoperative embolization may make subsequent surgical resection technically easier and safer. Staged embolization will decrease the risk of normal perfusion pressure breakthrough and reduce nidus size and pressure. If a large feeding pedicle arises deep into the nidus, surgical resection may be difficult, especially if large draining veins lay superficial to this structure. Ligation of these veins may cause nidus rupture unless the major arterial feeders are occluded. In many cases, a detachable silicone balloon can be placed in the deep arterial feeder prior to surgery. Test occlusion prior to detachment can be performed.

In large AVMs, the procedure is performed several days prior to surgical resection to allow the development of cerebral autoregulation. Figure 3 is from a 23-year-old female with frontal lobe hemorrhage and AVM. A large frontal polar artery supplies the AVM. Note the large superficial draining veins. A balloon was directed into the feeding pedicle and detached without deficit. The patient's surgical removal was technically easier and without incident. Both preoperative and intraoperative functional testing can be performed with Amytal or test occlusion and can define critical, eloquent regions that may alter surgical resections. Intraoperative embolization may make subsequent surgical resection easier. A postsurgical resection intraoperative angiogram may identify residual nidus.

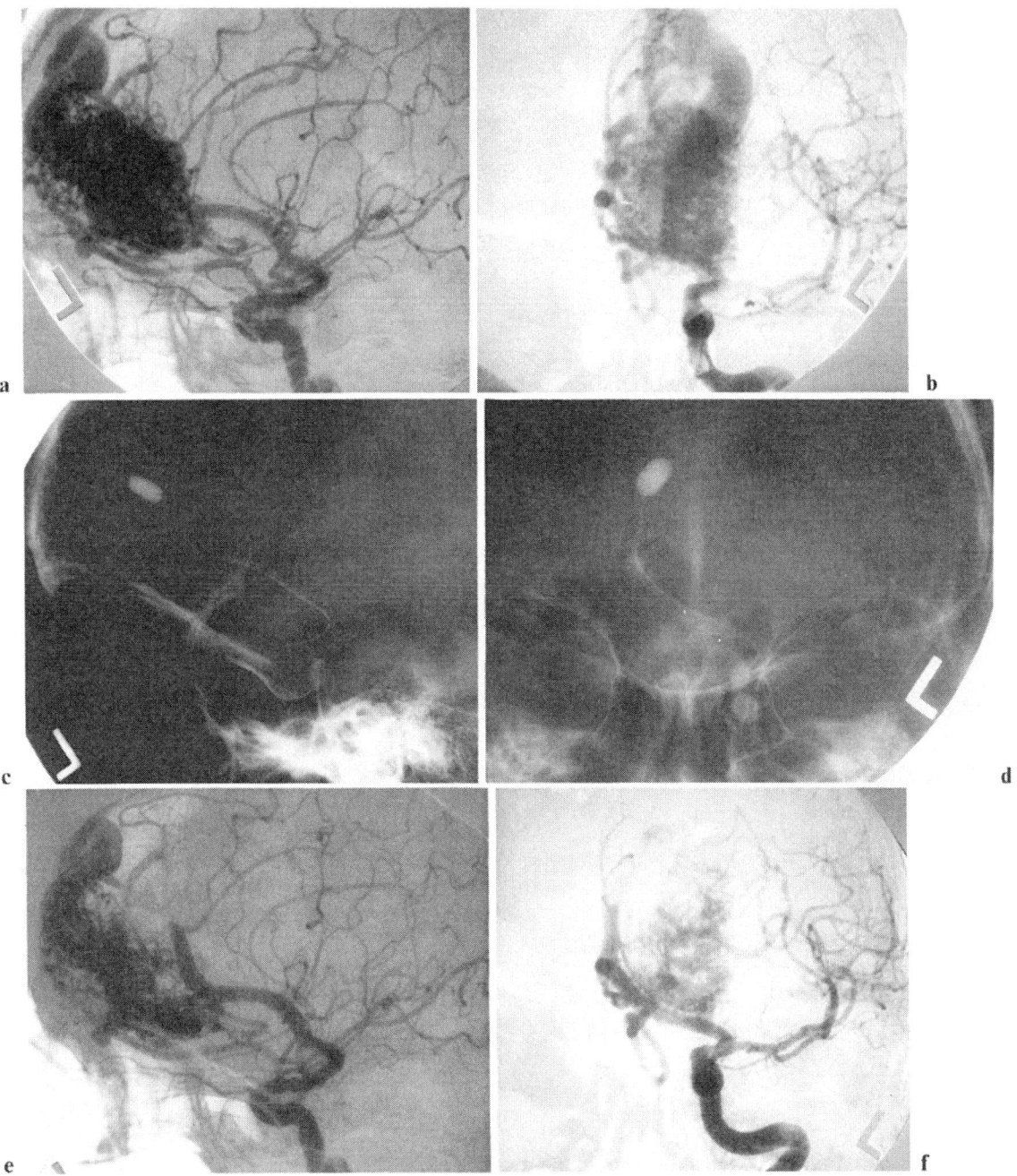

Fig. 3. a, b Internal carotid angiogram, lateral and AP view in young patient with hemorrhage. **c, d** Lateral and AP view during test occlusion of frontal polar branch supply to the AVM. **e, f** Lateral and AP view following detachment shows occlusion of the deep supply to the fistula

Conclusion

Embolization can alleviate some symptoms in selected patients. In some patients with clearly defined sources for hemorrhage, specific obliteration of that source can be of benefit. Embolization in conjunction with surgery or radiation therapy can diminish the risk from the disease. Each case deserves individual assessment of treatment risks and options, and a team approach is essential in the treatment of this difficult disease.

Aneurysmal Malformation of the Vein of Galen

Angioarchitecture, Clinical Pressentations, and Endovascular Treatment of 16 Patients Explored and/or Treated between 1983 and February 1987

P. Lasjaunias, K. TerBrugge, J. Comoy, H. Hoffman, J. Faivre, and R. Willinsky[1]

Introduction

Although rare, series of cerebral vascular malformations with dilatation of the vein of Galen (VG) have been reported for many years [3, 4, 6, 9]. However, the study of the associated anomalies of venous drainage was rarely analyzed, although its prognostic role in deep arteriovenous malformations (AVMs) was recognized for a long time [5, 8]. Imprecise anatomical and clinical analysis have led to the artificial regrouping of different lesions, making clinical and therapeutic research unreliable. From our analysis of a homogeneous series of 16 cases, for which one of us (PL) was involved between 1983 and February 1987, we have distinguished different population groups within the generic denomination of aneurysmal dilatation of the VG.

Material

Among the 16 cases reviewed, four different types of vascular lesions could be distinguished (Tables 1, 2; Fig. 1).

The AVMs of the VG. The arteriovenous shunt (nidus or direct AV fistula) was located within the wall of the VG. This type is rare, and a developmental anomaly of dural venous drainage at the VG (tentorial sinus, falcine sinus, or jugular foramen) was encountered in all our cases. The arterial supply to the AVM was mainly choroidal, and, additionly, frequently meningeal (Fig. 1c).

The parenchymal AVMs with ectasia of the VG. The arteriovenous shunt (nidus or direct AV fistula) is located in a territory of the VG tributary (Fig. 1a). The arterial pedicles of the AVM will depend on the territory in which the shunt

has developed. The posterior thalamic and tectal AVM can simulate a VG AVM. However, a characteristic angiographic feature confirms the parenchymatous nature of the lesion; transcerebral (diencephalic or mesencephalic) arterial feeders arising from the distal basilar artery (Fig. 1b). In this group, the ectasia of the VG is either developmental (mostly in pediatric forms) or acquired (mostly in adult forms). The acquired ectasias resulted from a thrombosis or stenotic kinking at the dural junction of the VG.

Developmental venous anomalies and pure dural lesions will not be considered here.

Clinical and Anatomical Discussion

Similar to dural lesion in children [1], the aneurysmal malformation of the VG (Table 3) poses two types of problems: the ectasia and the arteriovenous shunt (when it exists). The ectasia behaves like a giant aneurysm in the midst of parenchymal structures leaning dorsally on the rigid dura mater of the falx and tentorium. It acts as a pulsatile mass, compressing the aqueduct of Sylvius and thus causing a noncommunicating hydrocephalus. It is important to note that two of the spontaneous favourable evolutions in our series occurred after ventricular shunting at the hydrocephalic stage. Disappearance of the mass effect should not be expected if the aneurysmal dilatation is calcified. The arteriovenous shunt may produce three types of manifestations: systemic, local arterial, and local venous. The systemic manifestations can lead to cardiac insufficiency almost exclusively at the newborn age. In practice, there is not a simple relationship between the importance of the shunt and the presence of cardiac insufficiency. Apart from the possibly associated cardiovascular anomalies, certain newborns have a stronger cardiac status which is responsive to medical treatment, while others, with the same shunt, present with a severe cardiac failure that does not respond to medical therapy.

[1] Unité de Neuroradiologie Vasculaire, Hopital Bicetre Universite Paris XI, Le Kremlin Bicetre, France

Table 1. Aneurysmal malformation of the VG (1983–1987)

	Newborns	Infants	Adults	Total
VG AVM	5	2	0	7
Cere AVM VG ectasia	1	4	2	7
DVA + VG varix	—	—	1	1
VG DAVM	—	—	1	1
Total	6	6	4	16

VG vein of Galen, *AVM* arteriovenous malformation, *DVA* dural venous anomaly,
DAVM dural arteriovenous malformation

Table 2. Aneurysmal malformation of the VG (vascular architecture)

Vascular architecture	VG AVM	BAVM + VG ectasia	DVA + VG varix	VG DAVM
Development dural venous anomaly	+	+ (pediatric)	+	−
"Acquired" dural venous obstacle	−	+ (adult)	−	+
Cerebral parenchymatous shunt (nidus or fistula)	+	+	−	−
Transcerebral vascularization	−	In thalamotectal AVMs	−	−
Direct arteriovenous shunt within VG wall	+	−	−	+
Dural arteriovenous shunt at the VG-straight sinus junction	+ −	Possible if previous hemorrhage	−	+

+ present, − absent
BAVM brain arteriovenous malformation

In a newborn, four different scenarios can be distinguished: The first is severe cardiac failure with marked hepatomegaly into the right iliac fossa, tachycardia, edema, respiratory failure, severe hepatic insufficiency, and a poor or no response to medical treatment. These newborns are difficult to salvage even with embolization.

The second scenario is one of compensated cardiac failure or failure amenable to treatment, with frank hepatomegaly, moderate or no edema, and a tachycardia at <200/min, necessitating ventilatory assistance and fluid restriction, but stable for a few days. There is no hepatic insufficiency. With these patients, the endovascular approach gains a few months time with spectacular immediate results.

Thirdly are patients with compensated cardiac overload with moderate or absent cardiomegaly, hepatomegaly without edema, spontaneous ventilation but laboured breathing and sucking, and moderate tachycardia. An incomplete endovascular treatment permits one to wait several months or years.

In the fourth scenario, there is no cardiac effect. These patients will have the diagnosis delayed, since cranial auscultation does not represent a routine study in the newborn examination. The local arterial phenomena concern the classical and controversial steal phenomena of cerebral AVMs. These may result in an irreversible retardation of cerebral maturation, parenchymatous ischemia with cortical calcification, mental retardation, and neurological deficits. The venous constraints illustrate the effects of the venous obstacle. While the latter should theoretically protect the heart from volume overload, it actually provokes a significant retrograde hypertension in the cerebral veins. This reflux creates a retrograde congestion that compromises the hemodynamics of the cerebral capillary drainage. Non-pulsatile venous collateral circulation illustrates this phenomena. The venous reflux increases the pressure in the dural sinuses, which then compromises the CSF resorbtion, thus producing a communicating hydrocephalus.

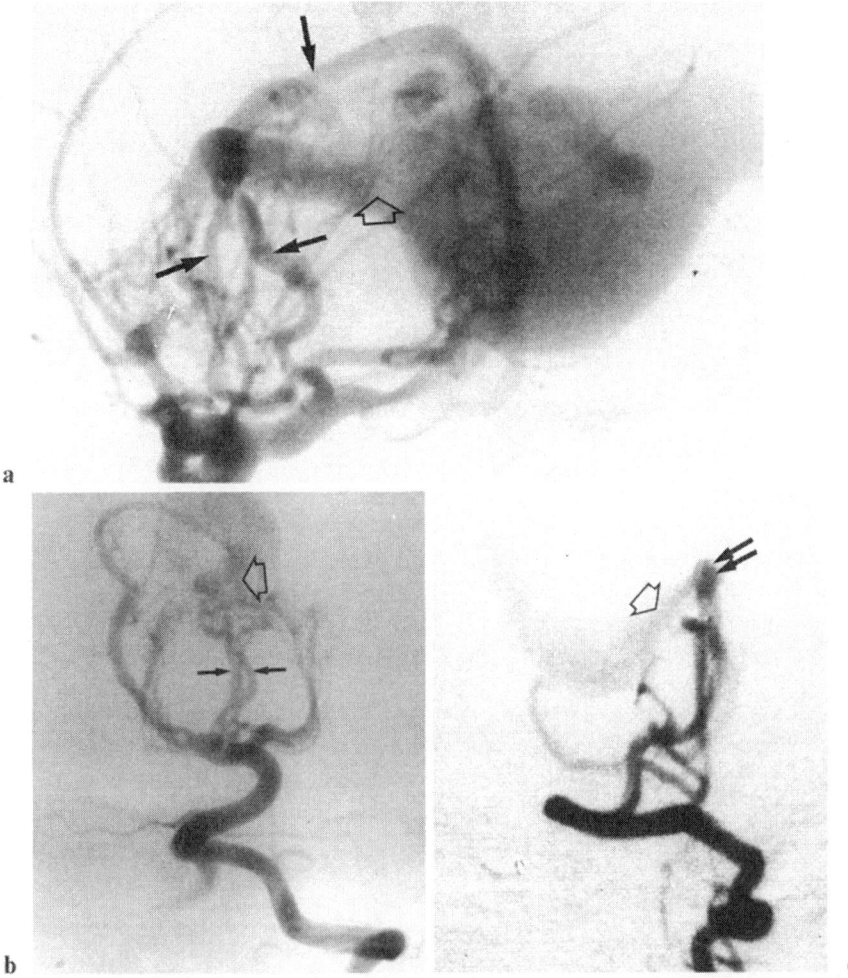

Fig. 1a–c. Different types of aneurysmal dilatations of the VG. **a** Arteriovenous fistula located at the foramen of Monro. The lenticulostriate and anteriorlateral choroidal arteries (*arrows*) rapidly fill the medial cerebral vein (*open arrow*) prior to the VG dilatation. **b** Tectal AVM with transmesencephalic arteries (*arrows*) feeding a parenchymatous nidus prior to the VG ectasia (*open arrow*). **c** VG AVM. Typical aspect of a direct opening of a choroidal artery (*double arrow*) into the VG dilatation (*open arrow*)

Therapeutic Discussion

Cerebral AVM treatment in 1987 must be multi-disciplinary (Table 3), and involve a properly experienced team. We shall only comment on the endovascular approach.

The endoarterial approach. As in surgery, the patient selection and the technical competence of the operators are the key factors. Our choice in newborns, for safety, reliability, and efficiency, consists of the systematic use of the femoral approach with a 4-F introducer, calibrated leak balloon, and isobutyl cyanoacrylate (IBCA) [7]. We have once used the carotid approach after failure of the femoral route due to multiple previous punctures. In this series, we have not had either definite technical failure or a complication related to the therapeutic method chosen and performed. One newborn could not be stabilized and died 8 days following embolization. In infants and adults, the technical therapeutic choices will be similar to those of the cerebral AVMs in general.

The intraoperative embolization. We have had no experience with arterial intraoperative embolizations, and, to our knowledge, there are no existing reports in the infant or newborn.

The venous technique [10] is indicated in the

Table 3. Aneurysmal malformation of the VG (material)

Sex	Age	Presenting symptoms	Treatment				Results and follow-up
			VG AVM (true)	Cere. AVM + VG ectasia	DVA + varix	VG DAVM	
M	2 d	Card. ins. + + + mod. hydroc.	Surg				Periop death
F	18 m	Failure to thrive,		Emb 1 (shunt)			Hydroc. post E1
*		fac. coll cir		Emb 2			excellent
M	8 m	Card. ins. + mild. hydroc, multi. shunts		Emb 1			Excellent 3 years
M	23 d	Card. ins. + + mod hydroc	Surg 1 Shunt				Neurol def periop
	5 y		Surg 2				death
M	5 d	Card. ins. + + mod hydroc. hep. ins. + + +	Emb 1 "Emb" 2				Occl. 40% failure
*		diff Hemor					dead E1 + 8d
M	21 y	Loss of consciousness			None		Asympt. 6 years
M	1 d	Neonatal Hem					Neur. seq.
	25 y	Hydroc + +		Shunt			improv.
	30 y	Prog. deficit headaches		Emb 1 Emb 2			impr. of symptoms
*				Emb 3			18 months
M	33 y	Subarac Hem.		Emb 1 Emb 2			Occl. 70% neuro norm 3 years
M	18 y	Hydroce + + subara hem 1, subara hem 2,		Shunt			Neur seq.
		subara hem 3		None			stable
M	3 m	Card. ins. + hydroc. mod.					
	7 y	Cerebell hem hemiplegia		Radiotherapy (proton)			Impr. neur.
	10 y	Growth retard		Emb 1			Hydroc
*				shunt			occl. 75%
F	15 m	Hydroc +	Vent. shunt				Spont. cure 20 months
M	6 m	Hydroc +	Vent shunt				Spont cure 14 months
M	5 d	Card. ins. + +	"Emb" 1				Failure
	18 d		Emb 1				Occl. 25%
	21 d		Emb 2 (per op)				Improv.
*							spect 8m.
F	1 m	Card. ins. + hydroc ?	Emb 1				Occl 40% Improv.
*							spect 9m.
M	3 m	Cardiac ins. fac coll cir		Medical treatment			Stabliz.
	11 y	Headaches mult. shunts		Emb 1			25% control
*		family cases					
F	62 y	Headaches, bruit, visual				Refuse Emb.	
*		seizures					

* Treatment still in process
d days, *m* months, *y* years

VG AVMs after failure of the arterial approach. We used it once with success, in the same newborn with whom we had to use the carotid approach. It is a dangerous technique in the case of AVMs with VG dilatation, where the shunt is far from the VG ectasia.

The objective of endovascular approach. If a complete occlusion of the shunt can be obtained by endovascular approach, it will be planed in a staged procedure. The therapeutic objective in the patients presenting with a secondary ectasia and a previous hemorrhage must be the anatomical cure by endovascular route, surgery, radiation therapy, or any combination. A reduction of the shunt and nidus by embolization, before radiotherapy, was chosen in one of our cases, and was considered nonsurgical. At this time, we have had an insufficient follow-up period to appreciate the efficacy of this combined treatment.

Conclusion

The traditional approach, with three different groups based on age, seems to us insufficiently adapted to modern therapeutic discussions. Instead, we have set out the means of differentiating the following groups: the AVMs of the VG, the secondary ectasia of parenchymal AVMs with congenital or acquired venous anomalies, the developmental venous anomalies with a varix of the VG, and the pure dural AVM of the VG.

The immediate results of the endovascular treatments are spectacular. However, the midterm neurological prognosis (5–10 years) is difficult to establish. The endovascular approach in the newborn and infant offers a unique therapeutic opportunity. As to the discussion of the endovascular approach in the adolescent or adult, its efficacy in the short term is reasonable but its benefits in the mid- or long-term remain to be proven.

References

1. Albright AL, Latchaw RE, Price RA (1983) Posterior dural arteriovenous malformations in infancy. Neurosurgery 13:129–135
2. Bedford THB (1934) The great vein of Galen and the syndrome of increased intracranial pressure. Brain 57:1–24
3. Clarisse J, Dobbelaere P, Rey C, D'hellemes P, Hassan M (1978) Aneurysms of the great vein of Galen: Radiological-anatomical study of 22 cases. J Neuroradiol 5:91–102
4. Diebler C, Dulac O, Renier D, Ernest C, LaLande G (1981) Aneurysms of the vein of Galen in infants aged 2–15 months: Diagnosis and natural evolution. Neuroradiology 21:185–197
5. Dobbelaere P, Jomin M, Clarisse J, Laine E (1979) Interêt prognostique de l'étude du drainage veineux des anévrysmes artérioveineux cérébraux. Neurochirurgie 25:178–184
6. Hoffman HJ, Chuang S, Hendrick B, Humphreys RP (1982) Aneurysms of the vein of Galen. J Neurosurg 57:316–322
7. Lasjaunias P, Terbrugge K, Chiu MC (1986) Coaxial balloon-catheter device for treatment of neoanates and infants. Radiology 159:269–271
8. Lasjaunias P, Terbrugge K, Lopez-Ibor L, Chiu M, Flodmark O, Chuang S, Gloasgnen J (1987) The place of dural obstacle in vein of Galen dilatation. AJNR 8:185–192
9. Massey CE, Carson LV, Beveridge WD, Allen MB, Brooks B, Yaghmai F (1982) Aneurysms of the great vein of Galen: Report of two cases and review of the literature. In: Vascular malformations. Raven, New York, pp 163–179
10. Mickle JP, Quisling RG (1986) The transtorcular embolization of vein of Galen aneurysms. J Neurosurg 64:731–735

Interventional Radiological Techniques in Cerebral AVMs

New Contrast Materials for Cyanoacrylate

Waro Taki[1], Yasuhiro Yonekawa[1], Jyokyu Gen[2], and Yoshito Ikeda[2]

Though surgical removal is the best treatment of cerebral arteriovenous malformation (AVM), many AVMs located in the dominant hemisphere or in the deep brain structure can hardly be removed. Also, huge AVMs are difficult to remove. Seventeen cases of those AVMs were treated with artificial embolization in our clinic. Percutaneous interventional technique, using detachable balloon with or without cyanoacrylate derivatives and Silastic spheres, were also used. One of the main problems was a technical difficulty in injection of cyanoacrylate derivatives which resulted in two mobility.

Among many materials used for artifical embolization of AVMs, cyanoacrylate derivatives (chiefly isobutyl 2-cyanoacrylate [IBCA]) have most effective embolizing results when applied properly and safely. Compared with particulate emboli, a large part of the nidus is occluded by a single injection of cyanoacrylate. Although this material is expected to be the only material that may lead to total embolization of AVMs, there are many technical problems in avoiding serious complications. Complications will be decreased if the mixture of IBCA and contrast material can be lowered in viscosity. A highly viscous mixture requires a high-pressure injection, which may lead to the accidental over-inflation of the ballon, rupturing the catheter as well as cerebral vessels. To decrease the chances of this complication, we are making an effort to develop new contrast materials for cyanoacrylate derivatives.

New Contrast Material for Cyanoacrylate Derivatives

The conventional contrast materials used for cyanoacrylate are iophendylate and Lipiodol.

Their viscosity is high and, thus, injection through superselective microballoon catheter becomes difficult. To decrease viscosity, we chose $CF_3CFBrCF_2Br$ (FPB2) and CF_2BrCF_2Br (FEB2), because they are low in viscosity and completely miscible with cyanoacrylate.

At first, radioopacity of the mixture of new contrast materials and IBCA was examined to see whether the mixtures could yield sufficient opacification under fluoroscopy. Four mixtures of new contrast (FPB2) and IBCA variable in their concentration were prepared and placed over the head of a volunteer for evaluation under the fluoroscopy. A mixture as low as 50% of FPB2 can give sufficient radioopacity. The 50% mixtures of both FEB2 and FPB2 were placed over the phantom and a plain X-ray film was obtained. The radioopacity of both mixtures was almost the same.

Viscosity

The viscosity of the new mixtures were examined by using BL-type viscogram. For contrast, the mixture of Lipiodol and IBCA was used. Viscocity of mixtures with variable concentration of contrast were plotted and listed in Fig. 1. The viscocity of pure Lipiodol was 35 cP, which was very high compared to a pure FEB2 and FPB2 viscocity of 2.5 cP. On the other hand, IBCA itself had a viscosity of 4 cP and had a higher value than FEB2 and FPB2. Therefore, by mixing FEB2 and FPB2, the viscosity of the mixture became lower than the pure IBCA. The 50% mixture of IBCA and Lipiodol showed a viscosity of 7 cP and the mixture of FEB2 and FPB2 were 2.5 cP, which was low enough and also sufficient for radioopacification.

Set Time of the Mixture

For lowering viscosity of the IBCA, the new contrasts are suitable, as long as they do not

[1] Department of Neurosurgery, Kyoto University Medical School, Kyoto, Japan
[2] Research Institute for Biomedical Material and Polymers, Kyoto University, Kyoto, Japan

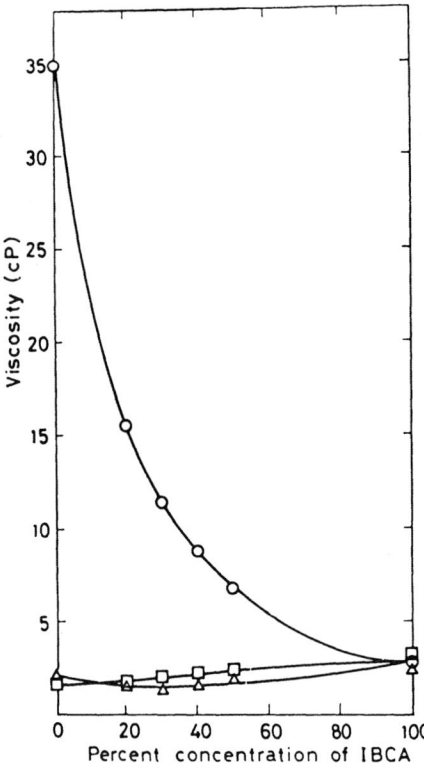

Fig. 1. Viscosities plotted against various concentrations of contrast medium and isobutyl cyanoacrylate (IBCA). Δ hexafluorodibromopropane, □ tetrafluorodibromoethane, o lipiodol ultra-fluide

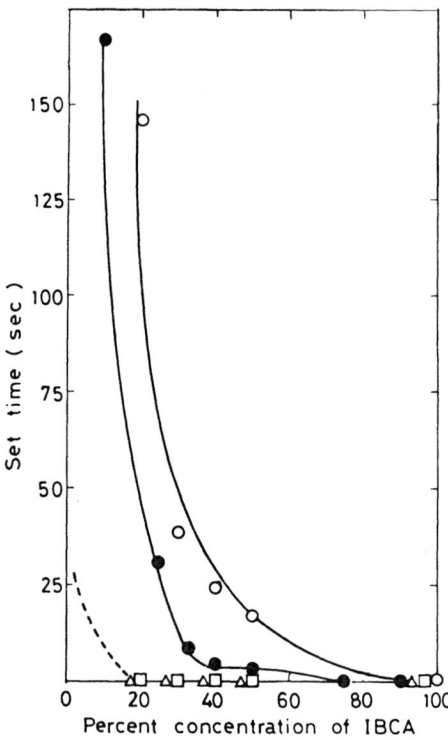

Fig. 2. Set times plotted against various concentrations of contrast medium and isobutyl cyanoacrylate (IBCA) (blood). Δ hexafluorodibromopropane, □ tetrafluorodibromoethane, o lipiodol ultra-fluide, ● iophendylate. After Cromwell and Kerber [1]

change the set time. Set time was measured by dropping the mixture onto human citrated blood (Fig. 2). The horizontal bar represents the ratio of mixture and the vertical bar represents set time. The mixture of Lipiodol and IBCA was plotted by an open circle, that of iophendylate by a blackened circle, that of FPB2 by an open triangle, and that of FEB2 by an open square. Since the stock of iophendylate in Japan was very small and hardly applicable for this experiment, the results of Cromwell and Kerber [1] were quoted. The set time of the mixtures was longest in Lipiodol and shortest in both FEB2 and FPB2. The set time of the 50% mixture of FEB2 and FPB2 was 2s.

Toxicity of New Contrast

Acute toxity of both materials was examined by parenteral administration to mice. The lethal dose for 50% of the group (LD_{50}) of FEB2 was 0.625–2.5 g/kg and the LD_{50} of FPB2 was

0.123–2.5 g/kg. These doses are smaller than the supposed maximum clinical dose of 2–3 g/60 kg. FEB2 appears to be safer than FPB2.

Conclusion

The new contrast materials are low in viscosity, have enough radioopacity, and appear to be suitable for transcatheter injection. Further examination of injection technique, the toxicity via other administration routes, and subacute effect should be made.

References

1. Cromwell LD, Kerber CW (1974) Modification of cyanoacrylate for therapeutic embolization: Preliminary experience. AJR 132:799–801
2. Taki W, Handa H, Yonekawa Y, et al. (1983) Embolization with cyanoacrylate derivatives: The Mt. Fuji Workshop on CVD 121–128

Nonsurgical Treatment of AVM: Development of New Liquid Embolization Method

Akira Takahashi and Jiro Suzuki[1]

For the recent development of intravascular surgery, it has become possible to treat the arteriovenous malformation (AVM) with percutaneous transluminal embolization. Because it is still difficult to achieve complete cure even with supreme techniques, it seemed to be mandatory to develop an ideal embolization method: superselective balloon catheters and embolization materials. First, we developed a silicone superselective balloon catheter with a floppy tip. Using this catheter, we could catheterize even into perforating branches of middle cerebral or posterior cerebral arteries. Second, we developed a new embolization method using new liquid materials. The materials which are used now consist of conjugated estrogen diluted in 25% ethanol and polyvinyl acetate. In this report, we present the process of the experimental and clinical development.

Materials and Methods

Experimental Studies

Extrogen diluted with 25% ethanol. We have reported the embolization method using conjugated estrogen in experiments. Because this method requires a continuous injection for 7–10 days in clinical cases, it is thought to be better to embolize the lesion with a one-shot infusion. Due to pure ethanol's strong effect on vascular walls and use for the embolization of renal cell carcinoma, it was added to enhance the effect of the estrogen. The experiment was planned to study the effect of this combination using the renal artery of a dog. A selective infusion of drugs was carried out through a double-lumen balloon catheter. The differences between the effect of estrogen (20 mg/ml; 0.3 ml/kg), 25% ethanol (0.3 ml/kg), and estrogen (20 mg/ml) diluted with 25% ethanol (0.3 ml/kg) were investigated angiographically and microscopically. The angiograms were estimated and graded according to following five-point scale: occlusion up to cortical arteries (grade I), occlusion up to interlobular arteries (grade II), occlusion up to interlobar arteries (grade III), occlusion up to main trunk arteries (grade IV), and occlusion up to the renal artery (grade V; Fig. 1). Sequential changes of the renal artery were also investigated.

Ethanol followed by polyvinyl acetate (PVac). After experience with clinical cases, it was recognized that embolization using ethanol induced some unwanted tissue reactions, such as edema or petechial hemorrhage. It was considered that these reactions were caused by the intact blood flow in proximal arteries which was damaged by ethanol. These unwanted reactions were pre-

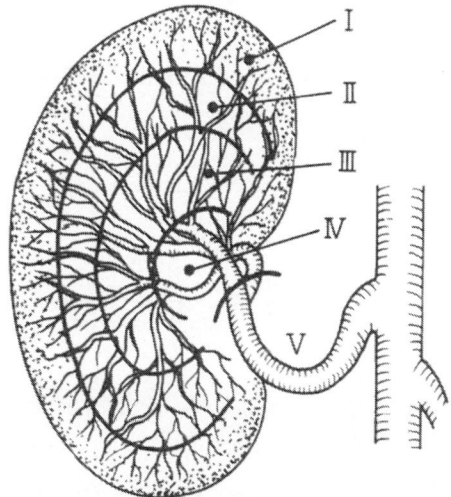

Fig. 1. Occlusion grade of renal angiogram. *I* occluded to cortical arteries, *II* occluded to interlobular arteries, *III* occluded to interlobar arteries, *IV* occluded to main trunk arteries, *V* occluded to the renal artery

[1] Division of Neurosurgery, Institute of Brain Diseases, Tohoku University School of Medicine, Sendai, Japan

vented by proximal occlusion using another material. PVac, diluted in an alcohol solution, becomes gelatinous in 1 s upon contact with water. The resulting substance does not adhere to the catheter. It is possible to make this material radiopaque using metrizamide. The final material consists of 190 mg/ml PVac, 340 mg/ml ethanol, 330 mg/ml distilled water, 200 mg/ml metrizamide, and 5 mg/ml propylene glycol. It has 100 mg/ml of radiopacity and a viscosity of 75 cP. Because of such low viscosity, this agent can be introduced through a tiny leak balloon (internal diameter 0.3 mm, 150 cm long). The effects on the renal artery of dog were examined in the same way. The injection of PVac was carried out during proximal occlusion using double lumen balloon catheter after a 20-min infusion of ethanol.

Clinical Cases

For the last 3 years, we have treated 15 AVMs in the central nervous system. These patients were assigned to three groups according to the embolization material (Table 1). Group I consisted of 11 cases who were treated with a continuous (cases 1–9) or one-shot infusion (cases 10, 11) of conjugated estrogen (chemical embolizing agent). Group II consisted of four patients who were embolized with a one-shot infusion of ethanol (case 15 was also assigned to group I and labelled case 9). Group III consisted of one case who was embolized with ethanol followed by an injection of PVac. Different infusion methods were used among the different groups, with group I, transaxillary or transfemorally introduced leak balloons were positioned in the feeders or their

Table 1. Summary of cases embolized with chemical agent

Case no.	Age/ sex	Clinical presentation	Location of AVM, feeding arteries	No. of emboli- zations	Emboli- zation (%)	Surgical resection	Complications and outcome
Group I: continuous or one-shot injection of conjugated estrogen							
1	10 F	Rt. cerebellar hemorrhage	Rt. cerebellum PICA, SCA, AICA	3	60	–	Extravasation of estrogen embolism in lt. PICA
2	19 M	IVH, ICH	Rt. thalamus med. post. ch	1	100	–	No neurological deficits
3	19 M	Seizures	Lt. frontal orbitofrontal, pre- frontal (AC, MC)	1	NC	+	Discontinued for catheter cut-off, anemia
4	30 F	ICH	Rt. thalamus med. post. ch, post. tp lat. post. ch	2	50	–	Lt. homonymous hemianopsia
5	45 F	Seizures	Rt. frontal orbitofrontal, pre- frontal (AC, MC)	2	5	–	Convulsion
6	45 F	SAH	Lt. occipital parietoccipital, calcarine (PC)	1	NC	+	Discontinued for catheter withdrawal, anemia, slight liver dysfunction
7	11 M	SAH	Spinal cord ascend. cerv. a	1	90	–	Preceded by unsuccessfull embolization with gelfoam
8	53 M	Seizures	Lt. occipital & corpus callosum lt. PC, MC, AC	1	NC	–	Discontinued for em bolism in lt P_2
9[a]	13 M	ICH, IVH	Lt. thalamus med. & lat. post. ch	1	60	–	Occlusion of lt. P_3 no neurological deficits
10	62 M	Seizures	Lt. occipital temporo-parietal post. temporal calcarine (PC)	1	NC	–	
11	23 F	IVH, ICH	Lt. thalamus med. post. ch, post. tp	1	60	–	

(Table 1 continued on following page)

Table 1 (*continued*)

Case no.	Age/ sex	Clinical presentation	Location of AVM, feeding arteries	No. of emboli- zations	Emboli- zation (%)	Surgical resection	Complications and outcome
Group II: one-shot injection of estrogen-alcohol
12	37 M	Hematomyelia SAH	Spinal cord C_2–C_5 lt. C_3–C_4 rad.a. blt. C_5–C_6 rad.a. ant. spinal a.	3	50	–	Symptoms improved, segmental embolization of ant. spinal artery
13	13 M	ICH, IVH	Lt. thalamus ant. ch, post. ch, thalamogeniculate	3	50	–	Rt. homonymous hemianopsia
14	10 F	Seizures	Lt. parieto-occipital lt. PC, AC, MC ant. ch, post. ch post. tp	4	50	–	Rt. homonymous hemianopsia, petechial infarction
15[a]	13 M	ICH, IVH	Lt. thalamus med. & lat. post. ch	1	80	–	Rt. homonymous hemianopsia, petechial infarction
Group III: combined injection of estrogen-alcohol and PVac
16	29 M	Seizures	Lt. fusiform gyrus post. temporal (PC, MC) occipitotemporal	1	90	+	Rt. homonymous hemianopsia

[a] Case 9 and case 15 are the same patient
lt left, *rt* right, *ICH* intracerebral hemorrhage, *IVH* intraventricular hemorrhage, *PICA* posterior inferior cerebellar artery, *SCA* superior cerebellar artery, *AICA* anterior inferior cerebellar artery, *med* medial, *lat* lateral, *post* posterior, *ch* choroidal artery, *AC* anterior cerebral artery, *MC* middle cerebral artery, *PC* posterior cerebral artery, *ascend.cerv.a.* ascending cervical artery, *tp* thalamoperforating artery, *rad.a.* radicular artery, *SAH* subarachnoid hemorrhage, *NC* no change

parent arteries. Continuous infusion of estrogen (100 mg/day) was carried out using an infusion pump under careful monitoring of neurological signs and angiography. In groups II and III, a superselective balloon catheter with a floppy tip was used to catheterize the feeders. Before the infusion, superselective angiograms via leak balloon under DSA monitoring and provocative tests by injection of amobarbital (20 mg) were performed in each case.

Results

Experimental Studies

Estrogen diluted with 25% ethanol. The enhancement effect of the alcohol was clearly shown on the angiograms taken either 1 h or 1 week after the embolization (Fig. 2a, b). Sequential microscopic changes of ethanol were characteristic;

whereas thrombosis was observed only in the intraglomerular capillaries 15 min after the infusion, occlusion of interlobular arterioles was observed 4 h later (Fig. 3a, b). Although we could not observe any edema or hemorrhage up to 4 h, there were focal necrosis, edema, and parenchymal petechial hemorrhages in some specimens 1 week after embolization (Fig. 3c).

Ethanol followed by PVac. Angiograms showed complete occlusion of the main trunks of the renal artery immediately after the embolization. No recanalization was observed in follow-up angiograms (Fig. 4). Four days after the embolization, we could not find the unwanted tissue reactions which were observed following ethanol embolization (Fig. 5a). Chronic follow-up examinations showed striking evidence of severe shrinkage of renal parenchyma and no cortical structures (Fig. 5b). There were no systemic toxicities or complications, such as pulmonary embolism or hemorrhage into the abdominal cavity.

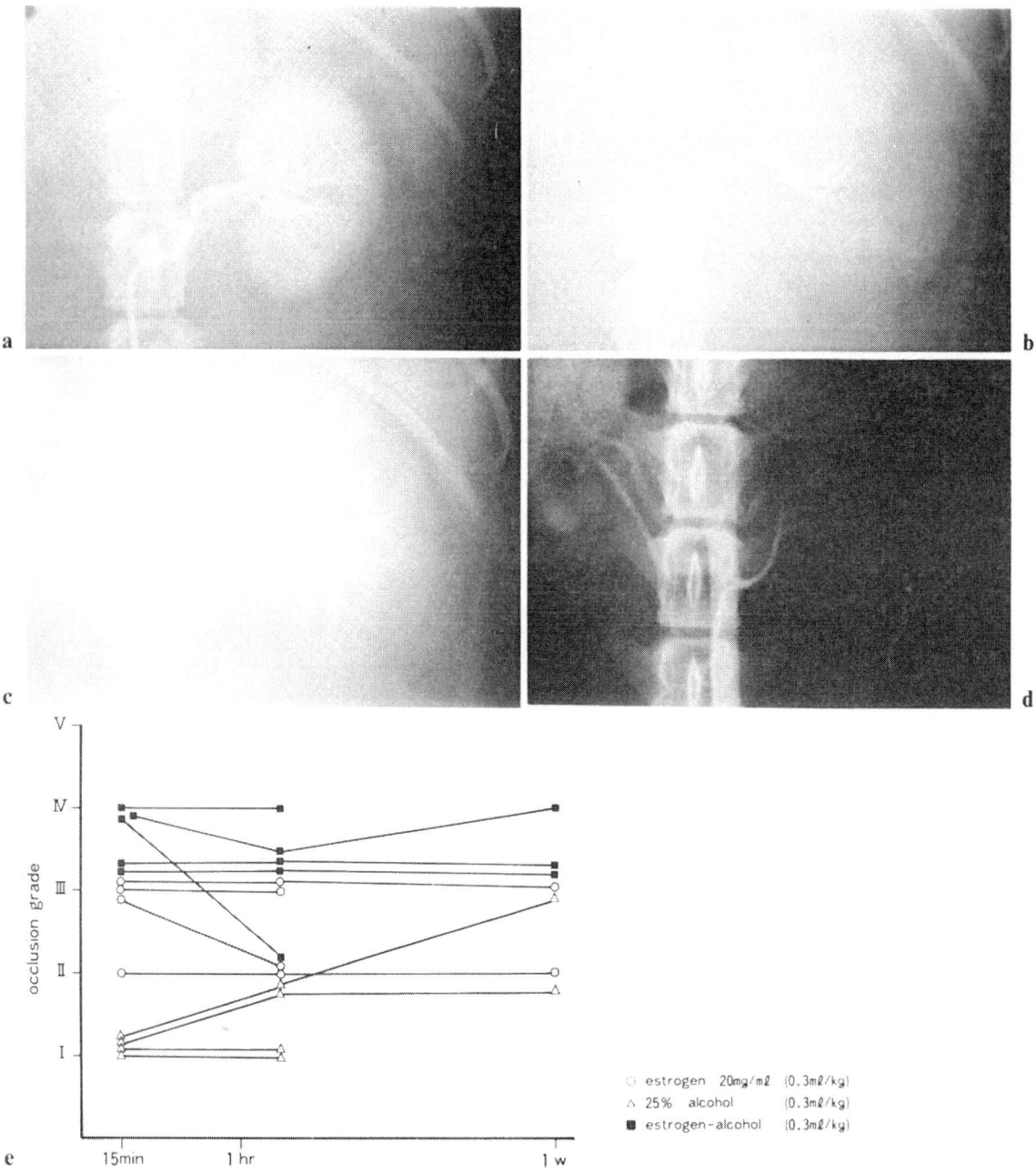

Fig. 2a–e. Embolization using estrogen-alcohol on left renal artery of dog. **a** Control angiogram before embolization. **b** Angiogram taken 15 min after the embolization, showing grade III occlusion. **c** Angiogram taken 1 h after the embolization, showing dilatation of arteries and grade II occlusion. **d** Angiogram taken 1 week after embolization, showing grade IV occlusion. **e** Effects of estrogen, 25% alcohol, and estrogen-alcohol. Combined infusion of estrogen-alcohol is superior to estrogen or 25% alcohol. *Occlusion grades* are the same as in Fig. 1

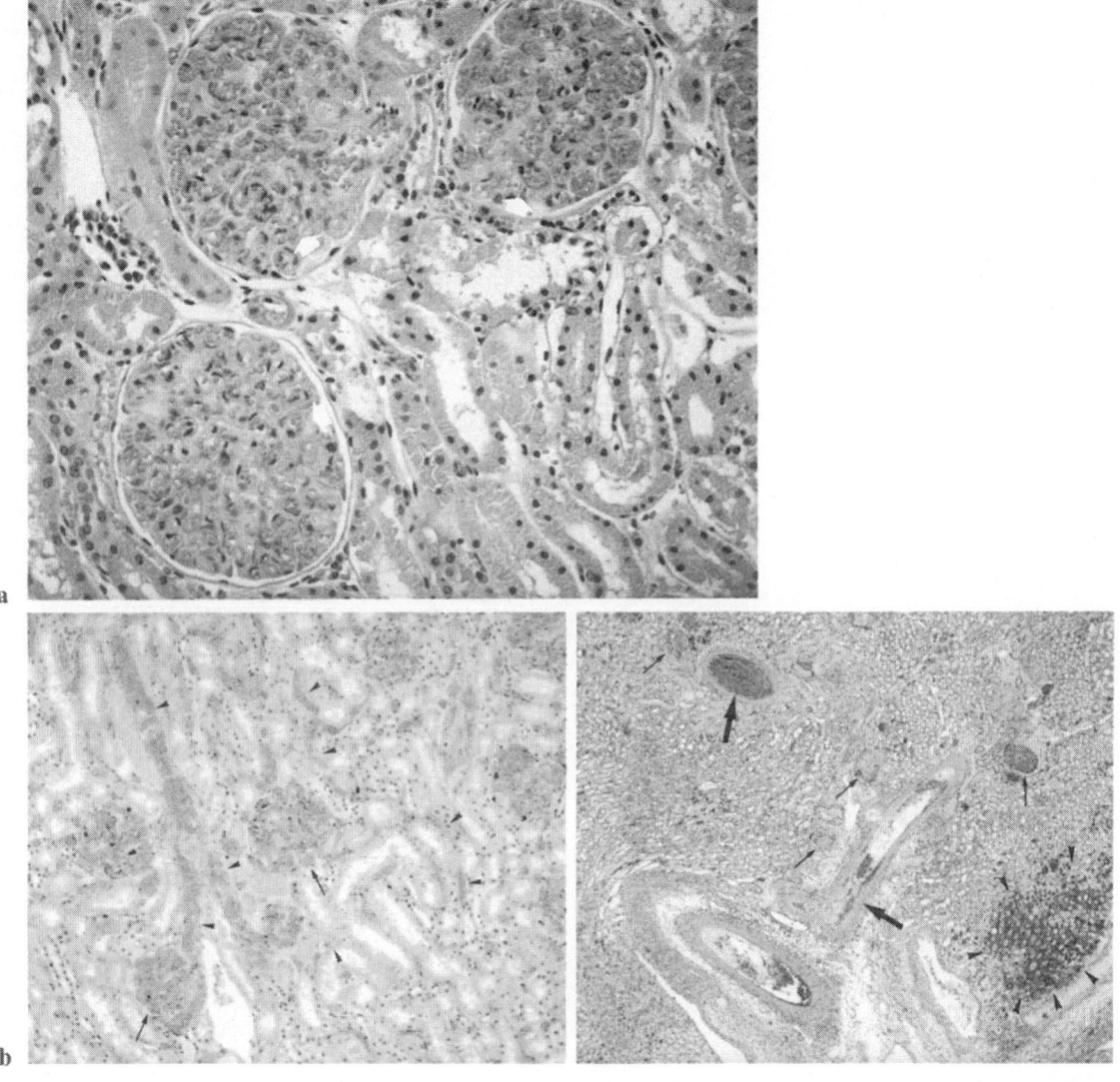

Fig. 3a–c. Microscopic preparations of kidney after embolization using estrogen-alcohol. **a** Fifteen minutes after the embolization. Diffuse thrombosis only in intraglomerular capillaries (*arrows*) is observed after perfusion fixation using 10% phosophate buffered formalin (H and E, × 260). **b** Four hours after the embolization. Diffuse thrombosis of intraglomerular capillaries and interlobular arterioles (*arrow heads*) with shrinkage of glomeruli (*arrows*) are observed. No tissue reactions are evident (H and E, × 100). **c** One week after the embolization. Hyalinization of glomeruli (*arrows*) and thrombosis of interlobar arteries (*large arrows*) are evident. Intraparenchymal petechial hemorrhages (*arrow head*) are also observed (H and E, × 50)

Clinical Cases

In group I, the nidus was totally obliterated in one case, subtotally obliterated in one, partially obliterated in five, discontinued the procedure in three, and remained unchanged in four (Figs. 6, 7). It was difficult to maintan the proper position of the catheter tip during continuous infusion. There were two cases of catheter-related embolic complications. In group II, 50%–80% of the nidi were obliterated in correlation to the feeders which were infused. Postembolization CT scan showed some perifocal edema and petechial hemorrhage. In group III, 90% of the nidus was obliterated without complication (Fig. 8). The remaining nidus was resected easily; there was no bleeding even during the transection of the nidus.

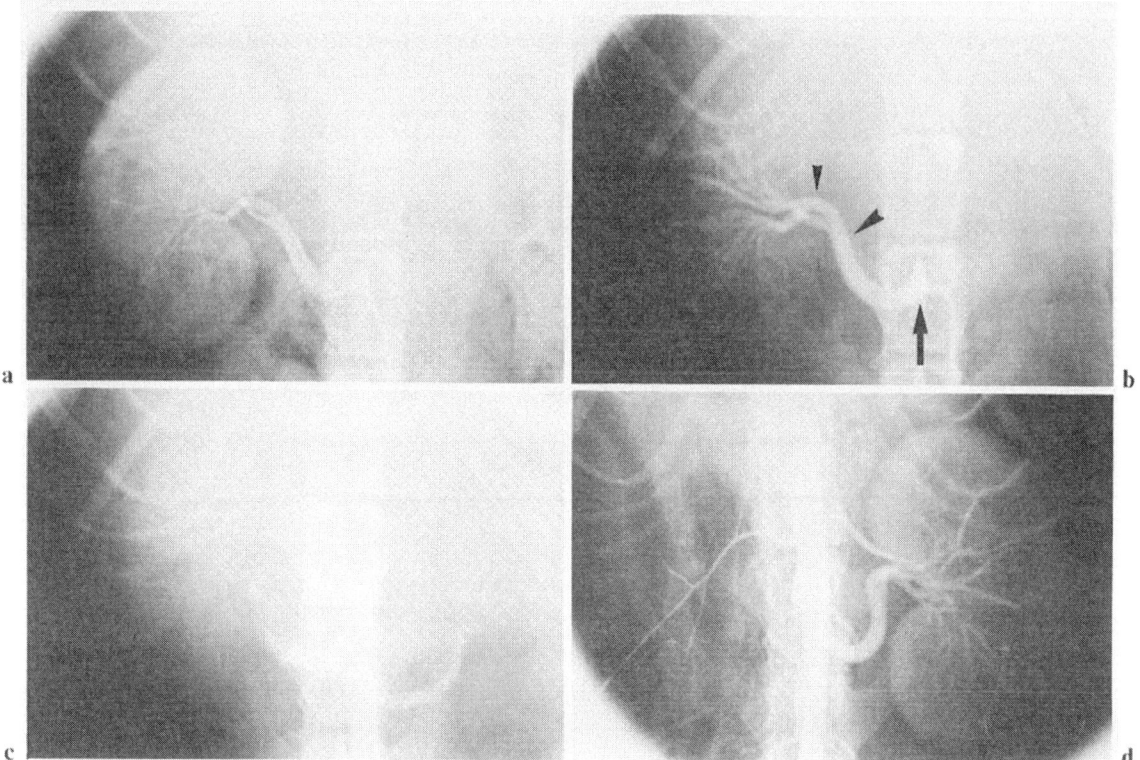

Fig. 4a–d. Embolization using estrogen-alcohol followed by injection of PVac of right renal artery of dog. **a** Control angiogram before embolization. **b** Plain radiogram immediately after the injection of PVac following infusion of estrogen-alcohol. Note the cast of PVac (*arrow heads*) and the proximal occlusion using double lumen balloon (*arrow*). **c** Angiogram taken 1 h after embolization shows complete occlusion of renal artery and decreased radiopacity of the cast of PVac due to parenchymal diffusion. **d** Aortogram taken 4 days after embolization shows no evidence of any trace of embolized renal artery or any collateralization of right kidney

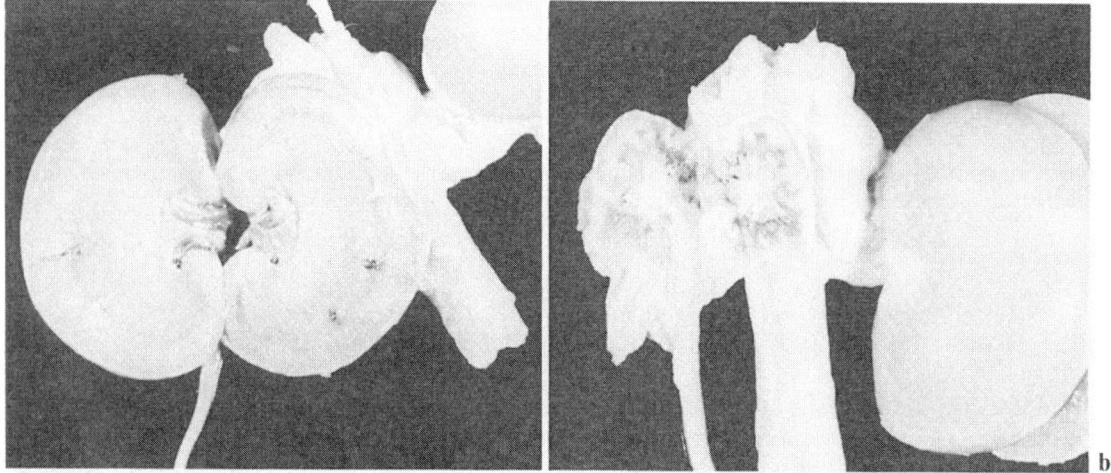

Fig. 5a, b. Macroscopic appearances of the dog kidney embolized by combined injection of estrogen-alcohol and PVac. **a** Four days after embolization. No evidence of unwanted tissue reactions are seen. The presence of the cast of PVac is shown in arcuate arteries at cortico-medullary junction and hilar arteries. **b** Three months after embolization. Marked shrinkage of right kidney is observed

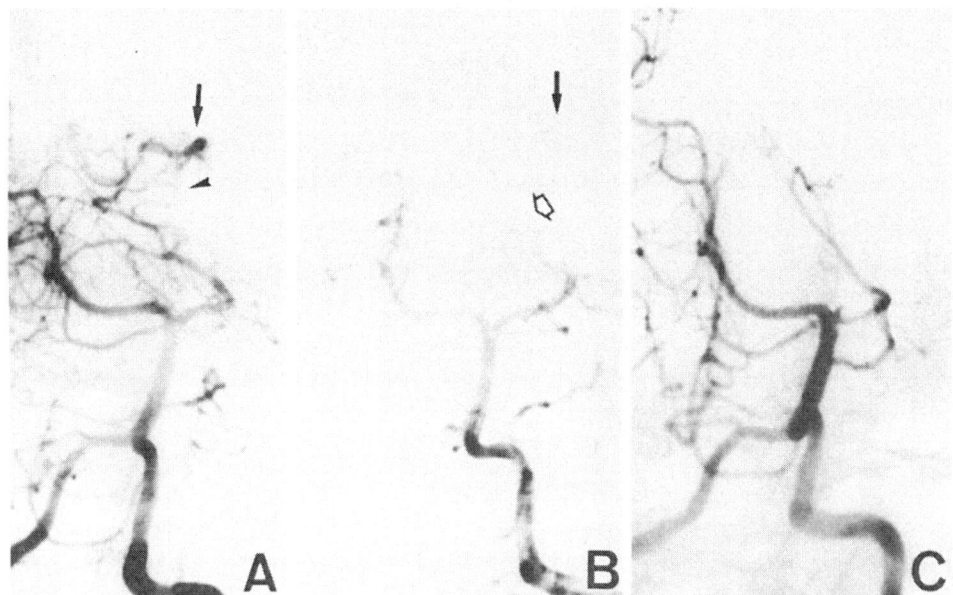

Fig. 6A–C. A 19-year-old male with left thalamic AVM (case 2). **A** Before chemical embolization (left VAG). Note the small thalamic AVM (*arrow*) fed by medial posterior choroidal arteries (*arrow head*). **B** Continuous infusion of estrogen into the left posterior cerebral artery for 5 days resulted in the disappearance of one feeder and diminished size of the nidus (*black arrow*). *Open arrow* indicates the other main feeder. **C** After embolization, note the disappearance of the nidus. In this case, the region of the left posterior cerebral artery was perfused by collateral circulation

Discussion

For the nonsurgical treatment of AVM, the role of intravascular surgery has become more important recently [1, 2, 7]. Among various embolization methods, it seems clear that a liquid embolizing agent injected through a calibrated leak balloon catheter is most effective and the only way to treat the lesion [1]. Many neuroradiologists are in favor of using isobutyl-2-cyanoacrylate (IBCA) as the promising liquid embolizing agent. In spite of the many advantages of this agent in completely obliterating the lesion, we think that there are many more technical difficulties and an incompleteness of the embolizing property. Recently, Vinuela et al. reported their critical review of long-term follow-up results in 30 partially embolized AVM cases [7]. They consider the main technical problem to be related to an inaccurate delivery of IBCA into the nidus of the AVM. This problem seems for us to be related to the characteristics of IBCA; its tendencies of polymerizing too quickly and of glueing the catheter. Therefore, this agent is thought to be difficult to control during the procedure. Moreover, Klara et al. reported the

morphological studies of AVM, which demonstrated a lattice structure and microchannels within the IBCA embolus [2]. This study indicates an incompleteness of the embolizing capability of IBCA. These disadvantages of IBCA made it seem mandatory to develop ideal embolizing materials.

We have reported the successful results of a chemical embolization method using conjugated estrogen [3, 5, 6]. This method has many advantages in embolizing the lesion from the capillary level with safety [3]. For the treatment of AVM in the central nervous system, it is better to improve this method which can be used with a one-shot injection. The enhancing effect of adding 25% ethanol as a diluent of estrogen is encouraging, but another problem occurred; unwanted tissue reactions. These reactions can be prevented by the additional use of another liquid embolizing material, PVac. This alcohol-soluble material was first reported in 1984 as an experimental renal embolization agent [4]. We tested it in vitro and in vivo and found the better combination with more diluted alcohol and metrizamide than the original combination with 95% alcohol and lipiodol respectively. The effect of the combina-

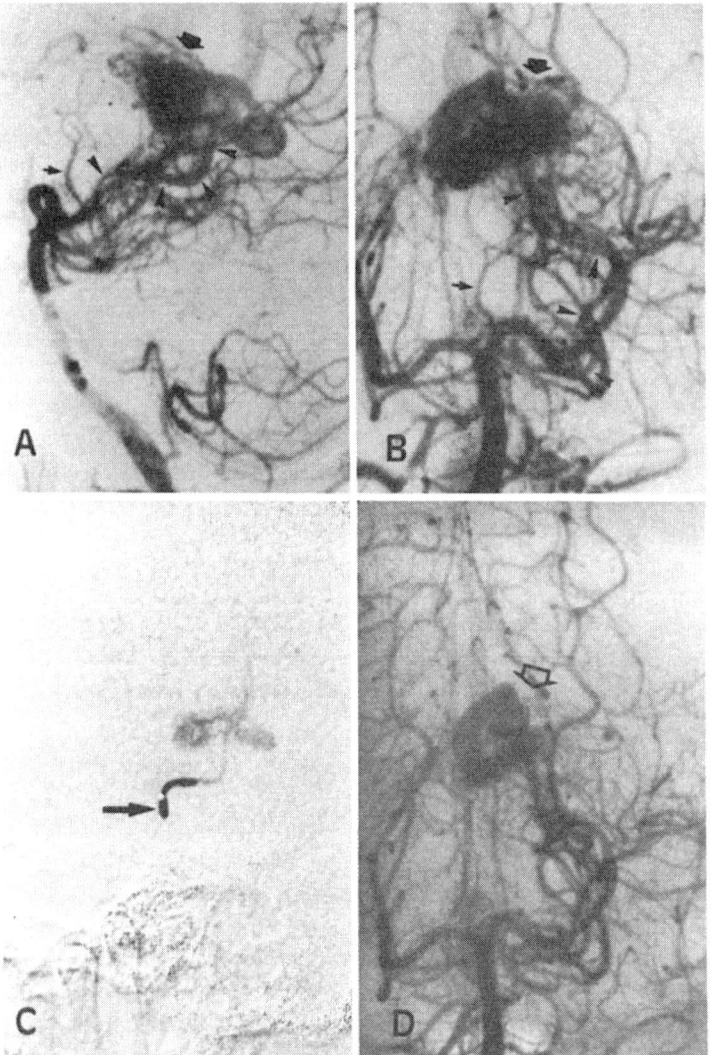

Fig. 7A–D. Angiograms of the AVM: 23-year-old female (case 11). **A** Left vertebral angiogram before embolization, lateral view, showing left thalamic AVM (*thick arrow*) mainly fed by medical posterior choroidal artery
(*arrow head*). *Small arrow* indicates posterior thalamo perforating artery, accesory feeder. **B** Left vertebral
angiogram before embolization, A-P view (*Arrows* indicate same above). **C** Superselective digital subtraction
angiogram of the medial posterior choroidal artery, lateral view, showing the correlation between this feeder and
the nidus. Infusion of estrogen was carried out immediately after this angiography. *Arrow* indicates superselective leak balloon **D** Left vertebral angiogram, A-P view, 1 week after the embolization. Lateral two-thirds
of the nidus (*open arrow*) was embolized

tion of estrogen-alcohol and PVac was strikingly
better in experimental renal artery embolization,
and the clinical experiences were encouraging.

Although we have not enough experience to
conclude about the usefulness of the combined
infusion of estrogen-alcohol and PVac, this new
method of embolization could fulfill the following prerequisites which are required for the
ideal embolization material for intravascular
treatment of AVM:

a) The material should be a liquid which is compatible with introduction through a tiny leak
balloon
b) This material should have high controlla-
bility, it must be radiopaque, infusion time
should be long enough to control the embolizing volume, and the material should not
adhere to the catheter
c) It should have the diffuse embolizing property from artery to capillary without propa-

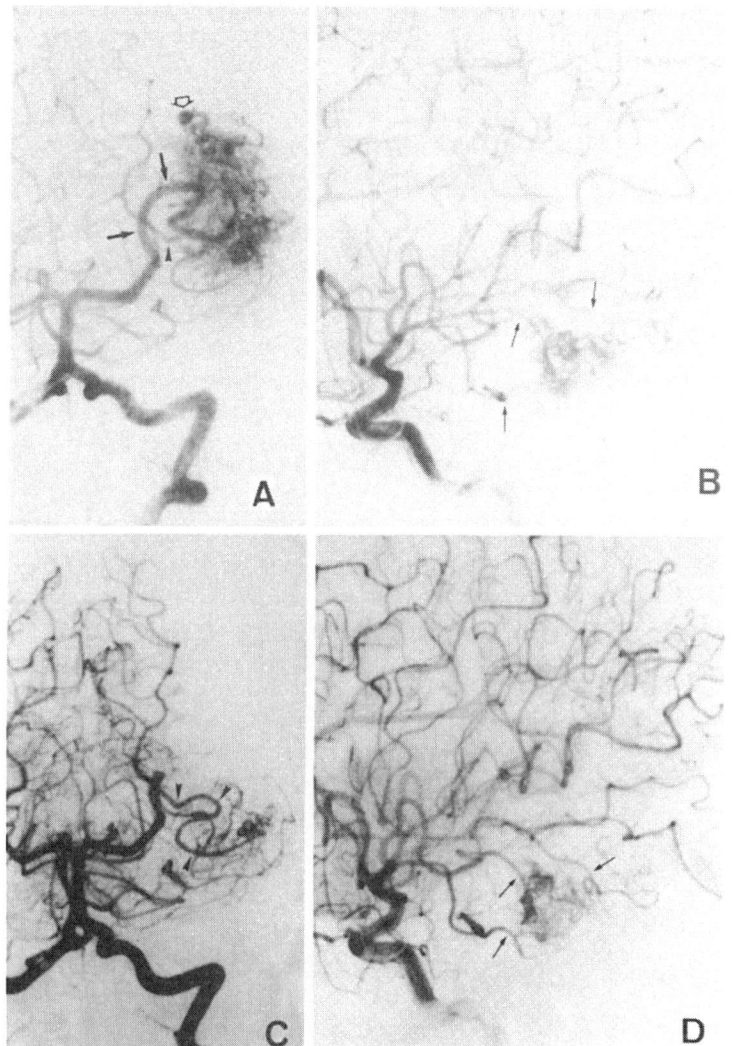

Fig. 8A–D. Angiograms of the AVM: 29-year-old male (case 15). **A** Left vertebral angiogram before embolization, A-P view, showing AVM (*open arrow*) in left fusiform gyrus fed by occipitotemporal artery (*arrows*) and posterior temporal artery (*arrow head*). **B** Left internal carotid angiogram before embolization, lateral view, showing supplemental supply from temporal branches of MCA (*arrows*). **C** Left vertebral angiogram 2 weeks after the embolization using estrogen-alcohol and PVac, A-P view, showing 90% of nidus obliteration with small amount of unembolized portion fed by posterior temporal arteries (*arrow heads*). **D** Left internal carotid angiogram 2 weeks after the embolization, lateral view, showing unchanged blood supply from temporal branches (*arrows*)

gation into veins and recanalization
d) It should be nontoxic, biologically inert, and less reactive with parenchyma
e) Embolized tissue should be resectable.

References

1. Debrun G, Vinuela F, Fox AJ, Drake CG (1982) Embolization of cerebral arteriovenous malformations with bucrylate: Experience in 46 cases. J Neurosurg 56:615–627
2. Klara PM, George ED, McDonnell DE, Pevsner PH (1985) Morphological studies of human arteriovenous malformations: Effects of isobutyl 2-cyanoacrylate embolization. J Neurosurg 63:421–425
3. Nagamine Y, Komatsu S, Suzuki J (1983) New embolization method using estrogen on microcirculation. Surg Neurol 20:269–275
4. Peregrin JH, Kaspar M, Vanecek R, Belan A (1984)

New occlusive agent for therapeutic embolization tested in dogs. Cardiovasc Intervent Radiol 7:97–101

5. Suzuki J, Komatsu S (1981) New embolization method using estrogen for dural arteriovenous malformation and meningiomas. Surg Neurol 16:438–442

6. Suzuki J, Nagamine Y, Takahashi A (1986) New embolization method for inoperable AVMs and vascular rich tumors: Chemical embolization using conjugated estrogen. In: Samii M (ed) Surgery in and around the brain stem and the third ventricle. Springer, Berlin, pp 223–230

7 Vinuela F, Fox AJ, Pelz D, Debrun G (1986) Angiographic follow-up of large cerebral AVMs incompletely embolized with isobutyl-2-cyanoacrylate. AJNR 7:919–925

Discussion

Commentator, *Symon* (London): A basic problem in dealing with arteriovenous malformations (AVM) is of course should they be treated? If the patient shows the three main indications, i.e., hemorrhage, fits, and intractable headache or advanced neurological deficit, the indication may be to treat them; however, the only absolute indication for treatment is recurrent hemorrhage. Our own experience is that almost every AVM will bleed sooner or later; statistics show that the bleed rate varies from about 3% to 5% over 7 years. Our own figures suggest that the bleed rate is not much different from that of previously unruptured aneurysms, though this is far from certain. Having decided that an AVM requires treatment, clearly the best way of doing this is to excise it if that is possible. But there are many AVMs that are so deep or so large that surgical excision involves an unacceptable risk, either of morbidity or of death. It is emerging I think from the studies of radiosurgery that the central neuraxial lesions, which are not very large, are probably adequately treated by this method, these create particular problems for balloon embolization since they may well be supplied with multiple perforating vessels. On the other hand, lesions that are supplied by single or multiple large arteries in the cerebrum or cerebellum are now amenable to microcatheterization. It is indeed remarkable that modern techniques have advanced so far that catheters can be put directly into AVMs or even aneurysms. Surgeons should be aware of balloon occlusion of major vessels in association with surgery; they should also be aware of reduction of high flow gradually before planned excision since this avoids the kind of complication described by Spetzler and others of undue brain swelling following reperfusion of previously ischemic tissue. The problem with embolization always remains that it is not difficult to embolize a great part of the malformation, but as the malformation's flow slows and preferential flow into the malformation is diminished the last piece becomes much more difficult. It is with the advances in glues, which will fill the entire malformation and prevent its possible recanalization, and the development of perfusion techniques that I feel progress will be made in the next few years.

Hosobuchi (San Francisco): As I said at the beginning there are two distinct approaches—the radiosurgical approach presented by Dr. Steiner and myself and glues and embolization. As a neurosurgeon what should be the selection criteria for the patients to be submitted to these nondirect surgical procedures?

Steiner (Stockholm): I think the position is as follows: the aim of surgery in AVM is to exclude the AVM from the circulation; the means by which this is achieved is not important as long as it is done with the minimum morbidity and mortality. It is clear as Prof. Symon pointed out that in deep-seated malformations, such as basal ganglia and brain stem malformations, radiosurgery is effective with lower morbidity and almost zero mortality. The mortality is not zero because during the long latency the patients can bleed and die as a result of this hemorrhage. At the moment, I have no final answer with regard to the indications for treatment. But my policy at present is the following. If the patient has never had a hemorrhage, I would perfer radiosurgery, irrespective of whether there is easy surgical accessibility to the malformation. If the patient has suffered a hemorrhage and the malformation is not in the basal ganglia or the brain stem I would prefer surgery. For a location in the basal ganglia or brain stem I would prefer radiosurgery. If the patient has had several hemorrhages I would prefer taking the higher risk of a surgical procedure.

Hosobuchi: Dr. Vinuela, what patients would you not consider for embolization?

Vinũela (Los Angeles): The more I become involved in the therapy for AVMs the more I realize that if there is an indication for surgery there is also an indication for embolization. The latter is a way of reaching the diseased area through the endovascular route. I do not think basically that either surgery or endotherapy is superior, though at present surgery would appear to be better, because of, for example, advances in microsurgical techniques. However, in the next few years, significant progress in endovascular therapy will be made. At present surgeons would appear to be benefitting greatly from advances in endovascular therapy in large AVMs which can be staged without surgical means.

Hosobuchi: Dr. Lasjaunias, you dealt with the very difficult problem of the surgical approach to the vein of Galen aneurysms, especially in young infants. Could you tell us about your selection criteria for these lesions?

Lasjaunias (Paris): In the series of patients referred to our center, two clear groups emerge. The first obviously requires surgical treatment and these patients have microlesions of the cortex with an intralobary hematoma; the patients are usually young and have no history of previous symptoms. The other group of patients are clearly more suited for an endovascular approach; these patients are newborns and infants with vein of Galen lesions. Of course, there are patients that do not conveniently fall into either group. Of our group of 15 patients, six were newborns, six infants, and three adults. There was one particular case of an AVM of the vein of Galen that we rejected for embolization. The patient was a newborn with high cardiac insufficiency. We felt that embolization would be of no benefit in this case even though the surgeon was of a different opinion. The patient died during the operation. Of the patients referred to us we only accept slightly more than 50%. We do not believe that simply because a lesion is embolizable that we should embolize it. A definite relationship has to be established between a morphological goal and a clinical objective. We try to select the clinical population in which we can be efficient. I think that the results of Prof. Steiner are related to the extreme severity of his selection of patients. This is what we also have to do. Our purpose is not to embolize all patients.

Mullan (Chicago): I would like to agree with Dr. Lasjaunias concerning the stenosis that exists

distal to the vein of Galen aneurysm. My series is that almost all of these dural AVMs begin with the thrombosis, which recanalizes and then becomes an AV fistula. And I would therefore disagree with Dr. Halbach who holds that turbulence caused that straight sinus thrombosis. My belief is that probably the thrombosis was primary. So I would like to ask Dr. Halbach in his total series of dural AVMs is there not very extensive evidence of a preexisting thrombosis? In my series, there certainly is this trend.

Halbach (San Francisco): I agree that the vein of Galen aneurysm is a specific entity and probably arises from thrombosis of the involved structures. In many of our AVMs, we can correlate the development of symptoms, particularly hemorrhage and neurological deficits, with acquired venous thrombosis; we have comparative angiograms on the more recent and symptomatic cases. So I would think that there is a component of congenital venous occlusion in some AVMs. But I believe that the acquired venous thrombosis is commonly associated with the symptoms. This has been well shown with the dural fistulas both by Drs. Vinũela and Lasjaunias.

Luessenhop (Washington): For 30 years, we have looked for some angiographic correlate for the type of AVM. I would like to ask Dr. Halbach how he assesses which AVMs will bleed at what rate and which AVMs will not bleed.

Halbach: We are currently reviewing the cases of AVMs that we have treated. The preliminary data suggest that there is a correlation between the degree of venous occlusive change and the risk of hemorrhage, though we have not yet reached the point where we can make a definitive statement in an individual case. With respect to small pseudoaneurysms within the nidus, it is very difficult with any imaging modality to identify that lesion. But patients with small pseudoaneurysms commonly have a history of repeated episodes of hemorrhage from a single location. With the hemorrhage that occurs there is often displacement of the peripheral vessels around the pseudoaneurysm, particularly in parenchymal malformations.

Flamm (New York): About 20% of malformation can be dealt with using nonsurgical techniques, but a great many more of them become subjected to partial occlusion. I would like to hear from the panelist about the role of embolization of a large malformation that has bled and cannot be removed surgically or obliterated by embolization. What is the advantage of partial embolization in such a case? If the answer is not known what methods do they see that we should take to establish a data-base for this?

Lasjaunias: We specifically examine the aneurysm and venous striction or thrombosis upstream or downstream of the AVM as a possible indicator of future risk to the AVM. Unfortunately, all this correlation can only be retrospective on the past history of the patient. However, we have found among our patients a significant relationship between the presence of aneurysm and venous stenosis of thrombosis and previous history of hemorrhage. This led us to try to assign to an incomplete embolization at least to change on these aneurysms and relief of venous pressure on stenoses. But we are very much aware that if either lesion can be removed it should be removed as long as the patient has bled. If we can relieve the situation by embolization we should do so, if not the patient should simply be operated upon; or the nidus should be reduced and the patient referred the radiosurgery.

Hosobuchi: Dr. Takahashi you have left some AVMs that are not totally occluded after your infusions. What do you think should be the next step?

Takahashi (Sendai): Usually, patients who bled once were totally resected afterwards, whereas those who had no bleeding but convulsion or headache were just followed up.

Vinuela: We have been following up our patients with incomplete embolization in eloquent areas of the brain, namely dominant hemispheres, motorsensory strips, and the area of the angular gyrus for an average period of $4\frac{1}{2}$ years. Among the 35 patients only three have rebled. We do not fully understand the significance of this at present. We are not increasing the rate of hemorrhage, we believe, but we are not sure if we are decreasing it. All statistics point to the fact that small AVMs bleed more than large AVMs. So we have tried to evaluate (weight) our techniques on this basis: Is bleeding from an AVM that has become reduced in size through embolization the same as bleeding from a small AVM in the course of its natural history? I would feel that we are helping these patients, but we do not know for certain. We have no statistical data-base for the answer to this. Perhaps with a double-blind study of 5000 cases in 10–15 years will provide the answer. We always make this clear to our patients that we do not really know if this change in the natural history is for the better. From the a priori finding that small AVMs bleed more than large AVMs we do not proceed very far. If we begin a study on endovascular therapy and AVMs becoming smaller and critically follow up the cases perhaps we will be the wiser.

Steiner: There is the contention that by irradiating a malformation without closing it completely the patient can be protected against bleeding. I recently reexamined my material using the same criteria as those who are of this belief: at least 1000 rads given to the whole malformation and at least 15 months latency between the radiation. This was supposed to protect the patient against new bleeding despite the fact that the malformation is not closed. However, on the basis of statistical analyses this is not true: An optimistic interpretation gives a hemorrhage rate of 2%/year; the pessimistic interpretation gives the rate at 4.8%/year. The average rate of 3% is that of the natural history. Only if the whole malformation is closed can the patient be protected against bleeding.

With respect to the price of the Gamma-Unit, it is over 2 million dollars.

RTD 5. Scientific Basis for Cerebral Infarction

Overview of Cerebral Ischemia: Rationale for Cerebral Protection

ROBERT F. SPETZLER, THOMAS W. GRAHM, and DANIEL G. NEHLS[1]

With the onset of profound cerebral ischemia, a complex chain of events is set into motion. If there is no intervention, irreversible damage occurs within several minutes. Although the primary insult of cerebral ischemia is a reduction in the supply of major nutrients, the depletion of cellular energy stores soon triggers a series of secondary events known as the "ischemic cascade." However, numerous factors influence the course of cerebral ischemia, and cell death is not necessarily the inevitable outcome. A simplified scheme of the progression of cerebral ischemia, with identification of possible sites for treatment, is presented in Figs. 1–3.

Two key factors in determining the outcome from cerebral ischemia are the depth and duration of ischemia. There are well-established thresholds of cerebral blood flow (CBF) for electrical failure and ion pump failure (Fig. 4) The earliest threshold is for electrical failure. In the cat, spontaneous electrical activity ceases at blood flows below 18 ml/100 g/min. In man, the EEG begins to flatten when cerebral blood flow falls below 16–17 ml/100 g/min. Somatosensory-evoked potentials are abolished in baboons at flows below 15 ml/100 g/min. At levels of electrical failure, the integrity of the ionic gradient is preserved. However, at lower levels of flow, these membrane ionic gradients cannot be maintained. In the baboon, ionic pump failure occurs at flows below 10 ml/100 g/min.

The critical levels of flow for infarction depend upon the duration of ischemia. Jones et al. [8] observed absolute thresholds for neurologic dysfunction in conscious monkeys undergoing middle cerebral artery occlusion and noted the reversibility of the deficit was a function of the duration of ischemia and the CBF. They formulated a relationship between thresholds of infarction, CBF, and duration of ischemia. Their concept of the time limits of reversible ischemia is represented in Fig. 5. Carter et al. [4] described similar time limits of reversible ischemia in cats studied at a number of different levels of local cerebral blood flow (lCBF). Within this framework, it is possible to devise strategies for cerebral protection. Such methods include elevating the blood flow above the threshold for infarction and lowering the infarction threshold itself.

Another important concept in understanding the rationale for cerebral protection is the "ischemic penumbra." With the complete cessation of CBF, there is a rapid reduction in phosphocreatine, glucose, and adenosine triphosphate (ATP). Cerebral function parallels the deterioration in cerebral energy state. In the clinical setting, however, ischemia is rarely complete due to collateral circulation. Within an ischemic region, there is a range of CBF. A dense ischemic core is surrounded by a zone of oligemia known as the ischemic penumbra. Within the ischemic penumbra, there is partial energy failure, and the fate of cells within this region depends upon the level of ischemia, its duration, and the differential vulnerability of each cell and region. This is the critical zone in which therapeutic intervention can raise the critical thresholds and prolong the time limits of reversible ischemia.

The metabolic rate for neurons differs from that of other cells. In addition to the energy expenditure for routine cellular functions, such as the maintenance of ionic gradients and the formation of cellular substrates, there is the energy demand imposed by electrical activity. The neuronal metabolic rate is a summation of a basic metabolic rate and an electrical metabolic rate, and is manifested in the separate thresholds for electrical and ionic pump failures. Measures designed to lower the cerebral metabolic rate for oxygen ($CMRO_2$) must take this fact into account. Agents, such as the barbiturates and isoflurane, affect only the electrical component of the $CMRO_2$ and are effective in lowering

[1] Barrow Neurological Institute, Phoenix, Arizona, USA

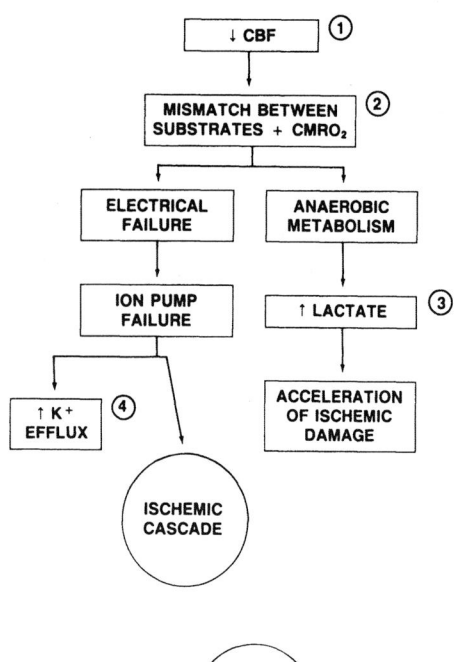

Fig. 1. Initial steps in cerebral ischemia. After Spetzler and Nehls [14], reprinted by permission of McGraw-Hill

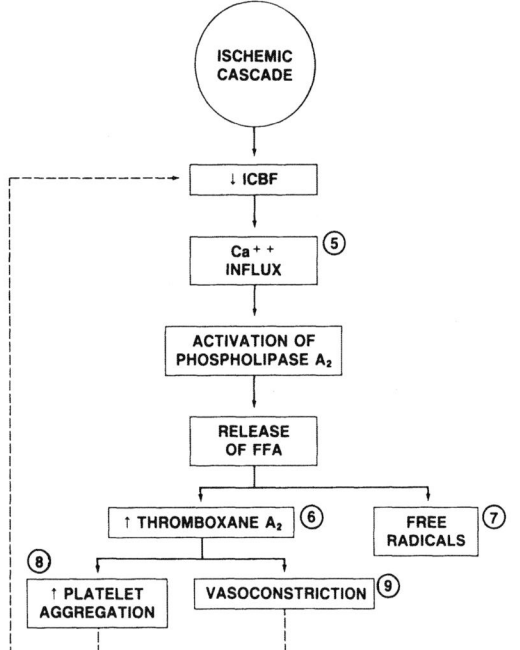

Fig. 2. Ischemic cascade (part 1). After Spetzler and Nehls [14], reprinted by permission of McGraw-Hill

cerebral metabolism before ischemic electrical failure.

Although the depletion of neuronal energy stores initiates the ischemic cascade, the rapid depletion of crucial metabolic substrates does not always terminate this chain of events. Once the ischemic cascade has begun, secondary processes can accelerate or modify the ischemic damage.

Hyperglycemia and elevated lactate may play an important role in accelerating ischemic dam-age. Rehncrona and colleagues [11] have studied the paradox that small amounts of blood flow may be more damaging than no flow at all. They found that this discrepancy could be explained on the basis of lactate accumulation due to the continued supply of glucose under the conditions of low flow. These authors felt that although high levels of lactate were not responsible for cell death, they accelerated the ischemic damage. Free radicals have also been proposed as triggers of the ischemic cascade. However, recent reports

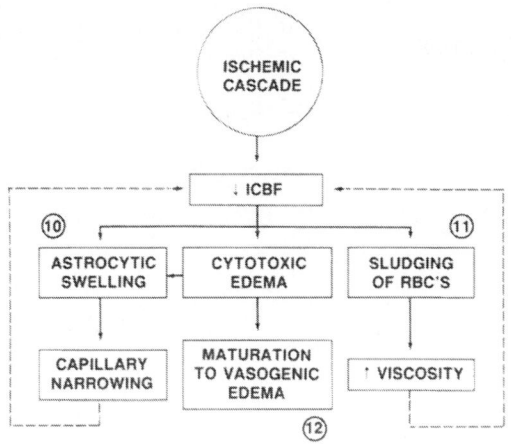

SITES FOR POSSIBLE THERAPEUTIC INTERVENTION

⑩ OSMOTIC DEHYDRATION (MANNITOL)

⑪ IMPROVE MICRORHEOLOGY (MANNITOL, FLUOSOL-DA)

⑫ STABILIZE BLOOD BRAIN BARRIER (STEROIDS, DMSO, BARBITURATES)

Fig. 3. Ischemic cascade (part 2), microcirculation. After Spetzler and Nehls [14], reprinted by permission of McGraw-Hill

question the validity of this mechanism [6, 7].

There is a growing body of evidence that calcium plays a major role in the pathophysiology of cerebral ischemia and is crucial in the final pathway for cell death. Ischemia impairs calcium homeostasis and leads to a large influx of calcium into the intracellular space. Earlier studies suggested elevation of intracellular calcium could activate phospholipase A_2 which releases free fatty acids (FFAs) from cell membranes and produces harmful agents, such as prostaglandins, leukotrienes, and free radicals. Rehncrona et al. [12] demonstrated no measurable breakdown of total or individual fatty acids or phospholipids following either complete or severe incomplete ischemia. They did note a rise in the free fatty acid content, but its release was not the result of peroxidative tissue damage.

Another event in the ischemic cascade is the development of cerebral edema. Two major forms of cerebral edema have been described by Klatzo [9]. Vasogenic edema results from leakage of plasma components into the extracellular space due to blood-brain barrier disruption and increased brain water content at the site of injury. Cytotoxic edema is a distinct entity caused by an impairment of membrane transport which leads to increased intracellular fluid. The edema produced by cerebral ischemia is complex. It initially resembles cytotoxic edema, with an increase of intracellular fluid due to membrane transport failure. This is followed by vasogenic edema as impairment of the blood-brain barrier develops. This process can occur over hours or days, with the peak increase in brain water occurring before disruption of the blood-brain barrier. Leukotrienes are lipoxygenase metabolites of arachidonic acid recently implicated in the path-

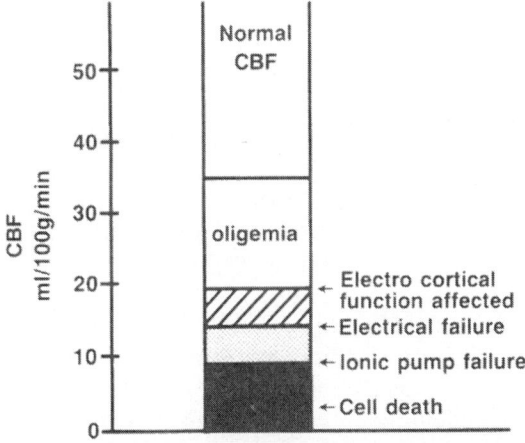

Fig. 4. Thresholds of cerebral ischemia. After Spetzler and Nehls [14], reprinted by permission of McGraw-Hill

ogenesis of cerebral edema. Black and Hoff [2] demonstrated an increase in brain water and blood-brain barrier permeability with direct injections of leukotrienes in the cerebral cortex. In a separate experiment, he demonstrated the presence of LTC_4 in the cortex surrounding human brain tumors [3]. Harris et al. [5] demonstrated that intravenous preloading of LTC_4 increased cerebral edema during severe incomplete ischemia in a primate model.

Corticosteroids have been shown to be effective in reducing vasogenic, but not cytotoxic, edema and are an accepted treatment of ischemic edema. Koide et al. recently reported a dramatic increase in cerebral damage after 10 min of reversible ischemia in animals which received chronic pretreatment with dexamethasone, and no improvement in animals who received

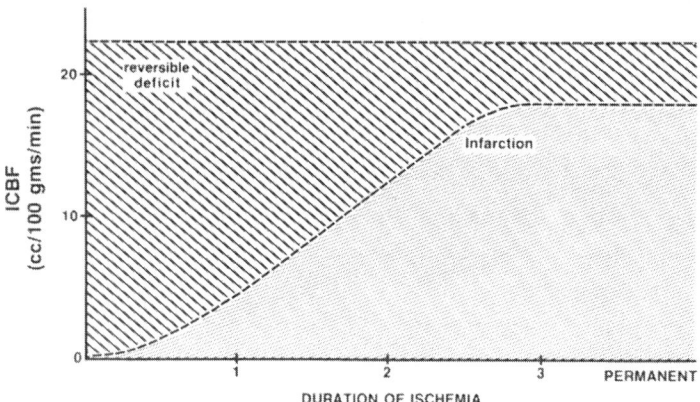

Fig. 5. Time limits of reversible ischemia. After Spetzler and Nehls [14], reprinted by permission of McGraw-Hill

steroids during the acute postischemic period [10].

Changes in the microcirculation can occur as a secondary effect of ischemia and can have profound effects upon its subsequent course. Ames et al. [1] were the first to demonstrate microcirculatory obstruction following profound ischemia and termed this the "no-reflow phenomenon." Others have studied this effect through morphological and CBF studies. Nonetheless, there are important changes in the microvasculature that occur during the primary phase of ischemia. Capillary narrowing, endothelial swelling, platelet aggregation, and erythrocyte cell sludging can lead to significant increases in blood viscosity and marked reductions in microcirculation.

Cerebral Protection

Cerebral protection can be divided into a number of categories. Therapy can be directed against the primary problem of ischemia: the mismatch between metabolic substrates (Fig. 1). Several methods of treatment are directed at this problem of increasing CBF and decreasing the metabolic rate. These forms of treatment are directed at the event that triggers the ischemic process itself and are truly protective. After the ischemic cascade has been initiated, other therapeutic techniques are necessary to combat secondary events. Cerebral edema and microvascular changes also require attention (Fig. 3).

In addition to actively treating cerebral ischemia, it is necessary to eliminate certain hazards which can increase the severity of the ischemic insult. Although raising the arterial oxygen tension above normal levels during cere-

bral ischemia does not lessen the ischemic damage, allowing hypoxia to occur can worsen the ischemic injury. Hypotension reduces the cerebral perfusion pressure and can diminish CBF. Hypertension can also be dangerous by exacerbating cerebral edema or causing hemorrhagic infarction.

Conclusions

Increasing blood flow to an area of cerebral ischemia can lessen the severity of the ischemia and can possibly raise lCBF to a level above one or more of the ischemic thresholds. Such techniques cannot be considered protective per se as they are directed at increasing the blood flow and not the primary or secondary events of cerebral infarction. Other techniques designed to augment blood flow include hypervolemic hemodilution and surgical revascularization. Induced hypertension is another method of supplementing blood flow and may be beneficial if begun early. Careful control of arterial pressure, volume status, hematocrit, and cardiac output to optimize the amount of blood flow that reaches an ischemic area via collateral circulation can dramatically influence the outcome.

Cerebral protection by therapeutic intervention of the ischemic cascade is primarily experimental. The role of hyperglycemia and tissue lactate remains controversial; a wide range of animal models have produced mixed outcomes. Whether mannitol improves microcirculation by reducing capillary edema, hemodilution, or other mechanisms, is also unclear. Investigations into the action of prostaglandins and leukotrienes during the ischemic cascade and cell death are in their infancy but exciting. Agents that improve rheology and oxygen delivery to the ischemic region have shown promise in both animal and clinical studies. Barbiturates, agents shown to be protective during the ischemic episode, may have another role besides reducing $CMRO_2$ [13]. Because of their ability to increase CBF and influence calcium fluxes, calcium antagonists were greeted by the medical community with great expectations. However, neither animal nor clinical studies have clearly demonstrated that calcium antagonists protect cerebral tissue. Even though corticosteroids have not been considered protective against ischemia, their use for the treatment of cerebral edema is now questioned. If steroids dramatically reduce cerebral tolerance for ischemia as recently demonstrated, their applications in clinical situations of delayed repetitive ischemia should be carefully studied. Clearly, the future holds great potential for defining the mechanisms of cerebral ischemia and cerebral protective agents.

References

1. Ames A III, Wright RL, Kowada M, Thurston JM, Majno G (1968) Cerebral ischemia: II. The non-reflow phenomenon. Am J Pathol 52:437–453
2. Black KL, Hoff JT (1985) Leukotrienes increase blood-brain barrier permeability following intraparenchymal injections in rats. Ann Neurol 18(3):349–351
3. Black KL, Hoff JT, McGillicuddy JE, et al. (1986) Increased leukotriene C_4 and vasogenic edema surrounding brain tumors in humans. Ann Neurol 19(6):592–595
4. Carter LP, Yamagata S, Erspamer R (1974) Time limits of reversible cortical ischemia. Neurosurgery 12:620–623
5. Harris RJ, Lindquist C, Kamiya K, et al. (1983) The role of leukotrienes in the formation of cerebral ischemic edema. J Cereb Blood Flow Metab 3(1):S285–S286
6. Ibayashi S, Fujishima M, Sadoshima S, et al. (1986) Cerebral blood flow and tissue metabolism in experimental cerebral ischemia of spontaneously hypertensive rats with hyper-, normo-, and hypoglycemia. Stroke 17(2):261–266
7. Jernigan J, Evans OB, Kirshner HS (1984) Hyperglycemia and diabetes improve outcome in a rat model of anoxia/ischemia. Neurology 34 (Suppl 1):262
8. Jones TH, Morawetz RB, Crowell RM, et al. (1981) Thresholds of focal cerebral ischemia in awake monkeys. J Neurosurg 54:773–782
9. Klatzo I (1967) Neuropathological aspects of brain edema. Presidential address. J Neuropathol Exp Neurol 26:1–14
10. Koide T, Wieloch TW, Seisjo BK (1986) Chronic dexamethasone pretreatment aggravates ischemic neuronal necrosis. J Cereb Blood Flow Metab 6:395–404
11. Rehncrona S, Folbergrova J, Smith DS, et al. (1980) Influence of complete and pronounced incomplete cerebral ischemia and subsequent recirculation on cortical concentrations of oxidized and reduced glutathione in the rat. J Neurochem 34:477–486
12. Rehncrona S, Westerberg B, Akesson B, et al. (1982) Brain cortical fatty acids and phospholipids during and following complete and severe incomplete ischemia. J Neurochem 38(1):84–93
13. Shiu GK, Nemoto EM, Alexander HL (1981) Brain free fatty acid changes during global ischemia with barbiturate anesthesia and hypothermia (Abstract). Br J Anaesthesiol 53:304
14. Spetzler RF, Nehls DG (1987) Cerebral protection against ischemia, chap. VII-D. In: Wood JH (ed) Cerebral blood flow: Physiology and clinical aspects. McGraw-Hill, New York

The Scientific Basis of Cerebral Infarction

Lindsay Symon[1]

In recent years the analysis of progression and irreversibility in brain ischemia has advanced considerably. Techniques of evoked response recording in relation to blood flow, of extracellular ionic analysis, and of tissue metabolism, either by detailed microbiochemical techniques from defined areas of ischemia or from in vivo analysis by spectrometric methods, have considerably increased our understanding of the disintegration in neural function occasioned by a progressive ischemia. We are further along the road to understanding the scientific basis of infarction then we were 10 years ago.

It has become apparent both from experimental and clinical analysis that an induced ischemic lesion will cause electrical failure in the area of brain distal to the occlusion. Abundant experimental evidence by inducing an ischemic lesion in known regions of the cerebral hemisphere by middle cerebral occlusion or basilar occlusion, the density of the ischemia being assessed by microcirculatory techniques such as the use of hydrogen electrodes, has indicated a threshold for failure of the evoked response of around 16 ml/100 g/min, normal blood flow being assessed at about 50 ml/100 g/min. Other laboratories have confirmed similar values, but it has been quite clear that failure of electrical activity does not necessarily apply infarction. Thus, the studies of Brierley and ourselves some years ago indicated that, following middle cerebral occlusion in the baboon, the area of infarction was considerably less than the area of electrical failure under acute circumstances and, although Jones and his colleagues have indicated that spreading of irreversible damage towards the threshold of electrical failure may occur, this has not been the experience in other laboratories. It appears

likely, therefore, that electrical failure is a reliable early signal of dangerous levels of ischemia, but not necessarily a signal of inevitable infarction.

Electrical function is closely related to cerebral blood flow (CBF). Originally, we felt that complete electrical failure below the ischemic threshold was due to synaptic depolarization possibly consequent to a release of potassium into the extracellular space. Other conditions, however, such as a change in neurotransmitter metabolism or tissue lactosidosis, have also been discussed in relation to complete electrical failure. In association with Lassen and Astrup some years ago, therefore, we tested the association between electrical function and extracellular ionic activity, potassium, and, subsequently, calcium and pH. The techniques of middle cerebral occlusion, hydrogen electrode recording of blood flow, and multi-barrel microelectrode recording of potassium and pH, or potassium and calcium, enables simultaneous ionic measurements in a single extracellular ionic pool in relation to blood flow.

When blood flow falls below 11 ml/100 g/min considerable and rapid increases in extracellular potassium levels indicate a failure of the ionic pump for potassium. At a slightly lower although statistically inseparable level, extracellular concentrations of calcium declined. Parallel experiments, using bicuculline-induced seizures in the rat, have indicated some biochemical correlates of this level of ionic failure. At the point of seizure interruption induced by a progressive reduction in the blood pressure in the bicuculline rat, extracellular potassium concentration remained low, indicating that sufficient energy remained for ionic pumping. This was verified by direct tissue analysis. Lactic acid was elevated and phosphocreatine decreased, but ATP remained close to normal. Correlates of our own baboon experiments with biochemical analysis by Bachelard's group in St. Thomas' Hospital have shown that significant phosphocreatine decreases occur

[1] Gough-Cooper Department of Neurological Surgery, Institute of Neurology, Queen Square, London, England

at levels of blood flow not yet associated with electrical failure or failure of the ionic pump, but that the other major constituents of the energy transport chain do not change until approaching the level of ionic failure.

Calcium has been of particular interest in relation to irreversible ischemia. The vital role of calcium in normal and pathological cellular function is evidenced by the calcium paradox reported by Zimmerman and Hulsmann in the heart. Heart perfused with a calcium free solution will loss its contractility but will remain able to maintain its electrical activity. Reperfusion after more than 2 min of calcium-free solution, however, caused disappearance of the electrocardiogram in association with a rapid irreversible loss of contractility. Shen and Jennings showed that reperfused myocardium could accumulate up to ten times its normal concentration of calcium, and other experiments have confirmed a rapid accumulation of calcium in reperfused myocardium, suggesting that calcium has an important role in tissue damage associated with a reduction of the ability of intracellular membranes to withstand or control certain ion fluxes and a failure of mitochondrial function by the physical effects of calcium uptake or deposition. Changes of calcium in the extracellular space of the brain was first shown by Nicholson in spreading depression and terminal anoxia in the cerebral cortex and cerebellum. Our own studies demonstrated that the flow threshold for disappearance of calcium from the extracellular space was slightly below that for potassium. Potassium and calcium transients were also seen which shed further light upon the relationship between both ions in the extracellular space. As in ischemia, extracellular potassium began to rise before calcium fell and baseline values of potassium 3.95 ± 0.8 mmol and of calcium 1.31 ± 0.01 mmol showed that extracellular potassium had to rise to levels of about 10.5 ± 3 mmol before calcium started to move. These relationships were exactly the same as what could be shown in progressive calcium and potassium movements in ischemia. Movements of potassium and calcium described in ischemia and in transient fluxes in the baboon are similar in characteristics to the onset of spreading depression studies by Kraig and Nicholson. At points of movement of calcium and potassium extracellular slow potential moves in a negative direction, probably indicating an increase in membrane permeability by depolarization of

ions slowing down their concentration gradients. Such depolarization-induced changes in membrane permeability are the possible cause of calcium movement both in ischemia and spreading depression.

The increase of extracellular potassium in ischaemia is undoubtedly due to a progressive overload of the potassium clearance mechanisms after increased leakage from the cells. The rapidity of onset of calcium influx could, therefore, be expected to relate to the rapidity of potassium movement, the time elapsing for potassium to climb to the critical levels of 13 mmol for calcium release being dependent upon blood flow. There is clearly a differential sensitivity of ion homeostatic mechanism to ischemia, although separate flow thresholds cannot really be established.

Anatomising these movements in greater detail, the rates of potassium efflux, expressed as minutes/pK, can be described by two functions: K^1 and K^2. Ca^1 describes the rate of fall of extracellular calcium as minutes/calcium. In this analysis, the relationship between K^1, K^2 and Ca^1 would suggest that, as an alternative to depolarization to explain calcium movement, availability of cellular energy may be of significance. K^2 is greater than K^1 in every case, suggesting that efflux of potassium increases at a time when the reduced cellular energy levels can no longer maintain ion homestasis, and that this is also the point when calcium begins to fall exponentially. Movement of calcium into the cells was corroborated to some extent by calculation of the extracellular calcium that would occur if all calcium were evenly redistributed between the intra- and extracellular compartments in ischemia. Assuming the compartment size reported by Hossmann and that there is no net change in total calcium, in our experiments the value obtained by extracellular calcium theoretically should be 0.25 mmol. The final extracellular calcium found in densely ischemic tissue with local cerebral blood flow of around 6 ml/100 g/min was 0.28 mmol. Calcium activity in the intra- and extracellular compartments is, therefore, likely to be in equilibrium. Adey's experiments further substantiated intracellular movement of calcium; although calcium was complexed in the membrane, the effect was undoubtedly modest. There is also a possible influence of change in the characteristic of the extracellular space. Rapid changes of the extracellular space (ECS) in ischemia have been demonstrated by impedance measurements or by the use of choline and tris buffer as markers. A decrease in the extracellular space without any net loss in calcium would explain the relatively slight increase in extracellular calcium while potassium rises to the threshold of 13 mmol. This is probably more likely than a change in the binding coefficient for calcium in the extracellular space.

Both Hass and Shanne have indicated the toxic effects of calcium in raised intracellular concentrations.

We do not feel that, with these data, it is possible to distinguish between depolarization and a critical reduction in energy levels as a cause for fall in calcium when potassium reaches 13 mmol. However, it seems clear that the recorded decrease of extracellular calcium indicates a progressive entry into the intracellular compartment to total equilibrium, and is of seriously damaging effect to the neuropil. It represents one of the major contributions to irreversible cell death in ischemia.

Effects of Dynorphin$_{1-13}$ on Opiate Binding and Dopamine and GABA Uptake in a Cat Model of Stroke

Y. Hosobuchi, H. Kuroda, and T. Matsui[1]

Opiates are best known for their analgesic properties, but they have many other effects on central nervous system (CNS) functions, including respiration, temperature control, and behavior. We have reported that certain opiates also may produce recovery from cerebral ischemia [1, 2, 4, 9]. Subsequent studies performed by others to confirm this finding in some [4, 9-11], although not all [6, 8], cases indicated that, in both experimental animals and in humans, opiate agonists exacerbate the symptoms of stroke, whereas opiate antagonists may prolong survival and, in some cases, ameliorate neurological deficits. Dynorphin$_{1-13}$, an endogenous opioid peptide with both agonist and antagonist properties [12, 13], also has been shown to improve survival in animals [3].

Although these findings have great clinical potential, the mechanisms of these actions are unknown. As several studies have indicated that opiates do not alter regional cerebral blood flow or systemic variables, such as blood pressure and heart rate [4], a direct action on the CNS seems a likely basis for the observed effects. In view of accruing evidence that endogenous opioids may act as a neurotransmitter or as modulators of a neurotransmitter [12], it is reasonable to hypothesize that opioid antagonists act on specific nervous pathways critical to survival or recovery from stroke. This conclusion is consistent with the findings in several studies demonstrating altered levels of endogenous opioids and of neurotransmitter uptake associated with stroke. For example, Brandt et al. [5] reported that β-endorphin was elevated in the cerebrospinal fluid (CSF) of a comatose patient with acute necrotizing encephalomyelopathy; similarly, we found a twofold increase in immunoreactive β-endorphin-like material (Ir-βE) and leucine-enkephalin in the CSF of one patient who had had a stroke. Focal elevations of Ir-βE have also been observed in the ischemic hemispheres of gerbils subjected to experimental stroke [9].

With regard to neurotransmitters, Weinberger and Cohen [14] reported differences in the sensitivity of dopamine (DA), gamma-aminobutyric acid (GABA), and glutamate uptake to stroke in gerbils, DA being the most sensitive.

In the present study, we explored these relationships further. We determined levels of both opiate-receptor binding and uptake of DA and GABA in various regions of brain in control, ischemic, and dynorphin$_{1-13}$-treated ischemic cats.

Materials and Methods

Cat Model of Stroke

Transorbital occlusion of the middle cerebral artery (MCA) in cats was performed. Briefly, adult male cats (3–5 kg) were anesthetized; the trachea was intubated, and each cat was placed in a stereotaxic device. The contents of the right orbit (except for the uptake studies, in which the left orbit was used) were removed, and a drill was used to enlarge the optic foramen. The MCA was accessible through an arachnoid dissection. The segment proximal to the lenticulostriate arteries was coagulated with bipolar forceps and transected with microscissors. The orbit was then filled with dental cement and the wound was closed with sutures.

The cats were fully awake within 1–2 h after the operation. We allowed an additional 4 h (for cats in uptake studies) or 6 h (for cats in binding studies) during which to assess their neurological status. If analgesia was necessary postoperatively, we administered 0.25% marcaine as a supraorbital and infraorbital nerve block. In specified experiments, dynorphin$_{1-13}$ (2 mg/kg) was injected intraperitoneally 1 h before the cat

[1] Department of Neurological Surgery, School of Medicine, University of California, San Francisco, California, USA

was killed.

This model of cerebral ischemia produced a highly consistent extent of infarction in studies of more than 80 cats. There was no significant difference in the size of the infarct produced among all control and treatment groups [3].

Preparation of Brain Tissue Fractions

The cat brain, less cerebellum and brain stem, was removed and divided into right and left halves. Each half was further divided into cortical and subcortical regions. Thereby, four regions were obtained from each cat brain. Each brain region was washed in ice-cold 0.32 M sucrose 25 mM N-2-hydroxyethylpiperazine-N'-2-ethanesulfonic acid (HEPES), pH 7.7, then homogenized in a Teflon^R glass homogenizer. The homogenate was centrifuged at 1000 g at 4°C for 10 min in a Sorvall RC2B centrifuge; the pellet was discarded and the supernatant processed to obtain either brain membranes (for binding experiments) or crude synaptosomes (for uptake studies). For brain membranes, the supernatant was centrifuged at 20 000 × g at 4°C for 20 min and the resulting pellet was washed once by resuspension in HEPES-sucrose and was centrifuged at 20 000 × g at 4°C for 20 min. The final pellet (p_2) was resuspended in HEPES-sucrose and was stored at −20°C. For synaptosomes, the supernatant was centrifuged at 27 000 × g at 4°C for 30 min and the pellet was retained. The pellet was then resuspended in Krebs-Ringer phosphate buffer (KRB), pH 7.4, containing 0.05 mM pargyline and 1.7 mM ascorbic acid at a concentration of 150 mg wet weight of tissue/ml. This preparation was used immediately for uptake studies.

Binding Experiments

In saturation experiments, 15 020 concentrations of [^{3}H] ethylketocyclazocine (EKC) ranging from 0.05 to 20 nM were used. The mixture also contained HEPES buffer (25 mM, pH 7.7) and 1 mg brain membrane protein. The mixtures were incubated in a shaking water bath at 37°C for 30 min and then in ice for 60 min, followed by filtration through glass fiber filters. Each filter was washed twice with 5 ml ice-cold HEPES buffer (5 mM), then placed into a polyethylene counting vial with 9 ml scintillation cocktail (Scintiverse II, Fisher Scientific). Radioactivity was counted in a Beckman LS-100C scintillation counter. Specific binding was determined as the

difference between the total brain membrane protein bound and that bound in the presence of 1 μM EKC. The binding data were analyzed by assuming two independent binding sites (high and low). All samples were analyzed in triplicate.

Uptake of Dopamine and GABA

Aliquots of crude synaptosomes were preincubated with KRB at 37°C for 10 min, then radioactive neurotransmitter in 100 μl was added to start the uptake. For DA uptake, the mixture contained 20 μl (100 μg) synaptosomes, 880 μl KRB and 50–600 nM DA. For GABA uptake, the mixture contained 40 μl (200 μg synaptosomes) in 760 μl KRB, 100 μl 10 mM B-alanine, and 4–64 μM GABA.

After 10 min at 37°C, the mixtures were passed through 0.65 μm DA Millipore filters. The filters were rapidly washed twice with 5 ml saline, placed into polyethylene counting vials in 9 ml scintillation cocktail and, 72 h later, were counted in a Beckman LS-100C scintillation counter. Specific uptake was determined as the difference between uptake determined at 37°C and that in samples incubated at 0°C throughout.

The KRB contained 118 mM NaCl, 4.7 mM KCl, 32.0 mM sodium phosphate (pH 7.4), 1.8 mM CaCl$_2$, 1.2 mM MgSO$_4$, 5.6 mM glucose, 1.3 mM ethylenedaminetetraacetate (EDTA), 1.7 mM ascorbic acid, and 0.05 mM pargyline. Radiolabeled neurotransmitters were obtained from New England Nuclear (Boston, Massachusetts): [^{3}H] DA (23.8 Ci/mmol) and [^{3}H] GABA (30.8 Ci/mmol). The [^{3}H]DA or [^{3}H] GABA was mixed with unlabeled DA or GABA. (The unlabeled DA and GABA were obtained from Sigma Chemical Company.)

Results

[^{3}H] EKC Binding

In each experiment, the Scatchard plot of [^{3}H] EKC was curvilinear, suggesting the existence of high-affinity and low-affinity binding sites. Figure 1 shows representative Scatchard plots for control and stroked cat brains. For subcortex, tissue from two identically treated cats was sometimes pooled in order to obtain enough material for assay. The plots for right and left cortices were virtually identical for control cats,

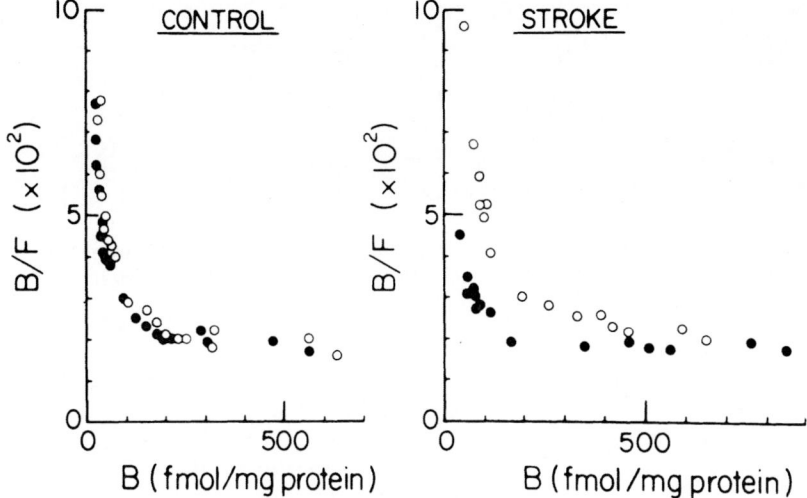

Fig. 1. Scatchard plots of tritiated EKC binding in control and stroked cat brain. [^{3}H]EKC binding was assayed as described in materials and methods. ● right cortex, ○ left cortex

Table 1. [^{3}H]EKC binding in control cat brain

	RC	LC	RS	LS
B_{max1} (fmol/mg protein)	47.7 ± 9.3	49.0 ± 4.9	42.1 ± 9.3	45.0 ± 15.8
K_{d1} (nM)	0.30 ± 0.001	0.30 ± 0.001	1.00 ± 0.005	1.01 ± 0.015
B_{max2} (fmol/mg protein)	200 ± 110	213 ± 99.6	205 ± 332	220 ± 57.2
K_{d2} (nM)	13.2 ± 2.6	12.0 ± 2.1	10.9 ± 0.7	9.3 ± 1.3

[^{3}H]EKC binding was determined as given in materials and methods. Each value represents mean $\pm$ SD. Data for cortex are based on eight separate experiments (one brain for each), and data for subcortex on four experiments (two pooled brains for each)
RC right cortex ($n = 8$), *LC* left cortex ($n = 8$), *RS* right subcortex ($n = 4$), *LS* left subcortex ($n = 4$)

Table 2. [^{3}H]EKC binding in stroked cat brain

	RC	LC	RS	LS
B_{max1} (fmol/mg protein)	58.5 ± 24.7	45.8 ± 16.5	49.6 ± 20.7	47.7 ± 20.0
K_{d1} (nM)	0.58 ± 0.32^a	0.30 ± 0.04	1.00 ± 0.04	1.01 ± 0.01
B_{max2} (fmol/mg protein)	313 ± 148	227 ± 84.3	317 ± 60.09	250 ± 56.0
K_{d2} (nM)	17.7 ± 10.7	12.8 ± 5.2	10.3 ± 3.1	10.6 ± 0.37

[a] $P < 0.01$ (two-tail test)
Number of determinations was 12 for cortex (C) and six for subcortex (S). Each value represents mean $\pm$ SD. A significant difference between stroke (R right) and nonstroke (L left) side is indicated by footnote [a]. Level of significance was determined by the paired Student's t-test. Right MCA was ligated, $n = 12$ (cortex), $n = 6$ (subcortex)

whereas there was a significant difference in the cat brains with stroke.

There was no significant difference in dissociation constant (K_d) and maximum binding capacity (B_{max}) between right and left halves in control cat brains (Table 1). In cats with stroke, the high affinity K_d of the right (ischemic) cortex was significantly ($P < 0.01$) more than that of the left (Table 2). There was no significant difference in other parameters or regions.

We also examined the effect of dynorphin$_{1-13}$ on [^{3}H] EKC binding in cats with stroke. Dynorphin$_{1-13}$ (2 mg/kg) was injected intraperitoneally 1 h before killing in six cats with

Table 3. [^{3}H]EKC binding in stroked cat brain treated with dynorphin$_{1-13}$

	RC	LC	RS	LS
B_{max1} (fmol/mg protein)	48.0 ± 9.1	50.2 ± 8.5	45.7 ± 16.6	53.2 ± 14.7
K_{d1} (nM)	0.31 ± 0.008	0.31 ± 0.008	0.90 ± 0.08	0.93 ± 0.05
B_{max2} (fmol/mg protein)	2.36 ± 41.5	236 ± 39.1	296 ± 87.7	326 ± 76.8
K_{d2} (nM)	12.0 ± 2.6	12.5 ± 3.6	11.6 ± 0.9	11.4 ± 2.5

Dynorphin$_{1-13}$ (2 mg/kg) was injected intraperitoneally 1 h before killing. Number of determinations for cortices (C) and subcortices (S) were six and four, respectively. Each value represents mean ± SD., $n = 6$ (cortex), $n = 4$ (subcortex)

stroke. This treatment abolished the difference in high affinity K_d between right and left cortex; the binding affinity in right cortex was now increased to the previous level in control (Table 3).

Dopamine and GABA Uptake in Control Cats

In the control cat brain, DA uptake was saturated with 600 nM DA in both cortex and subcortex. In either cortex or subcortex values, there was no significant difference in K_m or V_{max} between right and left halves (Table 4). GABA uptake was saturated with 64 μM GABA in both cortex and subcortex. Again, there was no significant difference between right and left halves of either cortex or subcortex (Table 4).

Dopamine and GABA Uptake in Cats with Stroke

All eight cats showed typical hemiplegia 4 h after left MCA occlusion. In the DA uptake study, the K_m was significantly reduced ($P < 0.001$) and the V_{max} was increased ($P < 0.05$) in the right cortex (nonoccluded side) as compared with that in the left cortex (Table 5). The latter values were not significantly different from right or left cortex values in control cats (Table 4). There was no significant difference in K_m or V_{max} between right and left subcortex. In the GABA uptake study, there was no significant difference in K_m or V_{max} between right and left sides either in cortex or subcortex, or between them and corresponding control values (Table 5).

In cats with stroke treated with dynorphin$_{1-13}$, the K_m of DA uptake in the right cortex was increased so that it no longer differed significantly from the corresponding value of the control cats (Table 4). However, the K_m of the left cortex in the dynorphin animals was also raised so that it was significantly higher than the control left cortex value (Table 6). The V_{max} value of the right cortex DA uptake was decreased

under these conditions so that it did not differ significantly from either control values or from the values for the left cortex for the same animal. Finally, the K_m of DA uptake of right subcortex was reduced in dynorphin$_{1-13}$-treated animals, relative to left subcortex or controls. There were no dynorphin-associated changes in GABA uptake parameters.

Discussion

In these studies, we used [^{3}H] EKC to assess opiate binding in control cats and cats with stroke. This opioid agonist binds to at least four major subtypes of opiate receptors found in the brain: mu, delta, kappa, and sigma [7]. We felt this lack of selectivity would be an advantage in our study, as we did not know which, if any, of these subtypes is affected by stroke.

When opiate binding was determined in this manner, the only significant effect of stroke was to increase the high-affinity K_d about twofold in ischemic cortex (Table 2). This effect was reversed by dynorphin$_{1-13}$ treatment, which otherwise had no effect (Table 3). Because EKC is nonselective under these conditions, it is conceivable that a single opiate receptor subtype is being affected by stroke to a much greater degree than is apparent from our data. As treatment of animals with irreversible alkylating agents selective for particular subtypes does not cause death, it seems unlikely that any magnitude of change in an opiate receptor by itself could be responsible for the debilitating effects of stroke. Nevertheless, the fact that dynorphin$_{1-13}$ was able to improve survival and reverse the change in EKC binding due to stroke suggests that this peptide plays a role in the process. Since the K_d change occurred in the high-affinity site of ischemic cortex only, and not in nonischemic cortex, it appears to be a direct reflection of ischemia, and

Table 4. Dopamine and GABA uptake in control cat brain

	RC	LC	RS	LS
DA uptake				
K_m (nM)	254 ± 39.5	237 ± 36.4	317 ± 64.0	329 ± 48.4
V_{max} (pmol/mg prot/10 min)	21.4 ± 3.2	21.5 ± 3.7	38.1 ± 7.0	34.6 ± 7.5
GABA uptake				
K_m (μM)	13.2 ± 3.5	12.9 ± 3.5	12.0 ± 2.7	11.5 ± 3.4
V_{max} (pmol/mg prot/10 min)	1091 ± 312	993 ± 217	1967 ± 512	2100 ± 446

Dopamine and GABA uptake were determined as given in materials and methods. Number of determinations for cortices (C) and subcortices (S) was nine. Each value represents mean $\pm$ SD, $n = 9$

Table 5. Dopamine and GABA uptake in stroked cat brain

	RC	LC	RS	LS
DA uptake				
K_m (nM)	181 ± 28.2^a	286 ± 64.4	337 ± 107	293 ± 75.3
V_{max} (pmol/mg prot/10 min)	26.1 ± 4.1^b	21.0 ± 3.8	33.4 ± 6.4	33.3 ± 14.3
GABA uptake				
K_m (μM)	11.5 ± 2.0	11.4 ± 2.1	9.9 ± 3.3	9.3 ± 2.9
V_{max} (pmol/mg prot/10 min)	1059 ± 268	1043 ± 310	2344 ± 61	1932 ± 671

[a] $P < 0.001$
[b] $P < 0.05$

Number of determinations for cortices (C) and subcortices (S) was eight. Each value represents mean $\pm$ SD. A significant difference between nonstroke (R right) and stroke (L left) side is indicated by footnotes [a] and [b]. Significance was determined by the paired Student's t-test. Left MCA was ligated, $n = 8$

Table 6. Dopamine and GABA uptake in dynorphin$_{1-13}$-treated stroked cat brain

	RC	LC	RS	LS
DA uptake				
K_m (nM)	246 ± 62.4	333 ± 70.6	227 ± 74.2	309 ± 116
V_{max} (pmol/mg prot/10 min)	21.9 ± 4.1	19.6 ± 4.3	37 ± 12.0	32.3 ± 9.3
GABA uptake				
K_m (μM)	11.4 ± 4.0	14.2 ± 5.8	10.6 ± 3.5	11.5 ± 4.5
V_{max} (pmol/mg prot/10 min)	1260 ± 269	1106 ± 231	2334 ± 480	2215 ± 614

Dynorphin$_{1-13}$ (2 mg/kg) was injected intraperitoneally 1 hour before killing. Number of determinations for cortices (C) and subcortices (S) was eight. Each value represents mean $\pm$ SD. A significant difference between nonstroke (R right) and stroke (L left) side is indicated by the asterisk. Significance was determined by the paired Student's t-test. Left MCA was ligated, $n = 8$

not a compensatory change.

We also found stroke-associated changes in DA uptake. In this case, it was the nonischemic cortex affected, with K_m significantly reduced while V_{max} was increased (Table 5). Thus, this could be a compensatory change in which healthy cortex adapts its functions in order to take over for injured tissue. Again, dynorphin$_{1-13}$ treatment reversed the effects, although the peptide raised the K_m in both cortices

so that the ischemic cortex K_m was significantly higher than control (Table 6). As with opiate binding, we observed no significant changes in DA uptake in the subcortex, except for a decrease in K_m, or right subcortex of stroked cats treated with dynorphin$_{1-13}$, and no changes in either cortex or subcortex of GABA uptake. In the latter respect, our findings thus agree with those of Weinberger and Cohen [14], who reported that DA uptake was most sensitive to stroke.

The possible relationship to stroke of changes in DA uptake, like that of opiate binding, is difficult to gauge. Because of the vital role that transmitter uptake plays in transmitter action, such changes could conceivably have significant effects on brain function. Be that as it may, the selectivity of the effect, with GABA uptake being unaffected, argues against its simply reflecting decreased energy availability. Furthermore, as with opiates, overall changes we observed may mask a larger change in a select group of neurons.

In summary, occlusion of the MCA induced changes in the opiate receptor and DA uptake systems in cats. Treatment with dynorphin$_{1-13}$ reversed these changes. We suggest that the action of dynorphin$_{1-13}$ must be specific because not all systems were affected. We previously reported that dynorphin prolonged survival in cats subjected to experimental stroke; 60% of treated cats survived for at least 7 days, whereas no untreated cat with stroke survived for more than two days. This rapid mortality for cats in the control condition prohibits controlled, long-term biochemical studies of dynorphin's effects. However, it could be that the biochemical changes we observed after 1 hour are merely initial changes, and prolonged study would show a greater potency of dynorphin in altering binding or uptake. Thus, we may be observing only a fraction of dynorphin's potency in altering binding or uptake.

References

1. Baskin DS, Hosobuchi Y (1981) Naloxone reversal of ischemic neurological deficits in man. Lancet 2:272–275

2. Baskin DS, Hosobuchi Y, Grevel JC (1986) Treatment of experimental stroke with opiate antagonists: Effects on neurological function, infarct size, and survival. J Neurosurg 64:99–103

3. Baskin DS, Hosobuchi Y, Loh HH, Lee NM (1984) Dynorphin (1-13) improves survival in cats with focal cerebral ischemia. Nature 312:551–552

4. Baskin DS, Kieck CF, Hosobuchi Y (1984) Naloxone reversal and morphine exacerbation of neurologic deficits secondary to focal cerebral ischemia in baboons. Brain Res 290:289–296

5. Brandt NJ, Terenius L, Jacobsen BB, Klinken L, Nordius A, Brandt S, Blegvad K, Yssing M (1980) Hyperendorphin syndrome in a child with necrotizing encephalomyelopathy. N Engl J Med 303:914–916

6. Cutler JR, Bredesen DE, Edwards R, Simon RP (1983) Failure of naloxone to reverse vascular neurological deficits. Neurology 33:1517–1518

7. Garzon J, Sanchez-Blazquez P, Lee NM (1984) [^{3}H]-ethylketocyclazocine binding to mouse brain membranes: Evidence for a kappa opioid receptor type. J Pharmacol Exp Ther 231:33–37

8. Holoday JN, D'Amato RJ (1982) Naloxone or the TRH fail to improve neurologic deficits in gerbil models of stroke. Life Sci 31:385–392

9. Hosobuchi Y, Baskin DS, Woo SK (1982) Reversal of induced ischemic neurologic deficit in gerbils by the opiate antagonist naloxone. Science 215:69–71

10. Iselin HA, Weiss P (1981) Naloxone reversal of ischemic neurologic deficit. Lancet 2:642–643

11. Jovaily J, Davis JB (1982) Naloxone partially reverses neurologic deficits in some but not all stroke patients. Neurology 32:A194

12. Lee NM, Smith AP (1984) Possible regulatory function of dynorphin and its clinical implications. Trends Pharmacol Sci 5:108–110

13. Talunay FC, Jen MF, Chang JK, Loh HH, Lee NM (1981) Possible regulatory role of dynorphin on morphine and β-endorphin-induced analgesia. J Pharmacol Exp Ther 219:296–298

14. Weinberger J, Cohen G (1982) The differential effect of ischemia on the active uptake of dopamine and aminobutyric acid, and glutamate by brain synaptosomes. J Neurochem 38:963–968

Does Glutamatergic Excitatory Synaptic Transmission Play a Role in Ischemia?

D. MILLER and S. J. PEERLESS[1]

Glutamate and aspartate have become increasingly accepted by neurophysiologists as endogenous neurotransmitters. These acidic amino acids mediate excitatory synaptic transmission throughout the central nervous system. Three dendritic, postsynaptic receptor subtypes are known; a fourth possibly exists at a presynaptic site. The major excitatory amino acid receptors are named on the basis of specific agonist binding: N-methyl-D-aspartate (NMDA or NMA), Kainate, and Quisqualate. The non-NMDA receptors mediate fast, all-or-none excitatory transmission within glutamatergic pathways, whereas the NMDA receptors mediate such complex neurophysiological functions as long-term potentiation, memory, and learning.

Evidence is accumulating that central excitatory synaptic transmission plays a major role in various CNS pathologies, including epilepsy, aging, chronic degenerative diseases, and hypoxic-ischemic disorders such as cerebral palsy and stroke.

Glutamate and its analogues are referred to as "excitotoxins" due to their capacity to cause axon-sparing, selective neuronal lesions upon intracerebral injection, and to cause neuronal culture cell death with topical application. Blockade of synaptic activity involving these excitatory amino acids has been shown to prevent cell death. Several studies have shown that ischemic neuronal cell death may be decreased or even prevented by either of two experimental methods: prior injection with an NMDA antagonist compound, or prior lesioning of the glutamatergic pathway. The exact pathophysiological mechanisms remain to be elucidated.

Concentration of excitatory amino acids within synapses is regulated solely by uptake mechanisms, mostly astrocytic but also neuronal (Fig. 1). Major differences exist between the NMDA and the non-NMDA receptors. NMDA receptors are normally blocked by a magnesium-dependent, voltage-gated mechanism, only responding to a neurotransmitter when unblocked; non-NMDA receptors are not gated and respond to any available excitatory neurotransmitter. NMDA receptors are found in high concentration in areas of selective vulnerability. NMDA receptors normally mediate physiological processes via a variety of intracellular metabolic cascades (Fig. 2). These are activated only by a barrage of dendritic synaptic input. NMDA receptors control receptor-operated calcium channels within the postsynaptic density which cause membrane depolarization, opening of dendritic low and high threshold voltage-operated calcium channels, and neuronal paroxysmal burst-firing. These NMDA receptors have other intracellular effects. Apparently, they stimulate other, second messenger systems besides calcium, i.e., cyclic guanosine monophosphate (GMP), cyclic adenosine monophosphate (AMP), and lipids. These membrane lipids play a significant role in signal transduction via the phosphatidyl-inositol-phosphate (PIP) system with subsequent production of arachidonic acid within the cell membrane.

In ischemia, both neuronal depolarization with neurotransmitter release and blockade of uptake mechanisms cause immediate massive elevation of excitatory amino acid neurotransmitter in the extracellular fluid (Fig. 1). Decreased extracellular levels of magnesium in ischemia may unblock neuronal NMDA receptors, making them available to respond to the abnormally elevated levels of excitatory amino acids. Intracellular metabolic cascades normally stimulated during transduction of the excitatory input via NMDA-receptors may, therefore, be hyperactivated early in ischemia. This could possibly be injurious to neurons via initiation of the process of depletion of essential energy stores and the disruption of energy utilization and perhaps compartmentalization. Excessive receptor

[1] Division of Neurosurgery, The University of Western Ontario, London, Ontario, Canada

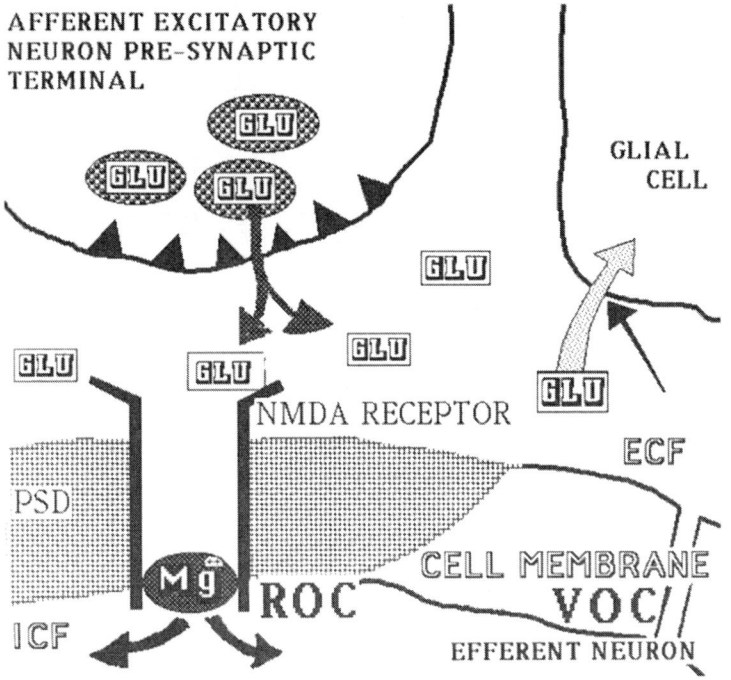

Fig. 1. Glutamatergic excitatory synapse. Presynaptic terminal depolarization releases large amounts of excitatory neurotransmitter into the synaptic cleft. High-affinity excitatory amino acid uptake mechanism (only means of removing neurotransmitter from synapse) is blocked. NMDA receptors are unblocked. *GLU* glutamate, *ECF* extracellular fluid, *ICF* intracellular fluid, MG^{++} magnesium, *NMDA* *N*-methyl-*D*-asparate, *PSD* postsynaptic density, *ROC* receptor operated channel, *VOC* voltage operated channel

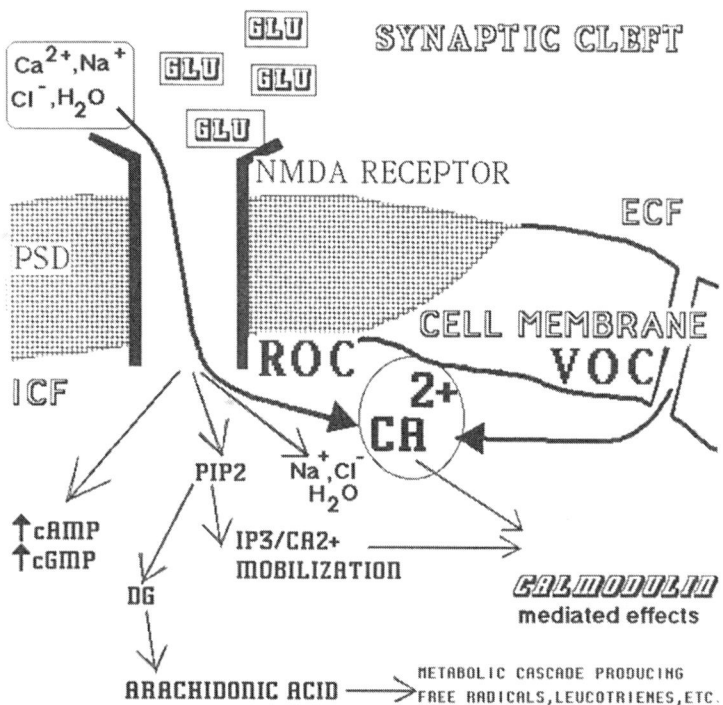

Fig. 2. Ischemic efferent neuron. Elevated levels of excitatory neurotransmitter in the ECF cause hyperactivation of unblocked NMDA receptors. Excessive activation of normal physiological intracellular processes has deleterious effects. IP^3 phosphatidylinositol triphosphate, *DG* diacyl glycerol, *cAMP* cyclic adenosine monophosphate, *cGMP* cyclic guanosine monophosphate, PIP^2 phosphatidylinositol 4,5-biphosphate, other *abbreviations* as in Fig. 1

stimulation could also cause rapid massive calcium influx with exhaustion of buffering mechanisms, leading to negative intracellular changes such as microtubular disruption and cytoskeletal modification via calmodulin overactivation, as well as uncoupling of oxidative metabolism along with many other effects (Fig. 2). The calcium toxicity theory of cell death could be mediated by NMDA receptors via these mechanisms alone, but they are also theorized to mediate cellular injury via chloride flux and intracellular swelling.

Other theories regarding the negative effects of arachidonic acid and free radicals are also compatible with mediation via NMDA receptors. Elevated levels of free fatty acid, especially arachidonic acid, occur immediately in ischemia and progressively increase. These are initially derived from the neuronal PIP signal transduction system. This is very likely due to hyperactivity of NMDA receptors with arachidonic acid production within the neuronal membrane, and with the subsequent production of deleterious compounds derived from its metabolism, such as free radicals, prostaglandins, and leukotrienes (Fig. 2). The rapid burst-firing seen immediately after the onset of ischemia, and also after recirculation, is probably mediated via NMDA receptors.

It is possible that, at the onset of ischemia, a hypermetabolic state is produced via hyperactivation of normal physiological processes. These could prove detrimental to the neuron, prior to significant energy failure.

The recent production of antagonist compounds for excitatory amino acid receptors has opened a new frontier for cerebral neurotransmitter and ischemia research. With further delineation of intracellular metabolic cascades, a more comprehensive knowledge of neurotransmitter physiology, development of potent excitatory amino acid antagonists capable of crossing the blood-brain barrier, and utilization in combination with other compounds directed towards specific pathophysiological mechanisms, it may be possible that drugs which block interneuronal glutamatergic excitatory transmission will prove clinically useful in combating cerebral ischemia in the future.

References

1. Benveniste H, Drejer J, Schousboe A, Diemer NH (1984) Elevation of the extracellular concentrations of glutamate and aspartate in rat hippocampus during transient cerebral ischemia monitored by intracerebral microdialysis. J Neurochem 43:1369–1374
2. Bosley TM, Woodhams PL, Gordon RD, Balazs R (1983) Effects of anoxia on the stimulated release of amino acid neurotransmitters in the cerebellum in vitro. J Neurochem 40:189–200
3. Dingledine (1986) NMDA Receptors: What do they do? Trends Neurosci 9:47–49
4. Excitatory Amino Acid Transmission, A Satellite Symposium to the XXX IUPS Congress, Abstract Volume, 20–23 July 1986
5. Fagg (1985) L-Glutamate, excitatory amino acid receptors and brain function. Trends Neurosci: 207–210
6. Fagg GE, Foster AC, Ganong AH (1986) Excitatory amino acid synaptic mechanisms and neurological function. Trends Pharmacol Sci 7:357–363
7. French ED, Aldinio C, Schwarcz R (1982) Intrahippocampal kainic acid, seizures, and local neuronal degeneration: Relationships assessed in unanesthetized rats. Neuroscience 7:2525–2536
8. Ikeda M, Yoshida S, Busto R, Santiso M, Ginsberg MD (1986) Polyphosphoinositides as a probable source of brain free fatty acids accumulated at the onset of ischemia. J Neurochem 47:123–132
9. Mayer ML, Westbrook GL (1987) Cellular mechanisms underlying excitotoxicity. Trends Neurosci 10:59–61
10. Meldrum B (1985) Excitatory amino acids and anoxic/ischemic brain damage. Trends Neurosci: 47–48
11. Meyer FB, Sundt TM Jr., Yanagihara T, Anderson RE (1987) Focal cerebral ischemia: Pathophysiologic mechanisms and rationale for future avenues of treatment. Mayo Clin Proc 62:35–55
12. Nicoletti FM, Iadarola JT, Wroblewski T, Costa E (1986) Exicitatory amino acid recognition sites coupled with inositol phospholipid metabolism: Developmental changes and interaction with 1-adrenoceptors. Proc Natl Acad Sci USA 83:1931–1935
13. Nicoletti F, Meek JL, Iadarola MJ, Chuang DM, Rothe BL, Costa E (1986) Coupling of inositol phospholipid metabolism with excitatory amino acid recognition sites in rat hippocampus. J Neurochem 46:40–46
14. Nicoletti F, Wroblewski T, Novelli A, Alho H, Guidotti A, Costa E (1986) The activation of inositol phospholipid metabolism as a signal-transducing system for excitatory amino acids in primary cultures of cerebellar granule cells. J Neurosci 6:1905–1911
15. Rothman SM, Olney JW (1986) Glutamate and the pathophysiology of hypoxic-ischemic brain damage. Ann Neurol 19:105–111
16. Schwarcz R, Foster A, French E, Whetsell Kohler C (1984) Excitotoxic models for neurodegenerative disorders. Life Sci 35:19–32
17. Schwarcz R, Meldrum, B (1985) Excitatory amino-acid antagonists provide a therapeutic approach to neurological disorders. Lancet 140–143
18. Siesjo BK (1984) Review article: Cerebral circulation and metabolism. J Neurosurg 60:883–908
19. Simon RP, Swan JH, Griffiths T, Meldrum BS (1984) Blockade of N-methyl-D-aspartate receptors may protect against ischemic damage in the brain. Science 226:850–852
20. Watkins JC, Evans RH (1981) Excitatory amino acid transmitters. Ann Rev Pharmacol Toxicol 21:165–204

The Possible Role of Free Radical Scavengers in the Mitigation of Ischemic Brain Damage

Takao Asano[1], Taku Shigeno[1], Hiroo Johshita[1], and Tetsu Hanamura[2]

Introduction

During the past decade, a considerable research effort has been directed toward substantiation of the hypothesized role of free radicals and lipid peroxidation in the occurrence of ischemic brain damage. Regarding the enhanced generation of active oxygens and the occurrence of lipid peroxidation during or following cerebral ischemia, however, experimental results have not been consistent. Although favorable effects of some free radical scavengers on ischemic brain damage were reported by some authors, the exact mechanism of action of each drug has remained uncertain. Therefore, the theory remains controversial as yet, and it seems justified to question what the real significance of free radical mechanism is in the occurrence of ischemic brain damage.

It has been well substantiated that living cells generate very small amounts of oxygen-free radicals and hydroperoxides. Also, there is no doubt that lipid peroxidation rapidly proceeds in incubated brain tissues. The most essential problem for the "free radical hypothesis" is whether or not an overt peroxidation of membrane lipids is induced by active oxygens at the time or after an ischemic insult so that the membrane function is irreversibly damaged. Whereas an immediate solution appears unlikely, it is possible to analyze this problem from an novel viewpoint, based on recent knowledge of the metabolic pathways of free arachidonic acid, i.e., the arachidonate cascade.

The brain is rich in the enzymes composing the arachidonate cascade. The production of a variety of biologically potent eicosanoids within the brain was shown to be increased under pathological conditions such as ischemia. Of particular relevance to the free radical mechanism is the fact that the arachidonate cascade liberates free radicals and that the tissue level of free radicals (ambient free radicals) affects the activity of key enzymes of the cascade such as cyclooxygenase and lipoxygenase [15]. Therefore, it can be postulated that an increased tissue level of free radicals may stimulate either one or both of the non-enzymatic (autoxidation) and enzymatic (the arachidonate cascade) pathways of lipid peroxidation. During the past several years, we have concentrated our research effort on the elucidation of the roles of free radicals and the arachidonate cascade in the occurrence of ischemic brain damage. In the present paper, pertinent findings are summarized and the rationale for the clinical application of free radical scavengers is discussed.

Relevance of Cyclooxygenase Products to Brain Edema and rCBF Following Prolonged Ischemia and Recirculation

Using the prolonged unilateral and transient bilateral carotid artery occlusion models in gerbils, Gaudet et al. [7, 8] showed a significant elevation in the brain level of prostaglandins (PGs) following ischemia. The increase in PGs was particularly marked following recirculation, the time course of which was almost parallel to the brain level of free arachidonic acid (AA) as we showed using a similar animal model [17]. Using the middle cerebral artery (MCA) occlusion model in cats, we recently determined the regional brain level of each PG which was topographically correlated to rCBF values (the hydrogen clearance method). Prolonged ischemia (rCBF < 30 ml/100 g/min) was associated with a moderate increase or each PG, and recirculation after 2-h ischemia was followed by an explosive elevation of PGE_2 and PGF_{2a}.

Regarding the relevance of cyclooxygenase products to edema formation due to prolonged ischemia, Gaudet et al. [8] reported that there

[1] Department of Neurosurgery, Saitama Medical Center, Saitama Medical School, Kawagoe, Japan
[2] Department of Neurosurgery, University of Tokyo Hospital, Tokyo, Japan

Table 1. The effect of each agent on the cortical specific gravity following prolonged ischemia[a] and recirculation[b]

	rCBF(ml/100g/min)	0–15	15–30
Prolonged ischemia	Saline (control)	$1.0353 \pm 4 \times 10^{-4}$ (24)	$1.0382 \pm 7 \times 10^{-4}$ (26)
	indomethacin	1.0353 ± 5 (20)	1.0357 ± 8 (16)[c]
	ONO 3144	1.0368 ± 7 (19)	1.0398 ± 8 (11)
	AVS	1.0400 ± 4 (22)[e]	1.0433 ± 9 (13)[e]
Recirculation	Saline	$1.0318 \pm 9 \times 10^{-4}$ (19)	$1.0365 \pm 12 \times 10^{-4}$ (18)
	indomethacin	1.0360 ± 10 (23)[d]	1.0382 ± 12 (20)
	ONO 3144	1.0355 ± 7 (29)[d]	1.0381 ± 11 (16)
	AVS	1.0346 ± 9 (19)[c]	1.0412 ± 1 (13)[d]

Cortical samples were divided according to the mean rCBF during MCA occlusion. The numbers in *parentheses* indicate the number of samples. Statistical analysis by U-test.
[a] Following 4-h MCA occlusion
[b] Following 2-h recirculation after 2-h MCA occlusion
[c] $P < 0.05$
[d] $P < 0.01$
[e] $P < 0.001$

was a poor correlation between the brain level of each PG and brain edema. We examined the effect of a cyclooxygenase inhibitor, indomethacin (4 mg/kg), on ischemic brain edema (the cortical specific gravity) and rCBF using the cat MCA occlusion model [3]. Indomethacin did not ameliorate and rather worsened edema. The rCBF during MCA occlusion was not affected (Table 1). This result is consonant to preceding studies showing that the cyclooxygenase products do not play a major role in edema formation due to prolonged ischemia. On the other hand, indomethacin markedly mitigated brain edema and improved rCBF following recirculation (Table 1; Fig. 1). Subsequent studies revealed that free radical scavengers such as ONO 3141 and AVS had similar effects to that of indomethacin. These results indicate that the hitherto known detrimental effect of recirculation is attributable to free radicals liberated from the arachidonate cascade. Thus, free radical scavengers seem to have a definite place in the therapy of cerebral ischemia when it is accompanied by recirculation.

Relevance of Lipoxygenase Products

It has been shown that the intracerebral injection of AA causes brain edema [1, 6], which is not suppressed by administration of indomethacin [6] as in the case of prolonged ischemia. Since intracerebrally accumulated free AA causes edema and since the conversion of free AA to lipoxygenase products is rather augmented by

indomethacin, it is tempting to speculate that the lipoxygenase products are involved in the occurrence of brain edema following prolonged ischemia. However, there is as yet a paucity in the literature concerning the brain level of lipoxygenase products in the normal or ischemic animals. Although a transient increase in leukotrienes (LTs) C_4 and D_4 was reported in the brains of animals exposed to transient ischemia, Subarachnoid hemorrhage (SAH), or trauma [12], LTs represent only a small portion of the whole spectrum of lipoxygenase products. Therefore, we undertook a study to determine the brain level of each lipoxygenase product (hydroxyeicosatetraenoic acid: HETE) using the rat MCA occlusion model.

The extent of cerebral infarction and the time-course of hemispheric edema following unilateral permanent MCA occlusion in rats were previously described [10, 11]. The content of each HETE in the affected hemisphere was determined by the use of high-performance liquid chromatography (HPLC) [16]. A significant and overall increase of HETEs was revealed as late as 72 h after MCA occlusion (Table 2). Although hemispheric edema became maximal at the same period in this model, it is not clear from this result whether the increased synthesis of lipoxygenase products was the cause or the result of brain edema. Therefore, we further investigated the alteration in the synthesis of lipoxygenase products following MCA occlusion within a particular fraction of the brain, i.e., brain microvessels.

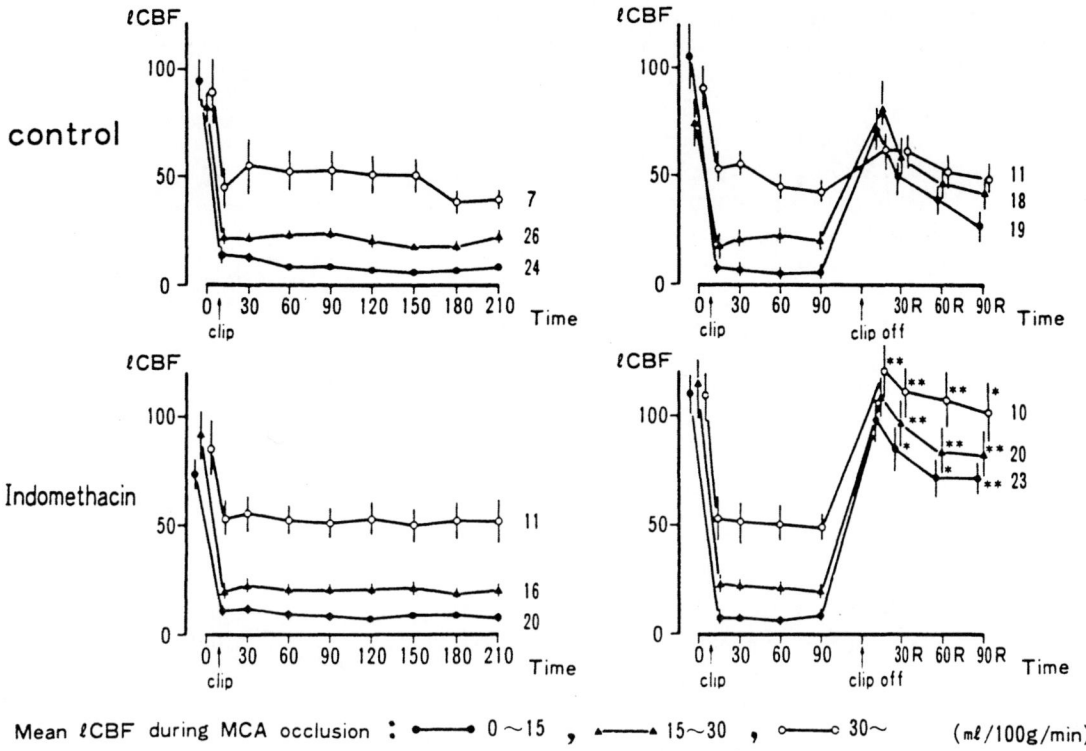

Mean ℓCBF during MCA occlusion : ●——● 0∼15 , ▲——▲ 15∼30 , ○——○ 30∼ (mℓ/100g/min)

Fig. 1. The effect of indomethacin on the rCBF during prolonged ischemia (*left*) and recirculation (*right*) in the CAT MCA occlusion model. Significance of the difference from the control was evaluated by the nonparametrical analysis (Wilcoxon test).* $P < 0.05$,** $P < 0.01$

Table 2. The hemispheric content (ng/g wet weight) of each HETE following MCA occlusion in rats

Duration of ischemia		5-HETE	9-HETE	8- and/or 12-HETE[c]	11-HETE	15-HETE
0 (control)	(n = 4)	0.0 ± 0.0	0.0 ± 0.0	0.0 ± 0.0	0.0 ± 0.0	2.1 ± 2.1
24 h	(n = 4)	0.0 ± 0.0	0.0 ± 0.0	0.0 ± 0.0	1.6 ± 1.6	9.1 ± 3.8
72 h	(n = 4)	18.3 ± 2.8[b]	16.6 ± 3.0[a]	23.7 ± 14.9	14.0 ± 3.4[a]	19.8 ± 5.5[a]

Each value represents the mean + SE for the number of independent determination indicated in the parentheses
Significantly different from the control at [a] $P < 0.05$, [b] $P < 0.01$
[c] 8- and 12-HETEs are in the same column because these were not separated by the HPLC used in the present study

Synthesis of Lipoxygenase Products in Brain Microvessels

Since the major function of the blood-brain barrier (BBB) resides in endothelial cells, it is clear that brain microvessels (MV) are involved in the pathogenetic mechanism underlying ischemic brain edema. The metabolically active MV was prepared from affected hemispheres by the use of nylon meshes and sucrose-density centrifugation. The eicosanoate synthetic capacity of the MV, i.e., the conversion from radiolabeled AA to each eicosanoids was determined by radiochromatography. A generalized increase in the synthetic capacity was revealed with each eicosanoids, and it was most pronounced with hydroxyacids (HETEs) [4]. Of particular interest is the fact that the synthesis of HETEs was greatest at 24 h after MCA occlusion, which was much earlier than the period when a significant increase in the hemispheric content of HETEs was detected in the same model. From this result, it may be surmised that the lipoxygenase pathway within a particular fraction of the brain, such as the MV, is stimulated early in the course of cerebral ischemia and participates in the formation of edema.

Regarding the chemical mechanisms involved in the increased synthesis of lipoxygenase products, we showed that a hydroperoxyeicosatetraenoic acid, 15-HPETE, caused a pronounced stimulation of the lipoxygenase pathway of the MV [13]. Other possible edema factors, such as monoamines, showed no significant effect. A free radical scavenger, AVS [1,2-bis(nicotinamide)-propane, Chugai Pharmaceutical Co.] inhibited the 15-HPETE-induced production of lipoxygenase products of the MV in vitro [13], and markedly mitigated brain edema following MCA occlusion in cats [2] and rats [10]. Taken together, these pieces of evidence indicate that the generation of free radicals and hydroperoxides, and the subsequent activation of a lipoxygenase pathway within the MV are involved in the pathomechanism underlying ischemic brain edema.

Effect of 15-HPAA on Membrane-bound Enzyme, Na$^+$, K$^+$-ATPase

It has been assumed that lipid peroxidation is harmful to cells because it damages the membrane-bound enzymes, such as Na$^+$, K$^+$-ATPase. Insomuch as the arachidonate cascade is a form of lipid peroxidation, our study, showing that the lipoxygenase products participate in edema formation, is apparently consonant to the above thesis. But, the study which was carried out to examine the possible damaging effect of 15-HPETE on Na$^+$, K$^+$-ATPase of the MV and synaptosomes revealed quite an unexpected result [14]. In relatively low concentrations ($< 10^{-5}$ M), 15-HPETE was found to increase the activity of the enzyme, whereas the agent significantly suppressed the enzyme activity of synaptosomes in higher concentrations. Since any hydroperoxide would scarcely exceed the concentration level of 10^{-5} M in vivo, it seems more likely that, in the living brain, the activity of MV-Na$^+$, K$^+$-ATPase is enhanced rather than suppressed by an increased level of hydroperoxides.

Role of Free Radicals, Hydroperoxides, Lipoxygenase Pathway, and MV-Na$^+$, K$^+$-ATPase in Occurrence of Ischemic Brain Edema

The above novel finding led us to reevaluate the role of sodium entry across the BBB in the pathogenesis of brain edema. As already re-

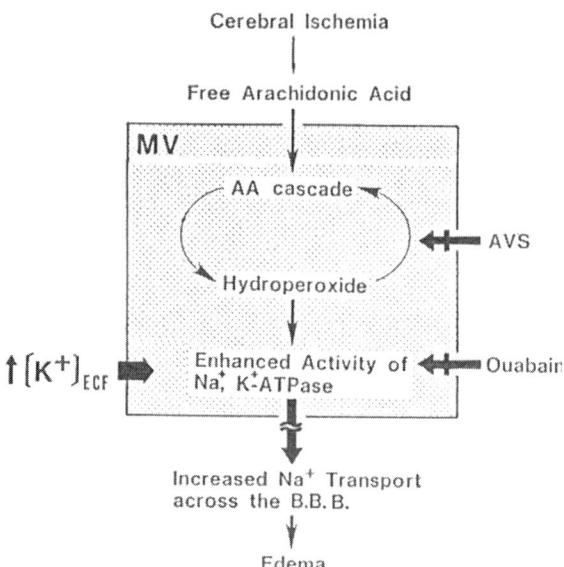

Fig. 2. The proposed biochemical mechanism underlying ischemic brain edema. The anti-edema effect of a free radical scavenger AVS may be due to the diminution of ambient free radicals which act to stimulate the AA cascade. *AA* arachidonic acid, *BBB* blood-brain barrier, *MU* microvessels

ported, a firm coupling between the sodium entry and the water entry was revealed throughout the evolution of ischemic brain edema following permanent MCA occlusion in rats [11]. The sodium movement across the BBB may be explained by either or both of the classical concepts of ultrafiltration in accordance with Gibbs-Donnan equilibrium and the novel concept of unidirectional active transport of sodium by Na$^+$, K$^+$-ATPase located in the antiluminal membrane of endothelial cells [9]. In this respect, the involvement of the latter mechanism was indicated by our recent study which showed that the edema formation following MCA occlusion in cats was significantly suppressed by the intraarterial perfusion with ouabain, a specific inhibitor of Na$^+$, K$^+$-ATPase [5]. Putting the above pieces of evidence together, we constructed a novel concept concerning the pathogenetic mechanism underlying ischemic brain edema as shown in Fig. 2

Conclusion

Role of Free Radical Scavengers in Therapy of Ischemic Brain Damage

It now seems evident that the in vivo effects of free radicals or hydroperoxides cannot always be regarded as destructive. As exemplified in the case of MV-Na$^+$, K$^+$-ATPase, hydroperoxides enhanced the enzyme activity and thus they might play a role in the regulation of the volume of brain extracellular fluid in physiological and pathological conditions. By the same token, the scavenging of free radicals may not always be beneficial. Administration of some free radical scavengers may interfere with the biological reactions of the brain or other organs to an ischemic insult, or may disturb the balance between the free radical generating system and the array of intrinsic free radical scavengers.

In conclusion, it still appears possible to manipulate for good or for bad those pathological sequences of events augmented by free radicals, by the use of free radical scavengers. Obviously, for such an agent to work, it must be accessible to the site of reaction, it must be specific to the free radical species involved, and it must attain the concentrations sufficient to cope with free radicals. Although there has not been any free radical scavenger which was shown to meet all these requirements, the importance of this research field is demonstraded and future development seems to be warranted.

References

1. Aritake K, Wakai S, Asano T, Takakura K (1983) Peroxidation of arachidonic acid and brain edema. Brain Nerve 35:965–973
2. Asano T, Johshita H, Koide T, Takakura K (1984) Amelioration of ischemic cerebral edema by a free radical scavenger, AVS, 1,2-Bis(nicotinamide)-propane: An experimental study using a regional ischemia model in cats. Neurol Res 6:163–168
3. Asano T, Matsui T, Basugi N, Tamura A, Takakura K, Sano K (1984) The effect of indomethacin on cortical specific gravity during regional ischemia and recirculation. In: Go KG, Baethmann A (eds) Recent progress in the study and therapy of brain edema. Plenum, New York, pp 617–626
4. Asano T, Gotoh O, Koide T, Takakura K (1985) Ischemic brain edema following occlusion of the middle cerebral artery in the rat: II. Alteration of the eicosanoid synthesis profile of brain microvessels. Stroke 16:110–113
5. Asano T, Shigeno T, Hanamura T, Koide T, Matsushita H, Watanabe E, Mima T, Johshita H, Usui M, Takakura K (1985) Alteration of brain

capillary function in cerebral ischemia: Role of capillary Na$^+$, K$^+$-ATPase in ischemic edema formation. J Cereb Blood Flow Metabol. 5 (Suppl 1): S63–S64
6. Chan PH, Fishman RA, Caronna J, Schmidley JW, Prioleau G, Lee J (1983) Induction of brain edema following intracerebral injection of arachidonic acid. Ann Neurol 13:625–632
7. Gaudet RJ, Alam I, Levine L (1980) Accumulation of cyclooxygenase products of arachidonic acid metabolism in gerbil brain during reperfusion after bilateral common carotid artery occlusion. J Neurochem 35:653–658
8. Gaudet RJ, Levine L (1980) Effect of unilateral common carotid artery occlusion on levels of prostaglandins D_2, F_{2a}, and 5-keto-prostaglandin F_{1a} in gerbil brain. Stroke 11:648–652
9. Goldstein GW, Betz AL (1983) Recent advances in understanding brain capillary function. Ann Neurol 14:389–395
10. Gotoh O, Koide T, Asano T, Takakura K, Tamura A, Sano K (1984) A model to study ischemic brain edema in rats and the influence of drugs. In: Go KG, Baethmann A (eds) Recent progress in the study and therapy of brain edema. Plenum, New York, pp 499–508
11. Gotoh O, Asano T, Koide T, Takakura K (1985) Ischemic brain edema following occlusion of the middle cerebral artery in the rat: I. The time courses of brain water, sodium, and potassium contents and blood-brain barrier permeability to ^{125}I-albumin. Stroke 16:101–109
12. Kiwak KJ, Moskowitz MA, Levine L (1985) Leukotriene production in gerbil brain after ischemic insult, subarachnoid hemorrhage, and concussive injury. J Neurosurg 62:865–869
13. Koide T, Gotoh O, Asano T, Takakura K (1985) Alterations of the eicosanoid synthetic capacity of rat brain microvessels following ischemia: Relevance to ischemic brain edema. J Neurochem 44:85–93
14. Koide T, Asano T, Matsushita H, Takakura K (1986) Enhancement of ATPase activity by a lipid peroxide of arachidonic acid in rat brain microvessels. J Neurochem 46:235–242
15. Lands WEM, Kulmacz RJ, Marshall PJ (1984) Lipid peroxide actions in the regulation of prostaglandin biosynthesis. In: Pryor WA (ed), Free radicals in biology, vol. 6. Academic, Orlando, pp 39–63
16. Usui M, Asano T, Takakura K (in press) Identification and quantitative analysis of hydroxyeicosatetraenoic acids in the rat brain exposed to regional ischemia. Stroke
17. Yoshida S, Inoh S, Asano T, Sano K, Kubota M, Shimaziki H, Ueta N (1980) Effect of transient ischemia on free fatty acids and phospholipids in the gerbil brain: Lipid peroxidation as possible cause of postischemic injury. J Neurosurg 53: 323–331

Biochemical Events in the Ischemic Brain and Pharmacological Basis of Mannitol, Vitamin E, Glucocorticoid, and Phenytoin

Shigeki Imaizumi, Hiroyuki Kinouchi, Teiji Tominaga, Takashi Yoshimoto, and Jiro Suzuki[1]

Introduction

Brain cell membranes are relatively enriched in polyphosphoinositides (PPI) which contain large amounts of arachidonic acid and stearic acid. Ischemia gives rise to severe energy depletion and the decomposition of PPI into diglyceride and inositol triphosphate by activation of phospholipase C. The subsequent hydrolysis of diglyceride accounts for free fatty acid (FFA) accumulation in the early stage of ischemia. Other general phospholipids are also hydrolyzed into lysophospholipids and FFA by activation of phospholipase A_2 with an increase of Ca^{2+}. On the other hand, free radical reaction is thought to be caused by active oxygens in the fatty acid carbon chain of phospholipids during ischemia, and is enhanced by Ca^{2+} which is mobilized by inositol triphosphate. The accumulated FFA in the ischemia is consumed as a substrate for propagation of free radical mediated peroxidation in the reperfusion period. This paper tries to attract attention to the PPI metabolism as a trigger of ischemic cell damage and participation of free radicals in the propagation of membrane lipid peroxidation. A study of preventive methods against the above pathophysiology was also made in the administration of mannitol, vitamin E, glucocorticoid, and phenytoin.

Experimental Materials and Method

Global cerebral ischemia was produced in male Wistar rats (220–250g) by occlusion of basilar and bilateral common carotid arteries [3].

The brain were frozen in situ at 1, 5, or 30 min of ischemia and 10, 30, or 60 min of recirculation following 30 min of ischemia. PPI, general phospholipids (PL) (phosphatidyl-inosital [PI],

-serine, -ethanolamine, -choline [PC] and sphingomyelin), lysophosphatidylcholine (LPC), 1,2-diacylglyceride (DG) and FFA were measured using high performance liquid chromatography (HPLC), thin layer chromatography (TLC), or gas liquid chromatography (GLC). Also, their acyl group compositions were determined.

The chemiluminescence (CL) emitted from the homogenate was detected with a CL Analyser OX-7 (Tohoku Electronics, Co. Ltd). The photon counts were recorded at intervals of 10 or 30 s and the mean of 10 measurements during the initial 5 minutes was used as the CL value. CL spectral analysis was carried out by using a filter spectrum analysis system [1, 2, 5].

In electron spin resonance (ESR) measurement, the time interval of killing was at 30 and 60 min of ischemia period, and 30 min after recirculation. After measuring the wet weight immediately, a brain homogenate was prepared by dilution in a fivefold volume of saline solution at 37°C under the constant flow of nitrogen gas. Next, 2.0×10^{-2} ml of brain homogenate was rapidly mixed with 2.0×10^{-4} M PBN, 0.6×10^{-6} M NADPH, and 1.0×10^{-6} M Fe-EDTA. From each brain sample, two such reaction mixtures were prepared—one to be incubated in air at 37°C, and one to be incubated in nitrogen gas under similar conditions for 20 min. ESR measurements were then undertaken [6]. The energy metabolism was measured by the enzymatic fluorometric methods of Lowry and Passonneau or by using HPLC.

The applied drugs (10 ml/kg 20% mannitol, 30 mg/kg vitamin E, 1 mg/kg betamethasone, and 10 mg/kg phenytoin) were administered intravenously 30 min prior to ischemic insult.

Results

Lipid Metabolism

During ischemia, phospholipids, including PI, decreased only subtly. But at the onset

---

[1] Division of Neurosurgery, Institute of Brain Diseases, Tohoku University School of Medicine, Sendai, Japan

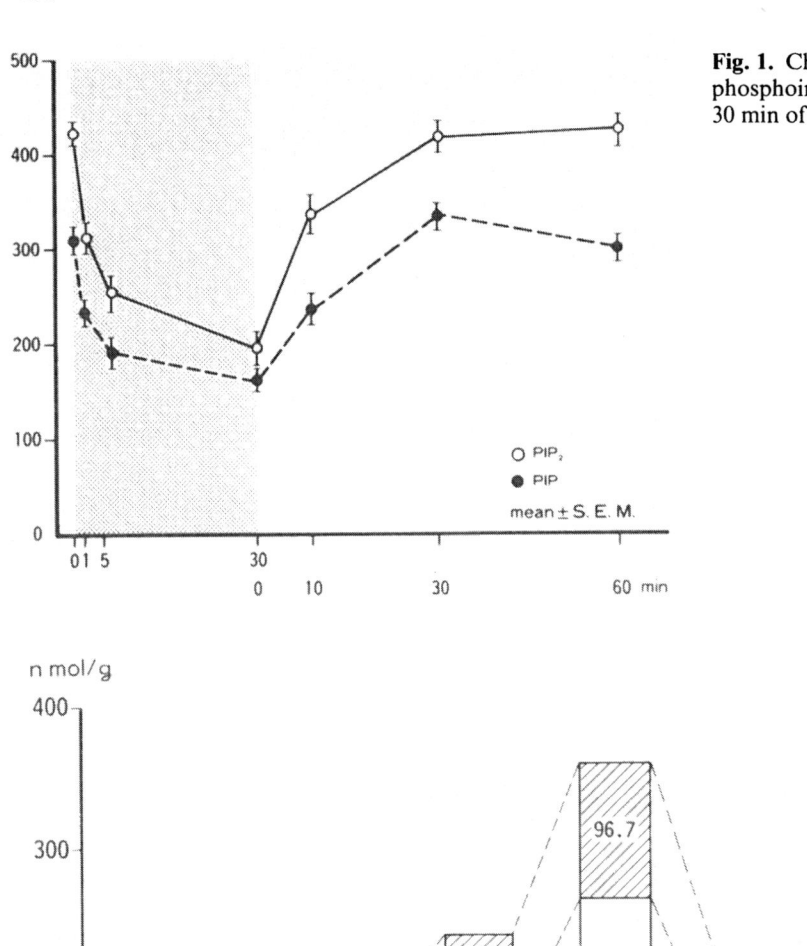

Fig. 1. Changes in the contents of poly-phosphoinositide during and following 30 min of ischemia

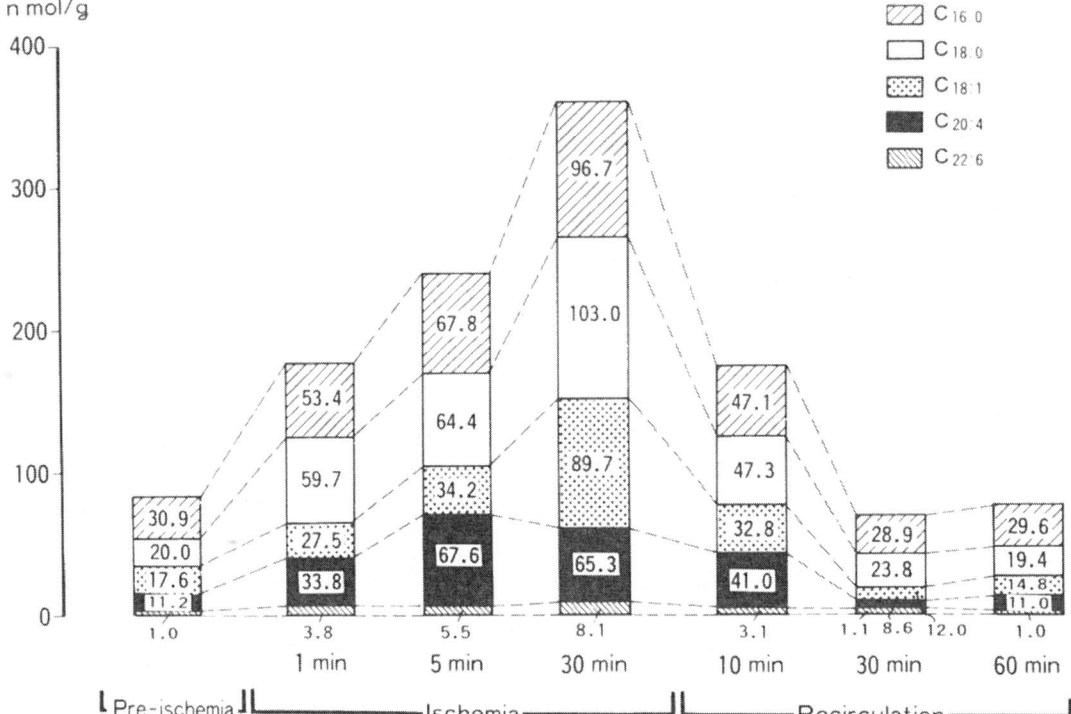

Fig. 2. Changes of fatty acid composition of diglyceride during 30 min of ischemia and after recirculation. *DG* diacylglyceride

of ischemia, triphosphoinositide (PIP2) and diphosphoinositide (PIP) rapidly decreased and DG increased symmetrically (Figs. 1, 2). PIP2, PIP and DG approached plateau values and about 30% of preschemic PIP remained unde-graded at 30 min of ischemia. In acyl group composition of DG, there were transient in-

creases of C18:0 and C20:4 with a decrease of C16:0 during 5 min of ischemia (Fig. 2). Re-covery of PIP2 and PIP were recognized in the recirculation—i.e., they increased to 85%–93% of preschemic levels at a recirculation, of 60 min (Fig. 1). Adversely, DG decreased by recircula-tion and returned to the preschemic value after

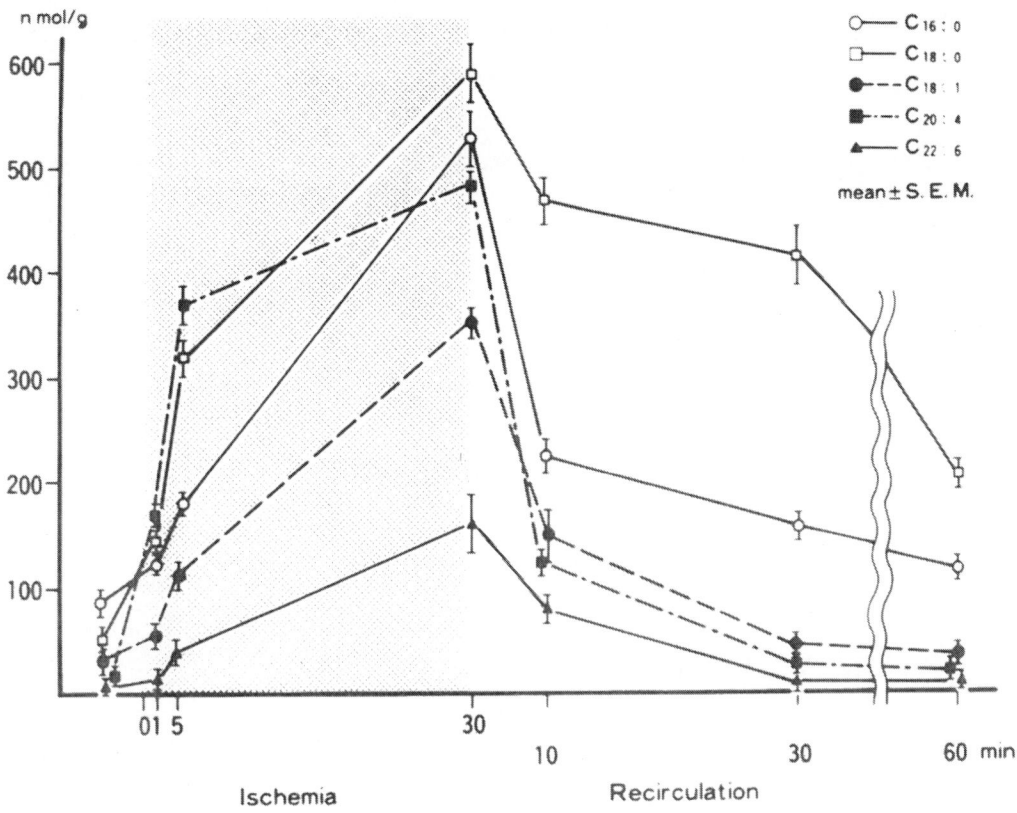

Fig. 3. Changes of FFA contents during and following 30 min of ischemia

recirculation for 30 min (Fig. 2). The amount of LPC increased twice during 5 min of ischemia followed by a steady decline in continuous ischemia. The level of LPC after recirculation for 30 min returned to the preischemic value. In FFA accumulated throughout ischemia, C18:0 and C20:4 increased rapidly during early stage, usually within 5 min. All individual FFA were decreased by recirculation, in which unsaturated FFA reduced more rapidly than the saturated type and returned to the preischemic value at a recirculation of 60 min (Fig. 3).

Inhibitory effects against the FFA accumulation was realized in the phenytoin-treated rats, in which the contents of C20:4, C18:0, and C16:0 were particularly attenuated (Fig. 4).

Free Radicals Alteration

Cl Value. The amount of CL per 30 s demonstrated a gradual increase from setting homogenate on the CL analyser in ischemic brain specimens. In contrast, normal brain homogenate demonstrated no significant increase within 40–60 min, even if they were similarly heated to 35°–36°C in room air. In the ischemic brain, the

CL value is higher in the recirculation period than in the ischemic period (Fig. 5).

CL spectral analysis. Spectral peaks were found at wavelengths of 480 nm, 520–530 nm, 570 nm, 620–640 nm, and 680–700 nm.

ESR measurement. In the three-vessel occlusion model, under both the air and nitrogen conditions, a BPN(N-tert-Butyl-α-phenylnitrone)-trapped radical, in which hyperfine splitting constants were $A_N = 16.2$–16.5 G and $A_\beta^H = 3.6$–3.8 G, was obtained (Fig. 6). Since the radical intensity was found to develop and grow with the duration of incubation at 37°C, the incubation time of the reaction mixture was fixed at 20 min for all experiments. The signal intensities obtained at each time period in the ischemic model were consistently stronger when the reaction mixture was incubated in air than when incubated in nitrogen gas.

Sequential changes in the relative intensity of BPN-trapped radical are shown in Fig. 7.

Effect of Sendai Cocktail No. 1 on CL value. When the combination of mannitol, vitamin E and betamethasone was administered in

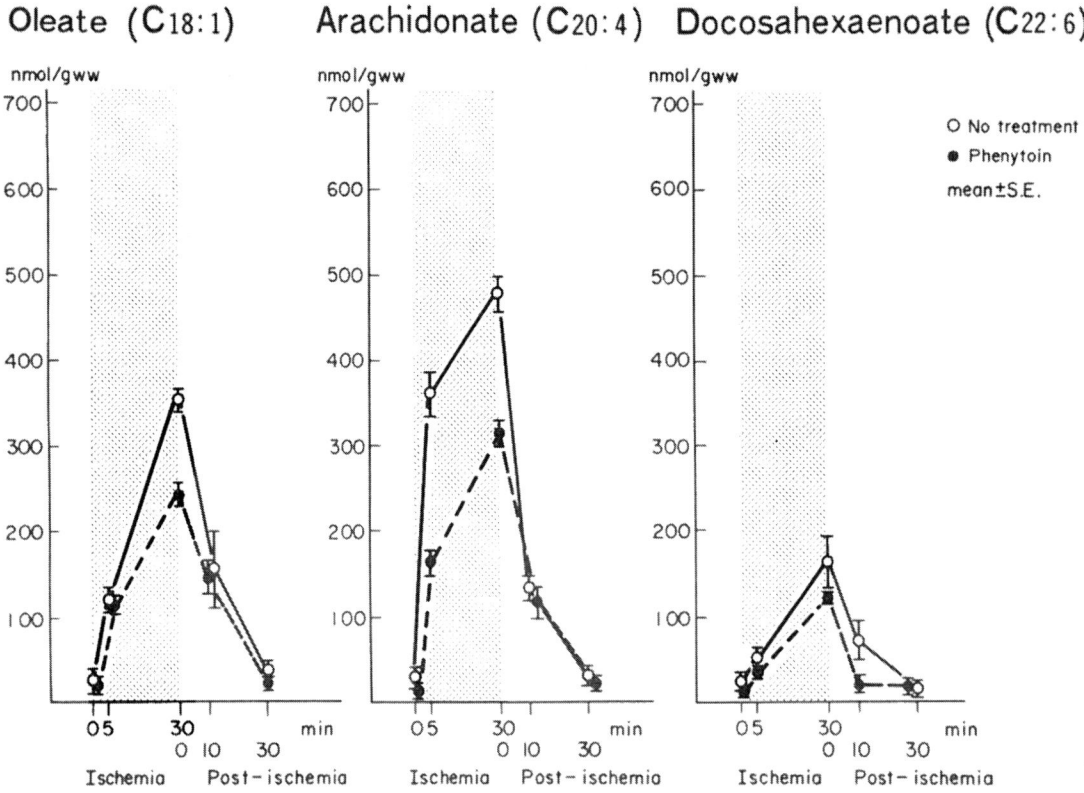

Fig. 4. Effects of phenytoin on unsaturated FFA accumulation in the ischemic brain

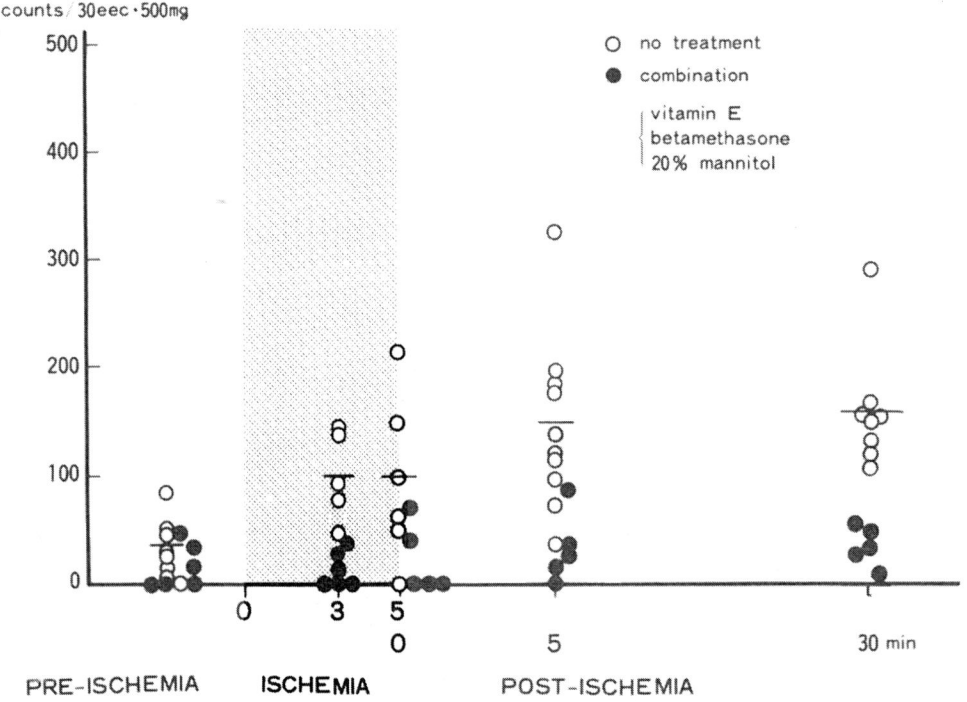

Fig. 5. Changes of CL values during and following ischemia and effects of combination therapy on CL values

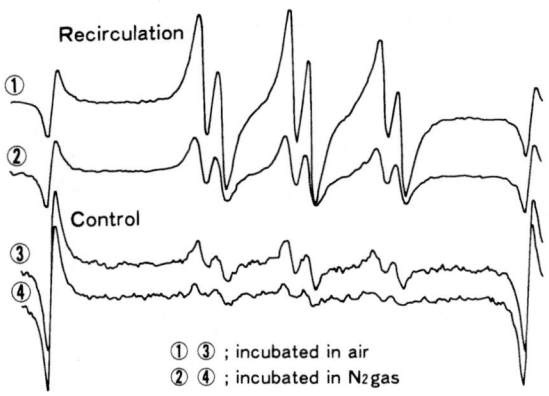

Fig. 6. The ESR spectra obtained when the reaction mixture was incubated for 20 min at 37 °C in air or nitrogen gas. *1, 2* were obtained from the recirculation group (30 min-recirculation following 30 min-ischemia) and *3, 4* were obtained from the control group

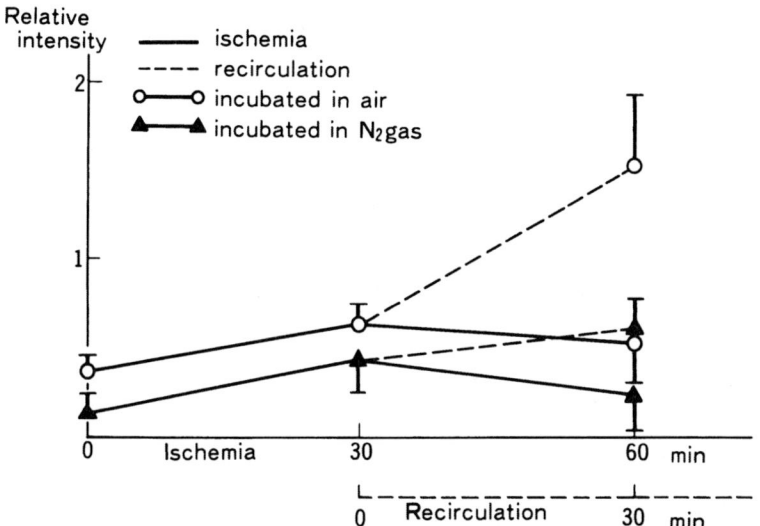

Fig. 7. The changes in relative intensity of ESR signal (mean $\pm$ SE)

the ischemic brain model, CL was suppressed throughout the 5-min-period of ischemia and 30-min of reflow (Fig. 5).

Energy Metabolism

Alterations of ATP, ADP, AMP, energy charge, glucose, and lactate in the global cerebral ischemia used for this study and the effects of combination therapy (Sendai Cocktail No. 1) are shown in Table 1. The effects of phenytoin in energy metabolism is shown in Table 2.

Discussion

PPI metabolism affected during ischemia has reversibility during recirculation. The increase of FFA (C18:0 and C20:4) during 5 min of ischemia may be derived from DG caused by the degradation of PIP2 and PIP. In the late period of ischemia, accumulated FFA are mainly due to the hydrolysis of other general phospholipids by phospholipase A2 and lysolipase. The status of LPC during ischemia is regulated by the combined action of phospholipase A2 and lysolipase, but the decrease of LPC after recirculation may be due to the activation of ATP-dependent reacylation. Accumulated DG during ischemia may be utilized for *de novo* synthesis of phospholipids, especially PPI, in recirculation.

The cerebral protective effect of phenytoin is caused by inhibition of phospholipase activity. There is also the possibility that the agent reduces intracellular Ca^{2+} by blockade of the Ca^{2+} channel into cytoplasma, or activation of Na^+, K^+-ATPase and an Na^+–Ca^{2+} exchange transport system.

The high levels of CL value found following the start of reflow or reoxygenation in the ischemic brain means that the propagation reaction has started together with the resupply of

Table 1. Movement of energy metabolism during and following 30 min of ischemia and the effects of combination therapy (mannitol, vitamin E and glucocorticoid)

	ATP	ADP	AMP	EC	Glucose	Lactate
Preischemia	2.74 ± 0.03	0.243 ± 0.019	0.031 ± 0.004	0.949 ± 0.003	3.51 ± 0.30	1.65 ± 0.32
Ischemia 5 min						
No treatment	0.38 ± 0.05	0.458 ± 0.014	1.308 ± 0.124	0.286 ± 0.012	0.51 ± 0.03	16.73 ± 1.36
Treatment	0.53 ± 0.07	0.452 ± 0.105	1.231 ± 0.039	0.306 ± 0.016	0.58 ± 0.06	6.45 ± 0.67[a]
Ischemia 30 min						
No treatment	0.05 ± 0.01	0.415 ± 0.065	1.252 ± 0.081	0.147 ± 0.017	0.06 ± 0.00	16.83 ± 0.83
Treatment	0.07 ± 0.04	0.376 ± 0.620	1.012 ± 0.050[b]	0.170 ± 0.010	0.18 ± 0.01[a]	4.81 ± 0.41[a]
Recirculation 30 min						
No treatment	1.52 ± 0.02	0.375 ± 0.031	0.308 ± 0.049	0.778 ± 0.022	4.05 ± 0.39	7.94 ± 0.60
Treatment	2.24 ± 0.10[c]	0.238 ± 0.043[c]	0.123 ± 0.048[b]	0.842 ± 0.047[c]	4.08 ± 0.04	3.98 ± 0.31[b]
Recirculation 120 min						
No treatment	1.76 ± 0.05	0.486 ± 0.028	0.357 ± 0.042	0.772 ± 0.011	3.58 ± 0.04	3.78 ± 0.31
Treatment	—	—	—	—	—	—

Difference from no-treatment, [a] $P < 0.001$, [b] $P < 0.01$, [c] $P < 0.05$
Mean $\pm$ SE: mmol/kg except EC
EC energy exchange

Table 2. Effects of phenytoin on energy metabolism movement during and following 30 min of ischemia

	ATP	ADP	AMP	Σ Ad	EC	Glucose	Lactate
Preischemia							
No treatment	2.77 ± 0.09	0.250 ± 0.022	0.034 ± 0.002	3.05 ± 0.08	0.951 ± 0.005	3.51 ± 0.30	1.65 ± 0.32
Phenytoin	2.67 ± 0.11	0.231 ± 0.010	0.058 ± 0.010	2.96 ± 0.12	0.952 ± 0.003	3.19 ± 0.19	2.03 ± 0.06
Ischemia 5 min							
No treatment	0.32 ± 0.04	0.305 ± 0.002	1.50 ± 0.05	2.16 ± 0.10	0.228 ± 0.021	0.67 ± 0.06	12.60 ± 0.93
Phenytoin	0.76 ± 0.12[b]	0.310 ± 0.020	1.35 ± 0.07	2.42 ± 0.17	0.363 ± 0.027[a]	1.04 ± 0.02[a]	9.84 ± 0.20[b]
Ischemia 30 min							
No treatment	0.08 ± 0.01	0.165 ± 0.020	1.67 ± 0.09	1.74 ± 0.12	0.076 ± 0.008	0.06 ± 0.02	14.83 ± 0.43
Phenytoin	0.13 ± 0.04[b]	0.179 ± 0.035	1.61 ± 0.03	1.91 ± 0.12	0.112 ± 0.008[b]	0.12 ± 0.01[b]	11.89 ± 0.45[b]
Recirculation 10 min							
No treatment	0.94 ± 0.02	0.280 ± 0.016	0.71 ± 0.06	1.93 ± 0.09	0.506 ± 0.045	3.88 ± 0.13	10.51 ± 0.24
Phenytoin	1.43 ± 0.05[b]	0.211 ± 0.014	0.50 ± 0.03[b]	2.14 ± 0.13	0.728 ± 0.022[b]	4.16 ± 0.53[b]	8.73 ± 0.27[a]
Recirculation 30 min							
No treatment	1.50 ± 0.05	0.202 ± 0.010	0.023 ± 0.001	1.72 ± 0.05	0.831 ± 0.005	4.05 ± 0.20	7.94 ± 0.60
Phenytoin	1.60 ± 0.06	0.223 ± 0.010	0.016 ± 0.002[b]	2.12 ± 0.03[b]	0.870 ± 0.010[b]	4.39 ± 0.11	6.32 ± 0.22
Recirculation 60 min							
No treatment	1.60 ± 0.08	0.212 ± 0.010	0.027 ± 0.002	1.83 ± 0.09	0.942 ± 0.006	4.50 ± 0.09	6.64 ± 0.32
Phenytoin	1.93 ± 0.02[b]	0.203 ± 0.001	0.021 ± 0.001	2.17 ± 0.01	0.946 ± 0.001	4.47 ± 0.13	4.54 ± 0.40[b]

Difference from no treatment, [a] $P < 0.01$, [b] $P < 0.05$
mean $\pm$ SEM, Σ *AD* Adenin pool, *EC* energy charge

oxygen. Suppression of CL value by combined therapy means this treatment has a scavenging effect on the ischemic brain (Fig. 5).

Subsequently, spectral analysis of CL was performed to learn the detailed mechanism. The spectral peaks found suggested the possibility that luminescence generated when singlet oxygen, i.e., $[^1\Sigma + g][^1\Delta g](0,0)$, $[^1\Delta g][^1\Delta g](2,0)$ $(1,0)$, $(0,0)(0,1)$, returned to ground state in the breakdown of lipid hydroperoxide was the substance of CL $(^1\Delta g + {}^1\Delta g \rightarrow 2^3o_2 + h\nu)$. Singlet

oxygen has a higher energy than triplet oxygen in the ground state.

In the ESR study, the signal intensity of the BPN-trapped radical ($A_N = 16.2$–16.5G, $A_\beta^H = 3.6$–3.8G) showed a gradual increase with a peak at about 30 min after the start of ischemia. Moreover, there was a marked increase in the radical intensity due to recirculation. The fact that a peak in the radical intensity due to ischemia was found demonstrates the possibility that a radical reaction occurs during ischemia. In other words, if an extremely small amount of oxygen molecules is present, the autoxidative reaction is initiated, and, if there is a sufficient supply of oxygen molecules, the reaction will progress. Consequently, it is thought that, in the ischemic brain, the resolved oxygen, which is the oxygen available during ischemia, has considerable importance. The changes in intensity of the PBN-trapped radicals in the present experiments may parallel the changes on consumption of resolved oxygen, possibly indicating a gradual increase followed by gradual decrease.

It was not so easy to identify the BPN-trapped radical obtained in this experiment which had hyperfine splitting constants of $A_N = 16.2-16.5G$ and $A_\beta^H = 3.6-3.8G$, because little fundamental data from lipid peroxidation systems have yet been found. Saprin and Piette [4] have demonstrated that two types of linoleic acid adducts of BPN obtained from liver microsome incubation system had hyperfine splitting constants of $A_N = 16.54G$, $A_\beta^H = 3.35G$ and $A_N = 15.8G$, $A_\beta^H = 3.75G$. They concluded that these signals were formed from the methyl group and alkoxy groups derived from linoleic acid. As is well known, the brain tissue content of FFA increases in ischemic conditions. It is likely, therefore, that the BPN-trapped radical obtained in this experiment is derived from FFA. Moreover, the oxygen demand in the generation of this radical suggests the possibility that it is involved in the process of FFA peroxidation reaction.

From these results, we can agree on the importance of PPI metabolism as a trigger of ischemic cell damage and that, during ischemia, the potential for oxygen radical formation does exist. Also, lipid peroxidation is propagated by oxygen resupply in the recirculation period. A strong link between energy metabolism and the initiation of free radical reaction was also demonstrated.

In other words, supplying oxygen without cerebral protection, such as scavengers or phenytoin, is rash for the ischemic brain.

References

1. Imaizumi S, Kayama T, Suzuki J (1984) Chemiluminescence in hypoxic brain—the first report: Correlation between energy metabolism and free radical reaction. Stroke 15:1061–1065
2. Imaizumi S, Suzuki J, Tominaga T, Uenohara H, Yoshimoto T (1985) Effect of free radical scavengers on cerebral ischemia and hypoxia evaluated by chemiluminescence. In: Spetzler RF (ed) Cerebral revascularization for stroke. Thieme-Stratton, New York, pp 299–306
3. Kameyama M, Suzuki J, Shirane R, Ogawa A (1985) A new model of bilateral hemispheric ischemia: Three-vessel occlusion model. Stroke 16:489–493
4. Saprin AN, Piette LH (1977) Spin trapping and its application in the study of lipid peroxidation and free radical production with liver microsomes. Arch Biochem Biophys 180:480–492
5. Suzuki J, Imaizumi S, Kayama T, Yoshimoto T (1985) Chemiluminescence in hypoxic brain—the second report: Cerebral protective effect of mannitol, vitamin E and glucocorticoid. Stroke 16:695–700
6. Tominaga T, Imaizumi S, Yoshimoto T, Suzuki J, Fujita Y (in press) Application of spin trapping study to NADPH-dependent lipid peroxidation in rat ischemic brain homogenate. Brain Res

Discussion

Pitts (San Francisco): Faden has recently suggested that dynorphin when given intrathecally in rats can cause hind limbs paralysis and his own current belief is that the kappaagonists, or kappaantagonists, are more likely to be useful. So to hear that dynorphin may show a beneficial effect would seem to be at odds with this. Could Prof. Hosobuchi comment on this.

Hosobuchi (San Francisco): I think this is because most of the dynorphin observations you are referring to were done at fairly high doses compared with ours. Certainly, the earlier experiment on the analgesic effect of dynorphin by intrathecal administration was at a far higher dose to cause the hypertonicity. This is very typical of many peptides that have a double effect, e.g., morphine has opposite effects according to the dose range. Dynorphin has a very clear bimodal effect. Thorough dose-response studies need to be done here. Secondly, I do not wish to make my points when Dr. Faden is not here, but his contention is that dynorphin was elevated during spinal cord injury, but close examination of his data reveals that the period of dynorphin elevation is the time when the rat's functions begin to return and the area of elevation is very specific. We cannot quite understand the direct significance of this to the return of the functions. But I think these opposite effects are based on dose response and typical of peptide activities.

van der Werf (Amsterdam): Some of my coworkers took advantage of our CSF drainage by cisternal drainage and we made daily measurements of catecholamines and enkephalins in the CSF after subarachnoid hemorrhage and they found that there was a significant drop from days 4 and 5 in met-enkephalins in patients with cerebral ischemia in contrast to those who did not show vasospasm or cerebral ischemia. We do not know if this is a cause or an effect of cerebral ischemia, perhaps with involvement of the hypothalamus in hypoperfusion. What does the panel make of this finding?

Symon (London): I think it is almost impossible to decide on cause and effect relationships. Many factors change in subarachnoid hemorrhages, for example, growth hormone changes and quite a few neuropeptides alter with some of the more severe types of hemorrhage. Your observation is interesting but I do not really know its significance.

Suzuki (Tokyo): Which anesthesic drug is best for stroke surgery?

Spetzler (Phoenix): I think there will be a lot of controversy here, but for a number of years in our institution we have used barbiturate anesthesia by the neuroanesthesiologists as a routine procedure. It has been used in many hundreds of cases. It is a very old but effective anesthetic that is monitored with the EEG down to burst suppression. It is very easily titrated. We use it in all patients who have the potential of vessel occlusion, including large tumors. It has some distinct advantages: It redistributes blood flow; it decreases blood flow and therefore decreases ICP and makes retraction somewhat easier. It is the one agent that has been shown in every laboratory to be protective. And since it is easily instituted, it is our agent of choice.

Peerless (Ontario): Which barhiturate do you use?

Spetzler: Pentathol by continuous intravenous administration. The difference between a short- and long-acting barbiturate becomes irrelevant after a certain amount has been given such that the other compartments are full. One of the problems of barbiturates of course is the inability to examine the patient immediately after surgery. But this does not last very long; brain stem reflexes are very very resistant to barbiturates. Evoked potentials remain easily discernible. Within a few hours the patient can be examined, even for a higher function.

Shigeno (Kawagoe): You described a very clear and interesting difference in the ICP course in both permanent occlusion and reperfusion. How does barbiturate affect the ICP pattern? Is there some effect of barbiturate in vasoconstricting cerebral vessels or is it just the result of the progression from edema? Did you actually measure brain water content in this situation?

Spetzler: We carried out many procedures. For example, we measured the blood flow, though obviously 10 min is not a very long time. We measured the blood flow using microspheres at various points during the ischemia. Three patterns occur with barbiturates: (a) There is a very small drop in the area of deep ischemia compared with the control side; (b) there is no change—the blood flow in the most severe area of the ischemia is the same as on the nonischemic side; (c) the most common pattern is that the blood flow increases very dramatically in the area of ischemia. I do not think that barbiturates have a specific effect on the blood vessel itself, rather they have a secondary effect of metabolic need: The blood flow in the rest of the brain is lowered so that what is accomplished with middle cerebral artery occlusion is no longer truly ischemic in the presence of barbiturates. With barbiturates, it is then very much a redistribution of blood flow. With permanent ischemia, this redistribution may actually be harmful, I am not really sure why this occurs. But obviously there are other effects of barbiturates, e.g., lowered blood pressure. Water content is very much increased in those that die from increased ICP.

Hung (Taipei): Are fluosol-like compounds of value in carrying oxygen to the brain?

Peerless: We are continuing to do work in this area, although we are not using the Japanese fluosol, we are investigating a drug made in the USA which has different chemical properties, although it does carry O_2 and CO_2 quite effectively. There is little doubt that the material will carry O_2 to areas of ischemic brain we presume by virtue of its ability to pass through cortical collaterals around an area of stenosis or occlusion. The effect is somewhat better than mannitol, though the difference is not striking. The problem with all these compounds is that the efficency of O_2-carrying capacity is closely related to the toxicity of the drug and it is a matter of balancing the two. I suspect that in the future these drugs will be of value. At present, a trial is about to begin on the perfusion of the human heart for heart transplantation purposes using a perfluoro compound. So no doubt these drugs are useful in isolated situations. Perhaps in future something

like the Sendai Cocktail may contain this material for administration perhaps in the operating room or in the ambulance or emergency room in situations of cerebral ischemia to gain a little more time. Unfortunately, with all these drugs, the presence of high levels or increasing levels of O_2 once the ischemic process begins is quite harmful to the brain; so that although they are useful in the beginning, the usefulness rapidly wears off and they can become quite troublesome. We have not solved this problem yet.

Symon: We repeated some experiments in the baboon that Dr. Peerless had done in cats using fluosol and we found that its major effect was a colloidal effect in that it reduced the shear rates and viscosity. Its effects could almost be replicated with low-molecular-weight dextran. So at the present we are a little disenchanted with it, though it well be something that is worth pursuing.

Weinstein (San Francisco): I'd like to ask Dr. Peerless about the location of NMDA receptors. Since most studies indicate that they are found in the selectively vulnerable hippocampal region, is there any evidence that suggests that these excitatory amino acid transmitter accumulations are present throughout the brain during ischemia? And if so might it not be the effect of deep barbiturate anesthesia acting as an anticonvulsant? In which case, the phenytoin as selected in the Sendai cocktail may be a less difficult agent to administer for protective purposes.

Peerless: These receptors are located throughout the brain but their concentration is much higher in those areas that the pathologists have long indicated have the highest selective vulnerability. We are working on the hippocampal slice, using this model in the same way as that used by the epileptologists: microelectrodes are employed intracellularly as well as to measure cell populations, because there are large concentrations of these receptors in that area. A question that has always troubled me is why is the brain so vulnerable to this anoxic insult? The composition of the cells is not so different to that of the heart for example, yet in transplantation the heart can be removed from the body, kept in a cooler for up to 5 h, and be implanted and work normally. One factor that is different, however, is the transmitter substances and receptors. This thus appears to be a crucial area. Barbiturates may well be related to this; barbiturates could interrupt the release of transmitter and stop the process at this point, although not as effectively as a specific antagonist.

RTD 6. Anterior Circulation Aneurysm

Anterior Communicating Aneurysm: Its Surgical Approach and Result

RAM. P. SENGUPTA[1]

The anterior communicating artery (ACOA) region is the most common site for ruptured intracranial aneurysms. These aneurysms lie deep within important brain structures, requiring a difficult surgical approach for obliteration. However, the management mortality and morbidity of patients with these aneurysms can be considerably reduced by appreciating their natural history, physiological factors of circulation, morphological features and the pathological changes involved following subarachnoid hemorrhage (SAH). Recurrent rupture remains more of a threat than ischemic problems from these aneurysms and their obliteration at the earliest possible time is not only feasible but helpful for an improved outcome.

The Natural History of Anterior Communicating Aneurysms

Incidence. The ACoA is the most common site of occurrence and, in the author's experience, 30% of ruptured aneurysms occurred at this site.

Age incidence. Comparatively young people tend to harbour these aneurysms. Fifteen percent of ruptured ACo aneurysms were seen in patient below the age of 30.

Sex preponderance. The male/female ratio is dramatically different in these aneurysms from those at other common locations. There is a slight preponderance of men over women, with a ratio of 56:44.

Association of anomalies in the circle of Willis. Anomalies in the anterior part of the circle of Willis are frequently associated with these aneurysms. This factor has considerable bearing on the management, surgical approach and outcome.

[1] Regional Neurological Centre, Newcastle General Hospital, Newcastle upon Tyne, England

Tendency to rupture. Of all the intracranial aneurysms, ACo aneurysms are notorious for their tendency to rupture. This is suggested by the fact that ruptured aneurysms at this site are usually small, and, when associated with other aneurysms, the source of bleeding is often at this site. Moreover, giant aneurysms are rarely seen and very seldom do they present with a clinical syndrome other than SAH. Incidental ACo aneurysms are less common.

Tendency to re-rupture. ACo aneurysms are prone to recurrent rupture. Once an ACo aneurysm has been identified as the source of rupture, recurrent hemorrhage will occur from it sooner or later.

Circulation Through the Anterior Part of the Circle of Willis

Norlen and Barnum (1953) drew attention to the different patterns of circulation through the anterior part of the circle of Willis in patients with ACo aneurysms, stressing their importance for the various surgical procedures. Knowledge of different types of circulation is also important in understanding the effects of vasospasm, as the available collateral supply differs. In an analysis of 100 patients with ACo aneurysms, Sengupta [1] noted four types of circulation and the aneurysms were classified accordingly.

Type I (ipsilateral) occurrence: 66%. In this type, the aneurysm and the distal anterior cerebral artery (A2) filled from one proximal anterior cerebral artery (A1):
1) Left anterior cerebral AC-ACo aneurysms. The pattern of circulation (Fig. 1) in these aneurysms may be as follows:
a) Left carotid injection fills the aneurysm and both A2 (Fig. 1a)
b) Left carotid injection fills the aneurysm and the left A2 (Fig. 1b)

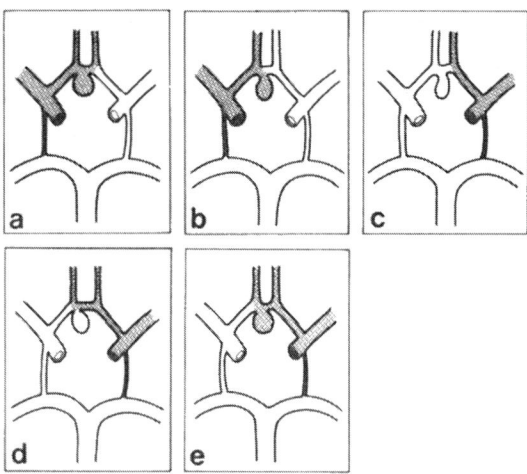

Fig. 1a–e. Type I, ipsilateral circulation

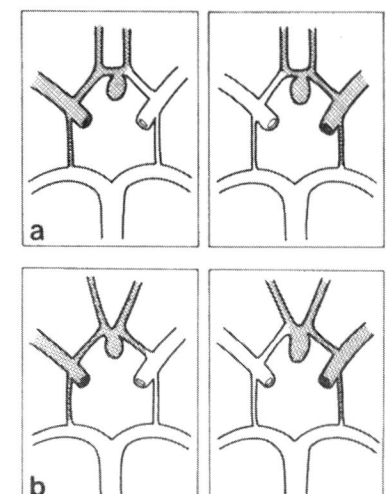

Fig. 2a, b. Type II, bilateral circulation. **a** Anterior communicating artery prominent; **b** anterior communicating artery rudimentary

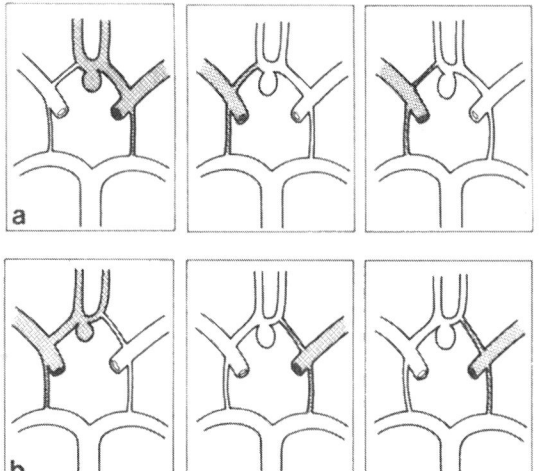

Fig. 3a, b. Type III, dominant circulation. **a** Dominant right anterior communicating artery; **b** dominant left anterior communicating artery

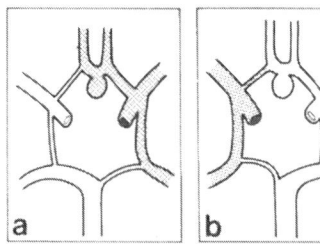

Fig. 4a, b. Type IV, dominant anterior communicating artery with fetal posterior cerebral artery. **a** Ipsilateral; **b** contralateral fetal posterior cerebral artery

c) Right carotid injection fills the right A2 only (Fig. 1c)
d) Right carotid injection with left carotid compression fills both A2, but not the aneurysm (Fig. 1d)
e) As in (d), but the aneurysm fills (Fig. 1e)
2) Right AC-ACo aneurysms. In these aneurysms the patterns of circulation are a mirror image of those of left AC-ACo aneurysms

Type II (bilateral) occurrence: 14%. In this type, the aneurysm and both ACA fill from both carotid injections (Fig. 2). This pattern of circulation is often associated with rudimentary ACoA. In fact, both ACA may be fused to each other. On the other hand, the ACoA may be seen as a prominent structure on the angiograms. The significance of this analysis is that in this type of circulation the region of the ACoA receives good collateral supply, and the effect of vasospasm is minimal. In cases of rudimentary ACoA, however, application of a clip may lead to kinking of both ACA, leading to severe ischemic problems.

Type III (dominant ACA) occurrence: 12%. In this type, the aneurysm arises from the axilla of the two A2, both of which are divisions of the dominant ACA, and the contralateral artery is hypoplastic (Fig. 3).

Type IV (dominant ACA with fetal posterior cerebral artery) occurrence: 8%. In this type, the circulatory patterns are like those in type III, but there are other associated anomalies in the circle (Fig. 4).

In types III and IV, the effects of postoperative vasospasm are considerable.

Morphological Anatomy of the Aneurysm

Location of the neck. These aneurysms rarely arise from the ACoA itself. Rather, their exact site of origin is usually close to its junction with one of the ACA. From the angiograms, the position of the neck of the aneurysm can be ascertained to a certain extent. Occasionally angiographic evidence is misleading, and the aneurysm may appear to have no clipable neck. The following variations (Fig. 5) in the location of the neck have been noted [1]:

a) Junction of the ACoA and the right A2 (Fig. 5a)
b) Junction of the ACoA and left A2 (Fig. 5b)
c) Junction of the ACoA and right A1 (Fig. 5c)
d) Junction of the ACoA and left A1 (Fig. 5d)
e) Junction of the right and left A2 in types III and IV circulation, as described before (Fig. 5e)
f) ACoA alone (Fig. 5f)

Relationship of the aneurysmal sac to major vessels. It is useful to know the precise relationship of the major vessels to the aneurysmal sac to avoid trauma to these vessels during dissection. In a study of 100 cases, the following relationships of the sac to the major vessels were found (Fig. 6):

a) No relationship to any major vessel (Fig. 6a)
b) ACoA alone (Fig. 6b)
c) ACoA and right A2 (Fig. 6c)
d) ACoA and left A2 (Fig. 6d)
e) ACoA and both A2 (Fig. 6e)
f) Right A2 (Fig. 6f)
g) Left A2 (Fig. 6g)

A Modified Approach for ACo Aneurysms without Exposing the A1

The modified approach for ACo aneurysms is based on two considerations [2]: The course of the ACA is such that, from the point of origin, it passes forwards and slightly upwards until it meets its fellow from the opposite side in the longitudinal fissure. Therefore, to expose an aneurysm of the ACo region, it is not necessary to dissect the carotid bifurcation, which is the deepest part of the circle.

Secondly, the A1 is the most important source of the vital perforating arteries, including

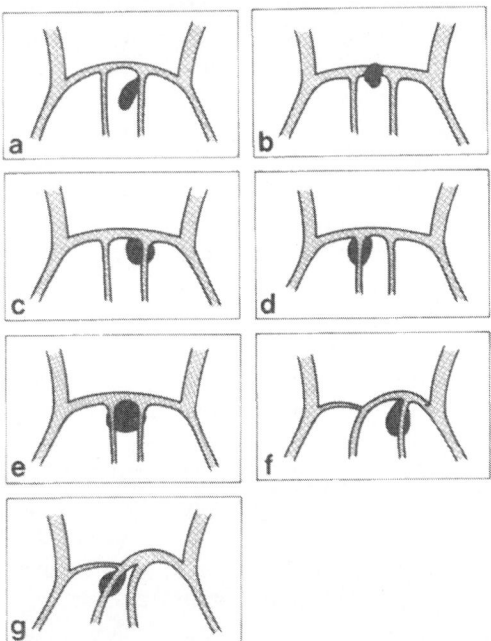

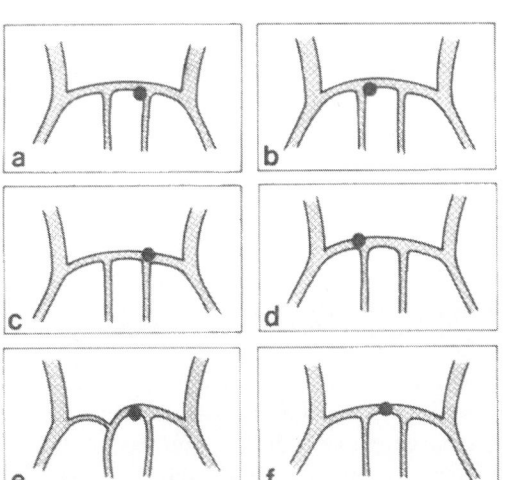

Fig. 5a–f. Locations of the neck

Fig. 6a–g. Relation of aneurysmal sac to major vessels

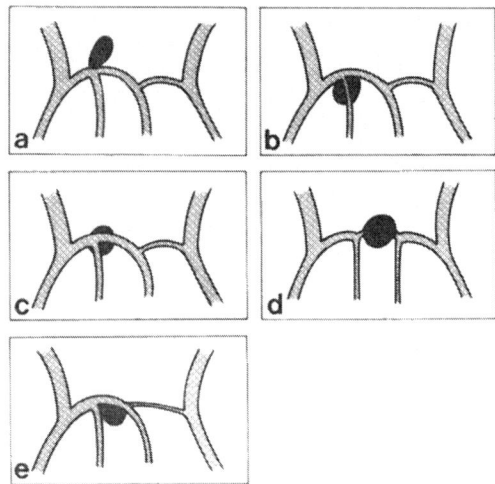

Fig. 7a–e. Surgical approach. **a–c** Left-sided; **d** staged bilateral; **e** right-sided for dominant left anterior communicating artery

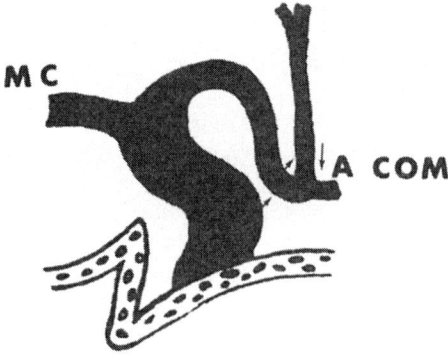

Fig. 8. Diagramatic scale (exaggerated) of the operative view through the pterional approach showing the route to the ACoA through the gyrus rectus. As the ICA bifurcation is in a much deeper plane, this route is much easier and less harmful

Heubner's artery, to the basal ganglia and the hypothalamus. Dissection of this artery can therefore produce harmful effects from vasospasm. With the use of hypotensive anesthesia, there is hardly ever any need for temporary occlusion of the proximal artery.

Side of craniotomy. It is generally accepted that ACo aneurysms should be approached through the right non-dominant side with the exception of a left frontal lobe hematoma or a dominant left ACA. In this approach, the side of the craniotomy is based on the position of the neck, the relationship of the sac, and the occasional need to expose the dominant ACA in large difficult aneurysms. Figure 7 clarifies the circumstances which decide the side of the craniotomy for these aneurysms. If the neck is located at the left A1-ACo junction (Fig. 7a), or if the sac is related to the left A2 segment (Fig. 7b, c), the approach should be left sided. In a situation with a large aneurysm (Fig. 7d), the approach should be bilateral. In Fig. 7e, although the dominant artery is on the left side, the approach is from the right, since the sac is intimately related to the right A2 segment. The position of the patient on the table is also crucial. The upper part of the table is elevated 15° and the head piece is slightly lowered. The shoulder on the side of the craniotomy is elevated on a sandbag. In this position, the floor of the anterior fossa can be approached with very little retraction. The craniotomy is centered on the pterion and the anterior border of the bone flap is made as low as

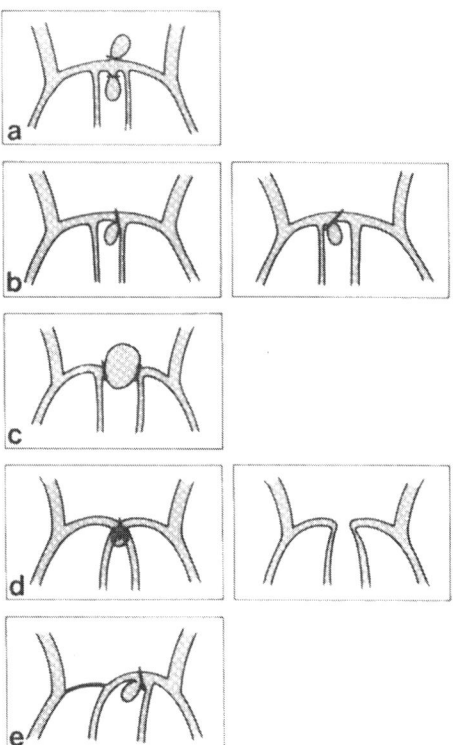

Fig. 9a–e. Placement of clips. **a** Clip on the neck (ideal); **b** clip on anterior communicating artery (harmless); **c** clip on anterior communicating artery at interval (minimal risk); **d** clip on anterior communicating artery (dangerous); **e** clip on anterior communicating artery (lethal)

possible. After separating the frontal lobe from the optic nerve and the internal carotid artery, the A2 in the longitudinal fissure is exposed through the gyrus rectus and further dissection is continued proximally until the ACoA is reached (Fig. 8).

Table 1. Outcome at discharge and follow-up[a]

Outcome	At discharge	At follow-up (6m–16 yr)
Good	166	178
Fair	42	16
Poor	5	3
Dead	8	[b]

[a] $n = 221$

[b] Sixteen patients could not be followed-up

Table 2. Grade at operation and outcome

Grades	Outcome				Total
	Good	Fair	Poor	Dead	
I, II	140	20	5	1	166
III, IV, V	26	22	0	7	55
	166	42	5	8	221

Table 3. Anomaly of circle of Willis and outcome

Type of circulation	Outcome (%)		
	Good	Fair	Poor/dead
I ($n = 91$)	79	15	9
II ($n = 37$)	92	5	56
III ($n = 40$)	62	25	22
IV ($n = 9$)	56	22	22

Table 4. Occupational status[a]

Status	Number
Employed	140
Capable but not employed	40
Unfit	17

[a] $n = 197$

Placement of the clip. Premature rupture from these aneurysms usually occurs during isolation of the neck from the ACoA. Application of a clip to the neck is the goal of direct surgery. However, with an appropriate circulatory pattern, the ACoA can be oblitered along with the aneurysm, if necessary, without any harmful effect. Considerable opinion has been expressed in recent years about the dangers of damaging small perforating vessels arising from the ACoA. From anatomical studies, we have found that a maximum of three perforating vessels arise from the ACoA. Moreover, embryological studies suggest that the purpose of the ACoA is primarily as a conduit for collateral channels rather than for nourishment of any particular area of the brain. When the artery is occluded, the perforating vessels may still receive blood from the opposite ACA. The possible effects of clipping this artery in various types of aneurysms with a differing circulatory pattern are shown in Fig. 9. Although a clip on the neck is ideal, occlusion of the ACoA along with the clip is harmless in some cases and lethal in others [1].

Control of intracranial pressure. Another significant step in this approach is to allow room for postoperative brain swelling by leaving the dura open. We have seen on many occasions that the bone flap rides during the first few postoperative days, due to swelling of the brain, and then subsides as the brain swelling disappears. In this way, the inevitable rise of intracranial pressure after surgical manipulation is controlled.

Results of Treatment

In a personal series of 703 patients, aneurysms of the ACoA. were present in 221. The surgical outcome in these patients is analysed in Tables 1–4. The overall mortality is 3.6% and severe morbidity is 2.2%. Sixteen patients could not be followed up since most of them died from other illnesses and an accurate history of any further haemorrhage was not available (Table 1). Table 2 shows that the result is very satisfactory in grade 1 and 2 patients, but in poorer grades also the outcome is appreciably better than the natural history. In Table 3 the surgical outcome is very much inferior when the aneurysm is associated with the anomaly of the circle. Table 4 shows that only 60% of the patients return to work. Since another 40 patients were capable of returning to work, their failure to do so may be due to social pension benefits available to them in this country following serious illness.

References

1. Sengupta RP (1977) Anterior communicating aneurysms. Thesis, Newcastle University, Newcastle
2. Sengupta RP, McAllister VL (1986) Subarachnoid hemorrhage. Springer-Verlag, Berlin, pp 204–213

Management of Carotid-Ophthalmic Aneurysms

Beniamino Guidetti[1]

A surgeon who has to treat carotid-ophthalmic aneurysms is confronted with several problems, some common to all aneurysms and others peculiar to aneurysms of this site. The first problem, common to all intracranial aneurysms, hinges on the patient's condition (grade I-V) and the length of the interval between hemorrhage and surgery. The second problem is what to do with a patient who has a subarachnoid hemorrhage from another aneurysm and who is found incidentally to have a carotid-ophthalmic aneurysm. The third problem is whether to opt for direct or indirect surgery by closure of the carotid at the neck.

Timing and Preoperative Care

The natural course of a carotid-ophthalmic aneurysm that has bled is the same as that of all intracranial aneurysms. The aim of surgery is to prevent further bleeding and, if the malformation is large and compresses neighboring nervous structures, to free them from compression by the sac.

The therapeutic philosophy at our institution for years has been that the patients meeting the criteria of Botterel grades I or II are offered definitive intracranial surgery early within 72 h after hemorrhage. More seriously ill patients are treated medically until their clinical condition seems stable, and then are subjected to surgical therapy. The only exceptions are patients in poor condition (grades III, IV, and V) who reach the hospital quickly after hemorrhaging. These patients undergo surgery at once in the hope of improving the prognosis, which usually is clearly bad. It is difficult to pass judgment on the value of immediate surgery in these seriously ill patients when the cases operated on within a few hours are so few. Usually, the great majority of these patients do not reach a neuro-surgical department for hours or days after rupture of the aneurysm; also, they are at a stage when the brain is edematous and its circulation is severly impaired.

Multiple Aneurysms

After identification of the ruptured aneurysm, which will be the operation target, there remains the problem of the carotid-ophthalmic aneurysm discovered incidentally at angiography.

We do not think any single rule is possible here. If a patient is not old, presents no serious signs of arteriosclerosis, is in good general condition, and if the brain is slack, the bleeding aneurysm has been closed with ease, and the intact aneurysm is of normal size and on the same side, a delicate attempt to exclude it from the circulation should be made. If the intact aneurysm is on the other side, it should be dealt with in a second operation after careful assessment of the site and size of the malformation, the status and age of the patient, and, most relevant, one's own experience. Much more complex and difficult is our attitude in the face of a giant aneurysm that has never bled and never caused neurological deficits. If it is on the side of the bleeder, a delicate attempt should be made to find the neck and close it, the above conditions permitting. If this maneuver proves arduous, it is better not to attempt it and to simply watch the course of the aneurysm.

When confronted by bilateral carotid-ophthalmic aneurysms, the surgeon must be guided always by their size and direction. If they are of normal size, they can be attacked from the same side, as we did in two cases.

Indirect or Direct Surgery

The third problem is whether to opt for direct or indirect surgery by closure of the carotid at the

[1] Department of Neurological Science, Roma University, La Sapienza Medical School, Rome. Italy

neck. Aneurysms less than 15 mm in diameter usually do not present distinct surgical problems. There no longer seems to be any place for indirect surgery in carotid-ophthalmic aneurysms of normal size but this method may still be indicated in some giant aneurysms provided that there are no aneurysms on the opposite side and no atheromatous stenosis of the contralateral artery.

The large bulbous and giant aneurysms, whatever their site of origin, present difficult problems with operating technique, arising partly from the size of the sac, the width of the neck (often greater than the diameter of the vessel that gives rise to it), the frequent presence of mural thrombi which complicate dissection, and the fact that these aneurysms, in the course of their development, often envelop the entire vessel of origin, which, on the angiograms and on the operating table, appears to run straight into the sac and to emerge from it after a course which sometimes defies the most careful dissection. Even in cases in which the carotid is not enveloped, it may adhere firmly to the walls of the aneurysmal sac and be extremely fragile and thinned because of the compression to which it has been subjected and the presence of arteriosclerotic changes. In addition to these difficulties common to all aneurysms of large size, there are those caused by the location of the aneurysm. This applies particularly to aneurysms developing toward the midline and upward and backward, and to those developing in the sella turcica. In the latter, the neck and sac often adhere to the dura mater of the base of the brain. Further, cases of intra- and supracavernous aneurysms are reported in the literature.

The above points explain the great technical difficulties that are encountered when isolating the carotid and the aneurysmal neck and their not infrequent rupture, and why it is incorrect to compare the results achieved in the surgical treatment of normal sized aneurysms with those achieved in the treatment of large and giant aneurysms.

Surgical Remarks on Large Bulbous and Giant Aneurysms

During the last years, in cases of large bulbous and giant aneurysms, we have systematically used the balloon occlusion test before operation. When balloon occlusion is planned, it is neces-sary to evaluate, by angiography, the cross-filling in the anterior and posterior cerebral arteries' complex. When collateral circulation seems adequate, test occlusion of the internal carotid artery (ICA) with a balloon close to the neck of the aneurysm is carried out for 20–30 min. During this time, the patient is awake and continuously tested neurologically. If temporary carotid occlusion and control of EEG is well tolerated, we can predict with reasonable confidence that the patient will not develop cerebral ischemia when the ICA will be temporarily or permanently occluded. If the patient tolerates well the test occlusion, the balloon is detached and inserted again during the operation. If the collateral circulation seems inadequate or the patient does not tolerate test occlusion, an extracranial-intracranial (EC-IC) bypass is performed, and balloon occlusion is attempted again a few days later after the patency of the graft has been demonstrated. Usually those aneurysms having supraclinoid development—in which the fundus of the sac digs a niche for itself in the orbital portion of the frontal lobe—can be controlled with no great difficulty, due to softness of the neck and wall. This proved to be feasible in all our cases with very good results. Aneurysms with supermedian or inferomedian development, often present one of the trickiest and most laborious phases of this procedure; that is, the separation of the carotid artery (often thin and fragile) from the sac with the risk of carotid rupture. In our experience, this occurred in the past in three patients and made it necessary—after vain attempts to spare the patency of the vessel—to close the carotid artery both below and above. Because of this painful experience, during the past few years we have used balloon occlusion of carotid artery close to the neck of the aneurysm. This lowers the pressure in the aneurysmal sac, enabling the surgeon, when necessary, to close the carotid artery above the neck of the aneurysm to reduce bleeding and eliminate the risk of distal thromboembolism. Blood pressure is raised during or following carotid occlusion and 500 ml of 20% mannitol is injected.

Once control of afferent circulation is ensured, the sac is opened and the soft thrombi are removed. The removal of hard thrombi that adhere to the thin wall of aneurysms may be done with hooks, dissectors, ultrasonic dissection apparatus, spoon, or scissors. To rebulk the aneurysm and collapse its sac, the neck has to be defined as accurately as possible and clamped temporarily with the tips of a forceps to see whether it is soft

Table 1. Summary of preoperative grade, method of surgical treatment, mortality, and morbidity in 76 patients

Treatment	No. of cases	Preoper. grade (Hunt)						No. of deaths	Results
		0	I	II	III	IV	V		
Neck occlusion (aneurysms evacuated)	57	14	25	10	6	1	1	4	10 improved vision—2 hemiparesis + 2 omolateral visual loss
Intracranial[a] trapping aneurysms evacuated	8	5	0	1	2	0	0	4	2 hemiparesis 1 omolateral visual loss
Aneurysm coated	4		2	2	0	0	0	0	Good
Combined extra-intracranial trapping	6	4	1	1	0	0	0	0	
Exploration only	1		1					1	
Total cases	76	23	29	14	8	1	1	9	

In our series, 18 aneurysms were giant and ten were of large size

[a] During dissection, the aneurysms are sheared off the carotid ten patients were operated also for associated omolateral aneurysms, two for contralateral aneurysm, one at the same stage for associated olfactory meningioma, one for adenoma and one for AV malformation. In two patients, a contralateral carotid-ophthalmic aneurysm was clipped

enough and whether there is any narrowing or kinking of the carotid artery. If the neck rigidity is associated with a mural thrombus, it has to be removed. If the neck appears to be soft and free of hard atheroma, an attempt is made to close it with one of the strongest clips available, usually Drake, Sugita or Yaşargil. In some instances, additional clips in tandem or at an angle to each other, are necessary. In cases in which the neck appears sclerotic, or the neck occlusion gives rise to kinking or deformity of the lumen of the carotid artery, it is preferable to leave a portion of the aneurysm base in situ wrapped with muslin, gauze, and adhesive. When neck exposure and clipping is thought impossible, direct surgery should be abandoned and the carotid artery should be closed above and below the neck of the aneurysm.

Long-term functional results are illustrated in Table 1.

References

1. Almeida GM, Shibata MK, Bianco E (1976) Carotid-ophthalmic aneurysms. Surg Neurol 5:41–45
2. Bengochea FG, Deland F (1975) Bilateral giant carotid-opthalmic aneurysms. J Neurosurg 42:589–592
3. Corradi M, Guidetti B, Riccio A (1959) Disturbi oculari negli aneurismi della carotide interna, tratto C2, ad estrinsecazione intra e soprasellare. Riv Neuropsichiat 5:345–360
4. Debrun G, Fox G, Drake C, Peerless S, Girvin J, Ferguson G (1981) Giant unclippable aneurysms: Treatment with detachable balloons. Am J Neurorad 2:167–173
5. Dolenc V (1985) A combined epidural subdural approach to carotid-ophthalmic artery aneurysms. J Neurosurg 62:667–672
6. Drake CG, Vanderlinen RG, Amacher AL (1968) Carotid-ophthalmic aneurysms. J Neurosurg 29:24–31
7. Drake CG (1979) Giant intracranial aneurysms: Experience with surgical treatment in 174 patients. Clin Neurosurg 26:12–95
8. Ferguson G, Drake CG (1980) Carotid-ophthalmic aneurysms: The surgical management of those cases presenting with compression of the optic nerve and chiasm alone. Clin Neurosurg 27:263–308
9. Ferguson G, Drake C (1981) Carotid-ophthalmic aneurysms: Visual abnormalities in 32 patients and the results of treatment. Surg Neurol 16:1–8
10. Guidetti B, La Torre E (1975) Management of carotid-ophthalmic aneurysms. J Neurosurg 42:438–442
11. Guidetti B (1985) Carotid-ophthalmic aneurysm. In: Fein J, Flamm E (eds) Cerebrovascular surgery, vol. III Springer, Berlin, pp 803–839
12. Handa H, Hashimoto N, Yonekawa Y (1982) Surgical treatment of giant aneurysms. Neurosurg Rev 5:169–172
13. Heros R, Nelson P, Ojemann R, Crowell R, De Brun G (1983) Large and giant aneurysms. Neurosurgery 12:153–163
14. Hosobuchi Y (1979) Direct surgical treatment of giant intracranial aneurysms. J Neurosurg 51:743–756
15. Ishii R, Tanaka R, Koike T, Takeda N, Takeuchi S, Sasaki O, Okada K (1983) Computed tomo-

graphic demonstration of the effect of proximal parent artery ligation for giant intracranial aneurysms. Surg Neurol 19:532–540

16. Iwabuchi T, Suzuki S, Sobata E (1978) Intracranial direct operation for carotid-ophthalmic aneurysms by unroofing the optic canal. Acta Neurochir 43:163–169

17. Kodama N, Suzuki N (1982) Surgical treatment of giant aneurysms. Neurosurg Rev 5:155–160

18. Lavyne MH, Klefield J, Davis KR, Ojemann RG, Crowell RM (1978) Giant intracranial aneurysms of the anterior circulation: Clinical characteristics and diagnosis by computed tomography. Neurosurgery 3:356–363

19. Meining G, Gunter R, Ulrich P, Suss W, Sommer B, Ludwig B, Schurmann K (1982) Reduced risk of ICA ligation after balloon occlusion test. Neurosurg Rev 5:95–98

20. Milenkovic Z, Gopic H, Antonic P, Jovicic J, Petrovic B (1982) Contralateral pterional approach to a carotid-ophthalmic aneurysm ruptured at surgery. J Neurosurg 57:823–825

21. Morley TP, Barr HWK (1968) Giant intracranial aneurysms: Diagnosis, course and management. Clin Neurosurg 16:73–93

22. Nakao S, Kikuchi H, Takahashi N (1981) Successful clipping of carotid-ophthalmic aneurysm through a contralateral pterional approach: Report of two cases. J Neurosurg 54:532–536

23. Onuma T, Suzuki J (1979) Surgical treatment of giant intracranial aneurysms. J Neurosurg 51:33–36

24. Peerless S, Ferguson G, Drake CG (1982) Extracranial-intracranial bypass in the treatment of giant intracranial aneurysms. Neurosurg Rev 5:77–81

25. Peerless J, Drake C (1982) Treatment of giant cerebral aneurysm of the anterior circulation. Neurosurg Rev 5:149–154

26. Pia HW, Zierski J (1982) Giant cerebral aneurysms. Neurosurg Rev 5:117–149

27. Sengupta RP, Gryspeerdt GL, Hankinson J (1976) Carotid-ophthalmic aneurysms. J Neurol Neurosurg Psychiatry 39:837–853

28. Sengupta RP (1982) Management of large and giant aneurysms. Neurosurg Rev 5:173–178

29. Soontag VKH, Yuan RH, Stein BM (1977) Giant intracranial aneurysms: A review of 13 cases. Surg Neurol 8:81–84

30. Spetzler R, Schuster H, Roski (1980) Elective extracranial-intracranial arterial bypass in the treatment of inoperable giant aneurysms of the internal carotid artery. J Neurosurg 53:22–27

31. Sundt TM (1982) Surgical technique of giant intracranial aneurysm. Neurosurg Rev 5:161–168

32. Suzuki J (1979) Cerebral aneurysms: Experience with 1000 directly operated cases. Tokyo Press, Tokyo, p 269

33. Thurel C, Rey A, Thiebaut JB, Chai N, Houdart R (1974) Anéurisms carotido-ophthalmiques. Neurochirurgie 20 (1):25–39

34. Yamada K, Haykawa T, Oku Y, Maeda Y, Ushio Y, Yoshimide T, Kaway R (1977) Contralateral pterional approach for carotid-ophthalmic aneurysm. Neurosurgery 15:5–8

35. Yaşargil MG, Gasser JG, Hodosh RM, Rankin TV (1977) Carotid-ophthalmic aneurysms: Direct microsurgical approach. Surg Neurol 8:155–165

Surgery for Pericallosal Aneurysms

JÁNOS VAJDA and EMIL PÁSZTOR[1]

Summary

Thirty patients with distal anterior cerebral artery aneurysm were operated on microsurgically in the last decade. Our technique has continuously been tailored to comply with the requirements of surgery of these lesions. A contralateral frontoparasagittal craniotomy and dissection of the neck are advised since these have been proved to make premature rupture of the often embedded sac less likely. Careful revision of all remaining arteries serves to prevent ischemic complications. We prefer to clip these aneurysms within 48 h after the first rupture if it has left the patient able to communicate, since fatal or disabling clinical vasospasm as well as early rerupture can be avoided this way.

Introduction

Although a distal anterior cerebral artery aneurysm should be defined as part of the aneurysms of the anterior circle of Willis, it has often been omitted from such materials or discussed separately as rare lesions. It often occurs as part of multiple aneurysms and when it does, it is usually responsible for the subarachnoid bleeding. The approach to these aneurysms is different from that to other aneurysms which raises difficulties when other aneurysms are also present and are attempted to be occluded. Their rupture may evoke severe clinical vasospasm causing more widespread brain edema or infarct than what would be expected in view of the relatively limited area supplied by the parent arteries. These are the peculiarities which make distal anterior cerebral artery aneurysms worth dealing with.

---

[1] National Institute of Neurosurgery, Budapest, Hungary

Clinical Material and Results

Thirty patients with distal anterior cerebral artery aneurysm were operated on in the last ten years in our Institute. None of them had mycotic or traumatic aneurysms. There were 20 females and ten males, their ages ranging from 30 to 64 years with a median of 39 years. Except for one case with a giant aneurysm, the sizes of the lesions were well under the average of sacs in other common localizations (5 mm). Half of the patients harboured multiple aneurysms, which is a very high ratio, though it agrees with data in the literature. There were three patients with double pericallosal aneurysms: "twin" distribution in two cases, and "mirror" distribution in the remaining. In 12 cases, other aneurysms were combined with pericallosal sacs: in nine cases the pericallosal sacs ruptured. Apart from three patients with multiple lesions in whom the pericallosal aneurysm never bled, there were three further cases with silent lesion presented with trauma, stroke, and frontal arteriovenous malformation (AVM) respectively. Six of 27 cases of subarachnoid hemorrhage suffered from two bleedings. The vast majority of the ruptures of distal anterior cerebral artery aneurysms were accompanied by loss of consciousness. A considerable amount of hematomas could be found in five cases.

Figure 1 shows the preoperative grading, according to Hunt and Hess, which all patients scored, in relation to the surgical results.

Vasospasm was evident on angiograms in two cases; both died after surgery from severe clinical vasospasm. Two other patients developed postoperative clinical vasospasm; one of them died. There was no strict timing policy applied in the first period targeted by this survey. All of our clinical vasospasm cases are now believed to be victims of inappropriate timing of admission and consequent surgery. None of our patients operated on within 48 h after the first bleeding developed vasospasm and they are all doing well.

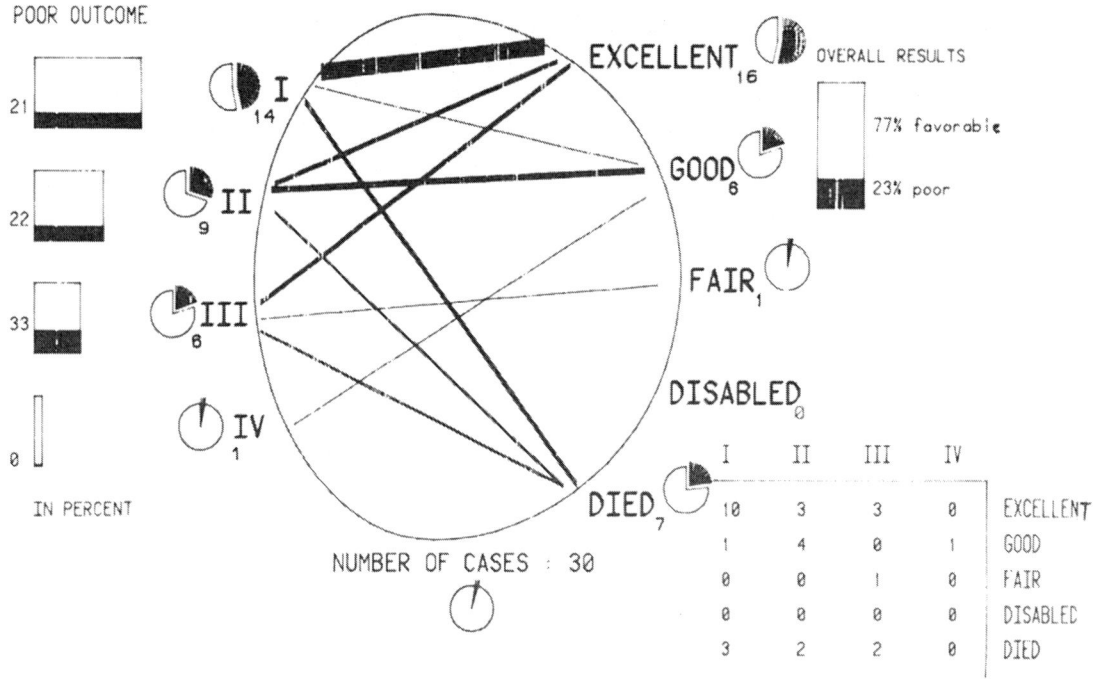

Fig. 1. Relationship between the preoperative condition and surgical results in cases with distal anterior cerebral artery aneurysms. The *width of lines* drawn between preoperative and recent states represents the number of patients in each group. The direction of the lines drawn corresponds to the change of clinical state of the patients. More groups of *wider lines* running upwards on the chart express better results. Poor outcome (disabled and died) expressed in percentage of each Hunt-Hess grade (*Roman numerals*) is shown. *White area of rectangles* belonging to each Hunt grade is in proportion to the number of patients cured of that grade. The *circle diagrams* show the number of patients in each clinical state as a percentage of all studied in this figure

We lost one case with silent pericallosal aneurysm who developed a huge frontal hematoma unrelated to surgery on the second postoperative day. The hematoma was removed immediately but she died two months later due to pulmonary infection and multiple cerebrovascular lesions.

The surgical technique we used has continuously been revised and improved as our experience has grown. In the earlier years of microsurgery, little attention was paid to the approach as such, and ipsilateral frontoparasagittal craniotomy was instituted as a rule. The arterial segments distal from the aneurysm (mainly the ascending branches of the callosomarginal artery) were firmly adhered to the falx by their arachnoid cover. Furthermore, it is the median cortex, which is mobilized and retracted during surgery, which most often contains the fundus. We speculated that these two pathoanatomical facts might have played a role in the premature rupture of the sac during dissection in seven of our 13 such cases which underwent ipsilateral

surgery. First, the head position was changed: its turn toward the craniotomy made less retraction necessary but increased the need of crossing the midline, i.e., the sagittal sinus, and of retracting the falx. In one of our later patients, however, the middle cerebral artery aneurysm on the left forced us to attack the ruptured pericallosal aneurysm on the right via a contralateral craniotomy. Dissection of contralateral vessels and the neck was surprisingly easier: almost no retracting or mobilization of nearby vessels were needed. The advantage of the contralateral approach became obvious in two patients with bilateral pericallosal aneurysms in whom the clipping of the lesion contralateral to our approach was more straightforward than that of the ipsilateral one, however silent. Seventeen cases with 19 aneurysms were operated on in the second period (Fig. 2). Premature rupture occurred in two cases: one of them had bilateral pericallosal aneurysm, and the bleeding came from the ipsilateral sac during retraction.

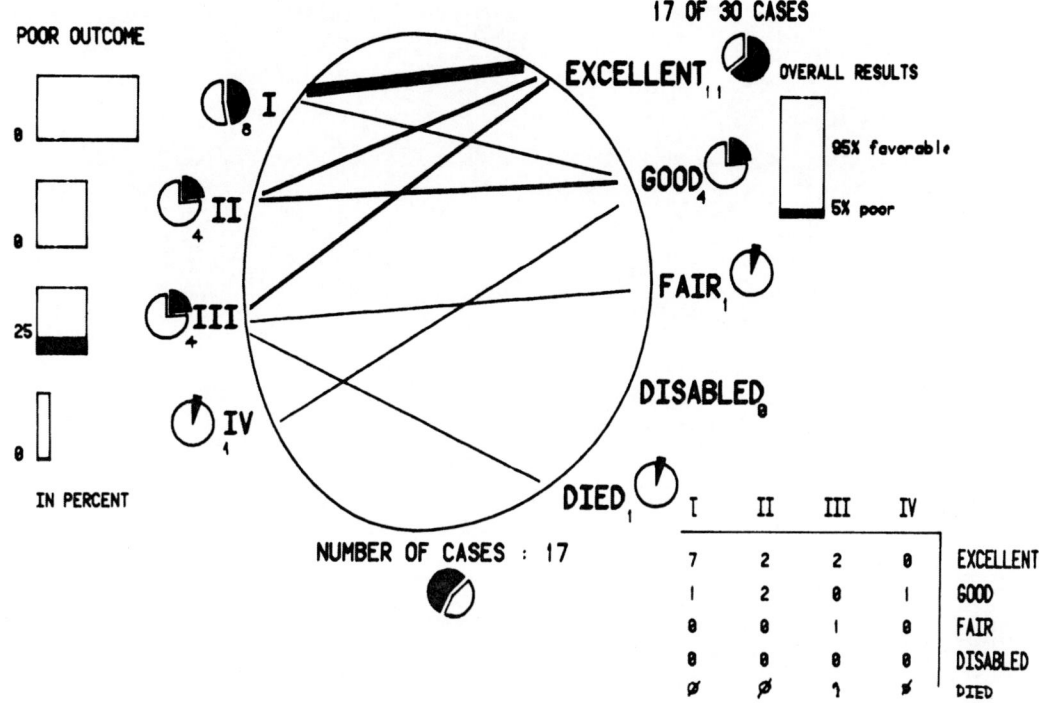

Fig. 2. Outcome of patients with distal anterior cerebral artery aneurysms (*DAAA*) who underwent surgery via contralateral approach. Note the better results compared with that of all cases. *Symbols are as in Fig. 1.* The number of cases studied in this figure is shown below as the percentage of all cases with distal anterior cerebral artery aneurysm

Surgical Technique

A curved incision is made above the hairline crossing the midline by 4 cm. The skin flap is turned frontally. Four burr holes are made. The two medial ones, near but not on the midline, are connected with Gigli's wire saw and pulled towards the contralateral side. This way the inner table of the sawn sloping surface of the skull still covers the sinus, while the outer table of its sawn surface is already over the contralateral side. With the inner, halved surface rongeured away, the result is a craniotomy which is extended across the sinus without endangering it and covered completely at closure by the bone flap. Then the dural flap is opened toward the midline and stiffened up to the falx. The interhemispheral fissure is this way immediately accessible. The frontomedian cortex is retracted gently, and we proceed along the falx down to the cingular region. A branch of the callosomarginal artery ipsilateral to the approach is sought and followed up to the bilateral callosomarginal trunks. The arachnoid may be torn easily and frequently during dissection due to previous bleedings and adhesions. The injured arachnoid often misleads the surgeon into the median parenchyma, causing unnecessary brain damage and further difficulties in dissecting the aneurysm. This mishap can mostly be avoided if arterial branches are used as guide to the interhemispheral fissure. After identifying the cingular cistern, only the side of the aneurysm contralateral to the craniotomy is looked at. The arachnoid is opened along the parent callosomarginal artery which is followed proximally up to the termination of the A2 segment of the anterior cerebral artery. This way the neck is easy to identify and handle. Since most of the sac is often embedded in the facing parenchyma, dissecting from the contralateral side around the neck is less dangerous and takes less time than from the ipsilateral side. It is the fissure between the sac and the callosomarginal artery which is usually seen better and is used, therefore, for clipping the neck in a plane perpendicular to the midline. The entire sac must then be freed and mobilized to exclude stenosis or occlusion of the pericallosal artery which often takes irregular curves at its origin (Fig. 3).

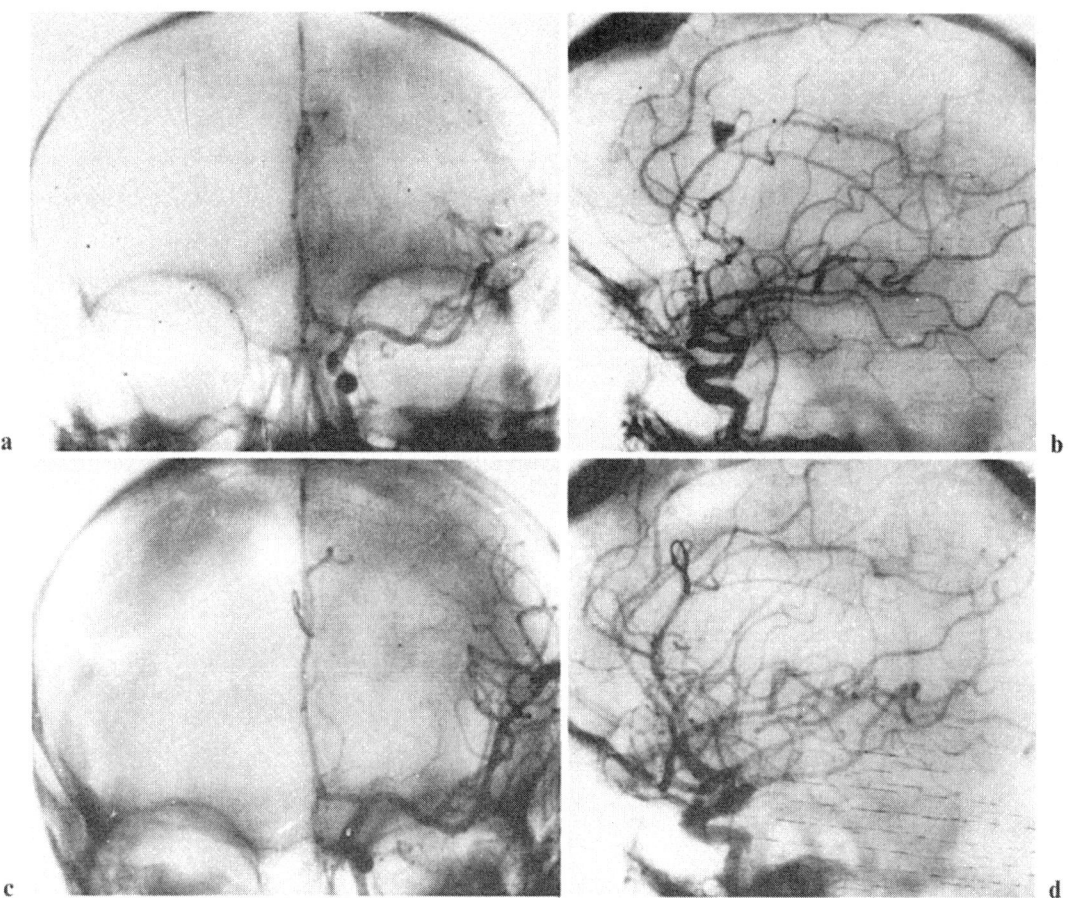

Fig. 3. a, b Preoperative carotid angiograms show an aneurysm on the left distal anterior cerebral artery. **c, d** Postoperative angiograms demonstrate the occlusion of the neck with a clip introduced via right frontoparasagittal craniotomy

Discussion

Reports on surgery for distal anterior cerebral artery aneurysms appeared scatteredly in the literature owing to their less frequent incidence. The number of such aneurysms are similar in the greater clinical materials reported lately. Our data confirm that neurosurgical centers receiving 150–200 aneurysm patients per year can expect four to eight cases with aneurysm in this localization with a further two to four cases in which a distal anterior cerebral artery aneurysm occurs as a part (most often the bleeding one) of multiple cerebral aneurysms. They incline to appear as mirror or twin aneurysms on bilateral arteries or at the same branching.

There is a higher incidence of multiple bleedings before admission with an obvious consequence of an even higher incidence of unconsciousness during the acute phase. This striking difference from our material to other aneurysms

may raise the question whether the rupture of these lesions is less obvious to recognize.

The subarachnoid bleeding they cause may result in severe, delayed, clinical vasospasm featuring widespread edema, intracranial hypertension, or basal ganglia lesion. This fact may seem to contradict the limited involvement of the pericallosal and the callosomarginal arteries in the cerebral circulation as a whole. One has to bear in mind, however, that cisternal bleeding in the midline can be unexpectedly voluminous and may accumulate in remote CSF compartments (Fig. 4). The axial subarachnoid clot certainly affects bilateral vessels and, when these arteries come to react by spasm, bilateral medial and deep areas may become ischemic. Correlation of results with preoperative grading alone revealed only minimal worsening of outcome among cases of inferior grading. An analysis of cause of deaths showed a high proportion of severe neurological deterioration leading to the breakdown of vegetative functions, attributable to vasospasm.

Three patients among those who died had undergone surgery between the 3rd and 7th days after the rupture and were presented with signs of initial vasospasm. The postoperative clinical course of these patients featured extreme bilateral brain edema in an area much larger than what would have been expected considering the volume of brain supplied by the parent arteries. The edema resulted from vasospasm of the distal anterior cerebral artery complex, and had spread as far as the bilateral temporal lobes. In the symptomatology, we found a subtle hypothalamic dysfunction followed by diencephalic syndrome with a gradual deterioration of consciousness. The process ended in all cases in untreatable intracranial hypertension.

Our results underline the importance of proper timing of surgery for distal anterior cerebral artery aneurysms, no matter if they are doubled or part of multiple lesions. Patients who had overcome the first bleeding in a relatively good condition benefited from surgery within 48 h unless there was some interference with the parent arteries at the definite clipping. This turned out to be an equally important factor.

Of course, all cerebral arteries bearing aneurysms are important enough to be saved during surgery. But the numerous irregularities, found in the region of the distal anterior cerebral arteries, make stenosis or occlusion of the origin of one of the remaining branches rather likely. This must be avoided by careful inspection of these vessels after the clip is applied and the sac emptied. Autopsy revealed severe stenosis in three cases, with distal thrombosis of the pericallosal artery in one case, due to improper clipping close to the origin of the pericallosal artery which, in all occasions, had unusual curved running as its proximal segment was hidden in the depths of the cistern. This explains why the surgeon could not notice the position of the artery, even if its distal segment seemed intact.

These important facets of distal anterior cerebral artery aneurysm surgery have been mentioned in the majority of papers. Description of surgical procedure, however, is nowhere detailed enough to discuss peculiarities.

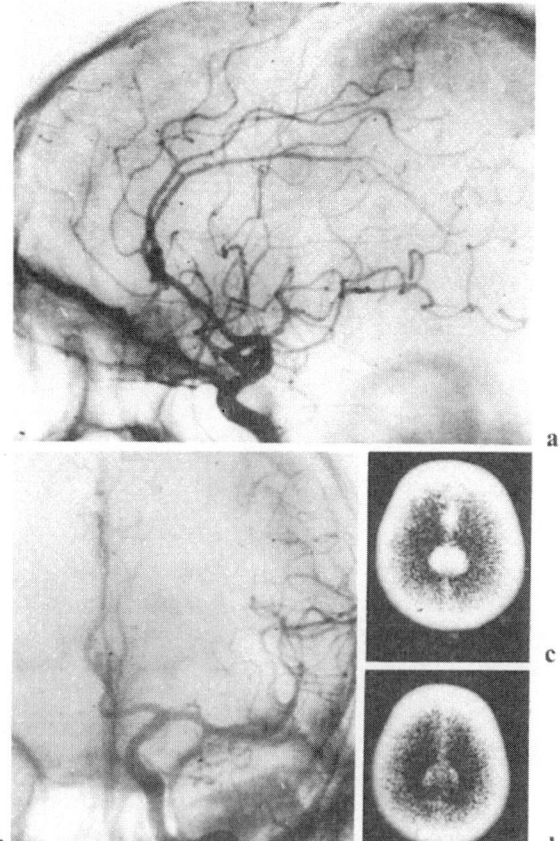

Fig. 4. a, b Preoperative left common carotid angriograms and **c** CT scan show an aneurysm at the origin of the callosomarginal artery and a considerable interhemispheral hematoma in the central region far distal to the site of the rupture (also clearly seen in the frontal area). **d** Postoperative CT demonstrates the spontaneous disappearance of the remote cisternal hemorrhage 7 days later

References

1. Becker DH, Newton TH (1979) Distal anterior cerebral artery aneurysm. Neurosurgery 4:495–503

2. Dechaume JP, Aimard G, Michel D, et al. (1973) Les anéurysmes de l'artère péricalleuse. Neurochir 19:135–150

3. Fleischer AS, Barrow DL (1985) Distal anterior cerebral artery aneurysms. In: Wilkins. RH, Rengachary SS (eds) Neurosurgery. McGraw-Hill, New York, pp 1383–1385

4. Horváth M, Vajda J, Juhász J (1979) Distal aneurysms of the anterior cerebral artery. Ideggy Szle 32:164–171 (in Hungarian)

5. Yaşargil MG, Carter LP (1974) Saccular aneurysms of the distal anterior cerebral artery. J Neurosurg 40:218–223

6. Yoshimoto T, Uchida K, Suzuki J (1979) Surgical treatment of distal anterior cerebral artery aneurysms. J Neurosurg 50:40–44

Results of the Surgical Treatment of Anterior Circulation Aneurysms

Nobuyuki Yasui, Akifumi Suzuki, Masahito Nemoto, Ken Asakura, and Masabumi Nagashima[1]

Introduction

Direct operative approaches for anterior circulation aneurysms have been commonly performed since the introduction of the operating microscope to neurosurgical operations. Consequently, operative results have improved. The results of anterior communicating artery (ACo) aneurysm could be cited as one good example of improvement [6, 7]. However, operative approaches and techniques are still the biggest problem in surgical treatment of intracranial aneurysms. Also, general complications can be troublesome, especially in older patients. These problems are closely matched to patient clinical outcome when compared with several secondary pathophysiological problems following subarachnoid hemorrhage (SAH). Pathophysiological problems include severe subarachnoid hematoma, intracerebral hematoma, vasospasm, etc.

In this paper, the causes of a poor clinical outcome, as well as problems related to surgery, will be discussed relative to cases of ruptured and nonruptured aneurysms of the ACo, internal carotid (IC), and middle cerebral (MC) arteries, where surgery was performed.

Materials and Methods

A total of 596 patients of intracranial aneurysm of the anterior circulation system, including ACo, IC, and MC arteries, were operated on at the Research Institute for Brain and Blood Vessels, AKITA, from April 1976 to December 1985. Patient ages ranged from 20 to 78, and the mean age was 53.7 years. There were 301 females and 295 males; 550 operations were performed for ruptured aneurysms, and 90 operations were done for nonruptured aneurysms. Background diseases in the cases with nonruptured aneurysms were one of the multiple aneurysms in the ruptured aneurysm, hypertensive intracerebral hematoma, and cerebral ischemia. The operative approach for the anterior communicating aneurysm was mainly performed using the anterior or basal interhemispheric (AIH or BIH) approach. Middle and IC aneurysms were performed by the transsylvian approaches. Evaluation of the severity of the condition of the patients was based on their level of consciousness and neurological symptoms. Clinical outcomes of the cases of ruptured aneurysms were classified as either fully recovered, self-managed, needing help, bedridden, or dead. The cases of nonruptured aneurysms showed either no change or a worsening when compared to the preoperative neurological condition.

The causes for a poor clinical outcome or worsening were investigated using CT scan, angiography, and operative records. Clinical courses, such as brain damage due to SAH, intracerebral hematoma, vasospasm, surgical procedures, and general complications, were also investigated. When a patient's condition worsened due to general complications where there was a prolonged disturbance of consciousness, the causes of those disturbances were regarded as the underlying factors resulting in a poor clinical outcome. When a patient's postoperative condition was worse than his preoperative state, the causes were judged as surgical complications.

Results

Clinical Outcome of Ruptured Aneurysms and the Causes of a Poor Clinical Outcome

Of 550 cases where operations were performed, 405 showed recovery to an independent state; 337 cases recovered fully. Seventy-one cases needed help, 29 cases were bedridden, and 45 cases died.

[1] Department of Surgical Neurology, Research Institute for Brain and Blood Vessels, Akita, Japan

Table 1. Level of consciousness before operation and clinical outcome in ruptured aneurysms

Consciousness	Fully recovered	Self-managed	Needed help	Bedridden	Died	Total
Clear	247 (83.2)	19 (6.4)	20 (6.7)	4 (1.3)	7 (2.4)	297
Drowsy	61 (55.5)	23 (20.9)	14 (12.7)	7 (6.4)	5 (4.5)	110
Confusion	12 (28.6)	10 (23.8)	6 (14.3)	3 (7.1)	12 (28.5)	42
Stupor	13 (30.2)	8 (18.6)	10 (23.3)	6 (14.0)	6 (14.0)	43
Semicoma	2 (4.7)	6 (14.0)	18 (41.9)	7 (16.3)	10 (23.3)	43
Coma	2 (14.3)	2 (14.3)	3 (21.4)	2 (14.3)	5 (35.7)	14
Total	337 (61.3)	68 (12.4)	71 (12.9)	29 (5.3)	45 (8.2)	550

Numbers in *parentheses* are percentages

Table 2. Site of the aneurysm and clinical outcome in ruptured aneurysms

Site of AN	Fully recovered	Self-managed	Needed help	Bedridden	Died	Total
ACo AN	127 (59.3)	28 (13.1)	25 (11.7)	15 (7.0)	19 (8.9)	214
IC AN	97 (63.8)	11 (7.2)	23 (15.1)	7 (4.6)	14 (9.2)	152
MC AN	113 (61.4)	29 (15.8)	23 (12.5)	7 (3.8)	12 (6.5)	184
Total	337 (61.3)	68 (12.4)	71 (12.9)	29 (5.3)	45 (8.2)	550

Numbers in parentheses are percent
AN aneurysm, *ACo* anterior communicating, *IC* internal carotid, *MC* middle carotid

Table 3. Causes of poor clinical outcome and site of ruptured aneurysms

Site of AN	VS	ICH	SAH	RA	BR	BO	NPH	GC	Total
ACo AN	31	4	5	6	2	2	0	9	59
IC AN	15	5	2	3	2	9	1	7	44
MC AN	12	16	0	1	4	2	0	7	42
Total	58	25	7	10	8	13	1	23	145

VS vasospasm, *ICH* intracerebral hemorrhage, *SAH* subarachnoid hemorrhage, *RA* rebleeding attack, *BR* brain retraction, *BO* branch occlusion, *NPH* normal pressure hydrocephalus, *GC* general complication

Of 297 cases, 247 (83.2%), being fully conscious before the operation, recovered fully, and 19 cases (6.4%) recovered to a self-managed state. Twenty cases (6.7%) needed help, four cases (1.3%) were bedridden, and seven patients (2.4%) died. A total of $76\frac{1}{2}$% of the patients in a drowsy state, 52.4% in confusion, 48.8% in a stupor, 18.7% in a semicoma, and 28.7% in a coma recovered to a state of being independent; $4\frac{1}{2}$% of the cases in a drowsy state, 28.5% in confusion, 14% in a stupor, 23.3% in a semicoma, and 35.7% in a coma died. The less severe the disturbance of consciousness, the better the clinical outcome was (Table 1).

The clinical outcome is slightly better in the cases with MC aneurysm, but there is no signifi-cant difference between the site of the aneurysm and the clinical outcome (Table 2). More than 70% of the cases recovered to an independent state and 6%–9% of the cases for each type of aneurysm died.

Vasospasm was the most frequent cause of a poor clinical outcome in ACo and IC aneurysms (Table 3). Intracerebral hematoma was a more frequent cause of a poor clinical outcome than vasospasm in the MC aneurysm cases. Brain damage caused by excessive brain retraction or brain contusion during operative procedures, branch occlusion, such as anterior choroidal artery or perforators, and general complications, such as massive GI bleeding, pneumonia, meningitis, and heart failure, were other important causes of a poor clinical outcome. Seven cases are included in the reattach group where rebleeding resulted from either a residual aneurysm or a slippage of the aneurysm clip after the operation.

Clinical Outcomes in Nonruptured Aneurysms and Causes of Postoperative Worsening

Sixty-five of 90 cases had no change and 25 cases became worse after operation. Sixteen of the 25 cases that worsened showed a transient neurological deficit caused either by operative complications or by transient deterioration because of general complications. Nine cases either resulted in a neurological deficit or died because of operative or general complications. The operative risk is higher in the group having ischemic disease (Table 4). The cases with permanent worsening are also significantly higher if they have ischemic disease. Direct technical problems, such as circulation disturbances of the perforating arteries, or brain damage caused by excessive brain retraction, form more than half of the causes of worsening (Table 5). Subdural effusions succeeded by preexisting brain atrophy are another important postoperative complication. Intracerebral hematomas which occurred apart from the operative procedures were found in two cases.

Discussion

Recently, results of the treatment for ruptured intracranial aneurysm have improved because of the introduction of microsurgery, as well as early operation and the development of perioperative management. Clinical results are not fully satisfactory in all cases, however. Many problems have been cited as causes of a poor clinical outcome. Among them, pathophysiological conditions, which are related directly to such bleeding attacks as intracerebral hematoma, severe SAH,

vasospasm, and so on, have been commonly discussed in relation to clinical results and the treatment of this disease [3–5, 8, 9].

Operative or general complications have been rarely discussed as the causes of a poor clinical outcome. The reason for this may be that these problems are too primitive to discuss as scientific problems. The clinical results of this study do not correspond with other reports. For example, although our series shows a higher incidence of severe cases, it shows better or equal clinical results when compared with the International Cooperative Study [2] or other such reports [3–5]. In spite of better clinical results in this study, more than one-third of the causes of a poor clinical outcome were related to operative or general complications. It may be possible that the incidence of these complications would increase in other reports if the influence of operative procedures and general complications were strictly appraised as they were in this study. This simply means that operative results could improve more by developing operative methods, or by pre- and postoperative management of today's patients.

Operative results of nonruptured aneurysms were also studied to solve these problems. Disturbance of blood flow caused by occlusion of the arteries (mainly perforating arteries), and brain contusion caused by excessive brain retraction are the main problems in the operative procedures of nonruptured aneurysm cases. Incidence of permanent neurological worsening is significantly higher in nonruptured aneurysm complicated with ischemic disease. Several reasons are listed as to why conditions are worse with ischemic disease cases. For example, the level of cerebral circulation is more critical and arteriosclerotic changes are more marked. Operative approaches have been developed so that brain retraction is at its minimum level in recent years. Some examples are the BIH approach for

Table 4. Background disease and clinical outcome

	No change	Worsening	
		Transient	Permanent
Ischemic cerebro-vascular disease	20 (64.5)	5 (16.1)	6 (19.4)
Hypertensive intracerebral hematoma	12 (75.0)	2 (13.3)	1 (6.7)
Nonruptured multiple aneurysm	33 (75.0)	9 (20.5)	2 (4.5)
Total	65 (72.2)	16 (17.7)	9 (10.0)

Numbers in *parentheses* are percentages

Table 5. Causes of postoperative worsening in nonruptured aneurysms

No.	Age (yrs)	Sex	Site of AN	BD	Severity	Cause of worsening
1	61	M	ACo	IS	Tr	Cerebellar hemorrhage
2	61	F	IC	IS	Tr	Branch occlusion (perforator)
3	49	F	IC	IS	Tr	Subdural effusion
4	63	M	IC	IS	Tr	Subdural effusion
5	64	M	MC	IS	Tr	Brain retraction
6	65	M	ACo	IS	P	General complication (pneumonia)
7	63	F	ACo	IS	P	Branch occlusion (perforator)
8	48	M	IC	IS	P	Brain contusion
9	63	M	IC	IS	P	Subdural effusion
10	63	M	MC	IS	P	Contralateral HIH
11	59	F	MC	IS	P	Branch occlusion (perforator)
12	59	M	IC	HIH	Tr	Brain retraction
13	64	M	MC	HIH	Tr	Meningitis
14	51	F	IC	HIH	P	Meningitis
15	66	F	ACo	MAN	Tr	Epilepsy
16	58	M	ACo	MAN	Tr	Subdural effusion
17	62	M	IC	MAN	Tr	Brain contusion
18	63	M	IC	MAN	Tr	Brain contusion
19	57	M	IC	MAN	Tr	Brain retraction
20	41	M	MC	MAN	Tr	Branch occlusion (perforator)
21	64	F	MC	MAN	Tr	Brain retraction
22	62	M	MC	MAN	Tr	Branch occlusion (perforator)
23	68	M	MC	MAN	Tr	Brain contusion
24	59	F	IC	MAN	P	IC trapping
25	59	M	MC	MAN	P	MC posterior trunk occlusion

AN aneurysm, *BD* background disease, *IS* ischemic cerebrovascular disease, *HIH* hypertensive intracerebral hematoma, *MAN* multiple aneurysm, *Tr* transient deficit, *P* permanent deficit, *IC* internal carotid, *MC* middle cerebral, *ACo* anterior communicating artery

anterior communicating aneurysm [10] and the zygomatic approach [11] for IC terminal aneurysm. Operative results were better for the BIH than the AIH in our series (unpublished data). There are some possibilities for improvement in the operative approach.

Another important problem is how to perform a complete neck clipping without disturbing cerebral circulation. Several methods have been recommended to assist complete neck clipping, especially in cases of giant, big, or broadly based aneurysms, such as systemic arterial hypotension at the time of clipping, temporary clipping of the aneurysm dome, multiple clipping method, and temporary occlusion of the parent arteries. Incidence of cases with surgical problems have decreased because of the development of microsurgical procedures at our institute. However, there have been some problem cases in spite of a combination of these methods. It is necessary that the effort to develop a safe, easy, and perfect clipping method should continue.

Conclusion

The author may overemphasize the importance of surgical and general problems in this paper. These may not be scientific problems, but are equal in importance to the pathophysiological conditions after SAH in clinical practice. It is also essential to discriminate these complications from pathophysiological factors after SAH for estimating the true pathophysiology of the disease.

References

1. Fujitsu K, Kuwabara K (1985) Zygomatic approach for lesions in the interpeduncular cistern. J Neurosurg 62:340–343
2. Kassell NF, Torner JC, Jane JA (1986) The International Cooperative Study on the Timing of Aneurysm Surgery. In: Kikuchi H, Fukushima T, Watanabe K (eds) Intracranial aneurysms: Surgical timing and techniques. Nishimura, Niigata, pp 184–189

3. Sano H, Jain VK, Tatou Y, Katada K, Kanno T (1986) Timing of surgery for ruptured aneurysms. In: Kikuchi H, Fukushima T, Watanabe K (eds) Intracranial aneurysms: Surgical timing and techniques. Nishimura, Niigata, pp 168–176
4. Sano K, Saito I (1982) Timing and indication of surgery for ruptured intracranial aneurysms with regard to cerebral vasospasm. Acta Neurochir (Wien) 63:163–174
5. Suzuki J, Yoshimoto T (1976) Early operation for ruptured intracranial aneurysms, especially the cases operated within 48 hours after the last subarachnoid hemorrhage. Neurol Surg (Tokyo) 4:135–141
6. Yaşargil MD (1969) Microsurgery applied to neurosurgery. Thieme, Stuttgart pp 126–130
7. Yaşargil MD, Fox JL, Ray MW (1975) The operative approach to aneurysms of the anterior communicating artery. In: Krayenbuhl H. (ed) Advances and technical standard in neurosurgery vol. 2. Springer, New York, pp 113–170
8. Yasui N, Ito Z, Ohta H, et al. (1982) Surgical problems and pathophysiology in severe cases with ruptured aneurysms in the acute stage. Acta Neurochir 63:163–174
9. Yasui N, Suzuki A, Sayama I, Kawamura S (1986) Indication and timing of surgery in the management of ruptured intracranial aneurysms. In: Kikuchi H, Fukushima T, Watanabe K (eds) Intracranial aneurysms: Surgical timing and techniques. Nishimura, Niigata, pp 157–167
10. Yasui N, Suzuki A, Sayama I, Kawamura S (1987) A new operative approach for anterior communicating aneurysm: Basal interhemishperic approach. Neurol Med Chir (Tokyo) 27:756–761

Bifrontal Interhemispheric Approach to Aneurysms of the Anterior Communicating Artery

KAZUO MIZOI and JIRO SUZUKI[1]

Introduction

Many approaches have been used in surgery on aneurysms of the anterior communicating artery (ACoA), but currently these diverse approaches can be subdivided into two main groups: an interhemispheric approach using a bifrontal craniotomy, and a pterional approach using a frontotemporal craniotomy. Although we have tried various surgical approaches, the majority of operations were performed using the interhemispheric approach, which we have come to believe is the safest and the most effective method for surgical treatment of such aneurysms.

In this paper, we review our experience with 651 cases of single aneurysms of the ACoA operated on directly during the 25-year period from 1961 to 1986, and describe the surgical technique we currently use [11].

Clinical Material

Between June 1961 and 1986, we performed direct operations in 200 cases of cerebral aneurysm. Among those cases were 651 (32.6%) aneurysms of the ACoA (Table 1). For analysis of the surgical results, we have classified the first 346 of these cases (those operated on between June 1961 and September 1975) as group 1, and the last 305 cases (those operated on between October 1975 and June 1986) as group 2. The group 1 cases were among the first 1000 cases of direct aneurysm surgery, whereas group 2 included those cases operated on in the period during which our surgical technique and indications for direct operations on aneurysms had become firmly established. All of the operations were performed by Suzuki.

[1] Division of Neurosurgery, Institute of Brain Diseases, Tohoku University School of Medicine, Sendai, Japan

Operative Techniques

The patient is placed in a supine position with the head immobilized facing forward and the jaw protruding slightly to facilitate an approach to the frontal lobes. A skin incision is made along the hairline of the forehead, four burr holes are drilled, and a bifrontal craniotomy is performed (Fig. 1). It is important to perform the craniotomy as close to the upper ridge of the orbita as possible. The frontal sinus is opened in most cases. The mucous membrane within the sinus is dissected and cauterized, and the internal lamina of the sinus is removed to decrease the dead space. The ostium communicating the nasal passage is closed with bone chips produced during craniotomy, and a small amount of bone wax is smeared firmly over the chips to completely block all communication with the nasal passage.

The dura is opened along the anterior bone edge as far forward as possible in order to minimize damage to the bridging veins. The falx cerebri is also cut as far forward as possible, and the severed end of the superior sagittal sinus is cauterized.

The olfactory tracts are dissected from the orbital surface of the frontal lobes bilaterally as far as the olfactory trigonal region. With this procedure, it is possible to preserve the olfactory tracts, and thus olfactory function, since traction will not be applied to the olfactory tract even if the frontal lobe is elevated during surgery [10]. After exposure of the internal carotid artery, the arachnoid membrane is opened over the base of the sylvian fissure, starting proximally. During removal of the subarachnoid blood clots, dissection is in a distal direction. Removal of the clots reduces brain volume, facilitating elevation of the frontal lobes and exposure of the A1 segments. It is important to expose both A1 segments initially because of the danger of premature aneurysm rupture.

The next step is to enter the interhemispheric fissure. At this stage the aneurysm is not ap-

Table 1. Aneurysm site and surgical results in 2000 patients (June 1961–June 1986, Tohoku University)

Site	No. of cases	Excellent	Good	Fair	Poor	Dead
ACoA	651	406	109	64	39	33 (5.1%)
ICA	455	286	78	35	32	24 (5.3%)
MCA	368	225	63	42	26	12 (3.3%)
ACA	86	61	7	6	8	4 (4.7%)
V-BA	68	32	13	7	10	6 (8.8%)
Multiple	372	188	83	43	24	34 (9.1%)
Total	2000	1198	353	197	139	113 (5.7%)

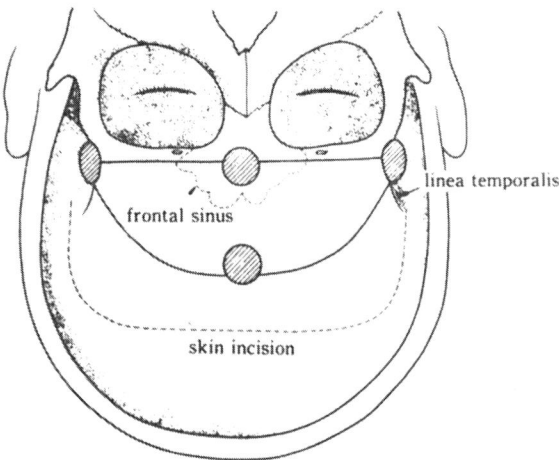

Fig. 1. Location of skin incision and craniotomy. The anterior edge of the bone flap is cut down frontally as close as possible to the orbital edge. *Shaded circles* represent burr holes

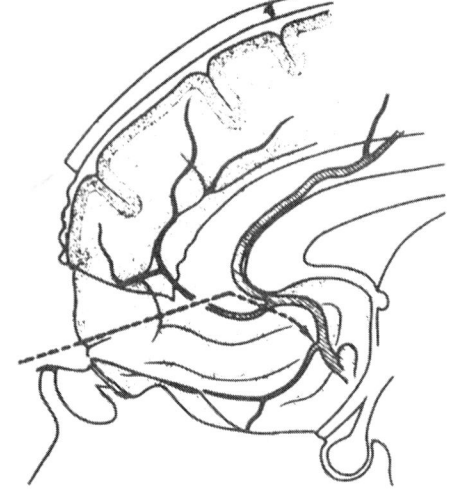

Fig. 2. Procedure for retrograde exposure of both A2 segments interhemispherically. At first, the distal A2 segments beneath the genu of the corpus callosum are approached, and then we proceed toward the AcoA complex. *Dotted line with arrow* indicates direction of approach

proached directly; instead, the distal A2 segments beneath the genu of the corpus callosum are approached in an "overhanging" manner (Fig. 2). In this way, both A2 segments are easily exposed, and blunt dissection is used from that point in proceeding toward the ACoA complex. Thus, damage to the medial surface of the cerebral hemisphere is minimized, the entire length of the A2 segment is exposed, and subsequent management of the aneurysm becomes easy.

If there is a danger of rupture as the aneurysm is approached following exposure of the A2 segments, a temporary clip should be placed on the dominant A1 segment. In the event of aneurysm rupture during dissection, application of temporary clips on the subdominant A1 and both A2

segments will allow treatment of the aneurysm in a bloodless field.

The aneurysm is then freed from the surrounding structures, and the aneurysm neck is exposed and ligated with 7–0 silk thread. The presence either of small arteries (such as the hypothalamic perforating vessels) behind the neck or of a fibrous adhesion sometimes make it possible to inadvertently produce kinking in feeding or draining vessels or to overlook the presence of a small aneurysm behind the larger one. Consequently, it is essential to completely dissect the aneurysm from all surrounding structures until it hangs loosely, thus allowing a direct view of the neck of the aneurysm during ligation. A clip is then placed on the ligated neck. If the clip were to

Table 2. Surgical results in 651 patients with anterior communicating artery aneurysms

Outcome	Group 1		Group 2		Total cases	
	No.	Percent	No.	Percent	No.	Percent
Excellent	197⎱	75.4	209⎱	83.3	406⎱	79.1
Good	64⎰		45⎰		109⎰	
Fair	39⎱	19.1	25⎱	12.1	64⎱	15.8
Poor	27⎰		12⎰		39⎰	
Dead	19	5.5	14	4.6	33	5.1
Total	346	100	305	100	651	100

Group 1: June 1961–September 1975
Group 2: October 1975–June 1986

Table 3. Preoperative grades and surgical results (June 1961–June 1986, Tohoku University)

Preoperative grade	Outcome					
	Excellent	Good	Fair	Poor	Dead	Total
0	7	4	0	0	1 (8.3%)	12
I	250	23	11	5	2 (0.7%)	291
Ia	6	9	5	2	1 (4.3%)	23
II	106	17	11	2	5 (3.5%)	141
III	36	50	28	16	18 (12.2%)	148
IV	1	6	9	14	6 (16.7%)	36
Total	406	109	64	39	33 (5.1%)	651

be applied at the outset, there is a danger of incomplete occlusion of the neck or of kinking or occlusion of the arteries. Therefore, it is advisable to clip the neck only after it has been ligated.

To prolong the permissible period of temporary vascular occlusion, we administer a combination of 20% mannitol (10 ml/kg), vitamin E (10 mg/kg), and phenytoin (10 mg/kg) by intravenous drip over 30–60 min [2]. Drug administration is timed so that it is completed just prior to application of the temporary clips. In the case of acute-stage surgery, it is also essential to institute continuous ventricular drainage and to remove as many subarachnoid clots as possible from the sylvian fissures and the interhemispheric fissure, as well as any intracerebral hematoma.

Operative Results

Surgical outcome was classified as follows: excellent (normal), good (minor neurological deficits, but normal social life possible), fair (neurological deficits, normal social life not possible),

poor (independent domestic life not possible), and dead.

Of the 651 patients in the total series, 406 (62.4%) were judged as having an excellent outcome at discharge, 109 (16.7%) as good, 64 (9.8%) as fair, 39 (6.0%) as poor, and 33 (5.1%) had died (Table 1). When group 2 is compared with group 1, it is seen that the mortality fell about 1% in group 2, and the number of patients capable of normal social lives (excellent and good outcome) rose about 8% in group 2 (Table 2).

The neurological condition of the patients at the time of operation was evaluated according to the classification of Hunt and Kosnick [1]. In the present series, there were 291 patients in grade 1, 141 patients in grade 2, 148 patients in grade 3 and 36 patients in grade 4. Ninety-four percent of grade 1 and 87% of grade 2 patients had an excellent or good outcome, while the mortality in these two grades was 0.7% and 3.5% respectively. Of the patients in grade 3, only 60% had an excellent or good outcome, and the mortality was as high as 12%. Six out of 36 patients who were in grade 4 died (16.7%; Table 3). The cause

Table 4. Surgical outcome in 101 cases operated on within 48 h after subarachnoid hemorrhage

Outcome	Group 1		Group 2		Total cases	
	No.	Percent	No.	Percent	No.	Percent
Excellent	5	25	48	59.3	53	52.5
Good	5	25	19	23.5	24	23.8
Fair	5	25	4	4.9	9	8.9
Poor	3	15	3	3.7	6	5.9
Dead	2	10	7	8.6	9	8.9
Total	20	100	81	100	101	100

Group 1: June 1961–September 1975
Group 2: October 1975–June 1986

of poor outcome in grade 3 and 4 patients was most commonly vasospasm. There was only one operative mortality in grade 0 patients. This case had a giant ACoA aneurysm; the A1 segment was buried in the aneurysm wall and was severed during resection of the wall. Hemorrhage was controlled by placing a silver clip on the A1 segment, but the patient died following a postoperative bleeding from the same site.

Among the 101 cases in groups 1 and 2 operated on within 48 hours following aneurysm rupture, nine (8.9%) died and 77 (76.3%) had an excellent or good outcome (Table 4). The mortality in group 2 was roughly the same as in group 1 (8.6% compared to 10%, respectively), but the percentage of patients experiencing a good or excellent outcome rose to 82.8% in group 2, indicating a notable improvement in the morbidity compared to group 1.

Discussion

The pterional approach is currently the most commonly used surgical procedure in cases of ACoA aneurysms [12]. However, this approach cannot be used without resection of the gyrus rectus when the aneurysm is located deep within the interhemispheric fissure, and particularly when it projects in a superior direction. Moreover, subarachnoid blood clots, which are the direct cause of postoperative vasospasm, not only are found in the basal cistern and interhemispheric fissure, but are also located bilaterally deep within the sylvian fissures. It is extremely difficult to remove clots from these regions when a unilateral pterional approach is used.

As a rule, it is important to dissect completely around the aneurysm before undertaking ob-

literation of the aneurysm neck. To insure safety, it is essential to prepare for the possibility of aneurysm rupture during surgery by identifying both the A1 and A2 segments bilaterally, which feed and drain the aneurysm, prior to dissection of the aneurysm itself. It is also essential to obtain a wide surgical field so that all the subarachnoid clots can be removed. We believe that these requirements are fulfilled by the interhemispheric approach in cases of ACoA aneurysms, and nearly all of our patients have been operated on using this approach.

The most unique feature of our surgical method is the use of temporary clips in nearly all cases. Particularly in early operations, when little time has elapsed since the original rupture, there is a possibility of rerupture during surgery. Therefore, we always apply temporary clips to the feeding and draining vessels prior to proceeding with treatment of the aneurysm. A key point in our surgical technique is that the aneurysm should be approached as follows: First, both A1 segments are identified by subfrontal approach. Next, the interhemispheric fissure is dissected, and both A2 segments are followed from the distal portion toward the ACoA complex. Before dissection of the aneurysm itself. temporary clips are placed on all four segments. If this is not possible, clipping of the dominant A1 segment should be performed at the very least. If the aneurysm should rupture during surgery, temporary clips can then be placed on the contralateral A1 and both A2 segments, thus allowing treatment of the aneurysm in a dry field.

It should be noted, however, that the use of temporary clips requires some measures for protecting the brain from ischemia. For this purpose, prior to 1971 we used moderate hypothermic anesthesia [5], and since then we have relied on the administration of mannitol. Our choice of this drug was based upon our experimental and clinical studies [7, 13, 14] which confirmed that mannitol has brain-protective effects. Since 1982, we have used a combination of mannitol, vitamin E, and steroids [3]. More recently, we administer a combination of 20% mannitol, vitamin E, and phenytoin. Using this method, we found that the permissible safety limit is a maximum of 40 min for occlusion of any combination of arteries within 100 min of drug administration. When more than 40 min of vascular occlusion is required, further occlusion can be performed following 5 min of recirculation.

With regard to the timing of surgery in cases of cerebral aneurysms, it has been believed for many years that surgical results are better if the operation is delayed 1 to 2 weeks after rupture. It was also recognized, however, that during the waiting period the condition of a considerable number of patients worsen or they die due to rerupture or vasospasm. To provide the most effective therapy for such patients, we advocated surgery as early as possible following rupture [6, 8], and we have been able to overcome virtually all of the problems entailed in early surgery. Details of the methods we use to resolve such problems have been reported elsewhere [4, 9, 11]. We believe that good therapeutic results can be obtained by means of ultra-early surgery (within 20 h, if possible), even in severe cases with ACoA aneurysms, provided that proper care is taken with regard to indication for surgery, choice of surgical technique, use of measures to prevent or supress vasospasm, and control of intracranial pressure. Use of ultra-early surgery results in fewer cases of deterioration or death during the waiting period, and a larger percentage of patients can be saved and returned to normal social lives.

References

1. Hunt WE, Kosnik EJ (1974) Timing and perioperative care in intracranial aneurysm surgery. Clin Neurosurg 21: 79–89
2. Suzuki J, Abiko H, Mizoi K, et al. (1987) Protective effect of phenytoin and its enhanced action by combined administration of mannitol and vitamin E in cerebral ischemia. Acta Neurochir 88: 56–64
3. Suzuki J, Fujimoto S, Mizoi K, et al. (1984) The protective effect of combined administration of anti-oxidants and perfluorochemicals on cerebral ischemia. Stroke 15: 672–679
4. Suzuki J, Kodama N, Yoshimoto T, et al. (1982) Ultra-early surgery of intracranial aneurysms. Acta Neurochir 63: 185–191
5. Suzuki J, Kwak R, Okudaira Y (1979) The safe time limit of temporary clamping of cerebral arteries in the direct surgical treatment of intracranial aneurysm under moderate hypothermia. Tohoku J Exp Med 127: 1–7
6. Suzuki J, Onuma T, Yoshimoto T (1979) Results of early operations on cerebral aneurysms. Surg Neurol 11: 407–412
7. Suzuki J, Yoshimoto T (1979) The effect of mannitol in prolongation of permissible occlusion time of cerebral artery: Clinical data of aneurysm surgery. Neurosurg Rev 1: 13–19
8. Suzuki J, Yoshimoto T (1978) Indication and timing in the surgery of ruptured cerebral aneurysm. Phronesis 36: 34–48
9. Suzuki J, Yoshimoto T, Kayama T (1984) Surgical treatment of middle cerebral artery aneurysms. J Neurosurg 61: 17–23
10. Suzuki J, Yoshimoto T, Mizoi K (1981) Preservation of the olfactory tract in bifrontal craniotomy for anterior communicating artery aneurysms, and the functional prognosis. J Neurosurg 54: 342–345
11. Suzuki J, Mizoi K, Yoshimoto T (1986) Bifrontal interhemispheric approach to aneurysms of the anterior communicating artery. J Neurosurg 64: 183–190
12. Yaşargil MG, Fox JL, Ray MW (1975) The operative approach to aneurysms of the anterior communicating artery. In: Krayenbihl H (ed) Advances and technical standards in neurosurgery, vol. 2. Springer, New York, pp 113–168
13. Yoshimoto T, Sakamoto T, Watanabe T, et al. (1978) Experimental cerebral infarction: III. Protective effect of mannitol in thalamic infarction in dogs. Stroke 9: 217–218
14. Yoshimoto T, Suzuki J (1979) Temporary clipping: Prolongation of the time of occlusion by mannitol. In Pia HW, Langmaid C, Zierski J (eds) Cerebral áneurysms. Springer, Berlin, pp 382–392

Discussion

Brock (Berlin): Like Prof. Lorenz, I think that with very few exceptions, premature ruptures are due to manipulation. In our last 100 cases of aneurysms of the anterior part, we had two premature ruptures. I had the opportunity today to see the interesting video tapes of Prof. Suzuki, and of the aneurysms he showed many ruptured probably due to the large exposure of the aneurysm and the manipulation of the vessels in order to clean the cisterns. This leads to the next subject—the use of temporary clips: If the aneurysm doesn't rupture temporary clips are not required. I would like the panel to comment on this.

Sengupta (Newcastle): The incidence of aneurysmal rupture during dissection is directly proportional to the experience of the surgeon, in my view. About 10–15 years ago, I experienced aneurysmal rupture during resection and at that time I used to depend on hypotension and took longer; with more experience, we use less hypotension and perform the resection faster and with a lower incidence of rupture. So I would say that if the surgeon does not perform many cases of this type, he should take more time and use more hypotension.

Brock: Could it also be due to technique, because Prof. Suzuki has extensive experience but still his patients develop ruptures intraoperatively?

Sengupta: Prof. Suzuki probably does not worry too much about ruptures; some surgeons feel that they should deliberately rupture the aneurysm to make sure that they have clipped or so they can apply the clip better. However, I feel that rupture of an aneurysm during surgery, particularly if you are not ready for it, is a thing to be avoided. It is better to have a clear field.

Guidetti (Rome): Personally, I think that with a well-prepeared vessel around the aneurysm rupture is not a problem: It is important to find precisely the neck of the aneurysm. If during the dissection the aneurysm ruptures, my opinion is that it is no problem whatsoever: Suction can be applied under the fundus of the aneurysm and the situation is easily resolved. However, if a rupture occurs before the vessels around the aneurysm have been prepared, this is a very bad situation.

Pásztor (Budapest): If the subarachnoid space is used with care there will be less incidence of premature rupture. If, however, premature rupture does occur we prefer suction and rarely use temporary occlusion. If all else fails we will resort to temporary occlusion.

Lorenz (Frankfurt): While fully agreeing with Drs. Sengupta and Pásztor I would add that in addition to experience the time elapsed between operation and hemorrhage is also a factor of importance. With an early operation the danger for rupture is higher than in an operation, say, 6 weeks after SAH.

Pásztor: That has not been our experience. We did not find a higher incidence of rupture with early operation. Early operation we take to mean within 48 h.

Brock: I would agree with that.

Yasui (Akita): I have only experienced two cases of premature rupture. Most ruptures occurred after approaching the aneurysm, at which time it is not so difficult to control bleeding: The blood can be removed by suction and the aneurysm body or dome can be clipped to stop the bleeding; the neck can then be dissected. Recently, I have preferred applying a body clip before a rupture can occur. It is easy to clip the neck. If a premature eruption does occur probably the best way of dealing with this is to open the dura and approach the aneurysm directly. In some cases, a temporary clip may be necessary, but I do not usually use a temporary clip for a parent artery.

Mizoi (Sendai): It should be stressed that we routinely use a temporary clip to prevent premature rupture of an aneurysm and to dissect the aneurysm neck completely and smoothly. We always apply a temporary clip before premature rupture, not after rupture.

Thomeer (Leiden): In my opinion, the chance of rupture of an aneurysm depends not only on the skill of the surgeon but also on the location of the aneurysm. I find that the anterior communicating and posterior communicating aneurysms are not cases of temporary clipping since if the neck only is dissected the chance of bleeding is small. On the other hand, with M1 and M2 aneurysms dissection of the whole fundus is necessary so as to ensure that none of the passing branches is clipped along with the aneurysm; in the latter case, I prefer to put a temporary clip on the neck for 1–2 min and then put a definite clip on the aneurysm.

Brock: With anterior communicating aneurysms, a little cortex can be sucked away, leaving the arachnoid on the sac. It's a gyrus rectus and really produces no symptoms. The aneurysm is attacked from behind. Leaving the arachnoid on the sac of course makes the sac stronger and not so liable to rupture. Prof. Lorenz, do you really feel it is necessary to remove the aneurysm? I sometimes puncture the aneurysm to empty it and be sure it is clipped. If the aneurysm has not been removed and the clip breaks the patient will develop an aneurysm again, but if the clip breaks and the aneurysm has been removed the patient will die.

Lorenz: It is not necessary to resect the aneurysm but I do it. In more than 350 cases, no new rupture occurred.

Giombini (Milan): Returning to premature rupture, it has been the experience of myself and others at my department that there is a difference between fissures and ruptures. Since the introduction of microsurgical techniques severe ruptures are no longer seen. Small fissures of the aneurysm are very well managed in our opinion without temporary clipping. I think it is very difficult to put a temporary clip on a parent vessel if a premature rupture has occurred. I would like some clarification on this from Prof. Sengupta; I see some difficulties in his approach

to the problem of premature rupture.

Brock: I think rupture is very rare; like Dr. Lorenz I have found that it is rather more frequent with operation in the acute phase not because the aneurysm is more fragile but because the brain is more swollen and greater force has to be applied. This difficulty can be circumvented by the use barbiturates, decreasing systolic pressure to about 70 mmHg, opening the cisterns, and if necessary applying a drainage. Occasionally, the operation has to be terminated and postponed. I think a temporary clip can be applied; it can be applied to the carotid near to the optic and to A1 as well as M1 with our approach. Though the problem then is in placing the final clip and removing the temporary one because there is little space; it takes more time but it can be done. How do the panel feel about the use of temporary clips?

Sengupta: As I said before, a temporary clip is very useful when the aneurysm looks as if it is about to burst under the tension or if the neck is difficult. With experience, the need to employ a temporary clip decreases, but I have no hesitation about using one if I feel there is danger of rupture. With the use of mannitol as introduced by Prof. Suzuki I feel that temporary clips can be applied longer.

Guidetti: Personally, I use them very very seldom. I think that today rupture of normal-size aneurysms is not really a problem. Problems only occur with timing and with giant aneurysms.

Pásztor: As I said before, we use temporary clips very rarely. Care should be taken not to put a clip on the neck but on the body of the aneurysm in a premature rupture. Then with a better field the attempt to put the clip on the neck can be made.

Brock: With regard to pericallosal aneurysms, when they are at the bifurcation between the pericallosal and callosomarginal I think an appraoch from the side of the aneurysm is essential since space will be required to separate the aneurysm from the bifurcation, otherwise it may be difficult to apply the clip.

Pásztor: Our experience with this contralateral approach is that the space obtained is exactly the same but that the approach to the neck and bifurcation is better. Premature rupture will perhaps be less frequent because the aneurysm need not be touched at all. The neck is approached from the opposite side and the surgeon tries to clip it. After the neck has been clipped, the three branches—pesicallosal, callosal marginal, and A2—can be examined to ensure that the clip is not on one of these arteries. This approach thus provides a better angle.

Lorenz: We only use temporary clips in exceptional cases—premature rupture.

Sengupta: I would like to comment on small craniotomies and the need for CSF drainage. With any manipulation, the brain is bound to swell up on the 2nd or 3rd postoperative day. So I always carry out a large craniotomy because of this swellings regardless of the cosmetic aspects; most of my patients are not too worried about the cosmetic appearance if they are alive and well. I leave the dura open in every case. When a check angiogram is performed, the bone flap of the craniotomy is seen to be quite high; later it falls back into place. So obviously the brain does swell and contract without this clinically being apparent. The large craniotomy is the one way in which the problem of vasospasm can be diminished, I believe, by overcoming the problem of raised intracranial pressure which invariably occurs after surgical intervention.

Lorenz: I must confess I do the contrary. I close the dura very carefully. In the past 2 years, I have used cisternal drainage more and more and I find that in the first few postoperative days it is beneficial for the patient; it makes for a smooth recovery.

Brock: I believe that the smaller craniotony is preferable; the brain is better protected. It has yet to be demonstrated that in a decompressive craniotomy leaving the dura open or removing the calvareum solves the problems of brain swelling and vasospasm. If the patient is kept under deep anesthesia for perhaps up to 2–3 days, recording the intracranial pressure, two things can happen: Either the pressure increases and the patient is lost or the pressure can be controlled and the prognosis is quite good. What we have not been able to show is that the intracranial pressure will stop increasing and the swelling be controlled by mechanical decompression; I think perhaps biochemical means should be used.

Commentator, *Svendgaard* (Lund): These lectures reflect the individualism characteristic of neurosurgeons. Each surgeon has his own approach to the same problem. Despite different techniques, each one achieves his goal. In fact, this session has demonstrated that the operative results with the techniques of today are so good that only minor improvements can be expected from technical advances.

Since the days of Prof. Lundberg, Lund has a tradition of intracranial pressure recording and ventricular CSF drainage. Personally, as a rule, I use CSF drainage in all patients with aneurysms in the midline, anterior communicating and basilar aneurysms. Due to the greater space achieved with drainage, less spatial pressure is required and in some cases it is not even necessary to resect the gyrus rectus. I also apply ventricular drainage very often in elderly patients with all kinds of aneurysms since they have a hard, inelastic brain and retraction easily causes edema, contusion, or hematoma. Using this technique, more multiple aneurysms can be operated at the same session. Via a bifrontal craniotomy, all anterior circulation aneurysms can be reached in one operation. To facilitate access to an aneurysm, I often strip off a vein 2–3 cm from the cortex. A routine procedure involves the use of tapered retractors with intermittent relief of the spatula pressure. Frequently, I apply a temporary clip on the aneurysm, 3–5 mm from the base, in order to facilitate the neck dissection and visualize parent arteries or perforators before applying the final clip. Concerning giant aneurysms in the sella region, because of the increased tendency for the development of spasm after surgery in that area, I have made it a rule not to remove and often not even to evacuate these aneurysms; they decrease in size spontaneously. The increased occurrence of spasm after operation of aneurysms close to the sella turcica may be elicited by manipulation of the hypothalamus. The results of my experimental work indicate that the median eminence is an effector organ in the genesis of spasm.

Finally, I would now like to draw attention to some of the problems of importance for the future. First, bringing the patients earlier to the neurosurgical unit and operating on grades I–III acutely in order to prevent rebleeding. Secondly, improving medical care for patients of grades IV and V. Thirdly, preventing late spasm or the effects of spasm.

With regard to the first point, during the last 10 years, we have received an increasing number of patients in the acute stage, as a result of lecturing at the district hospitals, writing letters to colleagues, and due to the fact that patients return to their local hospitals in good condition about 10 days after admission. Today, about 80% of the total number of operated patients are treated acutely; the rest are treated later, due either to patient or doctor delay.

Concerning the second point, greater knowledge of the pathophysiology is needed. Are the unsatisfactory results in groups IV and V due to primary or secondary brain damage? Does acute spasm occur in patients? What are the mechanisms behind the development of edema? In animal experiments, vasopressin has been found to be involved in the formation of edema in the acute stage. More research is needed in order to examine if vasopressin plays a similar role in humans. If that is the case, a vasopressin analogue may be useful in suppressing the secretion of vasopressin from the hypothalamus.

With reference to the third point, hypervolemia combined with hypertension is a good but demanding treatment. Calcium blockers may be of importance here. Future possibilities include, as far as I can see, investigations into fibrinolytic therapy or blockage of the neuronal pathways underlying vasospasm or suppression of certain hypothalamic functions.

RTD 7. Timing and Grading in Surgical Treatment for Aneurysm

Management of Supratentorial Saccular Aneurysms with Special Reference to the Timing and Results of Surgery

Series of 821 Cases

BERNARD PERTUISET[1], HIROTAKE NAKANO[2], MAENG KI CHO[3], and JEAN-PIERRE SICHEZ[1]

Recently, 821 workable records have been analyzed concerning patients admitted in la Pitié Hospital from 1 January 1972 to 1 January 1987 [10]. Operations were performed by a group of 5 neurosurgeons using the operating microscope, and aneurysmal necks were closed with Aesculap clips under a mean arterial pressure between 60 and 30 mmHg. We began to use CT scan in October 1977 and, at the same time, medicalized transportation of the patients was available day and night in the Paris area.

Three main groups have been considered (Table 1): group I—77 nonruptured aneurysms, group II—110 cases refused for surgery after rupture, and group III—634 ruptured cases cured by open surgery. Hunt and Hess clinical grading (I–V) was used.

Non Ruptured Aneurysms

Non ruptured aneurysms were divided into two groups: Aneurysms discovered by CT or angiography (61 cases) and those discovered in patients with neurological impairment from compression or repeated embolizations (16 cases). Of the aneurysms discovered by CT or angiography (61 cases), there were multiple aneurysms in 80% of the cases which were operated upon without mortality. Of the patients with aneurysms discovered due to neurological impairment from compression or repeated embolizations (16 cases), two died. One was a female of 68 years who had a giant aneurysm of the left middle cerebral artery giving recurrent episodes of hemiplegia and aphasia. She died of a pulmonary embolism two weeks after surgery. The other was a male of 47 years who had a compression of the right optic nerve by a carotid-ophtalmic aneurysm. The operation was difficult

after the intraoperative rupture of the sack and the patient died a week later from arterial vasospasm. We estimate that surgery of nonruptured aneurysms is indicated to prevent rupture, but the neurosurgeon must keep in mind that, for some patients, the risk of rupture must be balanced against the risk of surgery.

Ruptured Aneurysms Refused for Surgery

From 1972 to 1977 we refused surgery to 12 patients (of 231 admitted) with a mortality of eight (66.6%). From 1978 to 1986 98 patients (of 590 admitted) were refused surgery with a mortality of 78 (79.6%).

The increased number of patients refused for surgery after 1977 was the result of the day and night CT scan performance showing clearly the location and extension of cerebral hemorrhages. Therefore, refusal for surgery was based on the CT scan imagery, the clinical grading, the age of the patient, and the associated diseases.

Mortality happened in most of the cases during the first 3 days after admission, in spite of artificial ventilation and ventricular external drainage when the CT showed a ventricular hemorrhage. Regarding the 20 patients who survived, 60% did surprisingly well, and we estimate that our policy is better than early operation, which would leave patients in grade V costing too much to society and inducing family problems.

Operated Ruptured Aneurysms

Operated ruptured aneurysms can be divided into two groups: Those who were admitted after day 21 and could be considered as "cold lesions," necessitating, for a successful cure, a skilled neurosurgeon and modern facilities, and those who were admitted early during the 1st week after rupture, i.e., on day 1 or day 2.

---

[1] Clinique Neuro-chirurgicale de la Pitié, Paris, France
[2] University of Tokyo, Hongo, Tokyo, Japan
[3] University of Hallym, Hallym, Korea

Table 1. Selected mortality in a series of 821 saccular aneurysms

		No. of patients	Mortality	
			No.	Percent
Group I	Nonruptured aneurysms	77	2	2.5
Group II	Refused for operation	110	86	78.1
Group III	Operated ruptured aneurysms	634		
	Admitted before day 21	551		
	Clinical grades I, II, or III	485	40	8.2
	IV or V	66	32	48.4
	Admitted after day 21	83	0	0
Total		821		

We operated on 83 patients belonging to the first group without mortality (37 between 1972 and 1977; 46 between 1978 and 1986).

This is, for us, proof that the superb technique developed by Yasargil, and presented in 1969 to the International congress in New York, represented a giant step in the history of aneurysmal surgery.

There were 551 cases of the second group which were classified according to the clinical grading as follows: grades I–II–III, 485 cases; grades IV–V, 66 cases.

Most of the patients in grades IV and V had a cerebral hemorrhage, which explains a severe mortality of 32 (51.4%). Therefore, the most interesting group is the patients in grades I, II and III, the general mortality after surgery being 40 (8.2%); 47.5% of the deaths happened in ruptured aneurysms of the anterior communicating artery while 42% were provoked by arterial vasospasms.

Before giving our experience regarding timing of surgery, it will be of value to present our views with respect to the hemodynamic disorders occuring after rupture, and to the rebleeding problem.

Hemodynamic Disorders After Rupture

The rupture of an aneurysm induces a subarachnoid hemorrhage which will be at the origin of two hemodynamic disorders: brain swelling and arterial vasospasm.

Brain Swelling

Neurosurgeons who approach aneurysms during the first week after rupture have noticed a turgescence of the brain, the retraction of which is always difficult and sometimes impossible. From our experience, this brain swelling begins around 8 h after bleeding, is at its maximum on day 4, and has almost disappeared on day 8. Nevertheless, there are cases the brain swelling of which lasted 15 days.

The physiopathology of this brain swelling has been, for a long time, related to brain edema, but it was difficult to admit that dexamethasone alone was inefficient. More recently it was shown that such turgescence was due to disorders of the capacity for autoregulation of the brain arteries.

Voldby et al. [12] have monitored the cerebral blood flow after intravenous injection of Xe-133 in 11 patients between days 3 and 13. In all patients the cerebral blood flow (CBF) was under normal levels. Martin et al. [6] have evidenced the same phenomenon. Both authors have noticed a reduction of 30%–50% of the oxygen metabolism. In addition we have been able, with Ancri, to show a parallel increase of the blood volume using red cells taped with Tech 99 and a rotating gamma camera (ELSINT) [10].

It must be noted that Martin et al. [6] have observed such an increase of the blood volume parallel to a decrease of the blood flow in patients presenting a carotid stenosis. The increase of the blood volume suggest a reduction of the perfusion pressure, suggesting a dilatation of the small arteries and capillaries from a disorder of the arterial autoregulation mechanisms.

All these data are clearer in comatose patients. Figure 1 shows that the blood volume reflects the degree of the brain swelling. The increase of the blood volume provokes an elevation of the intracranial pressure as we have shown in 1981 [7]. Vold-by et al. [12] have recorded an intracranial pressure (ICP) between 10 mmHg and 20 mmHg in eight of eleven patients.

Is it possible to decrease during surgery the

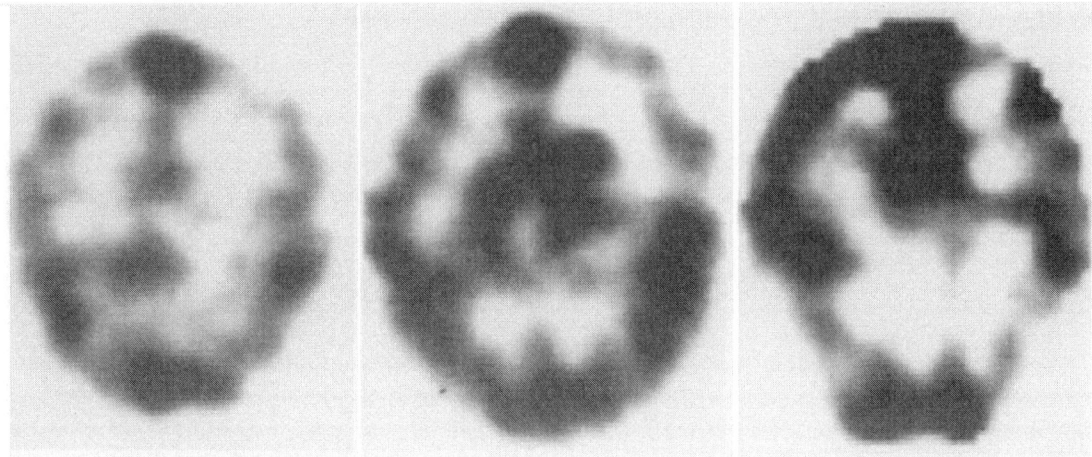

a, b   c

Fig. 1a–c. Variations of the blood volume after rupture of an anterior communicating artery aneurysm. **a** Day 20, grade II. **b** Day 25, grade IV, rebleeding. **c** Day 54, grade II, operation (rotating gamma-camera ELSINT)

brain swelling to facilitate the access to the base of the skull? The Sendai Cocktail, proposed by Suzuki et al. [11] (500 ml 20% mannitol, 300 mg vitamin E, and 30–50 mg dexamethasone) given as intravenous drip over 30–60 min can decrease the brain swelling.

We have used an infusion of Pentothal, associated or not with mannitol, and have been able to obtain enough reduction of the swelling to place a self-retaining retractor and, therefore, aspirate the CSF of the basal cisterns. This is not a comfortable situation, but it can help the surgeon pursue surgery. It must be noted that the same effect has been obtained on the brain swelling complicating radical surgery of arteriovenous malformations [7].

Arterial Vasospasm

Concerning arterial vasospasm, and looking back at the literature, there are factors which are known and others which are unknown.

Known factors. The arterial vasospasm which can provoke death occurs in ruptured aneurysms only. The presence of clots at the base of the brain is not the only factor to consider: there are deadly vasospasms in patients without clots at surgery, and around only 25% of the ruptured aneurysms gives a vasospasm. In addition vasospasm does not occur during the first 4 days after rupture.

There are families in which the vasospasm is especially frequent and there is reversibility of worse vasospasms [10].

Unknown factors. The intimate mechanism of the vasospasm remains unknown. When a vasospasm has been evidenced, it is not possible to predict its evolution: some will provoke death, some will provoke a hemiplegia, and some will keep the patient intact of neurological impairment.

Experience of la Pitié. In all of our patients, the diagnosis of vasospasm was obtained by comparing the angiogram on the day of admission to the angiogram on the eve of the operation. At first, preoperative vasospasm must be separated from postoperative ones.

Preoperative spasm. In 1985 [9], we found vasospasm in 60 cases among 265 patients (22.6%) at days 5 and 6. This percentage is close to Suzuki's, who, in 1973 observed 151 vasospasms in a series of 565 cases (26.7%).

In our present series [10] we observed 113 vasospasms (Table 2) in a series of 551 cases (20.5%). The mortality due to vasospasm was 33% between 1972–1977 and 13.9% between 1978–1986. This reduction of mortality came from our policy to postpone operation in patients with vasospasm.

The use of a calcium antagonist per os in 131 cases (1984–1986) was disappointing because we observed 26 vasospasms with a mortality of 23%. Moreover, it was clear that, in some patients, the day of vasospasm appearance was pushed from day 5 or 6 to day 9 or 10. Thus, the neurosurgeon was fooled into operating on a patient without vasospasm on day 6 but who was ready to develop one later on.

Table 2. Mortality of arterial vasospasms provoked by ruptured aneurysms

Years	Preop. vasospasm				Postop. vasospasm				Vasospasm in non-operated cases			
	No.	Percent	Dead	Percent	No.	Percent	Dead	Percent	No.	Percent	Dead	Percent
1972–1977	27/170	15.8	9/27	33	19/170	11.1	0	0	2/12	16.6	2/2	100
1978–1986	86/381	22	12/86	13.9	41/381	10.7	8/41	19.5	37/98	37.7	28/37	75.6
1984–1986 with nimo-dipin per os	26/131	19.8	6/26	23	18/131	13.7	2/18	11.1	10/16	62.5	7/10	70

According to our analysis, the preoperative vasospasm has been evidenced at a mean day of day 8 and, when the evolution was fatal, death appeared between days 12 and 20.

Postoperative vaso spasm. We observed postoperative vasospasm in 60 cases of 551 patients (10.9%) with a mortality of eight (13.3%) in our series. It is worthy to note that, between 1978–1986, mortality was 19.5%. It is our opinion that this increase was due to the use of a calcium antagonist which, per os, moved the day of appearance from day 6 to day 10. This is probably why, in 131 patients under nimodipin per os, we observed 19.8% of preoperative vasospasm with a mortality of 23% and 13.7% of postoperative vasospasm with a mortality of 11.1%.

Vaso spasm in nonoperated patients. It must be stressed that in nonoperated patients refused for surgery, mostly because of clinical grading and the presence of a hematoma, the percentage of vasospasm is higher: 27% with a terrific mortality of 87.8%. Nevertheless, in these cases, it was not always possible to be sure that death was due to the vasospasm.

In summary, vasospasm remains a dreadful complication of the aneurysmal rupture. Recently, Grotenhuis et al. [2] have opened the window of hope using a permanent infusion of nimodipin with an electrical syringe during a period of 14 days. This is certainly a better approach than the increased blood pressure with hypervolemia which has been very disappointing in our clinic after very early operations.

The severity of the vasospasm. Nowadays we do not have the capacity to predict if a vasospasm will be well endured or not by the patient. We tried the monitoring of somatosensory-evoked potentials and the topography of the vasospasm [9]: these two methods could not bring us a prediction before the clinical deterioration. We had the same results with an approach by ultrasonics and CBF.

There is no method with a 100% reliability. This is why, beginning on October 1977, we decided to postpone operation when a vasospasm was obvious on day 6 or 7 when compared with the angiogram at admission.

What we know is that when a vasospasm is located on the internal carotid artery (ICA) and its bifurcation, the prognosis is usually but not always poor (Table 3). It is the same when the striate arteries are not well injected or when a somatosensory-evoked potential cannot be evidenced (dislocated curve) [8, 9].

Timing of Surgery

It is necessary to consider the week of admission in the timing of surgery.

Admission during the 1st week. There are two policies. The first is ultra-early surgery (first 72 h). The advantage of this timing is the prevention of rebleeding. The disadvantage comes from the brain swelling which makes the operation difficult and thus increases the percentage of morbidity. In addition, it does not prevent vasospasm.

Ljunggren [5] has reduced mortality from 16% (1981) to 4% (1985), but in the same time, morbidity has increased from 10% to 20%: one of the causes is a difficult retraction of the brain. In our series, we decided only five times to operate during the first 72 h. All operations were difficult and one of the patients died from vasospasm while under per os nimodipin [8].

This policy of surgery from days 1 to 3 has been based upon two theoretical assumptions: At first the cisternal clots should be removed and the CSF should be drained to prevent vasospasm. We know now that the benefits of this procedure have not been proven.

The second assumption is that the main days of rebleeding are from days 1–7. We consider this view of Jane [3] Winn et al. [14], and Auer [1]

Table 3. Prediction of vasospasm mortality with respect to location: series of 60 cases of 265 (22%)

Localization of vasaspasm	Grading of spasm	No.	Mortality
ICA, ACA and MCA (33)	moderate 0.3	2	0
	severe <0.3	31 (93.9%)	13
ICA + ACA (13)	moderate 0.2	9	0
	severe <0.2	4	3
ACA + MCA (1)	moderate 0.2	1	0
	severe <0.2	0	0
ACA or MCA (9)	moderate 0.2	6	0
	severe <0.2	3	2
ICA (isolated) (2)	moderate 0.5	2	0
	severe <0.5	0	0
Pericallosal arteries (2)	moderate 0.2	0	0
	severe <0.2	2	2

Numbers in parentheses represent total number of patients in the group *ACA* anterior cerebral artery, *ICA* internal carotid artery, *MCA* middle cerebral artery

Table 4. Mean day of rebleeding from published series 15

Day 1	Between days 1 and 15	Between days 7 and 21
Winn (1982)	Hotta (1982) days 1 and 11	Gallhofer (1982) day 11
Auer (1985)	Sakurai (1979) days 1 and 8	Koos (1982) day 8
Jane (1977)	Nibbelink (1974) day 7	Pertuiset (1986) day 13
Jane (1985)		Locksley (1966) day 9
		Post (1977) day 9
		Aoyagi (1984) day 11
		Hudson (1968) day 7
		Fodstad (1982) day 12

as untrue. Table 4 reports the mean day of rebleeding in 15 published series. It is very clear that most of the authors have the experience of a rebleeding period timed between day 7 and day 21. We think that these views are probably based upon an incorrect estimation of day 1. It is correct that there are rebleedings on the day of admission, but it is probably already day 7–12. Waga [13], in 1975, and Leblanc [4] more recently have stressed the fact that there is often a fissuration before rupture, which, in fact, can be considered as a rebleeding.

Table 5 gives our experience regarding rebleeding which we have observed in 50 cases of 661 (7.5%). We have been very careful in evaluating day 1 and, in all cases, rebleeding has been proved by lumbar puncture or CT. It is very important to observe that, during the 1st week after rupture, the percentage of rebleeding has been 0.6% in grades I, II, and III patients and 3% in grades IV and V patients. Our second policy of surgical timing has been applied since 1977. We operate on patients after the decrease

of brain swelling and before the rebleeding period. In addition we postpone surgery when, on the eve of a scheduled operation, we observe a vasospasm on the angiogram. In other words, we operate at the end of the first week on days 7, 8, or 9. Table 6 gives the percentage of mortality with respect to this policy. Between 1978 and 1986 mortality has been 6.6% when operation was performed between day 7 and day 9. This has been the lowest mortality observed in our clinic.

Nevertheless, we advise a more early surgery in two instances: when the patient is hypertensive and cannot be controlled by clonidin, as well as when the patient has an intensive meningeal syndrome with permanent vomiting. In these cases, rebleeding can occur any time. During the waiting time before surgery, the patient is isolated in a room with music, if he likes, but without TV. He can have one visitor each day. He is given diazepam, Diphenylhydantoin, and clonidin when necessary. Since recently, we give a permanent infusion of nimodipin after stopping nimodipin per os.

Table 5. Rebleeding of 50 out of 661 ruptured aneurysms (7.5%)

	Grades I, II, and III		Grades IV and V		Nonoperated		Postop.		UnderVED		After A°	
Number	18/485	3.7%	8/66	12.1%	20/110	17%	1		1		2	
Mean day of rebleeding	day 15		day 12		day 13							
First week	3/485	0.6%	2/66	3%	4/110	0.3%						
Days 7–15	9/485	1.8%	3/66	4.5%	10/110	9%						
After day 15	6/485	1.2%	3/66	4.5%	6/110	5.4%						
Mortality 28/50 56%	3/18	8.5%	4/8	50%	17/30	85%	1	100%	1	100%	2	100%

VED ventricular external drainage, *A°* angiography

Table 6. Mortality percentage in 485 cases (grades I, II, and III) with respect to the timing of surgery

Days	1972–1977		1978–1986	
	No.	Mortality (%)	No.	Mortality (%)
Days 1–6	5/11	45.4	4/27	14.8
Days 7–9	3/40	7.5	11/165	6.6
Days 10–14	6/32	18.7	4/43	9.3
Days 15–21	3/44	6.8	4/49	8.0
After day 21	0/34	0	3/40	7.5
Total	17/161		26/324	

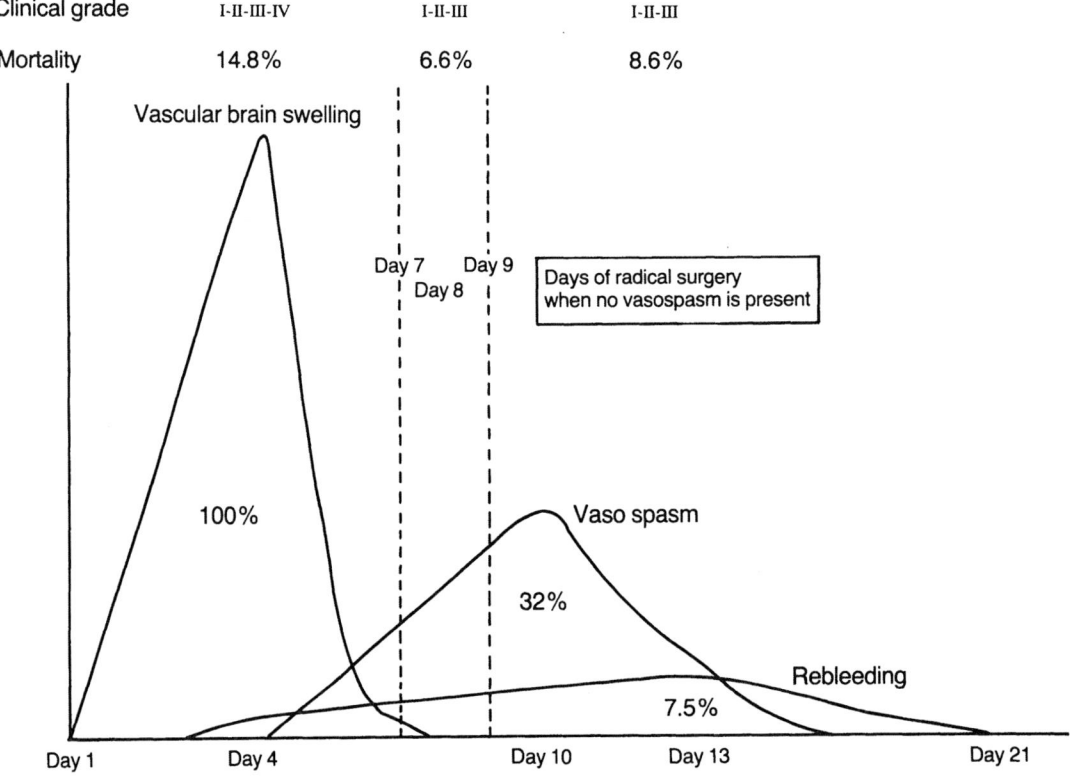

Fig. 2. Proposed timing of radical surgery in ruptured aneurysms

Operation is performed under induced hypotension, using neuroleptanalgesia and sodium nitroprusside when necessary, if, on the eve of operation, there is no vasospasm observed on the angiogram. We estimate that angiography could be replaced by ultrasonics in the future.

Admission during the 2nd week. Surgery must be performed as soon as possible because a rebleeding, the outcome of which is very serious, can occur any time. Nevertheless, the emergency must not drive the physicians to hasty surgery. The surgeon, the anesthetist, and the nurses must be skilled enough to give the patient the best chances to recover.

Admission during the 3rd week. Between days 14 and 18, the same policy must be followed. After day 18 we used to wait until day 21 or 22, when the operation is usually very easy without mortality and morbidity.

Conclusion

A saccular aneurysm is a benign lesion with a dreadful future. Once it has ruptured, hemodynamic disorders occur which we were not able to stop until now. Looking back at our experience [7–9], the staff estimates that the best time to operate a ruptured aneurysm is the end of the first week, i.e., days 7, 8 or 9. At this time, the brain swelling has disappeared or can be diminished by Pentothal and mannitol, the rebleeding period begins, and, if a vasospasm occurs, it can be evidenced by the angiogram on the eve of scheduled surgery (Fig. 2). This timing reduces morbidity to 4%.

In this series we never used antifibrinolytic therapy, which increases the percentage of ischemia and hydrocephalus.

References

1. Auer LM, Papaefthymiou G, Trittar T (1985) Early transportation organization of diagnosis and operation at the acute stage. In: Auer LM (ed) Timing of Aneurysm Surgery. Gruyter, Berlin, pp 635–640
2. Grotenhuis JA, Bettag W (1986) Prevention of symptomatic vasospasm after SAH by constant venous infusion of nimodipine. Neurol Res 8: 243–249
3. Jane JA, Kassel NF, Torner JC, Winn HR (1985) The natural history of aneurysms and arteriovenous malformation. J Neurosurg 62:321–323
4. Leblanc R (1987) The minor leak preceding subarachnoid hemorrhage. J Neurosurg 66:35–39
5. Lunggren B, Saveland H, Brandt L, Sygmunt S (1985) Early operation and overall outcome in aneurysmal subarachnoid hemorrhage. J Neurosurg 62:547–551
6. Martin WRN, Baker RP, Grubb RL, Raichle ME (1984) Cerebral blood volume, blood flow and oxygen metabolism in cerebral ischemia and subarachnoid hemorrhage: An in vivo study using positron emission tomography. Acta Neurochir 70:3–9
7. Pertuiset B, Ancri D, Lienhart A (1981) Profound arterial hypotension (MAP $\leqslant$ 50 mmHg) induced with neuroleptanalgesia and sodium nitroprusside (series of 531 cases): Reference to vascular autoregulation mechanism and surgery of vasculr malformations of the brain. In: Advances and technical standard in neurosurgery. Springer Berlin Heidelberg New York, pp 75–122
8. Pertuiset B, Sichez JP, Sermet A, Nakano H (1985) Ruptured supratentorial aneurysms (series of 143 cases operated by 5 neurosurgeons). In: Auer LM (ed) Timing of aneurysm surgery. Gruyter, Berlin, pp 217–226
9. Pertuiset B, Sichez JP, Lille F, Hazeman P, Nakano H, Chaumier E (1985) Evaluation and prediction of the vasospasm severity following a ruptured supratentorial aneurysm from angiography, clinical grade and somatosensory-evoked potentials. In: Auer LM (ed) Timing of aneurysm surgery. Gruyter, Berlin, pp 421–428
10. Pertuiset B, Sichez JP, Arthuis F (1987) Traitement chirurgical des anévrysmes artériels sacculaires supra-clinoidiens admis dans les trois semaines suivant la rupture. Neurochirurgie 33: (Suppl 1) 106
11. Suzuki J, Mizoi K, Yoshimoto T (1986) Bifrontal interhemispheric approach to aneurysms of the anterior communicating artery. J Neurosurg 64: 183–190
12. Voldby B, Enevoldsen E, Jensen FT (1985) Cerebrovascular reactivity in patients with ruptured intracranial aneurysms. J Neurosurg 62:59–67
13. Waga S, Ohtsubo K, Handa H (1975) Warning signs in intracranial aneurysms. Surg Neurol 3: 15–20
14. Winn HR, Richardson AE, Jane JA (1982) The late morbidity and mortality in ruptured single anterior circulation aneurysm treated by nonsurgical therapy. Acta Neurochir 63:71–81

Indications and Timing of Surgery on Ruptured Intracranial Aneurysms

RAM P. SENGUPTA[1]

Direct surgical obliteration of a ruptured intracranial aneurysm without the associated problem of subarachnoid hemorrhage (SAH) can be achieved with less than 2% mortality and 5% morbidity. This excellent progress, however, does not take into account two major aspects in the management of patients with SAH. First, a significant number of patients suffer secondary deterioration and never come to surgery. The outcome of these patients, when added to the surgical outcome, the management mortality, and morbidity, is still appalling. Second, and in my view more significantly, treatment of a patient with SAH over the last three decades has been identified with the control of the ruptured aneurysm, but treatment of the disease itself was largely ignored. This was primarily due to the fact that pathological changes associated with SAH were unrecognised and the method of identifying them with investigation, such as angiography, was itself harmful in a severely ill patient. With the introduction of the CT scan, Doppler ultra-sound, MRI and PET scan, it is now possible to assess the living pathology of SAH and specific treatment can be instituted. There is yet another challenge, not altogether at the control of the neurosurgeons, which awaits us for the future. As early as 1956, Walton [10] in Newcastle showed that one-third of these patients die from initial bleeding. This occurs even today. There is clear evidence from the study by Kassell and Drake [3] that two-thirds of these are due to ignored warning signs, misdiagnoses or late referral. An educational program illuminating the perils of SAH can aim to conquer the natural history of SAH from ruptured aneurysm.

In this communication, the author contends that the management mortality can be significant reduced, and the means of this reduction is discussed.

In the management of a patient with SAH, obliteration of the ruptured aneurysm is the dominant feature, since this is the most certain way of preventing rebleeding. Therefore, it is logical that the ealier a ruptured aneurysm is clipped, the less chance there is of rebleeding. In practice, however, indiscriminate surgical attempts on an aneurysm, without the understanding of the pathological process, produces a poor surgical result. On the other hand, when the storm of the SAH has subsided after the 1st week, the surgical outcome will be excellent, but a considerable number will suffer not only from recurrent bleeding but from the wrath of the initial bleeding. This dilemma can be resolved if we address the problem in aother way; by analysing each individual patient at the very moment he comes to the care of the neurosurgeon. Ideally, this should be on day zero, but more often than not, due to rarity of the condition and the system of referral, patients are brought to the neurosurgeon at varying time intervals. In Newcastle, we are able to admit only 10% of our patients within the first 3 days. Because of this, our instructions to the receiving hospitals are to refer the patient as quickly as possible, or to administer antifibrinolytic therapy as soon as a diagnosis of SAH is suspected.

Although we are probably in the minority in this regard, we believe that the place of antifibrinolytic therapy has been misguided. It has been shown by various studies that, while antfibrinolytic therapy reduces rebleeding, its benefit is offset by ischemic problems associated with this therapy. It must be appreciated that ischemic problems noted in these studies occurred when the drug had been used for at least 1 week or more. There is no study to suggest that these problems occur if the drug is used for less than 1 week. On the other hand, our own studies have convinced us that ischemic problems following SAH will occur if the patients, even in a favourable condition, are left unoperated. In a group of 76 patients who were treated medically

---

[1] Newcastle General Hospital, Newcastle upon Tyne, England

for 2 weeks without antifibrinolytic therapy, 31 patients were unsuitable for surgery, and eight of these suffered ischemic damage [8]. Allen et al. [1], in a controlled double-blind trial with nimodipine, treated 60 patients with placebo for 3 weeks. Of these, eight developed ischemic complications. In our view, ischemic sequelae of unoperated SAH has been unfairly credited to the antifibrinolytic therapy. Indications for aneurysm surgery and its timing will depend on several factors.

Initial Assessment

Clinical evaluation of the patient. Although this is essential for detecting progress or deterioration, it does not always indicate the suitability of surgery or the type of surgery suitable for the patient.

Pathological study of the brain with CT scan. Management depends largely on its findings in conjunction with the clinical condition of the patient. CT scan carried out within 5 days after SAH will show the following:
a) Evidence of mild or modest SAH without effect on the brain
b) Massive SAH
c) Massive ventricular hemorrhage
d) Significant hematoma with midline shift
e) Dilated ventricle with obstruction of CSF pathway
f) Swollen brain with squashed ventricle

Management According to CT Findings

Evidence of mild or modest SAH indicates immediate four-vessel angiography. A massive hemorrhage, if clinically favourable, will indicate a four vessel angiography. If the hemorrhage is clinically unfavourable, medical therapy should be performed. In cases of ventricular hemorrhage, ventricular lavage and external ventricular drain should be performed. When there is a significant hematoma with midline shift, limited angiography and evacuation of the hematoma with or without clipping of the aneurysm is indicated.

Dilated ventricle with CSF pathway obstruction indicates angiography with or without prior ventricular drain. In cases of swollen brain with squashed ventricle, if conditions are clinically favourable, angiography should be done. In clinically unfavourable cases medical therapy should

be performed.

The condition of those who require specific treatment before angiography is assessed daily to decide the timing of angiography.

Clinical Evaluation After Angiography

A small number of patients will suffer from this procedure. In most of the cases, however, immediate consideration can be given for definitive surgery. Definitive surgery on the ruptured aneurysm is based on several factors, and these are discussed in order of their importance [9].

Clinical condition. Clinical assessment is an essential step in the consideration of aneurysm surgery. Various grading systems have been advocated to classify the clinical status of the patient. This is not only useful to identify the changing status of the clinical pattern, but it helps to study the outcome. We follow a modified Hunt and Hess system of grading. However, it has been shown that there is a considerable amount of observer variability [4] and, more significantly, it does not always reflect the exact nature of pathology. For example, a patient may be obtunded from CSF pathway obstruction or from brain swelling. In both events there will be rise of CSF pressure. Whereas aneurysm surgery in the former is rewarding, it is harmful in the latter. Moreover, a patient with fixed neurological deficit may have recovered from the fire of SAH and can be subjected to aneurysm surgery without additional damage. Similarly, when patients are improving to a favourable grade, for example, from grade III to grade II, they suffer no harm from aneurysm surgery. On the other hand, on patients in grade II deteriorating to grade III, surgery will push them further down, or even to death. Therefore, the idea of aneurysm surgery on a definite grading system is not entirely satisfactory. It is the alertness of the patient and the improving slope of alertness which are essential in the determining of the suitability of surgery. In practice, grades I and II patients, stable grade III patients, and improving grades IV or V patients can be operated upon for obliteration of the aneurysm.

Anomalies of the circle of Willis. Anomalies of the circle of Willis are more common with intracranial aneurysms. These anomalies alter the area of supply of the major cerebral arteries and the collateral circulation is compromised. The surgical result is significantly affected in patients with vascular anomalies [7] The timing of surgery and method of treatment are influenced by these anomalies. These factors are not generally appreciated but, in my experience, they are potent factors in the propagation of ischemia from vasospasm.

Preoperative evaluation of vascular anatomy, minimal surgical manipulation, and the experience of the surgeon. In the early period of SAH, the worst period usually being the 3rd to 7th day, the brain is vulnerable to manipulation, and the exposure of too many vessels is likely to induce or propagate vasospasm. Vascular anatomy should be studied in the preoperative angiogram and surgical exposure should be limited to the neck of the aneurysm and its related vessels only. It is not the clipping of the aneurysm which is at stake; it is preventing or controlling its aftereffects. Here comes the experience in aneurysm surgery. A surgeon who is managing one aneurysm a week is likely to have a better overall result than one who sees an aneurysm once a month or less. Experience would also dictate what type of surgery, such as clipping or proximal ligation with bypass shunt, would be the most appropriate for a particular aneurysm, or even whether it would be best left alone. In this respect, it is significant to add that some rare aneurysms, such as a basilar aneurysm, are better served by pooling them into one regional centre where the cumulative experience of the surgical team would approach the aneurysm with much more confidence, resulting in a better outcome.

Neuroanesthesia. It is not sufficiently appreciated that progress in aneurysm surgery has come about with the improvement of neuroanesthesia. Unless the anesthesiologist understands the pathophysiological changes in the brain, associated with the induction of anesthesia, elective hypotension, unrecognised dehydration, and cerebral metabolism, the outcome of surgery will be adversely affected. There is a usual tendency for a drop in blood pressure during induction. This sudden drop in blood pressure is extremely harmful to the brain whose autoregulation has already been disturbed by the SAH. Similarly, sudden lowering of blood pressure during elective hypotension is harmful. The blood pressure should be lowered in a stepwise fashion so that the brain can adjust its cerebral perfusion. Brain swelling in an uncomplicated SAH during operation is often due to poor anesthesia.

Age. There is no doubt that, with advancing age, the cardiovascular and respiratory reserves diminish, and a formidable surgical undertaking and prolonged anesthesia impose greater risks. The benefit of surgery in such patients should be balanced against not only the natural history of the aneurysm, but also the increased probability of death from an unrelated illness. The effect of vasospasm is negligible before the age of 30, and the result of surgery between the ages of 30 and 65 is similar [9]. After that age, a certain restraint is necessary.

Associated medical illness. Like advancing age, associated chronic illness, such as hypertension, myocardial ischemia, and respiratory disease, imposes a greater burden. Provided special care is taken, there is no contraindication for surgery. In fact, early surgery is preferable on hypertensive patients.

Location and size of the aneurysm. These have considerable bearing on the technical aspects of surgery. For a difficult aneurysm in the basilar artery, or a giant aneurysm, manipulation of brain and blood vessels may be considerable. The timing of operation should be when the condition of the brain is favorable.

Angiographic vasospasm. If vasospasm causes a reduction in cerebral perfusion resulting in ischemia, the clinical condition is affected. Otherwise, it can be assumed that the area of the brain related to the spastic vessel has received sufficient collateral circulation to maintain its function. Surgery on a patient who is clinically in a favorable condition is not contraindicated on the basis of angiographic vasospasm alone.

Timing of Surgery

The timing of surgical treatment for a ruptured aneurysm is the most important consideration a neurosurgeon has to make in his surgical practice. To prevent recurrent hemorrhage, surgeons in the 1950s advocated early surgical obliteration of the aneurysm without appreciating the pathological changes which occur within the brain. However, it soon became obvious that the outcome of surgical treatment was far worse than no surgical treatment at all. Norlen and Barnum [5] obtained good results by delaying surgery for 2–3 weeks. As the natural history of aneurysms became apparent, surgery was advocated in the 2nd week before the period of highest rebleeding. During this waiting period, some patients will suffer recurrent hemorrhage and some others will continue to deteriorate from the effect

Table 1. Type of aneurysm versus outcome

Outcome	PComm	Other ICA	AComm	Other ACA	MCA	BV	Total
Good	126	78	166	16	104	21	511
Fair	24	24	42	1	33	11	135
Poor	6	3	5	—	1	2	17
Dead	10	6	8	4	6	6	40
	166	111	221	21	144	40	703

PComm posterior communicating artery, *ICA* internal carotid artery, *AComm* anterior communicating artery, *ACA* anterior cerebral artery, *MCA* middle cerebral artery, *BV* basilovertebral artery

Table 2. Age v. outcome

Age (years)	Good	Fair	Poor	Dead	Total
Below 30	80	9	—	—	89
30–59	381	103	14	32 (6%)	530
60 plus	50	23	3	8 (9.5%)	84

Table 3. Time of surgery v. outcome

Days	Good	Fair	Poor	Dead	Total
<4	72	21	—	5	98
5–7	116	19	5	6	146
8–11	115	28	2	12	157
12–14	52	8	4	7	71
15–18	37	13	2	1	53
19–21	14	3	2	1	20
21>	105	43	2	8	158

of the initial bleeding. Sano and Saito [6] advocated early surgery with the provision that it be avoided between the 5th and 8th days. Hori and Suzuki [2] advocated surgery within the first few hours if possible, and certainly within the first 3 days. They believe that the development of vasospasm may be prevented by removing blood clots from the subarachnoid cistern and around the major vessels at operation. From my own experience over the last 16 years, with personal series of over 800 aneurysms, I came to the view that a rigid timing of aneurysm surgery is unhelpful. Each patient must be judged individually, and a decision made as to when he is ready for definitive surgery. I shared the views of my Japanese colleagues that, in a large proportion of patients, aneurysmal obliteration can be achieved safely within the first few days before secondary changes occur within the brain. Moreover, I take the view that by early surgery some of the ill effects of SAH, particularly vasospasm, can be prevented. We do not know the initiating factor of vasospasm, but I believe that one of the most significant propagating factors is raised intracranial pressure. If this is controlled by early surgery, the ill effects of vasospasm can be prevented. There is no doubt that the amount and distribution of blood clots in the basal cistern have some bearing on the initiation of vasospasm, and that early surgery can remove the blood clots, but how effective this step is remains

Table 4. Condition at discharge versus follow-up (1970–1985)

At discharge	Total	At follow-up			
		Good	Fair	Poor	Lost/dead
Good	511	484	5	1	21
Fair	135	62	62	1	10
Poor	17		3	8	6
Dead	40				(40)
Total	703	546	70	10	37 (40)

to be judged. Although the earliest possible aneurysmal obliteration after SAH in the majority of patients is helpful, in practice it is not always possible to get them so early. Even then, definitive surgery is possible within the 1st week if other factors are favorable.

Results

With this philosophy, the author has operated upon 800 ruptured intracranial aneurysms since 1970. Unfortunately, he is unable to analyse all the patients with SAH during this period for serveral reasons. Some patients in grades 4 or 5 are not referred, and the system of medical practice is such that there is delay in referral to neurosurgery. Hence, some patients must have re-bleeding before being referred. Within these restrictions, however, the author has lost very few patients before surgery once they have been admitted, and these unoperated patients are now being analysed. Tables 1–4 analyse the outcome in the first 703 patients with intracranial aneurysm during the period 1970–1985.

Conclusion

The management outcome in patients with SAH can be improved by active intervention at the earliest opportunity. In a large number of patients, early surgery on aneurysm is not only possible but can help prevent secondary deterioration. In those who are deteriorating from an ischemicly swollen brain, additional manipulation is not only harmful but also unnecessary, as recurrent bleeding in this group of patients is uncommon.

References

1. Allen GS, Batty ER, Boone S, Chou S, Kelly D, Weir B (1982) Preliminary results of multicentral double-blind prospective study of Nimodipine in the prevention of delayed neurological deterioration from cerebral arterial spasm. Proceedings of the Congress of Neurological Surgery, Toronto, p 98
2. Hori S, Suzuki J (1979) Early intracranial operations for ruptured aneurysms. Acta Neurochir 46: 93–104
3. Kassell NF, Drake CG (1983) Review of the management of saccular aneurysms. Neurol Clin (1): 73–86
4. Lindsay KW, Teasdale GM, Murray L, Knill-Jones R (1980) Observer variability in grading patients with subarachnoid haemorrhage. Proceedings of the Autumn Meeting of the Society of British Neurological Surgeons, pp 61–67
5. Norlen G, Barnum AS (1953) Surgical treatment of aneurysms of the anterior communicating artery. J Neurosurg 10: 634–650
6. Sano K, Saito I (1978) Timing and indication of surgery for ruptured intracranial aneurysm with regard to cerebral vasospasm. Acta Neurochir 41: 49–60
7. Sengupta RP (1975) Anatomical variations in the origin of the posterior cerebral artery demonstrated by carotid angiography and their significance in the direct surgical treatment of posterior communicating aneurysms. Neurochirurgia 18: 32–42
8. Sengupta RP, So SC, Villare jo-Ortega FJ (1976) Use of epsilon aminocaproic acid (EACA) in the preoperative management of ruptured intracranial aneurysms. J Neurosurg 44: 479–484
9. Sengupta RP, McAllister VL (1986) Subarachnoid hemorrhage. Springer, Berlin, pp 193–196
10. Walton JN (1956) Subarachnoid hemorrhage. Livingstone, Edinburgh

Management of Patients with Ruptured Cerebral Aneurysms

Some Considerations from Recent Experience

LUDWIG M. AUER

Introduction

As the recent international cooperative aneurysm study again shows the old problems of aneurysm surgery are the same as the present problems. Who should be operated upon? Who should be operated upon early and who should undergo delayed operation? Is rebleeding really a significant problem influencing prognosis and, hence, worth consideration in the timing of surgery? Does early rebleeding really exist and thus justify acute management of patients after subarachnoid bleeding? Is delayed ischemia from vasospasm really a significant problem or are these patients a hidden pool of surgical complications?

The results of the international cooperative study have indeed shown that both rebleeding and vasospasm are still significant problems despite early surgery. Recently, besides surgical prevention of vasospasm by early evacuation of subarachnoid blood, calcium antagonists of the dihydropyridine group have been used to prevent vasospasm and improve overall outcome. Presently, the question being asked is whether calcium antagonist treatment is an achievement or just another drug therapy for drug therapy believers. This paper aims at an overview of a variety of studies and an outlook for our decisionmaking in the future.

Does early Surgery Influence the Incidence of Preoperative Rebleeding?

Since the beginning of 1982, our department has made considerable efforts to admit and operate early on patients with subarachnoid hemorrhage (SAH) from ruptured cerebral aneurysms. For the 224 patients who were admitted to hospitals

Department of Neurosurgery, University Hospital, Graz, Austria

and were diagnosed as having subarachnoid hemorrhage until the end of 1986, we were successful in 70% of cases. A total of 159 patients were transferred to neurosurgery within the first 24–28 h; of these, 75% arrived within the first 24 h.

Among the early referrals, rebleeding before operation occurred in 18 (11%). The detailed circumstances are shown in Table 1.

Among the 64 patients admitted during the same period of time but too late for early surgery, preoperative rebleeding occurred in 25%; six patients died from rebleeding and ten were operated after this rebleeding.

These present data indicate that rebleeding is still a significant problem, not only when a delayed surgical procedure is considered, but also for patients who are considered for early neurosurgical repair. In accordance with the results of the international cooperative aneurysm study, our results indicate that rebleeding within the first 48 h is frequent and therefore justifies acute management of patients with SAH on a non-emergency basis: All diagnostic and therapeutic steps should be performed as early as possible, but without hurry, by an experienced team.

Table 1. Preoperative rebleeding in 18 patients planned for early aneurysm operation

Rebleeding	No. of patients
Dead from preoperative rebleeding	5
Rebleeding during early phase of operation, clipping impossible	2
Operated upon after preoperative rebleeding	
In peripheral hospital before transport	2
During transport	3
During angiography	4
During induction of anesthesia	2
Total	18 (11% of 159 patients)

Vasospasm Despite Early Surgery: Are Calcium Antagonists of Help?

Despite early surgery and evacuation of subarachnoid blood, the incidence of delayed ischemic neurological deficit from vasospasm has remained more or less the same. In recent analyses of different groups of patients, this complication still occurs in around 30% of the cases [7, 8, 10, 12, 14–16]. Following a variety of experimental studies on the effect of the dihydropyridine calcium antagonist nimodipine [3, 6], this latest effort to prevent ischemic symptoms from vasospasm has been carried into clinical neurosurgery. While Allen [1] carried out a controlled multicenter study of peroral treatment with nimodipine and showed a significant reduction in the incidence of symptomatic vasospasm, the first pilot studies in Europe showed a marked reduction of symptomatic vasospasm in only a small percentage using intravenous preventive treatment combined with initial cisternal treatment [2]. In addition, a European open multicenter trial on intravenous nimodipine resulted in 2% incidence of symptomatic vasospasm [5].

Since the beginning of 1982, a protocol of early surgery and intracisternal as well as intravenous nimodipine [2] was used on our consecutive series of 150 patients: their preoperative Hunt-Hess grades are indicated on Table 2. Among these patients, delayed ischemic symptoms developed in four and were reversible in two, and irreversible in two, with significant neurological deficit.

Do these open studies really show a lower incidence of delayed ischemic symptoms from vasospasm due to treatment with nimodipine, or due to the transfer of more patients into the category of surgical complication instead of the category of complication due to vasospasm because of a thorough analysis of the postoperative course in early operated patients? The answer from recent controlled studies of preventive nimodipine treatment is that nimodipine does in fact lead to a significant reduction of poor outcome from symptomatic vasopasm [11, 13].

Among our 64 patients admitted too late for early surgery who received the regimen of intravenous nimodipine treatment and were operated at various periods of time after SAH the incidence of symptomatic vasospasm with unfavorable outcome was 7%.

Prognosis After Early Surgery and Preventive Nimodipine

Delayed ischemic symptoms from vasospasm were the cause of unfavorable outcome in only one of the 150 patients (Table 3). The analysis of unfavorable outcomes after early surgery and preventive nimodipine treatment thus shows that vasospasm ranks among the rare complications, while the initial event of the hemorrhage is the most frequent cause of poor outcome (15% in the whole series, 65% among all patients with unfavorable outcome). Surgical complication ranks second among the causes of unfavorable outcome with 8% in the whole series and 32% among all unfavorable outcomes. Table 4 details the complications during operation in these 12 patients.

Table 3. Early aneurysm surgery 1982–1986: causes of unfavorable outcome

	Number	Percent
Initial hemorrhage	24	65
Surgical complication	12	32
Delayed ischemic symptoms, irreversible	1	3
Total	37	100

Patients were considered as having an unfavorable outcome when they had moderate or worse neurological deficits were dead at 6 months after operation

Table 2. Early aneurysm surgery 1982–1986

Hunt-Hess grade	No. of patients
I	34
II	36
III	39
IV	24
V	17
Total	150

Table 4. Early aneurysm surgery 1982–1986: surgical complication and unfavorable outcome

Complication	No. of patients
Hemorrhagic infarction (spatula pressure)	1
Premature rupture, hemorrhage	4
Brain swelling, brain resection	4
Occlusion of major arterial branch	2
Unidentified	1
Total	12

Table 5. Causes of unfavorable outcome in patients operated early and late

Cause of unfavorable outcome	Timing of operation	
	Early (%)	Late (%)
Preoperative rebleeding	11	25
Vasospasm	0.7	7

Table 6. Aneurysm surgery 1982–1986: early versus late

6-Month outcome	Preoperative Hunt-Hess grade		
	I–II	III–IV	V
Good	91 (76)	75 (30)	12 (0)
Poor	6 (9)	8 (40)	12 (33)
Dead	3 (15)	17 (30)	76 (67)

The numbers indicate percentages of patients in Hunt-Hess grades I–II, III–IV and grade V. Numbers in *parentheses* indicate patients with late operation

Causes of Unfavorable Outcome After Early Versus Late Surgery

In the early operated group, the rate of unsatisfactory outcomes (moderate deficit or more) among the patients in preoperative Hunt-Hess grades I–III was 9%, all caused by surgical complications. In the group of delayed operation, unsatisfactory outcomes occurred in 40% of patients in Hunt-Hess grades I0III.

Among patients in preoperative Hunt-Hess grade IV, unsatisfactory outcome after early surgery occurred in 50%, while it occurred in 62% of patients in the late operation group. The rate of preoperative rebleeding was 11% before early and 25% before late operation. Unfavorable outcome from vasospasm occurred in 0.7% of early operated patients versus 7% in patients in the delayed operation group (Table 5). Patients in preoperative grades III or IV are especially better after early surgery, with a good outcome rate of 75%, versus 30% in patients operated late (Table 6).

A View into Epidemiology: Are We Improving Overall Outcome in a Referral Area?

Analysing all reports of SAH which occurred between the years 1981–1985 in our referral area (Harusch and Auer, unpublished data), 291 events of SAH were detected. Data were collected in cooperation with all peripheral hospitals and by studying all protocols of post-mortem examinations in the whole referral area. Figure 1 analyses the course of the disease: 9% of patients did not even reach a hospital, but died from the primary event of fatal SAH. Forty additional patients, among those who were admitted to a hospital, died for various reasons before they were operated (Table 7).

About 50% of preoperative mortality appears avoidable when considering the high number of undiagnosed cases who died from rebleeding as well as diagnosed cases who died from rebleeding during slow management. One can also assume that immediately lethal SAH, as observed in 9% of this series, is preceeded by warning leaks in about 50% of the cases [4].

Altogether, not more than about 50% of all patients with ruptured aneurysm arrive in our department for early diagnosis and treatment. Operation is delayed in one-fourth of these patients, a procedure which harbors the previously mentioned risk of 25% preoperative rebleeding and 7% vasospasm, together roughly a 30% risk of secondary preoperative deterioration.

What are we doing hence to improve the prognosis of aneurysm patients in a referral area, in our efforts to treat patients early and prevent their symptomatic vasospasm with calcium antagonists? A good outcome, i.e., outcome with no or minimal deficit, is still limited to 57% of patients; mortality is as strikingly high as 40%. Comparing these results to those of Kassell and Drake [9], where less than one-third of patients are believed to have a useful outcome, a considerable improvement seems to be achieved by early management and prevention of vasospasm, following the present protocol. However, the overall outcome of this group of patients is still very unsatisfactory.

Conclusion

To date, we can say that delayed management of patients following SAH from a ruptured cerebral aneurysm still harbors an unacceptably high risk of rebleeding. The observation that about 50% of rebleeding in our recent series occurred within 48 h justifies acute management of patients.

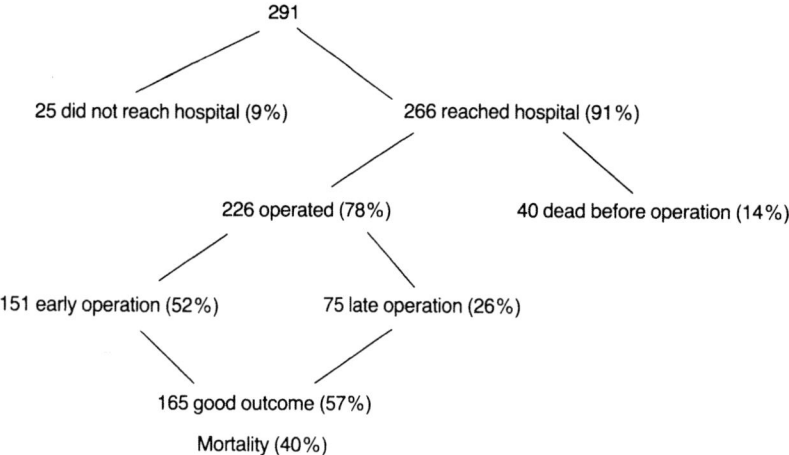

Fig. 1. Epidemiological aneurysm study 1981–1985. Within 5 years, a total number of 291 patients with subarachnoid hemorrhage was discovered in our referral area

Adequate sedation for transportation and diagnostic procedures may be of additional help.

Delayed ischemic neurological deficit from vasospasm remains a significant prognostic factor despite early surgery and the assumed washout of subarachnoid blood. Preventive treatment with the dihydropyridine calcium antagonist nimodipine minimizes this risk to a small percentage. The major factor for poor results in a whole patient population, however, is still the appreciable incidence of misdiagnosis, delayed diagnosis, or delayed transfer to a neurosurgical center.

The rate of unsatisfactory outcomes in 9% of patients preoperatively graded I, II, or III irrespective of preoperative morphological findings justifies recommending early management of these patients. As for the reason of unsatisfactory outcomes in patients preoperatively graded IV or V, the vast majority of cases showed a combination of deep-seated intracerebral hemorrhage from an aneurysm of the anterior circulation. Since 63% of these patients do not survive after early surgery, such surgery is contraindicated in most circumstances.

Apneic patients are almost unavoidably lost; their early transportation is therefore contraindicated. Patients with spontaneous respiration should undergo computerized tomography. In patients with deep-seated devastating intracerebral hemorrhage, above all elderly patients with this finding, there is no indication for early surgery.

Patients in poor clinical grades, but with only SAH or an additional subdural hematoma, can

Table 7. Preoperative death from subarachnoid hemorrhage: epidemiological aneurysm study 1981–1985

	No. of patients
Comatose, apnea	12
Undiagnosed, rebleeding	10
Diagnosed SAH, rebleeding after 1–7 days	4
Admission to neurosurgery	14
Admitted after day 3, rebled until day 8	4
Admitted after day 3, vasospasm	2
Arrived early, apneic	2
Inoperable for other reasons	2
Preoperative rebleeding	4

have a good prognosis and should be operated upon in the acute stage . The major neurosurgical problem at present is thus an adequate medical education and postgraduate informaion in order to achieve a high rate of diagnosed warning leaks. There is no doubt that, even viewed from a socioeconomic point of view, mild clinical symptoms justify a CT scan.

References

1. Allen GS, Ahn HS, Preziosi TJ, Battye R, Boone SC, Chou SN, Kelly DL, Weir BK, Crabbe RA, Lavik PJ, Rosenbloom SB, Dorsey SC, Intram CR, Mellits VE, Bertsch LA, Voisyert DPJ, Huntley MB, Johnson RK, Strom JA, Transou CR (1983) Cerebral arterial spasm: A controlled trial of nimodipine in patients with subarachnoid hem-

orrhage. N Engl J Med 308:619–624
2. Auer LM (1983) Acute surgery of cerebral aneurysms and prevention of symptomatic vasospasm. Acta Neurochir 69:273–281
3. Auer LM (1985) Timing of aneurysm surgery. Second International Symposium on Cerebral Aneurysm Surgery in the Acute Stage, 1984, Graz. Gruyter, Berlin
4. Auer LM (1986) Management of patients with subarachnoid hemorrhage from ruptured cerebral aneurysms: What remains to be done? 1st International Workshop on Intracranial Aneurysms, 1986, Tokyo
5. Auer LM, Brandt L, Ebeling U, Gilsbach J, Groeger U, Harders A, Ljunggren B, Oppel F, Reulen HJ, Saeveland H (1986) Nimodipine and early aneurysm operation in good condition SAH patients. Acta Neurochir 82:7–13
6. Auer LM, Heppner F, Symon L (1982) Aneurysm surgery in the acute stage. First International Symposium on Cerebral Aneurysm Surgery in the Acute Stage, 1981, Graz. Acta Neurochir 63:1–306 Springer, Vienna
7. Kassell N (1986) Timing of surgery: Results in cooperative aneurysm study. First International Workshop on Intracranial Aneurysms, 1986, Tokyo
8. Kassell NF, Boarini DJ, Adams HP Jr, Sahs AL, Graf CJ, Torner JC, Gerk M (1981) Overall management of ruptured aneurysm: Comparison of early and late operation. Neurosurgery 9:120–128
9. Kassell NF, Drake CG (1982) Timing of aneurysm surgery. Neurosurgery 10:514–519
10. Kassell NF, Torner JC (1984) The international cooperative study on timing of aneurysm surgery: An update. Stroke 15:566–570
11. Mee EW, Dorrance DE, Low D, Neil-Dwyer G (1986) Cerebral blood flow and neurological outcome: A controlled study of nimodipine in patients with subarachnoid hemorrhage. J Neurol Neurosurg Psychiatry 49:469
12. Ono H, Mizukami M, Kitamura K, Kikuchi H, and the Cooperative Study Group in Japan (1983) Preventive effect of ticlopidine on cerebral ischemia due to cerebral vasospasm following ruptured aneurysm: A double-blind cooperative study. 52nd Annual Meeting of the American Association of Neurological Surgeons, 24–28 April 1983, Washington, DC
13. Philippon J, Grob R, Dagreou F, Guggiari M, Rivierez M, Viars P (1986) Prevention of vasospasm in subarachnoid haemorrhage: A controlled study with nimodipine. Acta Neurochir 82:110–114
14. Yamamoto I, Hara M, Ogura K, Suzuki Y, Nakane T, Kaneyama N (1983) Early operation for ruptured intracranial aneurysms: Comparative study with computed tomography. Neurosurgery 12:169–174
15. Taneda M (1982) Effect of early operation for ruptured aneurysms on prevention of delayed ischemic symptoms. J Neurosurg 57:622–627
16. Taneda M (1982) The significance of early operation in the management of ruptured intracranial aneurysms: An analysis of 251 cases hospitalized within 24 hours after subarachnoid haemorrhage. In: Auer LM, Heppner F, Symon L (eds) Proceedings of the symposium on aneurysm surgery in the acute stage. Acta Neurochir 63:201–208

Timing and Grading in the Surgical Treatment for Aneurysm

Bengt Ljunggren, Lennart Brandt, and Hans Säveland[1]

A total of 149 patients were subjected to acute stage aneurysm clipping following subarachnoid hemorrhage (SAH). In 57 individuals, the ruptured aneurysm originated from the anterior cerebral artery complex (ACA). In 39, it was located on the internal carotid artery segment (ICA), and, in 44 patients, the ruptured aneurysm arose from the middle cerebral artery (MCA). Ninety patients were in a favorable condition prior to surgery (within 72 h after hemorrhage), while 28 were either confused, had minor neurological deficit, or both (equivalent to Hunt-Hess neurological grade III). Twenty-two individuals were in poor condition. In addition, all patients received an intravenous infusion, with the calcium channel blocker nimodipine, during the critical period for symptomatic vasospasm or delayed ischemic deterioration. The overall success rate was 76% good neurological recoveries and the mortality was 5%. The success rate was 95% in the grade I patients, 87% in the grade II patients, 64% in the grade III patients, and 36% in the poor grade patients.

Introduction

The immediate mortality following aneurysmal SAH is approximately 17% [15]. Nothing can be done for these individuals. In another 8%, the aneurysm rupture besides the SAH results in an associated massive intraparenchymal hemorrhage. These patients are almost without exception in a poor condition upon early hospital admission. Of the total population of victims of ruptured intracranial aneurysms, another 25% appear severely devastated by the first bleed. Thus, only every other patient suffering from rupture of an intracranial aneurysm will pass the initial stage in a good or fairly good condition. Aside from the direct effect of the initial bleed, most of the long-term death and disability can be traced to either recurrent bleeding or cerebral vasospasm.

Early Admitted Patients in a Favorable Condition

In the region covered by our clinic in Lund, serving a population of 1.46 million, there remains approximately 42% of the total population of victims who are admitted early and who show a primary "recovery" in the first days after the bleed and who are at great risk to rebleed and/or develop secondary SAH-induced cerebral vasospasm [15]. These individuals provide the target group for an immediate management program aiming at the prevention of rebleeds and secondary ischemic deterioration.

Recurrences occur frequently within the first weeks. In a 1962 report, 55% of patients who were alive upon admission to hospital eventually rebled, with a 75% mortality [23]. In another series of patients subjected to conservatie treatment during the first 6–8 weeks, there was a 60% mortality from the second bleed; three-fourths of the recurrences occurred within the first 8 weeks [17].

During the 1950s, it gradually became clear that many patients did not die from rebleeding but from ischemic complications related to the hemorrhage, and the frequent occurrence of coexisting intracranial arterial spasm became recognized. When the occurrence of intracranial arterial spasm was recognized, it seemed logical to assume that additional intraoperative brain retraction might cause further cerebral hypoperfusion resulting in infarction. With this background, most neurosurgeons preferred delayed operation for ruptured intracranial aneurysms.

While awaiting surgery, many patients die or become disabled from recurrent hemorrhage(s), vasospasm, or both. Thus, even if delayed sur-

[1] Department of Neurosurgery, University Hospital, Lund, Sweden

gery is safer as an operative procedure, the complications during the waiting period contribute to the prevailing, unacceptably high management morbidity and mortality. Ropper and Zervas [19], in 1984, reported that also in selected cases subjected to conventional late surgery, i.e., after 12–14 days, the ultimate outcome was unsatisfactory in almost 50% of their initially good-risk patients when viewed from a wider perspective.

The cause of cerebral vasospasm remains obscure. During the last two decades, an immense number of studies have been undertaken to elucidate the pathophysiology of cerebral vasospasm and delayed ischemic dysfunction after aneurysmal SAH, but they "have produced more questions than answers." [20] A large number of different substances have been suggested to account for the pathogenesis of delayed cerebral hypoperfusion, and the list has grown as new vasoactive agents have been discovered [27]. Because of the numerous substances incriminated in delayed vasoconstriction, a variety of drugs have been tried in an effort to prevent or treat cerebral vasospasm, but, despite many promising preliminary reports, the results of clinical trials have been disappointing. Among other mechanisms suggested to be involved in the pathogenesis of cerebral ischemic dysfunction are lesions in the arterial wall, including endothelial damage and enhanced platelet aggregability leading to thrombus formation.

In 1957, it was already suggested that subarachnoid blood clot may cause and maintain narrowing of cerebral vessels and elicit serious ischemia [10]. With the introduction of CT scan, a relationship between the amount of extravasated blood in the subarachnoid space and the subsequent development of vasospasm and delayed ischemic cerebral dysfunction was established [7, 18]. Though many surgeons still favor delayed operation as being a safer operative procedure, early surgical intervention is increasingly proposed not only with a view to improve the overall outcome by preventing rebleeding but also in an attempt to prevent ischemic complications by removal of subarachnoid blood.

The belief that the outcome from late surgical intervention is superior to that of early operation has been contradicted by several studies focused on results of substantial amount of individuals subjected to early operation [13, 16, 21] So far, however, there is no randomized study to document the outcome of patients undergoing early aneurysm surgery versus the outcome with delayed treatment. In a study published in 1981 [13] comprising 81 grade 1–III (Hunt-Hess [8]) patients subjected to early operation (within 3 days after SAH), a comparison was made with the outcome in a group of 55 similar patients undergoing delayed operation. The comparison showed that early operation, resulting in 74% good neurological recoveries, 10% morbidity, and 16% mortality, was superior to delayed management, which resulted in 56% good neurological recoveries, 18% morbidity, and 26% mortality [13]. The latter outcome corresponded well with that reported the same year from North America for similar patients undergoing late operation, which had resulted in 51% good neurological recoveries, 22% morbidity, and 27% mortality [11].

We studied the incidence of symptomatic vasospasm or delayed ischemic deterioration (DID) leading to permanent neurological deficit or death and found a 13% rate of such DID in 137 grade I–III patients subjected to early operation without specific anti-ischemic treatment [14]. In conclusion, DID is not abolished by early operation although it may be reduced by early washout of blood-contaminated cerebrospinal fluid (CSF) and clots.

Subsequent studies in the 1980s have made the timing of surgical intervention less controversial. Recently, Milhorat and Krautheim [16] compared two series of 100 consecutive patients, each subjected to delayed and early operation, respectively. The overall survival rate was 35% in the first series (delayed surgery) as compared to 80% in the other (early surgery).

Several studies have revealed a pronounced cerebrovascular dilatatory effect of calcium channel blockers of the dihydropyridine group, including experiments on human cerebral arteries in vitro [1, 6], as well as in vivo [3–5]. It has also been shown that the dilatatory effect of these drugs in vivo are inversely proportional to the resting vessel caliber [3, 5], and subsequent experimental studies on the dihydropyridine derivative nimodipine have revealed a relatively predominant cerebrovascular dilatatory effect [3, 12]. The mechanisms behind this selectivity have not been established, but may be related to a greater dependency in cerebral than in peripheral vessels on extracellular calcium for the smooth muscle activation [2].

Since all contractile substances incriminated in cerebral vasospasm are more or less dependent of calcium for their contractile effect, a reasonable approach to the problem of cerebral vasospasm would be to interfere with the final step in the vascular smooth muscle contraction mechanism. Consequently, it has been proposed that calcium antagonists might be useful to counteract *any* late cerebral vasoconstriction following subarachnoid extravasation of blood [1, 3–6, 12].

It has been shown that cerebral vasospasm associated with neurological deterioration observed several days following aneurysmal SAH is unaltered by pharmacological agents directed against the proposed increase in vascular smooth muscle tone [26]. Almost every drug that might have a vasodilatatory effect has been tried, and animal experiments have also demonstrated that the chronic phase of vasospasm is unaltered by vasodilators such as aminophylline, nifedipine, or papaverine [24]. This evidence of irreversibility by pharmacological agents is consistent with findings of structural alterations in the vascular wall in patients with chronic vasospasm. It is therefore reasonable to believe that it is only the early phase of increased smooth muscle tone that can be affected by vasodilators. For this reason, it has been suggested that any treatment of delayed ischemic deterioration associated with cerebral vasospasm should be prophylactic. Apart from the vasodilatatory properties of the dihydropyridines, inhibitory effects on platelet aggregation might be involved [22].

Results of Early Surgery Combined with Intravenous Nimodipine

A total of 149 individuals were subjected to acute stage clipping for a ruptured supratentorial aneurysm combined with nimodipine treatment. Nimodipine was administered as follows: topical intraoperative application on exposed arterial segments immediately after clipping of the aneurysm within 72 h after rupture followed by continuous intravenous administration of approximately 0.5 μg/kg body weight/min (2 mg/h) for at least 10 days. During the intravenous infusion, the mean plasma concentration was 26.6 + 1.8 ng/ml (range: <3 − 38.8 ng/ml) [25]. Nimodipine assay was through the use of high-pressure liquid chromatagraphy with UV detection at 254 nm.

The preoperative status of the patients is given in Table 1 and the outcome assessed at least 3 months later is presented in Table 2. The overall incidence of DID with permanent neurological deficit (PND) was 3% (Table 3). The occurrence of DID with PND in relation to location of ruptured aneurysm is given in Tables 4–6 [14].

Conclusion

It may be argued that the lowered incidence of DID in the recent series of early operated patients may be ascribed to increased surgical skill only. However, surgical expertise eventually approaches an asymptote. It is therefore not very

Table 1. Preoperative condition (Hunt-Hess neurological grade) in 140 patients subjected to acute stage aneurysm clipping combined with intravenous nimodipine

Grade	Number
I	20
II	70
III	28
IV	12
V	10
Total	140

Table 2. Preoperative condition and outcome in 140 patients subjected to acute stage aneurysm clipping combined with intravenous nimodipine

Preop grade[a]	Good recovery	Fair outcome	Poor outcome	Dead	Total	Success rate (%)
I	19		1		20	95
II	61	5	3	1	70	87
III	18	4	2	4	28	64
IV	6	3	2	1	12	50
V	2	2	5	1	10	20
Total	106	14	13	7	140	76

[a] Hunt-Hess neurological grading system

Table 3. Incidence of delayed ischemic deterioration with permanent neurological deficit in patients subjected to acute stage aneurysm clipping with and without intravenous nimodipine

Preop grade	Without nimodipine		With nimodipine	
	No. of patients	With DID	No. of patients	With DID
I	43	1	20	0
II	61	10	70	3
III	33	7	28	1
IV–V			22	1
Total	137	18 (13%)	140	5 (3%)

DID delayed ischemic deterioration

Table 4. Incidence of delayed ischemic deterioration with permanent neurological deficit following acute stage clipping of ruptured anterior cerebral artery complex aneurysm with and without intravenous nimodipine

Preop grade	Without nimodipine		With nimodipine	
	No. of patients	With DID	No. of patients	With DID
I	20	0	6	0
II	27	5	32	3
III	14	1	13	1
IV–V			6	1
Total	61	6 (10%)	57	5 (9%)

DID delayed ischemic deterioration

Table 5. Incidence of delayed ischemic deterioration with permanent neurological deficit following acute stage clipping of ruptured middle cerebral artery aneurysm with and without intravenous nimodipine

Preop grade	Without nimodipine		With nimodipine	
	No. of patients	With DID	No. of patients	With DID
I	6	0	8	0
II	15	2	15	0
III	8	3	7	0
IV–V			14	0
Total	29	5 (17%)	44	0 (0%)

DID delayed ischemic deterioration

Table 6. Incidence of delayed ischemic deterioration with permanent neurological deficit following acute stage clipping of ruptured internal carotid artery aneurysm with and without intravenous nimodipine

Preop grade	Without nimodipine		With nimodipine	
	No. of patients	With DID	No. of patients	With DID
I	17	1	6	0
II	19	3	23	0
III	11	3	8	0
IV–V			2	0
Total	47	7 (15%)	39	0 (0%)

DID delayed ischemic deterioration

likely that this should be the prime reason for the marked reduction of DID, and it is consequently suggested that intravenous nimodipine provides an additional anti-ischemic protective effect following aneurysmal SAH and early operation.

Following the natural course of aneurysmal SAH, only 18% of all victims may be expected to be alive and well after 10 years [9]. The overall outcome following early surgical intervention combined with additional nimodipine treatment resulted in 42% good neurological recoveries, 19% morbidity, and 39% mortality [15]. Despite recent improvements with elimination of rebleeds by early surgical intervention in good grade patients and a pronounced reduction of DID in such patients who initially are in a favorable condition following rupture of an intracranial aneurysm, the overall outcome remains hampered by all those individuals who are permanently devastated as a result of the initial bleed.

References

1. Allen GS, Banghart SB (1979) Cerebral arterial spasm: IX. In vitro effects of nifedipine on serotonin-, phenylephrine-, and potassium-induced contractions of canine basilar and femoral arteries. Neurosurgery 4:37–42.
2. Andersson KE (1986) Role of calcium ions in the excitation-contraction coupling mechanisms of brain vessels. In: Owman C, Hardebo JE (eds) Neural regulation of brain circulation. pp 67–79
3. Auer LM, Oberbauer RW, Schalk HV (1983) Human pial vascular reactions to intravenous nimodipine-infusion during EC-IC bypass surgery. Stroke 14:210–213
4. Brandt L, Andersson KE, Bengtsson B, Edvinsson L, Ljunggren B, McKenzie ET (1979) Effects of nifedipine on pial arteriolar calibre: An in vivo study. Surg Neurol 12:349–352
5. Brandt L, Ljunggren B, Andersson KE, MacKenzie E, Tamura ET, Teasdale G (1982) Effects on feline cortical pial microvasculature of topical application of a calcium antagonist (nifedipine) under normal conditions and in focal ischemia. J Cereb Blood Flow Metab 3:44–50
6. Edvinsson L, Brandt L, Andersson KE, Bengtsson B (1979) Effect of a calcium antagonist on experimental constriction of human brain vessels: Possible efficacy in cerebrovascular spasm. Surg Neurol 11:327–330
7. Fisher CM, Kistler JP, Davis JM, (1980) Relation of cerebral vasospasm to subarachnoid hemorrhage visualized by computerized tomographic scanning. Neurosurgery 6:1–9
8. Hunt WE, Hess RM (1968) Surgical risk as related to time of intervention in the repair of intracranial aneurysms. J Neurosurg 28:14–19
9. Jennett G, Galbraith S (eds) (1983) An introduction to neurosurgery, 4th edn. Heinemann London, p 187
10. Johnson RJ, Potter JM, Reid RG (1958) Arterial spasm in subarachnoid hemorrhage: Mechanical considerations. J Neurol Neurosurg Psych 21:68
11. Kassell NF, Adams HP Jr., Torner JC, Sahs AL (1981) Influence of timing of admission after aneurysmal subarachnoid hemorrhage on overall outcome: Report of the cooperative aneurysm study. Stroke 12:620–623
12. Kazda S, Towart R (1982) Nimodipine: A new calcium antagonistic drug with a preferential cerebrovascular action. Acta Neurochir (Wien) 63:259–265
13. Ljunggren B, Brandt L, Kågström E, Sundbärg G (1981) Results of early operations for ruptured aneurysms. J Neurosurg 54:473–479
14. Ljunggren B, Säveland H, Brandt L (1983) Causes of unfavorable outcome after early aneurysm operation. Neurosurgery 13:629–633
15. Ljunggren B, Säveland H, Brandt L, Zygmunt S (1985) Early operation and overall outcome in aneurysmal subarachnoid hemorrhage. J Neurosurg 62:547–551
16. Milhorat TH, Krautheim M (1986) Results of early and delayed operations for ruptured intracranial aneurysms in two series of 100 consecutive patients. Surg Neurol 26:123–128
17. Pakarinen S (1967) Incidence, etiology, and prognosis of primary subarachnoid hemorrhage. Acta Neurol Scand 43 (Suppl. 29):1–128
18. Pasqualin A, Rosta L, Da Pian R, Cavazzani P, Scienza R (1984) Role of computed tomography in the management of vasospasm after subarachnoid hemorrhage. Neurosurgery 15:344–353
19. Ropper AH, Zervas NT (1984) Outcome 1 year after SAH from cerebral aneurysm: Management morbidity, mortality, and functional status in 112 consecutive good-risk patients. J Neurosurg 60:909–915
20. Sundt TM Jr, Davis DH (1980) Reactions of cerebrovascular smooth muscle to blood and ischemia: Primary versus secondary vasospasm. In: Wilkins RH (ed) Cerebral arterial spasm, vol. 1. Williams and Wilkins, Baltimore, pp 244–250
21. Suzuki J, Onuma T, Yoshimoto T (1979) Results of early operations on cerebral aneurysms. Surg Neurol 11:407–412
22. Takahara K, Kuroiwa A, Matsushima T, Nakashima Y, Takasugi M (1985) Effects of nifedipine on platelet function. Am Heart J 109:4–8
23. Tappura M (1962) Prognosis of subarachnoid hemorrhage: A study of 120 patients with unoperated intracranial arterial aneurysms and 267 patients without vascular lesions demonstrable in bilateral carotid angiograms. Acta Med Scand 1 (Suppl 392):1–75
24. Varsos VG, Liszczak TM, Han DH, Kistler JP, Vielma J, Black PM, Heros RC, Zervas NT (1983) Delayed cerebral vasospasm is not reversible by aminophylline, nifedipine, or papaverine in a "two-hemorrhage" canine model. J Neurosurg 58:11–17
25. Vinge E, Andersson KE, Brandt L, Ljunggren B,

Nilsson LG, Rosendal-Helgesen S (1986) Phar-macokinetics of nimodipine in patients with aneu-rysmal subarachnoid hemorrhage. Eur J Clin Pharmacol 30:421–425

26. Wilkins RH (1980) Attempted prevention or treatment of intracranial arterial spasm: A survey. Neurosurgery 6:198–210

27. Wilkins RH (1986). Attempts at prevention or treatment of intracranial arterial spasm: An update. Neurosurgery 18:808–825

Timing and Risk Factors in Surgery of Ruptured Cerebral Aneurysms

Isamu Saito, Hiromu Segawa, and Koichi Aritake[1]

Introduction

The decision whether to operate or not in cases with ruptured cerebral aneurysms in the acute stage is still a controversial problem [1, 2, 5, 6]. Since the beginning of 1970, microsurgery has been utilized in our operations on cerebral aneurysms and we have actively performed early operations after rupture. In this paper, we will analyze 248 consecutive cases of ruptured cerebral aneurysms admitted within one week after subarachnoid hemmorhage (SAH) and detail the risk factors producing unfavorable surgical results.

Clinical Material and Methods

During the last 12 years (1974–1986), a total of 248 cases with cerebral aneurysms were admitted within 7 days after SAH to the care of Saito at Mitsui Memorial Hospital and Fuji Brain Institute and Hospital. Within one week of SAH, 206 cases (83%) were operated on, 22 (9%) were submitted to surgery later than 1 week after SAH, and the remaining 20 cases (8%) were treated conservatively: 19 of them died before surgery.

The status of patients was evaluated 6 months after the aneurysm rupture, classifying them as "independent" or "dependent." Independent means that the patient was working or independent in his daily live. In the dependent state, the patient was bedridden or needed help in his daily life.

Results

Overall Mortality and Morbidity

In Table 1, the overall mortality and morbidity

---

[1] Department of Neurosurgery, University of Tokyo, Tokyo, Japan

of all 248 cases with ruptured cerebral aneurysm admitted within 7 days after SAH is shown according to the modality of treatment and grade of patient (Hunt-Hess) at admission. Six months after SAH, 65% were in an independent state, 9% were in a dependent state, and 26% had died. The grade at admission and final outcome are also shown in Table 1. When patients in grades 1, 2, and 3 were characterized as being in a favorable condition at admission, 150 (79%) of 190 cases were independent and 28 (15%) had died within 6 months after SAH.

Timing of Surgery and Risk Factors Producing Unfavorable Results

Surgery Within First 3 days (days 0–2)

Age of patient. In early operations on the ruptured cerebral aneurysm, surgical results did not always depend on the grade of the patient. Table 2 shows the surgical results of cases in grades III and IV operated on within 3 days after SAH, in two age groups below and above 60 years of age. Younger patients showed statistically better neurological condition ($P < 0.005$) in the follow-up. As for patients in grades I and II, there was no perceptible difference in surgical results among these two age groups.

Location of aneurysm. Overall results according to the location of aneurysm are shown in Table 3. Cases with vertebrobasilar aneurysms demonstrated significantly more unfavorable results compard with cases in other locations. Of seven patients with vertebrobasilar aneurysms who died before surgery, six were patients with basilar aneurysms admitted in grades III, IV, or V.

Diffuse extensive cisternal clots. Surgical results of patients in grade IV operated on within 3 days of SAH varied and were not favorable, particularly in patients with extensive cisternal clots. In patients whose neurological symptoms were due to diffuse and extensive cisternal clots, washout of clots was often not complete and postopera-

Table 1. Overall mortality and morbidity in 248 cases admitted within 1 week after SAH

		Independent	Dependent	Died
Cases operated on within 1 week of SAH	206	142 (69%)	20 (10%)	44 (21%)
Cases operated on later than 1st week	22	18 (82%)	2	2
Nonoperated cases	20	1	0	19 (95%)
Total	248	161 (65%)	22 (9%)	65 (26%)
Grade at admission and final outcome[a]				
Grade I–II	132 (1)	112 (1) = 85%	6	14 = 11%
III	58 (7)	38 = 66%	6	14 (7) = 24%
IV	35 (2)	10 = 29%	7	18 (2) = 51%
V	23 (10)	1	3	19 (10) = 83%
Total	248 (20)	161 (1)	22	65 (19)

[a] Numbers in parentheses represent nonoperated cases

tive vasospasm could not be prevented sometimes.

In our early operations on ruptured aneurysm, the cisternal clots were sucked as much as possible (early washout) during surgery. Furthermore, since 1983, we have been trying a cisternal irrigation system for a more efficient washout of clots and vasoactive substances after surgery. A pair of silicone tubes were inserted into the cisterns, one in the prechiasmatic cistern and the other in the sylvian fissure. From a bottle at 30–40 cm above the head of the patient, 500 ml saline or Ringer solution with 24 000 units urokinase and 50 mg gentamycin was dripped through one catheter and drained from the other. Irrigation continued for as long as 15 days, using 1500 ml of solution per day [3].

Up to now, a total of 42 cases operated on within 3 days after SAH have been submitted to this cisternal irrigation and, in 19% of these cases, particularly in cases with diffuse cisternal clots on preoperative CT, postoperative vasospasm developed in spite of washout during and after surgery. The internal carotid artery or the M1 portion of the middle cerebral artery did not demonstrate vasospasm. Postoperative vasospasm was sometimes seen in the M2 or M3 portion of the middle cerebral artery or the A2 portion of the anterior cerebral artery. These results are due to the fact that the saline fluid was effective in carrying the blood clots away from the area between the prechiasmatic cistern and the sylvian fissure, whereas irrigation was not so effective in the posterior part of the sylvian fissure, the subarachnoid space of the cerebral convexity, and the interhemispheric fissure.

Operation During Days 3–7

Diffuse extensive cisternal clots. The follow-up results of cases in grade III operated on within 7 days after SAH also varied. The independent group of cases (36%; four of 11 cases) operated on between day 3–7 was statistically low ($P < 0.025$) as compared with cases operated on earlier (75%; 24 of 32 cases; Table 4).

Meanwhile, patients in grade IV, admitted within one week after SAH, usually showed severe neurological symptoms preoperatively. Nevertheless, surgical results in cases with intracerebral hematomas were relatively good, whereas patients in grade IV with severe SAH or intraventricular hematoma showed poor results due to the development of postoperative vasospasm.

Whether washout of blood clots in this period (delayed washout) was too late to prevent postoperative vasospasm or not was examine in 36 recent cases operated on from day 3 to day 7. In 17 cases of no high-density area (HDA) or a diffuse, thin HDA on preoperative CT, postoperative vasospasm was rare and mild, if it occurred at all. Of 14 cases with localized HDA, severe vasospasm developed in five cases, particularly in the cerebral arteries of the posterior part of the sylvian fissure and cerebral convexity, where washout of clots was not feasible by surgical procedure. In the diffuse, thick groups (five cases), it was usually impossible to washout completely and all showed postoperative vasospasm; four of them died from severe vasospasm.

Based upon these results, it seems possible that even delayed washout in days 3–7 can also prevent vasospasm, if it is complete.

Table 2. Surgical results according to age groups regarding cases in grades 3 and 4 operated on within days 0–2

		Independent	Dependent	Died
Under 60 years old	42	30 (71%)[a]	5	7 (17%)
60 years and over	15	4 (27%)[a]	2	9 (60%)

[a] $P < 0.005$

Table 3. Overall mortality and morbidity according to locations of cerebral aneurysms

		Independent	Dependent	Died
V-B	17 (7)	4[a] = 29%	1	12 (7) = 71%
Others	231 (13)	157 (1)[a] = 68%	21	53 (12) = 23%

[a] $P < 0.001$
Numbers in *parentheses* represent non-operated cases
V-B vertebrobasilar aneurysms

Preoperative diffuse vasospasm. In 10 of 58 cases operated on in days 3–7, a symptomatic vasospasm was observed preoperatively. In five cases, vasospasm migrated to more distal portions of the cerebral arteries such as the sylvian segment or the ascending branches of the middle cerebral artery. However, preoperative vasospasm of the internal carotid artery or the M1 portion of the middle cerebral artery was relieved or disappeared after blood clots were surgically removed from these areas and 4% papaverine was applied topically. In three cases, vasospasm remained unchanged postoperatively. In the remaining two cases with preoperaive diffuse vasospasm, a severe brain swelling occured during operative intervention and the postoperative CT demonstrated a large low density area with an extensive mass effect. Both patients died.

Discussion

Our 12 years' experience of early operations on ruptured cerebral aneurysms indicated to us that the following risk factors exert crucial influence upon overall results of treatment of ruptured aneurysms in the acute stage: Age over 60 years location of aneurysm in vertebrobasilar artery, diffuse extensive cisternal clots, and diffuse symptomatic vasospasm.

As for vertebrobasilar aneurysms, and particularly for basilar aneurysms, we did not perform surgery in the acute stage and postponed it until 2 weeks after SAH. In surgery of vertebral aneurysms, however, retraction of the brain is minimal and operations could be carried out safely with as good results as in aneurysms of the anterior circulation. Meanwhile, operation on the basilar aneurysm has been avoided because of the necessity of extensive retraction. However, almost all cases with basilar aneurysms in grades III–V have died due to rerupture or development of vasospasm. This would seem to indicate that early surgery on basilar artery aneurysms be tried hereafter.

In early surgery, not only the clipping of aneurysms, but the removal of blood clots has been carried out to prevent vasospasm. Until 1983, we settled a silicone catheter into the basal cisterns, for removal of residual clots and vasospasmogenic substances, continuously after surgery. However, this method could decrease the incidence of vasospasm by only 10% compared with the incidence of vasospasm (45%) occurring in the natural course. Since 1984, we have been trying cisternal irrigation for more effective washout of cisternal clots as mentioned above. Of 42 cases submitted to this method, only 19% of them developed symptomatic postoperative vasospasm. In these cases, vasospasm did not occur in the internal carotid arteries or the M1 portions of the middle cerebral arteries. When vasospasm developed, particularly in cases with diffuse, thick cisternal clots on preoperative CT, it was restricted to the peripheral branches of the cerebral arteries. When compared with previous cisternal drainage methods, this system of cisternal irrigation is expected to be a more effective procedure for prevention of postoperative vasospasm.

Table 4. Surgical results according to grade and timing of surgery

Grade	Day 0–2				Day 3–7			
	Cases	Independent	Dependent	Died	Cases	Independent	Dependent	Died
I–II	82	70 (85%)	3	9	41	33 (80%)	3	5
III	32	24[a] (75%)	3	5	11	4[a] (36%)	4	3
IV	24	10 (42%)	4	10	3	0	0	3
V	10	0	4	6	3	0	0	3
Total	148	104 (70%)	14 (10%)	30 (20%)	58	37 (64%)	7 (12%)	14 (24%)

[a] $P < 0.025$

Our division of the 1st week after SAH into two periods is associated with the possibility of preventing vasospasm by operation [4]. In the natural course of SAH, vasospasm never occurred before day 4 and developed frequently around day 7 after SAH.

As shown in this paper and reported before, patients in grade III operated on in days 3–7 did worse than those operated on within 3 days after SAH. These results were explained as follows: The vasospasm-causing substances are probably produced in the latter half of the 1st week after SAH and the cerebral arteries are inclined to vasospasm in this period. Therefore, operations between the 4th and 7th day after SAH enhance the anticipated vasospasm. In operations performed by the 3rd day after SAH, on the other hand, extravasated blood clots can be easily removed by suction during the operation and by continuous postoperative irrigation and drainage before the degradation of blood clots occurs. One of the causes of cerebral vasospasm is thus removed from the area of the cerebral arteries, and the postoperative vasospasm is not apt to develop. For the first 6 years (1974–1980), we rarely operated on cases admitted on days 3–7 in grade III. During this period, 13 cases in grade III were admitted on days 3–7, and surgery on their aneurysms was postponed. Six (46%) of them died before surgery; four due to severe vasospasm, one due to rebleeding and the sixth one from pulmonary edema. Seven cases were operated on later than one week after SAH: five (38%) were independent in the follow-up whereas two (15%) were dependent.

During the last 4 years, we have again actively operated on cases previously characterized as poor candidates for surgery, because the overall results of the delayed surgery method were not good and some other effective methods of treat-

ment for vasospasm, such as hypervolemia and hypertension, have become available. However, as shown in Table 3, only four of eleven cases showed favorable results. These four cases demonstrated an intracerebral hematoma or localized vasospasm preoperatively. On the other hand, the other seven cases displayed diffuse cisternal clots on the preoperative CT or diffuse preoperative vasospasm, and were in a poor condition or died after surgery.

In this paper, we have also examined whether washout of blood clots around the cerebral arteries during surgery performed between days 3 and 7 was too late to prevent postoperative vasospasm or to relieve preoperatively developed vasospasm. It was shown that there is a possibility of preventing vasospasm by washout of blood clots in this period (delayed washout). Vasospasm did not occur in the cerebral arteries where blood clots were removed. However, in cases with diffuse, thick blood clots, displayed on the preoperative CT, washout of blood clots was usually not complete and vasospasm always developed, particularly in the peripheral arteries, such as the M2 or M3 portion of the middle cerebral artery and the A2 portion of the anterior cerebral artery.

This study has reinforced our inclination towards early operation on ruptured aneurysms, but our experience of 12 years has caused us to make some changes in the policy of treatment of ruptured aneurysms in the acute stage [5]. Three new principles, particularly in the treatment of ruptured aneurysms within one week of the SAH, have been developed.

For cases in grades I or II, microsurgery can be safely indicated. During the first 3 days (days 0, 1, and 2), grade III cases can be submitted to clipping of the aneurysmal neck and removal of the subarachnoid clots. In grade IV cases with intracerebral hematoma, surgery is also indicated, and the prognosis will depend on the site of the hematoma. However, for grade IV patients in severe neurological condition due to diffuse and extensive cisternal clots or intraventricular rupture, washout of the cisternal clots is often not complete, and postoperative vasospasm usually occurs. Patients in grades III or IV and aged over 60 years should be treated conservatively.

During days 3–7 after SAH, cases in grades III and IV can be safely submitted to surgery only when patients show hydrocephalus, local vasospasm, or intracerebral hematoma. Delayed washout of blood clots in this period can also prevent and relieve vasospasm, if the washout is complete. However, when patients show symptomatic diffuse vasospasm, an operation on the aneurysm will always produce brain swelling. Therefore, other therapy, such as the administration of barbiturates, should be tried.

References

1. Adams HP Jr, Kassell NF, Torner JC, et al. (1981) Early management of aneurysmal subarachnoid hemorrhage: A report of the Cooperative Aneurysm Study: J Neurosurg 54:141–145
2. Kassel NF, Drake CG (1982) Timing of aneurysm surgery. Neurosurgery 10:514–519
3. Saito I, Segawa H, Nagayama I, Nihei H (1985) Prevention of postoperative vasospasm by cisternal irrigation. In: Auer LM (ed) Timing of aneurysm surgery. Gruyter, Berlin, pp 587–594
4. Saito I, Ueda Y, Sano K (1977) Significance of vasospasm in the treatment of ruptured intracranial aneurysm. J Neurosurg 47:412–429
5. Sano K, Saito I (1978) Timing and indication of surgery for ruptured intracranial aneurysms with regard to cerebral vasospasm. Acta Neurochir 41: 49–60
6. Weir BK, Aronyk K (1981) Management mortality and timing of surgery for supratentorial aneurysms. J Neurosurg 54:146–150

Results of Ultra-Early Surgery on Intracranial Aneurysms by the Sendai Group of Neurosurgeons

Yoshiharu Sakurai[1], Takehide Onuma[2], and Jiro Suzuki[3]

Introduction

Since the early 1970s, we have been advocating ultra-early surgery for ruptured cerebral aneurysms, and have reported on its therapeutic effectiveness [8, 11]. In 1985, however, Nishimoto, et al. reported [4] that the surgical results in ruptured cerebral aneurysm cases from various neurosurgical clinics in Japan were quite poor when the operation was performed within 48 h of onset. Even for relatively mild grades I and II cases, the mortality was said to be 26.6%, and it was notably poor for more severe cases: 35.6% in grade III, 55.2% in grade IV, and 79.1% in grade V cases. We are consequently concerned that such results using early stage surgery can only have caused a complete loss of confidence in this procedure in the West.

In the present study, we report the surgical methods used by the Sendai group of neurosurgeons, who have performed such surgery using a consistent policy for operative procedures and postoperative care. The essential points required for successful ultra-early stage surgery are emphasized.

Clinical Materials

Over the 8-year period from 1978 to 1985, we experienced a total of 1122 patients who were hospitalized within 3 days of the last rupture of an aneurysm of the anterior half of the circle of Willis. Among those cases, intracranial radical surgery was performed in 843 (75.1%), and 565 of the operated cases (67.0%) were operated in the ultra-early period (within 3 days of the last

bleeding episode; Fig. 1). These 565 cases constitute the materials for the present study.

The locations of the aneurysms were as follows: 199 anterior communicating artery (AcomA) cases (35.2%), 29 anterior cerebral artery (ACA) cases (5.1%), 136 internal carotid artery (ICA) cases (24.0%), and 201 middle cerebral artery (MCA) cases (35.5%). The ages of the patients ranged from 13 to 80 years, with a mean age of 51.0. Indication for radical surgery was determined by us from the patient's state of consciousness and its course. If the patient was at least in a stuporous state and capable of responding to his name, and, provided that the state of consciousness is not taking a notably downhill course, the patient is judged as suitable for the radical treatment [7, 8].

Surgical Method

The type of craniotomy is determined by the site of the aneurysm and the extent of the intended

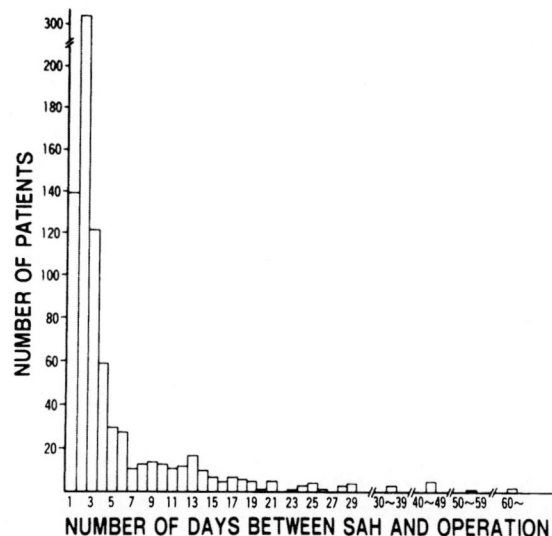

Fig. 1. Timing of operation. *SAH* subarachnoid hemorrhage

[1] Division of Neurosurgery, Sendai National Hospital. Sendai, Japan
[2] Sendai City Hospital, Sendai, Japan
[3] Institute of Brain Disease, Tohoku University School of Medicine, Sendai, Japan

extirpation of the subarachnoid hematoma, which will be required to prevent the occurrence of delayed postoperative vasospasm. Specifically, craniotomy with extirpation of a subarachnoid hematoma is decided upon if CT numbers in excess of 65 are found in CT scans taken immediately prior to surgery [10]. Prior to the intracranial procedures, a continuous ventricular drainage is inserted into the anterior horn of the lateral ventricle. Cerebral spinal fluid (CSF) is aspirated and, consequently, the brain becomes slack.

The preoperative CT scans are referred to and, while taking care not to damage cerebral veins, the subarachnoid space is opened. The hematoma is removed and the subarachnoid space rinsed as thoroughly as possible. After complete aspiration, the subarachnoid space is packed with cotton plaglets, which have been soaked in 10–50 mmol sodium nitrite ($NaNO_2$). The sodium nitrite acts to convert oxyhemoglobin into methemoglobin, which is known to be a much weaker vasospastic agent [6]. For dissection of the aneurysm and treatment of the aneurysmal neck, temporary clips are placed on the feeding artery, and sometimes on the feeding and draining arteries, under administration of the Sendai Cocktail [1, 12]. As a rule, the entire aneurysm in then completely dissected, and neck ligation and clipping are done. Efforts are always made to stop all hemorrhaging and thus prevent the occurrence of postoperative vasospasm caused by the bleeding. The ventricular drainage is left in place and used postoperatively. If postoperative removal of the drainage is deemed undesirable, a ventricul peritonial (V-P) shunt operation is done.

From an early postoperative period, the alpha-blocker, Plazocin, is administered to prevent delayed cerebral vasospasm [2]. However, if symptoms of cerebral ischemia appear, the Sendai Cocktail is administered and induced hypertension therapy, using angiotensin II, is undertaken as a first choice. In cases where there is still no improvement in symptoms, cervical sympathectomy [3] is then done.

Therapeutic Results

The severity of preoperative neurological symptoms was evaluated using Hunt and Kosnik's classification, and the operative results at the time of discharge were classified into the following five categories: excellent (normal), good

Table 1. Pre-operative grade and results of operation within three days after the last SAH (April 1978– December 1985)

Grade	Ex	G	F	P	D	Total
I	26	4	1			31
II	223	40	21	6	14	304
III	67	34	19	7	19	146
IV	13	24	17	15	12	81
V		1		1	1	3
Total	329	103	58	29	46	565
	76.5%		15.4%		8.1%	

SAH subarachnoid hemorrhage, *Ex* excellent, *G* good, *F* fair, *P* poor, *D* dead

(mild neurological deficits, but normal social life still possible), fair (neurological deficits, such that normal social life is not possible), poor (independent domestic life not possible), and dead (Table 1).

Favorable outcomes (excellent or good) were obtained in 293 of the 335 cases (87.5%) which had been operated on while the patient was in relatively good condition (grades I or II). Unfavorable outcomes (fair or poor) were obtained in 28 of these patients, with a morbidity of 8.4%, and there were 14 deaths (4.2%).

Among the 146 patients who were grade III preoperatively, favorable outcomes were obtained in 101 (69.2%), 26 were in a morbid state (17.8%), and there were 19 fatalities (13.0%). Among the 81 grade IV cases, favorable outcomes were obtained in 37 (45.7%), and the morbidity and mortality rates were 39.5% (32 cases) and 14.8% (12 cases), respectively. Three of the cases which were grade V preoperatively had intracerebral hematomas due to rerupture of MCA aneurysms while in hospital, but two were discharged in good condition and one in poor condition. There was one fatality.

In summary, favorable outcomes were obtained in 432 of the 565 cases undergoing radical surgery (76.5%), whereas 87 (15.4%) were discharged in a morbid state, and there were 46 deaths (8.1%). Symptomatic cerebral vasospasms, diagnosed from postoperative CT scans and symptomatology, were found in 129 patients (22.8%; Table 2). Among these patients, the symptoms due to vasospasm had nearly disappeared by the time of discharge, due to the above-mentioned therapies, in 62 cases (10.9%). Moderate sequelae were present in 48 patients (8.4%), who required rehabilitative therapy. Death due to cerebral vasospasm occurred in 19

Table 2. Preoperative grade and incidence of postoperative symptomatic vasospasm

Grade	Severity of symptoms					Total
	Negative	Slight	Moderate	Fatal	Uncertain	
I	29	2				31
II	249	35	16	2	2	304
III	104	18	15	8	1	146
IV	48	7	17	8	1	81
V	2			1		3
Total (%)	432	62 (10.9)	48 (8.4)	19 (3.3)	4	565
	76.5%		22.8%		0.7%	

cases (3.3%).

The cause of death among the 46 fatalities was most commonly due to cerebral vasospasm (19 cases or 41.3%), followed by systemic disorders, such as gastrointestinal bleeding or pneumonia (13 cases or 28.3%), central nervous system (CNS) disorders, such as postoperative meningitis (nine cases or 19.6%), troubled operations in three cases, and the postoperative rupture of an undetected aneurysm in two cases.

Discussion

It was once believed that better surgical results could be obtained from intracranial surgery on ruptured cerebral aneurysms if the operation were delayed 1 or 2 weeks after the onset of the disease. At the same time, however, it was fully acknowledged that the condition worsens in a considerable number of patients during this period of waiting, due to rerupture or cerebral vasospasm.

During the current era of neurosurgery, in which a means for protective therapy of rerupture and cerebral vasospasm has not been firmly established, we concluded that acute stage surgery might be a means of solving this problem. We have consequently developed and advocated so-called ultra-early stage operations [8, 11]. Specifically, we perform intracranial direct surgery as early as possible following rupture of the aneurysm, generally within 48 h of onset and, if possible, within 20 h [11].

The reason for performing ultra-early stage operations stems from the fact that swelling of the brain increases with time following the subarachnoid hemorrhage, and the danger of intracranial surgery increases proportionately. There are, however, certain essential points which must be noted if favorable surgical results are to be obtained in acute stage operations.

The first is that strict criteria for surgical indication must be adhered to. We believe that grade V patients are not indicated for surgical treatment. Moreover, at the present time, we believe that patients whose state of consciousness is comatose or semicomatose (all grade V and some grade IV cases), or patients whose state of consciousness is taking a notably downhill course, are unsuitable for radical surgery, but all other cases are indicated [8].

All cases which are thought unsuitable for surgery on admission are administered the Sendai Cocktail and accelerators of cerebral metabolism intravenously, and continuous ventricular drainage is instituted in order to induce improvements in the state of consciousness. If such improvements are found, such that the patient falls within the criteria for radical surgery, the intracranial operation is immediately undertaken. With regard to the relationship between the patient's age and indication for surgery, it must be said that each case requires individual study to determine the severity of the arteriosclerosis. Moreover, we consider all patients over the age of 70 as unsuitable for the radical operation unless they are in good condition (grades I or II) preoperatively.

Next, we will discuss several important points concerning surgery on ruptured cerebral aneurysms in the ultra-early stage. The first point regards the method employed for aspiration of the subarachnoid hematoma. As discussed above, we decide upon the method of craniotomy based upon the CT findings obtained immediately prior to surgery [10]. That is, in nearly all cases, the CT scans in the acute period following rupture show high-density areas (HDAs) in the subarachnoid space. In recent years, it has been widely acknowledged that oxyhemoglobin, released due to the hemolysis occurring within the subarachnoid hematoma, is a powerful spasmogenic substance [6]. One of the major objectives in the aspiration of the hematoma during surgery is, consequently, the elimination of that substance.

Simultaneously, however, there is a danger of causing further brain damage due to the wide opening of the subarachnoid space and the removal of blood clots. Therefore, the minimal aspiration of the subarachnoid space, which suffices for removal of the hematoma, should be done. For this reason, we decide upon the regions requiring aspiration in light of the CT numbers of the subarachonoid hematoma.

The aspiration itself must be undertaken with great care, using an aspirating tube and continually adjusting the strength of the aspiration, such that arterioles and venules are not damaged in the process. It is particularly important to aspirate as fully as possible those hematomas which completely envelope and are adherent to vascular walls. During such procedure, however, venous hemorrhaging sometimes occurs, and there may arise difficulty in controlling the bleeding. Control can normally be regained simply by raising the position of the patient's head. At the completion of aspiration of subachnoid clots, the subarachnoid space should be packed with cotton pieces which have been soaked in $NaNO_2$. Since the oxyhemoglobin released during the aspiration procedure can be the cause of postoperative vasospasm, these precautionary steps convert the oxyhemoglobin into the relatively inactive methemoglobin [6] and prevent the flow of blood to deep-lying sites, if premature rupture during the aneurysm treatment should occur.

The second important point concerns the control of the intracranial pressure. In order to reduce the size of the brain prior to the intracranial procedure, we insert a continuous ventricular drainage into the anterior horn of the lateral ventricle and extract CSF. Provided that sufficient fluid can be removed and the volume of the brain reduced, this measure can greatly facilitate the subsequent intracranial procedure. Postoperative care is also facilitated if the drainage is left in place following the operation. In mild cases, where the postoperative need for ventricular drainage is thought to be minimal, the drainage tube can be removed in an early period postoperatively. When continued control of the intracranial pressure using this technique is required for more than 2 weeks, the drainage should be replaced by a V-P shunt, because there is a danger of infection if the drainage is left in

place.

The third and final point concerns the dangers involved in dissecting the aneurysm. The possibility of a premature rupture of a cerebral aneurysm during the acute stage operation must be treated as a virtual certainty. In order to prevent such an incident, therefore, the feeding and draining arteries of the aneurysm must first be identified and temporary clips placed on them. This procedure should be done under the administration of the Sendai Cocktail [12], which has been shown in both animal experiments [5] and clinical trials [13] to have cerebral protective effects. Having reduced the internal pressure of the aneurysm to zero, the treatment of the aneurysm can be completed in a dry field, even if aneurysm rupture were to occur.

Dissection of the aneurysm must include not only the aneurysmal neck, but also the dome of the aneurysm and its backside, and the aneurysm must be separated from any small vessels in its vicinity. After identification and treatment of the neck region, the neck should be ligated and a permanent clip placed on it. Care must be taken not to bring about kinking of the parent artery when treating the aneurysmal neck.

In order to avoid damage to the vascular walls due to application of the temporary clips, we have developed a clip with a reduced blade pressure of 40–50 g [9], which we habitually use. At sites where severe arteriosclerosis is evident, however, there is a danger of releasing an atheroma plaque following damage to the vascular wall, and thereby causing vascular occlusion. In such cases, the temporary clips should be placed elsewhere.

It is essential that complete hemostasis be achieved in this operation. For this reason, after completion of the entire procedure for aspirating the hematoma, aspiration of the blood clots found deep in the subarachnoid space and those adherent to vascular walls should be done once more, thus preventing the postoperative occurrence of cerebral vasospasm.

As discussed in detail above, in the ultra-early stage operation on ruptured cerebral aneurysms, several essential points must be kept in mind: (a) the criteria for indication for surgery must be strictly observed, (b) the acute stage surgical method must be perfected, (c) steps necessary for the prevention of postoperative vasospasm must be taken, and (d) means for controlling the intracranial pressure must be employed. If all of these conditions are met, then one can be confident that favorable surgical results will be obtained.

Conclusion

Over the 8-year period since 1978, the Sendai group of neurosurgeons has performed ultra-early stage radical operations (within 3 days of the last rupture) on a total of 565 ruptured cerebral aneurysms located on the anterior portion of the circle of Willis. These cases included 335 with a preoperative grade of I or II, 146 grade III, 81 grade IV, and three grade V. Good outcomes and a return to normal social living was possible in 432 cases (76.5%). A morbidity rate of 15.4% (87 cases) and a mortality rate of 8.1% (46 cases) were obtained at the time of discharge from hospital.

Symptoms indicative of postoperative cerebral vasospasm were found in 129 cases (22.8%): approximately one half (62 cases) of them had transient symptoms and 3.3% (19 cases) were fatal. We have discussed our surgical method for ultra-early stage operations and have indicated the essential points which will allow for favorable surgical results.

References

1. Abiko H, Suzuki J, Mizoi K, Ohba M, Yoshimoto T (1986) Protective effect of phenytoin and its enhanced action by combined administration of mannitol and Vitamin E in cerebral ischemia. Brain Nerve (Jpn) 38:328–335
2. Ishibashi Y, Konda R, Yoshimoto T, et al. (1984) The effect of prazosin hydrochloride on cerebral vasospasm—an experimental study. No Shinkei Geka 23:133–139 (in Japanese)
3. Kodama N, Hori S, Kamiyama K, et al. (1980) Cervical sympathectomy for cerebral vasospasm after aneurysm rupture. In: Wilkins RH (ed) Cerebral arterial spasm. Williams and Wilkins, Baltimore, pp 680–684
4. Nishimoto A, Ueta K, Onbe H, et al. (1985) Nationwide cooperative study of intracranial aneurysm surgery in Japan. Stroke 16:48–52
5. Seki H, Yoshimoto T, Ogawa A, et al. (1983) Effect of mannitol on rCBF in canine thalamic ischemia—an experimental study. Stroke 14:46–50
6. Sonobe M, Suzuki J (1978) Vasospasmogenic substance produced following subarachnoid haemorrhage and its fate. Acta Neurochir 44:97–106
7. Suzuki J, Yoshimoto T (1978) Indication and timing in the surgery of ruptured cerebral aneurysm. Phronesis 36:34–48
8. Suzuki J, Onuma T, Yoshimoto T (1979) Results of early operations on cerebral aneurysms. Surg Neurol 11:407–412
9. Suzuki J, Kodama N, Homma M (1979) New clip and flexible clip forceps for neurosurgery. In: Suzuki J (ed) Cerebral aneurysms. Neuron, Tokyo, pp 386–388
10. Suzuki J, Komatsu S, Sakurai Y, Sato T (1980) Correlation between CT findings and subsequent development of cerebral infarction due to vasospasm in subarachnoid hemorrhage. Acta Neurochir 55:63–70
11. Suzuki J, Kodama N, Yoshimoto T, et al. (1982) Ultra-early surgery of intracranial aneurysms. Acta Neurochir 63:185–191
12. Suzuki J, Fujimoto S, Mizoi K, et al. (1984) The protective effect of combined administration of antioxidants and perfluorochemicals on cerebral ischemia. Stroke 15:672–679
13. Yoshimoto T. Suzuki J (1979) Temporary clipping—prolongation of the time of occlusion by mannitol. In: Pia HW, Langmaid C, Zierski J (eds) Cerebral aneurysms, Springer, Berlin, pp 382–392

Discussion

Commentator, *Sano* (Tokyo): Two years ago, we reviewed our series of 1130 cases submitted to surgery. We used the chi-square test and Man-witness U test; the latter we regard as particularly important since it takes into account both morbidity and mortality. The following gradings are all preoperative Hunt-Hess gradings without modification. Grade I and II patients consistently showed good results regardless of the timing of surgery. So, early surgery would be preferable in these patients to prevent rebleeding. With grade IV and V patients, the results were always poor with surgery. With these patients, it is better to delay surgery until the grade of the patient improves. Timing is also, therefore, not important in grade IV and V patients. Grade III patients, however, did show statistically significant differences according to the timing of surgery. In grade III patients, surgery performed within 3 days of onset showed the best results. In these patients, early surgery is indicated if logistical considerations permit. Age is an important factor in patients of grades II–V, patients in these grades aged 65 years and over showed bad results. Age is not important in grades I and II. Our principles for timing of surgery as follows: Surgery is indicated for grade I and II patients at any time. Patients of grade III less than 65 years of age may also be submitted to surgery during the first 3 days. Surgery for older grade II patients and patients of grades IV and V should be postponed until the patients show neurological improvement. With respect to cases where vasospasm is already present, the 2nd week after the onset of vasospasm we have found to be the optimal timing of surgery. If intracerebral hematoma is present, immediate surgery—clipping of the aneurysm and removal of the hematoma—is indicated, otherwise the patient cannot be saved. This morning's speaker did not say too much about the grading of patients. Grading is currently being discussed by the Grading Committee of the World Federation of Neurosurgical Societies. I would now like to revise the simple grad-

ing system I proposed at the Graz meeting. Grades I and II have a Glasgow-Coma score of 15. (We use the Glasgow-Coma score since it is internationally recognized.) Grade I patients are neurologically intact; grade II patients have headache and/or neck stiffness. Grade III has a Glasgow-Coma score of 13–14; grade IV has a Glasgow Coma score of 7–12; grade 5 has a Glasgow Coma score of 3–6. Previously, we gave Glasgow Coma score of 3–7 for grade V and 8–12 for grade IV. We revised our grading on the basis of a statistical analysis of our results. Of course, since this grading is very simple the information and prognosis are less satisfactory. So a modification of this grading would seem to be required. If paralysis is present this should be indicated by *RP* if on the right, or *LP* if on the left. If aphasia is present, the word *aphasia* should be added. If the patient is 65 years or older *aged* should be added. If CT shows high density, Fisher's classification should be added, e.g., *Fisher's group 3*. There are many classifications of CT and so far I have found no really satisfactory one. This point could be revised later, but for the time being I would suggest the use of Fisher's classification. Even in grades I and II, many patients later show vasospasm, but this can be modified on the basis of CT findings. There is no ideal grading system. If a lot of information is put into a grading system it will become very complicated and even then it cannot forecast completely the appearance of vasospasm or other complications. A simpler one would therefore appear to be preferred.

Schisano (Naples): I quite agree with Dr. Sengupta that antifibrinolytics should be used only if the patient did not undergo early surgery and that they should be used just for a short time. But I would like to hear his comments about dosage. I think that the dosage need is rather high. From the hematological literature, it is evident that even in generalized fibrinolysis the doses commonly used are much lower than those in neurosurgery and neurology. I think the 10%–11% recurrence reported by Dr. Kassell can also be achieved with very low doses. The important point here is to administer the drug every 6–8 h but at the lowest possible dosage. I would like to hear your comments on this.

Sengupta (Newcastle): I do not wish to give the impression that I would advocate antifibrinolytic therapy instead of early surgery. However, I would agree with you that based on the results of the study on antifibrinolysis under various circumstances for a period of 2 weeks or so, often with the addition of hypotensive therapy, that ischemia has been shown to result. Little work seems to have been done on the best dose to be used. I would agree with you that we can perhaps use doses lower than the present ones.

Brock (Berlin): In several patients, we have been forced to discontinue the administration of nimodipine because of a very marked drop in arterial pressure associated with an increase in both central venous and intracranial pressure. I would like to hear from the panelists who have experience with this drug about the incidence of this phenomenon and the measures they take when it occurs.

Auer (Graz): This point has been raised a number of times. We have not experienced such a case with a complicated course since 1981. Hypotension is a matter of debate. There are studies which show that on average patients with and without nimodipine treatment showed a similar course and there was the same incidence of hypotension in both groups. This means that low blood pressure of about 80 mmHg will be encountered in bed-ridden patients irrespective of nimodipine treatment. This parallel increase in central venous and intracranial pressures together with hypotension has been occasionally reported. We have not observed such a case ourselves. It may be an increase in cerebral blood volume that raised intracranial pressure in these cases. I am not sure about the dosage given. As far as I know the background in these cases and the additional complications that may have been the real cause of the problem are not really known.

Ljunggren (Lund): I would completely agree with Prof. Auer. We have had complications of severe hypotension in over 150 patients. There was a case recently where a nurse accidentally administered a whole bottle of nimodipine at a high dose into a patients over a period of a minute. The patient's blood pressure fell from 150 to 110 mmHg, but there were no side effects and the patient was all right. A possible explanation of the occurrence of hypotension reported by other colleagues may be interaction with other drugs. During the intravenous infusion of nimodipine, we do not give our patients any other drug, such as steroids or anticonvulsants. With respect of antifibrinolytic treatment, we think this is extremely dangerous.

Al Mefty (Jackson): There is apparently a difference in the value of early surgery between the Lund and American studies. How would the panelists explain these differences?

Kassell (Virginia): I think that the difference is the effectiveness with which vasospasm is treated. If we had been effective in treating vasospasm in the overall group of 3521 patients, the favorable outcome would have been 75%, which is the figure given in every report presented today. In the series of Drs. Drake and Peerless and myself, we do not use calcium channel-blocking agents, but we do very aggressively treat our patients with hypertensive and hypervolemic therapy, when ischemic deficits occur, the overall favorable outcome is 75%. I think the standard has been set today that whether the ischemic consequences of vasospasm are prevented or reversed hemodynamically overall favorable results of 75% should be possible to achieve. In the cooperative study the results were in the region of 58%–60% and this reflects the fact that vasospasm was not effectively treated in those patients.

Sano (Nagoya): It has been said that with grades I and II there are no problems, with grade III there are some indications for early surgery, and that with grade IV there are no indications for early operation. No one has reported poor results following a delay in surgery in grade IV patients. However, following advances in neurosurgery, it may be possible for grade III patients to be treated. But next time we will treat grade IV. If we say there are no indications for early operation in grade IV patients shall you stop the early operation in grade IV? I would think not. How do the panelists feel about this?

Sakurai (Sendai): Dr. Sano has been operating on grade IV patients but has reduced the number of surgical cases. The patient response to name calling shows whether surgery is indicated, and this accounts for about half of grade IV patients.

Saito (Tokyo): Grade IV patients with intracerebral hematoma or focal vasospasm show good results, but patients with diffuse cisternal clot always show poor results whether they are operated upon or not. The latter patients are the most difficult to treat. However Drs. Auer and Ljunggren have indicated the effectiveness of nimodipine.

Zierski (Giessen): Does anyone still believe that angiographic investigation in a patient with asymptomatic vasospasm on, say, day 3 or 4 after bleeding has any influence on the surgical decision. For example, in a patient who has a vasospasm on Doppler sonography on the 3rd, 4th, or 5th day after bleeding but who is in good condition?

Saito: A patient with diffuse vasospasm very often shows enhancement of vasospasm after the operation. But where the spasm is localized in an artery, e.g., the internal carotid or the M1 portion of the middle cerebral artery, quite good results are seen following surgery even between days 3 and 7.

Ljunggren: We rarely see patients at that stage since most of our patients arrive within 48 h. But I certainly agree that with patients with disturbed hemodynamics on Doppler flow or with established vasospasm there is the risk of deterioration through surgical trauma.

Suzuki (Sendai): I will perform an operation in spite of asymptomatic vasospasm, though of course during the surgery sodium nitrite has to be used to convert oxyhemoglobin to metohemdglobin. The main cause of vasospasm is oxyhemoglobin; metahemoglobin only causes vasospasm to a very small extent. Many neurosurgeons use a combination of hypotension and drugs, however using the Sendai Cocktail the use of hypotension, which can be dangerous in older patients, is avoided.

RTD 8. Surgical Treatment for Atherosclerotic Extracranial Lesion

Total Management of Cerebral Atherosclerosis

Sean Mullan[1]

Cerebral atherosclerosis is only one aspect of a systemic disease. It is clearly recognized that coronary occlusion is a major morbidity factor in those who suffer from carotid atherosclerosis. If the neurosurgeon is to assume a role other than that of the arterial technician, then he must assume total responsibility for bringing the maximum available total treatment to his patient. Though risk factors are now well known, and methods for minimizing them are well established, most papers on surgical management of atherosclerosis do not report an optimum concomitant medical regimen.

The epidemiological evidence for the overwhelming role of diet is long established. It is derived from the experience of both world wars, from the details of the spontaneous incidence in many countries with differing lifestyles and diets, and from studies of controlled diet, as in Finland [2, 11, 12]. The essential message is that the elimination of saturated fats reduces the incidence of atherosclerotic catastrophe, and that serious reduction of fat and calorie intake further minimizes it. Since the fat-soluble vitamins can be easily substituted, there is no nutritional need to consume fats. Their use is a matter of choice and of custom. Animal experiments have long since demonstrated that, despite fat deprivation, simple carbohydrate intake will result in ample accumulation of body fat. The need for caloric restriction must be emphasized, as existed in the world war epidemiology experience and as recommended in the recent article in the Journal of the American Medical Association, which, for longevity, recommends a body weight of 10% (or perhaps 20%) below previously accepted standards [7].

Essential protein is best obtained from ocean, preferably cold-water, fish, which contain Omega III fat. This apparently not only lowers low-density lipoprotein (LDL) but increases high-density lipoprotein (HDL) and probably affects platelet adhesiveness [3].

There is now sufficient evidence to incriminate cigarette smoking as a risk factor, so that total abstinence is recommended. A modest alcohol consumption is not deleterious and might even carry some mildly ameliorating influence [4]. The role of an antihypertensive regimen is too well known to require further mention, as is the role of aspirin and persantine in inhibiting platelet adhesion [8].

The drugs used in lowering LDL and in raising HDL include cholestyramine and colestipol, nicotinic acid, probucol, chlofibrate, and gemfibrozil. Lovastatin (Mevinolin) is a new and promising one still under study [1, 5, 6, 9, 10, 13]. Since 1960, it has been known that the quaternary ammonium amine exchange resonance lowered blood cholesterol. This is brought about by at least two mechanisms. It combines with the bile salts, glycocholine, and taurocholine, which, instead of being reabsorbed, are excreted. These, utilized by the liver as building blocks for cholesterol, are lost. The liver is, of course, an efficient synthesizer of the relatively simple cholesterol molecule, and it simply makes more, but there is a tendency not to keep up, especially if alternate mechanisms are also interfered with. The second mechanism also depends upon the bile sequestration property. This, by interupting the necessary emulsification of ingested fat, limits absorption. The reduced saturated fat intake will reduce the stimulus to produce more LDL. A combined effect results in a substantial fall in blood LDL without much change in the very low-density lipoprotein (VLDL) fraction. Since cholestryramine, which is a very large molecule, is neither broken down nor absorbed, it can be administered in very large doses (24–36 gm daily). It has a grainy texture and is something like flavored clay. Its greatest problem is a marked tendency towards constipation. A theoretical malabsorption of fat soluble vitamins has not appeared, probably due to supplementary in-

[1] Department of Neurosurgery, University of Chicago Medical Center, Chicago, Illinois, USA

take. It may interfere with administration of warfarin, digitalis, and thyroxin, and possibly with other drugs. If anticoagulation is necessary, cholestyramine should be discontinued. The great importance of cholestyramine is that in the very rigorous Lipid Research Clinics Coronary Primate Prevention Trial study, a decrease of 8% in total cholesterol resulted in a 19% decrease in coronary heart disease risk over a period of 7.4 years. Most other studies have depended upon correlating a drug with a lowered serum cholesterol but without the clinical correlation, or else the numbers involved were not sufficient to be truly impressive.

Colestipol is quite similar to cholestyramine but is slightly less expensive. It has been recently associated with Lovastatin in the most spectacular cholesterol reduction trial to date.

Nicotinic acid, or niacin, is a vitamin widely found in food, of which we need 100 mg daily. Lack of it (due to deficient diet) causes pellagra. Its derivative, nicotinamide, also controls pellagra but has nothing to do with cholesterol. In a dose up to 9 g daily, that is 90 times the daily requirement, it will effectively lower LDL as first reported in 1955. At these higher levels, it may interfere with liver function, causing an increase in uric acid, a change in glucose, and, eventually, change in liver enzymes. The effect is reversible. Immediately after ingestion, there may be a flushing of the skin of brief duration due to a wide opening of the small blood vessels in the skin, producing a type of hot flash. This can be reduced or eliminated by one aspirin tablet daily. Occasionally, a dermatitis can result. Numerous clinical studies attest to its ability to lower both LDL cholesterol and triglycerides, but no long-term controlled clinical study has yet been done to prove that it will limit the clinical progression of atherosclerosis.

Probucol is another drug of potential merit. It too has a significant cholesterol lowering effect, but VRLD may be lowered more than LDL, and HDL is usually lowered more than LDL. It is, therefore, probably inadvisable in those patients who already have a low HDL. It increases the excretion of fecal bile acid: it may also decrease the early cholesterol synthesis. There is some evidence that it induces arrhythmias in animals given an atherogenic diet, but only a prolonged Q-T interval has been noted in humans. It should not be taken unless the patient is on a low fat diet and is free from cardiac arrhythmias. Its efficiency in lowering cholesterol is well documented, but, in controlling clinical atherosclerosis, it remains unproven.

Chlofibrate, first reported in 1962, is probably more effective in dealing with raised triglycerides than a high LDL fraction. It has been used in England and in Scotland, and a significant effect in controlling incidence of stroke has been reported. On occasion it produces a change in liver enzymes. There may be gastric symptoms, and an altered response to antiarrhythmic drugs and anticoagulant drugs has been reported.

A very recent study on the combined use of lovastatin (mevinolin) and colestipol has given a 48% reduction in LDL levels and a 17% increase in HDL levels. Further studies will be necessary to determine both the ultimate safety of this new medication and the ultimate influence upon atherosclerosis progression [12].

Probably the best combination of drugs now available to reduce cholesterol is that of cholestyramine or colestipol and niacin. A problem exists as to what is the optimum figure. Over the years, the standards have become more rigorous. Earlier standards were based upon averages in Western society, in which 50% of the population died of atherosclerosis. More recently, a figure of 160 mg/ml, which is in the low normal range in Japan, is accepted. Not much thought has been given to the possibility of an even more desirable 120 mg. Since HDL has an apparently ameliorating effect, we seek a figure in the high range of about 60 mg/ml. A total cholesterol (TC) divided by an HDL figure of less than three or an LDL divided by HDL of less than two is sought. Patients who carry the Lp (a) lipoprotein apparently have a hereditary disposition to atherosclerosis even when the cholesterol is in the low normal range. Perhaps we should aim at a subnormal figure for these indivduals.

In medical decisions, we like to have evidence that is quite precise or seems to be quite precise, such as an arteriogram, even though, as we have found in the EC/IC bypass, apparent precision may not reveal precise truth. We tend to distrust imprecise evidence even when the accumulative impact is, indeed, substantial. Much of the evidence for medical management is derived by analogy from studies of coronary atherosclerosis, not cerebral atherosclerosis. Does this mean that we should passively accept the annual 6% increment that is inherent in the uncontrolled state without medical intervention? Should we advise token medical control such as the now discredited "Prudent" diet, or should we not clearly point out to the patient the options that are now available? Frequently we underestimate the patient's resolve. The majority, when absolutely confronted with the prospect of cascading strokes and heart attacks, are quite prepared to make radical changes in their lifestyle. They will accept medications which will alter known risk factors, even though the long-term, carefully controlled clinical studies have not yet been carried out. Since these medical regimens are based upon sound presumptive evidence of control, and since they involve no known dangers, it would appear ethically improper to make them unavailable just because proper statistical studies may still be a decade away.

The major problem is what to do with a patient who has a cholesterol level within the low normal range. It is well recognized that cholesterol is not the only factor in atherosclerosis, but it is a final factor in all cases. The presumption exists that a figure lower than normal should be effective, and it would be reasonable to aim for a 25% reduction below that which is generally considered normal. This would be especially true if HDL was low, in which case the aim would be to produce a more favorable LDL/HDL ratio.

References

1. Borhani NO (1985) Prevention of coronary heart disease in practice. JAMA 254, 2:257–264
2. Keys A (1975) Coronary heart disease. Atherosclerosis 22:149–192
3. Kromhout D, Bosschieter EB, Coulander D (1985) The inverse relation between fish consumption and 20-year mortality from coronary heart disease. J Engl J Med 312, 19:1205–1209
4. Lieber CS (1984) To drink (moderately) or not to drink? N Engl J Med 310, 13:846–7
5. Lipid Research Clinics Program (1984) The lipid research clinics coronary primary prevention trial results: I. Reduction in incidence of coronary heart disease. JAMA 251, 3:351–364
6. Lipid Research Clinics Program (1986) The lipid research clinics coronary primary prevention trial results: II. The relationship of reduction in incidence of coronary heart disease to cholesterol lowering. JAMA 251, 3:365–373
7. Manson JE, Stampfer MJ, et al. (1987) Body weight and longevity: A reassessment. JAMA 257, 3:353–358
8. Mettinen TA, Juttlunen JK, Kaukkarinen V, et al. (1985) Multifactorial primary prevention of cardiovascular diseases in middle-aged men. JAMA 254, 15:2097–2102
9. Rhoads GG, Dahlen G, Berg K, et al. (1986) Lp (a) lipoprotein as a risk factor for myocardial infarction. JAMA 256, 18:2540–2544
10. Schaefer EJ, Levy R (1985) Pathogenesis and management of lipoprotein disorders. In: Flier JS, (ed) Seminars in medicine of the Beth Israel Hospital, Boston. N Engl J Med 312, 20:1300–1310
11. Turpeinen O (1979) Effect of cholesterol-lowering diet on mortality from coronary heart disease and other causes. Circulation 59:1–7
12. Vartiainen I, Kanerva K (1947) Arteriosclerosis and war-time. Ann Med Fenn 36, 3:748–758
13. Vega GL, Grundy SC (1987) Treatment of primary moderate hypercholesterolemia with lovastatin (mevinolin) and colestipol. JAMA 257, 1:33–38

Surgical Management of Extracranial Atherosclerosis: Indications and Timming

W. Richard Marsh and Thoralf M. Sundt, Jr.[1]

Operative treatment of all types of occlusive cerebrovascular disease is undergoing an agonizing reappraisal of operative indications. Carotid endarterectomy is no exception. Optimal information on the natural history of carotid occlusive disease is obtained from population-based surveys in which an entire community can be under medical surveillance for a long period of time. In this way, a determination of stroke incidence and survival following transient ischemic attack can made. Such data from the population of Rochester, Minnesota have been obtained and analysed. This analysis shows that the probability of survival following first transient ischemic attack is 91% at 6 months, 88% at 1 year, and 50% between 7 and 8 years. Actuarial assessment of the probability of stroke among patients following first transient ischemic attacks shows an 8% probability of stroke at 1 month, 10% probability of stroke at 6 months, 13% probability of stroke at 1 year, and a 40% probability of stroke at 8 years. Thus, in order to improve upon this natural history by any operative treatment, the morbidity and mortality of each proposed treatment must be low. In a series of 1935 patients operated upon by our department from 1972 to 1984, the overall mortality was 1.3%, major morbidity 1%, and minor morbidity 1%. Using the Sundt grading schema, the combined morbidity/mortality was less than 1.0% in grade I, 1.8% in grade II, 4.0% in grade III, and 8.5% in grade IV. We believe carotid endarterectomy can be an effective operation for patients with symptomatic carotid stenosis [1].

Optimal therapy for many human diseases is lacking. Ideally, complete understanding of the biochemistry and pathophysiology would lead to preventive medicine or at least treatment directed at the cause of the disease. Realistically,

however, this is not possible for many human conditions, of which cerebral atherosclerosis is ore. Consider only that it is one aspect of a condition affecting the entire organism and that often it is neither symptomatic nor even the chief threat to life or limb for an individual patient. Nevertheless, the potential disability to an individual is often great from cerebral infarction due to atherosclerosis.

More than any other event or observation, it was the recognition that episodes of transient focal cerebral ischemia were often the prelude to a serious, potentially disabling stroke that stimulated interest in developing means of treatment that might prevent or at least delay serious incapacity from cerebral infarction. Fisher first suggested the term transient ischemic attack, or TIA, to describe this situation. Further understanding has shown that there are many possible causes for such transient cerebral dysfunction, large extracranial vessel disease being only one (Table 1). Before the efficacy of carotid endarterectomy as therapy for patients with TIA can be evaluated, an understanding of the natural history of TIA occurring in patients with known carotid occlusive disease is necessary. Ideally, this would be done in a randomized, controlled manner, with a contemporary control group of

Table 1. Categories of pathophysiological mechanisms of TIA

1. Large artery atherosclerosis with or without ulceration
2. Intracranial artery atherosclerosis with or without ulceration
3. Hemodynamic decrease in blood flow associated with focal intracranial or extracranial arterial stenosis or occlusion
4. Small arterial or arteriolar disease
5. Migraine (vasospasm?)
6. Arterial dissection with or without thrombosis
7. Inflammatory arterial disease
8. Cardiac disease

[1] Department of Neurological Surgery, Mayo Clinic, Rochester, Minnesota, USA

Table 2. Actuarial estimation of probability of survival (TIA, Rochester, Minnesota, 1955–1969)

Years after diagnosis	Persons alive at start of interval	Survival rate (%)	Adjusted normal survival rate (%)	Mortality ratio
1/12	184	96	99.6	9.6
6/12	176	91	97.5	3.6
1	170	88	95	2.4
2	161	82	90	1.8
3	151	75	85	1.6
4	138	70	80	1.5
5	129	63	75	1.5
6	113	58	71	1.5
7	100	52	66	1.4
8	81	46	62	1.4

Table 3. Actuarial estimation of probability of stroke, given survival prior to stroke (TIA, Rochester, Minnesota, 1955–1969)

Years after diagnosis	Persons alive and free of stroke at start of interval	Probability of stroke, given survival (%)	Expected probability of stroke (%)	Observed to expected ratio
1/12	184	8	0.067	120
6/12	167	10	0.4	25
1	159	13	0.8	16
2	151	19	1.6	12
3	137	25	2.4	10
4	122	26	3.2	8
5	114	29	4	7
6	99	31	4.8	6
7	88	36	5.6	6
8	69	40	6.4	6

optimal medically treated patients and a treatment group with patients undergoing operation. At this point in time, such information is, of course, not available. However, we do have retrospective data regarding the natural history of TIA from which some inferences can be drawn regarding the value of carotid endarterectomy.

Population-based studies are optimal for defining the natural history of TIA. The population of Rochester, Minnesota is an excellent resource for such study because the medical record system at the Mayo Clinic and the record linkage system to the community provide a continuing medical record of each patient in the community who seeks medical care. This population has provided the most complete information to date on the natural history of TIA.

The average annual incidence rate of TIA in Rocheser is 31 per 100 000 population for all ages. This rate increases with age such that, in the decade age 65–74 years of age, the incidence is 220 per 100 000 population per year. Prevalence rates for the same population show that about 1% of persons in the 65–74 age group and 2% over age 75 were alive and had not had a stroke after one or more TIA's.

The two major areas of importance, with respect to the natural history of TIA, are probability of survival and probability of stroke following the first TIA. The probability of survival following the first TIA and the expected survival for a normal population of the same age and sex distribution is seen in Table 2. The 50% survival is between 7 and 8 years. Review of the data shows a greatly increased probability of death in the first 4–6 weeks and that, by 2 years, the death rate approaches 1.5 times the normal population. The primary cause of death is cardiac disease since nearly 50% of the deaths were of cardiac origin. Stroke, both ischemic and hemorrhagic, was also an important contributor to mortality, with 29% of deaths being due to some type of stroke.

Actuarial estimates of the probability of stroke

Table 4. Results of carotid endarterectomy for primary stenosis—1 January, 1972 to 31 December, 1984

Grade	Cases	Neurological complications					Mortality			
		Transient deficit	Ischemic stroke		Intracerebral hemorrhage		Ischemic stroke	Intra-cerebral hemorrhage	Myocardial infarct	Other
			Minor	Major	Minor	Major				
I	632	5	4	1	0	0	0	1	0	0
II	402	6	4	2	0	1	0	0	0	0
III	549	10	3	4	1	1	0	1	9	2
IV	352	14	8	8	0	3	3	5	2	2
Total	1935	35	19	15	1	5	3	7	11	4

Overall, mortality approximates 1.3%; major morbidity is 1.3% and minor morbidity is 1% in patients with primary carotid stenosis. This does not include the grade V group of 37 patients with preoperative occlusion and hemiplegia nor the group of 57 cases with recurrent disease

are shown in Table 3. Most of the 10% stroke probability in the first 6 months after TIA occurred in the 1st month. No significant difference was noted between carotid and vertebrobasilar TIA.

Among the 777 Rochester patients who had their first cerebral infarct between 1955 and 1969, only 9% were known to have a prior TIA. This is in contrast to all patients with cerebral infarction seen at the Mayo Clinic from outside Rochester. In this group, 30% of the patients had experienced a TIA. This is another example of the subtle selection process for patients seen at referral centers.

From the above data it can be concluded, firstly, that a patient experiencing a TIA is at significantly increased risk of a fatal myocardial event in the 1st year after the TIA, secondly, that there is a substantially increased risk of stroke in the first several months after TIA but, following this "window of vulnerability," the risk diminishes appreciably, and, thirdly, that a majority of cerebral infarcts occur without a warning TIA. If a given patient's cause for TIA is carotid stenosis and carotid endarterectomy is the treatment, then the risk of operation— including morbidity and mortality—must be lower than the actuarial probability of stroke in the untreated population experiencing TIA. While the above data lumps patients with TIA from all causes and does not separate patients out with TIA from carotid stenosis, nevertheless, it does suggest that the combined morbidity and mortality from any procedure must be less than 5% for any appreciable benefit from operation to accrue to the patient.

The experience at our institution would sug-

Table 5. Morbidity and mortality by grade

Grade	Mortality/morbidity
I	<1.0%
II	1.8%
III	4.0%
IV	8.5%

gest that these figures for morbidity and mortality are achievable. From 1 January 1972 to 31 December 1984, 1935 carotid endarterectomies were performed for primary stenosis of the extracranial carotid artery. Patients were classified preoperatively into four grades based on a combination of risk factors, including medical, angiographic, and neurological factors. All patients underwent cerebral angiography prior to operation. Surgery was performed under general anesthesia with a volatile anesthetic agent. A variety of anesthetic agents were employed: early in the series halothone was used predominately but, in recent years, isothrome has been employed. All patients were monitored with continuous intraoperative electroencephalography (EEG) and measurements of cerebral blood flows (CBF). We feel these techniques allow the operation to be performed in an expeditious but unhurried fashion. An indwelling shunt is used, depending upon the information obtained from the EEG and CBF measurements. The patient is heparinized for the period of temporary carotid occlusion and the heparin is not reversed at the end of the case. Most of the vessels are not closed primarily but with the use of a saphenous vein patch graft. We feel there is at

Table 6. Grade of patient with primary stenosis v. type and frequency of complication

Grade of patients	No. of cases	Type of complication									
		Post-operative occlusion	Intra-operative emboli	Post-operative emboli	Occlusion time ischemia	Infarct con-tralateral carotid or VB	Migraine variant	Seizures	Intra-cerebral hemorrhage	Myocardial[a] infarction	Other[b]
I	632	4	3	1	1		1		1		
II	402	3	3	2	1		3	1	1		
III	549	4	3	4		1	2	2	3	10	2
IV	352	4	6	3	3	3	4	10	8	2	2
Total	1935	15	15	10	5	4	10	13	13	12	4

[a] Includes only those complications leading to neurological symptoms or death
[b] For example, mesenteric artery occlusion
VB vertebrobasilar

least a fourfold reduction in acute postoperative occlusion by this technique and believe that it may reduce the rate of restenosis at the operative site.

The overall mortality approximates 1.3% with major morbidity of 1.3% and minor morbidity of 1% (Tables 4, 5). When the combined mortality and major morbidity is analyzed by preoperative grade, we see the figure for grade I is less than 1%, grade II is 1.8%, grade III is 4.0%, and grade IV is 8.5%. The major types of complications and instances observed were as follows (Table 6): acute postoperative occlusion in 15 cases (0.8%), intraoperative emboli in 15 (0.8%), postoperative seizure in 13 (0.7%), intracerebral hemorrhage in 13 (0.7%), myocardial infarct in 12 (0.6%), and postoperative emboli in 10 (0.5%).

We have further analyzed a subgroup of 151 conservative patients who had transient focal cerebral ischemia in one carotid arterial system and who underwent carotid endarterectomy on the side corresponding to the symptoms. Long-term stroke morbidity was less than would have been expected for a comparable group of patients with TIA, and the percentage of deaths due to a cardiac cause was higher than expected,

owing to a relative shift from stroke mortality to cardiac mortality.

Operative treatment of all types of occlusive vascular disease is undergoing a reappraisal of indications for operation. We look forward to the results of the proposed Canadian Symptomatic Cooperative Study in which patients suffering a TIA, nondisabling stroke, or reversable ischemic neurological deficit, will be randomized to medical and surgical therapy. Close attention must be paid to that part of the study population eligible but not randomized and also the morbidity/mortality figures for the surgical arm of the study. On the basis of our own retrospective data, we believe carotid endarterectomy performed by an experienced surgical team on selected patients with ipsilateral carotid system transient ischemia can reduce subsequent stroke morbidity.

References

1. Sundt TM (ed) (1987) Occlusive cerebrovascular disease: Diagnosis and surgical management. Saunders Philadelphia

Pitfalls During Carotid Endarterectomy

Fernando G. Diaz and James I. Ausman[1]

Carotid endarterectomy has been used in the management of patients with arteriosclerotic cerebrovascular occlusive disease since it was described by Carrea et al. in 1956 [5]. DeBakey [7] made considerable efforts toward making this procedure safe and acceptable in the management of patients with cerebral ischemic symptoms. Most use the procedure for patients presenting with unilateral cerebral ischemic symptoms which result from arteriosclerotic lesions in the ipsilateral carotid artery [1–4, 12, 18, 23, 24]. These patients, in general, should have presented with transient ischemic attacks, reversible ischemic neurological deficits, or mild cerebral infarctions which have resolved, leaving only a minor or no residual deficit [3, 6, 12, 13]. The carotid lesions considered suitable for surgical excision are stenotic lesions which encompass 80% or more of the cross-sectional diameter of the artery as seen on biplane angiography, and/or lesions which are ulcerated with or without significant associated stenotic lesions [1, 10, 12, 13, 18, 19, 21]. The types of ulcers found most likely to result in embolic phenomena are the C-type lesions described by Moore et al. [15]; these are large and irregular ulcerated lesions.

Great controversy exists over whether an asymptomatic carotid lesion should be excised prophylactically [9, 16, 17, 22, 23, 25, 26]. In general, most would agree that stenotic lesions which are greater than 80% of the cross-sectional diameter of the vessel, or which progress rapidly to that degree of stenosis, carry an increased risk of developing a cerebral infarction and should, therefore, be considered suitable for prophylactic removal [9, 16, 17, 23]. There is no data available regarding the potential for cerebral infarction in patients harboring an asymptomatic carotid ulceration. Many believe that far too many carotid endarterectomies are being performed in the United States, and that perhaps this procedure is overutilized [25, 26]. However, no definitive data has been reported in the literature to objectively support this argument.

Arterial Problems

The carotid artery may present several problems during the course of a carotid endarterectomy. These problems include anatomical variables as well as technical problems [1, 4, 14, 18]. The anatomical variables which may be a problem include different sites of origin for the carotid bifurcation in the neck, elongations or rotation of the vessels in the neck, and different calibers for the carotid artery. The technical problems to consider include the possible perforation of a very thin carotid artery wall in a site different than the one where the endarterectomy has been performed, tearing of the wall of the carotid artery during the closure of the arteriotomy from excessive pressure on the suture line or from a very thin carotid artery wall, stenosis on the carotid artery lumen secondary to a constrictive surgical repair, kinking or torsion on the origin of the internal carotid artery, residual intraluminal tags in any of the vessels which were endarterectomized, intimal flaps in the distal ends of the plaque on either end of the vessel, and occlusion of the vessels which were endarterectomized from the development of a dissection of the intima or from a stenosing arterial closure [4, 8, 12, 14, 18].

Most problems which arise from variations in the normal anatomy of the carotid artery can be handled by having a clear understanding of the anatomy of the carotid artery and its surrounding structures. It cannot be overemphasized that the planning for the operation has to take place during the evaluation of the angiographic studies in the days preceding the operation. Through careful analysis of the angiographic anatomy, the surgeon can best draw an operative plan

---

[1] Department of Neurosurgery, Henry Ford Hospital, Detroit, Michigan, USA

based on the images seen: the surgical approach can then be tailored to the anatomy found [10, 14, 18]. A high or low carotid bifurcation can then be approached with an appropriately placed incision, rotation or kinking on the carotid arteries can be anticipated and appropriate steps taken to make the correct identification of the vessels once they have been exposed, and potentially small arteries can receive the required prosthetic or autologous vein patch which must be secured prior to the performance of the endarterectomy [4, 18, 21].

The technical problems which may be encountered generally result from deviation from basic surgical principles in the course of the carotid endarterectomy. Thinning of the arterial wall which may lead to the development of perforations or tears on the arterial wall usually result from a vigorous removal of the plaque. Care must be taken to remove as much of the plaque as possible to perform a satisfactory operation, but being overzealous in the removal of the plaque may be unwise, since the vessel wall may become damaged in the process. The removal of the plaque may be started in a variety of ways, depending on the surgeons training and practice. What we consider important in the process is to make sure that the plaque is sectioned proximally flush with the arterial wall so not to leave a flap which may become raised and may stenose the proximal lumen of the endarterectomy [8]. The dissection of the plaque may then be continued distally on the common, internal, and external carotid arteries, with care not to enter the most peripheral layers of the media. The distal ends of the endarterectomy may then be removed in one of two ways: they can be removed under direct vision with the direct transection of the plaque where it feathers with the vessel wall [14, 20] or; when the plaque is thick and well-developed, it may be removed through an intussusception technique, everting the vessel and then removing the plaque. The advantage of the former method to the open method is that the terminal ends of the plaque may be visualized, and any small dissections of the distal intima may then be fixed to the vessel wall directly prior to the closure of the endarterectomy [12, 13, 14, 20]. The intussusception method does not permit the internal fixation of the distal intima, and many surgeons would prefer not to use this method of excision for this reason. The disadvantage of the open method is that it requires a longer period of carotid clamping: since it requires the opening of the internal

carotid artery, it also requires its closure, with the potential development of stenosis [4, 8]. The clamping of the carotid artery is usually much less with the intussusception technique, and the potential for stenosis of the internal carotid artery does not exist since this artery is never opened.

Distal occlusion of the carotid artery has occurred with either of the two techniques described, and generally results from inadequate fixation of the distal intima [8, 14, 21]. During the open procedure, one must insure that the distal intima will not be elevated by the jet of blood by placing tacking sutures holding the intima to the vessel wall. During the intussusception technique, one cannot place intimal sutures, and the surgeon must confirm on the operative table that the vessel will remain patent at the end of the operation by either measuring flow in the different vessels with a doppler, obtaining a transoperative dopscan, or performing an arteriogram. We have found some patients who have required the reopening of their endarterectomy for fixation of distal points of dissection. The time required for the reopening of the vessel, the excision of the intimal tags, and the fixation of the distal intima has not resulted in any additional morbidity in our patients.

The carotid artery plaque may not end in the neighboring area of the endarterectomy in some cases, but continue with a long tail into the more distal internal carotid artery. When this occurs, it is necessary to transect the tail end, which extends further up into the carotid artery, and fix that end to the vessel wall so that it will not become detached. This can only be done through the open procedure.

The vessel lumen is generally large, even in patients who have had a stenotic plaque for many years. However, in some patients, the caliber of the artery is very small; even after the endarterectomy, little additional lumen is gained by the force of the arterial pressure over the vessel wall. This can sometimes be anticipated preoperatively and measures can be taken to harvest a vein for patch grafting of the carotid artery [4, 12, 14, 18]. When this has not been planned beforehand, the patch may be fashioned with any number of synthetic materials available for arterial repair [21]. To perform either one of these patching procedures, or, in many cases, for a conventional endarterectomy, many have recommended the routine use of an intraluminal shunt to prevent the development of transoperative ischemia [2, 12–14, 19, 20].

A number of problems may arise from the use of an intraluminal shunt [2, 12, 14, 19, 21], including the introduction of emboli into the cerebral circulation, which may be either air, cholesterol, or thrombotic material. The shunt, when introduced into the vessel lumen, may dissect the endothelium from the luminal surface of the vessel wall and create either an intimal flap or evolve into a complete dissection or occlusion of the artery. The shunt may get kinked inside the vessel lumen or may become obstructed if it is pressed against the vessel wall. When this happens, the purpose of the shunt is defeated, since the brain would not get any more blood than without the shunt. The only way to prevent the inadvertent occlusion of the shunt would be to use a shunt that has, incorporated in its wall, a blood flow recording system to monitor and insure flow through the shunt once it has been placed. Without this attachment, the placement of the shunt may give a false sense of security, since there would not be any definitive certainty that the shunt is really functioning.

Stenosis of the arterial lumen of the internal carotid artery may develop when the incision is extended into the internal carotid artery, especially when the artery is of small caliber to begin with. When the arteriotomy is closed by primary intention, the only way to minimize the potential for stenosis of the internal carotid artery is to make sure that the absolute minimum amount of arterial wall edge is used for the closure of the arterial opening. Using mostly or only the adventitial portion of the wall is not adequate because it will result in the development of a pseudo-aneurysm at the suture line [8]. When the caliber of the artery is too small, the only alternative is to use a patch to close the arterial wall [1, 4, 8, 14]. Stenosis of the arterial wall may also occur when a long arteriotomy defect is closed with a single running suture. The tendency in this situation is to pull the suture too tightly, which will result in the development of purse stringing at the suture line with wrinkling and stenosis at the distal end of arterial closure. To prevent this problem, one may have to use two or three different running sutures interrupted at short intervals.

Nerve Problems

The normal anatomical relationship of the carotid artery to many cranial and peripheral nerves makes any surgical procedure directed to its treatment subject to the potential risks of damaging any one of these nerves. The problems most commonly seen result from traction or dissection of the superior laryngeal nerve, which is usually found deep and medial to the internal carotid artery as it separates from the vagus nerve high in the neck. The inadvertent manipulation, traction, or laceration of this nerve will result in moderate hoarseness. In contrast with this observation, lesions to the inferior or recurrent laryngeal nerve are less common and usually result from traction on the trachea as the sternocleidomastoid muscle is separated from the medial structures. Lesions to the recurrent laryngeal are more common on the right side because the nerve is shorter and more superficial than on the left side. The severity of the dysphonia is much greater than on patients who have suffered lesions to the superior laryngeal nerve [1, 14, 21].

The mental branch of the facial nerve is sometimes damaged by retraction applied to the mandible, resulting in the development of retraction of the inferior margin of the lower lip on the ipsilateral side. This is usually a subtle finding, but it can be very disturbing to some patients, especially women. The branch may get traumatized when it swings below the edge of the mandible, especially when the dissection is carried out high in the neck requiring retraction applied near the horizontal portion of the mandible [1, 14].

Horner's syndrome is infrequently observed in patients after a carotid endarterectomy [1, 14]. This usually results from trauma to the ascending sympathetic chain in the retrocarotid space. When the dissection of the carotid artery is extended posteriorly beyond the carotid sheath and the sympathetic nerves are manipulated, retracted, or transected, one may observe Horner's syndrome. These patients have their neurological problems usually for short periods of time, and their symptoms usually resolve completely.

Lesions to the phrenic nerve, to the cervical root nerves, or to the brachial plexus branches are possible but very infrequent. The dissection of the cervical structures has to be carried out too far laterally to reach these nerves: unless they have an anatomical anomaly in their location, one would not expect to see any lesions to these nerves resulting from the procedure. Upper extremity symptoms of peripheral nerve involvement may be seen in some patients, resulting from pressure applied on the ulnar nerves from inadequate padding of the elbows [1].

Wound Problems

Local wound problems, such as infections and hematomas, may also develop after a carotid endarterectomy [1, 14]. A wound infection may mean a very big problem because of the potential for the development of a periarterial abscess with the possibility for dehiscence of the suture line and blowout of the arteriotomy [1, 14, 21]. Any wound infection after a carotid endarterectomy must be treated very aggressively. Any areas of suppuration must be immediately drained and the patients should receive antibiotic therapy. Most of these infections generally resolve rapidly and heal uneventfully.

Wound hematomas are usually the result of inadequate hemostasis on the periarterial tissues, which may frequently be complicated when these patients have received antiplatelet agents preoperatively. In some of these patients who were treated with antiplatelet agents, hematomas will develop in spite of very meticulous hemostasis. Some of these hematomas may become very large and could compromise respiration by displacing the trachea [1, 11, 14, 18]. When this happens, endotracheal intubation is generally all that is needed while the hematoma resolves spontaneously. In very few cases, it has been necessary to return the patient to the operating room for surgical removal of the hematoma. Some patients who develop bleeding from the suture line do require the surgical closure of the leaking site because the hemorrhage is occurring under arterialized pressure. Hematomas in these patients usually expand very rapidly, and respiratory distress develops in the immediate postoperative period [11].

Chyle fistulas or chyle cysts may be seen in some patients when the dissection is extended too far down near the base of the neck, especially on the left side near the site of drainage of the thoracic duct [1, 14]. The duct is generally visible and must be sutured to prevent leakage from its lumen. When the duct is transected inadvertently, one can readily identify the chyle fluid by its milky character. Suture of the leaking site is then imperative to prevent any further leakage of chyle. When the leak is not identified until the postoperative period, pressure dressings may be effective in controlling the leakage if its small. A temporary drain with a low fat diet has been effective in some individuals, but, in general, these fistulas are very indolent and require operative surgical correction.

References

1. Allen GS, Preziosi TJ (1981) Carotid endarterectomy: A prospective study of its efficacy and safety. Medicine 60:298–309
2. Baker WH, Dorner DB, Barnes RW (1977) Carotid endarterectomy: Is an indwelling shunt necessary? Surgery 82:321–326
3. Blasisdell WF, Clauss RH, Galbraith JG, Imparato AM, Wylie EJ (1969) Joint study of extracranial arterial occlusion: IV. A review of surgical considerations. JAMA 209:1889–1895
4. Callow AD, Matsumoto G, Cossman D, Stein A (1977) Early restenosis after carotid endarterectomy. Stroke 8:14
5. Carrea R, Molins M, Murphy G (1955) Surgical treatment of spontaneous thrombosis of the internal carotid artery of the neck. Acta Neurol Latinoam 1:71–78
6. Cartlidge NEF, Whisnant JP, Elveback LR (1977) Carotid and vertebral basilar transient cerebral ischemic attacks. Mayo Clin Proc 52:117–120
7. DeBakey ME (1975) Successful carotid endarterectomy for cerebrovascular insufficiency: 19 year follow-up. JAMA 223:1083–1085
8. Diaz FG, Patel S, Boulos R, Mehta B, Ausman JI (1982) Early angiographic changes after carotid endarterectomy. Neurosurg 10:151–161
9. Durward AJ, Ferguson GG, Barr HWK (1982) The natural history of asymptomatic carotid bifurcation plaques. Stroke 13:459–464
10. Eisenberg RL, Nemjek WR, Moore WS, Mani RL (1977) Relationship of transient ischemic attacks and angiographically demonstrable lesions of carotid artery. Stroke 8:483–486
11. Erwin D, Pick MJ, Taylor GW (1980) Anaesthesia for carotid artery surgery. Anaesthesia 35:246–249
12. Ferguson GG (1982) Extracranial carotid artery surgery. Clin Neurosurg 29:543–574
13. Jauid M, Taylor C (1978) Neurosurgical experience with carotid endarterectomy at university hospitals. Wisconsin Med J 77:65–68
14. Matsumoto GH, Cossman D, Callow AD (1977) Hazards and safeguards during carotid endarterectomy: Technical considerations. Am J Surg 133:458–462
15. Moore WS, Boren C, Malone JM, Roon AF, Eisenberg R, Goldstone J, Mani R (1978) Natural history of nonstenotic asymptomatic ulcerative lesions of the carotid artery. Arch Surg 113:1352–1359
16. Quinones-Baldrich WJ, Moore WS (1985) Asymptomatic carotid stenosis: Rationale for management. Arch Neurol 42:378–382
17. Roeder GO, Yanglois YE, Jager KA, Primozich JF, Beach KW, Phillips DJ, Strandness DE (1974) The natural history of carotid artery disease in asymptomatic patients with cervical bruits. Stroke 15:605–613
18. Sundt TM, Sandok BA, Whisnant JP (1975)

Carotid endarterectomy complications and preoperative assessment of risk. Mayo Clin Proc 50: 301–306

19. Sundt TM, Sharbrough FW, Piepgras DG, Kearns TP, Messick JM, O'Fallon WM (1981) Correlation of cerebral blood flow and electroencephalographic changes during carotid endarterectomy with results of surgery and hemodynamics of cerebral ischemia. Mayo Clin Proc 56:533–543

20. Thompson JE (1979) Complications of carotid endarterectomy and their prevention. World J Surg 3:155–165

21. Thompson JE, Garrett W (1980) Peripheral arterial surgery. NEJM 302:491–503

22. Toole JF, Janeway R, Choi K, Cordell R, Davis C, Johnston F, Miller HS (1975) Transient ischemic attacks due to atherosclerosis: A prospective study of 160 patients. Arch Neurol 32:5–12

23. West H, Burton R, Roon AJ, Malone JM, Goldstone J, Moore WS (1979) Comparative risk of operation and expectant management for carotid artery disease. Stroke 10:117–121

24. Whisnant JP, Sandok BA, Sundt TM (1983) Carotid endarterectomy for unilateral carotid system transient cerebral ischemia. Mayo Clin Proc 58:171–175

25. Yatsu FM, Fields WS (1985) Asymptomatic carotid bruit, stenosis or ulceration: A conservative approach. Arch Neurol 42:383–385

26. Ziegler DK (1983) Carotid lesions—to operate or not to operate? Current Concepts Cerebrovasc Dis 18:7–10

Surgical Treatment of Atherosclerotic Extracranial Lesions

Is There an Indication for Carotid Endarterectomy?

Sydney J. Peerless and Henry J.M. Barnett[1]

Introduction

The most common disease of the brain causing death, serious disability, and prolonged suffering is ischemic stroke. Although the incidence of ischemic stroke has declined markedly in the past 30 years, the prevention of stroke continues to be a major concern of neurologists, neurosurgeons, and, indeed, the whole medical community.

Carotid endarterectomy, as a therapy to prevent stroke, has been practiced since the mid-1950s and is being performed with increasing frequency. In 1971, 15000 carotid endarterectomies were done in the United States; by 1982, 82000 were performed and an estimated 125000 were done in 1984. It has been estimated that the hospitalization and medical care related to the procedure costs the US health care system 2.1 billion dollars annually [10–12]. This increase in the number of endarterectomies has occurred despite the fact that the incidence of stroke has gone down by at least 40% in the same period of time due, in part, to improved management of risk factors and the use of platelet antiaggregates. At the same time, improved surgical technique, anesthesia, and intensive care measures have undoubtedly combined to make carotid endarterectomy safer and possibly more effective as a prophylactic procedure.

There have been two previous attempts at randomized controlled clinical trials to determine the benefit of carotid endarterectomy. Neither of these trials could be claimed to be definitive, and both concluded that the procedure was not better than medical therapy. It is highly possible that both trials, because of imperfect design or execution, overlooked a benefit of the surgical procedure.

The uncertainty as to the value and indications for carotid endarterectomy arises from the fact that we do not know what the outlook is for patients with extracranial atherosclerotic occlusive disease without surgery, particularly in the face of modern medical management [3, 4, 8, 20, 21, 23, 24, 27, 37]. We are also uncertain as to the risk for stroke in certain selected subgroups of patients (e.g., degree of carotid stenosis, ulceration of the atherosclerotic plaque, tandem lesions). Moreover, we are very aware that any possible surgical benefit is highly dependent on the perioperative risks of the surgical procedure, which may vary considerably among surgeons and units [2, 7, 13, 16, 17, 26].

What is the risk for stroke and stroke death in patients with symptomatic extracranial atherosclerotic carotid artery disease? One can arrive at an answer in only a most approximate fashion. The populations that have been studied vary considerably in such factors as age, sex, the extent of complicating cerebral arterial disease, coexisting heart disease, hypertension, and diabetes. As well, there is little data on patients who are symptomatic and who have had complete cerebral angiography to document clearly the degree and extent of their atherosclerotic occlusive disease. In a joint study [15], 149 patients randomized to the medical group with cerebral ischemic symptoms had carotid artery lesions which were not necessarily appropriate to their symptoms, but experienced a stroke rate of 13% and a combined stroke and death rate of 26% in the 42 months of follow-up.

In those patients not receiving aspirin [5] who entered with symptoms of transient cerebral ischemia and minor stroke in the Canadian platelet antiaggregant trial, the risk of stroke and death combined was 13% in the first year, 22% by the end of the second year, and 30% by the end of the three years. The French trial of aspirin demonstrated that 15% of a similar group of patients suffered stroke or fatal stroke after 3 years [6]. A 10-year follow-up of the London, Ontario center's contribution to the Canadian aspirin study included 158 patients, of whom 94% had arteriography. These patients had a

---

[1] Divisions of Neurosurgery and Neurology, The University of Western Ontario, London, Ontario, Canada

total ischemic stroke rate of 5.5% per year, of which 2.9% were ipsilateral to their original symptoms, and 2.6% in other territories. In this same group of patients, 80 patients had surgically accessible internal carotid artery lesions and were not operated upon. When these potential surgical patients were reexamined with a view to determine whether the degree of stenosis of their carotid artery was a predictor of subsequent stroke, it was found that 21% of the patients with severe stenosis (greater than 70%) had suffered a stroke and 27% of those with less than 70% stenosis had suffered stroke in the 10 years of follow-up [22].

Control of risk factors and the use of either anticoagulants or antiplatelet agents have been the mainstay of medical management of patients at risk for cerebral stroke. The use of anticoagulants has declined markedly in the past decade, since the introduction of platelet antiaggregating agents. Aspirin is now an established therapy for the prevention of subsequent cerebrovascular events based on five prospective double-blind studies. In these studies, the annual stroke rate is 3% per year, and stroke and/or death is 5% per year in those patients treated with aspirin. These scientifically credible trials have shown that stroke and stroke death were reduced by one-third to one-half in those patients receiving aspirin as compared to the control group [5, 6, 14, 30].

It is also clear that, in addition to aspirin, the optimal management of elevated blood pressure decreases the risk of subsequent stroke. The control of serum lipids and the cessation of cigarette smoking also reduce the risk of stroke, but these measures are more difficult to achieve because of the lack of patient compliance [34, 39].

What is the evidence that certain subgroups of patients are particularly benefited by carotid endarterectomy? It is suggested that frequent, or crescendo, transient ischemic attacks (TIAs), like unstable angina, are clear indication for endarterectomy because of the high likelihood of the patient going on to suffer a stroke which can be prevented by removing the stenosing carotid plaque. Convincing data to support this popular notion is not available. Indeed, in the EC-IC Bypass Study [31, 32], 80% of the medical patients and 78% of the surgical patients had experienced a reduction of 50% or more of their frequent TIAs. Moreover, studies carried out by Atcheson and Hutchison [1], Marshall [23] and Baker [4] did not detect a statistically significant

difference in the number of strokes after medical treatment in patients who presented with many ischemic events, as opposed to those that presented with few.

Urgent surgery has also been suggested in patients presenting with transient ischemia or progressing stroke and the detection of intraluminal thrombus in the carotid artery at the time of angiography. The reports which suggest that this is an emergent surgical indication, document few patients without controls [9, 33]. A recent review of 31 patients in our institution, of whom 23 had severe carotid stenosis proximal to an intraluminal thrombus, suggested a better outcome for the 14 patients treated initially by anticoagulants than for the 17 patients treated with urgent surgery. There were no new strokes nor worsening of infarction in the medically treated patients, as compared with five episodes of new or larger infarction in the surgically treated patients. Of the 14 patients who were initially treated with anticoagulants, six underwent delayed surgery and one suffered a fatal cerebral infarction [18]. Based on these observations in nonrandomized patients, who may well be dissimilar, one cannot be certain that urgent surgery in the presence of radiologically visualized intraluminal thrombus is justified.

Because of surgeon's preoccupation with flow and the hemodynamic theories of stroke, it has been generally held that the tighter the stenosis, the more dangerous is the atherosclerotic lesion [29]. This notion is supported by evidence of follow-up studies of patients with asymptomatic disease indicating that their prognosis for subsequent ischemic events increases when the narrowing has reached more than 80%. This data has not been supported in follow-up of symptomatic patients. Similarly, conflicting evidence regarding the significance of angiographically demonstrated ulcerative lesions has also been reported. To our knowledge, there is no data available to indicate that either degree of stenosis, with or without ulceration, constitutes a firm indication for carotid endarterectomy [22, 25].

Finally, the manner of presentation of patients has not been shown to be a good guide to select patients who will benefit from the operation. Harrison and Marshall [19] reported on 215 patients with TIA, reversible ischemic neurological deficit (RIND), or partial stroke, with angiographically confirmed carotid lesions. Treatment, not determined by any statistical study design, involved endarterectomy in 61, EC-IC bypass in one, anticoagulants in 91, acetylsalicylic acid (ASA) only in 22, and other therapies to manage risk factors alone in 40. Of these, 188 patients were followed until death, or for a mean period of 4.1 years, and the risk of stroke and death was not significantly different among the therapeutic groups [19]. However, the prognosis for both stroke and death was worse in those patients with occluded carotid arteries than in those with normal arteries. The outlook for stroke-free survival was the same in those patients with carotid arteries that were only irregular and not significantly stenosed as in those with significantly narrowed carotid arteries.

Because we have such fragmentary data on the natural history of extracranial atherosclerotic occlusive disease, and because surgical morbidity and mortality figures are derived from populations that certainly differ from the overall population at risk, it is not possible to determine the effect of surgery on producing stroke-free survival in patients presenting with symptomatic or asymptomatic carotid occlusive disease. Walow [35], using data from 18 reports over a 20 year period, compiled the morbidity and mortality in patients presenting with TIA and undergoing endarterectomy. The combined operative stroke and death risk in this aggregate of 2097 patients ranged between 2.5% and 24.4% with an average of 7.4%. Similar figures can be obtained from small and large consecutive series of surgical patients from community hospitals and from units with specialized expertise in cerebrovascular disease. All of these reports lack a clear definition and systematic documentation of perioperative stroke and other intraoperative complications, and the factors used to select or reject those patients for surgery.

A survey of North American vascular surgeons and neurosurgeons, active in the performance of carotid endarterectomy in the year 1981, has been reported by Fode, Sundt, Robertson, et al. [17]. Data derived from 46 institutions, involving 3328 patients submitted to endarterectomy, demonstrated an average combined postoperative mortality and significant morbidity of 6.4%. Whisnant, Sandok, and Sundt [38] studied a consecutive series of 151 patients operated on at the Mayo Clinic and documented a 4%, 30-day, operative morbidity and mortality. This prospective but uncontrolled study is unique in its careful attention to methodological detail combined with independent neurological examination.

It is clear that endarterectomy must be performed with careful pre- and postoperative management, as well as expert anesthetic and operative skill. To be an effective treatment, endarterectomy must be done with an operative risk which is sufficiently low that, within a few years, the benefit to these surgically treated patients can be demonstrated to be clearly superior to medical therapy alone.

Two previous randomized evaluations of carotid endarterectomy have been done. Both trials suffer from insufficient numbers. The Joint Study [15] randomized 316 patients with documented carotid stenosis, but only 55% had symptoms referable to their carotid disease, and 45% presented with vertebrobasilar symptoms. During the 42-month follow-up period, the 169 patients assigned to surgery suffered a stroke rate of 12% and a combined stroke and death rate of 27%. The 147 patients assigned to the medical group experienced a 13% rate of stroke and 26% rate of stroke and death. The 30-day perioperative stroke and death rate was 11%, and suggests that it would require more than 4 years before any benefit could be expected by the survivors. Only 94 patients, with only unilateral carotid stenosis, were randomized. Only 45.4% of the surgical group and 50.3% of the medical group had appropriate carotid symptoms. Although a reduction in TIA was noted in those patients undergoing endarterectomy, a significant benefit in stroke prevention was not demonstrated.

A small British randomized study [28] was flawed with a 35% operative morbidity and mortality after only 41 patients had been entered. The trial was abandoned because it was evident that there was no hope of proving efficacy of the endarterectomy over medical therapy.

In 1981, a British-European randomized trial of endarterectomy was undertaken [36]. By 1986, a total of 850 patients had been entered, with three patients being randomized to surgery for every two patients randomized to medical therapy alone. There is concern that the British-European trial may not satisfy the demands for endarterectomy in North America for three reasons. First, the procedure is done much less frequently in Britain and Europe. Second, the British-European protocol allows centers to exclude patients with major stenosis from the trial and, finally, the relatively few patients in the British-European trial will not permit the identification of a possible important subgroup who might benefit from the procedure.

Conclusions

It would seem clear that, although carotid endarterectomy is a frequently performed operation and is increasing in its use, the therapy is unproven and should be scientifically evaluated for its efficacy. This is particularly true in that the incidence of stroke continues to decline dramatically, making it essential to reexamine the benefit-to-risk ratio of any therapy designed to prevent stroke and stroke-related death. Moreover, previous attempts to assess carotid endarterectomy have not shown a benefit from the procedure, but these studies have not been definitive. It is certain that the medical management of stroke has changed substantially since carotid endarterectomy was first used, but, at the same time, the safety of anesthesia and the surgical procedure has also improved, increasing the likelihood of the overall efficacy.

We believe that the probability is that carotid endarterectomy, when carried out by a well trained expert surgeon in an optimum clinical setting, is a beneficial therapy for some patients who are yet to be defined. There is then the need for a credible randomized study to determine if there is a favorable risk-to-benefit ratio for carotid endarterectomy in patients with carotid stenosis and transient cerebral ischemia or partial stroke.

There are three specific questions that must be answered. Does the addition of carotid endarterectomy to optimal medical care reduce the risk of subsequent stroke and stroke-related death and improve stroke-free survival over time in patients with TIA or partial stroke and appropriate carotid stenosis? Does the degree of carotid stenosis, with and without ulceration, affect outcome and which of these subgroups of patients most benefit from carotid endarterectomy? Will the functional status of the patient, following carotid endarterectomy, remain the same, deteriorate, or improve with time in comparison to patients who are not operated upon?

We hope to answer these important questions with a North American carotid endarterectomy trial which will begin to randomly assign patients to the medical or surgical arms of the study in September 1987. Fifty-two centers in Canada and the USA, involving an equal number of vascular surgeons and neurosurgeons with documented experience and skill in the procedure, have agreed to collaborate with the research plan. The trial will involve 3000 patients entered over a 2-year period and followed for an average of 5 years by an independent neurologist. In all centers, nonrandomized patients will be reported and characterized. A system of alerting rules will ensure that the study will be stopped if there is evidence of harm patients because of unexpected morbidity or mortality from the endarterectomy, or because significant benefit is detected in the surgical group or major subgroup thereof.

We hope to show that carotid endarterectomy will alter the clinical course of atherosclerotic carotid stenosis in an enduring way by arresting the advancing disease, enhancing health by preventing stroke, improving function, and postponing death. To prove this with scientific credibility will be of great value to all of our patients.

References

1. Acheson J, Hutchinson EC (1964) Observations of the natural history of transient cerebral ischemia. Lancet II: 871–874
2. Allen GS, Preziosi TJ (1981) Carotid endarterectomy: A prospective study of its efficacy and safety. Medicine 60:298–309
3. Anderson GI, Whisnant JP (1982) A comparison of trends in mortality from stroke in the United States and Rochester, Minnesota. Stroke 13:804–809
4. Baker RN, Ramseyer JC, Schwartz WF (1968) Prognosis in patients with transient cerebral ischemia. Neurology 18:1156–1165
5. Barnett HJM (1979) The Canadian Cooperative Study of platelet-suppressive drugs in transient cerebral ischemia. In: Price TR, Nelson E (eds). Cerebral diseases. Raven, New York, pp 211–236
6. Bousser MG, Eschwege E, Haguenau M, et al. (1983) "AICLA" controlled trial of aspirin and dipyridamole in the secondary prevention of athero-thrombotic cerebral ischemia. Stroke 14:5
7. De Weese JA, Rob CG, Satran R, et al. (1971) Endarterectomy for atherosclerotic lesions of the carotid artery. J Cardiovasc Surg 12:299–308
8. Dixon S, Pais SO, Raviola C, et al. (1982) Natural history of nonstenotic asymptomatic ulcerative lesions of the carotid artery. Arch Sur 117:1493–1497
9. Donnon GA, Bladin PF (1979) The stroke syndrome of long intraluminal clot with incomplete vessel occlusion: Clinical and experimental. Neurology 16:41–47
10. Dyken M (1986) Personal communication
11. Dyken ML, Calhoun RA (1983) Changes in stroke mortality: Effects on evaluating and predicting outcome for therapeutic studies. In: Reivich M, Hurtig HI (eds) Cerebrovascular diseases. Raven, New York, pp 51–55
12. Dyken ML, Pokras R (1984) The performance of

endarterectomy for disease of the extracranial arteries of the head. Stroke 15:948–950

13. Easton JD, Sherman DG (1977) Stroke and mortality rate in carotid endarterectomy: 228 consecutive operations. Stroke 8:565–568

14. Fields WS, Lemak NA, Frankowski RF, Hardy RJ (1977) Controlled trial of aspirin in cerebral ischemia. Stroke 8:301

15. Fields WS, Maslenkiov V, Meyer JS, et al. (1970) Joint study of extracranial arterial occlusion: V. Progress report of prognosis following surgery or non-surgical treatment for transient cerebral ischemic attacks and cervical carotid artery lesions. JAMA 211:1993–2003

16. Fleming JFR, Griesdale DE, Schutz H, Hogan M (1977) Carotid endarterectomy: Changing morbidity and mortality. Stroke 8:14

17. Fode NC, Sundt TM, Robertson JT, et al. (1986) Multicenter retrospective review of results and complications of carotid endarterectomy in 1981. Stroke 17:370–376

18. Gates PC, Buchan AM, Barnett HJM (1985) Luminal thrombus in the cerebral circulation. Stroke 16:140

19. Harrison MJG, Marshall J (1982) Prognostic significance of severity of carotid atheroma in early manifestations of cerebrovascular disease. Stroke 13:567–569

20. Harward IRD, Kroener JM, Wickbom IG, Bernstein EF (1983) Natural history of asymptomatic ulcerative plaques of the carotid bifurcation. Am J Surg 146:208–212

21. Kannel WB, Wolf PA (1983) Epidemiology of cerebrovascular diseases. In: Russell RW (ed) Cerebral arterial disease, 2nd edn. Churchill-Livingstone, Edinburgh

22. Lauzier S, Cote R, Ogunyemi A, et al. (1986) Predictive value of cerebral atheroma in 158 patients—a ten year follow-up. Stroke 17:5

23. Marshall J (1964) The natural history of transient ischemic cerebrovascular attacks. Quart J Med 33:309–324

24. Matsumoto N, Whisnant JP, Kurland LT, Okazaki H (1973) Natural history of stroke in Rochester, Minnesota, 1955 through 1969: An extension of a previous study, 1945 through 1954. Stroke 4:20–29

25. Moore WS, Boren C, Malone JM, et al. (1978) Natural history of nonstenotic asymptomatic ulcerative lesions of the carotid artery. Arch Surg 113:1352

26. Nunn DB (1975) Carotid endarterectomy: An analysis of 234 operative cases. Ann Surg 182:733–738

27. Roederer GO, Langlois YE, Jager KA, et al. (1984) The natural history of carotid arterial disease in asymptomatic patients with cervical bruits. Stroke 15:605

28. Shaw DA, Venables GS, Cartlidge NEF, et al. (1984) Carotid endarterectomy in patients with transient cerebral ischemia. J Neurol Sci 64:45–53

29. Sundt TM, Sharbrough FW, Piepgras DG, et al. (1981) Correlation of cerebral blood flow and electroencephalographic changes during carotid endarterectomy with results of surgery and hemodynamics of cerebral ischemia. Mayo Clinic Proc 56:533–543

30. The Canadian Cooperative Study Group (1978) A randomized trial of aspirin and sulfinpyrazone in threatened stroke. New Engl J Med 299:53–59

31. The EC/IC Bypass Study Group (1985) The international cooperative study of extracranial/intracranial arterial anastomosis (EC/IC bypass study): Methodology and entry characteristics. Stroke 16:397–406

32. The EC/IC Bypass Study Group (1985) Failure of extracranial-intracranial arterial bypass to reduce the risk of ischemic stroke. Results of an international randomized trial. New Engl J Med 313:1191–1200

33. Thompson JE, Austin DJ, Potman RD (1970) Carotid endarterectomy for cerebrovascular insufficiency: Long-term results in 592 patients followed 13 years. Ann Surg 172:663–679

34. Tuomilehto J, Nissinen A, Wolfe E, et al. (1985) Effectiveness of treatment with antihypertensive drugs and trends in mortality from stroke in the community. Br Med J 291:857–861

35. Warlow C (1984) Carotid endarterectomy: Does it work? Stroke 15:1068–1076

36. Warlow C (1986) Personal communication

37. Whisnant JP, Matsumoto N, Elveback LR (1973) Cerebral ischemia attacks in a community. Mayo Clinic Proc 48:194–198

38. Whisnant JP, Sandok BA, Sundt TM Jr. (1983) Carotid endarterectomy for unilateral carotid system transient cerebral ischemia. Mayo Clinic Proc 58:171–175

39. Wolf PA (1986) Cigarettes, alcohol and stroke. New Engl J Med 315:1087–1089

Surgical Treatment of Extracranial Internal Carotid Malformations

Giampaolo P. Cantore[1]

Extracranial internal carotid malformations (EICM) are usually congenital, but are often worsened, and sometimes caused, by arteriosclerotic lesions. EICM may be responsible for cerebrovascular insufficiency by embolic or hemodynamic mechanisms. In the former case, they produce changes in blood flow with turbulence and vortexes that are the causes of embolism formation as a result of platelet aggregation. In the latter case, there are hemodynamic alterations from temporary occlusion of the vessel during head movements or from hypotensive attacks [1]. Obviously, a malformed vessel is more likely to cause problems of cerebrovascular insufficiency when associated with anomalies of other epiaortic vessels and/or the circle of Willis, or with stenosing arteriosclerotic alterations of other epiaortic or cerebral vessels. While the incidence of cerebrovascular insufficiency from atheromatic alterations of the epiaortic vessels is greatest in people age 50–60 years, in EICM the most frequently involved age group is 30–50 [6].

By EICM, we mean course anomalies, wall alterations, which may often be associated with one another, and carotidojugular fistulas. More precisely, course anomalies consist of tortuosity, coiling, and kinking. Wall alterations consist of aneurysms and fibromuscular dysplasia. Tortuosity is an undulation of the internal carotid artery's course, which assumes an S or C form; coiling is elongation and redundancy of the internal carotid, resulting in an exaggerated S-shaped curvature or in circular configuration. Kinking is the angulation of one or more segments of the internal carotid [9]. These three alterations may be associated with atheromatic plaque. By aneurysm, we mean a circumscribed dilatation, either saccular or fusiform, of the arterial wall that is often secondary to dysplasia in the neck vessels. Fibromuscular dysplasia is an alteration of the artery wall due to a defect in

development; these walls may undergo various modifications.

The incidence of course anomalies (coiling and kinking) varies from 5% to 24%, if we refer to radiological case series [1]. In surgical case series, the course anomalies alone in endarterectomies vary from 4.8% to 34.6% [1]. In our case analysis, the percentage of EICM operated (including all types of malformations) with respect to endarterectomy was 14.4%. From an etiopathogenetic point of view, we have divided EICM into congenital and acquired groups, even though there is no common agreement on this. Tortuosity, coiling, and dysplasia are considered congenital. In the embryo, the internal carotid is normally angled and the artery assumes its normal straight morphology when the fetal heart and the large vessels descend into the mediastinum. In some cases, this process is probably not completed, so that the curvature of the embryonic period persists and, as a result, produces a varying grade of angulation, undulation, and tortuosity. The association between intracranial aneurysms and course anomalies of the internal carotid of the neck, the frequent finding of tortuosity and coiling in young patients who do not suffer from arterial hypertension or arteriosclerosis, as well as the very frequent bilaterality of the lesion, all testify in favor of the congenital theory. Moreover, these malformations, which are not only bilateral but are also equidistant from the bifurcation [1], may be associated with course anomalies of the vertebral arteries and, less frequently, with arteriovenous fistulas of the extracranial vessels or with intracranial angiomas. Fibromuscular dysplasia is a multifocal angiopathy whose etiology is unknown, and which may cause multiple concentric stenoses and/or aneurysmal dilatation. Recent studies suggest that its origin is multifactorial with minimal congenital lesions of the smooth muscle cells and the internal elastic membrane, favoring an anomolous fibroproliferative response to circulatory or mechanical stimulation. On the other hand, the pathogenesis of kink-

[1] Department of Neurological Sciences, University of Rome, Rome, Italy

ing seems to be an acquired condition. Saphir [7] considers kinking to be due to arteriosclerosis which results in dilatation and stretching of the artery. Florin, as quoted in Weibel and Fields [9], found that the wall of the artery was thinner at the level of the kinking and believes a defect of the media associated with arteriosclerosis to be responsible.

In our opinion, all these factors play an important role in the formation of kinking, especially when there is already redundancy of the carotid, as in the case of congenital tortuosity. Aneurysms may be congenital or acquired: when there is a dysplasic alteration of the wall, they are of a congenitally acquired nature: if they are posttraumatic, mycotic, or degenerative, then they are acquired [8].

Once the ischemic nature of the neurological syndrome has been determined and other possible embolic origins excluded by echocardiogram and Holter, the diagnostic iter consists of Doppler sonography and echotomography of the epiaortic vessels, and EEG recording, which later serves as a comparison with intraoperative and postoperative parameters. However, for surgical indication, angiography is essential. The most comprehensive data is supplied by traditional selective angiography with a complete study of the four epiaortic vessels, in the various head positions and possibly in different projections. This method also shows any delays in transit of contrast medium at the level of the malformation. However, neither the selective angiography nor the digitalized angiography are able to show changes in intima in the form of plicae, which are often present in coiling or kinking and play an important role in the formation of platelet aggregation. In EICM with a middle or high localization, it is helpful to temporarily occlude the internal carotid during selective angiography by means of a balloon catheter with the patient awake and with simultaneous EEG recording, as a means of evaluating the efficiency of the compensatory circulation and foreseeing the necessity of using the intraoperative internal shunt. To reduce the risks connected with selective angiography, we follow Fox's protocol [4]. When selective angiography is contraindicated or is difficult to perform, digitalized angiography may be carried out as an alternative. If this does not give sufficient information, then it is essential to resort to direct puncture of the common carotid, against the current if possible.

Surgery of EICM began together with endarterectomy but has not gained the same popu-

larity due to three main difficulties: the first is encountered in trying to reach EICM with middle or high localization, the second in the use of temporary internal shunt (when necessary), and the third in the incidence of postoperative occlusions. Any surgeon about to perform this type of operation must be well aware of these problems and face them one at a time, beginning with treatment of the more straightforward EICM and, in the case of those with a high localization, deciding to operate only if certain they are responsible for the attacks of cerebral ischemia in patients who have already been treated with antiaggregants and, sometimes, anticoagulants, or only if the EICM has caused hemorrhage, compression of the cranial nerves, or cerebral circulation steal.

The surgical approaches designed to give exposure of the internal extracranial carotid, from the carotid bifurcation to the carotid canal, are diverse and become increasingly more difficult the higher up they reach. Although the bifurcation does not correspond to the same vertebral level in all patients, and although one type of malformation may not always have the same characteristics, in order to simplify things we will divide EICM into low, middle, and high, according to their localization. The low localization refers to those below C3, the middle localization to those between C3 and the lower limit of the body of C1, and the high localization comprises those from the lower limit of C1 to the carotid canal.

Starting from the bottom and going upwards, we have used a variety of approaches either singly or combined, such as the tradiional approach along the anterior border of the sternocle idomastoid muscle, with eventual cutting and tendinous suture of the digastric muscle, and possible dislocation of the mandible, as described by Fry and Fry, for treatment of traumatic carotid lesions [5]. We also have used the approach described by Sundt for treatment of aneurysms of the extracranial carotid [8], and the "type A" infratemporal approach proposed by Fisch for the treatment of chemodectoma and for aneurysms of the carotid canal [3]. Exposure of low EICM does not present difficulties, even though it is sometimes necessary to cut the digastric muscle and dislocate the mandible, both procedures being decided intraoperatively, with the sole precaution of intubating the patient through the nose [2].

For surgery of middle EICM, it is often sufficient to cut the digastric muscle and dislocate the mandible, but sometimes Sundt's approach [8] is necessary. This must be planned preoperatively because it necessitates pre- and retroauricular incision, anterior exposure of the parotid and the seventh cranial nerve (CN) distally to the stylomastoid foramen, cutting of the descending branch of the twelfth CN, cutting of the occipital artery, sectioning of the digastric muscle and the styloid muscles, sectioning of the stylomandibular ligament, and exposure of the ninth, tenth, and eleventh CN.

In the case of high EICM, Sundt's approach is sometimes sufficient for exposure, but more frequently Fisch's approach is necessary. This must be planned preoperatively in as much as it requires moving the pavilion of the ear forward by means of a retroauricular incision, cutting of the external auditive canal, exposure of the parotid and seventh CN distally to the stylomastoid foramen, mastoidectomy, removal of the tympanic membrane, anvil, and hammer, exposure and arterior transposition of the seventh CN from its canal and, finally, exposure of the intrapetrous tract of the internal carotid artery. Before considering direct surgical attack on EICM, the certain and/or possible damage deriving from these approaches should be carefully evaluated. While neither cutting and tendinous suture of the digastric muscle nor intraoperative dislocation of the mandible present inconvenience for the patients, Sundt's approach carries a moderate incidence of disturbances of deglutition, phonation, and facial paresis which are, in general, transitory. Fisch's approach causes permanent transmissive-type deafness, and possibly deglutition and phonation disturbances, and facial paresis, generally transitory.

The choice of approach depends not only on the localization of the malformation but also on the need to use the internal intraoperative shunt, and on the complexity of the operation we intend to perform on the carotid. In low EICM and in some of the middle ones, the use of the shunt can be decided during surgery, while for the middle-high localizations, it is advantageous to know beforehand, using a balloon catheter, whether the shunt is needed, because, in this case, the surgical approach must make allowances for sufficient exposure of the carotid above the malformation. Intraoperatively, the need for shunt is decided on the basis of the parameters regarding stump pressure, EEG, and somatosensory-evoked potentials. For further cerebral protection during surgery, general anesthesia is carried out by means of neuroleptoanalgesic, keeping the PCO_2 around values of 30–40 torr: barbiturate protection is given during carotid clamping. Routinely, the radial artery is cannulated for continuous monitoring of systemic arterial pressure, keeping the pressure at preoperative values. We prefer the Heyer-Schulte-Sundt-type shunt or the Heyer-Schulte one with a balloon on the tip. We advise inserting the shunt through an incision of the common carotid or the internal carotid at more than a centimeter below the carotid stump, beneath the malformation: this will facilitate removal of the shunt and the application of Derra-Cooley forceps once anastomosis is completed.

Surgery of EICM should aim at total removal of the malformation and successive correct alignment of the carotid with nonstenosing anastomoses. The best results are obtained when, after removal of a course anomaly (tortuosity, kinking, coiling), direct anastomosis of the two stumps of the internal carotid is possible. If this is not possible, then we can resort to interposition of a tract of saphena taken from the patient's thigh, avoiding the use of heterologous material, which is the most frequent cause of postoperative occlusion, even after many months. In coiling and kinking with high localization, as an alternative to total removal of the malformed tract when there are technical difficulties and especially when the internal shunt is necessary, we can completely unwind the malformation and shorten the normal tract of carotid interposed between the bifurcation and the malformation. This technique aims at straightening and normalizing the course of the carotid, but there is still the problem of the plicae in the intima, often present in the malformed tract. This problem can be partly solved by angioplasty, using metallic dilators with progressive diameters. In such cases, when the internal shunt is necessary, the dilators can be inserted through the incision through which the shunt has been removed, alternating brief periods of clamping of the carotid artery with longer periods of restored blood flow, with application of Derra-Cooley forceps. With the exception of a few particular cases, the mere unwinding of the malformation, without shortening, and solely transposing the digastric muscle and/or suspending it from the sternocleidomastoid muscle to avoid a new angulation of the redundant vessel, is not advisable. In general, this technique does not ensure good alignment and, moreover, preserves the malformed tract together with any possible plicae.

Surgical treatment of internal extracranial carotid aneurysms should also aim toward complete substitution of the affected tract of vessel, because there are usually considerable full-thickness changes of the carotid wall on which the aneurysm has formed: the neck is often inexistent and numerous thrombi inside the sac often appear in the carotid lumen. For these reasons, the use of long clips for giant aneurysms is not advisable: they also tend to slide down towards the carotid after application, thus causing stenosis.

Complete removal of the malformation should be carried out for dysplasias as well, unless the initial results with angioplasty force us to change our opinion in the future. In the case of arterovenous fistulae of the carotid circulation with subtraction of blood to the cerebral area, for the middle-high localizations, treatment with inflatable and detachable balloon according to Debrun's technique is indicated, with surgical completion when needed.

Finally, in cases where the patient is very much at risk whether he is directly operated for EICM or not operated at all, complete closure of the internal carotid at the bifurcation may be considered, performing a good canalization between the common carotid and the external carotid, providing that the ophthalmic artery gives good compensatory circulation. After closure of the carotid, other alternatives may be STA-MCA bypass or bypass with interposition of saphena vein between the extracranial and intracranial carotids. Obviously, in surgery for EICM, when there is atheromatic plaque at the bifurcation, careful endarterectomy of both the internal and external carotids should be performed. Similarly, when we plan a normal endarterectomy and find ourselves faced with tortuosity of the first tract of the internal carotid, the advantages of shortening should not be ignored because the tortuous carotid, as a result of its loss of rigidity after endarterectomy and its detachment from the surrounding tissues, may be subject to angulation or postoperative occlusion.

The third problem regarding EICM surgery is the incidence of postoperative carotid occlusion which makes it necessary to employ several technical devices and introduce a suitable anticoagulant therapy. The devices advised are: magnifying glasses, anastomosis performed with a very oblique angulation, use of 5/0 and 7/0 suture thread/silk according to the width of the wall, temporary aneurysm clips on the internal carotid and suitable clamping forceps regulated at not more than 120 g of closing/pressure, graft

of saphenous vein avoiding the use of heterologous material, periodic intraoperative declamping of the upper stump of the internal carotid, and frequent Doppler-sonographic checks of the ophthalmic artery postoperatively. The anticoagulant therapy which we currently use, after various past protocols, consists of calcic heparin administered subcutaneously 48 h before surgery at an initial dosage of 8000 IU, three times a day, with repeated checks of partial thromboplastin time values on the second postoperative day. Indirect anticoagulants are associated with the heparin therapy: heparin is suspended when the prothrombin time international wormalaized Ratio value is between 2 and 3.5. Anticoagulants are continued for 3 months in order to allow complete endotherlization of the vessel. At the end of this period, anticoagulants are replaced by antiaggulants. Previously, other protocols of the type used in cardiac surgery for coronary bypass were used, with continuous endovenous infusion of the heparin by micropump; but several complications of the operative wound and one death due to hemoperitoneum persuaded us to give up this method.

From 1974 through 1986, we operated on 72 EICM in 63 patients, nine of which were bilateral. Over the last 2 years we have operated on 30 patients using approaches to reach middle and high malformations. Since 1974, we have operated on 27 coilings, 27 kinkings, four tortuosities associated with atheromatic plaque, eight aneurysms, four fibromuscular dysplasias, one case of coiling associated with chemodectoma, and one carotid-jugular fistula which was treated first by a detachable balloon method and then surgically. In 34 cases, the approach used was traditional, in 29 anterior dislocation of the mandible associated with cutting of the digastric muscle in nine, Sundt's approach in six, and Fisch's approach in three. The malformation was removed in 43 cases with end-to-end suture between the two vessel stumps; in six the malformation was straightened out; in two cases the ICA was closed and the common carotid canalized into the external carotid: one after application of a long giant aneurysm clip which caused thrombosis of ICA, and another for a dissecting aneurysm of the internal carotid extending up to the carotid canal. During 1974, in the first six cases, the malformation was replaced by heterologous material, and, in the next 14, by saphenous vein. Temporary internal shunt was used in eight cases (11.1%). One patient died 24 h after surgery because of severe hemi-peritoneum. Eight patients presented dysphonia, transitory in all but one, five presented transitory dysphagia, two had transitory, and one other permanent, deficits of the seventh CN, in addition to permanent transmissive deafness in three patients operated by Fisch's approach. Two patients had transitory hemiparesis congruous with the operated side. Follow-up varied from 2 months to 12 years with an average of 4.2 years. Of the 63 patients operated for EICM, 55 were postoperatively checked by angiography and eight by echotomography. Of the former, 49 showed good alignment of the operated vessel without stenosis at the level of suture. Six patients, in all of whom the malformation had been replaced by heterologous material, had carotid thrombosis: three within the 1st month and three within 18 months. In two other cases, the internal carotid was closed and external carotid canalized. Three patients had new ischemic attacks 6 months, 1 year, and 3 years after surgery: angiographic control showed good visualization of the operated vessel without stenosis in all three while CT revealed ischemic areas at the cerebellar level in one case and was negative in the other two. On the basis of our results, we believe that EICM, responsible for CVI attacks, should always be surgically corrected, while those adjacent to the carotid canal should only be considered for surgery in selected cases. In fact, the approach required for these malformations causes a greater incidence of deficits of cranial nerves and, therefore, we think surgery is justified only when the vascular alteration is very stenosing, when anticoagulant therapy does not protect the patient from new ischemic attacks, or when there is hemorrage or compression of the cranial nerves.

References

1. Cantore GP, Delfini R, Ciappetta P, Santoro A, Oppido P, Zanette E, Buttinelli C (1986) Le malformazioni della carotide interna extracranica. 3rd Meeting Nazionale della Società Italiana di Neurosonologia. 24–25 October 1986, Turin
2. Cantore GP, Delfini R, Mariottini A, Santoro A, Cascone P Anterior displacement of the mandible for better exposure of the distal segment of the extracranial carotid artery. Acta Neurochirurg (in press)
3. Fisch U (1970) Transtemporal surgery of the internal auditory canal: Report of 92 cases, technique, indications, and results. Adv Oto rhinolaryng 17:203–204
4. Fox AJ (1981) Cerebral angiography in TIA and stroke. In: Barnett H, Paoletti P, Flamm E, Brambilla G (eds) Cerebrovascular diseases: New trends in surgical and medical aspects. Elsevier North-Holland, Amsterdam pp 107–121
5. Fry RE, Fry WJ (1980) Extracranial carotid injuries. Surgery 88:581–587
6. Leipzig TG, Dohrmann GJ (1986) The tortuous or kinked carotid artery: Pathogenesis and clinical consideration. A historical review. Surg Neurol 25:478–486
7. Saphir O (1935) Serpentine aneurysm of the internal caroid artery. Arch Pathol 20:36–45
8. Sundt TM, Pearson BW, Piepgras DG, Houser OW, Mokri B (1986) Surgical management of aneurysms of the distal extracranial internal carotid artery. J Neurosurg 64:169–182
9. Weibel J, Fields WS (1965) Tortuosity, coiling and kinking of the internal carotid artery: I. Etiology and radiographic anatomy. Neurology (Minneap) 15:7–18

Surgical Treatment of Extracranial Atherosclerotic Lesions

Hirohisa Ono[1]

Extracranial atherosclerotic lesions have long been treated with carotid endarterectomy and various arterial bypass graft procedures. The bypass procedures have been proven to provide no beneficial effect in prevention of stroke recurrence. However, the EC/IC bypass study raised serious questions and admonitions against the traditionally accepted belief that stroke can be prevented by simply restoring loss of blood flow in the brain. Moreover, the randomization of structural abnormalities, such as angiographic abnormalities, may not be enough to predict outcome of functions. The carotid endarterectomy may follow the same fate if future studies are designed to randomize stroke patients solely upon the degree of carotid stenosis and ulceration by angiogram. It is well known that results of many randomization studies contradict each other. This may reflect inadequacies in factors randomized, or incapability of these structural randomizations in prediction of functional outcome. The latter may be analogous to so-called used car evaluation pessimism. The pessimism relates to the difficulty in predicting durability of the car, even with the most elaborate mechanical and structural evaluation. The mechanical and structural evaluation does not include the handling and the maintenance of the car, which can be more decisive in determination of the prognosis of the car. No such functional factors are randomized in stroke studies, such as physical activities, psychological stresses, personal characteristics, socioeconomic status, working conditions and hours, and many others. Accordingly, in order to have the current randomization method be able to overcome the pessimism, the mechanical or structural abnormality has to be analysed with more precision and should be presented in such a way as to include reflection of some of the functional aspects. In addition, the mechanical factors have to be more grave than the functional factors.

The major question is whether carotid occlusive lesions or ulcerations are universally grave indicators in prediction of stroke recurrence, as compared to the patient's lifestyle. It is well known, though, that complete obstruction, severe stenosis, and ulcerations are not the only decisive factors, simply because these angiographic findings are seen frequently in asymptomatic patients or in the contralateral side of the symptomatic patients. It is quite conceivable that if another randomized study is designed based upon these angiographic findings only, the result of the study will be to negate the benefit of carotid endarterectomy. We have attempted in the past to obtain more detailed angiographic findings which can reflect prognostic factors. In addition, functional aspects of the carotid disease were evaluated with cerebral blood flow study and blood chemistry. This paper intends to identify and summarize some of these factors.

Materials and Methods

Repairability of Carotid Ulcer and Atheroma Surface

We analysed the angiographic findings in relation to pathological findings, particularly for the repairability of ulcers and atheroma surface. Our hypothesis was that if the abnormality seen in preoperative angiogram is completely covered with newly proliferated endothelial area after a defined time of antiplatelet treatment, the abnormality will be repaired and, hence, the prognosis of the patient will be benign. If the region still showed loss of endothelial cells with active thrombus formation, the lesion was not cured and was assumed to be capable of triggering recurrence of stroke symptoms with poor prog-

[1] The Oregon Health Sciences University, Sunnyside Medical Center, Portland, Oregon, USA, and University of Nagasaki School of Medicine, Nagasaki, Japan

nosis. Pathological specimens were taken during carotid endarterectomy, usually 4 weeks after the onset of stroke symptoms (transient ischemic attack [TIA], reversible ischemic neurological deficit [RIND], minor stroke). During the 4 weeks, the patient was treated with standard doses of aspirin. Carotid plaques and ulcers were immediately irrigated with heparin solution after the arteriotomy was performed for the endarterectomy. Then the plaque was removed, without damaging the surface, and provided for scan electron microscopic study. The same specimen was studied subsequently with transmission electron microscope for three-dimensional evaluation for identification of endothelial cells.

Cerebral Blood Flow Study

The cerebral blood flow was measured pre- and postoperatively by conventional radioisotopic technique. Intraoperatively, the common carotid artery blood flow was measured by electromagnetic flow meter. These data were combined and utilized to analyze the role of stenotic lesion at the carotid bifurcation, and also to assess the adequacy of intracranial collateral circulation. The patients who were chosen for conservative treatment were evaluated, as much as possible, with a follow-up cerebral blood flow study.

Angiographic Evaluation of Amaurosis Fugax Patients

Forty-three patients were selected from consecutive cases to match age and sex, and divided into two groups of patients according to who had a history of amaurosis fugax and who did not. Angiographic findings, such as the degree of stenosis, ulceration of the carotid bifurcation, and configuration of ophthalmic arteries, are included for evaluation.

Results

Repairability of Carotid Ulcer and Atheroma

Sixty-two carotid plaques were examined under electron microscope. The preservation of the carotid plaque in 20 cases (32%) was not adequate for ultrastructural observation. In nine (22%) of the remaining 41 plaques, the surface of the plaque was totally covered with endothelial cell layers. In most of these plaques, however, multiple areas of abnormal arrangements and irregular schooling of endothelial cells were seen.

These areas were distinctively different from an ordinary arrangement and parallel schooling of normal endothelial surfaces. In addition, the size of the endothelial cells varied significantly in these areas from the surrounding areas. No aggregation or adhesion of the platelet was seen. Five of these eight plaques showed a smooth elevation of the surface angiographically and a rather mild degree of stenosis (average degree of stenosis was 62%). In three of these plaques, there was an area of significant depression, which indicates that this was a well-healed ulcer.

In 32 (78%) carotid plaques, the endothelial surface was disrupted and either partially or entirely covered with aggregated platelets or erythrocytes with fibrin formation. Some of the surface was covered only with aggregated platelets. The latter findings are usually seen in small areas of approximately 5–20 endothelial cell sizes. The former findings were common in the middle of the ulcer. At the periphery of the ulcer, the endothelial cells were very irregular in shape, size, and arrangements. Three-dimensional analysis of the specimen indicated that one end of the endothelial cell body was frequently elevated from the subendothelial layer underneath. This finding was not seen in the nonatheromatous portion of the specimen. Some of the elevated cell bodies appeared almost detached from the surface. The configuration and the uniformity of the direction of the elevation suggested that the blood flow was the culprit of the abnormality.

Pre- and Postoperative Cerebral Blood Flow Study and Intraoperative Electromagnetic Flow Study

Pre- and postoperative cerebral blood flow study and intraoperative electromagnetic flow study were performed in 18 cases. In another 11 cases, cerebral blood flow was performed, but no surgery was done.

Operative cases. In most of the operated cases, electromagnetic flow of the common carotid artery, proximal to the operative site, increased at the end of the endarterectomy. The increase varied in a wide range 0%–160%, compared to the value measured before the removal of the plaque. The degree of increase was not linearly related to the degree of stenosis of the carotid artheromatous lesions.

Cerebral blood flow was decreased preoperatively in all of the cases at least in one region of 8–16 hemispheric regions measured (more than 15% reduction of the contralateral value). Postoperative cerebral blood flow studies showed various degrees of increase. The increase was divided into four groups, according to the number of regions which showed flow increase after surgery. The increase was defined as excellent (increasing more than five regions), moderate (three to five regions), mild (one to two regions), and no increase. No increase occurred in six cases, while excellent, moderate, and mild increases were observed in three, eight, and one case(s), respectively. However, the degree of increase was not parallel to the change in the intraoperative electromagnetic blood flow study. During a follow-up period of 2–5 years, no recurrence of stroke symptoms occurred in these cases.

Nonoperative cases. In 11 of the nonoperative cases, five patients showed no flow decrease or minor change. In six patients, severe reduction of blood flow occurred, and three of these six patients developed recurrent TIA or minor stroke, while no patient in the group of no blood flow reduction suffered from the recurrence of stroke symptoms.

Angiographic Analysis of Amaurosis Fugas Patients

Eleven cases of amaurosis fugax patients (60% of total amaurosis fugax patients), as well as 11 cases of patients without amaurosis fugax (44% of total nonamaurosis fugax patients), had a large and irregular ulceration at the carotid bifurcation as seen by angiogram. The difference was not significant statistically (x^2, 0.16). Severe degree of stenosis at the carotid bifurcation (more than 75% occlusion) was more frequently present in amaurosis fugax patients as compared to nonamaurosis fugax patients (15 patients or 68% of total amaurosis fugax patients v. eight patients or 36% of total nonamaurosis fugax patients). The difference of the incidence was significant statistically (x^2, 5.01).

The configuration of the ophthalmic artery takeoff was evaluated by the location of the takeoff and the angle of the takeoff from the internal carotid artery. When the angle was less than 90°, or opposite to the direction of the internal carotid artery blood flow at the C3 portion of the internal carotid artery siphon, this was designated as retrograde takeoff. When the angle of the takeoff was greater than 90°, and the direction of the blood flow was parallel to the blood flow of the internal carotid artery, at least at the beginning of takeoff, this group of patients

was classified as antegrade bifurcation. The incidence of antegrade bifurcation was 60% in amaurosis fugax patients and 31% in the nonamaurosis fugax group. The difference was statistically significant with an x^2 value of 3.08. The location of the ophthalmic artery bifurction tends to be more distal in amaurosis fugax patients as compared to nonamaurosis fugax patients. However, this difference was not statistically significant. When the distal takeoff was combined with the antegrade bifurcation, the incidence was 52% v. 20% in the amaurosis fugax group and in the nonamaurosis fugax group, respectively. This difference was statistically significant.

Discussion and Conclusion

The prognosis of patients with the extracranial atherosclerotic vascular lesion is difficult to predict, but it may be feasible to assess more accurately by carefully investigating multiple factors, as mentioned above. Carotid endarterectomy is indicated only when the results of this analysis indicate the poor prognosis and high risk of recurrent symptoms or developing major stroke. Good prognosis of the lesion should include predictable repairability of the plaque by its configuration and location. This repairability would be accelerated by controlling blood pressure, hyperlipidemia, and smoking, and administration of antiplatelet regimen. Although postoperative cerebral blood flow increased in slightly more than half of the endarterectomized patients, the prognosis was excellent as a whole. The same excellent prognosis was observed among the patients who had no reduction of cerebral blood flow and never underwent endarterectomy, despite severely stenotic carotid plaque. These findings suggest that endarterectomy increased circulatory reserve of the brain, which may be the explanation for the good prognosis. The same explanation may be applied in nonoperative cases. Good prognosis of severely stenotic carotid artery was suggested if the endothelial cells maintained their function, and this may be enhanced with sufficient circulatory reserve of the brain. However, no measurement of the CBF reserve was done in this study.

Severely stenotic lesions were more frequently found in amaurosis fugax patients in this study. Contradictory results in the previous studies [1, 2] may be due to the prevalence of less severe pathologies found in these studies. Since the ulcer with less severe stenosis was not a characteristic finding for amaurosis fugax patients in this study, other causes should be investigated if amaurosis fugax is the sole clinical symptom. If the ulcer is associated with severe stenosis, or a steep type with poor repairability and spontaneous healing is not foreseen because of systemic factors, then carotid endarterectomy in indicated. We have reported elsewhere [3] that carotid plaques of the Japanese patient were more abundant with ω-3 fatty acids as compared to Caucasian plaques. These included eicosapentanoic acids (C20:5ω3) and docosahexaenoic acid (C22:6ω3). The former was about ten times and the latter was approximately six times higher in the Japanese plaques than they were in the Caucasian plaques. Since the Japanese plaque demonstrated complete healing of the ulcer, lipidemic studies may add another dimension to the predictability of the carotid pathology prognosis.

Summary

Current evaluation of carotid bifurcation pathology is not sufficient to differentiate high risk pathology from benign pathology. The author has proposed more detailed evaluation for the configuration and the location of the pathology by angiogram. For the study of functional aspects of the patient, cerebral blood flow study may add another dimension to surgical treatment of extracranial cerebral atherosclerotic lesions. In addition, blood chemistry analysis for long chain and saturated fatty acid may assist in differentiating the prognosis of carotid pathology. These multifactorial evaluations are needed to avoid indiscriminate surgery of carotid pathology, which still appears to be dominant in surgical practice.

References

1. Eisenberg RL, Mani RL (1978) Clinical and arteriographic comparison of amaurosis fugax with hemispheric transient attacks. Stroke 9:254–255
2. Harrison MJG, Marshall J (1986) Arteriographic comparison of amaurosis fugax and hemispheric transient attacks. Stroke 16:795–796
3. Ono H, et al. (1981) Carotid occlusive disease: Differences in a Japanese population from an American population. Exerpta Medica International Congress Series (Abstr) 548:31–32

Carotid Endarterectomy without Internal Shunt in 83 Cases

Shunro Endo and Akira Takaku[1]

We have experienced 83 cases of carotid end-arterectomy without internal shunt. These operations have been performed over the last 5 years and have been follow-up after more than 1 year. The operative mortality and morbidity rate was 0% in this series. No unconventional operative techniques or anesthesia besides the administration of 20% mannitol before and during carotid artery occlusion were employed. This report presents three subjects: characteristic clinical features of atherosclerotic extracranial carotid lesion in Japanese, the significance of administering 20% mannitol, and the surgical indication for cases with severe stenosis and showing progressing neurological symptoms.

Characteristic Clinical Features in Japanese

In Japanese this disease is not so common. In my clinic, about 30% of the ischemic cerebral symptoms found in our patients are suspected to be caused by this disease. Symptomatically, the appearance of amaurosis fugax is rare [3]; only three patients showed amaurosis fugax in this series. Anatomically, the frequency of the lesion located in high cervical level is relativery high. The carotid bifurcation of 38 cases were located above the C3 vertebra in this series. The operation was performed in the cases in which the distal end of the stenotic lesion is located below the upper verge of the C2 vertebra.

The Significance of Administering 20% Mannitol

First, I will present the investigation concerning internal carotid artery stump pressure and angiographical findings examined in the first 23 cases in this series [4–9]. These 23 cases were classified into four groups according to the collateral circulation with respect to the circle of Willis (Fig. 1): Type A had collateral supply from the contralateral carotid artery through the anterior communicating artery, type P had collateral supply from the vertebrobasilar system through the posterior communicating artery, type A + P had both collateral supplies of type A and type P, and type (−) was without collateral supply through the circle of Willis.

Stump pressure, systolic blood pressure during occlusion, occlusion time, and the amount of mannitol used in the examined 23 cases are summarized in Table 1. In 11 cases with collateral circulation (type A, type P, type A + P), the value of stump pressure in all cases was more than 40 mmHg, but individual differences were seen. The postoperative course was uneventful in these 11 cases. In 12 cases without collateral circulation (type (−)), on the other hand, the value of stump pressure was less than 35 mmHg in all cases: the minimum value was 6 mmHg. The amount of mannitol ranged from 300 to 800 ml. Two patients, cases 13 and 23, showed transient neruologucal deficit for a couple of hours just after the operation. In these two cases, only 300 or 500 ml of mannitol were administrated. Thus, we speculated that the appearance of these neurological symptoms was probably related to an insufficient amount of mannitol.

After this experience, we determined the optimal amount of mannitol on the basis of this data. For cases expected to have collateral circulation on the preoperative angiograms, 300 ml is administrated before occlusion and 200 ml is added during occlusion when the stump pressure is less than 50 mmHg. In cases where collateral circulation is unexpected, 500 ml is administrated before occlusion and 300 ml is added only in cases showing the stump pressure less than 30 mmHg. If the collateral circulation and stump pressure is not confirmed, mannitol is administrated according to the worst estimated condition. The courses of the other 60 cases, operated in such a manner, was uneventful.

[1] Department of Neurosurgery, Toyama Medical and Pharmaceutical University, Toyama, Japan

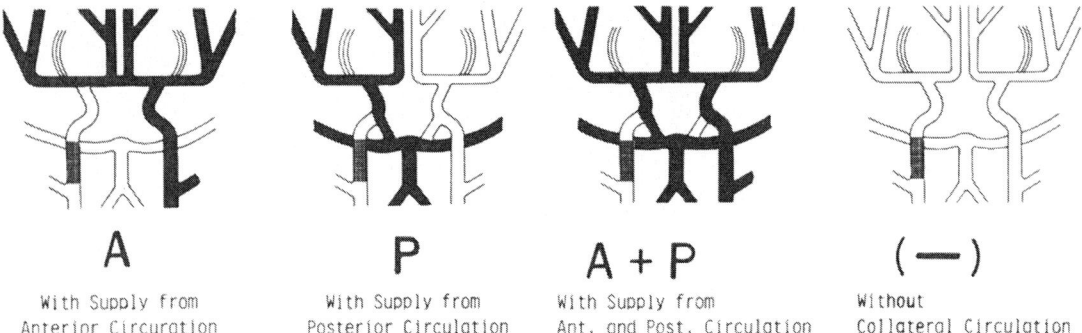

Fig. 1. Four types of collateral circulation about the circle of Willis, expected from angiographical findings in cases with internal carotid artery stenosis. *Block shading* expected collateral circulation, *crosshatched shading* stenosis of internal carotid artery

Table 1. Stump pressure, systolic pressure, occlusion time, and amount of mannitol in 23 cases of carotid endarterctomy without internal shunt

Type of CC	Case	Age (yrs)	Sex	Stump pressure	Systolic pressure	Occlusion time	Mannitol
A	1	74	M	40	150	35	800
	2	68	M	60	120	30	300
	3	66	M	60	160	39	500
	4	57	M	70	170	30	300
	5	56	M	90	140	37	300
P	6	51	M	40	100	32	400
	7	65	F	45	150	45	500
	8	77	M	60	140	34	500
	9	65	M	70	110	48	800
A + P	10	78	M	50	135	40	300
	11	57	M	60	120	33	500
(−)	12	60	F	6	140	32	800
	13	64	M	15	160	34	500
	14	59	M	15	160	38	700
	15	58	F	20	140	30	800
	16	72	F	20	150	32	800
	17	62	F	25	120	29	600
	18	60	F	25	120	30	700
	19	64	M	30	165	40	600
	20	64	M	30	150	32	500
	21	70	M	30	180	30	600
	22	59	M	35	180	32	500
	23	69	M	35	180	32	300

CC collateral circulation

Surgical Indication for Cases with Severe Stenosis and Showing Progressing Neurological Symptoms

In 17 cases in this series, the internal diameter of the stenotic portion was less than 0.5 mm (greater than 95% stenosis) on the angiograms [1, 2, 10]. Symptoms were frequent transient ischemic attacks in eight cases and progressing mild or moderate neurological deficits in nine cases. On the other hand, three nonoperated cases with such a severe stenosis were experienced. The clinical course and angiographic findings in these 20 cases are presented in Fig. 2. On the occasion of carotid endarterectomy, ipsilateral superior cervical ganglionectomy was

Carotid Endarterectomy without Internal Shunt in 83 Cases

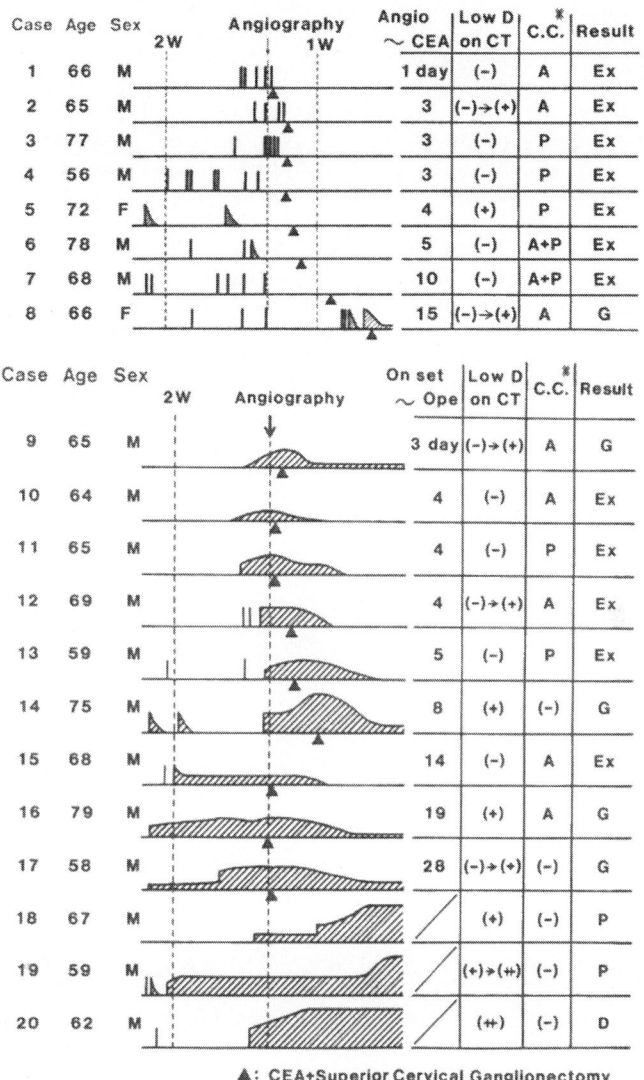

Fig. 2. Clinical course, type of collateral circulation and prognosis in 20 cases with severe stenosis. Symptoms are frequent transient ischemic attacks of eight cases (*upper*) and progressing neurological deficits of 12 cases (*lower*). *Low D* low density area, *CEA* carotid endarterectomy

▲: CEA+Superior Cervical Ganglionectomy
∗ C.C.: Collateral Circulation

performed simultaneously. The postoperative course of these 17 cases was symptomatically uneventful. The appearance of small high-density-areas on postoperative CT scans were observed in two cases, but these changes were restricted in the preoperative low-density area and any affects upon the clinical course were not observed. Twelve cases showed full recovery, and mild neurological deficits remained in five cases. Three cases without surgical treatment grew worse and one of them died due to cerebral infarction. The relationship between prognosis and angiographical collateral circuration in 20 cases is summarized in Table 2. The existence of collateral circulation is very important for a good

Table 2. Summary of prognosis and type of angiographical collateral circulation in 20 cases with severe internal carotid artery stenosis

Prognosis	Collateral circulation			
	A + P	A	P	(−)
Ex	2 ●●	5 ●●●●●	5 ●●●●●	
G		3 ●●●		2 ●●
P				2 ○○
D				1 ○

● CEA
○ medical treatment
CEA carotid endarterectomy

prognosis, but it is dangerous to overestimate it.

These results suggest that the emergent operation in the cases with severe stenosis is more effective, even though the symptoms are progressive.

References

1. Barnett HJM, Plum F, Walton JN (1984) Carotidendarterectomy—An expression of concern: Stroke 15:941–943
2. Duke LJ, Slymaker EE, Lamberth WC, Wright CB (1979) Carotid arterial reconstruction: Ten years experience. Am Surg 45:281–288
3. Gaul JJ, Marks SJ, Weinberger J (1986) Visual disturbance and carotid artery disease. Stroke 17:393–398
4. Jafar JJ, Johns LM, Mullan SF (1986) The effect of mannitol on cerebral blood flow. J Neurosurg 64:754–759
5. McKay RD, Sundt TM, Michenfelder JD, Gronert GA, Messick JM, Sharbouth FW, Piepgras DG (1973) Internal carotid artery stump pressure and cerebral blood flow during carotid endarterectomy: Modification by helothane, enflurane, and innovar. Anesthesiology 45:390–399
6. Ott DA, Cooley DA, Chapa L, Coelho A (1980) Carotid endarterectomy without temporary intraluminal shunt: Study of 309 consecutive operations. Ann Surg 191:708–714
7. Spetzler RF, Martin N, Hadley MN, et al. (1986) Microsurgical endarterectomy under barbiturate protection. J Neurosurg 65:63–73
8. Sundt TM, Sharbrouth FW, Anderson RE, Michenfelder JD (1974) Cerebral blood flow measurements and electroencephalograms during carotid endarterectomy. J Neurosurg 41:310–320
9. Suzuki J, Yoshimoto T (1979) The effect of mannitol in prolongation of permissible occlusion time of cerebral artery. Neurosurg Ren 1:13–19
10. Whisnant JP, Sandok BA, Sundt TM Jr (1983) Carotid endarterectomy for unilateral carotid system transient cerebral ischemia. Mayo Clin Proc 58:171–175

Discussion

Commentator, *Guidetti* (Rome): I was impressed with all the papers but particularly with the views of Drs. Mullan and Peerless: A comparative study with a wide range of material is required. I hope that Dr. Peerless will do the same job here as he did for bypass. In carotid endarterectomy there is the need for a randomized clinical trial. I agree with Dr. Mullan that atherosclerosis is a medical disease; we cannot simply treat the carotid and ignore the heart and kidney. By means of medical therapy and diet, atherosclerosis can be reduced remarkably. The indications and contraindications for surgery should be closely examined: I am not really sure whether surgery is useful or not and I think many of the audience may well feel the same. The indication for surgery should be quite strict. Surgery is perhaps indicated if an ulcerative plaque is present; in the case of stenosis, however, there is a lot of collateral circulation and I believe an operation is contraindicated, unless the stenosis is very heavy and the circulation poor. With an ulcerative plaque steps should be taken to prevent embolization.

The neurological morbidity of carotid endarterectomy arises from: (a) intraoperative embolization, (b) cerebral ischemic injury during the period of carotid artery clamping, (c) postoperative embolization or thrombosis originating at the endarterectomized segment, (d) postoperative intracerebral hemorrhage. Intraoperative embolization can occur during exposure of the carotid artery probably due to the dislocation of thrombotic or atherosclerotic material. This complication is early identified by a very dramatic change in EEG and can be avoided by meticulous attention to technical detail in surgery. We insert a shunt at the time the vessels are occluded in those patients in whom a major EEG change is observed and stump pressure is less than 25 mmHg. We have no experience with barbiturate, which seems to protect the brain and improve tissue tolerance to ischemia.

Ischemia during the period of carotid artery clamping is a potential cause of neurological complications. The major debate that exists with respect to intraoperative cerebral protection in patients undergoing endarterectomy is whether an intraluminal shunt or selective shunt in those patients identified as having poor collateral blood flow. Some authors do not use a shunt at all; some use it routinely; some use it selectively.

The monitoring systems used to select patients at major risk of ischemia arising from cross-clamping include monitoring of neurological function using regional anesthesia, measurement of carotid artery stump pressure, continuous measurement of regional blood flow. Unfortunately, this technique is only adequate to identify reliably those patients who require shunting to avoid infarction.

The plaque must be removed meticulously from the vessel with no leak to the intima distally and no stump of the external carotid artery. The use of an operative microscope enables more accurate removal of a plaque and the fragments of atherosclerotic material; heparinized saline irrigation also be used.

Residual fragments of atherosclerotic plaques, intimal flags, and vessel stenosis cause blood flow abnormalities but in principle does not intravascular thrombus formation, embolization, and occlusion. In order to prevent postoperative thrombic events 250 mg aspirin every 8 h and 75 mg dipiridamol every 8 h are administered pre- and postoperatively in our patients.

Heparin is only administered prior to carotid artery clamping and stopped after vessel occlusion. With respect to the operative microscope, it is possible to perform a more precise separation and more complete removal of more fragments of a plaque and less intimal damage, thus reducing postoperative embolization and thrombosis. In the case of intracerebral hemorrhage in patients with high-grade carotid stenosis and history of recent cerebral infarction, the patients show evidence of marked cerebral hyperperfusion after endarterectomy. The occurrence of warning signs such as migraine, headache, and focal seizure should prompt judicious blood pressure reduction and discontinuation of anti-aggregant drugs. Relapse, whether symptomatic or not, with varying grades of stenosis of the carotid occurs in about 10% of operated patients within the first 10 years of surgery.

A useful preventive measure is to keep the patient under constant antiaggregant therapy. If stenosis occurs, a evolutive operation should be performed. After surgery, the patient should be given a full medical checkup every 3 months to begin with, and then every 6 months. The above are our recommendations for use in very select cases. But I would say that the proposals of Drs. Peerless and Mullan are to be followed closely.

Commentator, *Gentili* (Toronto): Dr. Guidetti has already made many of the points that I was going to make. As noted by Dr. Peerless, the results of carotid endarterectomy have been subject to scrutiny and criticism for the reasons he outlined. While the results from particular surgeons and institutions with extensive experience in this field indicate that the procedure can, with careful attention to operative detail, be carried out with minimal morbidity and mortality (e.g., in our own series of over 1200 cases the combined mortality and major morbidity was 2.6%), these data cannot be extrapolated to represent management results in general. Though many of us who carry out this procedure regularly are convinced that it is indeed of value and can show decreased stroke rate on long-term follow-up compared with historical controls, we are also aware that this lacks scientific validity. Therefore, I think that most doctors now would agree with Dr. Peerless that a randomized clinical study is indeed essential to dispel the uncertainties associated with the procedure.

I would like to ask the panel if they think there is ever an indication for endarterectomy in an asympotomatic carotid lesion.

Ausman (Detroit): Many studies have been carried out, primarily by vascular surgeons, which indicate that if the endarterectomy is performed it will prevent the patient from having a stroke. I do not think we really have an idea whether surgery is of any value in the prevention of what may be a stroke. A randomized study currently underway is testing whether operating or not operating is better in such a case. We occasionally receive patients with very severe stenosis of the internal carotid artery at the bifurcation and would consider carrying out an endarterectomy, but I do not know that this is the best procedure.

Marsh (Rochester): Like Dr. Ausman, we do not really know at our institute what to do in such a case. There is one study by Dr. Moore which suggests that patients with a deeply ulcerated plaque upon angiography may show a somewhat higher incidence of subsequent stroke in follow-up. But even in these cases, the margin of benefit of surgery is small compared with the studies I mentioned and totally relies on a very low mortality and morbidity from any operative procedure. At our own institution, a randomized trial is underway for patients with asymptomatic but hemodynamically significant lesions as measured by OPG and Doppler.

Peerless (Ontario): As has been said, there is a trial that will shortly begin, probably this autumn, in the United States run by a neurologist of Bowman-Gray University, on the question of asymptomatic stenosis and its treatment. The results of this trial will be very interesting. Perhaps the best study we have today has come from Toronto together with the collaboration of some other hospitals; this study indicates that high-grade stenosis, i.e., >90% area stenosis, that is asymptomatic runs a risk of stroke which is less than 2%/year; <90% stenosis, it is less than 1%/year stroke. So the surgery has to be carried out with extreme care to beat those risks. I would predict that it would be difficult to show that surgery is beneficial. The real answer is of course that we do not know. In the face of Dr. Mullan's very important comment that the biggest risk for death is myocardial infarction by a factor of V, unless total medical care is instituted to these patients the likelihood of this operation altering their long-term outcome is very poor indeed.

Ono (Nagasaki): I would advise the patient to take aspirin immediately until sympotomatic neurological deficits develop. We have had only one case, as I mentioned, in which we performed endarterectomy for asymptomatic bruit. The patient had very bad bruit such that he could not sleep at night which was why we performed surgery.

Hwang (Mitaka): Could Dr. Ausman comment on the differences between coumadin and aspirin treatment in patients with TIA?

Ausman: I think this has been studied and, to the best of my knowledge, not found to be any value over the natural history of the disease. This is a risk of coumadin therapy itself. I do not think many neurosurgeons have gone to coumadin therapy beyond aspirin therapy. We would not use it.

Mullan (Chicago): I would certainly give coumadin for the initial period, though not for long—only for a few weeks. If there seems to be a recent TIA I think a short course of coumadin would be quite appropriate.

Ausman: Could Dr. Mullan give more details about his aggressive dietary management.

Mullan: This is obviously speculative rather than based on a controlled series. It is possible to control saturated fat intake totally and reduce it to zero, reduce cholesterol to zero. A recent article in the New England Journal of Medicine suggests that the average weight as accepted by insurance companies is 10% too high in terms of longevity. Currently available, there is the use of 6–8 g/day niacin and 24–36 g/day cholestyramine or colestipol, two quaternary resins. For patients with a high triglyceride level, chlofibrate may be used. So the medical regimen is tailored according to the specific blood pattern in terms of HDL, LDL, and LPA. The ideal medication of lovastatin is becoming more popular. A recent study shows that a combination of lovastatin, which is an anti-cholosterase drug, and the colestipol has reduced the LDL by 48% and has raised the HDL by 17%. If these figures can be extended into a statistical series of survival this would present a completely new approach to the treatment of this disease.

Guidetti: Does anyone have experience of urokinase and similar drugs?

Ausman: We have attempted this in six patients who had almost hopeless conditions and in five cases the radiologists infused the urokinase intra-arterially at the site of the embolus and there was some alteration in one or two patients; in one patient, there was a reduction in the embolus, in fact opening of the basilar artery, and the patient died of a brain stem hemorrhage. There was one case where there was not complete occlusion but what appeared like basilar artery symptoms and some defect in the arterial wall and these conditions diminished after urokinase treatment. To my knowledge, there were some studies I believe

that were published in 1974 in Neurology and the major problem was hemorrhage produced in the parenchyma after its introduction. The problem was I think the timing of the drug, which was after a number of hours. There is some interest in the use of this treatment.

Ono: As Dr. Endo said, the incidence of carotid disease is very low in Japan. I investigated this about 5 years ago in the Nagasaki area, which has a population of about one million; there were 75 cases over 5 years of carotid disease, whereas in Portland, Oregon, which has a similar population, these were 1800 cases. What is the reason for this difference? One suggestion may be the difference in the amount of encosapentanoic acid and other unsaturated fatty acids: the amount in plaque in Japanese is about three times higher than in Caucasians. The eating habits too are completely different. From these kind of findings, I think Dr. Mullan's ideas is very interesting.

Peerless: However, in Japan the incidence of extracranial carotid disease and coronary heart disease is rising with the change toward more Westernized eating habits.

Suwanwela (Bangkok): I would like to ask the panel if they think there is any place for angioplasty in extracranial carotid stenosis?

Peerless: We know that our colleagues in France are doing a good number of such operations with some considerable success. I was quite surprised to see figures of 100 cases with only one complication. We have not done any in our institution though we are very often asked by the radiologists if they can insert the balloon since they do the vertebral and subclavian arteries and the base vessels in that area. Our concern has been with distal thromboembolization from the fragile plaque. We understand that in both France and the USSR they use a double balloon that can expand the plaque and then withdraw material back into the proximal circulation, allowing it to go back into the arms. It may well be a surgical treatment that can outstrip traditional surgical treatments in the future.

Mullan: In the animal, carotid atherosclerosis can be prevented by simply removing the bifurcation, i.e., eliminating the external, which just leaves a simple tube that does not become subject to atherosclerosis. That would be a different form of angioplasty.

RTD 9. Vasospasm

Progress in the Approach to Vasospasm

V.A. Fasano[1], E. Levi[2], R. Urciuoli[1], W. Liboni[3], P. Pignocchino[2], P. Bolognese[1], M. Egidi[1], M.M. Fontanella[1], A. Bulla[2], G.F. Lombard[1], R. Clemens[4], and M. Davico[1]

Prediction of Vasospasm

Preoperative Vasospasm

Progress has been substantial in the prediction of vasospasm. Even if the agents with a specific spasmogenic effect have not yet been determined, reliable predictions can be made by combining the findings offered by instrumental investigations.

The prediction of vasospasm can be made within the first 2 days of the onset of subarachnoid hemorrhage (SAH) by CT evidence of intracisternal bleeding and fibrin/fibrinogen degradation products (FDPs) in excess of 80 μg/ml in the CSF; if these are found with slow EEG rhythms in the same period, there is a strong probability of the occurrence of secondary ischemia [7].

Transcranial Doppler (TCD) is quite a new instrument and we have direct experience of its use in more than 50 cases. This noninvasive method permits an evaluation of a vessel's diameter by means of the assessment of changes in the rate and characteristics of the velocity of the blood flow in the major intracranial vessels. There is a correlation between the angiographic and TCD pictures, but noninvasive techniques are potentially superior to angiography in hemodynamic assessment, even though only the latter can provide morphological data. This noninvasive method particularly helps the physician to quantify the stenosis and follow the effects of pharmacological treatment.

Most of the present authors maintain that vasospasm exists when the mean rate of blood flow is more than 90 cm/s, while more than 129 cm/s is probably indicative of subcritical stenosis. A rate higher than 200 cm/s is certain evidence of critical stenosis. In these cases, the frequency of symptomatic vasospasm is considerably higher [1]. Some of us maintain that TCD yields valuable information about the planning of early surgery. Practically, early operation should be performed before the spasm starts to develop. No operations should be carried out during the high phases of the velocity curves. Even if there is a clear and constant correlation between increasing velocity values and decreasing vessel diameter, the onset and the gravity of the ischemia cannot be reliably correlated. In fact the onset of ischemia is dependent on other factors besides vasal narrowing: the degree to which compensation can be provided by the collateral circulation, preservation of the capacity of microcirculatory autoregulation, and various systemic and local differences between one patient and another (intracranial pressure, viscosity, hypertension, etc.). However, a more increased velocity and its rapid progression, while it certainly reflects progressing reductions in vessel diameter, does not always predict the onset of ischemia. Our series includes cases where rates more than 120 cm/s, even with the presence of rapid increment, were not accompanied by symptomatic vasospasm (Fig.1a), as well as others in which ischemic deficits were present despite a flow rate of less than 80 cm/s (Fig.1b).

We are presently investigating whether evaluation of the diastolic rate and its derivative parameter—systolic/diastolic ratio, Pourcelot' index, pulsatility index—enhances the prediction of symptomatic vasospasm before its clinical appearance.

Topographic EEG mapping is more valuable in studies of subclinical cortical ischemia than normal EEG. Abnormalities are revealed significantly more often in the region of cortical impairment, which is more clearly defined. Topographic extention of ischemia can be controlled

[1] Institute of Neurosurgery, University of Turin, Turin, Italy
[2] Banca del Sangue e del Plasma, Fondazione G. Strumia, Turin, Italy
[3] Institute of Neuroradiology, University of Turin, Turin, Italy
[4] Klinische Forschung, Behringwerke, Marburg, Federal Republic of Germany

(Fig. 2).

The best approach to the prediction of symptomatic vasospasm must be found through multidisciplinary collaboration and the formation of a medical and paramedical team trained for continuous clinical and instrumental checking on the patient.

Postoperative Vasospasm

We have used the microvascular Doppler (MVD) in more than 150 cases. It must be distinctly pointed out, however, that since surgery was usually postponed in the presence of serious symptomatic vasospasm, its intraoperative assessment was very infrequent in percentage terms. Nonetheless, MVD permitted evaluation of angiographic segmentary vasospasms in 20% of cases. MVD was mostly utilized to evaluate the results of topical treatment with nimodipine on intact and spastic vessels (Fig. 3).

Investigating comparative effects on ruptured and intact aneurysms, we noted that only parent vessels of the former may react with spasm as a result of surgical manipulation.

Laser Doppler exploits the Doppler effect with a low-power laser beam, whose high frequency permits investigation of the microcirculation over restricted, superficial areas. We have started using this instrument to check the effect of drugs on the microcirculation (Fig. 4), in order to evaluate the possibilities of autoregulatory compensation to the incipient ischemia.

Prevention of Vasospasm

Preoperative Vasospasm

Multidisciplinary research on the part of hematologists, angiologists, and radiologists is indispensable to the solution of these problems. A normovolemic or slightly hypervolemic hemodilution as a preventive treatment encourages better release of oxygen to the ischemic tissues, washout of potentially spasmogenic substances from the site of injury, and an increase in the supply of drugs.

The rationale for this technique during ischemia is to recover the "penumbrae," i.e., areas of relative ischemia, which can only be done by prompt reestablishment of an adequate flow [6]. When ischemia is present, the mechanisms of cerebral autoregulations are partly or totally abolished:

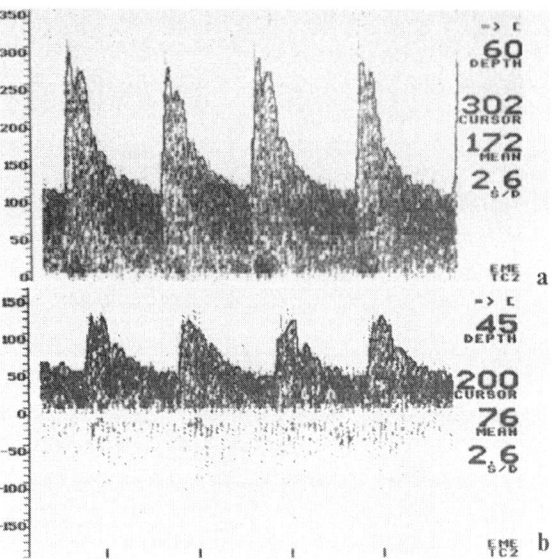

Fig. 1. a Critical spasm of right MCA, 8 days after SAH (38-year-old male). High mean velocity and pathological s/d ratio (normal, 2–2.2) are evident. **b** Clinical spasm of left internal carotid artery (ICA) 7 days after SAH (42-year-old female). Mean velocity is quite normal while spectral analysis shows turbulent phenomena (Transcranial Doppler imagery)

the blood passively responds to changes in pressure and viscosity. Therefore, hemodilution steps up this flow into the "penumbrae".

Our small series confirms Ender's 1981 results; vasospasm is delayed until the 14th–16th day. Treatment was unsuccessful in about 18%–20% of the cases. Researchers are in the progress of taking the biochemical etiological model into consideration. We are currently investigating the effectiveness of the combined use of eicosapentenoic or linoleic acid, with regard the use of eicosapentenoic or linoleic acid for 8–10 days—a duration correlated to the mean life of platelets—it has been suggested that there is an alteration in the CSF equilibrium between the concentration of metabolites of arachidonic acid acting as vasoconstrictors (TXA2, PGF2alpha, PGD2), which are enhanced, and those acting as vasodilatators (PGI2), which are depressed. This imbalance probably reflects the combined effect of both depressed synthesis of PGI2 on the part of the injured endothelium and an increase in the TXA2 released by activated platelets in the lesion site. Theoretically, a proper vasoconstrictor/vasodilatator ratio could be obtained by replacing spasmogenous TXA2 by non-spasmogenous TXA3 through the augmentation of the dietary

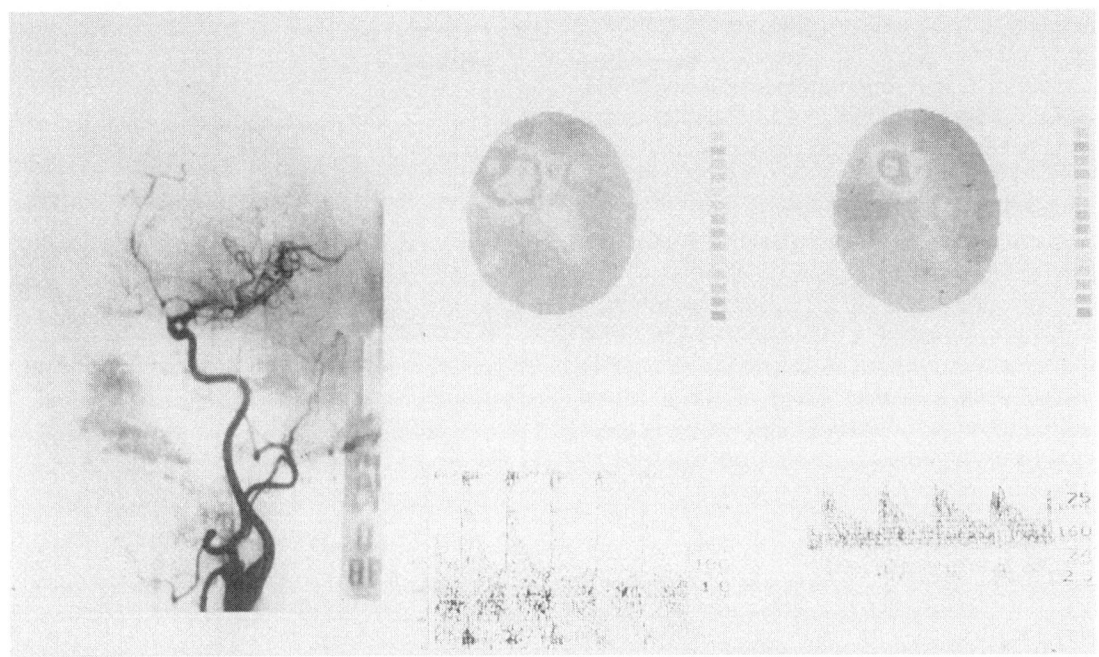

Fig. 2. EEG mapping. Evolution of left frontal ischemic area correlated with dynamic data of TCD and morphological data of angiography, which demonstrate an ACA vasospasm

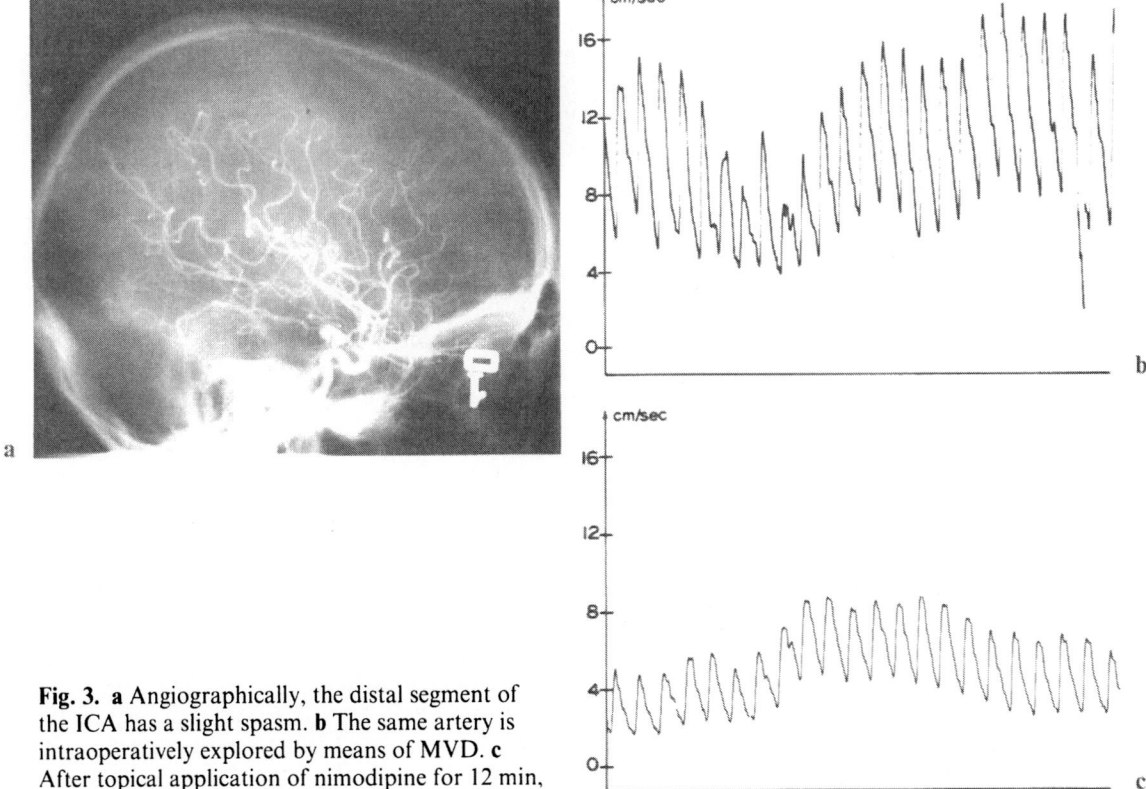

Fig. 3. a Angiographically, the distal segment of the ICA has a slight spasm. **b** The same artery is intraoperatively explored by means of MVD. **c** After topical application of nimodipine for 12 min, the doppler patterns are normalized

intake of the polysatured acids mentioned above [3].

Vitamin E and superoxide-dismutase (SOD), possibly associated with catalase, should reduce the concentrations of lipid peroxides and other free radicals in the CSF which are responsible for the damage to the cell membranes [9].

Calcium channel blocking agents [2] can also help prevent vasospasm. Contraction of the smooth muscle cells of the vessel (the ultimate cause of vasospasm) is regulated by the intracellular concentration of calcium. Changes in this concentration may occur as the result of either the entry of extracellular calcium (promoted *inter alia* by potassium, norepinephrine and serotonin) or its release (promoted by platelet TXA2 and PGF2alpha). Therefore, it is useful to prevent the increase of the intracellular concentration. Nimodipine (2 mg/kg/h i.v. or 360 mg/day per os) has been administered for the prevention of vasospasm immediately on admission and then for 21 days in 44 patients (Hunt-Hess grades I–IV). At the end of treatment, we considered the efficacy in the prophylaxis of ischemic neurological deficits: 38 patients were completely free from symptoms or had only very slight neurological deficits. There were three patients with severe disablement; three patients died during the treatment.

The limited effectiveness of these drugs could be due to their insufficient capacity to inhibit the mobilization of intracellular Ca^{2+}. It is known that the calcium channels modulate exchanges between cells and extracellular liquids and thus have only an indirect effect on cytoplasmic Ca^{2+}, which is under the control of calmodulin, the enzyme that serves as the intracellular Ca^{2+} ionophore. Better results could perhaps be achieved by associating nimodipine with a Calmodulin inhibitor: Chlorpromazine seems to be particularly indicated for this purpose, since it also possesses a slight adrenolytic action [8].

Studies of the treatment with chlorpromazine plus nimodipine are in progress in hypertensive patients under continuous pressure monitoring. We do not use continuous intracisternal infusion of nimodipine. Washout of the accumulated blood in cisterns did not influence the rate of velocity registered by TCD or reduce the incidence of postoperative symptomatic vasospasm.

Postoperative Vasospasm

B-scanning and MVD are currently used for preventing the ischemia dependent for manipulation

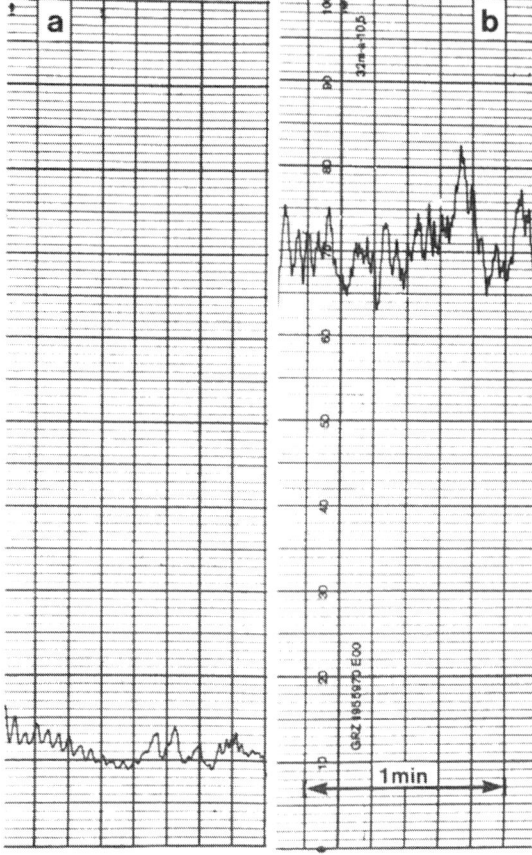

Fig. 4a, b. Intraoperative analysis of the cortical microcirculation by Laser Doppler; **a** Normal basal pattern; **b** After systemic imput of mannitol; a flux increase and a different shape of the record are evident

of the tissue. B-scanning shows the real shape of the aneurysm and demonstrates the site of rupture visualizing the adjacent clot and the extent of SAH [4] (Fig. 5). MVD (high-frequency pulsed) explores the lumen through minimal detection windows. This method enables us to distinguish an iatrogenic stenosis due to lateral clipping from a superimposed spasm (Fig. 6).

Treatment of Vasospasm

The resolution of the narrowing of the vessels was attempted with the administration of nimodipine topically and by intravenous perfusion. We used nimodipine topically (4 ml of 0.02% solution for 12 min) in eight cases. Modifications in caliber of the vessels and in flow of the parent vessels, checked with MVD, were variable. In one patient who showed aggiographic, clinical,

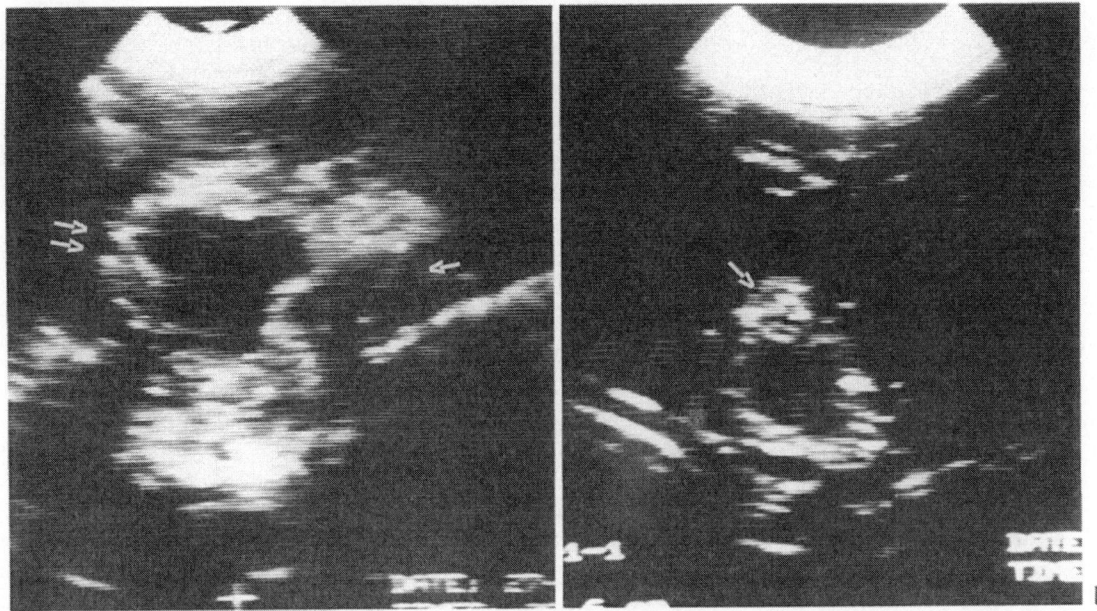

Fig. 5. a Anterior communicating artery aneurysm; the shape and real dimension of the aneurysm, the endoluminal thrombus, the thick (*arrow*) and thin (*double arrow*) portion of the aneurysmatic wall, and the extension of SAH, are evident. **b** Anterior cerebral artery aneurysm, the shape and the dimension of the aneurysm, and the blood clot next to the break point (*arrow*), are evident (B-scan)

and MVD evidence of vasospasm, an immediate MVD flow normalization was registered though not associated with clinical improvement.

Nimodipine does not influence angiographic vasospasm or block the evolution of correlative serious ischemia.

The effects of 2 mg/kg per hour i.v. nimodipine used for 2 days in the course of vasospasm for preventive neuronal protection was evaluated on the clinical course in 36 patients with ongoing angiographically-demonstrated vasospasm. In grades I–III subjects with more than a 50% reduction in vessel diameter, a clinical improvement was observed in 66%, whereas in those with less than a 50% narrowing and a comparable clinical picture, improvement only occurred in 20%. Only 10% of grave IV progressed to a lower grade. All patients underwent surgery on the 8th day after SAH. This seems to confirm that drug protection is more frequent in those cases in which the hemodynamic situation is more critical.

The risk of vasospasm has been demonstrated in the course of treatment with anti-fibrinolytic drugs (AFL) to prevent recurrence. The reduction of this risk can also be attempted by the administration of factor XIII [5]. This drug produces stabilization of the clot, activating the

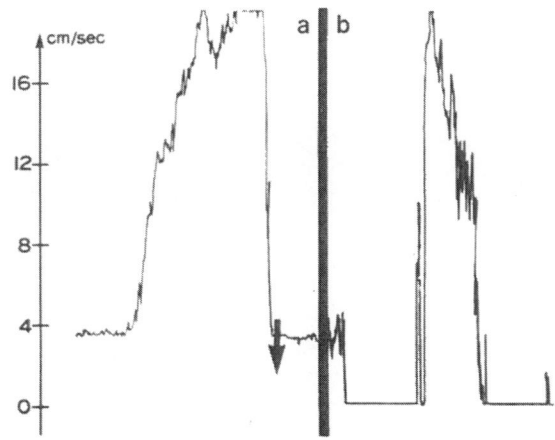

Fig. 6a, b. The vessel lumen is directly measured by shifting the detection gate of MVD. **a** Lateral clipping of a parent artery; the steeper portion corresponds to the clipping point. **b** Vasospasm superimposed to lateral clipping; the lumen is very narrowed

healing processes by means of fibroblastic activity (Fig. 7). AFL can block the reticuloendohelial system and indirectly block the FDP clearance increasing the risk of vasospasm. We treated 58 cases with factor XIII; rebleeding was ob-

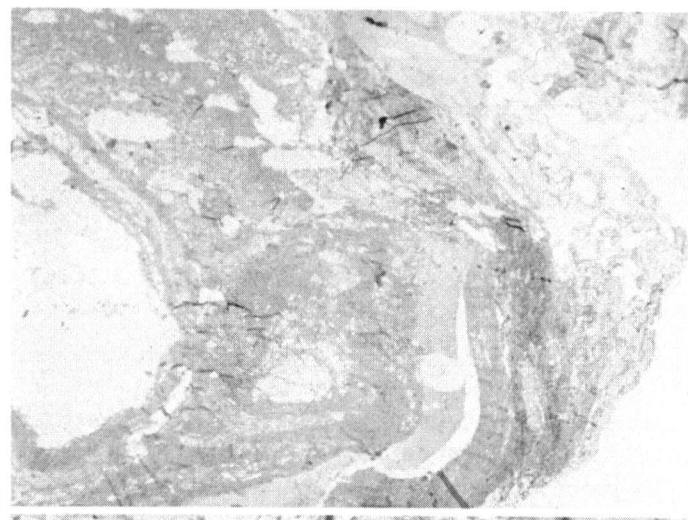

Fig. 7a, b. Factor XIII. Visualization by immunohistochemical means of action site of factor XIII on aneurysmatic dome **a** Factor XIII disposition on rupture site (*left*). **b** The same image in detail

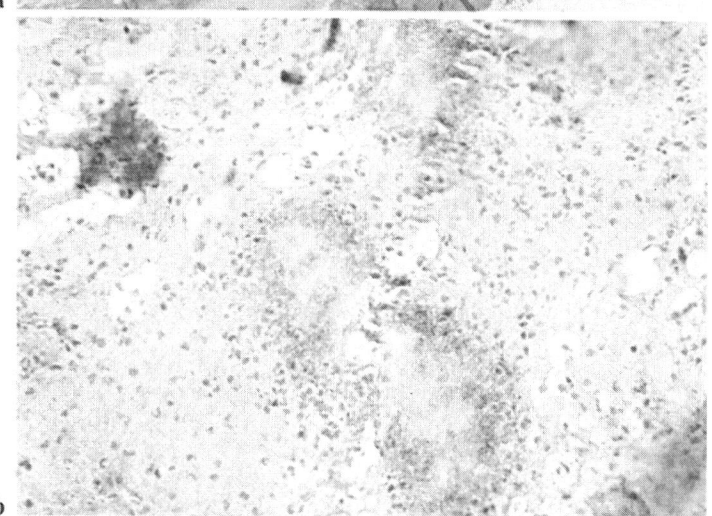

served in four cases, symptomatic vasospasm appeared in four patients (postoperatively in one), while, in 24 patients treated with antifibrinolytics (tranexamic acid), rebleeding was noted in three cases and vaosopasm appeared in nine.

References

1. Aaslid R (ed) (1986) Transcranial doppler sonography. Springer-Verlag, Vienna
2. Allen GS, et al. (1983) Cerebral arterial spasm: A controlled trial of nimodipine in subarachnoid hemorrhage patients. New Engl J Med 308:619–624
3. Chan RC, et al. (1984) The role of the prostacyclin-thromboxane system in cerebral vasospasm following induced SAH in the rabbit. J Neurosurg 61:1120–1128
4. Fasano VA, et al. (1986) Uso intraoperatorio combinato di A-mode e B-mode in neurochirurgia. Acta Chir Italica 42:4
5. Fasano VA, et al. (1986) Premières observations sur l'activité du Facteur XIII dans le traitement des hémorragies sous-arachnoidiennes. Workshop International Facteur XIII, 6 June 1986. Lyon
6. Grotta JC, et al. (1985) Baseline hemodynamic state and response to hemodilution in patients with acute cerebral ischemia. Stroke 16(5):790–795
7. Landau-Ferey J, et al. (1984) Apport de l'EEG au diagnostic de vasospasme après rupture d'anéurisme intra-cranien. Neurochirurgie 30:25–29
8. Nakano M, et al. (1984) Effects of chlorpromazine on experimental delayed cerebral vasospasm. J Neurosurg 61:857–863
9. Sakaki S, et al. (1986) Biological defense mechanism in the pathogenesis of prolonged cerebral vasospasm in the patients with ruptured intracranial aneurysms. Stroke 17(2):196–201

Current Topics in Cerebral Vasospasm

Eugene S. Flamm[1]

Prediction of Cerebral Vasospasm

Although considerable improvement in operative mortality and morbidity has been made in the past 15 years in patients with subarachnoid hemorrhage (SAH) from cerebral aneurysms, many reports document the lack of similar improvement in case morbidity and mortality [1, 3]. A major contributing factor to the persistently high morbidity of SAH is the development of cerebral vasospasm and ischemia which leads to progressive ischemic neurological deficits during the first 5–9 days after SAH [1, 3, 4, 5]. Vasospasm is found by angiography in as many as 70% of patients, and symptomatic vasospasm develops in 20%–30% of patients following SAH. Cerebral vasospasm with secondary ischemia is the leading cause of death and disability among patients with aneurysmal SAH [9].

The major predictor of cerebral vasospasm is the amount of blood in the subarachnoid space, which is best assessed on the first CT scan obtained after the subarachnoid hemorrhage. Since subarachnoid blood is less likely to be seen on CTs obtained 48 h after SAH, it is important to have an early CT to use as a predictor. In spite of this, it is still difficult to determine which patients will develop symptomatic cerebral vasospasm. There is no clear correlation between the occurrence of symptomatic cerebral vasospasm and aneurysm site, age of the patient, or other types of vascular disease such as hypertension.

Symptomatic vasospasm can be suspected by looking for early clinical changes. Symptoms included a slight increase in headache, low-grade fever, or meningismus, with an onset 4–12 days after SAH. Fluctuating or gradually evolving focal neurological signs usually then develop. CT and other studies should be used to confirm the presence of cerebral infarction and to eliminate other causes of neurological deterioration.

Prevention of Cerebral Vasospasm

At present, management of cerebral vasospasm is limited to attempts to reverse focal ischemic deficits with a regimen of drug-induced hypertension and hypervolemia-hemodilution to improve cerebral perfusion [10]. There is no established method of preventing cerebral vasospasm. The timing of surgery, an issue that is still far from completely resolved, seems to be an independent variable. The incidence of cerebral vasospasm is not increased by early surgical intervention, although the presence of symptomatic cerebral vasospasm is a contraindication for surgery until the cerebral perfusion has improved. At the present time, we do not have a uniform policy regarding the timing of aneurysm surgery. In those patients who are grade I and ready for surgery within 5 days of their SAH, surgery is carried out on a regularly scheduled day. Only those aneurysms that are non-complex and will not require extensive dissection of the adjacent vessels are managed in this fashion. This is based on the hypothesis that extensive dissection of the cerebral vessels is a possible contributing factor to the development of postoperative cerebral vasospasm. Surgery is delayed until a later time if vasospasm is noted on the angiogram, if the patient has any focal or nonfocal neurological deficit, or if the aneurysm will require considerable manipulation of exquisite areas of the brain. If surgery is to be delayed, a regimen that addresses itself to such problems as control of blood pressure, sedation, and antifibrinolytic therapy is required. Utilizing this regimen, our incidence of rebleeding has been maintained at 6%.

At the present time the most widely used regimen for prevention of cerebral vasospasm is through the use of volume expansion and prevention of too low blood pressure. No attempt

[1] Division of Neurosurgery, University of Pennsylvania School of Medicine, Philadelphia, Pennsylvania, USA

should be made to restrict fluid intake in patients with SAH. The usual daily intake is 2500–3000 ml per day, either orally or intravenously. This is particularly important in patients who develop cerebral vasospasm either with or without clinical signs of ischemia.

We prefer to carry out angiography soon after the patient is admitted. This is done when the full neuroradiological team is available and not on an emergency basis. Although a second study prior to delayed surgery will be necessary, the first angiogram provides an early diagnosis which is of obvious importance for managing the patient. If spasm is present on the follow-up angiogram, surgery is delayed until repeat studies show the spasm is beginning to resolve. It is not necessary to wait until the spasm has completely cleared.

The prevention of postoperative cerebral vasospasm requires a diligent continuation of the preoperative regimen. The goals of postoperative care are to maintain adequate cerebral perfusion, reduce any postoperative cerebral swelling or increase in intracranial pressure, and to prevent the occurrence of seizures. These aims can be accomplished by continuing the preoperative medical regimen of corticosteroids, anticonvulsants, and maintenance of an expanded plasma volume through the liberal use of fluids and colloid. In those patients who undergo early surgery, it is important to remember that may not be at risk for cerebral vasospasm until a week has passed and at a time when discharge is being considered.

Current Use of the Calcium Channel Blocker Nicardipine

Recent work has centered on the control of calcium by the use of drugs that increase the binding of intracellular calcium or decrease the entry of calcium into vascular smooth muscle. The ideal calcium channel blocking drug for the treatment of vasospasm should have its major effect on cerebrovascular smooth muscle, penetrate the blood-brain barrier, be given intravenously, and have minimal or no side effects. We have recently completed a phase II study utilizing nicardipine (2,6-dimethyl-4- [3-nitro-phenyl]-1, 4-dihydro-pyridine, 3, 5-dicarboxylic acid 3- [2-(N-benzyl-N-methyl amino)] ethyl ester 5-methyl ester hydrochloride), an agent that meets most of these criteria. At the start of this study, nicardipine had not been reported for the treatment or prevention of clinical cerebral vasospasm. Since then, this drug has been used in Japan in a study utiliz-

Table 1. Nicardipine dosage schedule

Level	BSA Dose $(mg/m^2/h)$	Weight dose $(mg/kg/h)$	Hourly dose (mg/h)	No. of patients
I	0.42	0.01	0.8	3
II	0.83	0.02	1.6	3
III	1.67	0.04	2.9	4
IV	2.50	0.06	4.3	4
V	3.33	0.08	5.8	17
VI	4.50	0.11	7.8	3
VII	6.00	0.15	10.4	33

Treatment period, 14 days after SAH
BSA body surface area

ing very low doses [7].

Experimental data suggests that nicardipine exhibits preferential binding to cerebral vascular smooth muscle and has effects similar to other dihydropyridine calcium channel blockers in reversing experimental vasoconstriction and preventing ischemic damage [6, 8]. It is clear from the literature on cerebral protection that beneficial effects are not seen with all types of calcium channel blockers [2]. This emphasized the need for a preliminary phase II study prior to establishing a randomized clinical trial of different calcium channel blocking agents. We, therefore, carried out a dose escalation study to determine the maximally tolerated dose of nicardipine and studied the possible therapeutic response to a high dose.

Patients between the ages of 18 and 75 admitted to NYU Medical Center and the University of Iowa within 7 days of SAH from a documented cerebral aneurysm were entered into the study after fulfilling certain criteria. Cerebral angiography was performed before entry to demonstrate the presence of a saccular aneurysm and the *absence* of vasospasm. Patients were excluded if they were deeply comatose or had a large intracerebral hemorrhage, if they had a non-aneurysmal cause of SAH, if they had a traumatic or mycotic aneurysm, if they had a severe neurological deficit from another cause that would confound neurological examination, or if vasospasm was found on the initial arteriogram.

In the course of this study we have been able to increase the dose of nicardipine from 0.01 to 0.15 mg/kg per hour (Table 1). Thirty-three patients have been treated at the highest level. From this study we have been able to show that the drug can safely be given at this level with minimal side effects; that there appears to be a reduction in the

Table 2. Entry characteristics

Age	25–72, Mean, 50
Male:female	32:35
Blood pressure:	
Systolic	96–252
Diastolic	60–140
Neurological deficit	
WFNS 1 and 2	50/67 (75%)

WFNS World Federation of Neurological Surgeons

Table 4. Site of aneurysm responsible for SAH

Site	No. of patients
PCA	22
ACA	21
V-B	10
MCA	8
ICA	6
Total	67

PCA posterior communicating artery, *ACA* anterior cerebral artery, *V-B* vertebral-basilar artery, *MCA* middle cerebral artery, *ICA* internal carotid artery

Table 3. Grade on admission

	Levels I–VI ($n = 34$)	Level VII ($n = 33$)
WFNS		
I	11	15
II	13	11
IIIA	6	3
IIIB	1	1
IV	2	3
V	1	0
		8

WFNS World Federation of Neurological Surgeons

Table 5. Outcome (GOS) and vasospasm

GOS	Present	Absent
1	21	31
2	6	2
3–5	4	3
Total	31	36

GOS Glasgow Outcome Score

incidence of angiographic cerebral vasospasm and, more importantly, symptomatic cerebral vasospasm. The feasibility of using this drug in a randomized clinical trial has been demonstrated, and such a multicenter trial is soon to begin.

The patients' average age was 50 years. Thirty-five patients were women and 32 were men. The intervals from SAH until treatment were 0–1 days for 25 patients, 2–3 days for 14 patients, and 4–7 days for 28 patients. The entry characteristics are summarized in Table 2. The clinical grades upon admission are in Table 3. Sites of the ruptured aneurysms are listed in Table 4.

Declines in blood pressure were observed at several dose levels, but they were more common among patients treated with the highest dose. This dosage (approximately 10 mg/h) is much higher than that used for treatment of either heart disease or hypertension. It is also approximately 25–40 times higher than the dose given in the only other clinical trial of nicardipine in patients with SAH [7]. We believe that this dose of nicardipine (6.0 mg/m^2/h) is safe. It is close to the maximal dose that will be tolerated by patients. Escalation to a much higher dose will be accompanied by increased risk of symptomatic hypotension.

Of the 67 patients that have been treated, 31 (46%) have developed angiographic evidence of

vasospasm while on nicardipine and 11 patients have developed clinical signs of ischemia. This represents 16% of the total group and includes patients at all dose levels. However, of the 33 patients treated at level VII, only two patients developed symptomatic cerebral vasospasm, an incidence of 6%.

Of the 31 patients who developed angiographic cerebral vasospasm, 21 (68%) had an excellent outcome (Glasgow Outcome Score—GOS 1), six were fair (19%) (GOS 2), and four (13%) had a poor outcome (GOS 3–5) (Table 5). Of the 36 patients who did not develop vasospasm, 31 (86%) had an excellent outcome.

Although no overall conclusions can be made at this time, several preliminary observations are appropriate. Nicardipine administered in a range from 0.01 to 0.15 mg/kg/h has been well tolerated. No adverse effects or unexpected reactions to the drug have been encountered. The anticipated problem of hypotension has not produced any deleterious effects with the inclusion of volume expansion in the regimen.

We have also determined a possibly effective dose of nicardipine in preventing vasospasm and cerebral ischemia. In comparing the results of treatment in the seven dose levels, we noted fewer ischemic symptoms and a much lower rate of vasospasm among patients treated with the highest dose. Outcomes at 3 months were also favorable in more than 75% of the patients. We noted no deaths due to vasospasm.

Approximately 25% of the patients treated in levels I–VI developed symptomatic vasospasm. However, only 6% of patients treated at level VII developed cerebral ischemic symptoms. Neither patient had permanent sequelae. We believe that this dose of approximately 6.0 mg/m^2 per hour is the potentially optimal dose.

Clearly, other variables must be accounted for before any conclusions about efficacy of nicardipine can be made. It is not the purpose of a preliminary study such as this to establish the effectiveness of the drug, but rather to determine a safe and possibly effective dose that might be utilized in a controlled study. Certain other parameters are yet to be analyzed. A correlation between outcome and serum and/or CSF levels must be examined. Only in this way will we be able to determine if the suggested dose response relationship exists. Based on these preliminary results, there are strong indications for a randomized clinical trial.

References

1. Adams HP Jr, Kassell NF, Torner JC, Nibbelink DW, Sahs AL (1981) Early management of aneurysmal subarachnoid hemorrhage: A report of the Cooperative Aneurysm Study. J Neurosurg 54:141–145
2. Clarke B, Grant D, Patmore L, Whiting RL (1983) Comparative calcium entry blocking properties of nicardipine, nifedipine and P4108068 on cardiac and vascular smooth muscle. Br J Pharmacol 79:333
3. Drake CG (1981) Management of cerebral aneurysm. Stroke 12:273–283
4. Flamm ES (1986) The timing of aneurysm surgery 1985. Clin Neurosurg 33:147–158
5. Flamm ES (1986) Vasospasm and the timing of aneurysm surgery: Have we progressed? Neurosurg Rev 9:71–76
6. Grotta J, Spydell J, Pettigrew C, Ostrow P, Hunter D (1986) The effect of nicardipine on neuronal function following ischemia. Stroke 17:213–219
7. Handa J, Matsuda M, Nakasu Y, Nakasu S, Kidooka M, Watanabe K (1984) Early operation of aneurysmal subarachnoid hemorrhage use of nicardipine, a calcium channel blocker. Arch Jpn Chir 53:619–630
8. Handa J, Yoneda S, Koyama T, Matsuda M, Handa H (1975) Experimental cerebral vasospasm in cats: Modification by a new synthetic vasodilator YC-93. Surg Neurol 3:195–199
9. Kassell NF (1985) Cooperative study on timing of aneurysm surgery. American Association of Neurological Surgeons Annual Meeting, 23 April 1985, Atlanta
10. Kassell NF, Peerless SJ, Durward QJ, Beck DW, Drake CG, Adams HP (1982) Treatment of ischemic deficits from vasospasm with intravascular volume expansion and induced arterial hypertension. Neurosurg 11:337–343

Preliminary Experience with the Treatment of Intracranial Vasospasm by Transvascular Balloon Angioplasty

Van V. Halbach, Grant B. Hieshima, Randall T. Higashida, and Peter Yang[1]

Microneurosurgical advances have greatly decreased the morbidity and mortality associated with ruptured intracranial aneurysms, particularly in patients with good clinical status. In patients with poor clinical status, the devastating effects of hemorrhage on the cerebral circulation can result in ischemia and infarction. Early neurosurgical clipping allows more aggressive postoperative management of delayed cerebral vasospasm with volume expansion and hypertension. Early surgery has shown a decreased incidence of delayed vasospasm if the clot surrounding the cerebral vasculature can be removed [8]. In patients with delayed cerebral vasospasm with an untreated aneurysm, treatment with hypertension and volume expansion can increase the risk of rehemorrhage. In the United States, as many as 11% of patients with ruptured aneurysms will die secondary to the ischemic consequences of vasospasm, and considerably more will be permanently disabled [7].

Despite a myriad of pharmacological agents that have been utilized to prevent or reverse the effects of delayed cerebral vasospasm [1–3, 6, 9], it remains the primary cause for delayed deterioration in patients who survive their initial subarachnoid hemorrhage.

Zubkov and colleagues were the first to describe the treatment of delayed cerebral vasospasm by transvascular balloon angioplasty techniques [10]. Our earliest experience with the transvascular dilatation of vasospasm was in patients with ruptured aneurysms in whom transvascular balloon embolization of the aneurysm was being performed [4, 5]. The vasospasm occurred in the parent artery proximal to the aneurysm, and the patients were not symptomatic from the arterial narrowing. The areas of narrowing were dilated to a normal caliber with a silicone balloon. The aneurysms were subsequently treated by balloon embolization with complete obliteration of the aneurysm. Follow-up angiograms at 3, 6, and 24 months have demonstrated that the segment of arterial narrowing (vasospasm) treated by balloon dilatation remained normal in caliber on all subsequent examinations.

Since then we have treated several patients with symptomatic delayed vasospasm following subarachnoid hemorrhage. All had ruptured unclipped cerebral aneurysms; their poor clinical status precluded neurosurgical clipping. All had failed standard medical treatment for delayed vasospasm (hypertension and hypervolemia). The procedures were performed with local anesthesia from a femoral arterial access to allow continuous neurological monitoring. A diagnostic angiogram is first performed to determine the location and severity of the vasospasm. Because dilatation of cerebral vessels often improves cerebral perfusion to both ischemic vascular territories, as well as to the recently ruptured aneurysm, a subsequent plan for definitive aneurysm occlusion by surgery or balloon embolization must be formulated. Close interaction with neurosurgical colleagues is essential for a favorable outcome.

The catheter system utilized for balloon angioplasty consists of a triaxial polyethylene catheter with a 7.3-F polyethylene outer catheter system with a 4- and 2-F inner coaxial system. The balloon utilized for dilatation is constructed of silicone and its inflated diameter is matched to the normal caliber of the vessel to be dilated (Interventional Therapeutics Corporation, Santa Barbara, California). The balloon is valveless and firmly attached to the 2-F catheter by a friction fit. Silicone is many times softer than latex and allows vessel dilatation with less risk of vessel rupture or vascular damage. The balloon is usually flow-directed by gentle inflation and deflation: however, special curves can be placed in the 2-F catheter to allow flow in a direction independent of the balloon system. Because of

[1] Departments of Radiology and Neurological Surgery, UCSF Medical Center, San Francisco, California, USA

the cerebral ischemia in the vascular territory being treated, occlusion times during dilatation of the segment of artery narrowed are kept to a minimum, usually under 8 s. During dilatation, the soft silicone material often conforms to the branches and shapes of the parent vessel. Following dilatation of stenosed segments of artery, restenosis had not been observed unless the patient rehemorrhaged. Adjacent segments of narrowing that were untreated remain constricted on follow-up angiograms.

Our experience with vasospasm associated with neurological deficits of recent onset is that dramatic improvement and recovery in neurological function can occur immediately following balloon dilatation of the segment of artery responsible for the symptoms. An example is of a middle-aged man who suffered a subarachnoid hemorrhage from an aneurysm arising between the posterior cerebral and superior cerebellar arteries. Two weeks following a rehemorrhage, his clinical status deteriorated to deep coma. An angiogram demonstrated severe narrowing of the entire vertebral-basilar system with a slow circulation time. A balloon dilatation procedure was performed of the entire right vertebral and basilar artery to a point just below the origin of the ruptured aneurysm. Despite improved caliber of the vessels dilated, the patient remained in deep coma. Therefore, the remainder of the basilar artery and the proximal right posterior cerebral arteries were dilated. Several minutes after this dilatation, the patient awoke and remembered all events subsequent to the dilatation of the distal basilar and posterior cerebral arteries. The presumed mechanism for this patient's dramatic recovery in function is a reversal of critical midbrain ischemia. Similiar results with dramatic reversal in neurological deficit have occurred in other vascular territories following balloon angioplasty.

In one patient with a poor clinical status for several days, no improvement in function occurred despite dramatic radiographic improvement after dilatation of severe spasm. The several days of symptomatic spasm may have resulted in cerebral infarction. This may indicate the neccessity for early intervention of balloon dilata-

tion in symptomatic patients.

Our preliminary experience suggests that, in selected patients with cerebral vasospasm refractory to medical treatment, balloon dilatation may dramatically improve neurological deficits and reduce morbidity. Controlled studies are necessary to prove the effectiveness of this new treatment modality. The possible role of transvascular balloon dilatation procedures on early vasospasm should be explored.

References

1. Allen GS, Banghart SB (1979) Cerebral arterial spasm, Part 9: In vitro effects of nifedipine on serotonin-, phenylephrine-, and potassium-induced contractions of canine basilar and femoral arteries. Neurosurgery 4:37–47
2. Cummins BH, Griffith HB (1971) Intracarotid phenoxybenzamine for cerebral arterial spasm. Br Med J 745:382–383
3. Handa J, et al. (1973) Effect of intracarotid phenoxybenzamine on CBF and vasospasm: A clinical study. Surg Neurol 1:229–232
4. Hieshima GB, Higashida RT, Halbach VV, Cahan L, Goto K (1986) Intravascular balloon embolization of a carotid-ophthalmic artery aneurysm with preservation of the parent vessel. Am J Neuroradiol 7(5):916–918
5. Hieshima GB, Higashida RT, Wapenski J, Halbach V, Cahan L, Bentson J (1986) Balloon embolization of a large distal basilar artery aneurysm. J Neurosurg 65(3):413–416
6. Ishii S, Chigasaki H, Nonaka T, et al. (1977) Clinical usefulness of haptoglobin in the treatment of vasospasm following SAH. Neurosurgery 1:65–66
7. Kassell NF, drake CG (1982) Timing of aneurysm surgery. Neurosurgery 10(4):515–519
8. Mizukami M, Kawase T, Usami T, et al. (1982) Prevention of vasospasm by early operation with removal of subarachnoid blood. Neurosurgery 10(3):301–307
9. Sundt TM Jr, Onofro BM, Merideth J (1973) Treatment of cerebral vasospasm from subarachnoid hemorrhage with isoproterenol and lidocaine hydrochloride. J Neurosurg 38:557–560
10. Zubkov TN, Nikitrov BM, Shuitin VA (1984) Balloon catheter technique for dilatation of constricted arteries after aneurysmal SAH. Acta Neurochir 70:65–79

Management of Subarachnoid Hemorrhage

Experience with 360 Patients (1980–1986)

Dries J.M. van der Werf, Rob Dreissen, Louise Hageman, Demetrios Velis, Wouter Schievink, K. Albrecht, and O.C. van Gent[1]

Introduction

Faced with a high rate of recurrent bleeding after subarachnoid hemorrhage (SAH)—highest in the first 24 h, accumulating up to 20% in the first 2 weeks—and with the increasing incidence of delayed cerebral ischemia, particularly after the use of antifibrinolytics, we started to operate on ruptured cerebral aneurysms as early as possible (usually within 72 h after the bleeding) since 1979. We assumed that the higher operative mortality and morbidity of early surgery would still be an improvement over the increased mortality and morbidity from recurrent bleeding and an increased rate of delayed cerebral ischemia in delayed surgery.

If antifibrinolytics would be as effective as early surgery in preventing rebleeding after the first 24 h, and if, at the same time, delayed ischemia could be prevented by conservative means like hypervolemia, calcium antagonists, lowered blood viscosity, or other methods, delayed or late surgery would be the best treatment. This implies that the increased incidence of hydrocephalus observed with this conservative treatment should also be prevented by some other means. The high mortality and morbidity of conservative treatment thusfar has not convinced us of its effectiveness [4, 5, 7]. Even if one assumes that recurrent bleeding within 24 h after the initial SAH can sometimes be prevented by the use of antifibrinolytics and never by early surgery, there remains a substantial percentage of rebleeding thereafter; nor has delayed cerebral ischemia been prevented up to now by hypervolemia, hemodilution, control of blood viscosity, or calcium antagonists preoperatively. Most authors agree that the amount of blood in the basal cisterns is related to the development of delayed ischemia, hypovolemia, hyponatremia, and hydrocephalus, the latter by obstruction of CSF pathways. Since this cisternal blood is by far the most important prognostic factor, it must be removed as soon as possible after the bleeding unless its consequences can be avoided by conservative means. Narrowing of conductive vessels is not or only very partially prevented by the use of calcium antagonists as shown by control angiography. Perhaps small vessels do react and brain cells can be protected against ischemia by these drugs. Fibrinolytics that might dissolve blood and fibrin clot and thereby reopen CSF pathways carry a high risk of rebleeding: in fact the use of antifibrinolytics prevents such resolution. Restoration of CSF pathways necessary for CSF circulation and resorbtion, and for washout of blood and fibrin surrounding basal vessels, cannot be expected from conservative treatment. Only surgical intervention with direct removal of blood and fibrin clot, wide opening of the cisterns and their connections, and postoperative CSF drainage can remove, to a large extent, the deadly threat of secondary vasculopathy and hydrocephalus.

Once the aneurysmal neck is secured, we feel free to increase cerebral perfusion as much as necessary to reverse the neurological deficit without the risk of rebleeding. Cerebral perfusion can be increased by raising the pulmonary wedge pressure, hypervolemia, and hemodilution. In resistant cases, the mean systemic blood pressure may be raised by 15%–20% or more until the neurological deficit disappears. The peripheral resistance may be decreased by lowering the blood viscosity with Rheomacrodex, mannitol, human albumin, and by bleeding. If the intracranial pressure is kept at a normal level by preventing or treating hydrocephalus, the optimum cerebral perfusion is obtained. We have seen a paretic arm rise again with a raise in blood pressure or after bleeding the patient and hemodilution.

In order to detect patients who are at risk of developing delayed ischemia in both operated and nonoperated cases (i.e., late referrals)

---

[1] Department of Neurosurgery, Academic Medical Center, Amsterdam, The Netherlands

we perform the following daily investigations: blood-viscosity and hematocrit, blood sodium content, and transcranial Doppler blood flow velocity measurement.

Control of Blood Viscosity after Aneurysmal SAH

Cerebral perfusion depends on the systemic arterial pressure, the intracranial pressure, the diameter of cerebral conductance vessels, and the peripheral vascular resistance. The latter is influenced by the blood viscosity, i.e., the inherent resistance of blood to flow, among other things.

In 17 patients with aneurysmal SAH (grades I and II) operated within 5 days after the hemorrhage, blood viscosity and hematocrit were measured 12 h after admission, before angiography, and at daily intervals for an average of 12 days. Three shear rates—low, middle, and high—were determined.

We found blood viscosity to be significantly higher when the level of consciousness was low, or in the presence of neurologic deficit. For the prevention and treatment of cerebral ischemia after SAH, control of the blood viscosity and hematocrit during treatment with hypervolemic hemodilution, venisection, mannitol, and high molecular dextran was found to be very useful [6].

Hyponatremia

In a well-documented study, Wijdicks showed that, in patients not yet operated for aneurysmal SAH, the incidence of cerebral infarction was significantly higher in patients who developed hyponatremia (defined as a sodium level lower than 135 mmol/l on 2 consecutive days), and that there was an associated decrease in plasma volume [9]. In our patients, we found a similar drop in plasma sodium content postoperatively, preceding clinical signs of cerebral ischemia by several days. Despite large amounts of extra sodium infusions, it proved to be very difficult to raise the plasma sodium content, and it took an average of 14 days after the bleeding for that content to become normal. Perhaps the addition of fludrocortisone to increased salt intake decreases further natriuresis, as suggested by Wijdicks. The concomitant hypovolemia was combatted by generous albumin, plasma, and Rheomacrodex infusions.

Transcranial Doppler Examination

Cerebral blood flow velocities can be measured transcranially [1]. In 42 patients with SAH, daily transcranial Doppler examinations were performed. In 34 patients, reliable data were obtained. Of these, 19 showed no significant rise in the mean flow velocity. In 15 patients, however, a rise to 200 cm/s or more was found. The peak velocity in these patients was reached between 5 and 7 days after the bleeding; the steep rise usually started at day 3 or 4, which was well in advance of the appearance of clinical symptoms. These symptoms were found in 12 of 15 patients. Three cases showed musical murmers. Blood flow velocities decreased more markedly after CO_2 inhalation in patients with clinical vasospasm than in normal controls.

Since high mean velocities and the pulsatility index $\left(\dfrac{Vmax - Vmin}{Vmean} \right)$ may be the same in patients with high maximum velocities (Vmax) and low minimum velocities (Vmin) as in those with maximum and minimum values close to the same mean, we esteem that the descending slope of the Doppler curve and other characteristics of the curve have more to say about the peripheral vascular resistance and the flow capacity than the mean flow velocity values themselves. The mathematic processing of the curves is now the object of a further study.

Clinical Material and Methods

Since 1980, a short time after we started to operate on cerebral aneurysms in the acute stage, we have treated a consecutive series of 360 patients admitted with a proven diagnosis of SAH. The diagnosis was verified by lumbar puncture and/ or CTscan. Three- or four-vessel angiography was done in 340 patients.

A total of 287 patients were operated. Of these, 148 underwent early surgery (within 72 h after SAH), 33 were operated between days 4 and 8, and the remaining 106 were operated more than 8 days after the last bleeding (Table 1). Forty-one patients were not operated for various reasons. In 32 (11%) of 280 patients admitted during the years 1982–1986, no aneurysm could be found despite a complete four-vessel angiography. The fate of these patients and the possible origin of the bleeding will be discussed elsewhere.

Results

Early operations. Of a total of 287 patients, 148 (51%) were operated within 72 h after the last SAH. The outcome after at least 3 months was, for grades I–III patients on admission, good in 81.7%, moderately disabled in 8.7%, and dead in 9.5%; none were severely disabled. For all grades (I–V) these figures were good in 71%, moderately disabled in 7.4%, severely disabled in 1.3%, and death in 20.1% (Table 2).

Delayed surgery. These results were approximately the same as in the early operated patients (Table 3).

Late surgery (more than 8 days after SAH). These patients faired slightly better; less were severely disabled or dead and more were moderately disabled (Table 4).

As cause of death in the operated cases we noted the following:

a) Faulty operative technique, such as incorrectly placed clip, occlusion of major vessel, clipping of aneurysm that had not bled, tear of major bloodvessel, slipping of clip post-operatively, or partial occlusion of the neck

b) Postoperative delayed ischemia and infarction

c) Uncontrolable rise in intracranial pressure, hematoma, and herniation (all grades IV or V)

d) Other complications, such as pneumonia, pulmonary embolism, or thrombosis of venous sinuses

The causes of death for the different groups of patients according to the timing of surgery are shown in Table 5.

Table 1. Patients admitted with SAH (1980–1986)

			No. of patients
Operated	Early	(<3 days)	148
	Delayed	(4–8 days)	33
	Late	(>8 days)	106
			287
Not operated			41
No aneurysm found			32

$n = 360$

Table 2. Outcome after early aneurysmal surgery (1980–1985)

	Good	Moderately disabled	Severely disabled	Dead
Grades I–III	81.7%	8.7%	0%	9.5%
All grades (I–V)	71%	7.4%	1.3%	20.1%

$n = 148$
Surgery was performed within 3 days after SAH

Table 3. Outcome after delayed aneurysmal surgery (1980–1986)

	Good	Moderately disabled	Severely disabled	Dead
Grades I–III	83.8%	3.2%	3.2%	9.7%
All grades (I–V)	78.8%	3.0%	3.0%	15.2%

$n = 33$
Surgery was performed in days 4–8 after SAH

Table 4. Outcome after late aneurysmal surgery (1980–1986)

	Good	Moderately disabled	Severely disabled	Dead
Grades I–III[a]	82.9%	11.4%	2.9%	2.9%

$n = 106$
Surgery was performed more than 8 days after SAH
[a] There was only one grade IV patient and no grade V patients in this group

Table 5. Causes of death in operated patients and timing of surgery

	Operative technique	Ischemia or infarction	Rise in ICP or herniation	Other
Early (<3 days)	9	4	13	1
Delayed (4–8 days)	2	5	—	
Late (>8 days)	1	—	—	1
Total	12	9	13	2

ICP intracranial pressure

Table 6. Outcome of clinical ischemia after aneurysmal surgery in relation to CT scan and nimodipine treatment

	Nimodipine		No nimodipine	
Amount of blood on initial CT	+ +(+)	+	+ +(+)	+
Outcome				
Good	7	1	11	4
Moderately disabled	3	1		1
Severely disabled				1
Dead	1	2	4	2

n = 39

Table 7. Time of recurrent bleeding after first SAH

Outcome	Intervals after admission					
	<24 h	2 days	3 days	4 days	8–10 days	>14 days
Good	2	2	1	1		
Dead	12	3	2		3	2
Total	14	5	3	1	3	2

Clinical Ischemia

Of 287 patients, 39 (13.6%) developed clinical signs of ischemia. Symptomatic ischemia developed six times preoperatively and 24 times postoperatively. The onset of clinical symptoms took place mostly on days 5, 6, or 7 after the last hemorrhage, to which it was more related than to the day of surgery. Twenty-six patients were operated early (before 3 days) seven between days 4 and 8, and six after day 8. Nine patients died of cerebral infarction; four after early surgery (2.7%), and five after delayed surgery (15%). The relationship between the amount of blood on the initial CT scan and the treatment with or without nimodipine is represented in Table 6.

Recurrent Bleeding

Recurrent bleeding is one of the most important complications after SAH besides delayed cerebral ischemia and hydrocephalus. It is generally believed to occur mostly within the first 24 h after the initial hemorrhage. Thereafter, the incidence is thought to decrease gradually. Of 303 patients admitted after their first bleeding, 30 (10%) had a rebleed after their admission. After 24 h, only 284 patients were alive due to 12 fatal recurrences and seven deaths from initial bleeding: Of these 284, 16 (5.6%) had a later recurrent bleeding of whom ten died. Two could be attributed to an incorrectly placed clip (Table 7). We consider this low recurrent rate (5.6%) the benefit of our early surgery policy.

Hydrocephalus

Acute hydrocephalus, requiring any form of drainage, occurred only six times in 360 patients. Delayed hydrocephalus was found in 51 patients (14%). Internal shunting was necessary in 34 patients (approximately 10%). We feel that this relatively low percentage may be related to our policy of early surgery, removal of blood clot, and opening of CSF pathways, on the one hand and postoperative cisternal drainage—a practice adopted during the last years—on the other hand (Table 8).

Not Operated Patients with Aneurysmal SAH

As mentioned before, 41 patients were not operated for various reasons. Three were technically inoperable, four were in bad general condition. Recurrent bleeding occurred within 24 h in 14 patients and seven were dead within 1 day of the first bleeding. Delayed ischemia and/or recurrence occurred in 12 patients. One patient was not operated for unknown causes. Of the 40 patients, all but one died.

Overall Management Results

Of all 328 patients admitted with aneurysmal SAH 220 (67.1%) finally were in excellent or good condition, 25 (7.7%) in moderately disabled condition, six (1.8%) in severely disabled condition, and 77 (23.4%) died.

References

1. Aaslid R (ed) (1986) Transcranial Doppler sonography 1986 Springer, Vienna
2. Ausman JI, Diaz FG, Malik GM, Fielding AS, Son CS (1985) Current management of cerebral aneurysms: Is it based on facts or myths? Surg Neurol 24:625–35

Table 8. Incidence of hydrocephalus after SAH

Number of patients	360
Hydrocephalus (all forms)	57
Drainage: External	5
Internal	34
Acute hydrocephalus (<5 days)	6
Internal shunt	4
External drainage	2
Good recovery	4
Recurrent SAH	2 (died)

3. Gent OC van, Velis DN (1987) Serial quantitative EEG in patients with subarachnoid hemorrhage. J Neurophysiology (submitted for publication)
4. Hydra A (1986) Aneurysmal subarachnoid hemorrhage: A clinical and CT study of complications and outcome. Thesis, University of Amsterdam
5. Milhorat, Krautheim M (1986) Results of early and delayed operations for ruptured intracranial aneurysms in two series of 100 consecutive patients. Surg Neurol 26:123–128
6. Schievink WI, Hageman LM, Velis DN, Werf AJM van der, Hardeman MR, Goedhart PT (1987) Relationship between blood viscosity and cerebral ischemia after surgical treatment of ruptured cerebral aneurysms. Surg Neurol 27
7. Vermeulen M, Lindsay KW, Murray GD, Cheah F, Hydra A, Muizelaar JP, Schannong M, Teasdale GM, Crevel H van, Gijn J van (1984) Antifibrinolytic treatment in subarachnoid hemorrhage. N Eng J Med 311:432–437
8. Werf AJM van der (1986) Spasme vasculaire et ischémie cérébrale après hémorragie meningée par rupture anéurysmale. Neurochirurgie 32:1–22
9. Wijdicks EFM (1987) Hyponatremia, volume status, and blood pressure following aneurysmal subarachnoid hemorrhage. Thesis, Rotterdam University

Cerebral Microthrombosis, Synthesis Imbalance of TXA$_2$-PGI$_2$, and Subarachnoid Focal Acidosis in the Pathogenesis of Symptomatic Cerebral Vasospasm

Shigeharu Suzuki[1], Hiroki Ohkuma[1], Takashi Iwabuchi[1], and Noriaki Yoshimura[2]

Numerous investigations of cerebral vasospasm (hearafter referred to as vasospasm) confirm the pathogenesis to be various and complicated. In accounting for the pathogenesis of vasospasm, it is our contention that subarachnoid focal acidosis resulting from anaerobic changes in subarachnoid clots may play a role in inducing multiple cerebral microthrombosis, which in turn induces cerebral ischemia or infarction by platelet aggregation caused by an imbalance in the synthesis of TXA$_2$ and PGI$_2$ (Fig. 1) [6–9]. In this paper, we tried to corroborate that contention in clinical studies focussed firstly on the pH of intracranial irrigation fluid for aneurysmal surgery during the vasospasm predilection period and, secondly, on the effectiveness of TXA$_2$ synthetase inhibitors in the prevention of symptomatic vasospasm, and in histopathological studies of the brains of patients who died of subarachnoid hemorrhage.

Introduction

With regard to the involvement of the TXA$_2$ synthesis system and the participation of cerebral microthrombosis, we cite here the results of our previous clinical studies on the effectiveness of TXA$_2$ synthetase inhibitors in the prevention of symptomatic vasospasm [7, 9]; we also cite the results of a double-blind comparative clinical study on the same compound, completed and published only quite recently in Japan [2], and histopathological evidence of microthrombosis in the brains of patients who had suffered typical vasospasms, compared with an autopsy specimen where the primary cause of death was hydrocephalus. We stress the role of subarachnoid

Departments of Neurosurgery[1] and Pathology[2], Hirosaki University School of Medicine, Hirosaki, Japan

focal acidosis in the pathogenesis from a clinical viewpoint, centering on the pH of intracranial irrigation fluid for aneurysmal surgery during the vasospasm predilection period.

Participation of Prostaglandins Synthesis System

The involvements of both the prostaglandins (PGs) synthesis system and microthrombosis in the pathogenesis were suggested by the result of our previous in vitro experiments: we found that the vasocontractility of the CSF blood mixture is higher in anaerobical than in aerobical incubations, and this contractility was attenuated much more by the PGs synthesis inhibitor mecrofenamate than by phenoxybenzamine [6]. We also encountered a significant number of cases with asymptomatic vasospasm or with marked cerebral ischemic symptoms where the arterial narrowing was not particularly severe [7]. These observations led us necessarily to focus upon TXA$_2$, which is the principal metabolite of the PGs synthesis system and a potent platelet aggregator. TXA$_2$ synthetase inhibitors were thus studied clinically in the prevention of this disease (Table 1).

Initially, a pyrimidine derivative (trapidil) was tested independently in our department in 20 reported cases [7], and on 17 additional patients with ruptured cerebral aneurysms. We determined that this drug was not always effective for angiographical vasospasms but was considerably effective for cerebral ischemic symptoms. An imidazole derivative (OKY-046) was then tested cooperatively at ten neurosurgical services, on a total of 82 patients and similar results were obtained [9].

Recently, a double-blind controlled study of OKY-046 for the prevention of delayed cerebral ischemia after aneurysmal rupture was conducted cooperatively in 48 neurosurgical services in Japan [2]. In this study, 80 mg/day or 400

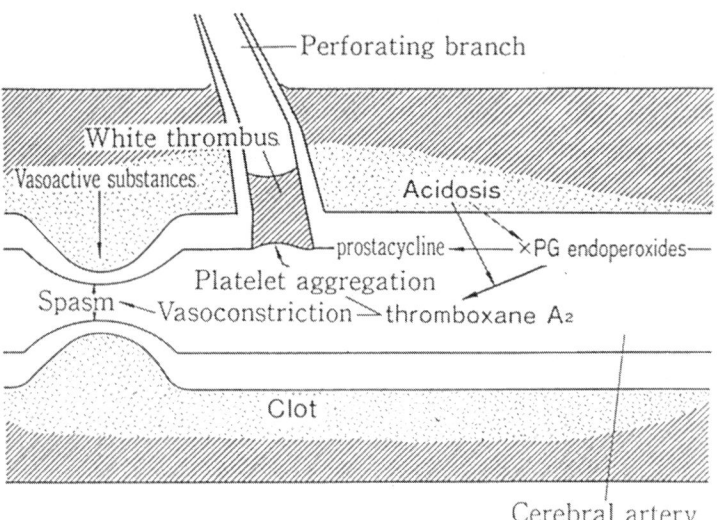

Fig. 1. Schematic of the hypothetical pathogenesis of cerebral ischemia after subarachnoid hemorrhage

Table 1. Clinical studies on prevention of cerebral vasospasm with TXA_2 synthetase inhibitors

Compounds	Type of study	Participating centers	Subjects	Doses	Efficacy
Pyrimidine derivative (trapidil)	Open	1	10	300 mg/day	Ischemic symptoms
			27	450 mg/day	
			37		
Imidazole derivative (OKY-046)	Open (cooperative)	10	34	2 μg/kg/min	Ischemic symptoms
			18	5 μg/kg/min	
			30	10 μg/kg/min	
			82		
Imidazole derivative (OKY-046)	Double-blind (cooperative)	48	86	Placebo	
			84	80 mg/day	Either ischemic symptoms or cerebral vasospasm
			86	400 mg/day	
			256		

mg/day of the compound or a placebo were administered to the patients who underwent direct aneurysmal surgery until the 3rd SAH day, and 256 patients in total were studied for clinical evaluation. The incidences of low-density area (LD) on CTs and angiographical vasospasms were significantly lower in the groups receiving the compound. The functional prognosis after one month of SAH among those cases with severe preoperative clinical grades, or with high grade high-density areas (HD) in the initial CTs, was clearly better for the group receiving 80 mg/day of the drug than for the placebo group.

Multiple Cerebral Microthrombosis in Symptomatic Cerebral Vasospasm

The participation of microthrombosis caused by platelet aggregation in this pathogenesis is urged by two findings: first, there are clinical cases in which the grades of angiographical vasospasm and ischemic signs are not parallel [7], which suggests the involvement of some intraarterial factors in the completion of cerebral ischemia. Second, as described above, the synthetase inhibitor of TXA_2 (a potent platelet aggregator) was proved effective in the prevention particu-

Table 2. Summary of autopsies performed on SAH fatalities by aneurysmal rupture

Cases	Sex	Age (yrs)	Site of aneurysms	Angiographical Vasospasms	LD in CT	Microthromosis
1	F	63	A Com A	Lt ACA (+ + +)	(+)	(+)
				Lt MCA (+ + +)	(+ + +)	(+ + +)
				Rt ACA (+ + +)	(−)	(±)
2	M	61	Rt MCA	Lt (no angiography)		(+)
				Rt ACA (+ + +)	(+ + +)	(+ + +)
				Rt MCA (+ + +)	(+ + +)	(+ + +)
3	M	71	A Com A	Lt ACA, MCA (+ + +)	(+ + +)	(+ + +)
				Rt ACA, MCA (+ + +)	(+ + +)	(+ + +)
4	F	73	Lt ICPC	Lt ACA, MCA (+ +)	(−)	(+)
				Rt (no angiography)	(−)	(±)

A Com A anterior communicating artery, *MCA* middle cerebral artery, *ICPC* internal carotid-posterior communicating artery, + + + high grade, + + moderate, + slight, ± barely positive, − negative

larly of ischemic symptoms rather than of angiographical vasospasm per se after SAH.

We have previously demonstrated [8] histologically that multiple microthrombi were a major cause of cerebral infarction in the autopsied brain of a patient who died from the rupture of a cerebral aneurysm followed by typical vasospasm. Two similar cases and a fatality resulting mainly from advanced hydrocephalus after SAH were autopsied thereafter (Table 2). Case 1 in the table was previously reported [8]. Case 2 was a 61-year-old male who had suffered SAH with intracerebral hematoma (ICH) due to the rupture of a right middle cerebral aneurysm. Moderate vasospasms in the right anterior and middle cerebral arteries had already been observed in the angiograms taken on the 5th SAH day when the patient was transferred to our hospital, but craniotomy and aneurysmal neck clipping were performed on the same day because of the massive ICH. LD areas in the regions of spastic arteries were revealed in the CTs taken on the 8th SAH day; the patient died on the 15th SAH day. Histopathological examinations of the brain revealed that microthrombi had multiplied to a much greater extent in the right cerebral hemisphere. Case 3 was a 71-year-old male who died on the 8th SAH day from the rupture of an anterior communicating aneurysm followed by severe symptomatic vasospasms in the bilateral anterior and middle cerebral arteries, which were confirmed by angiographies performed on the 5th and the 6th SAH days and by CTs taken on the 6th SAH day, in which extensive bilateral LDs were delineated. This patient was not operated upon because his preoperative grade was too poor. Multiple fibrin thrombi were seen dif-

fused through all the regions of the autopsied brain, which we suspected to have induced even a disseminated intravascular coagulation in this case. No confirmation, however, could be obtained because the autopsy was permitted only for the brain. In case 4 (a 73-year-old female), on the other hand, SAH itself was severe enough, and no consciousness level better than semicoma was observed from the rupture of a left internal carotid-posterior communicating broad neck aneurysm to the patient's death on the 9th SAH day. As her initial CTs showed marked hydrocephalus together with severe SAH, ventricular drainage was commenced on the day of the onset. On the 2nd SAH day, the aneurysm was clipped, although no improvement was seen clinically. Right carotid angiography performed the next day, however, revealed diffuse moderate vasospasms on both the right anterior and middle cerebral arteries. Repeated difficulties in drainage were followed by rapid aggravation of hydrocephalus, but no definite LD was seen even in CTs taken two days before the patient's death. Histopathological examination of the brain evidenced fibrin thrombi, in very low incidence, in the capillaries and venules of the left cerebral hemisphere.

Participation of Subarachnoid Focal Acidosis

Our investigations lead us to believe that subarachnoid focal acidosis resulting from anaerobic changes in subarachnoid clots may also play a role in the pathogenesis of vasospasm [1, 8, 10].

Physiological saline solution has generally

Table 3. Clinical changes after aneurysmal surgery performed during vasospasm predilection period (4th–11th SAH day) in cases with pre- or postoperative cerebral vasospasm: Comparison of two groups treated with physiological saline solution and with pH 8.0 Hartmann solution

	Cases treated with physiological saline solution	Cases treated with pH 8.0 Hartmann solution
Cases with preoperative vasospasm		
Deteriorated	9 (100.0%)	2 (22.2%)
Unchanged	0	3
Improved	0	4
Total	9	9
Cases with postoperative vasospasm		
Deteriorated	6[a] (66.7%)	3[b] (30.0%)
Unchanged	3	5
Improved	0	2
Total	9	10

[a] Three of the six patients showed clinical deterioration 2, 4, and 20 h respectively after operation
[b] Clinical deterioration occurred 2–3 days after the operation
All other clinical deteriorations were already observed as the patients emerged from anesthesia

been used for intracranial irrigation during craniotomy, including aneurysmal surgery. The pH value of the physiological saline we have been using is 6.401 ± 0.122 (n = 11). There are opinions, on the other hand, that vasospasm has a predilection period extending from the 4th to the 11th SAH day, the peak falling on the 7th [10], and that the results of aneurysmal surgeries performed around this period are poorer than those performed earlier or late [3–5].

Given this, it is possible that introducing physiological saline with its lower pH to the cerebral arteries—which are at the time acidotic—could in fact trigger the onset of vasospasm. Therefore, we now use pH 8.0 Hartmann solution (H-solution) instead of physiological saline for intracranial irrigation during aneurysmal surgery, particularly on the 4th–11th SAH days.

Direct surgery upon ruptured cerebral aneurysms has been performed in 499 cases in our department so far. Two groups of these patients were operated on between the 4th and 11th SAH day, using physiological saline in 40 cases and H-solution in 43 for intracranial irrigation. We studied these two groups clinically and comparatively, focussing mainly on the effects of the operation itself upon clinical symptoms and vasospasms (Table 3).

Preoperative vasospasms were confirmed in nine patients each in both the physiological saline and H-solution groups. The vasospasms were symptomatic in all nine patients in the former group and in seven of the patients in the latter, but were asymptomatic in the remaining two patients in the H-solution group. Occurrences of postoperative vasospasms were confirmed in nine patients in the total physiological saline group and ten in the total H-solution group. To evaluate the direct effects of the operation itself on these cases, we compared their immediate pre- and postoperative clinical conditions.

Among the cases with preoperative vasospasms, all nine patients treated with physiological saline deteriorated clinically through the operation and showed aggravated clinical grades immediately thereafter. Of nine patients treated with H-solution, two showed clinical deterioration, not immediately, but 1 and 2 days respectively after the operation. Another three patients were unchanged, and the remaining four showed some improvement. As no particular operative damage was incurred, all clinical deteriorations were considered to have been caused by the aggravation of the vasospasm itself.

Postoperative vasospasms in the physiological saline group were asymptomatic in three of the nine patients, but were symptomatic in another six (66.6%) incurring postoperative clinical deterioration. Three of the six patients with symptomatic vasospasms suffered clinical deterioration already observable as they emerged from anesthesia, and vasospasms per se were confirmed by cerebral angiographies performed several days later. In the remaining three patients, the deteriorations occurred 2, 4, and 20 h respectively after the operation and were confirmed by angiographies. Among the ten patients

Table 4. Comparative clinical outcome at discharge of two groups treated with physiological saline solution and with pH 8.0 Hartmann solution

Clinical outcome	Cases treated with physiological saline solution	Cases treated with pH 8.0 Hartmann solution
0	12 (30.0%)	25 (58.1%)[a]
1	7 (17.5%)	6 (13.9%)
2	1 (2.5%)	1 (2.3%)
3	2 (5.0%)	3 (7.0%)
4	1 (2.5%)	3 (7.0%)
5	5 (12.5%)	1 (2.3%)
6	2 (5.0%)	0
7	1 (2.5%)	1 (2.3%)
8	9 (22.5%)	3 (7.0%)[b]
	40	43

0 normal, *1* almost normal, *2* slight neurological deficit, *3* unaided daily life, *4* assisted daily life, *5* can leave bed with assistance, *6* confined to bed, *7* vegetative state, *8* deceased
[a] $P < 0.01$
[b] $P < 0.05$

in the H-solution group, five were unchanged clinically, and another two showed postoperative improvement. In the remaining three (30.0%) patients the vasospasms were symptomatic; this manifested itself somewhat later than for those in the physiological saline group, at 2–3 days after the operation.

Functional outcome at the time of discharge was expressed in nine grades, from 0 (normal) to 8 (deceased), and the two groups were compared (Table 4). Twelve patients in the physiological saline group were graded 0 (30.0%), as were 25 (58.1%) in the H-solution group ($P < 0.01$); nine patients (22.5%) and three (7.0%) respectively were graded at 8 ($P < 0.05$). Significantly better outcomes were thus obtained in the H-solution group.

Summarizing the above, we can say that intracranial irrigation with low pH solution during the vasospasm predilection period (the supposed peak of the subarachnoid focal acidosis) tends to cause immediate induction or aggravation of the vasospasm. The possible participation of subarachnoid acidosis is thus emphasized.

Conclusion

Our contention regarding the pathogenesis of cerebral vasospasms that subarachnoid focal acidosis, synthesis imbalance of TXA_2 and PGI_2, and multiple microthrombosis in the peripheral cerebral vessels may play an important role in inducing symptomatic vasospasm, is

emphasized here again. The details and discussion of each step in this hypothesis are contained in papers we have previously submitted [6–10]. In treating patients with ruptured cerebral aneurysms, however, we insist here that operations should be performed as soon as the patient's condition permits, to prevent either aneurysmal rerupture or vasospasm. A TXA_2 synthetase inhibitor should be administered on the earliest possible occasion for the prevention of symptomatic vasospasm, physiological or alkaline solution should be used for intracranial irrigation during craniotomy, and, when vasospasm occurs, therapeutic measures against thrombosis should also be taken, together with induced hypertension, particularly be hypervolemic treatment [1].

References

1. Kudo T, Suzuki S, Iwabuchi T (1981) Importance of monitoring the circulating blood volume in patients with cerebral vasospasm after subarachnoid hemorrhage. Neurosurgery 9:514–520
2. Sano K, Handa H, Suzuki S, Asano T, Tamura A, Yonekawa Y, Ono H, Tachibana N, Hanaoka K (1986) Therapeutic usefulness of a thromboxane synthetase inhibitor, OKY-046 Na, in cerebral vasospasm and delayed ischemic neurological deficits after aneurysmal rupture. Igakuno Ayumi (Japan) 138:455–469
3. Saito I, Ueda Y, Sano K (1977) Significance of vasospasm in the treatment of ruptured intracranial aneurysms. J Neurosurg 47:412–429
4. Shephard RH (1983) Ruptured cerebral aneurysms:

Early and late prognosis with surgical treatment. A personal series, 1958–1980. J Neurosurg 59:6–15

5. Suzuki J, Kodama N (1980) Grading and timing of surgery for cerebral aneurysm. In: Wilkins RH (ed) Cerebral Arterial Spasm. Williams and Wilkins, Baltimore pp 438–446

6. Suzuki S, White RP, Chapleau CE, Robertson JT (1980) An experimental evaluation of anaerobic condition in the pathogenesis of cerebral vasospasm associated with subarachnoid hemorrhage: A preliminary report. Hirosaki Med J 32:48–56

7. Suzuki S, Sobata E, Iwabuchi T (1981) Prevention of cerebral ischemic symptoms in cerebral vasospasm with trapidil, an antagonist and selective synthesis inhibitor of thromboxan A_2. Neurosurgery 9:679–685

8. Suzuki S, Suzuki M, Iwabuchi T, Kamata Y (1983) Role of cerebral microthrombosis in symptomatic cerebral vasospasm: With a case report. Neurosurgery 13:199–203

9. Suzuki S, Iwabuchi T, Tanaka T, Kanayama S, Ottomo M, Hatanaka M, Aihara H (1985) Prevention of cerebral vasospasm with OKY-046, an imidazole derivative, and a thromboxane synthetase inhibitor: A preliminary cooperative clinical study. Acta Neurochir 77:133–141

The Therapeutic Methods for Cerebral Vasospasm

Prevention and Treatment

TAKASHI YOSHIMOTO and JIRO SUZUKI[1]

Introduction

Vasospasm of cerebral vessels is known to occur between the 4th and 14th days following the rupture of a cerebral aneurysm, and to lead to ischemic symptoms of varying severity, sometimes to death. A variety of therapies have been employed to treat such vasospasm, but little success has been achieved. In the present paper, we discuss our current therapeutic techniques and recent results, based upon our experiences of direct operations on more than 2000 cases of ruptured cerebral aneurysm.

The Mechanism of Onset of Cerebral Vasospasm

It is thought that the primary causes of cerebral vasospasm are the inducing substances produced by the ongoing biochemical changes in blood components which have been released into the subarachnoid space due to aneurysm rupture. Endo, Sonobe, and colleagues from our department have performed a series of experiments on cerebral vasospasms using the basilar artery of the adult cat [1, 5]. They found that a mixture of fresh arterial blood and cerebrospinal fluid (CSF) produces the strongest vasospasm after seven days of incubation (Fig. 1). From biochemical analysis of the incubate, they demonstrated that oxyhemoglobin (oxyHb), released from erythrocytes following hemolysis, induced severe and persisting vasospasm. It was also shown that the level of oxyHb increased sharply three days following the hemolysis, reached a peak after 7 days, and was nearly converted to methemoglobin (metHb) after 15 days. Once oxyHb had been converted to metHb, the severity of the cerebral vasospasm was markedly reduced.

Those experimental results are in excellent agreement with clinical findings, both with regard to the timing of the vasospasm and the pattern of induction. Such results have led us to conclude that the vasospasm in most clinical cases is due to oxyHb. Moreover, electron-microscopic studies have shown that, in those vessels which are constricted due to oxyHb, the oxyHb is brought to the vessel via the sympathetic nerve terminals [4] which are densely distributed on the vascular adventitia. It was also demonstrated that the severity of vasospasm due to oxyHb in brain vessels which have been denervated by means of cervical sympathectomy is greatly reduced [2] (Fig. 2).

Prevention and Treatment for Cerebral Vasospasm

Acute Stage Hematoma Removal

Prevention of cerebral vasospasm can be accomplished by removal, at as early a stage as possible following the aneurysm rupture, of the hematoma in the subarachnoid space, which is the primary cause of vasospasm. We have obtained good results by means of hematoma removal and treatment of the aneurysmal neck within 48 h of rupture [7, 8, 10]. Particular attention must be paid to the fact that, clinically, the substance which brings about vasospasm is not the liquid blood CSF, but is the blood clots in which oxyHb is most abundant, particularly blood clots adherent to the internal carotid artery (ICA) M1, M2 and A1, A2 portion. Excision of such clots must be done as thoroughly as possible.

When surgery is performed 3 or more days after the aneurysm rupture, hemolysis will have already progressed and oxyHb will have been released from erythrocytes. As a consequence, the oxyHb may be brought into contact with blood vessels and, postoperatively, cerebral

---

[1] Division of Neurosurgery, Institute of Brain Diseases, Tohoku University School of Medicine, Sendai, Japan

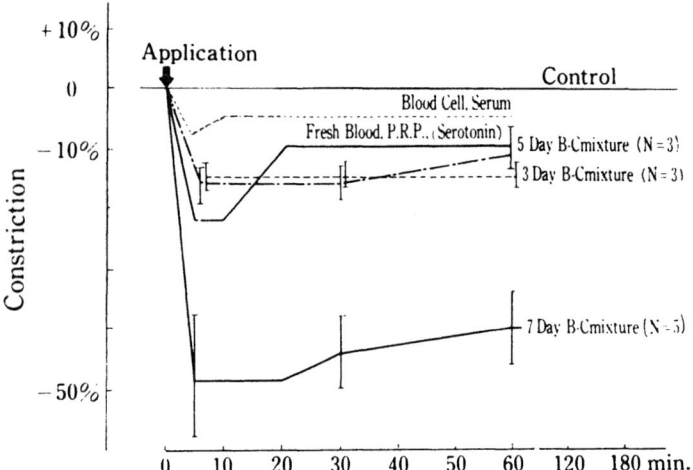

Fig. 1. Vasoconstriction of the basilar artery in the cat after the application of several substances. *P.R.P* platelet-rich plasma, *B–C* blood cell

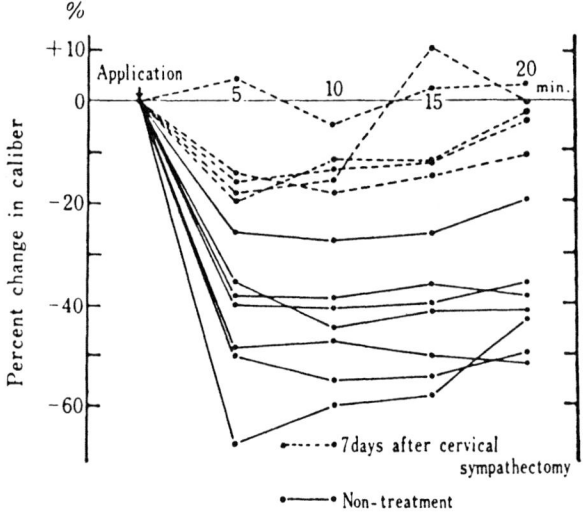

Fig. 2. The effect of cervical sympathectomy on vasospasm. In five cases undergoing cervical sympathectomy 7 days before induced vasospasm by the blood and CSF mixture incubated for 7 days in a cat's basilar artery

vasospasm may occur. In this manner, the patient's condition may actually be aggravated by the surgical operation. For this reason, surgery undertaken in the acute stage should be done while covering all blood clots and surrounding areas with cotton swabs soaked in 10 mmol $NaNO_2$. By so doing, the oxyHb will be converted to metHb and its vasospasmogenic effects neutralized.

CT Prediction of Vasospasm

It is possible to predict the occurrence and site of cerebral vasospasm using sequential CT scans by noting the high-density areas (hematomas) in the subarachnoid space following the aneurysm rupture [6]. Specifically, in cases where a hematoma with a CT value in excess of 65 is seen immediately following rupture, there is a strong prob-

ability that vasospasm will develop in that region. In cases where there is a sudden decrease in the high-density area after the 2nd day, however, the likelihood of vasospasm is low. If CT values in excess of 60 persist through the 5th or 6th day, there is a danger of severe vasospasm (Fig. 3).

Treatment for Cerebral Ischemia due to Vasospasm

Even when acute stage excision of a hematoma is performed and $NaNO_2$ is used in the surgery, it is often not possible to prevent completely the occurrence of vasospasm. Moreover, there are patients who are admitted to the hospital around the 7th day following rupture, when the vasospasm is at its peak. In either case, steps must be taken to treat the symptoms of cerebral ischemia which are brought about by the vasospasm.

Our first measure is to administer the so-called Sendai Cocktail (10 ml/kg 20% mannitol, 10 mg/kg vitamin E, and 10 mg/kg phenytoin)—a mixture of drugs which we have shown to be effective in reducing the damage due to cerebral ischemia [9]. When necessary, hypertensive therapy, using controlled administration of Hypertensin, is also done. If these measures are thought unlikely to avert the vasospastic crisis, cervical sympathectomy is also done to reduce the severity of subsequent vasospasm [3]. During the sympathectomy, care must be taken not to put pressure on the ICA or to cause a decrease in blood pressure, but the single most important point with regard to treatment is that it should be started at an early stage in the course of the disorder, while symptoms are mild, and prior to the development of severe and irreversible pathology. At the latest, therefore, the cervical sympathectomy should be done prior to the patient's having succumbed to a "drowsy" state of consciousness.

In place of these surgical techniques, we are currently studying the possibility of preventing cerebral vasospasm by means of oral administration of the selective alpha-prime blocker, prazosin hydrochloride, during the early stage following aneurysm rupture (Fig. 4).

Further, the control of intracranial pressure during ischemia is of particular importance. We have found that simple and effective control of that pressure can be obtained by leaving the ventricular drainage tube, which is inserted during radical surgery, in place for subsequent use.

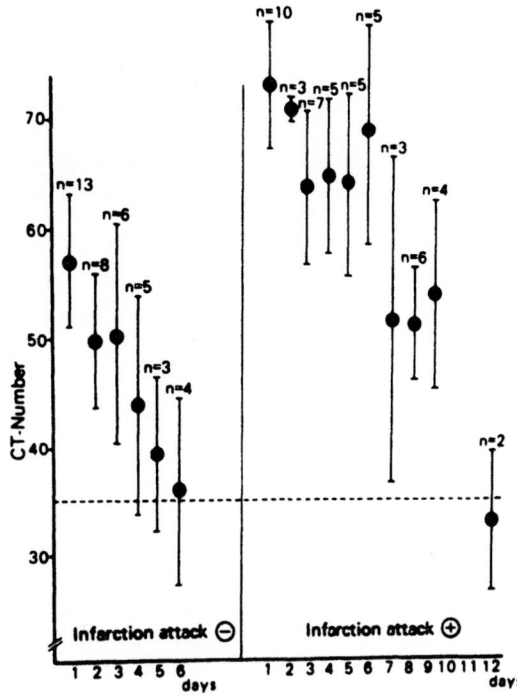

Fig. 3. Correlation between change in the highest density area and the occurrence of cerebral vasospasm. *Dotted line* Hounsfield number of normal thalamus

The Occurrence of Vasospasm in Clinical Cases

At the Division of Neurosurgery of Tohoku University, we have performed intracranial radical surgery on ruptured cerebral aneurysms in 208 cases during the 3-year period from 1983 to the end of 1985. For the present analysis, we used

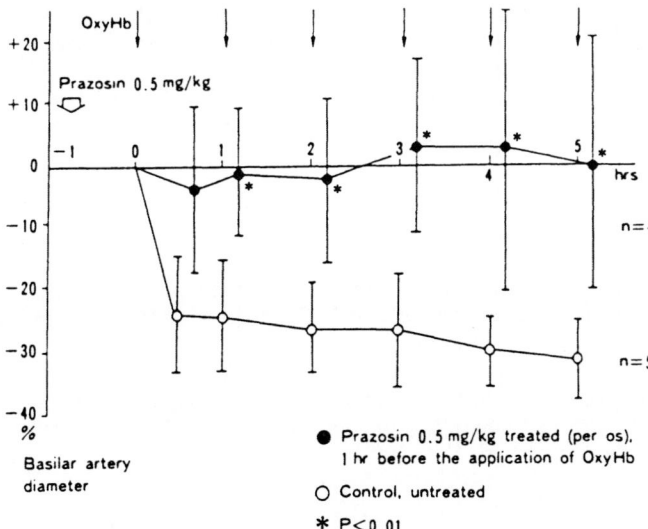

Fig. 4. Change in the basilar artery diameter during vasospasm induced by hourly application of oxyHb. *OxyHb* oxyhemoglobin

Table 1. Incidence of vasospasm per number of days from direct aneurysm surgery

SAH → Surgery	No. of cases		Spasm		
Day 0	18		6		33%
1	61	103	15	25	25%	24%
2	24		4		17%
3–7	37		7		19%
8–14	31		9		29%
14–	37		7		19%
	208		48		23%

103 cases in which radical surgery was performed within two days of the subarachnoid hemorrhage and in which, moreover, removal of the hematoma was possible (Table 1). Among these 103 cases, symptoms of cerebral ischemia due to cerebral vasospasm arose in 25 cases (24%).

These cases included four of the nine patients who were over the age of 70 (44%): vasospasm was found to be progressively less frequent in the patients in their 50s and 60s. The relationship with the preoperative grade was that none of the six grade I cases showed symptoms of vasospasm, but 22% of the grade II, 28% of the grade III, and 38% of the grade IV patients had vasospasm. Vasospasm was also found to have occurred in three of the 35 anterior communicating artery (AComA) aneurysm cases (9%), 11 of the 30 ICA aneurysm cases (37%), and nine of the 33 middle cerebral artery (MCA) cases (27%). The relatively low incidence of vasospasm among the AComA cases is thought to be due to the fact that, in all such cases, bifrontal craniotomy was used and the hematoma was thoroughly removed from the bilateral sylvian fissure and the interhemispheric fissure [10].

In the 25 cases in which ischemic symptoms arose due to vasospasm, there was complete disappearance of the symptoms in 16 cases, remaining neurological deficits in seven cases, and death due to the cerebral ischemia in two cases (Table 2).

Table 2. The outcomes of 25 cases in which ischemic symptoms due to vasospasm arose

No. of cases	Outcome
16	Normally recovered
7	Remaining neurological deficits
2	Death due to cerebral ischemia

References

1. Endo S, Suzuki J (1977) Experimental cerebral vasospasm after subarachnoid hemorrhage: Development and degree of vasospasm. Stroke 8:702–707
2. Endo S, Suzuki J (1979) Experimental cerebral vasospasm after subarachnoid hemorrhage. Participation of adrenergic nerves in cerebral wall. Stroke 10:703–711
3. Owada K, Hori S, Suzuki J (1979) Results of cervical sympathectomy for cerebral vasospasm following aneurysm rupture. In: Suzuki J (ed) Cerebral Aneurysms. Neuron, Tokyo, pp 435–441
4. Sato S, Suzuki J (1975) Anatomical mapping of the cerebral nerve vasorum in the human brain. J Neurosurg 43:559–568
5. Sonobe M, Suzuki J (1978) Vasospasmogenic substances produced following subarachnoid hemorrhage and its fate. Acta Neurochir 44:97–106
6. Suzuki J, Komatsu S, Sato T, et al. (1980) Correlation between CT finding and subsequent development of cerebral infarction due to vasospasm in subarachnoid hemorrhage. Acta Neurochir 55:63–70
7. Suzuki J, Kodama N, Yoshimoto T (1982) Ultra-early surgery of intracranial aneurysms. Acta Neurochir 63:185–191
8. Suzuki J, Yoshimoto T, Kayama T (1984) Surgical treatment of middle cerebral artery aneurysms. J Neurosurg 61:17–23
9. Suzuki J, Fujimoto S, Mizoi K, et al. (1984) The protective effect of combined administration of anti-oxidants and perfluorochemicals on cerebral ischemia. Stroke 15:672–679
10. Suzuki J, Mizoi K, Yoshimoto T (1986) Bifrontal interhemispheric approach to aneurysms of the anterior communicating artery. J Neurosurg 64:183–190

Discussion

Pitts (San Francisco): I would like to ask Dr. Kassell if he thinks there is a relationship between the length of time antifibrinolytics are used and the likelihood that they will lead to the ischemic complications attributed to them? Because in the studies where complications are reported the antifibrinolytics were used for prolonged periods of time—2 weeks or so. Do you think there is a dose response between the length of time of pharmaceuticals and vasospasm? I also have a general question for the panelists who have stopped using antifibrinolytics: If there were an effective treatment for ischemia would you go back to using antifibrinolytic agents?

Kassell (Virginia): I think in general that antifibrinolytic therapy has been used too long; a duration of 5–7 days is probably optimal. In the past, I do not think that a loading dose has been used and this should perhaps be employed to try and eliminate the early rebleeding.

Flamm (New York): I am encouraged by the data I presented to you: In two-thirds of the patients who received both the calcium-channel blocker and antifibrinolytic agents, the incidence of symptomatic vasospasm in what we think is a useful dose was only 6%. I think we have the ability to take advantage of antifibrinolytic activity and at the same time reduce the incidence of ischemic events. In patients that I do not operate on early, and these represent a fairly large number of my patients, I continue to use antifibrinolytic agents in combination with calcium-channel blocker.

van der Werf (Amsterdam): There is a study currently being carried out by the Utrecht and Rotterdam group on the use of antifibrinolytics for 3–4 days; this is a randomized double-blind study, like the former one, for 4 weeks. We are awaiting the results here. I am inclined to use antifibrindytics for 24–48 h when I am forced to delay the operation.

Takakura (Tokyo): There are similar ways of treatment—medication, such as factor XIII or nicardipine. And there are new ways of treatment such as transluminal angioplasty. I would like to ask the panelists what they think about medication.

Fasano (Turin): The problem with factor XIII is this: We found that the method that repairs a fissure on the aneurysm only acts locally; it does not affect all the antifibrinolytic function. It does not, therefore, involve the reticuloendothelial system. The decrease in the degradation of fibrin is much lower. We now have to evaluate whether this method is useful in a large, nonselected series of patients.

Shi (Taichung): Do you think that angiography itself can induce vasospasm? For example, if you receive a patient who is comatose or semicomatose in grade IV or V with a lot of subarachnoid hemorrhage on CT scan would you perform the angiography immediately or defer this until the patient has improved? If you do carry out angiography, do you think that four-vessel angiography is necessary?

Flamm: Yes, I do think that four-vessel angiography is necessary: One should not undertake the treatment of any aneurysm without it. The first part of your question I would rather ask Dr. Halbach, who is a radiologist. I think that a mechanical irritation can be produced with a catheter, but I do not think that delayed ischemic events can be produced or increased by the use of an angiogram unless there is some other angiographic complication. I use the angiogram when I need it.

Yoshimoto (Sendai): We attach a great deal of importance to CT scans. Of course, four-vessel angiography using Seldinger's method is ideal. We examine the CT scans for the distribution of clots and then carry out angiographic study on the basis of the results of CT scanning.

Suzuki (Hirosaki): During the period when vaso-spasms occur, we do not like to perform angio-grams, since we do not wish to disturb the intima.

Flamm: I would like to ask Dr. Halbach how he views the data presented by Dr. Suzuki, since I feel it is a very limited view of vasospasm after subarachnoid hemorrhage that it only deals with the circle of Willis. I think it is a much more diffuse process involving vessels that are not seen angiographically; it is important to focus on the whole brain circulation and not just the vessels.

Halbach (San Francisco): Yes, I totally agree. It would be very pleasing if noninvasive therapy could be maintained. The patients we treat have failed standard medical therapy. I think the mechanism is probably that there are ischemic changes from narrowing of both large and small vessels and that by dilating part of the large base of the brain, which is technically accessible, we may improve the inflow and perfusion in the ischemic area. I believe that there probably is vasospasm involving even the smaller vessels, and technically of course we cannot reach these at present.

Commentator: *Ishii* (Tokyo): Prof. Kassell, through an analysis of the results of the International Cooperative Aneurysm Study, summarized the risk factors for predicting the occurrence of vasospasm following subarachnoid hemorrhage; they include CT finding of subarachnoid blood, age, sex, location of aneurysm, preexisting blood pressure. Profs. Fasano and van der Werf also added Doppler and EEG findings. However, there was no disagreement among the discussants that the CT finding of a subarachnoid clot, particularly diffuse and with high density, is the most reliable predictor. All the panelists mentioned their efforts to prevent or reverse the cerebral vasospasm; the drugs and

measures they employ can be divided as follows: (a) Dilation of the cerebral arteries by drugs, gas, cervical sympathectomy, or even angioplasty; (b) increase of cerebral flow by reducing blood viscosity, increasing the circulating blood volume, or raising the systemic blood pressure; (c) protection of the brain against the ischemic insult by calcium-channel blocking agents or other drugs, such as the Sendai Cocktail or thromboxin A2 synthesis blocking agent; (d) removal of the subarachnoid clot by early surgery followed by cisternal drainage. Most of these means do not necessitate a new trial. Prof. Fasano mentioned the usefulness of factor XIII; it can reduce the rate of rebleeding without any unfavorable effect on the occurrence of vasospasm. If so, it may give us a freer hand in selecting the time of surgery. An excellent report made by Prof. Flamm on the therapeutic use of nicardipine, a potent calcium blocker, appears very promising. As he mentioned, our Japanese group also made significant studies with this drug a few years ago, but unfortunately the result was negative. However, the does of nicardipine used was approximately 1/20 that used by Flamm et al. We will repeat our studies. Dr. Halbach reported a trial with transluminal angioplasty to dilate a spastic artery. As has already been discussed, angiographically demonstrated narrowing of the large arterial lumen is not necessary related to the clinical signs of vasospasm. However, he found a dramatic improvement in the clinical grading in a limited number of patients, so we look forward to their future findings. With regard to the WFNS meeting in Toronto, I would like to repeat something said by Dr. Heros: "After many years of intensive research, the only therapy of substantial value currently available for vasospasm is so far symptomatic, namely improvement of cerebral perfusion pressure." This is not too encouraging but I hope that in a year or two we will know more.

RTD 10. Treatment for Intracerebral Hemorrhage

Endoscopic Evacuation of Intracranial Hematomas

Ludwig M. Auer[1]

Introduction

Neurosurgical endoscopy has gained new interest due to the availability of ultrasound and laser technologies. The present paper summarizes experiences with endoscopic burr hole evacuation obtained since 1983.

Methods and Patients

The rigid endoscope, with an outer diameter of 6 mm, harbors a suction irrigation system, a channel for a 600-μm or a 400-μm neodymium Yag microlaser tube, the optical system for visual control on a videoscreen via an attached miniaturized TV camera, and an instrument channel for the introduction of microinstruments such as a biopsy forceps. The instrument is introduced via a burr hole under intraoperative ultrasound control, as recently described in detail [1-3].

Placement of the trepanation depends on the location of the hematoma: subcortical hematomas are approached either via the cortical area, where they reach nearest to the surface, or in the longitudinal direction of the hematoma, which can always be done either through a frontal, a temporal, or an occipital burr hole. Basal ganglionic hemorrhage was operated either via a frontal or a temporal burr hole, depending on their predominant extension. Thalamic hemorrhage was mostly done through an occipital burr hole via the posterior horn, so as to be able to evacuate ventricular clots at the same time, and to approach the thalamic hematoma through its site of rupture into the ventricle in the region of the pulminar thalami. Ventricular clots without intraparenchymal hemorrhage, in cases of disturbed CSF circulation, were evacuated via a frontal burr hole. Cerebellar clots are approached via a trepanation on the occipital plane over a cerebellar hemisphere.

Following CT diagnosis, angiography was considered mandatory in all cases in order to exclude patients with aneurysms, arteriovenous (AV) malformations, or apoplectic brain tumors.

A total of 120 consecutive patients with spontaneous intracerebral hematomas, admitted within 48 h after stroke, were subjects of a randomized study of endoscopic surgical versus medical treatment.

Exclusion criteria for the randomized study were age below 30 or above 80 years, unproportionally high anesthesiological risk due to recent myocardial infarction or other causes, aneurysm, AV malformation or brain tumor, a bleeding event more than 48 h before possible start of surgery, hematoma volume below 10 cm^3, or patient neurologically intact on admission. Following sequential randomization by aid of a computer program, and following treatment, clinical and CT scan controls were done until 6 months after stroke. Final outcome was estimated at 6 months.

Six criteria were used for randomization, in the following rank order: volume of hematoma above or below 50 cm^3, location of hematoma (subcortical, basal ganglionic, or thalamic), state of consciousness (alert, somnolent, soporous, or comatose), left or right hemisphere, and age of the patient. Besides spontaneous intracerebral hematomas, traumatic intracerebral and cerebellar hematomas were operated upon. In total, 112 patients were operated by the endoscopic technique.

Results and Conclusion

Overall Results

There was no surgical mortality attributable to the surgical procedure. Two patients deteriorated postoperatively due to rebleeding into the

---

[1] Department of Neurosurgery, University of Graz, Graz, Austria

hematoma cavity. Other complications did not occur. Complete evacuation of clot was possible in 44% of patients. In 56% of cases, evacuation was difficult due to toughness of the clot, and not more than 50%–70% of the hematoma could be evacuated. On the average, operation time was below 1 hr.

In a preliminary evaluation of the first 100 patients in the randomized study, there was significantly less mortality within 6 months after treatment in the surgical group ($P < 0.01$), significantly more patients made a good outcome following surgery ($P < 0.05$). Moreover, excellent outcome with no deficit whatsoever occurred significantly more often in the surgical group ($P < 0.01$). However, this result was entirely due to a better outcome in the group of patients with subcortical hematomas.

Subgroups

Localization versus outcome. In the group of subcortical hematomas, significantly less ($P < 0.05$) patients died after surgery and significantly more operated patients ($P < 0.01$) made an excellent outcome (Table 1). In patients with basal ganglionic or thalamic hemorrhage, there was no difference between the treatment groups.

Prognosis versus volume of hematoma. In the operated group, there was no difference in survival or survival quality between patients with hematomas smaller than 50 cm^3 and patients with larger hematomas. In the medically treated group, however, significantly more patients died with hematomas larger than 50 cm^3.

Comparing surgical versus medical treatment, significantly more patients with small hematomas made an excellent outcome, but there was no difference in mortality. In patients with large hematomas, significantly more patients died with medical than with surgical treatment. Survival quality was not influenced by the mode of treatment.

Prognosis versus age. Significantly less patients up to 50 years of age died after surgical treatment compared to the older age group ($P < 0.005$).

With medical treatment, age made no difference for the outcome. Comparing surgical versus medical treatment in younger patients, significantly more patients died with medical treatment ($P < 0.01$), and significantly more operated patients made an excellent or good outcome ($P < 0.05$) (Table 2). In the older age group, operated

Table 1. Outcome in 45 patients with subcortical hematomas

Outcome	Treatment	
	Endoscopic (%)	Medical (%)
Full recovery	29[a]	0
Dead	33[b]	71

[a] $P < 0.01$
[b] $P < 0.05$

Table 2. Outcome in 51 patients aged under 60 years

Outcome	Treatment	
	Endoscopic (%)	Medical (%)
Full recovery	18.5[a]	0
Dead	26[b]	64

[a] $P < 0.05$
[b] $P < 0.01$

patients made an excellent outcome significantly more often ($P < 0.05$): there was no difference in mortality.

Prognosis versus consciousness. In the surgical group, significantly more patients in a preoperatively soporous or comatose state died compared to the group of alert or somnolent patients ($P < 0.01$). Significantly more patients made a good outcome when preoperatively in a better state of consciousness ($P < 0.05$). In the medically treated group, significantly more patients died despite an initially better state of consciousness ($P < 0.05$): there was, however, no difference regarding survival quality.

Comparing surgically and medically treated patients in an initially alert or somnolent state, mortality was significantly lower in the operated group ($P < 0.01$), and an outcome without deficit was significantly more frequent in the operated group ($P < 0.05$).

In the soporous and comatose patients, there was no difference regarding mortality or survival quality comparing surgically with medically treated patients. The completeness of clot evacuation did not influence mortality or survival quality.

In conclusion, an ultrasound-guided endoscopic evacuation of intracranial hematomas through a burr hole can be considered as a low risk alternative to conventional methods. Patients with subcortical hematomas of the present study made a significantly better outcome compared to medically treated patients. As a further advantage, the operation time is shorter than medical treatment. However, a whole scale of high-tech instrumentation is necessary.

References

1. Auer LM (1985) Endoscopic evacuation of intracerebral haemorrhage: High-tech surgical treatment—A new approach to the problem? Acta Neurochir 74:124–128
2. Auer LM (1987) Endoscopic evacuation of intracranial hematomas. Neurosurgeons 6:381–388
3. Auer LM, Holzer P, Ascher PW, Heppner F (1988) Endoscopic neurosurgery. Acta Neurochir 90:1–14

Spontaneous Intracerebral Hemorrhage

BENIAMINO GUIDETTI[1]

The present paper provides a review of personal attitute towards the problem of spontaneous intracerebral hematoma treated in our service after introduction of computerized tomography. (CT), which has considerably influenced the indications for medical or surgical treatment. Consequently, our survey of cases will not include patients treated before 1975, presented at a workshop held in Giessen-Bad Nauhein in 1979. In evaluating our cases, it is necessary to note that our institute is a specialized hospital where we preferably hospitalize selected patients in whom there is the possibility of surgical treatment. In this way we have no true way of comparing the results of surgical and conservative treatment.

Clinical Material

The basis of this contribution is 140 consecutive patients affected by spontaneous intracerebral hematoma not caused by detectable vascular malformations, trauma, or neoplasm, observed in the last 10 years. The series comprises 71 males and 59 females, with the greatest frequency in patients aged 50–60 years old. Only 68 patients presented with an arterial systolic pressure above 150 mmHg. CT was performed in all cases immediately upon hospitalization of the patients and was repeated in successive days. Angiography was performed only in young patients and in cases in which existed the clinical doubt that the hemorrhage was caused by the rupture of a vascular malformation. In 15 patients, the extradural intracranial pressure was recorded continuously for some days in order to take a decision in favor of surgical or conservative treatment.

The data furnished by the neuroradiological examinations, by the clinical state, and by the surgeon's medical reports have allowed us to

classify the hematomas, as has been done by other observers, as lobar (74 cases) and capsular (66 cases), in which the hematomas prevalently implicate the deep-seated structures. This information about the location and size of the hematoma, the presence or nonpresence of herniation of midline structures under the falx and/or the tentorium, and the level of consciousness were used to decide our strategy. As a general rule, patients in whom the hematoma involved the basal nuclei without gross shift were usually subjected to conservative treatment. The majority of these patients reach us in a state of profound stupor or coma and surgery seemed of dubious value. Those patients with large lobar hematomas and with increased intracranial pressure were mainly subjected to surgical treatment. In young patients with hematoma of noteable dimensions, intervention was thought to be advisable, even if the hematoma was capsular.

From the point of view of the operative technique employed, we preferred, in all cases, to practice a small osteoplastic flap centered in the cortical area where the hematic collection appeared more superficial, naturally avoiding damaging the area of noteable functional importance. The hematoma was evacuated through a small cortical incision. The wall of the cavity was accurately probed to research an eventual pathological tissue, the cavity washed abundantly with physiological warm solution, and drained through a silicone catheter. The drainage has the advantage of also measuring the intracranial pressure.

Results

To assess our results we used the grading system of Hunt and Hess. Table 1 classifies patients operated on or treated conservatively in five groups according to their condition. It shows that more than half (40 of 72) of the patients not operated on were classified in grades IV and V, which were the cases of moribund or grave pa-

---
[1] Department of Neurological Science, Roma University La Sapienza Medical School, Rome, Italy

Table 1. Results in relation to grade (Hunt and Hess)

Grade	No. of cases	Results							
		Excellent		Good		Poor		Dead	
		Surg.	Cons.	Surg.	Cons.	Surg.	Cons.	Surg.	Cons.
I	22	8	10	1	2	1	0	0	0
II	28	12	7	4	2	1	1	1	0
III	34	11	4	8	2	3	3	2	1
IV	25	0	1	2	1	4	6	4	7
V	31	0	0	0	1	2	4	4	20
Total	140	31	22	15	8	11	14	11	28

Surg. surgical treatment, *Cons.* conservative treatment, *Excellent* regained prehemorrhagic state, *Good* some neurological deficits, *Poor* severe neurological deficits

Table 2. Results in relation to anatomic localization

Results	Basal ganglia		Lobar	
	Surgical	Conservative	Surgical	Conservative
Excellent	2	0	29	22
Good	4	4	11	4
Poor	10	10	1	4
Died	10	26	1	2
Total	26	40	42	32

tients reaching the hospital more than 24 h after hemorrhage. Twenty-seven patients died at various times from their admission to the clinic, and autopsy performed in 16 proved the futility of surgical treatment. Of the 72 patients who underwent conservative treatment, the hemorrhage was classified as lobar in 32 and as capsular in 40 (Table 2). In another 32 patients who underwent conservative treatment, operation was thought to be unjustified either because the hemorrhage was of modest dimension, or because there was a clinical picture of continuous and progressive improvement associated with normal intracranial pressure.

Of 68 patients who underwent surgical treatment and were observed for a period of 1–9 years, 11 died after the intervention and, of these, eight belonged to grades IV and V and two to grade III. Of another 57 patients the results can be considered excellent in 31 (the patients regained their prehemorrhagic state), good in 15 (some neurologic deficit of minor importance), and poor in 11 (marked and invaliding neurologic deficits).

Concerning the location of hematoma (Table 2), it can be seen that the cases operated on, the

hematoma was lobar in 42 and capsular in 26. Of 46 patients discharged in excellent or good condition, the hematoma was lobar in 40 and capsular in 6. Among those discharged with grave neurological deficits the hematoma was lobar in only one, while in ten it was capsular. In relation to the time during which surgery was carried out we have observed that, of 22 patients operated on during the first 3 days, six died, while of 46 patients operated on after this period, five died.

Discussion and Conclusion

Our neurosurgical department is dealing with a selected group of patients and so we have no chance to compare the real results of surgical or conservative treatment. Many of our patients arrived at the hospital many hours or days after bleeding and in this way we lost the opportunity inherent in very early operation (first 12 h after the bleeding). With these limitations, it appears clear that the therapeutic indication varies according to the location and size of hematoma, the rapidity of its evolution, the level of consciousness, and the presence of signs of herniation. Age, hypertension, arteriosclerosis, coagulation deficits, and disturbances of heart, lung, liver, and kidney functions additionally influence therapeutic indications.

On the basis of our experience, we feel that patients with hematoma who are alert, stable or improving, and are absent of any gross shifts, should be treated conservatively. The same attitude is advised in patients with hemorrhage involving the basal ganglia and/or brain stem with the absence of any gross shifts. Massive hemorrhage, involving the basal nuclei occurring acutely in grades IV and V patients from the onset, should be treated conservatively. Surgical treatment does nothing but aggravate the damage already made by the hemorrhage. In general, there is no indication for operating upon intraventricular hemorrhage. Patients of grades I or II with large clots mainly collected in the white substance and marked midline shifts should be operated as soon as possible. Young patients, grade III and IV, who reach the hospital in the first few hours after bleeding, with large clots and gross shifts, should be submitted to surgical treatment. The most favorable results were observed in cases operated on within the first few hours. If these patients reach the hospital 12 h after the hemorrhage, a operation is indicated only if brain compression and shifts increase in spite of intensive conservative treatment. A rapid deterioration or a quick transition to a decerebrate state is a contraindication to surgery. Concerning late operation (1–2 weeks after bleeding), surgery is indicated only if intracranial pressure measurements show pathological pressure waves.

References

1. Garde A, Bohmer G, Selden B, Neiman J (1983) One hundred cases of spontaneous intracerebral hematoma. Eur Neurol 22:161–172
2. Gillingham J (1980) Conservative and surgical management. In: Pia HW, Langmaid C, Zierski J (eds) Spontaneous intracerebral hematomas. Springer Berlin, pp 391–392
3. Guidetti B, Gagliardi FM (1980) Experiences with operation in 149 cases of spontaneous ICH (1966–1977). In: Pia HW, Langmaid C, Zierski J (eds) Spontaneous intracerebral hematomas. Springer, Berlin, pp 251–256
4. Kanaya H, Yokawa H, et al. (1980) Grading and the indications for treatment in ICH of the basal ganglia. In: Pia HW, Langmaid C, Zierski J (eds) Spontaneous intracerebral hematomas. Springer, Berlin, pp 264–267
5. Kaneko M, Tamaka K, Shimada T, et al. (1983) Long-term evaluation of ultra-early operation for hypertensive intracerebral hemorrhage in 100 cases. J Neurosurg 58:838–842
6. Kanno T, Sano H, Shinoniya Y, Katada K, Nagata J, Hoshino M, Mitsuyama F (1984) Role of surgery in hypertensive intracerebral hematoma. J Neurosurg 61:1091–1099
7. Loew F, Jaksche H (1980) Surgical treatment. In: Pia HW, Langmaid C, Zierski J (eds) Spontaneous intracerebral hematomas. Springer, Berlin, p 326
8. Nath F, Nicholls D, Fraser J (1983) The prognosis of intracerebral hemorrhage. Acta Neurochir 67:29–35
9. Pasztor D, Afra D, Orosz E (1980) Experiences with the surgical treatment of 156 ICH. In: Pia HW, Langmaid C, Zierski J (eds) Spontaneous intracerebral hematomas. Springer, Berlin, pp 251–256
10. Pertuiset B, Yacoubi A, Sichez J, Gardeur D (1980) Prognostic factors in the first 48 hours in ICH and spreading hemorrhaes. In: Pia HW, Langmaid C, Zierski J (eds) Spontaneous intracerebral hematomas. Springer, Berlin, pp 294–300
11. Suzuki J, Sato T (1980) Grading and timing of operation in putaminal ICH. In: Pia HW, Langmaid C, Zierski J (eds) Spontaneous intracerebral hematomas. Springer, Berlin, pp 274–278
12. Suzuki J, Sato T (1980) Trans-sylvian approach in putaminal ICH with mild symptoms. In: Pia HW, Langmaid C, Zierski J (eds) Spontaneous intracerebral hematomas. Springer, Berlin, pp 345–347
13. Volpin L, Cervellini P, Colombo F, et al. (1984) Spontaneous intracerebral hematoma: A new proposal about the usefulness and limits of surgical treatment. Neurosurgery 15:663–666

The Evolution of Our Surgical Approach in Hypertonic Hematomas

Vladimír Beneš[1]

In the rich history of surgical treatment of hypertonic intracerebral hematomas, a basic note can be ascribed to the work of Cushing who, in his paper on brain hemorrhage, described the increase of systemic pressure with the increase of intracranial pressure: the so-called Cushing phenomenon.

French neurosurgeons have greatly contributed to the postwar development of surgical treatment. The neurosurgical departments in Czechoslovakia have been engaged in the systematical surgical treatment of hematomas since 1960. At first, we operated on 8–12 patients at the neurosurgical clinic in Prague each year, and, in the whole of Czechoslovakia, with a population of over 15 million, we operated an annual average of 60 patients. Since 1975, there has been a steady decrease in the number of operated cases, although, according to official statistics, the number of hospitalized patients with sudden cerebrovascular accidents has shown an ever increasing tendency. Only since 1981 has there been an obvious decrease in the number of cerebral hemorrhage in Czechoslovakia (Table 1). It has been ascertained that this is due primarily to preventive treatment, and, only in the second place, to the treatment of atherosclerosis and hypertension.

During the past 25 years, we have used several surgical methods successively. We shall deal with them chronologically as they represent changes in our opinion concerning the pathophysiology of the disease as verified by us in the clinical, anatomical, morphological, and experimental work outlined in my book [4].

Types of Operations

Our first patients were operated very shortly after the stroke, irrespective of their clinical state, on the basis of neurological examination and angiography. We carried out large, usually frontal, craniotomies and evacuation of the hematoma under visual control. The limited number of operations sufficed to draw the conclusion that the results were not distinctly superior to those obtained by conservative treatment. This was also in accordance with the well-known work of McKissock et al. [7, 8].

Inspired by Zülch's work on the most frequent source of hypertonic hemorrhage from the striate arteries, and his remark that the zone of question is perfectly known to stereotactic neurosurgeons, we have developed our own original method by using Guiot's frame (Fig. 1). We have arrived at the conclusion that this method could be applied at any hospital equipped with a standard X-ray, thus obviating the necessity of transferring the patient to some distant neurosurgical department. However, the operation lasted about one hour and did not result in a substantical reduction of the operational time. With almost all patients, we succeeded in reaching the hematoma and evacuating it, but the results proved as bad as in the cases of craniotomy. We were probably the first to use the stereotactic technique, and were surely the first to give it up.

Table 1. Mortality of CVD in Czechoslovakia (population 15 million)

Year	CVD	ICH
1979	28 576	7 424
1980	30 893	7 717
1981	29 347	5 966
1982	30 316	5 825
1983	31 041	5 624
1984	30 595	4 980

CVD cerebrovascular disease, *ICH* intracerebral hemorrhage
International classification of diseases: CVD, 430–438; ICH, 431

[1] Neurosurgical Department, Hospital of Pediatric Faculty of Charles University, Prague, Czechoslovakia

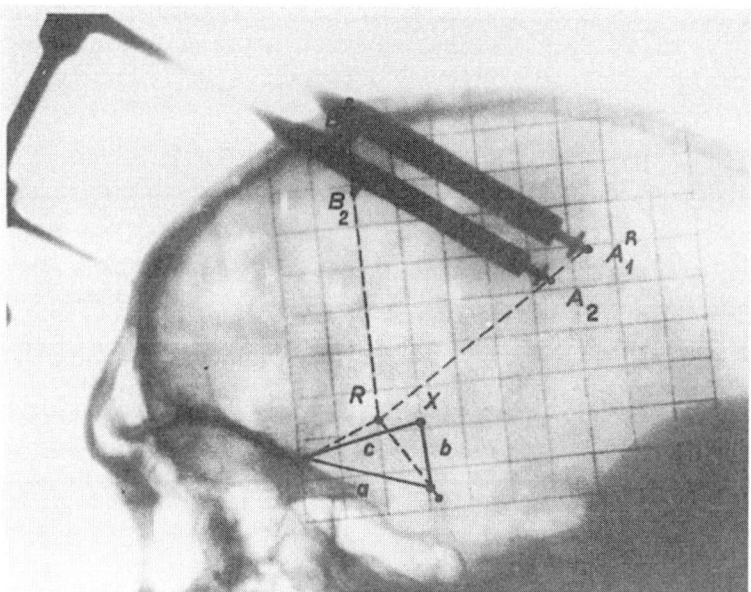

Fig. 1. Stereotaxic method used B, B_1, B_2, R, c, a, b, X, A_2, A_2

In order to shorten and simplify the surgical method, we carried out a mathematical calculation of the target point by applying external bone reference points. By a statistical evaluation of 20 X-ray pictures and comparison of them with the stereotactic atlas, we determined the rectangular reliability zone for anterior commissure (Fig. 2), the lateral projection of which is the zone of striate arteries.

We related this zone to the coronal suture and meatus acusticus externus. On the basis of our estimates, we have constructed a simple stereotactic single-purpose apparatus in which the centering arm outside the skull at the meatus acusticus focused the suction cannula in the swingbolt precisely to the target zone. We operated by this method on only five patients. We always reached the hemorrhage, but the results again proved unsatisfactory (Fig. 3).

We abandoned this method as we had carried out, in the meantime, anatomical, experimental, and pathological work which clarified to us the pathophysiology of cerebral hemorrhage of hypertonics and thus explained to us the failures of our operations.

We have carried out a detailed analysis of 100 brains of patients deceased after hemorrhage. We became convinced that the hemorrhage could be classified in two types: destructive hemorrhage and limited hemorrhage. The first shatters the total zone of basal ganglia with the thalamus, and frequently breaks into the ventricles. Destructive hemorrhage is clinically correlated

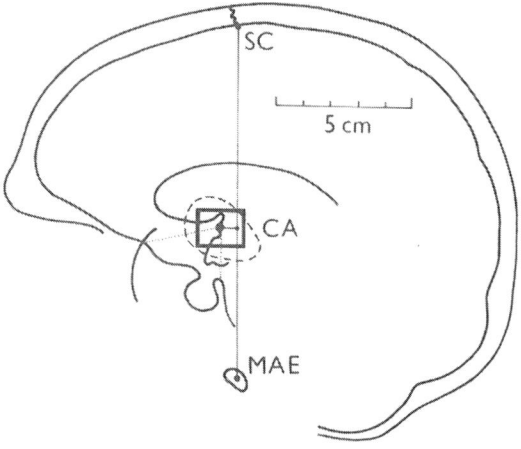

Fig. 2. Zone of the striate arteries in correlation to external bone points. *SC* coronal suture, *CA* anterior commissure, *MAE* external auditory meatus

with sudden, deep unconsciousness and vegetative failures. Limited hemorrhage has a round or drop-like shape with a narrower diameter in the hemorrhagic zone and a wider orientation towards one of the lobes as a result of the hematoma's spreading in the direction of the radiation. This classification has won the approval of most authors engaged in hemorrhage studies, but they apply differing terminology. Thus, our destructive hemorrhage corresponds to Pia's medial type or Pertuiset's and Arseni's hemorrhages. Its very process conforms to the thalamic hemorrhage of the Japanese. The limited type is

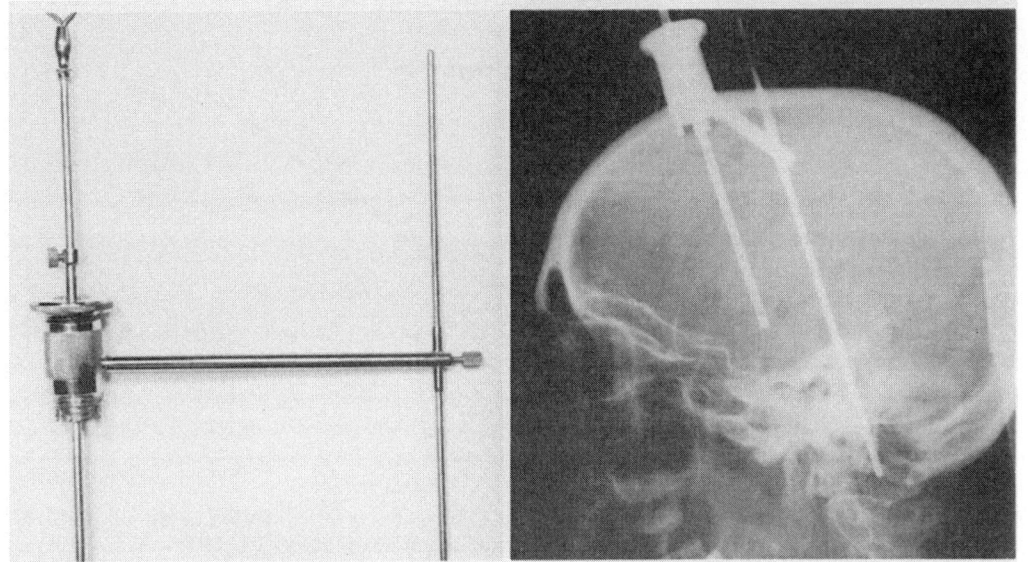

a   b

Fig. 3a, b. Single purpose apparatus for evacuation of hematomas

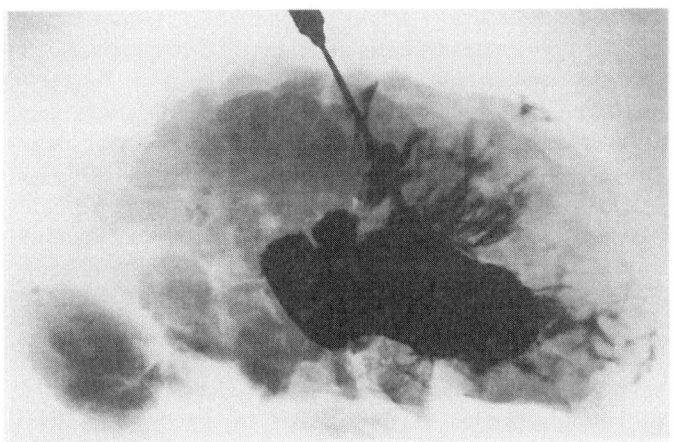

Fig. 4. Simulated limited hematoma

classified by Pia as lateral hematoma, by Pertuiset and Arseni simply as hematoma, and corresponds to the putaminal type mentioned by Japanese authors. The distinction of hemorrhage and hematoma is only of didactic importance as we deal with the same event of different intensity.

We have carried out experiments by simulating hematoma with contrast medium into partially hardened brains. At a steady flow of 1 ml/min, we measured the pressure at the target zone and took repeated X-ray pictures. We found that, at this slow flow, there arises a hematoma with drop-like propagation into the frontal lobe and, after 20–30 min, the flow of the contrast medium stops (Fig. 4). A further increase of pressure or flow results in a rupture into the ventricles

or in a local shattering of the brain. According to our experiments, verified by studies with radioisotopes, the hemorrhage is a single-phase event which stops spontaneously. We consider the assumption of repeated or continuous hemorrhage incorrect.

This was confirmed also by our analysis of 100 postmortem protocols. A deterioration of the clinical state and the death several days after the stroke were never caused by repeated hemorrhage, but were due to an extracerebral cause, most frequently pneumonia. The patients checked by us did not die at a later stage as a result of repeated brain hemorrhage, but of a cardiac infarct.

In a second experiment, conserved blood

under steady pressure was infused into a fresh cadaver brain. The flow stopped after 50 ml in all studied cases (Fig. 5). We thus obtained the confirmation of a well-known finding; the volume reserve of the intracranial space is about 50 ml and in fact, the rupture into the ventricles opens this reserve so that it is not always a fatal sign, as we previously assumed. In our opinion, death is not caused by the tamponade of ventricles, but by the excession of the volume reserve and, thus, also of intracranial pressure. The proposed puncture and drainage of ventricles is important only from the point of view of decreasing intracranial pressure.

From the analysis of 100 postmortem protocols, we could critically estimate the number of deceased who might have been saved by an operation. We came to the conclusion that an operation was indicated in about 13% of hypertonics with brain hemorrhage. We plotted the results of our analysis compared with clinical experiences on the line segment of a graph (Fig. 6) in which we depicted the groups according to the grading of the clinical state and the localization of the hematoma. It has been clearly revealed that it is not necessary to operate on patients who are in a good clinical state without disturbances of consciousness and with a small hematoma on CT. Nor is the operation indicated in group V patients with serious disturbance of consciousness and vegetative symptoms, as all patients die.

There remain only groups II, III, and IV, in which the indication is influenced also by other factors such as age, blood pressure, other simultaneous diseases and lateral localization. According to Japanese authors, an operation may save the lives of patients of these groups, but mostly at the price of a deep neurological deficit.

The introduction of CT marked a new criterium for surgical indications. Some went so far as to indicate an operation on the basis of the measured size of hematoma and its localization. I shared the opinion that the number of operated persons would increase owing to the possibilities offered by CT. This was the case in the early stages, but today it has become obvious that CT, on the contrary, leads to a decrease in the number of operated patients as smaller hematomas can be monitored and followed as the density diminishes to a final small cyst; in the case of destructive hematomas, CT contraindicates operation. However, CT is only an auxilliary method for determing indication. Of decisive importance remain the clinical state and the evaluation of disturbance of consciousness. Basing our opin-

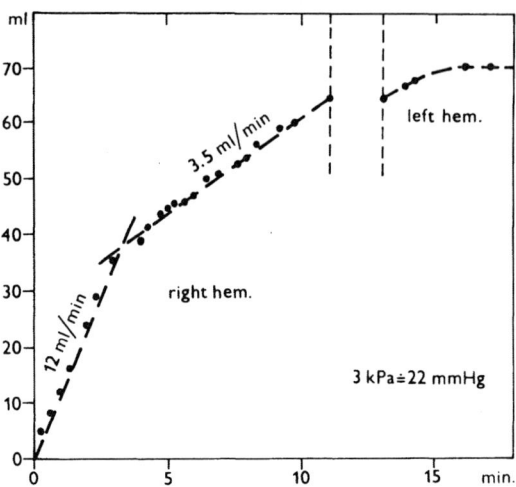

Fig. 5. Simulation of hematoma determining the intracranial volume reserve

ions on the comparison of our experiments and clinical experiences during the last 25 years, we believe that the surgical indications in hypertonic haematomas are, at present, fairly clearly determined.

The timing is determined by a complex of factors, most importantly the level of consciousness. We consider as disadvantageous the use of a different evaluation in the cases of brain trauma, and a different one in subarachnoidal hemorrhage, and yet another one in intracerebral hemorrhage. The mechanism of the failure might be different, but the result is always the same. Consequently, the disturbance of consciousness should be evaluated according to the same scheme. In our opinion, in the cases of deep disturbance of consciousness with vegetative symptoms, it would be preferable to administer aggressive medical treatment until the patient's state becomes stabilized and the eventual surgery can be reconsidered later.

Acute operations do not bring better results than medical treatment. I consider the frequently repeated axiom that a deterioration of patient's state is an indication for operation as a mistaken notion. A worsening of state after a longer period following the stroke is, according to our research, almost always due to extracerebral causes, and an operation only aggravates the state. If the aggravation continues from the moment of the stroke, then it is a sign of a rapid increase of intracranial pressure with brain herniation and direct brain damage as well: surgery is useless. In our opinion, on the contrary, a stagnation of the clinical state of a patient with limited hematoma

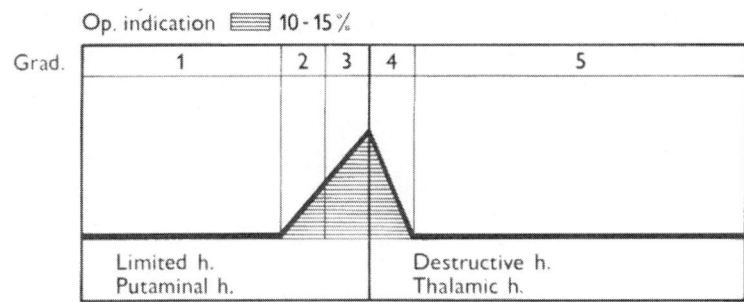

Fig. 6. Scheme of surgical indications. *h* hematoma, *Op.* operative, *Grad.* grade

revealed by CT represents an indication for surgery. If the patient's failure of consciousness becomes repaired after a short time and, thus, the focal symptoms come to the forefront, such as hemiparesis which do not improve, then the surgery becomes absolutely indicated as it can accelerate the return of functions which would occur slower and probably to a lesser extent even with conservative treatment. A slow reconvalescence, however, represents a danger of secondary complications. It is necessary to repeat again that not a deterioration, but a stagnation of the clinical state is, in our opinion, an indication for operation.

Our opinion on surgical indication, as outlined, explains our failures in all types of operations used. No operation of hypertonic hematomas can be successful if it is incorrectly indicated. On the contrary, if correctly indicated, every method of operation can bring good results. The surgical technique is not decisive. From our conclusion that the hemorrhage is a single-phase short event, we have come to think that no operation has so far confirmed that it could stop the bleeding of an artery, if we consider, according to the old theory of Charcot-Bouchard, the rupture of a miliary aneurysm of striate arteries as the cause of the hemorrhage. When we found, during or shortly after the operation, signs of fresh bleeding, we were always compelled to admit frankly that we had caused the hemorrhage ourselves by manipulating the inside wall of the cavity or by tearing the thrombus.

That is why, after many years of experience, we have returned to craniotomy which we localize according to the CT finding, to small cerebrotomy in the deaf cerebral zone, and to the careful removal of the whole hematoma, mostly under a microscope which illuminates the cavities well.

The modern stereotactic method is effective, yet we are of the opinion that a small hematoma, which would necessitate stereotaxy to be reached, does not need to be operated, and a large hematoma can be punctured directly without stereotaxy. Our experiences have shown that only a small part of the hematoma can be evacuated by a cannula. At a subsequent open operation, or at a section, we became surprised by the large size of the hematom left in the cavity after the suction. Therefore, some recur to whirling the hematoma by a small propeller. This has, however, the same disadvantages as a careless evacuation, namely tearing off of tamponing thrombi. Furthermore, the proposed complex apparatuses are rather costly.

Summing up our 25 years of experience, we have come to the conclusion that the number of hypertonic hemorrhages is decreasing, and, consequently, also that of their operations, the indications of which in recent years have become very precise, thanks to pathophysiological advances and the use of CT.

A correct indication, not the method of operation, is of decisive importance for the result of the operation. We have returned to the removal of hematoma after a small targeted craniotomy.

References

1. Auer LM (1985) Endoscopic evacuation of intracerebral haemorrhage. High-tech surgical treatment—a new approach to the problem? Acta Neurochir 74:124–128
2. Beneš V, Vladyka V, Zvěřina E (1965) Stereotaxic evacuation of typical brain haemorrhage. Acta Neurochir 13:419–426
3. Beneš V, Koukolík F, Obrovská D (1972) Two types of spontaneous intracerebral haemorrhage due to hypertension. J Neurosurg 37(5):509–513
4. Beneš V (1983) Intracerebral haemorrhage of hypertonic. Avicenum, Prague
5. Cushing H (1903) The blood-pressure reaction of acute cerebral compression, illustrated by cases of intracranial hemorrhage. (1984) Amer J med Sci 125:1027–1044
6. Matsumoto K, Hondo H (1984) CT-guided stereotaxic evacuation of hypertensive intracerebral hematomas. J Neurosurg 60:803–813

7. McKissock W, Richardson A, Walsh L (1959) Primary intracerebral haemorrhage. Results of surgical treatment in 244 consecutive cases. Lancet II 7105:683–686

8. McKissock W, Richardson A, Taylor J (1961) Primary intracerebral haemorrhage: A controlled trial of surgical and conservative treatment in 180 unselected cases. Lancet II 7196:221–226

9. Luyendijk W, Schoen HR, (1964) Intracerebral haematomas: A clinical study of 40 surgical cases. Psychiat Neurol Neurochir 67:445–468

10. Mitsuno T, Kanaya H, Shirakata S, Ohsawa S, Ishikava I (1966) Surgical treatment of hypertensive intracerebral haemorrhage. J Neurosurg 24:70–76

11. Shivers JA, Adcock DF, Faustino CG, Radcliffe WB (1974) Radionuclide imaging in primary intracerebral hemorrhage. Radiology 11(8):211–212

12. Suzuki J, Sato T (1972) The new transinsular approach to the hypertensive intracerebral hematoma. Jpn J Surg 2:47–52

Aspiration Surgery for Hypertensive Brain Hemorrhage in the Acute Stage

Keizo Matsumoto, Hideki Hondo, and Keisuke Tomida[1]

Introduction

Hypertensive brain hemorrhage (HBH) occurs most commonly in the basal ganglia, the subcortex, the thalamus, the pons, and the cerebellum. Although its exact source and pathology are still controversial, it has been considered to be due to the pathological rupture of small arteries resulting from longstanding hypertension. The angiopathy involved has been named lipohyalinosis, hyaline arteriosclerosis, fibrinoid necrosis, or angionecrosis associated with milliary microaneurysm [8]. In many patients, HBH is associated with various complications, such as diabetes mellitus, pulmonary disorders, renal or heart failure, or gastrointestinal bleeding. Besides clinically manifested brain hemorrhage and these complications, we should be aware of other latent hypertensive angiopathies that many provoke additional unfavorable conditions in patients postoperatively.

Judging from these considerations, it is clear that the hematoma of the brain must be evacuated as rapidly as possible under surgical conditions that do not cause progress or exaggeration of the complications or latent underlying angiopathy of the patients. Our method of aspiration surgery (AS), which is to evacuate the hematoma gradually through a burr hole under local anesthesia in the acute stage, seems preferable to conventional surgery (CS), in which the hematoma is exposed by craniotomy under general anesthesia and removed completely at one time under an operating microscope. AS can be applied to hematomas at any site or stage, even in poor risk patients with minimal tissue damage, with the exception of cases of progressing hemorrhage: CS can be applied only to subcortical, putaminal, and cerebellar hemorrhages in good risk patients.

[1] Department of Neurological Surgery, School of Medicine, The University of Tokushima, Tokushima, Japan

Operative Method of Aspiration Surgery

Evacuation of the hematoma. First, a burr hole is made under local anesthesia [5]. Then, under observation by computed tomography (CT), the center of the hematoma is tapped and partially aspirated by the needle or probe of our specially designed "ultrasonic hematoma aspiration system," which will be described later. After this initial aspiration, a drainage tube is placed in the hematoma cavity and 3–5 ml urokinase solution of 6000 IU to 20 000 IU is infused. About 4–6 h later, the liquefied hematoma is sucked out by syringe under CT observation and urokinase solution is again infused through the drain, taking care to avoid an abrupt change of intracranial pressure. This procedure is repeated until the hematoma has been evacuated completely. In most cases, hematomas can be evacuated completely within 3 or 4 days (Fig. 1). The systemic blood pressure should be reduced to normal before surgery by drip infusion of trimetaphan, and maintained at a normal level postoperatively while drainage is continued. The antifibrinolytic agent tranexamic acid cannot be used because it inhibits the action of urokinase.

CT-controlled stereotactic method. A CT-controlled stereotactic method has been developed for accurate insertion of the needle into the center of the hematoma [6]. First, two slice CT images are taken, one involving the target point (T) of the center of the hematoma and the other involving the center of the exposed cortex (H) at the burr-hole. The spatial coordinates of T (X_t, Y_t, Z_t) and H (X_h, Y_h, Z_h) are obtained with values of the X and Y axes as cursor numbers in the CT images and values of the Z axis as sliding table indices (Fig. 2). The aiming angles, α and β, and depth of the probe can be calculated from the spatial coordinates of T and H provided CT gantry is perpendicular to the sliding table, as follows:

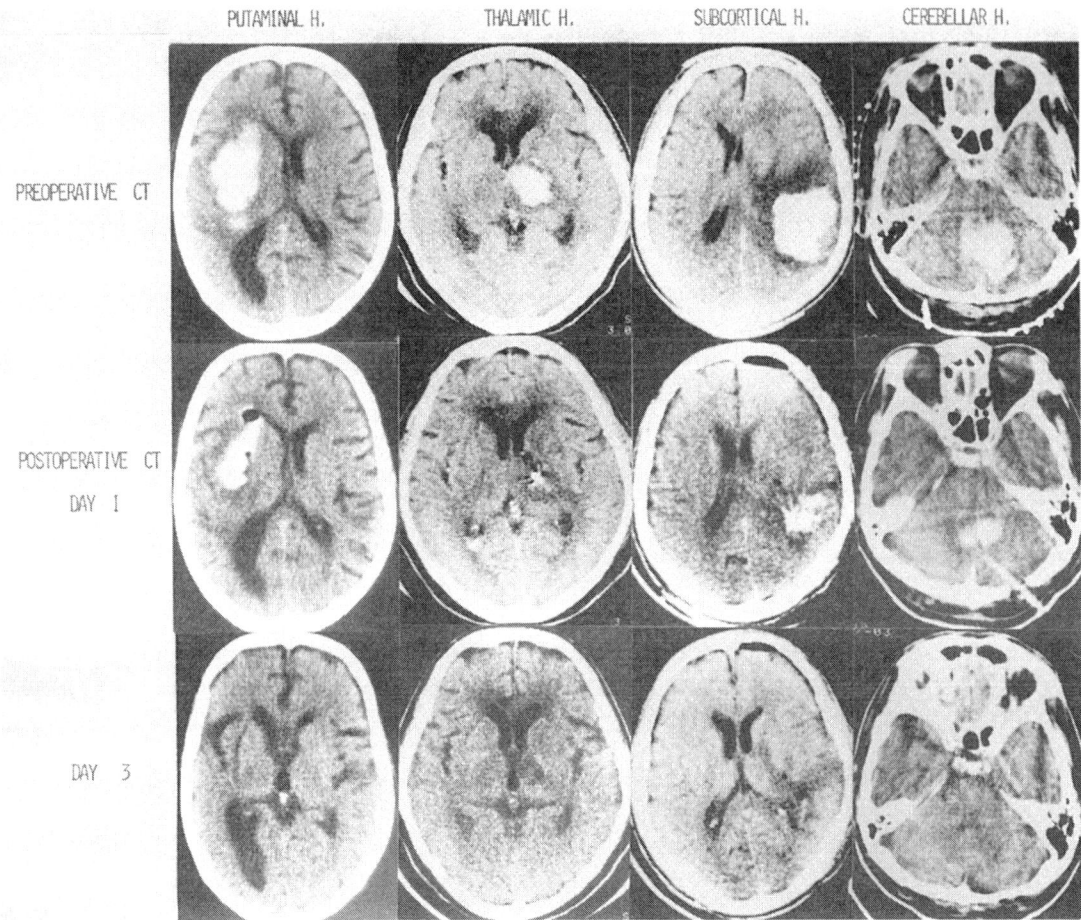

PUTAMINAL H.   THALAMIC H.   SUBCORTICAL H.   CEREBELLAR H.

PREOPERATIVE CT

POSTOPERATIVE CT
DAY 1

DAY 3

Fig. 1. Preoperative and postoperative CT in cases of aspiration surgery

$$\alpha = \tan^{-1}\left(\frac{R(X_h - X_t)}{Z_h}\right) \quad (1)$$

$$\beta = \tan^{-1}\left(\frac{R(Y_h - Y_t)}{\sqrt{R^2(X_h - X_t)^2 + Z_h^2}}\right) \quad (2)$$

$$D = \sqrt{R^2[(X_t - X_h)^2 + (Y_t - Y_h)^2] + Z_h^2} \quad (3)$$

where α = angle α, azimuth of the probe to the target at the burr hole, β = angle β, elevation of the probe to the target at the burr-hole, D = distance from the center of the exposed cortex at the burr-hole to the target, R = value of the deviation ratio that transforms the cursor number to millimeter length. Our CT scanner has a scan field of 240 mm^2, which is divided by a 320 × 320 grid. R = 240/320 = 0.75.

The direction of the probe is confirmed and readjusted precisely after placing its tip on the cortex at the burr-hole with angles α and β as follows. Two slices of CT images are made at the optional two points (N_1 and N_2) of the fixed probe, and values of spatial coordinates with N_1

(X_1, Y_1, Z_1) and N_2 (X_2, Y_2, Z_2) are obtained (Fig. 2). Values of the coordinates of the X and Y axes in the plane of the chosen target (X_0 and Y_0) are calculated with the values of the coordinates of N_1 and N_2 as follows:

$$X_0 = \frac{X_1 Z_2 - X_2 Z_1}{Z_2 - Z_1} \quad (4)$$

$$Y_0 = \frac{Y_1 Z_2 - Y_2 Z_1}{Z_2 - Z_1} \quad (5)$$

where X_0, Y_0 = values of coordinates (X, Y) of the aiming point of the fixed probe in the axial CT image of the chosen target.

Values of X_0 and Y_0 should be concordant with those of the chosen target, X_t and Y_t, respectively.

We have created a software program of Eqs. (1)–(5), so we can obtain solutions to these equations automatically by simply inputting requested values of coordinates into the computer (Fig. 3). We have also devised a prototype of a

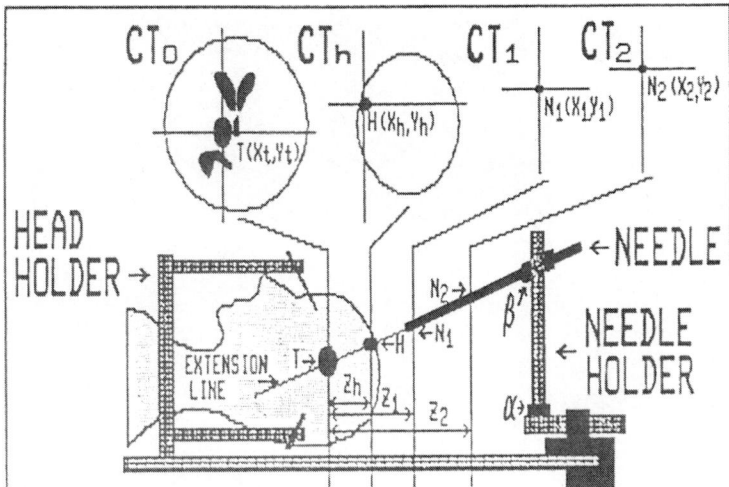

Fig. 2. Principle of CT-controlled stereotaxy. Four fundamental CT slices and coordinates

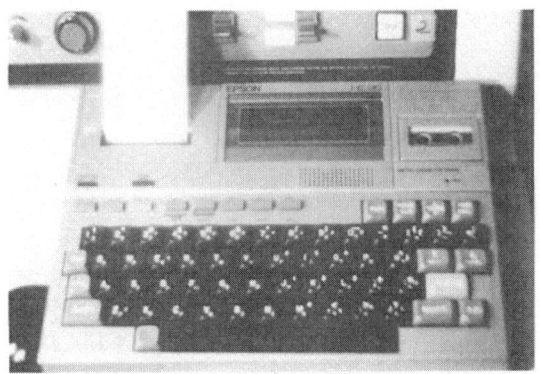

Fig. 3. A small personal computer in which equations are loaded as software

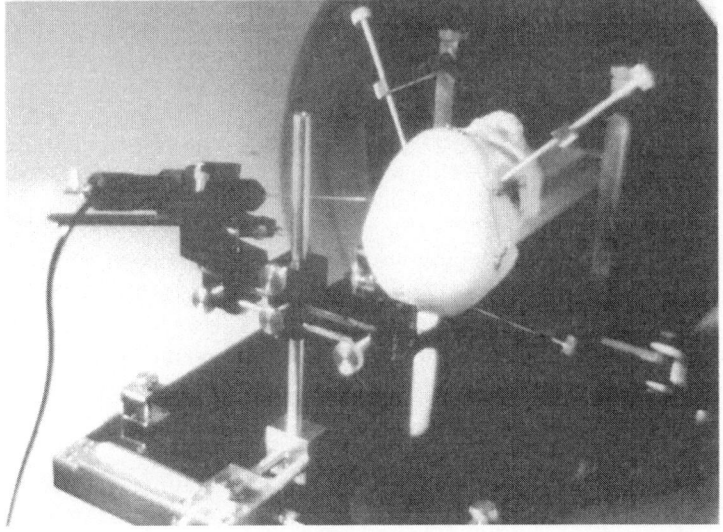

Fig. 4. Our stereotactic apparatus for the CT-controlled operation

stereotactic apparatus for this CT-controlled method (Fig. 4).

Ultrasonic hematoma aspiration system. The instrument consists of a gas-sterilizable surgical handpiece and a control box for regulating the power of suction and ultrasound [7]. The needle of the handpiece is 20 cm long. The needle is available in two sizes; 2.0 mm and 2.4 mm outer diameter. The maximal vacuum is 720 mmHg. On-off controls of ultrasound and suction are

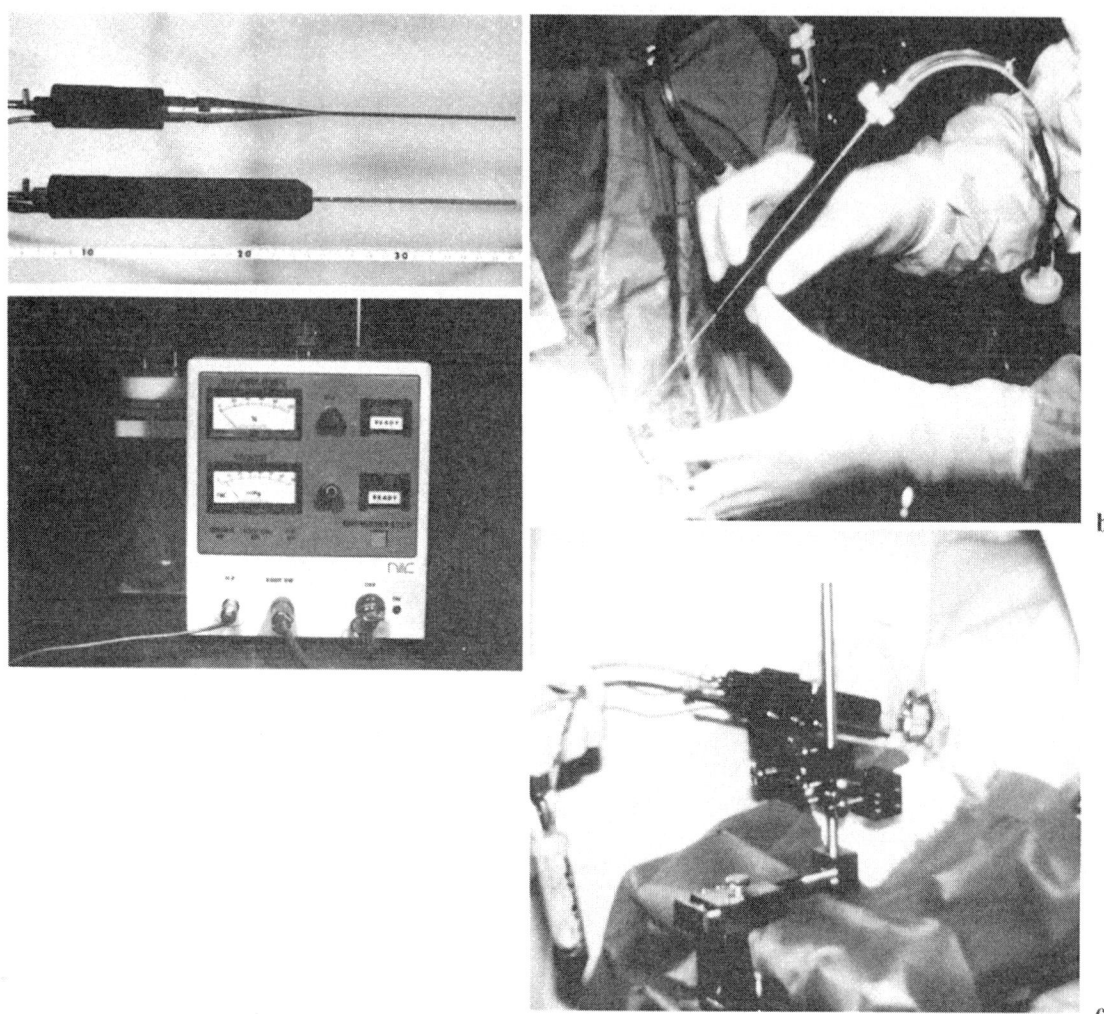

Fig. 5a–c. Our specially deviced ultrasonic hematoma aspiration system. **a** Control box and probes. **b** Manual use. **c** Use in the stereotactic apparatus. Specifications: Type of vibrator, electrostrictive transducer (PZT); oscillation frequency, 40 kHz; ultrasonic power output, 0–10 W; maximum tip amplitude, 40 μ; maximum aspiration pressure, 72 cmHg; hand piece length 27 cm, diameter 2.6 cm, weight 120 g; probe length 12 cm, 1. outer diameter 2 mm, inner diameter 1 mm, 2. outer diameter 2.4 mm, inner diameter 1.6 mm; control box dimensions 19 × 29 × 21 mm (W × D × H), weight 14 kg; power supply 100 V, 50/60 Hz, 2 A

achieved with foot switches. The handpiece can be fixed to our stereotactic apparatus or used manually by the surgeon (Fig. 5).

This system has been applied successfully for initial aspiration of the hematoma after careful animal experiments for confirmation of its safety and utility.

Results

From December 1980 to April 1986, we used AS in 375 cases of HBH: 244 basal ganglionic hemorrhages, 63 thalamic hemorrhages, 50 subcortical hemorrhages, and 18 cerebellar hemorrhages.

Operations were done in the acute stage, within 3 days after the onset of hemorrhage, in 341 of these 375 cases (Table 1). The operations on the 228 cases of acute basal ganglionic hemorrhage were done within 6 hours in 76 cases (33%), within 12 h in 128 cases (56%), and within 24 h in 190 cases (83%; Table 2).

Preoperative neurological grading, CT classification, and the 6-month postoperative outcome were evaluated by the criteria proposed by the Japanese Ad Hoc Committee in 1978 [2] (Tables 3–5). For the clinical evaluation of the AS technique for basal ganglionic hemorrhage, we compared the postoperative outcomes in our patients with those of patients after CS throughout Japan (H. Kanaya, K. Mizukami, M. Kaneko et al., personal communication), and those after conservative treatment, reported in 1986 by Waga et al. [9] (Figs. 6, 7).

First, the results of AS were compared with those of CS. In cases of AS, the mortality rates were 3%, 10%, 12%, 39%, 68%, and 90% for grades 1, 2, 3, 4a, 4b, and 5, respectively. On the other hand, the respective mortality rates in CS were 14%, 15%, 22%, 36%, 68%, and 83% (Fig. 6). Thus AS seems to be better than CS in grades 1–3. The prognosis of the functional state after AS also seemed to be better than that after CS in grades 1–3. There was no statistical difference in the mortalities or activities of daily living (ADL) after operations by the two methods.

However, it does not seem appropriate to compare the two methods in this way, because more older and poor risk patients were treated by AS than by CS. Therefore, the cases were divided into three groups: cases with good risk preoperatively who could have been treated by CS, cases of over 70 years old, and cases of high risk with poor general condition who could not have been treated by CS. The outcomes in these groups are presented graphically in Figs. 8–10.

The outcomes of AS in good risk patients were better than those for all patients in Japan after CS (Fig. 8) and comparable to those of Kaneko's cases [3] of grades 2 and 3, who underwent CS after very strict preoperative case selection (Fig. 9). In high aged patients, the outcome of AS was also better than that for all patients in Japan

after CS (Fig. 10). It is interesting that even in eight poor risk patients (35%), the outcome of AS was good.

Second, the results of AS were compared with those of conservative treatment (Fig. 7). The mortality rates of the respective grades were 6%, 13%, 29%, 69%, 77%, and 100% on conservative treatment. With respect to mortality, AS seemed to be better than conservative treatment in grades 3, 4a, and 4b. The prognosis in terms of function also seemed to be better after AS than after conservative treatment in grades 3, 4a, and 4b. There was a statistical difference in the mortality rates of cases of grade 4a after AS and conservative treatment.

Rebleeding during initial aspiration occurred in four cases and was fatal in two. Reaccumulation after initial aspiration was noted by repeat CT in 17 cases who had been treated successfully by continuous drainage of the initial hematoma.

Table 1. Types of HBH treated by aspiration surgery (1980–1986)

	Acute stage[a]	Overall
Basal ganglia	228	244
Thalamus	59	63
Subcortex	39	50
Cerebellum	15	18
Total	341	375

[a] Operation within 3 days after the onset
HBH hypertensive brain hemorrhage

Table 2. Interval from onset to aspiration of hematoma in 228 consecutive cases of acute basal ganglionic hemorrhage

NG	Interval					Total (cases)
	<6 h	6–12 h	12–24 h	24–48 h	48–72 h	
1	3	7	11	4	4	29
2	18	11	19	12	2	62
3	16	19	12	5	8	60
4a	8	7	12	1	0	28
4b	24	7	6	1	1	39
5	7	1	2	0	0	10
Total	76 (33%)	52 (23%)	62 (27%)	23 (10%)	15 (7%)	228

128 (56%)
190 (83%)
213 (93%)
228 (100%)

NG Neurological grading

Table 3. Criteria of Japanese Ad Hoc Committee (1978): Preoperative neurological grading system

Grade	Criteria[a]
1	Alertness or confusion
2	Somnolence
3	Stupor
4a	Semi-coma without herniation signs
4b	Semi-coma with herniation signs
5	Deep coma

[a] Herniation signs: (a) uni- or bilateral mydriasis (over 5 mm) and no reaction to light, or (b) uni- or bilateral decorticate or decerebrate rigidity

Table 5. Criteria of Japanese Ad Hoc Committee (1978): Code for postoperative evaluation of patients

Code	Description
ADL 1	Well (full work)
ADL 2	Minimal disability (self-sufficient)
ADL 3	Partial disability (partially self-sufficient)
ADL 4	Total disability (bedridden)
ADL 5	Vegetative
Died	

ADL activity of daily living

Table 4. Criteria of Japanese Ad Hoc Committee (1978): Classification of basal ganglion and thalamic hemorrhage on CT scan

Class	Type
Basal ganglionic hemorrhage	
I	Localized outside internal capsule
II	Extending to anterior limb
IIIa	Extending to posterior limb without MVH
IIIb	Extending to posterior limb with MVH
IVa	Extending to anterior & posterior limbs without MVH
IVb	Extending to anterior & posterior limbs with MVH
V	Extending to thalamus or subthalamus
Thalamic hemorrhage	
Ia	Localized in thalamus without MVH
Ib	Localized in thalamus with MVH
IIa	Extending to internal capsule without MVH
IIb	Extending to internal capsule with MVH
IIIa	Extending to hypothalamus or midbrain without MVH
IIIb	Extending to hypothalamus or midbrain with MVH

CT computerized tomography, *MVH* massive ventricular hemorrhage

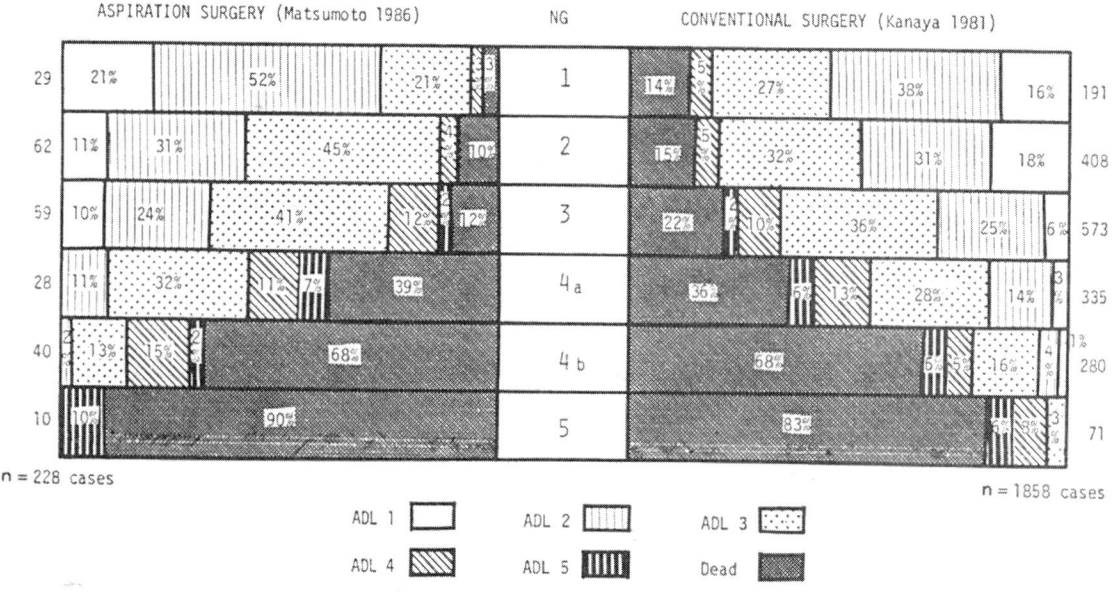

Fig. 6. Six-month postoperative outcomes of basal ganglionic hemorrhage of AS and CS. *NG* neurological grade, ADL grades are defined in Table 5

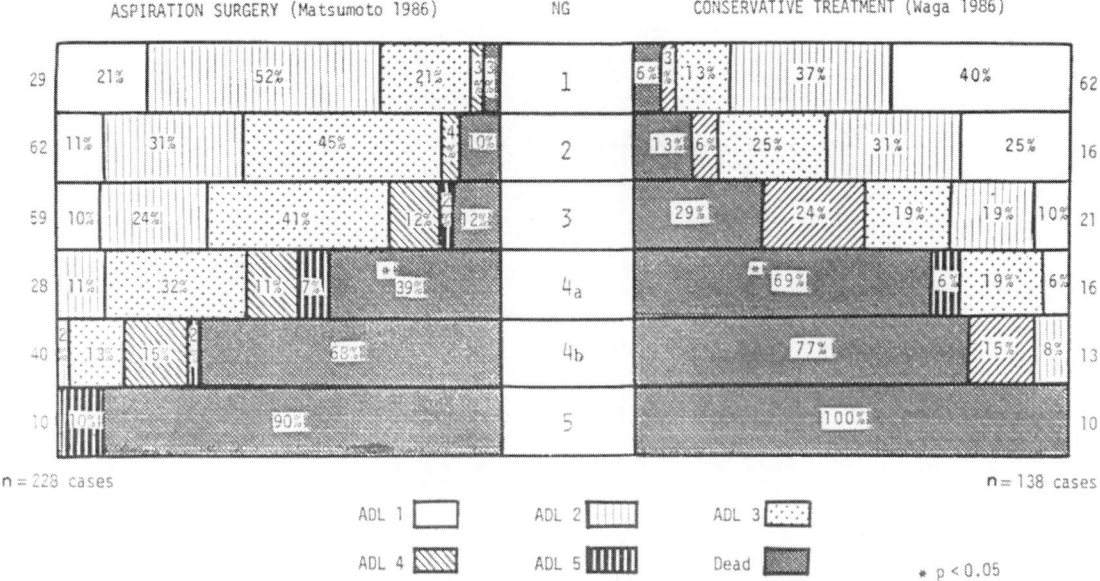

Fig. 7. Six-month postoperative outcomes of basal ganglionic hemorrhage of AS and conservative treatment. *ADL grades* are defined in Table 5

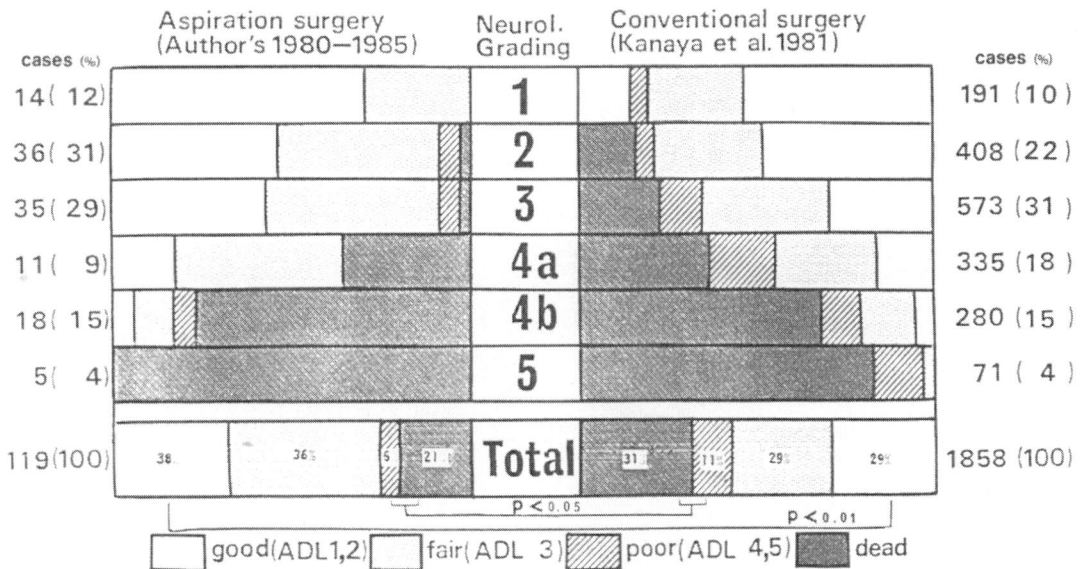

Fig. 8. Six-month postoperative outcomes of AS with good risk and Kanaya's CS (throughout Japan). *ADL grades* are defined in Table 5

Discussion

Almost all these cases showed abrupt elevation of the systemic blood pressure when rebleeding occurred.

Recently, CT-guided stereotactic operations have been used for evacuation of intracerebral hematomas or cystic lesions, for biopsy of deep seated brain tumors, and for brachytherapy of brain tumors. However, for most of these operations, a stereotactic localizing frame is used for determination of the coordinates of the target point. This paper reports the principles and actual operative procedures of a new operative method for stereotactic surgery using the coordinate system of the CT apparatus itself. This

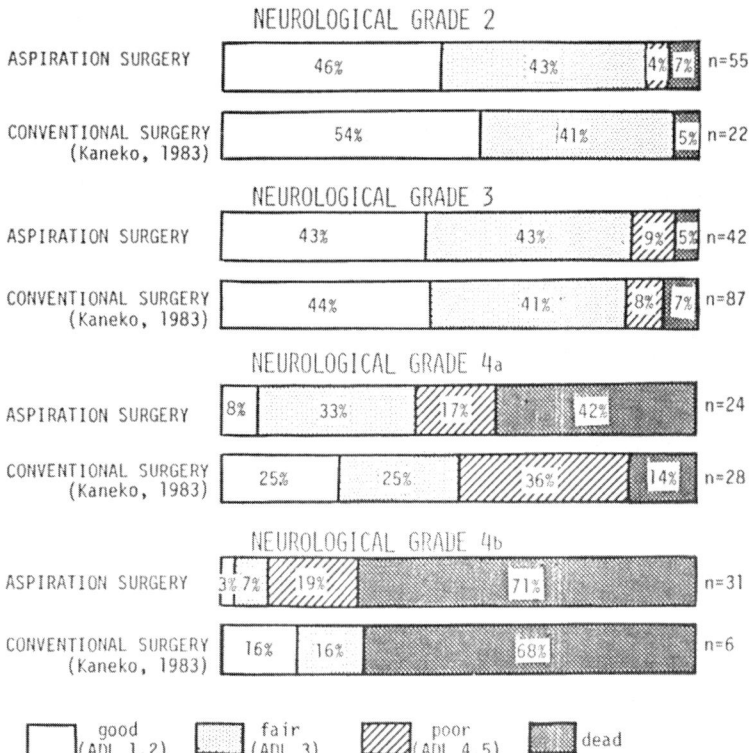

Fig. 9. Six-month postoperative outcomes of AS in good risk patients and Kaneko's CS in grades 2, 3, 4a, and 4b. *ADL grades* are defined in Table 5

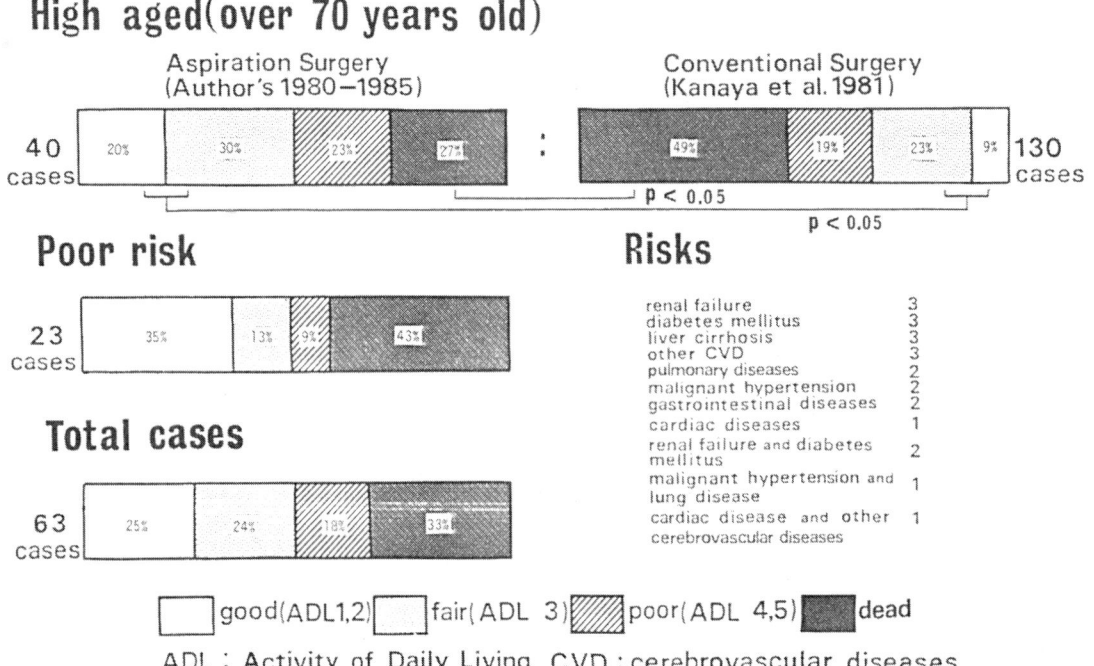

Fig. 10. Six-month postoperative outcome of AS in high aged and poor risk patients and Kanaya's CS. *ADL grades* are defined in Table 5

method is called "CT-controlled stereotactic surgery", because the procedure is performed with the intraoperative use of a CT scan [6]. This new method needs no special accessory frame and is highly accurate in hitting the target.

Backlund and von Holst [1] first proposed a new instrument for evacuation of hematomas; since then, several devices for aspiration of the bulk of a deeply located intracerebral hematoma have become available. However, in some of these, a blood clot may obstruct the cannula or tube and interfere with continuous aspiration. To overcome this problem, we have designed a new ultrasonic surgical aspirator for the stereotactic aspiration of hematomas that facilitates aspiration of a dense clot in the acute stage.

The management of HBH, and especially basal ganglionic hemorrhage, is still controversial. There are recent reports of no significant difference in the outcomes of patients with hypertensive basal ganglionic hemorrhage after CS and conservative treatment [4, 9]. AS did not cause progress of neurological deterioration or increase of perifocal edema after initial aspiration, even in cases of a large hematoma, whereas CS caused transient postoperative deterioration and an increase of intracranial pressure, which necessitated removal of bone flap or administration of mannitol as routine managements. This is a great advantage of AS. The development of AS for HBH in the acute stage [5] provides a new approach to management of this condition.

However, there are still controversial technical aspects of AS, such as optimal initial amount of evacuation of the hematoma, indication for a small hematoma, the optimal dosage of urokinase, indications for use of the stereotactic apparatus, and choice of the trajectory to approach a pontine hemorrhage. Precise clinical evaluation of the efficacy of AS in comparison with that of CS and conservative treatment is also necessary.

Conclusion

Aspiration surgery for HBH was formerly thought to be ineffective and to be associated with poor results in CS. However, CT-controlled stereotactic aspiration surgery has proved effective and so provides a new method for surgical treatment of HBH.

References

1. Backlund EO, von Holst H (1978) Controlled subtotal evacuation of intracerebral hematomas by stereotactic technique. Surg Neurol 9:99–101
2. Kanaya H, Yukawa H, Itoh Z, et al (1978). A neurological grading for patients with hypertensive intracerebral hemorrhage and a classification for hematoma location on computed tomography, In: Proceedings of the 7th Conference of Surgical Treatment of Stroke. Tokyo, Neuron pp 265–270 (in Japanese)
3. Kaneko M, Koba T, Yokoyama T (1977) Early surgical treatment for hypertensive intracerebral hemorrhage. J Neurosurg 46:579–583
4. Kanno T, Sano H, Shinomiya Y, et al. (1984) Role of surgery in hypertensive intracerebral hematoma: A comparative study of 305 nonsurgical and 154 surgical cases. J Neurosurg 61:1091–1099
5. Matsumoto K, Hondo H (1984) CT-guided stereotactic evacuation of hypertensive intracerebral hematomas. J Neurosurg 61:440–448, 1984
6. Matsumoto K, Shichijo F, Masuda T, Miyake H (1985) Computer tomography-controlled stereotactic surgery. Appl Neurophysiol 4:39–44
7. Matsumoto K (1986) Treatment with stereotactic needle aspiration: II. Aspiration surgery for hypertensive intracerebral hemorrhage in acute stage. The Mt. Fuji Workshop on CVD 4:117–123 Kodama, Tokyo (in Japanese)
8. Ooneda G (1974) Pathogenesis of cerebral hemorrhage. Bunkodo, Tokyo (in Japanese)
9. Waga S, Miyazaki M, Okada M, et al. (1986) Hypertensive putaminal hemorrhage: Analysis of 182 patients. Surg Neurol 26:159–166.

Stereotactic Evacuation of Hypertensive Intracerebral Hematoma Using Plasminogen Activator
Surgical Technique and Long-Term Results

Toru Itakura, Norihiko Komai, Ekini Nakai, and Eiji Doi[1]

Introduction

Treatment of hypertensive intracerebral hemorrhage has generally been carried out using either surgical evacuation by craniotomy or by conservative therapy. In 1974, Komai et al. [9] demonstrated for the first time that intracerebral hematoma can be safely evacuated by stereotactic technique, and suggested that stereotactic evacuation may become an applicable surgical procedure for hypertensive intracerebral hematoma. In 1980, we reported, for the first time, an extensive series of intracerebral hematomas treated by stereotactic evacuation using a plasminogen activator [1]. This new surgical procedure has since been acknowledged by other authors to be a safe and valuable treatment method for hypertensive intracerebral hematoma [7]. Since 1978, we have treated 241 intracerebral hematomas using the stereotactic approach. We herein report an analysis of our series and offer discussion on several controversial points in the surgical treatment of this disease.

Materials and Methods

From 1978 to 1986, 241 patients with hypertensive intracerebral hematomas were treated by the stereotactic procedure in our department. Of 241 intracerebral hematomas, 144 were putaminal, 63 were thalamic, 12 were cerebeller hemorrhages, 12 subcortical, and ten were pontine hemorrhages (Table 1). The present study is confined to analysis of putaminal and thalamic hemorrhages. Analyses of cerebellar and pontine hemorrhage has been published elsewhere.

Procedure in Stereotactic Surgery

The stereotactic apparatus devised by Komai was used [4–6]. The instrument consists of a head frame and an arm, made of aluminous alloy, bearing a cannula. The head frame has four pins for fixation to the skull. It also has an attachment of a coordinate system and the arm (Fig. 1a). The coordinate system is comprised of nine vertically and two obliquely oriented cylindrical aluminum rods inserted into a plastic plate. The operation is usually performed under a local anesthesia. After the head frame is fixed to the patient's head, the coordinate scale and patient's head are imaged simultaneously by a CT scanner (Fig. 1b, c). Then the coordinate system is removed from the head frame and the arm frame is attached to the ring. A small linear skin incision and burr hole are made under local anesthesia. A cannula made of stainless steel (3 mm in outer diameter) is inserted into the target point (the center of the hematoma cavity), and the hematoma is aspirated through the cannula. Then, a small (3 mm in outer diameter) silastic tube is introduced into the cavity through the same track. The skin is sutured, leaving the drainage tube in place. After the operation, the plasminogen activator (6000 IU urokinase in 2–5 ml saline) is injected into the hematoma cavity two or three times a day. Drainage and urokinase injections are continued until the hematoma can no longer be observed under CT scan.

Table 1. Number of cases treated by stereotactic procedure

Location	No. of cases
Putaminal hemorrhage	144
Thalamic hemorrhage	63
Subcortical hemorrhage	12
Cerebellar hemorrhage	12
Pontine hemorrhage	10
Total	241

[1] Department of Neurological Surgery, Wakayama Medical College, Wakayama, Japan

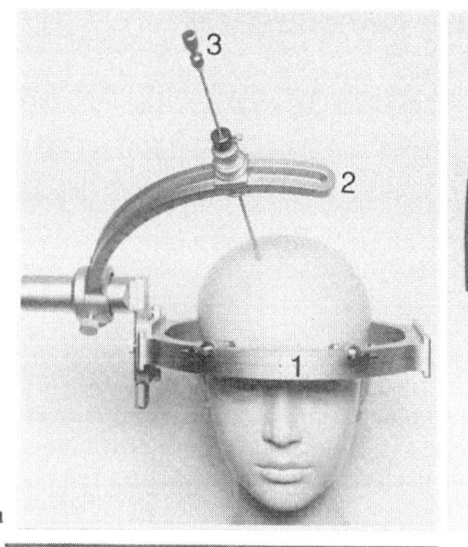

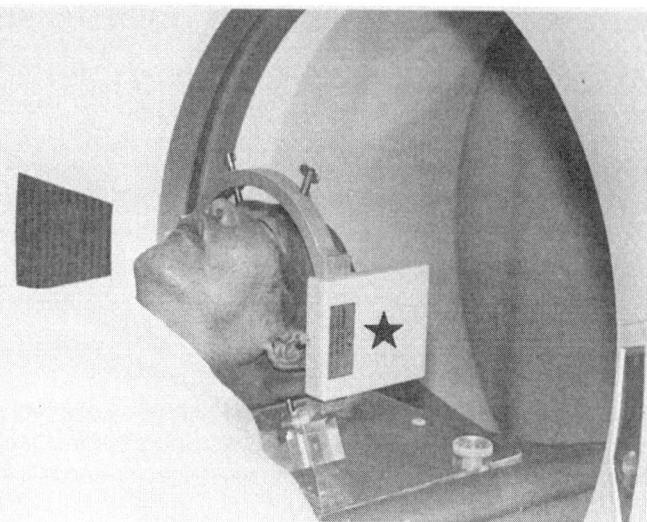

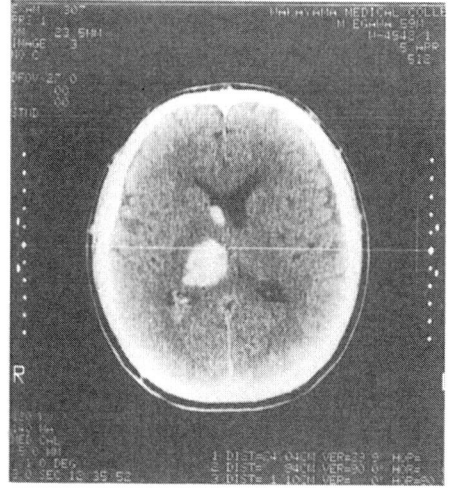

Fig. 1. a Komai's CT-stereotactic apparatus, *1* head frame, *2* arm, *3* cannula. **b** The coordinate scale (*asterisk*) and patient are imaged simultaneously by CT scanner. **c** CT scans of patient's brain and the coordinate scale. The target is selected by the CT images

Evaluation of Patient Status and Prognosis

Preoperative neurological grading, CT classification of the hematoma, and patient outcome were evaluated by the criteria of the Japanese Ad Hoc Committee on Hypertensive Intracerebral Hemorrhage. Briefly, the preoperative neurological grading was evaluated on admission as follows: grade 1 as alertness or confusion, grade 2 as somnolence, grade 3 as stupor, grade 4a as semicoma without herniation signs, grade 4b as semicoma with herniation signs, and grade 5 as deep coma.

Grades of putaminal hemorrages were classified under CT scan as follows: I as localized outside internal capsule, II as extending to anterior limb, IIIa as extending to posterior limb without massive ventricular hemorrhage, IIIb as extending to posterior limb with massive ventricular hemorrhage, IVa as extending to anterior and posterior limbs without massive ventricular hemorrhage, IVb as extending to anterior and posterior limbs with massive ventricular hemorrhage, and V as extending to thalamus or subthalamus. Grades of thalamic hemorrhage were classified under CT scan as follows: Ia as localized in thalamus without massive ventricular hemorrhage, Ib as localized in thalamus with massive ventricular hemorrhage, IIa as extending to internal capsule without massive ventricular hemorrhage, IIb as extending to internal capsule with massive ventricular hemorrhage, IIIa as extending to hypothalamus or midbrain without massive ventricular hemorrhage, and IIIb as extending to hypothalamus or midbrain with massive ventricular hemorrhage.

Results of the treatment were evaluated on the basis of activity in daily living (ADL) 3 months after the operation, as follows: good, indicating full recovery to social life or independent home

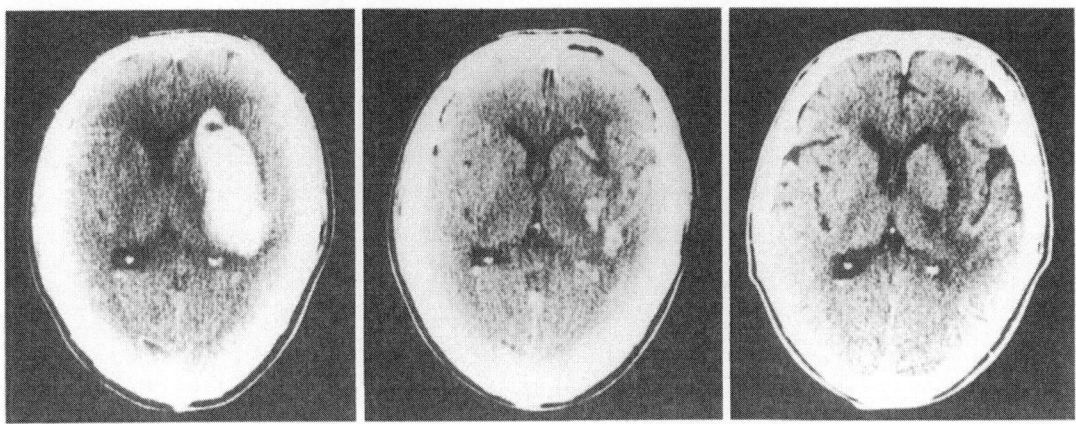

a, b
c

Fig. 2a–c. CT scan of a representative case of putaminal hemorrhage. **a** Before operation; **b** just after operation; **c** 20 days after operation

life with self-care or partial recovery to social life; fair, meaning dependent home life requiring some help for daily life, usually ambulatory with a cane; poor, signifying bedridden but conscious or vegetative; and died.

Results

Evacuation of the Hematoma

The hematoma volume in each patient was estimated under preoperative CT image. Aspiration rate (hematoma volume aspirated by operation divided by the preoperatively estimated hematoma volume) was calculated. Total evacuation rate was also calculated (hematoma volume aspirated by operation plus hematoma volume drained by urokinase after operation divided by the preoperatively estimated hematoma volume).

Putaminal hemorrhage. Figure 2 shows a representative case of a putaminal hemorrhage evacuated by the stereotactic procedure. The hematoma was completely evacuated by this method. The aspiration rate of the hematoma was averaged to be 63.9%, and the total evacuation rate was averaged at 84.9%. Table 2 shows the correlation between preoperative hematoma volume and aspirated hematoma volume. Most hematomas, except those of more than 60 ml in volume, were well aspirated by the operation (54.8%–75.1%), and the total evacuation rate was also quite high (77.8%–89.9%; Table 2). Table 3 summarizes the correlation between tim-

ing of the operation and the evacuation rate. In operations carried out early (within 5 days), the aspirated hematoma volume at operation averaged 59.3%. In contrast, in hematomas operated on 6–15 days after onset, the aspirated hematoma volume was approximately 72%. However, the total evacuation rate showed no variation with regard to timing of the operation.

Thalamic hemorrhage. Figure 3 shows a representative case of thalamic hemorrhage treated by the stereotactic procedure. The average hematoma volume in thalamic hemorrhage was estimated at 12.4 ml. The aspiration rate was 67.5%, and total evacuation rate was 84.5%. As the hematoma volume increased, the aspiration rate decreased slightly, but no significant difference was noted in total evacuation rates of small and large hematomas (Table 4). Table 5 summarizes the correlation between timing of the operation and evacuated hematoma volume. Early (within 5 days) and later (after 5 days) operations showed almost the same aspiration rate. In this analysis, the total evacuation rate showed no significant difference with regard to early and late operations (average 84.5%).

Prognosis of the Patients Treated by Stereotactic Procedure

The outcome in cases of intracerebral hemorrhage is influenced by several variables, notably the size and location of the hematoma, and clinical status of the patient on admission. These factors were analyzed in putaminal and thalamic hemorrhage.

Table 2. Hemorrhage volume, aspiration volume of hematoma at operation, total evacuation volume, and ADL at 3 months after operation in putaminal hemorrhage

Hematoma volume (ml)	No. of cases	Estimated volume of hematoma (ml)	Aspiration volume of hematoma at operation (ml)	Total evacuation volume of hematoma (ml)	ADL			
					Good	Fair	Poor	Died
−10	8	7.9	4.1 (54.8%)	6.3 (80.5%)	7	1	0	0
10.1–20	37	16.0	10.6 (68.4%)	14.2 (89.9%)	23	13	1	0
20.1–30	36	24.7	16.5 (63.5%)	22.0 (84.9%)	26	8	2	0
30.1–40	32	35.4	21.9 (62.3%)	29.5 (82.9%)	13	15	4	0
40.1–50	14	47.1	27.2 (58.5%)	36.6 (77.8%)	3	8	2	1
50.1–60	11	56.1	41.0 (75.1%)	48.5 (82.8%)	3	6	1	1
60.1–	6	78.7	38.2 (49.9%)	50.5 (57.4%)	0	3	3	0
Total	144	29.9	20.0 (63.9%)	25.1 (84.9%)	75	54	13	2

ADL activity in daily living

Table 3. Timing of operation, aspiration volume of hematoma at operation, total evacuation volume, and ADL at 3 months after operation in putaminal hemorrhage

Timing of operation (day)	No. of cases	Estimated volume of hematoma (ml)	Aspiration volume of hematoma at operation	Total evacuation volume	ADL			
					Good	Fair	Poor	Died
−5	59	31.2	19.5 (59.3%)	26.1 (84.0%)	22	25	10	2
6–10	33	31.5	21.8 (72.1%)	28.3 (87.5%)	19	12	2	0
11–15	27	29.8	20.8 (71.5%)	24.8 (88.3%)	19	7	1	0
16–20	16	26.8	14.6 (53.4%)	23.5 (85.4%)	11	5	0	0
21–	9	25.6	15.0 (58.2%)	17.9 (71.0%)	4	5	0	0
Total	144	29.9	20.0 (63.9%)	25.1 (84.9%)	75	54	13	2

ADL activity in daily living

Putaminal hemorrhage. Hematoma volume, location of the hematoma, and neurological grading correlated well with the outcome. However, timing of the operation did not necessarily influence the patient outcome (Tables 2, 3).

Thalamic hemorrhage. The hematoma volume and location of the hematoma correlated well with the outcome. For example, 66.7% of the patients with small thalamic hemorrhage (less than 10 ml) resulted in good ADL, but only 43.5% of those with large hematomas (more than 10.1 ml) resulted in good ADL. In the CT classification, 87.5%, 55.2%, and 14.3% of the patients with hematomas classified as I, II, and III, respectively, showed good ADL. The neurological grade on admission also correlated well with patient outcome. Of patients showing grades 1, 2, and 3, 78.9%, 45.4%, and 44.4%, respectively, revealed good outcomes. In contrast, timing of operation did not influence the patient prognosis (Table 5).

Complications

As a complication, postaspiration hemorrhage was encountered in five cases (3.5%) in putaminal and three (4.8%) in thalamic hemorrhage. Bleeding during urokinase injection into the hematoma cavity was not encountered in our series. No infection was found during aspiration or drainage.

Discussion

Since 1974, when Komai et al. [9] reported that intracerebral hematomas were safely evacuated by a stereotactic procedure, we have carried out stereotactic evacuation in 241 cases of intracerebral hematoma: 144 putaminal, 63 thalamic, 12 subcortical, 12 cerebellar, and ten pontine hemorrhages. The total evacuation rate of the hematoma was 84.9% in putaminal, and 84.5%

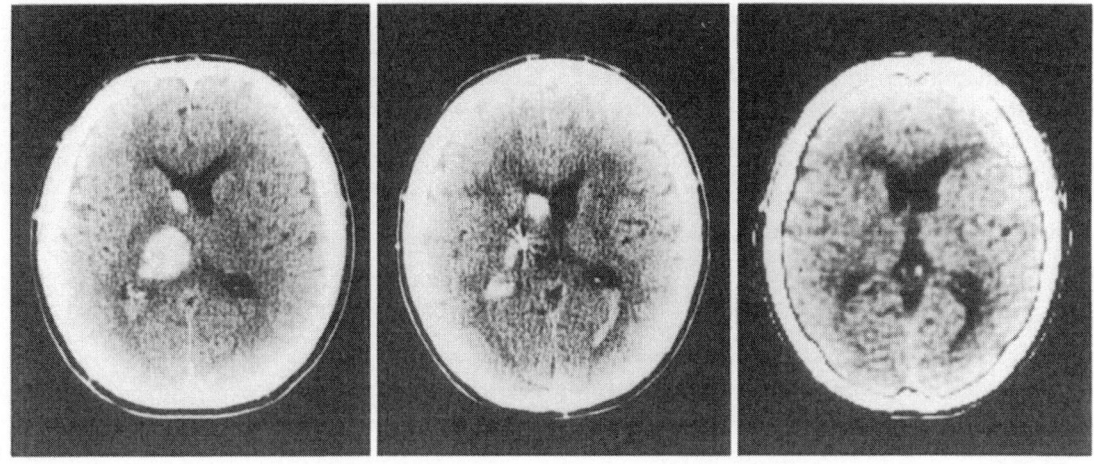

a, b   c

Fig. 3a–c. CT scan of a representative case of thalamic hemorrhage. **a** Before operation; **b** just after operation; **c** 20 days after operation

Table 4. Hematoma volume, aspiration volume of hematoma at operation, total evacuation volume and ADL at 3 months after operation in thalamic hemorrhage

Volume of hematoma (ml)	No. of cases	Estimated volume (ml)	Aspiration volume at operation (ml)	Total evacuation volume (ml)	ADL			
					Good	Fair	Poor	Died
−5.0	4	5.0	3.8 (75.0%)	4.5 (90.0%)	2	2	0	0
5.1–10.0	28	8.3	5.8 (71.5%)	7.0 (84.2%)	16	11	0	1
10.1–15.0	15	13.2	8.5 (63.9%)	10.2 (82.2%)	6	8	1	0
15.1–20.0	11	17.8	11.9 (66.9%)	15.5 (87.2%)	3	4	2	2
20.1–	5	32.9	15.6 (51.2%)	25.2 (83.7%)	3	1	0	1
Total	63	12.4	8.1 (67.5%)	10.5 (84.5%)	30	26	3	4

ADL activity in daily life

Table 5. Timing of operation, aspiration volume of hematoma, total evacuation volume and ADL at 3 months after operation in thalamic hemorrhage

Timing of operation (day)	No. of cases	Estimated volume (ml)	Aspiration volume at operation (ml)	Total evacuation volume (ml)	ADL			
					Good	Fair	Poor	Died
−5	28	12.3	8.1 (70.1%)	9.6 (84.3%)	9	14	2	3
6–10	8	13.0	9.6 (72.8%)	10.8 (82.0%)	5	3	0	0
11–15	9	9.3	7.3 (66.1%)	8.6 (78.6%)	5	4	0	0
16–20	11	12.6	5.9 (61.6%)	11.4 (88.9%)	7	3	0	0
21–	7	16.0	10.7 (63.0%)	14.9 (89.0%)	4	2	1	0
Total	63	12.4	8.1 (67.5%)	10.5 (84.5%)	30	26	3	4

ADL activity in daily life

in thalamic hemorrhage. The stereotactic procedure enables exactly reaching anyplace in the brain without imparting obvious damage in the trajectory. Thus, we have safely evacuated hematomas not only in the putamen and cerebellum, but also in the thalamus and pons. In comparison with conventional craniotomy [2], the stereotactic procedure revealed a better outcome in our series. For example, the mortality in cases of thalamic hemorrhage was 34% using craniotomy, but only 6.8% in this series. In neurological grades 1 and 2 patients, craniotomy resulted in a good outcome in 16.6% of the cases, but a good outcome was obtained in 66.7% of the same grade patients in this series. The marked difference in mortality and morbidity may be attributable to the differing degrees of invasion of the underlying normal brain in these two methods.

In the present study, the aspiration rates of the hematomas were 63.9% in the putaminal and 67.5% in the thalamic hemorrhage. However, the total evacuation rate increased to 84.9% in putaminal and 84.5% in thalamic hemorrhage. These data strongly suggest that injection of urokinase into the hematoma cavity might be effective for lysing the residual hematoma. Narayan et al. [8] reported that clot lysis was achieved in 90% of intracerebral hematoma in rabbits by 3 h injection of urokinase as compared with 14% of that in controls. The present clinical data also suggest the safety and efficacy of utilizing urokinase in lysing of the residual hematoma after aspiration.

Our clinical data clearly showed that duration from onset to operation did not necessarily influence the evacuation rate of the hematoma, suggesting that hematoma can be successfully evacuated at any time. However, it has been shown that the affected arteries are still bleeding within 6 h after the onset [3]. Taking this into consideration, together with our data, the hematoma can probably be safely evacuated at any time from 6 h after onset. However, it is also suggested that surrounding brain tissue compressed by the hematoma may be successfully revived by performing operation early. Considering these clinical viewpoints, we recommend that hypertensive intracerebral hematoma should be operated on from 6 h to 3 or 4 days after the onset. From the present analysis of the patient outcome, the most important factors influencing the patient outcome were as follows: the location of the hematoma (CT classification), neurological grade on admission, and volume of the hematoma. In contrast, the timing of the operation was found to be a factor of less importance.

References

1. Doi E, Moriwaki H, Komai N (1980) Stereotactic operation for hypertensive intracerebral hemorrhage, especially for thalamic hemorrhage. Neurol Med Chir 20 (Suppl): 124–125 (abstract)
2. Kanaya H, Saiki I, Ohuchi T, Kamata K, Endo H, Mizukami M, Kagawa M, Kaneko M, Ito Z (1983) Hypertensive intracerebral hemorrhage in Japan: Update on surgical treatment. In: Mizukami M, Kanaya H, Kogure K, Yamori Y (eds) Hypertensive intracerebral hemorrhage. Raven, New York, pp 147–163
3. Kaneko M (1983) Timing of surgery for hypertensive intracerebral hemorrhage. In: Mizukami M, Kanaya H, Kogure K, Yamori Y (eds) Hypertensive intracerebral hemorrhage. Raven, New York, pp 249–253
4. Komai N (1984) CT-guided stereotactic operation. Nihon Rinsho 42:954–974
5. Komai N (1986) CT-stereotaxy. No Shinkei Geka 14:123–133
6. Komai N, Doi E, Moriwaki H, Nakai E (1986) Stereotactic evacuation of hypertensive thalamic hematoma using plasminogen activator (urokinase). No shinkei Geka 14:249–256
7. Matsumoto K, Hondo H (1984) CT-guided stereotactic evacuation of hypertensive intracerebral hematomas. J Neurosurg 61:440–448
8. Narayan K, Narayan M, Katz A, Kobnblith L, Murano G (1985) Lysis of intracranial hematomas with urokinase in a rabbit model. J Neurosurg 62: 580–586
9. Shimamoto Y, Komai N, Nishina H, Kido T, Hamada T, Yabushita R, Kobayashi R, Taketsuna S, Koshimichi S (1974) Stereotactic removal of space-occupying lesions in the brain. J Wakayama Med Soc 25:391

CT-Guided Stereotaxic Aspiration of Intracerebral Hematoma on 168 Cases

Hiroshi Niizuma and Jiro Suzuki[1]

Introduction

Together with the proliferation of CT-guided stereotaxic systems, there has been a rapid increase in stereotaxic operations for intracerebral hematoma [1-9, 11]. We have performed the aspiration of spontaneous intracerebral hematomas on 212 cases using Leksell's CT-stereotaxic system since 1983, and the 168 cases were followed up for 6 months. This paper reports upon our method and results of these 168 cases.

Clinical Materials and Methods

The patients ranged in age from 28 to 81 years. Nineteen (11.3%) of our 168 cases were over 70 years of age. A history of hypertension was found in 128 cases (76.2%). Preoperative consciousness levels and sizes of the hematomas are shown in Tables 1 and 2.

In cases of putaminal or thalamic hematoma, patients with obvious hemiparesis of grade 2 or less, according to DeJong's classification, were submitted to stereotaxic operation after waiting at least 6 h from the time of onset. Patients with large size hematomas of more than 40 ml, admitted within 5 h from onset, were treated by craniotomy, that is, the transsylvian approach [10]. Those with coma or semicoma with herniation signs were excluded from surgical interventions. In the case of subcortical hematoma, more than 20 ml of hematoma with neurological symptoms was aspirated stereotaxically. Aspiration of the cerebellar hematoma was performed in the cases with more than 16 ml of hematoma or cases with 11-15 ml of hematoma in which conservative therapy had been used, but recovery from symptoms was slow. The time from onset to operation is shown in Table 3. Operation was performed within 24 h from onset in 43.5% of the cases.

Operations were performed in the CT room under local anesthesia with intravenous injection of pentazocin and diazepam. The three dimensional coordinates of the target point were directly measured from the CT using Leksell's CT-stereotaxic system. Aspiration of supratentorial hematoma was done by the following three methods: a frontal approach, in which a burr hole is made near or slightly anterior of the coronal suture, a parietal approach, in which a burr hole is made over the parietal area along the long axis of the hematoma, and double-track aspiration (Figs. 1, 2). The double-track aspiration technique is used when the parietal approach is deemed inappropriate for long hematomas extending in an anterior-posterior direction [9]. The supine-lateral retromastoid approach was used for the aspiration of posterior fossa hematoma [8].

Aspiration of the hematoma was done manually using a syringe and a lengthened Dandy ventricular cannula (3 mm in diameter, 220 mm in length). After initial aspiration, a sylastic drainage tube was inserted into the hematoma cavity and 6000 units of urokinase dissolved in 2-3 ml saline solution was injected 3-12 h after the operation. Twelve to twenty-four hours later, the dissolved hematoma was aspirated through the drainage tube. If required, injection of urokinase can be repeated at bedside one to two times a day until the bulk of the hematoma has been removed.

Results

By initial aspiration, more than 80% of the estimated hematoma could be removed in 58 cases (34.5%), and between 50% and 79% could be removed in 61 cases (36.3%). In 39 of these successfully aspirated cases, urokinase was not used because the bulk of the hematoma was removed

[1] Division of Neurosurgery, Institute of Brain Diseases, Tohoku University School of Medicine, Sendai, Japan

Table 1. Site of the hematoma and preoperative consciousness level

Site of hematoma	Preop. consciousness level					Total
	Alert	Confusion	Somnolence	Stupor	Semicoma	
Putamen	22	43	18	17	8	108
Thalamus	9	12	10	5	3	39
Cerebellum	2	4		2	2	10
Subcortex	3	6				9
Pons					2	2
Total	36	65	28	24	15	168

Table 2. Site of hematoma and estimated hematoma volume

Site of hematoma	Estimated hematoma volume (ml)							Total
	6–10	11–15	16–20	21–30	31–40	41–60	61–132	
Putamen	4	9	14	25	23	21	12	108
Thalamus	16	11	2	6	1	3		39
Cerebellum		2	2	4	2			10
Subcortex				3	1	4	1	9
Pons	2							2
Total	22	22	18	38	27	28	13	168

during operation. Between 30% and 49% of the hematoma was removed in 35 cases (20.8%) and less than 29% in 14 cases (8.3%) (Table 4). In the first ten cases, there were five cases in which aspiration of less than 29% was possible. In the following 158 cases, those in which less than 29% was removed numbered only nine: the blood clot was too hard to aspirate in these nine cases.

Rebleeding occurred in ten cases (5.9%). Reaccumulated hematomas were larger than preoperative hematomas in five cases (major bleeding), and smaller in five cases (minor bleeding). Three of the major bleeding cases underwent conventional craniotomy, while the others received continued aspiration or were treated conservatively. Rebleeding during operation was seen in only two cases. In the other eight cases, rebleeding occurred while urokinase was being used postoperatively. Rebleeding seems to have been due to the excessive aspiration and changes in the position of the drainage tube while urokinase was being used postoperatively.

Finally, more than 80% of the hematoma was removed in 123 cases (73.2%). Between 50% and 70% of the hematoma was removed in 31 cases (18.5%). Twenty of these 31 were the cases with the estimated hematoma of less than 20 ml. Between 30% and 40% of the hematoma was

Table 3. Time of operation

Onset prior to operation	No. of cases
4–5 h	3[a]
6–24 h	70
2 days	34
3 days	18
4–7 days	21
8–14 days	18
15–31 days	4
Total	168

[a] Cerebellar hematoma cases

removed in nine cases (5.4%). Three were the cases with rebleeding and the remaining six were the cases with hard clot.

In comparison with conservative treatment or conventional craniotomy, the postoperative recovery following stereotaxic aspiration is rapid in many cases, and more than two-thirds of our patients showed improvement in symptoms within several days after operation. The drainage tube was left in place for 1–6 days. Postoperative meningitis occurred in two cases, on whom ventricular drainage was also performed for acute hydrocephalus.

Follow-up results at 6 months showed 91

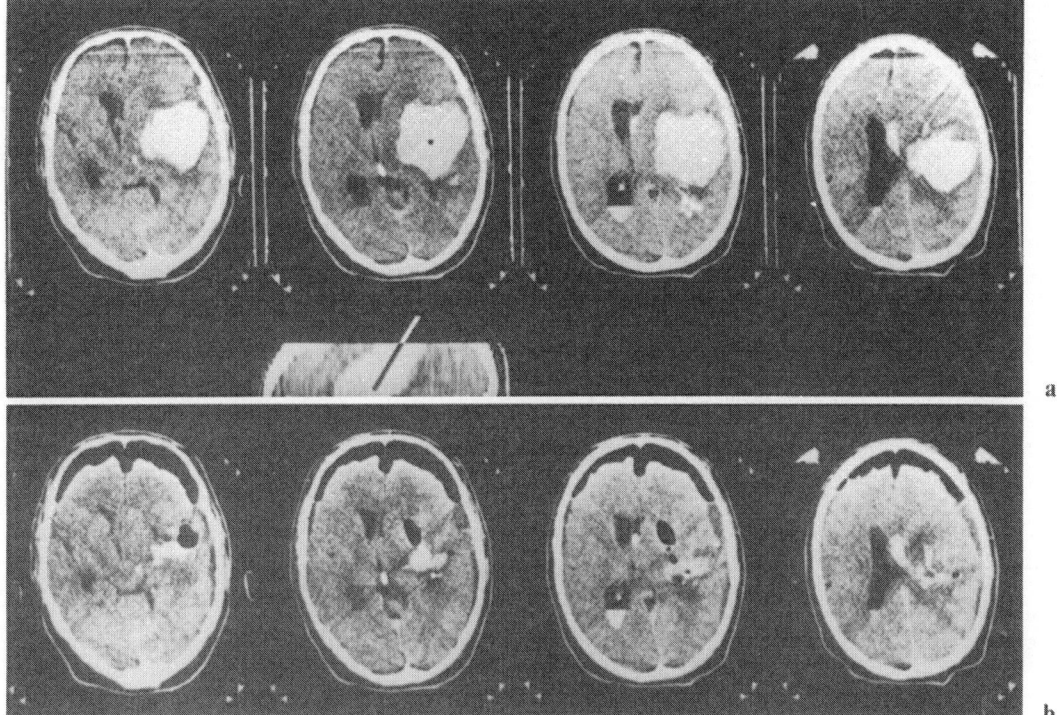

Fig. 1a, b. Parietal approach. **a** Before aspiration, **b** after aspiration

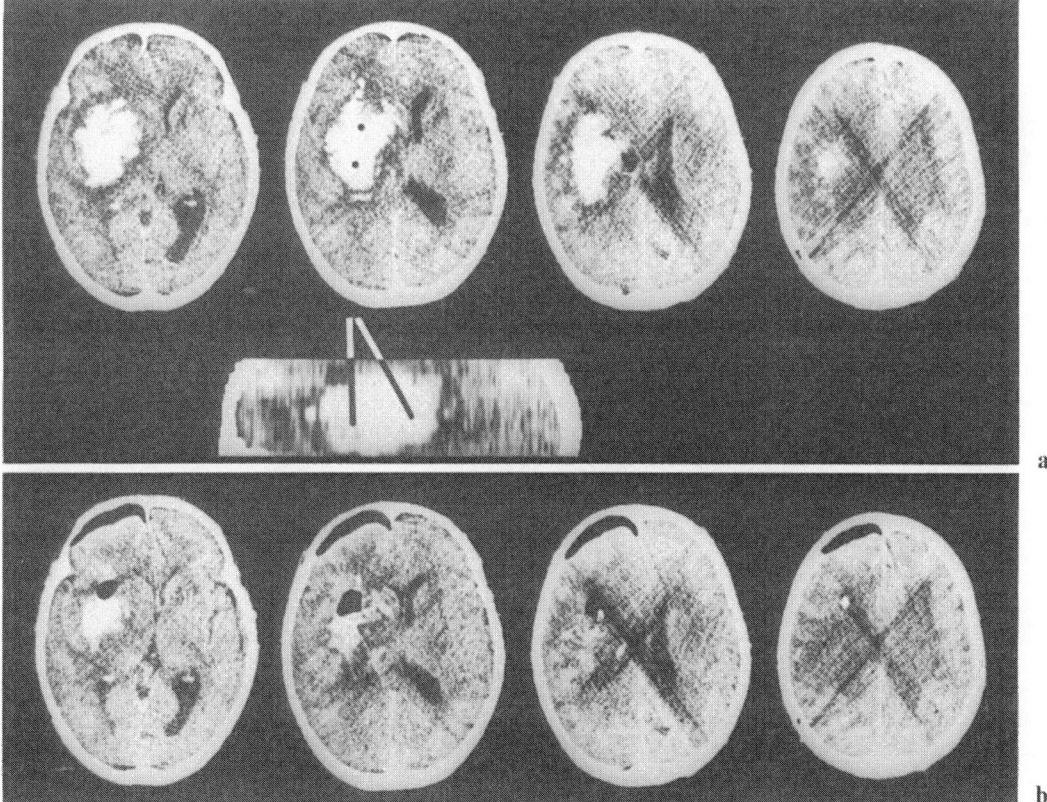

Fig. 2a, b. Double track aspiration. **a** Before aspiration, **b** after aspiration

Table 4. Initial aspiration rate

Initial aspiration rate	Site of hematoma					Total (%)
	Putamen	Thalamus	Cerebellum	Subcortex	Pons	
More than 80%	44	8	3	3		58 (34.5)
50%–79%	37	15	5	3	1	61 (36.3)
30%–49%	19	10	2	3	1	35 (20.8)
Less than 29%	8	6				14 (8.3)
Total	108	39	10	9	2	168

Table 5. Site of hematoma and follow-up results at 6 months

Site of hematoma	Excellent		Good		Fair		Poor		Dead		Total
	No.	Percent	No.	Percent	No.	Percent	No.	Percent	No.	Percent	
Putamen	23	21.3	38	35.2	31	28.7	8	7.4	8	7.4	108
Thalamus	4	10.3	13	33.3	17	43.6	4	10.3	1	2.6	39
Cerebellum	4	40.0	2	20.0	2	20.0	2	20.0			10
Subcortex	5	55.6	2	22.2	1	11.1	1	11.1			9
Pons							1	50.0	1	50.0	2
Total	36	21.4	55	32.7	51	30.4	16	9.5	10	6.0	168

Table 6. Age and follow-up results at 6 months

Age (yrs)	Excellent		Good		Fair		Poor		Dead		Total
	No.	Percent	No.	Percent	No.	Percent	No.	Percent	No.	Percent	
28–39	3	33.3	4	44.4	2	22.2					9
40–49	9	28.1	12	37.5	8	25.0	2	6.3	1	3.1	32
50–59	13	21.7	25	41.7	19	31.7	2	3.3	1	1.7	60
60–69	8	16.7	12	25.0	17	35.4	4	8.3	7	14.6	48
70–81	3	15.8	2	10.5	5	26.3	8	42.1	1	5.3	19
Total	36	21.4	55	32.7	51	30.4	16	9.6	10	6.0	168

excellent or good cases (54.2%; Table 5). The rate of excellent outcome was high in subcortical hematoma (55.6%) and cerebellar hematoma (40.0%), and low in thalamic hematoma (10.3%). The rate of poor outcome and mortality were 9.5% and 6.0%, respectively. Four deaths during hospitalization were caused by rebleeding, pneumonia, myocardial infarction, and cerebral infarction of the contralateral side. Six deaths at follow-up were attributed to primary brain damage in three cases and other combined diseases in the remaining three cases. Sixteen cases of poor outcome consisted of eight cases of over 70 years of age, seven cases with large hematoma. Outcome at 6 months from the onset were

bad in the cases of over 60 years (Table 6). In the cases of over 70 years, eight of the 19 cases (42.1%) were poor, and one (5.3%) was dead. The result seems to show the deterioration of reversibility in aged patients.

Discussion

CT-guided stereotaxic technique makes the stereotaxic operation a safer and minimally invasive method. Since the operation can be performed without general anesthesia, it is relatively easy to perform even in aged patients or patients with serious combined diseases, though the operative result is not necessarily so good. When the CT - guided stereotaxic operation was performed in the CT room, special aspiration instruments such as a rotating helical mandrel [1, 4] or an ultrasound aspirator (developed by Matsumoto) seemed to be rarely necessary. When the initial ten cases are excluded, more than 30% of the estimated hematoma could be aspirated at operation in 94.3% of our 158 cases. If a hematoma can be approached along its long axis, or double track aspiration is employed, more than 50% of the hematoma can be aspirated at operation in most cases, even in the acute stage. By following the injection of urokinase to dissolve the residual hematoma, the majority of hematoma can be finally removed.

The greatest disadvantage of this technique is that, when rebleeding has been brought about, it is then difficult to begin treatment other than craniotomy to counteract the hemorrhage. Nonetheless, by means of careful handling of the site and control of blood pressure, a fatal outcome from the hemorrhage is thought to be unlikely. CT-guided stereotaxic aspiration is believed to be very useful method for treatment of intracerebral hematoma.

References

1. Backlund EO, Holst H (1978) Controlled subtotal evacuation of intracerebral hematomas by stereotactic technique. Surg Neurol 9:99–101
2. Broseta J, Gonzalez-Darder J, Barcia-Salorio JL (1982) Stereotactic evacuation of intracerebral hematomas. Appl Neurophysiol 45:443–448
3. Doi E, Moriwaki H, Komai N, et al. (1982) Stereotactic evacuation of intracerebral hematomas. Neurol Med Chir 22:461–467
4. Higgins AC, Nashold BS (1980) Stereotactic evacuation of large intracerebral hematoma. Appl Neurophysiol 4:96–103
5. Kandel EI, Peresedov VV (1985) Stereotaxic evacuation of spontaneous intracerebral hematomas. J Neurosurg 62:206–213
6. Matsumoto K, Hondo H (1984) CT-guided stereotaxic evacuation of hypertensive intracerebral hematomas. J Neurosurg 61:440–448
7. Niizuma H, Otsuki T, Johkura H, et al. (1985) CT-guided stereotactic aspiration of intracerebral hematoma—Result of a hematoma-lysis method using urokinase. Appl Neurophysiol 48:427–430
8. Niizuma H, Suzuki J (1987) Computed tomography-guided stereotactic aspiration of posterior fossa hematoma: supine lateral retromastoid approach. Neurosurgery 21:422–427
9. Niizuma H, Suzuki J (1988) Stereotactic aspiration of putaminal hemorrhage using a double track aspiration technique. Neurosurgery 22 (in press)
10. Suzuki J, Sato S (1972) The new transsylvian approach to the hypertensive intracerebral hematoma. Jpn J Surg 2:47–52
11. Tanikawa T, Amano K, Kawamura H, et al. (1985) CT-guided stereotactic surgery for evacuation of hypertensive intracerebral hematoma. Appl Neurophysiol 48:431–439

Discussion

Commentator: *Kanaya* (Morioka): Aspiration surgery with stereotactic CT-guided and echo-guided instruments will be a valuable method for treating hypertensive intracerebral hematomas. The advantage of aspiration surgery is the less invasive effect on the brain and the whole body by accurate positioning of the instrument into the hematoma cavity without giving rise to bleeding from the brain; this is achieved by means of a small burr hole and local anesthesia. This method is suitable, therefore, for older patients and those at high risk.

With respect to rebleeding after aspiration, the incidence is reported to be 4%–6% and even higher in the acute stage within 6 h or in patients with hemorrhagic diasthesis such as platelet reduction and liver function disorders. Also, it is very important to prevent rebleeding by controlling the blood pressure during operation using hemostatic agents because these methods involve blind surgery. When the larger hematoma occurs it is very important to evacuate the hematoma by craniotomy as soon as possible and to stop the bleeding immediately after aspiration.

With respect to aspiration of the hematoma, though the best method is to evacuate the hematoma totally from the point of view of surgical results the aspiration rate of the hematoma is 60%–70%, being lower in hard hematomas. It is better to use urokinase for the remaining hematoma and to increase the aspiration rate by the use of various–sized needles and devices such as echoencephalography during operation, the ultrasonic aspirator developed by Dr. Matsumoto, and endoscopic aspirator developed by Dr. Auer are employed. These instruments are excellent for aspiration surgery. We look forward to further developments in this type of instrument and technological advances in evacuating the hematoma.

Echo-guided aspiration is a valuable method for early location of rebleeding and increasing the aspiration rate from intraoperative monitoring in real time.

The following is an update of surgical treatment of hypertensive intracerebral hemorrhage in Japan. The surgical indications are limited in the case of patients over 70 years of age, with stupor or semicoma, and marked mass effect on CT in putaminal hemorrhage. Aspiration surgery is a valuable method for hypertensive intracerebral hematoma but there remain some problems, particulary the prevention of rebleeding after aspiration and surgical indications compared with the results of evacuation surgery with craniotomy and conservative treatment.

Auer (Graz): Two pictures seem to have emerged from the papers presented. The first is the quite clear picture of the trend toward miniaturized approaches to the treatment of hematomas, whether in stereotactic aspiration or in an endoscopic technique; the instrument was a few millimeters in diameter that entered the hematoma and diminished the volume of the hematoma rather than evacuating it completely. The rest is resolved by urokinase—in my view a very good idea. The second picture was the rather unclear one concerning the best time to operate upon a hematoma; what are the indications? Even in the recent literature, opinions are very divergent: Some colleagues believe the only indication is for subcortical hematomas; others say it is rather for the one or the other putaminal hemorrhage than for anything; some authors even believe that there is a certain group of thalamic hemorrhages in which surgery is indicated.

Hegde (Bangalore): Is it necessary to aspirate the hematoma completely or would it be sufficient to aspirate partially and stop aspiration once the mass effect in CT scan has subsided or the ICP has returned to normal? My second question is: Is there any additional risk of rebleeding with complete aspiration and the use of clot–lysing agents?

Auer: In answer to your first question, we statistically analyzed the outcome with complete and incomplete evacuation and there was no difference.

Itakura (Wakayama) I do not think it is necessary to aspirate the total volume of the hematoma by surgery. It is very dangerous because of the risk of rebleeding. Only 60% of the volume of the hematoma should be aspirated; urokinase is then injected into the hematoma cavity and this will make it possible to remove the total volume of the hematoma a couple of days after the operation.

Auer: With regard to the second question posed, the figures presented here for rebleeding are from less than 1% to 6%. We had 2 of 120 cases; it was half–deteriorated but it was more than 2 days after evacuation of the hematoma. When these figures are compared with those for the spontaneous course in medically treated patients, the rate of postoperative rebleeding is not seen to be higher.

Kanno (Toyoake): Nowadays, we can use cortical spinal direct response during surgery. Using this means of monitoring, it can be seen that if 50% of the hematoma is evacuated the response improves, but if 100% of the hematoma is removed the response becomes much better. So if all the hematoma is not removed at that time this chance to improve the motor function may be missed.

Auer: This is an interesting phenomenon; it may, however, be time dependent: what is immediately observed in cases of total evacuation may be seen later on in partial evacuation.

Schisano (Naples): I would like to hear the panel's comments on operative indication. In my opinion, indication for operation is given by a typical clinical–radiological condition: The clinical signs are deterioration of the patient and the radiological signs are the alterations in the CT—all the alterations that show a distortion of the brain stem, e.g., dilatation of the contralateral ventricle. I would also like to add that there appears to be a difference between Western and Japanese neurosurgeons with regard to the indications for surgery in very deep hematomas.

Auer: I feel that what we need primarily here are clear–cut data, indicating from control trials where a better outcome exists.

Guidetti (Rome): Personally, I feel the shift of the midline structure is very important. If the hematoma has a moderate or no shift I will not operate but just follow it by CT scan. I think the worst thing that can happen during surgery is hemorrhage, but there is very little chance of hemorrhage if the hematoma is removed without causing a shift. If there is a shift in the contralateral part, the midline structure can be saved by removing the hematoma.

I can perhaps justify aspiration in older patients, but in young patients I want to see if there is some arteriovenous malformation inside the cavity. So in younger patients, I think it is no problem to open the cavity, remove all the hematoma, and observe the wall to see if there is any malformation.

Matsumoto (Tokushima): In Japan, we deal rather differently with this kind of patient. We perform the operation very early and midline shift is quite uncommon in this very acute stage. Therefore, indications for surgery cannot always rely upon the existence of the midline shift. In my presentation, I showed the case of a patient with a large hematoma but who was still alert; there was no shift on CT. In a case where the shift developed 2–3 days later, we should have operated much earlier. The indications are not so very clear cut here.

Guidetti: I do not feel it is too late if the patient is followed with a CT scan, because in a small hematoma there is no shift.

Steiner (Stockholm): I think the only indication for surgery on the basis of the data we have today is to save life. The author speaks in terms of the clinical condition and I spoke in terms of the quantification of the volumes of the hematoma, though these really amount to the same thing. If there is a mass effect, if the hematoma is more than 70 ml the patient will be in a poor condition and the hematoma must be operated upon. In this way, as I said, the indication to save life is absolutely clear; what is not clear is whether we can improve the quality of life, i.e., whether the neurological condition of the patient can be improved. In my experience, surgery does not improve the neurological condition of the patient more than conservative treatment. My policy is as follows: If the patient is in a critical condition I will use stereotactic evacuation to reduce the volume of the hematoma, thereby changing the status of the patient form high to low risk. If the patient is in better condition I prefer using microsurgery with a stereotactic guide.

Niizuma (Sendai): It has been said that the neurological condition cannot be improved, but when the hematoma was about 20–50 ml, improvement of the paresis was identified within a week after stereotaxic aspiration surgery in one-third of the patients. In addition, if disturbances of consciousness existed, these improved after surgery in almost cases.

Ramamurthi (Madras): In thalamic and putaminal hemorrhage, is surgery better than medical treatment? I would like to hear from the panel what the mortality and morbidity are in surgery versus medical treatment.

Auer: My brief answer would be our randomized study has shown that in thalamic and putaminal hemorrhages surgery is of no value.

Matsumoto: We are conducting a randomized study into this at the moment and shall have the results soon.

Steiner: In our experience we have not seen improvement in patients with thalamic hemorrhages following surgery, nevertheless I cannot now completely rule out surgery; a randomized study is due.

Beneš (Prague): I think most patients with thalamic or putaminal hemorrhages are in grade 4 or 5 and, therefore, we should not operate.

Guidetti: In my experience thalamic and putaminal hemorrhages should not be operated upon, especially if they are not so large and do not show a big shift. If you save the life of the patient, the quality of life is very poor.

Itakura: I have the strong impression that a patient treated by stereotactic surgery improves and the results are better than in medically treated patients. But I agree that an international study into this is required.

Niizuma: We have found that the results with thalamic hematomas are not so good as in putaminal hematomas. This is due to both sensory and motor disturbances: Some patients show good motor function but sensory impairment leads to a poor outcome.

Ohtsuki (Sendai): I worked on the same project with Dr. Niizuma and we presented the results in another session. With thalamic hematomas of medium size (20–40 ml), the rehabilitation score at the end of rehabilitation was better in operated than in medically treated patients. With small hematomas, the results following surgery were not so good; with large hematomas, neither surgery nor medical treatment gave good results.

Auer: This would be exactly in keeping with the data I presented today, i.e., with hematomas of 20–50 ml the operative treatment is better.

Volpin (Vicenza): Some years ago, I presented some results which showed that volume of the hematoma is an indication of the prognosis. I found that when the volume of the supratentorial hematoma was less than 25 ml, the patients outcome was favorable and no surgical treatment was required; where the volume of the hematoma was greater than 80 ml, the prognosis was bad for both surgical and nonsurgical patients. For a hematoma volume of 25–80 ml, surgery may be of use in patients with a low level of consciousness—almost comatose.

Lee (Seoul): Though hematomas progressively decrease in Hounsfield number and size on follow-up CT scanning, do hematomas act toxically upon the surroundings when they stay longer in the brain?

Beneš: I think it is indeed toxic and this was also indicated in the book "Spontaneous Hematoma" by a Japanese author.

Matsumoto: We have conducted experiments in which we inserted a hematoma into a dog brain and it was toxic in terms of histological changes.

Lee: Do you think the toxic effect comes from changes in the chemical components?

Matsumoto: I do not know, but signs such as thicker granulation are seen. If evacuation is carried out earlier the reactive tissues are very thin.

Auer: Elevated intracranial pressure or compartmental pressure has been measured in a very small number of patients and it has been shown that the pressure of the tissue surrounding the hematoma is higher than the intracranial pressure in the rest of the cavity; so a compartmental pressure distribution is present.

Pan (Taipei): I started using stereotactic surgery to evacuate hematomas 3 years ago. The indication for surgery I use is a deep-seated hematoma bigger than 30 ml threatening the life of the patient. I only select patients where the deep-seated hematoma is in the basal ganglia or putaminal region. I have only a small series of 18 patients, of whom only one died; the others recovered satisfactorily. I had three cases of rebleeding, where I had to reoperate by craniotomy. It is my impression the improvement in consciousness and motor function is better with this procedure than with conventional craniotomy. I use a modified version of Backlund's design with the Archimedes screw, but I never use urokinase. So I would like to ask the panel about the urokinase dosage: How much do you give and at what time intervals?

Niizuma: 6000 units.

Itakura: 6000 units in 5–10 ml saline twice a day.

Matsumoto: I use the same.

Kanno: We have checked changes in the neurotransmitter at the marginal zone of the hematoma in experiments in dogs. The neurotransmitter decreased very rapidly, due I think to the toxicity of the clot. The hematoma clot itself therefore appears to have toxicity. My second comment concerns the reason why the surgical indication for putaminal hemorrhage is still controversial; it is due to the kind of method used to compare medically and surgically treated groups. The method differs among neurosurgeons. If the two groups are compared in terms of daily living, surgery of some types of hematoma is indicated. But if the groups are compared in terms of damage to higher brain functions, such as social adjustment, intellectual ability, verbal activity, no difference in outcome can be seen. If each case is assessed by evoked potential during operation, most operated cases showed good improvement. So even using the same material, different conclusions can be arrived at according to the method of comparison.

Raja (Multan): We assess these patients in terms of the clinical condition, the size of the hematoma, and whether the mass effect is present. If the patient is alert and the clinical condition is good even if the total hematoma is 20–25 ml and there is very little mass effect, perhaps 1–2 mm, we treat the patients conservatively. Obviously we use CT to see whether the clot size is increasing or not, but this has to be correlated with the clinical condition of the patient. In cases of massive, deep-seated bleeding of grades 4 or 5, we are not really sure whether operative treatment has the edge over nonoperative treatment. However, at times we come under pressure from, say, the patients' relatives who feel we ought to operate; I am not sure though that results following operation are any better than those after medical treatment.

Beneš: I think following this discussion it is clear that first of all we need to unify the nomenclature and definitions before the next randomized study.

Auer: To date we know that it is useful to operate on a certain number of patients with subcortical hematomas; this is evident both from personal experience and statistical results. However, regarding thalamic and putaminal hemorrhages, we are awaiting definite indications and criteria. The point to be settled here is whether our aim is a higher rate of survival or a better quality of survival; with respect to the indications, these are two completely different goals. This needs to be settled by a large multicenter controlled trial.

RTD 11. Surgical Treatment for Deep-Seated or Large AVMs

Management of Deep-Seated Cerebral AVMs
Report on 28 Cases

Madjid Samii and Walter Bini[1]

Introduction

Cerebrovascular malformations may be present anywhere in the cranial cavity [6]. Even though the advances in surgical techniques and instrumentation, along with better anesthesia characteristic of the progress in the last decade, have improved the general results of surgery of vascular malformations, the surgical treatment for deep-seated angiomas, as well as for extensive cortical lesions, remains a challenge to neurosurgeons [1–3, 9, 16, 18–20]. This type of pathology is, therefore, a primary topic in modern day neurological surgery.

The existence of these malformations has been known for over a century and still there exists discussion on such fundamental questions or aspects as classification, pathogenesis, and natural history. The therapeutic strategy has also originated diverse opinions [2, 7, 9–11, 18, 21–25].

We report on our experience in the surgical treatment of deep-seated AVMs, with consideration of the 28 cases operated in our clinic during the past 8 years.

The general policy has been to carry out operations in AVMs which had had an episode of bleeding, to prevent further hemorrhage. In other cases, surgery was indicated in view of advancing neurological symptomatology, and, in one case, because of intractable headaches (Table 1). The age, general health status, and site and size of the AVM were taken into account.

Clinical Material and Method

From January 1978 until December 1986, 28 patients with deep-seated AVMs were admitted, studied, and surgically treated in our clinic. In

Tables 1 and 2 is the summary of the clinical presentation and findings, as well as localization (postdiagnosis) and age distribution. The most common mode of presentation in our series, as in the other major series reported (14, 16–18, 21), was intracranial bleeding, which occurred in 18 cases (64.3%). Nine cases (32.1%) were located in the brain stem and another nine cases (32.1%) in the lateral ventricle. Of our patients, 17 (60.7%) were between the ages of 10–30 years. The diagnostic routine included CT, four-vessel angiographies, and, with increasing frequency, magnetic resonance imaging (MRI). By means of MRI, we acquired important data towards planning the surgical approach, for it delimits, as no other method, the area of functional brain tissue surrounding the angioma, as no functional tissue is present in the malformation itself.

The indication for operation was made in every case by considering the clinical presentation with the neurological status, age general condition, and the site and extent of the lesion. General indications include repeated subarachnoid hemorrhage (SAH), intracerebral hematoma, progressive neurological disability (i.e., uncontrollable seizures), AVM in a favorable localization (asymptomatic), AVM in functionally important regions with SAH, and repeated SAH without angiographical proof of AVM. The alternative methods reported for treatment of these vascular lesions in most cases fail to obliterate the lesions completely, the limiting factors being the size, number of feeders, and location. Even with embolization with bucrylate, a complete "wipe-out" rate is achieved only in 9% of the cases, and a size reduction in 50%–75%. The other method which can achieve good results is the Bragg proton beam therapy [7]. Using stereotactic means, a high success rate of AVM obliteration has been obtained in cases of small malformations whose radius measures 25 mm [22, 23]. Nevertheless, a long-term follow-up is necessary.

In establishing our indication for surgery, we

[1] Neurosurgical Clinic, Nordstadt Hospital, Hannover, Federal Republic of Germany

Table 1. Clinical presentation and symptomatology in 28 cases of deep-seated AVMs

Clinical presentation		Symptomatology	
Intracranial bleeding	18	Hemiparesis	12
First bleeding	11	Psychosyndrome	5
Num. bleedings	7	"Steal" phenomenon	4
Intractable headaches	1	Headaches	7
Progressive neurological disability	9	Cranial nerve palsy	6
		Seizures	3
		Aphasia	1
		Decreased visual acuity	2
		Decreased concentration	1

were confronted with the controversial and still obscure natural history of these lesions. According to the literature, and the three major series [4, 14, 17], angiomas generally present a risk of bleeding of 47% in 20 years if they have bled before, and of 39% during the same time span without previous bleeding. The mortality increases with the number of hemorrhages (recurrences). It is about 10% after the first bleeding, 13% after the second, and 20% after the third episode [4, 14, 17].

The overall morbidity caused by hemorrhage from deep-seated AVMs is not known: some authors report a mortality of 100% in these cases in which the hemorrhage extends to the ventricular system [2].

The only method of avoiding hemorrhage is a complete microsurgical excision of the angioma by direct approach. Therefore, there is justification for surgery in order to influence the natural history of this pathology. Surgery is also indicated when the symptoms and neurological deficits progress and, of course, we agree that direct surgery is the only acceptable strategy in AVMs which occupy space and create severe blood shunting or increased intracranial pressure.

The problem lies in the large angiomas which might need a staged operation and, therefore, the risk of hemorrhage or iatrogenic neurological deficits increases. All these factors influenced us to operate on our 28 patients.

Surgical Strategy

The operative technique is based on the microsurgical techniques and the standard procedures of brain relaxation. A controlled hypotension of 70–80 mm systolic is advisable, but we didn't use severe hypotension in any of our cases. Bipolar cautery is indispensable, and our strategy is the

Table 2. Localization and age in 28 cases of deep-seated AVMs

Localization	No. of cases
Corpus callosum	1
Thalamus	2
Lateral ventricle	9
Pineal region	2
Brain stem	9
CPA	1
IV ventricle	3
III ventricle	1

Age	No. of cases
less than 10 years	1
10–30 years	17
31–50 years	8
over 50 years	2

CPA cerebello-pontine angle

step by step resection removing the malformation as a tumor, due to the presence of a pseudocapsule. We prefer to preserve the major cerebral arteries and draining veins until the end of the surgical procedure. The total removal of the angioma should be the aim. Special attention should be given to the angioma bed and to the bleeding which might come from the area. Small angiomatous vessels in the periphery are responsible and should be coagulated. In two of our cases, the Nd: YAG laser was used during parts of the operation. Preliminary advantages can be seen using a defocused mode on these small pathological rest vessels. The surgical approaches used in our series are listed in Table 3. Here one must point out that the patient operated by subfrontal approach was diagnosed preoperatively as having a craniopharyngioma, our only case of preoperative false diagnosis (3.6%).

Table 3. Deep-seated AVMs: Surgical approaches (n = 28)

Approach	No. of cases
Cortical/transventricular	11
Transcallosal	2
Subtemporal	5
Suboccipital supra/infratentorial	4
Infratentorial (IV ventricle)	5
Subfrontal	1

Results and Discussion

In our series, we obtained good results (were able to return to a normal social and, in great part, professional life) in 23 cases (82.1%). In five patients, the results can be considered as fair, for the preexisting neurological deficits were accentuated postoperatively. Two of these patients became disabled and needed help in their daily lives, and one died suddenly 3 weeks after successful removal of a large angioma with brain stem extension and good postoperative neurological status, due to a massive pulmonary embolism. Total removal was achieved in 24 cases. Partial removal was a compromise in four AVMs, due to size and location. These patients have done well in the follow-up and have not experienced added neurological deficits (Tables 4–7).

Operative mortality was 0%, and no case of rebleeding was observed. The overall morbidity due to the operation was 46.4%. In 60.7%, no complications resulted from the surgical treatment.

Conclusion

It is important to differentiate between cerebral AVMs which might be located in the cerebral convexities and the deep-seated malformations. Their natural history, even though somewhat similar, differs as far as degree of severity. One fact supports this observation; the morbidity and mortality associated with the first hemorrhage of the deep-seated malformations ranges between 80% and 90%.

The deep-seated AVMs are, in essence, the last of the intracranial malformations to be managed successfully by surgeons, even though the first one to be removed was in 1932. Since the revolution occurred after the introduction of microsur-

Table 4. Operative results of 28 cases of deep-seated AVMs

Operative results	No. of cases
Good	23
Fair	5[a]

[a] Of the fair group, one patient died of a nonsurgical cause

Table 5. Postoperative angiography in 28 cases of deep-seated AVMs

Postoperative angiography	No. of cases
Total removal	24
Partial removal	4

Table 6. Complications in 28 cases of deep-seated AVMs

Complications	No. of cases
Transient aphasia	2
Hemiparesis (transient)	5 (1)
Seizures	1
Hemianopsia	2
Cranial nerve palsy	1
Pulmonary embolism	1
No complications	17
Recurrent bleeding	0

Table 7. Postoperative results in 28 cases of deep-seated AVMs

Result	Percent
Operative mortality	0
Operative morbidity	46.4
Recurrent bleeding	0
Total removal	85.7
Total results	
Good	82.1
Fair	17.9

gical techniques, there is now hope for these dangerous lesions, which are literally time bombs. The acceptable rate of morbidity/mortality is also reported by others [3, 12, 16, 26]. In experienced hands and with modern day instrumentation, surgery seems to be the ideal treatment for deep-seated malformations. The passive approach leaves the patient with the risk of a recurrence and fatal hemorrhage. Embolization techniques are hazardous. Reported experiences are still too few [8, 10, 11, 20], and some attempts have had fatal consequences [5]. The lesions tend to be too distal and most of the arterial supply (90%) comes from channels that originate from the basilar and vertebral arteries. Radiation may be effective in small angiomas, but sometimes it leaves the patient exposed to bleeding in the time between treatment and obliteration, and the effect on nearby tissue (radionecrosis) is still in discussion. Our results have shown that, with a complete preoperative diagnostic preparation, which should include analysing size, feeders, general condition, and possible approaches, and by means of microsurgical techniques, results can be positive in as many as 82.1% of the patients, with total removal of these lesions, which are often still considered inoperable, in 85.7% of the cases.

In these closing remarks, one must highlight three aspects. First of all, MRI has added a new dimension to the diagnosis as well as operative concept in relation to cerebral angiomas. With this method, we acquire important data to support what we have observed with the microscope, which is that there is no functional tissue inside the angioma or a pseudocapsule around the nidus due, in part, to micro- or macrohemorrhages, and to shunting, delimiting the area of lesion. The law of supply and demand is also valid here. The AVM is a network of tangled arteries, veins, and capillaries, even though these latter ones are not actually represented and, therefore, no O_2 is used for brain tissue exchange. The brain tissue around this area will be replaced by gliosis. This allows us to remove these lesions like tumors, and, if one remains in the angioma, no added neurological deficit will result from the operation.

Therefore, it is our opinion that the decisive factors for deep-seated AVM surgery are the size and location but, more fundamentally, the way or approach necessary to reach these lesions and the intrinsic vascular supply which, in areas such as the brain stem, is highly complex, vital, and selective.

Even though selective catheterization, flow-directed microcatheters, and intraoperative techniques might improve in the near future, the controversy regarding the hemodynamic principles of AVMs is still to be solved [5, 13, 15]. The significance of each individual feeding vessel is not fully unmasked, and a more functional angiography is necessary to reveal the actual dynamic relationships of each vessel to the angioma and to the nearby tissue. Of our four partial removals, two were known and were a compromise due to size, but the two other cases were revealed later by means of a control study. This clearly shows the advantage and indication of intraoperative angiography, especially when dealing with angiomas in delicate regions.

The best therapeutic attitude for handling AVMs in deep-seated areas is the direct surgical and radical removal of the lesion, if possible.

References

1. Batjer H, Samson D (1986) Arteriovenous malformations of the posterior fossa. J Neurosurg 64:849–856
2. Davis C, Symon L (1985) The management of cerebral AVM's. Acta Neurochirurgica 74:4–11
3. Drake CG, Friedman AH, Peerless SJ (1986) Posterior fossa AVM's. J Neurosurg 64:1–10
4. Forster DMC, Steiner L, Hakanson S (1972) Arteriovenous malformations of the brain. A long term clinical study. J Neurosurg 37:562
5. Fox JL, Al Mefty O (1977) Embolization of an AVM of the brain stem. Surg Neurol 8:79
6. Kaplan HA, Aronson SM, Browder EJ (1961) Vascular malformations of the brain. An anatomical study. Harvey Cushing Society Meeting (Presentation)
7. Kjellberg RN, Poletti CE, Robertson GH, Adams DA (1978) Bragg peak proton beam treatment of AVM's of the brain. In: Carrea R (ed), Neurological surgery. Proceedings of the 6th International Congress of Neurological Surgery, Sao Paulo, 19–25 June 1977. Excerpta Medica, Amsterdam, pp 181–187
8. Kricheff II, Maydayag M, Braunstein P (1972) Transfemoral catheter embolization of cerebral and posterior fossa AVM's. Radiology 103:107
9. Kunc Z (1972) Surgery of AVM's in speech and motor sensory regions. J Neurosurg 103:107–111
10. Luessenhop AJ (1975) Artificial embolization of inoperable AVM's. In: Pia HW, Glaeve JRW, Grote G, Zierski J (eds) Cerebral angiomas: Advances in diagnosis and therapy. Springer, Heidelberg, pp 198–205
11. Luessenhop AJ, Presper J (1975) Surgical embolization of cerebral AVM's through internal, carotid and vertebral studies: Long term results. J Neurosurg 42:443
12. Martin NA, Stein BM, Wilson CB (1984) Arteriovenous malformations of the posterior fossa. In: Wilson CB, Stein BM (eds) Intracranial arteriovenous malformations Williams and Wilkins, Baltimore pp 209–221
13. Mullan S, Brown FD, Patronas NJ (1979) Hyperemic and ischemic problems of surgical treatment of AVM's. J Neurosurg 51:757–764
14. Nibbelink DW (1975) Cooperative aneurysm study in cerebral vascular disease. Ninth confer-

ence. In: Whismant JP, Sandok BA (eds) Grune and Stratton, pp 155–165

15. Nornes H, Grip A (1980) Hemodynamic aspects of cerebral AVM's. J Neurosurg 53:456–464

16. Parkinson D, Bachers G (1980) Arteriovenous malformations. J Neurosurg 53:285–299

17. Perret C, Nishicka H (1983) Report on the cooperative study of intracranial aneurysms and SAH. AVMs in analysis of 545 cases of cranio-cerebral AVMs and fistulae reported to the Coop Study. J Neurosurg 25:467–490

18. Pertuiset B, et al. (1983) Radical surgery in cerebral AVM's. In: Advances and technical standards in neurosurgery, vol 10. Springer, Heidelberg, pp 81–143

19. Ramina R, Samii M (1983) Operative Behandlung von tiefliegenden Angiomen mit Eindringen in das Ventrikel-System. Arbeitstagung Mikrochirurgie Hamburg

20. Sano K, Jimbo M, Saito I, et al. (1973) Artificial embolization of inoperable angioma with polymerizing substance. In: Pia HW (ed) Cerebral angioma. Springer, New York, pp 222

21. Solomon RA, Stein BM (1986) Management of arteriovenous malformations of the brain stem. J Neurosurg 64:857–864

22. Steiner L, Leksell L, Forster DMC (1974) Stereotactic radiosurgery in intracranial AVM's. Acta Neurochir (Suppl) 21:196–209

23. Steiner L (1984) Treatment of AVM by radiosurgery. In: Wilson CB, Stein BM (eds) Intracranial arteriovenous malformations. Williams and Wilkins, Baltimore pp 295–311

24. Veerapen RJ, et al. (1986) Surgical treatment of cryptic AVM's and associated hematoma in the brain stem and spinal cord. J Neurosurg 65:188–193

25. Wilson C, Hoi Sang U, Dominique J (1979) Microsurgical treatment of intracranial vascular malformations. J Neurosurg 51:446–454

26. Yaşargil MG, Jain KK, Antic J, et al. (1976) Arteriovenous malformations of the anterior and middle portion of the corpus callosum: Microsurgical treatment. Surg Neurol 5:5, 67

Surgical Treatment for Deep-Seated or Large AVMs

Alfred J. Luessenhop[1]

Introduction

Excluding patients with primarily dural or intra-orbital arteriovenous malformations (AVMs), our experience over the past 25 years includes approximately 480 patients with AVMs, primarily in the brain. The size distribution of these is approximately as follows: 50% were 3 cm or less, 20% were 4 cm, 15% were 5 cm, 10% were 6 cm, and 5% were greater than 6 cm. This distribution is probably tilted toward larger AVMs because many of our patients were referred when their lesions was considered not amenable to surgical excision.

From our cases and the literature, the age incidence of a first symptom, hence probable diagnosis, indicates that the cerebral AVMs become progressively symptomatic during the second decade of life and, after the third decade, at least 80% will have been diagnosed. However, approximately 10% will escape diagnosis until the sixth decade of life (Fig. 1). With present imaging techniques, it can be anticipated that a larger number will be found incidentally even earlier in life.

The most accurate assessment of the spontaneous bleeding rate is 2%–3% per year with an increase to 6% during the first year following a clinically evident hemorrhage [1]. Each clinically evident hemorrhage carries approximately a 10% mortality and 30% morbidity. The likelihood of spontaneous bleeding for any single patient relates to the remaining years of risk exposure (Figs. 2,3) [4]. This is an important consideration when selecting patients for surgery after the sixth decade of life.

Progressive neurological deficit, not obviously related to bleeding, is more common with large AVMs in critical locations. The deficit steadily progresses over many years, with occasional pro-longed intervals of stabilization. In general, however, the prediction of deficit progression is not perfectly reliable [5].

Small But Deeply Seated AVMs

I would place AVMs approximately 3 cm or less in diameter in this category. Unless critically located, AVMs of the this size are not likely to produce a significant neurological deficit, and the treatment consideration is primarily for prevention of spontaneous bleeding. Our experience to date suggests that most of these are suitable for surgical obliteration which should be carried out with a mortality and morbidity very close to zero [2, 4].

The breaking-off point between large and small AVMs is whether or not the AVM can be obliterated primarily by bipolar coagulation in situ with induced hypertension. When situated deep within a cerebral hemisphere, the approach is through a sulcus following the feeding arteries and draining veins (Figs. 4–6). Those primarily on the medial surface of the hemisphere can be approached by retraction of the hemisphere and

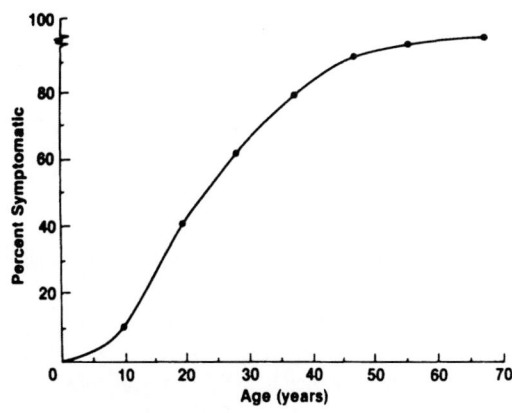

Fig. 1. Estimated rate of first appearance of symptoms with cerebral AVMs

[1] Georgetown University Hospital, Washington, DC, USA

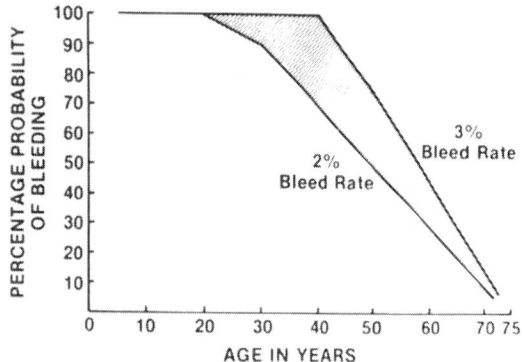

Fig. 2. Probability of bleeding v. age in cases of cerebral AVMs

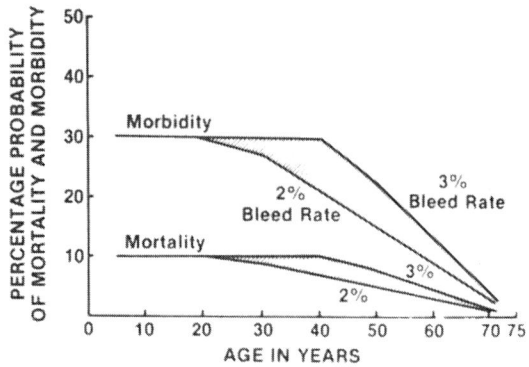

Fig. 3. Probability of mortality and morbidity V. age in cases of cerebral AVMs

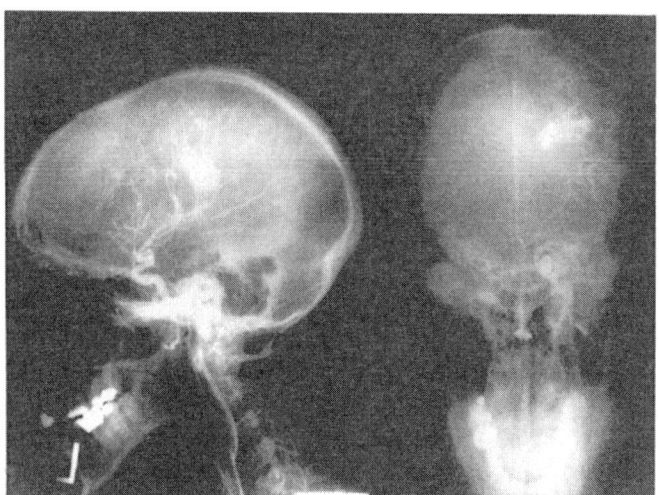

Fig. 4. A small AVM located deep in the middle of the left cerebral hemisphere

those within the walls of the lateral ventricles approached transcallosally (Figs. 7, 8). When the AVM is compact, surgical obliteration by the coagulation technique can be considered in areas adjacent to speech production or within the motor and sensory cortices. However, after the sixth decade of life, surgery is not always advisable by this technique because in the remaining projected years of life, the risk of mortality and morbidity from spontaneous hemorrhage rapidly declines (Fig. 3).

For us, the major pitfalls in dealing with these smaller AVMs have been incomplete obliteration requiring a second operation during the same hospitalization and postoperative bleeding within the cavity of the obliterated AVM. At present, we routinely perform CT studies on the 1st–3rd postoperative day. Many patients experience a transient neurological deficit of varying degree during the 1st postoperative week.

The Large Cerebral AVMs

We consider AVMs 4 cm or larger in diameter as belonging in this category. As a rule, these cannot be managed by in situ coagulation and require marginal or block resection. Even when primarily on a cortical surface, there is extension to the deeper hemispheric structures, including the internal capsule, basal ganglia, and thalamus, and participation of the deep penetrating arteries of the circle of Willis (Fig. 9) [2]. For a few AVMs primarily restricted to the cortex, total excision is usually possible by block or marginal resection and, when the lesion is very compact, damage or destruction of adjacent normal functional brain can be minimal (Figs. 10–12).

For the more common large AVM in the combined territories of deep penetrating arteries and surface arteries, total excision is only occasionally possible. In a few who have accumulated a

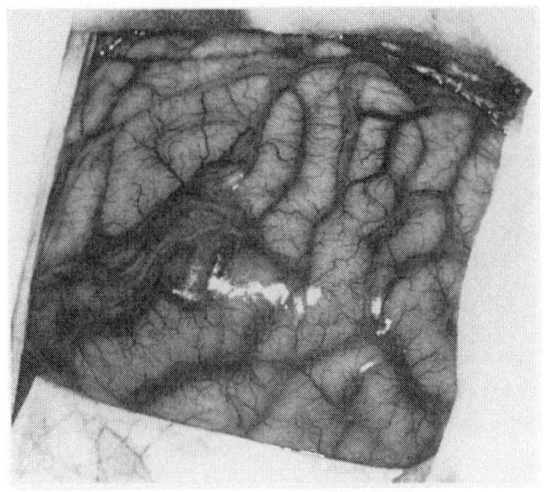

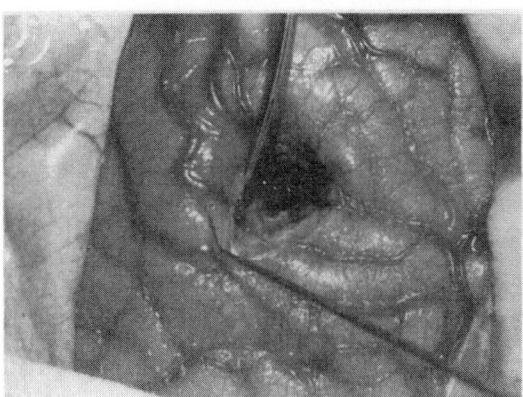

Fig. 6. The AVM of Fig. 2 is obliterated by bipolar coagulation *in situ* at the depth of the sulcus

Fig. 5. The cortical presentation of the AVM in Fig. 4 showing feeding arteries and draining veins passing into a cerebral sulcus

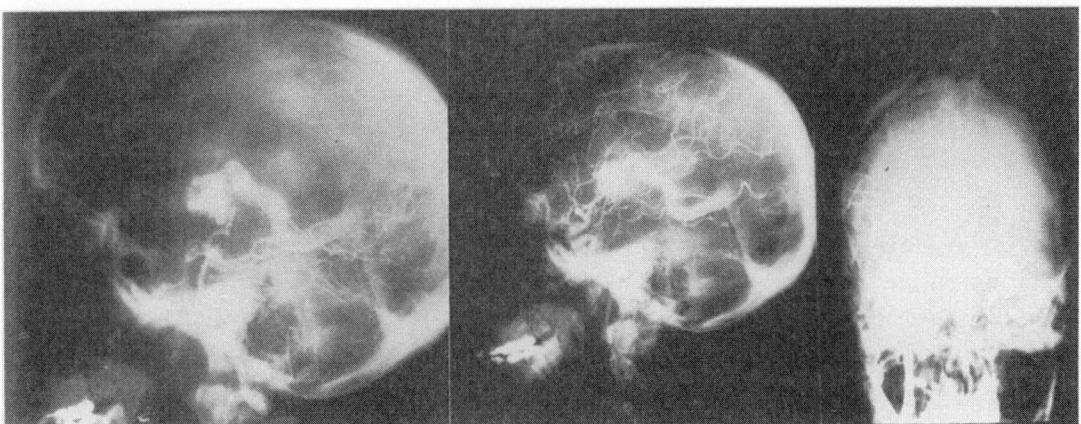

Fig. 7. An AVM in the wall and floor of a lateral ventricle

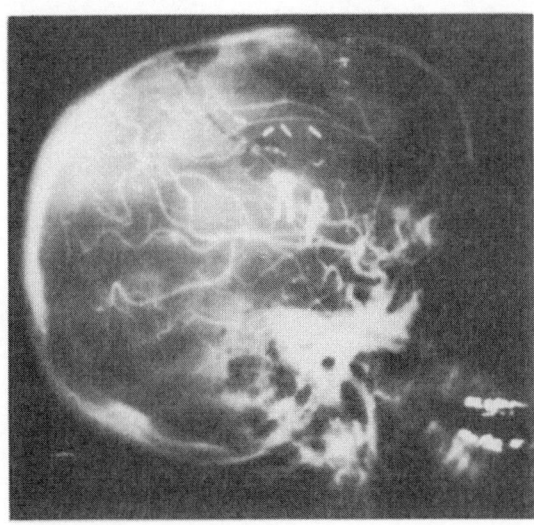

Fig. 8. A postoperative angiography following surgical obliteration by a transcallosal approach for the AVM of Fig. 7

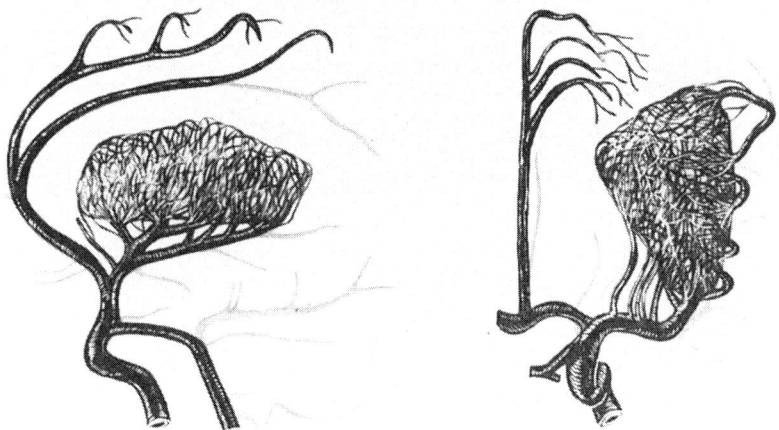

Fig. 9. A diagramatic representation of a large AVM showing the typical medial extension to incorporate contributions from the penetrating arteries arising from the middle cerebral artery trunk

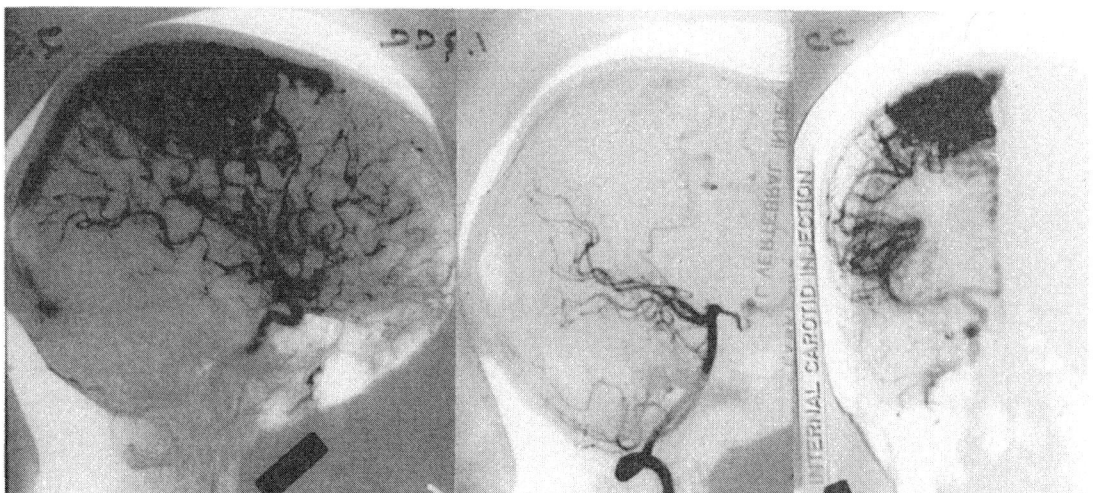

Fig. 10. A large AVM of the cortical surface with very little projection to the middle of the cerebral hemisphere and only a minor contribution from the deeper vasculature

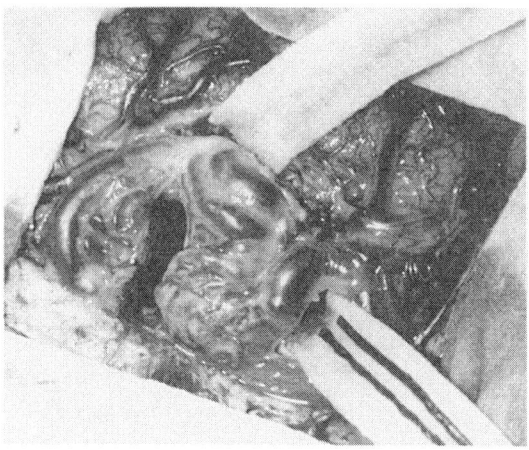

Fig. 11. Marginal resection of the AVM shown in Fig. 10

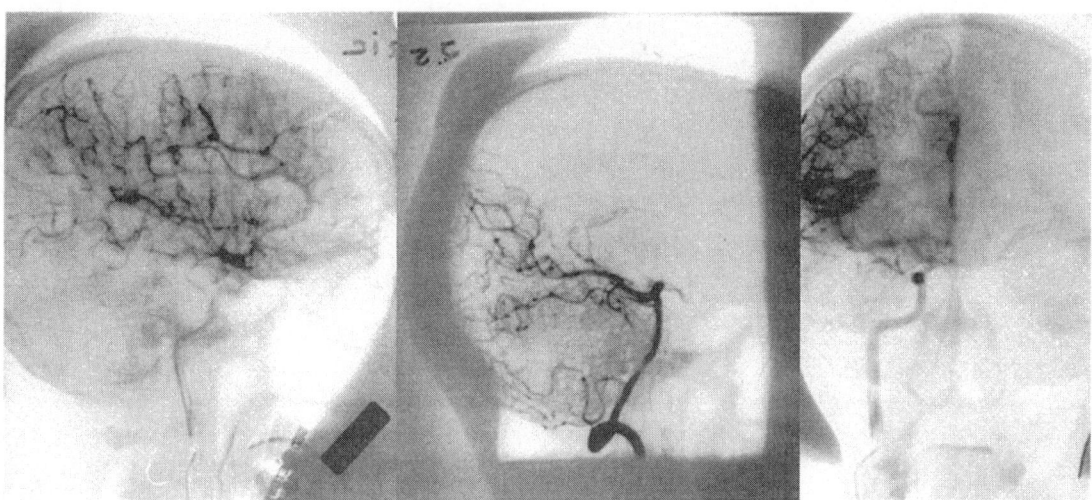

Fig. 12. Postoperative angiography of the AVM shown in Fig. 10

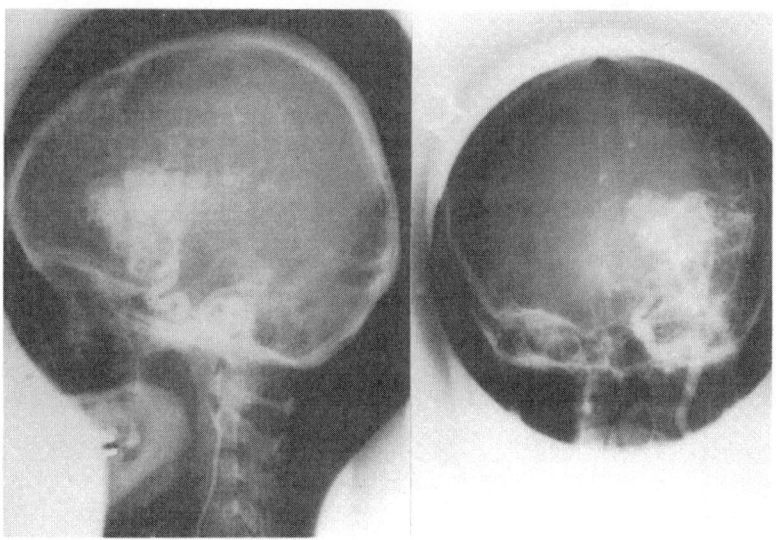

Fig. 13. A large AVM, primarily in the territories of the penetrating arteries at the base. A severe deficit had accumulated by prior hemorrhages

significant deficit, we have removed the lesions following embolization to obstruct the major feeding trunks (Figs. 13, 14). In others with less severe deficits, we have only occasionally achieved total eradication with both embolization and surgery (Figs. 15, 16). For the large AVMs primarily in the territory of the penetrating arteries, we have employed direct surgery only sparingly, to occlude selectively some of the major feeding arteries for example. For the most part, we have used embolization to selectively occlude the various arterial trunks, principally the middle cerebral. As we have shown, this will not necessarily produce an increased deficit in

these large lesions (Figs. 17–19) [3]. In our view, this does not reduce the threat of future bleeding, but there is some suggestion that this may abort or delay the progression of a neurological deficit.

Similar to the small AVMs, the pitfalls have been incomplete removal by follow-up angiography and recurrent hemorrhage in the immediate postoperative period. We do not regard circulatory breakthrough as a significant problem. This is most apt to occur in lesions with large shunts and for these we use preliminary embolization, staging, and continuation of controlled hypertension during the first 4–6 days postoperatively.

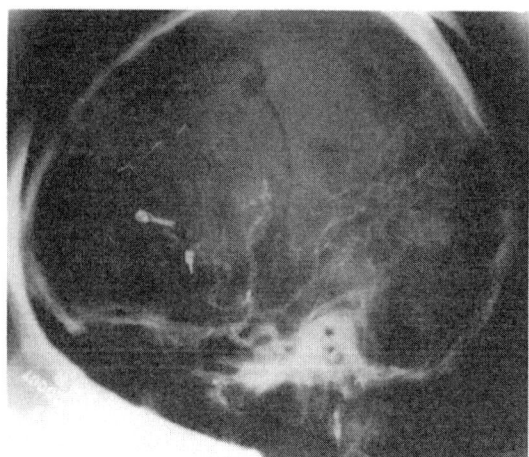

Fig. 14. Postoperative angiography of the AVM shown in Fig. 13 following presurgical embolization and staged surgical removal. There was no increase in the preexisting neurological deficit

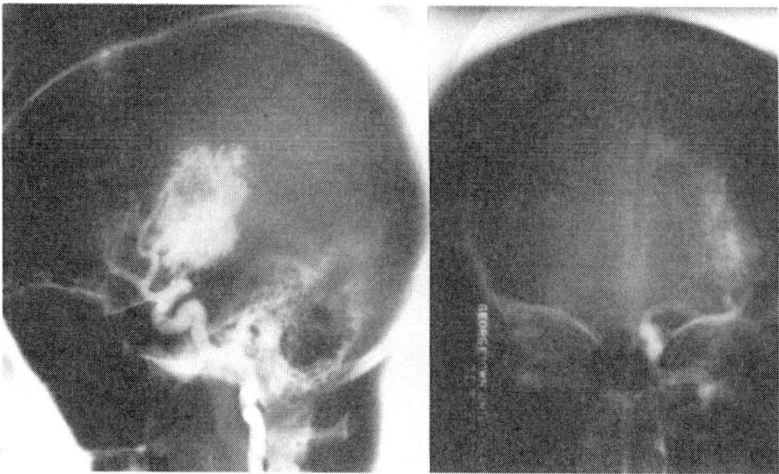

Fig. 15. A large AVM, principally in the territories of the surface sylvian arteries and the penetrating vessels from the middle cerebral trunk. A minor deficit had accumulated

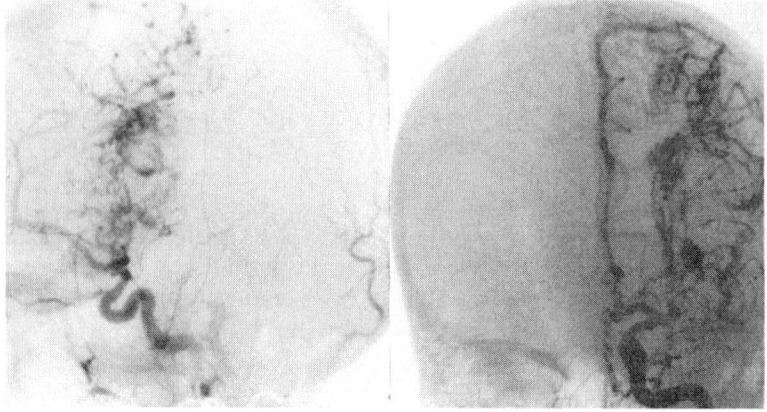

Fig. 16. Postoperative angiography of the AVM in Fig. 15 showing residual portions of the AVM deep within the cerebral hemisphere

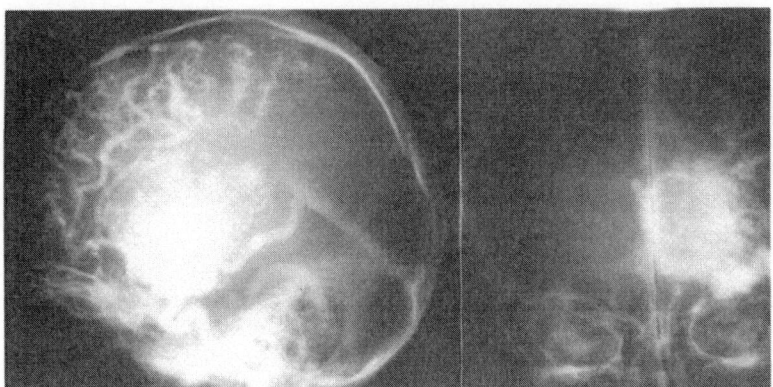

Fig. 17. A large AVM solely within the territories of the penetrating arteries from the circle of Willis. The patient had accumulated a moderate hemiparesis and had intractable seizures

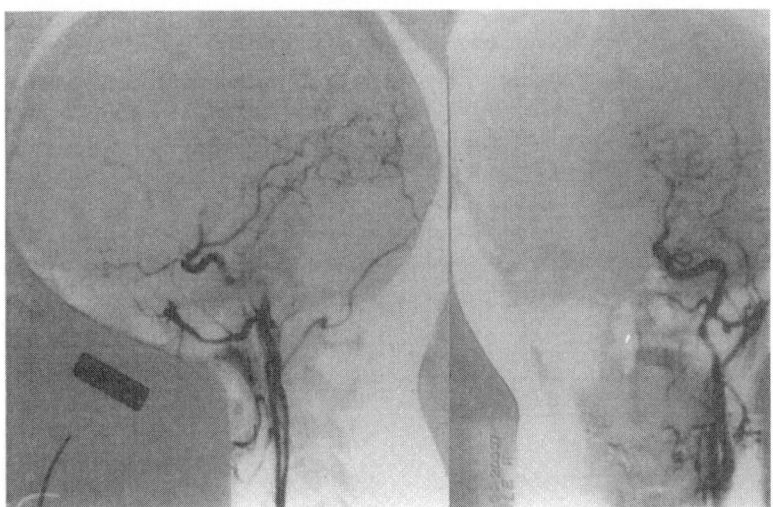

Fig. 18. Postembolization angiography of the AVM shown in Fig. 17. The middle cerebral trunk was obstructed without altering the preexisting neurological deficit

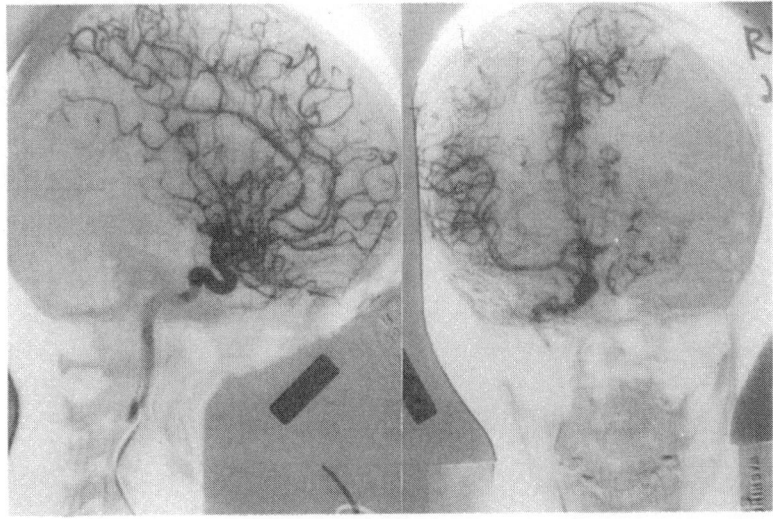

Fig. 19. Postoperative angiography from the opposite side of the AVM shown in Fig. 17. The A-1 segment had been clipped to prevent cross-filling of the residual AVM

Conclusions

At the present stage of our technical development, at least 60%, and perhaps 70%, of all cerebral AVMs, when first diagnosed, are amenable to surgical excision with the anticipation that the mortality and morbidity will be better than natural history, particularly for patients under the age of 50 years. Nearly all of the smaller lesions, irrespective of location, are candidates for surgical removal. Intravascular technique may curtail progression of a neurological deficit in large lesions not within the surgical realm. Whether or not combinations of surgery and intravascular techniques will curtail the progression of the large lesion solely within territories of the penetrating arteries is uncertain at present.

References

1. Graf CJ, Perret GE, Torner JC (1983) Bleeding from cerebral arteriovenous malformations as part of their natural history. J Neurosurg 58:331–337
2. Luessenhop AJ, Gennarelli TA (1977) Anatomical grading of supratentorial arteriovenous malformations for determining operability. Neurosurgery 1 (1): 30–36
3. Luessenhop AJ, Mujica FH (1981) Embolization of segments of the circle of Willis and adjacent branches for management of certain inoperable cerebral arteriovenous malformations. Neurosurg 54:573–582
4. Luessenhop AJ, Rosa L (1984) Cerebral arteriovenous malformation, indications for and results of surgery and the role of intravascular techniques. J Neurosurg 60:14–22
5. Luessenhop AJ, (1984) Natural history of cerebral arteriovenous malformation. In: Wilson CB, Stein BM (eds) Current neurosurgical practice. William and Wilkins, Baltimore, pp 12–23

Radical Open Surgery of Supra-Tentorial Arteriovenous Malformations
Series of 268 Cases

Bernard Pertuiset[1], Daniel Ancri[2], François Arthuis[1], and Siddiq Ahmed Siddiqui[3]

Nowadays radical excision of an arteriovenous malformation (AVM) is the unique procedure which is able to remove the lesion totally, giving the patient a final cure. It must be stressed that a remaining 10% of the lesion is sufficient to severely impair the future of the patient.

It is not an easy surgery; it can be a dangerous surgery. There are cases which cannot be operated upon because the AVM is too large, the patient is too old, or there are associated diseases. Fortunately, the CT scanner has allowed discovery of more and more AVMs in young patients after one or two seizures. In these cases it is very gratifying to see surgery give the patient a new start in life.

Evidently, the aim of the neurosurgeon is to cure his patient without mortality and morbidity. For this purpose, starting our clinical research in 1976, we have classified, according to anatomical and hemodynamic factors [11, 12], the AVM on which the radical excision looked possible. All technical procedures described in this paper are in this classification.

Classification for Surgery

Volume of the AVM

The volume can be evaluated from the lateral and AP views of the angiogram. More recently, the volume has been estimated from a rotating gamma camera using red cells tagged with Tech 99, as well as from a magnetic resonance imaging (MRI) investigation. AVMs have been divided into three groups:

Group A volumes over 40 cm^3. In our series are cases with volumes from 40 cm^3 to 100 cm^3

Group B volumes between 20 and 40 cm^3

Group C volumes under 20 cm^3

These groups have been determined from experience.

Feeders of the AVM

We discovered that the knowledge of the number of feeders entering the lesion was not very useful. It was more important to know the degree of participation of both internal carotid arteries and the basilar system from selective angiograms.

In group A AVMs, there is always more than one of the big arteries participating in the vascularization. Either both carotid systems, one carotid artery and the basilar artery, or all three systems participate. In group B AVMs, usually no more than two systems are implicated: either both carotid arteries or one carotid artery and the basilar artery. In group C AVMs, only one system is feeding the AVM.

There is, of course, a relation between the number of big feeders and the location of the AVM. For instance, an AVM of the parietal lobe will be vascularized by the homolateral carotid artery and, usually, the basilar artery. In addition, the contralateral carotid artery can participate via the pericallosal artery.

In one case of our series of 268 AVMs, the external carotid system was seriously participating. Usually small feeders coming from the dura do not represent a challenge to the surgeon.

Relation with the Lateral Ventricle

This is very well known since we are using the CT scanner with an i.v. contrast media.

It is very seldom that an AVM does not extend to the ventricle wall, where there is always a pedicle with arteries and draining red veins. It must be stressed that the surgeon must find this pedicle during operation; otherwise, a postoperative hematoma can develop and eventually kill the patient.

[1] Clinique Neuro-Chirurgicale de la Pitié, Paris, France
[2] Service de Biophysique et de Médecine Nucléaire, La Pitié, Paris, France
[3] University UTESA of Santo Domingo, Dominican Republic

Small Feeders Around the AVM

We do not know of an investigation which is able to evidence all small arteries entering the nidus, in which lies the high velocity shunt.

We know from experience that these small arteries exist and can challenge the tenacity and patience of the most skilled surgeon. They can provoke a profuse bleeding when the hemodynamic factors have not been investigated prior to surgery, leading to the most appropriate surgical tactic.

Hemodynamic Factors

Two of these factors have to be investigated prior to surgery: the blood flow passing through the shunt and the capacity of the brain arteries to evacuate the surplus of blood once the shunt has been excised.

Blood Flow in AVM

Until now, a method does not exist which is able to measure the quantity of blood passing through the AVM per minute.

We have approached the flow by recording the velocity of the red cells in both internal carotid arteries and in both vertebral arteries using a pulsed Doppler Mark 500 of ATL (Advanced Technology Laboratory-Seattle).

In order to take into account the systolic as well as the diastolic velocity, Ancri has established a diastolic rate [1]:

$$D.R. = \frac{(DV)^2}{SV} = cm/sec$$

We have been lucky enough to demonstrate that when a carotid system is excluded from feeding the AVM, after clipping the anterior communicating artery, for instance, the diastolic rate which was over 20 cm/s goes down to 10 cm/s or less. The same is true when comparing the values of the diastolic rate before and after radical excision of the AVM (Tables 1, 2). Therefore, the surgeon, from this investigation, can evaluate the risk of a profuse bleeding and take the appropriate technical measures to reduce the flow before approaching the lesion.

We know that, in normal individuals, the diastolic rate into the internal carotid artery must be under 15 cm/s. Between 15 cm/s and 20 cm/s, the values are under discussion. Over 20 cm/s, the flow velocity is abnormal. Regarding the vertebral arteries, figures vary from one individual to

the other and from one side to the other.

Nevertheless, when the basilar system is implicated, as in the ampula of Galen AVMs, the values of the flow velocity in the vertebral arteries can go up to 70 cm/s, as we observed in two children.

There is a close relationship between the level of the flow velocity and the volume of the AVM as stated previously.

Capacity for Autoregulation of the Brain Arteries

As it has been shown in 1909 by Bayliss on the animal, brain arteries have the capacity to regulate their diameter maintening at a constant value the blood flow for protecting the brain. Thus the caliber of the arteries increases when occur an arterial hypotension [2].

Since 1976, we have demonstrated, during an episode of induced hypotension, that there was normally an increase of the blood volume recorded with a gamma camera after tagging the red cells with Tech 99 [9, 10]. In large AVMs, this capacity for autoregulation can disappear or there can be disorders of this autoregulation phenomenon. In other words, the blood which enters the brain after excision of the shunt can provoke a vascular brain swelling comparable to the breakthrough described in the animal by Spetzler et al. [13]. Therefore, there is a relationship between the volume, the flow, and the disorders of vascular autoregulation. Nevertheless, there are small AVMs with disorders of capacity for autoregulation and large AVMs with normal or instable ones.

We recommend clearly establishing these hemodynamic factors before advising surgery.

Postocclusive Effect

In 1980, Nornes and Grip [4] described a very important phenomenon. When a clip is placed on the main artery of an AVM, even of small size, there is an increase of 50% of the arterial pressure up to the clip. Then a small collateral can rupture in the ICU and provoke a fatal hematoma. This observation is consistent with the angiographic one by Norlen [3]. After operation, the arteries which were feeding the AVM increase their caliber for about 1 week.

This postocclusive effect will not represent a danger if a temporary clamp is placed on the common carotid artery in the neck, reducing its caliber and, therefore, the flow during the first 24 h after surgery.

Table 1. Diastolic rate $\left(\dfrac{DV^2}{SV}\right)$ in both internal carotid arteries before and after clipping of the anterior communicating artery in cerebral AVMs ($n = 16$)

	AVM side	Opposite side
Before clipping	30.25 ± 8.84	19.6 ± 5.42
After clipping	34.59 ± 8.01	10.42 ± 4.35

Values are means $\pm$ SD

Table 2. Diastolic rate $\left(\dfrac{DV^2}{SV}\right)$ in the internal carotid artery before and after radical surgery in cerebral AVMs ($n = 22$)

	AVM side	Opposite side
Before surgery	25.41 ± 11.27	15.56 ± 7.34
After surgery	9.60 ± 6	8.93 ± 3.62

Values are means $\pm$ SD

General Principles for Surgery

Patients must be psychologically prepared for surgery. It is absolutely necessary to obtain a trustful cooperation and advise the patient that, for instance, he or she will keep the tracheal tubing for 24 h.

Anaesthesiology

The general anaesthesia will be a neuroleptanalgesia with a permanent recording of the pulmonary pressure, by a Swan Gantz tubing, and of the mean arterial pressure.

The operation will be performed at a mean arterial pressure (MAP) of 50 mmHg, which can only be obtained by neuroleptanalgesia [7–9]. There are cases in which it is necessary to use a permanent infusion of sodium nitroprusside.

After losing a patient from an air embolism, we have adopted an anti-gravity inflated suit. Since then we have not recorded air in the pulmonary artery.

When a vascular brain swelling begins, the patient is given penthotal. When this drug is given at the beginning of the swelling, the effect is striking.

We want to emphasize the importance of the anaesthetist, who must be dispassionate, like the surgeon, and give the necessary information, no more.

It is better to elevate the head of the patient above the level of the table.

After closure at a MAP of 100 mmHg of the wound, the patient will remain on the operating table, anaesthetized, for 3 h without manipulating him with a normal MAP.

If, after this period, the patient is well, he will be taken to the ICU where he will remain intubated for 24 h. Since we have adopted this policy, we have stopped the occurence of acute intracranial hematomas.

Technical Facilities

In the operating room, there must be two machines for suction and two coagulators, because this is the type of operation which cannot be interrupted by failure of a facility. It is absolutely necessary to be able to use an operating microscope, which will enable the surgeon to complete a difficult hemostasis or to remove a deep-seated AVM.

Self-retaining retractors are absolutely necessary, and we advise using those which are placed on the operating table to avoid epidural hematomas. We have made striking progress since we began using string clips, especially for closure of the small arteries. We use only Aesculap phynox clips and, recently, the Caspar forceps, which we consider the best.

These operations can last a long time: therefore, it is absolutely necessary to have an air conditioning system of great fiability.

In these cases of AVM, prediction of the amount of intraoperative bleeding is impossible, unless the AVM is group A. Therefore, such patients must be operated in a hospital which has a blood bank for replacing the blood loss in case of profuse bleeding.

Recently we began using a cell-saver, which allows auto-blood infusion, reducing the amount of injected foreign blood.

Resection of the AVM

A large bone flap is necessary, extending beyond the limits of the angiographic imagery. There are cortical malformations which do not appear on the X-rays.

Coagulation of the abnormal vessels facilitates the dissection of the AVM and preserves the normal brain tissue. This coagulation can use mono- or bipolar coagulation. We personnally prefer monopolar coagulation unless the AVM is near the hypothalamus or the brain stem; this is possible only when the MAP is at the 50 mmHg level.

The general rule in neurosurgery is to remove the lesion without impairing the normal brain, when it is a benign one, and retraction of the brain must provide a permanent and equal pressure on it.

Tactics of Surgery According to Classification

Group C

The total excision of the lesion will begin from the arterial pole when the main feeding artery is located in a fissure such as the interhemispheric fissure. When the AVM is embedded in the cortex, it is safer for the brain to begin with the drainage pole and terminate with the arterial pole, in order to clip the feeding arteries at the junction between the brain and the AVM, as was proposed in 1968 [5].

The malformation will be coagulated under induced arterial hypotension and, for these small AVMs, we advise the use of an operating microscope. The only danger lies in the postocclusive effect, especially when the AVM is located in the parietal lobe and fed by the long and straight middle cerebral artery branches. In such cases, we advise placing a clamp on the homolateral common carotid artery and reducing the flow to 50% of its value for 24 h [11]. This reduction of value will be checked by an ultrasonic evaluation of the flow velocity in the internal carotid artery. Some neurosurgeons may think that such a measure is not necessary. They must be taught that AVMs are vicious lesions and it is more difficult to succeed in 100 removals than to be the hero of one.

Group B

In this group are two types of AVMS: the first is those which are vascularized by only one of the main arteries. When this artery is from the carotid system, the AVM can be removed in one operation. It will be better to place a clamp on the common carotid artery before operation and reduce its caliber when the diastolic rate is over 20 cm/s. The clamp will be opened after 24 h when the patient is well, and removed after 36 h.

When the basilar system is involved, the tactic will differ according to the location. If the AVM is located in the internal part of the occipital lobe,

it can be removed in a one-stage operation. Most unfortunately, it is not possible to control the diameter of the basilar artery. Therefore, we advise operating the patient in the transatlantic position. It is absolutely necessary to use an anti-G suit to prevent air embolism.

When the AVM is located in the occipito-temporal area, it might be necessary to program two operations: at first, the clipping of the posterior cerebral artery on the brain stem (pterional flap) and, three weeks later, the radical excision of the AVM. The second type of AVM is those vascularized by two main systems. In the case of these AVMs, it might be safer to program two operations. If both carotid systems are involved, we begin by placing a clip on the anterior communicating artery when the diastolic rate is between 15 and 20 cm/s in both ICA. This operation, which we have now performed 16 times, is very efficient and leaves one carotid only for controlling the blood flow.

Then, during a second and final operation, the AVM is removed under a reduction of the caliber of the common carotid artery (CCA). If there is involvement of one carotid system and the basilar system, procedure depends upon the value of the diastolic rates. When it is high in the vertebral arteries, it is safer to clip the posterior cerebral artery first. We are not very happy with the clipping of the posterior cerebral artery. On the one hand, it is efficient in reducing the flow into the AVM; on the other hand, it provokes a lateral homonymous hemianopsia in 80% of the cases. It is actually the price payed for safety: new techniques must be invented.

Group A

These AVM are the most dangerous to approach. They must *always* be removed in multiple-staged operations (from 3 to 6) [9, 10]. The principle is to progressively reduce the amount of blood passing through the AVM before radical excision. We shall take, as an example, a large parieto-occipital or parieto-motor AVM vascularized by the three main arteries. The first operation will eliminate the flow coming from the hetero-lateral carotid system. It will be performed easily, by clipping the anterior communicating artery. This must be done through a pterional flap located on the side opposite the AVM. In addition to this clip, we usually place a second clip on the pericallosal artery over the Heubner artery on the side of the AVM. This operation reduces to normal the diastolic rate into the ICA opposed to the AVM side.

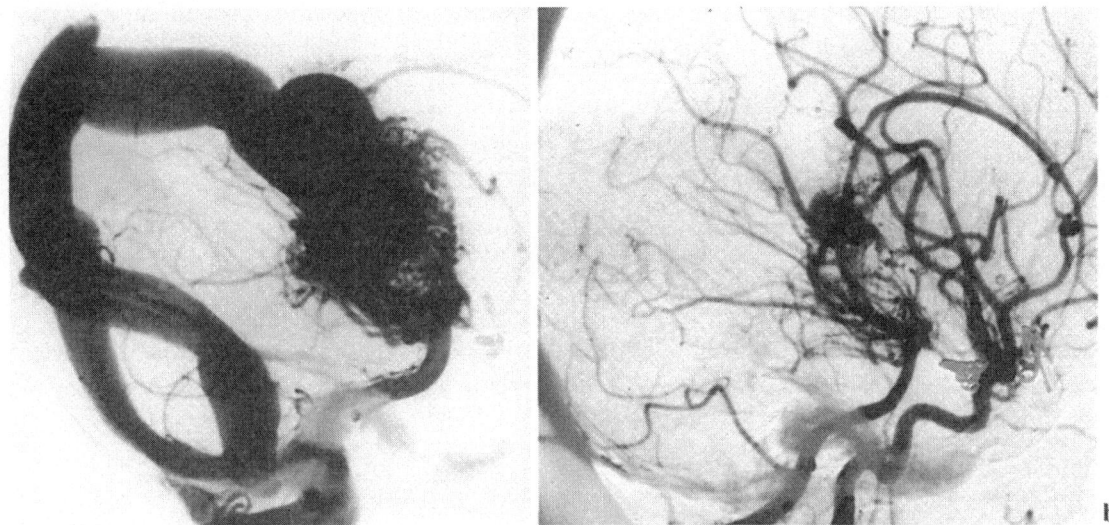

Fig. 1. AVM of the upper brain stem with isolated drainage in the superior sagittal sinus through a dilatated Galen ampulla (September 1985). **b** Cure after ligation of the superior sagittal sinus (December 1985)

The second operation will eliminate the flow coming from the basilar system. Therefore, a clip will be placed on the posterior cerebral artery on the side of the AVM through a pterional flap. Actually, we place the clip on the artery after it has turned around the peduncle. However, we doubt the wisdom of this placement, as two patients developed a hemiparesis. Therefore, we advise clipping this artery more posteriorly, even if one branch arising up to the clip is not eliminated.

During the third operation, the superficial collaterals of the middle cerebral artery will be clipped and, when possible, a cleft 2–3 cm deep will be created around the AVM. The fourth operation will remove the AVM. A clamp will *always* be placed on the CCA, and a reduction of the caliber will be performed with a checking of the flow velocity into the ICA by using a pulsing Doppler.

In fact, programing of surgery will depend upon the angiographic control, which will be performed after each operation. Each operation must be separated by 3 or 4 weeks in order to let a new equilibrium establish itself. Until now we have not had to perform more than six operations. It is time consuming and hard to accept for the patient and his family but, finally, it is gratifying to cure, for good, a young patient. I advise the patient be discharged at least one or two weeks, to raise moral courage. One must realize that every patient, as well as every AVM, is different. Therefore, each case must be discussed and the best tactic must be defined.

Special Cases

Gray Nuclei AVM

We have the experience of working on lenticulocaudate and thalamic AVMs. In both cases, as it was presented for the first time in Sao Paulo, we approached these lesions through the lateral ventricle, anterior or posterior to the motor area [6].

We found that these lesions were easier to cure than the cortical ones. Coagulation of the AVM, under a mean arterial pressure of 50 mmHg, can be performed using the operating microscope. Dissection from the normal brain is obtained by easing the clipping of the small vessels coming from the bed of the AVM.

With respect to the lenticulocaudate AVM, it is necessary to know before operation if the anterior perforated space arteries going to the AVM are surrounded by normal arteries going to the brain. We have lost a patient in whom all perforated arteries were feeding the AVM. Thus, this is a contraindication to surgery.

AVM Drained into the Ampula of Galen

In two cases presenting an AVM of the peduncle, drainage was into the ampula of Galen and, posteriorly, into the superior sagittal sinus. We have been able to demonstrate that closing the arterial drainage could provoke a coagulation into the malformation as well as a striking reduction of the diastolic rate from 70 cm/s in the vertebral arteries to 6–10 cm/s (Figs. 1, 2).

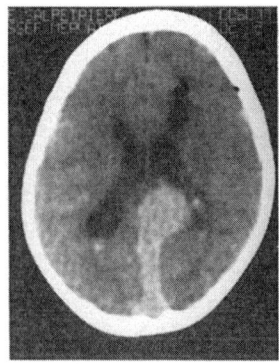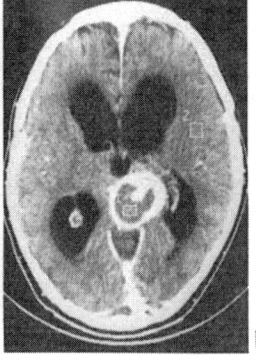

a   b

Fig. 2a, b. AVM of the upper brain stem with drainage into the ampulla of Galen. CT **a** before (September 1985) and **b** after (December 1985) ligation of the superior sagittal sinus

Table 3. Mortality after open radical surgery in 268 cases of supratentorial AVMs (1958–1986)

	1958–1978 ($n = 162$)	1979–1982 ($n = 51$)	1983–1986 ($n = 55$)
Mortality	18	7	2
Conscious patients	6.9%	13.7%	4%
Comatose patients	41.1%	–	–

These two cases demonstrate a third hemodynamic factor; the importance of the aspiration from the venous system. This has been already demonstrated in dural AVM. This means that, if possible, all AVM should be cured by simply closing all drainages. Unfortunately, this is not possible, especially because of deep drainages into the lateral ventricle or into the vein of Rosenthal.

Conclusion

We have tried to clarify our views concerning open surgery of AVM. Some results have been already published [8–11] and the reader will be able to find them in Table 3. The fatalities from 1983 to 1986 were related to group A.

References

1. Ancri D, Pertuiset B (1985) Measure des vitesses sanguines instantanées dans les malformations artério-veineuses cérébrales. Neurochirurgie 31: 1–5
2. Bayliss WM (1902) On the local reactions of the arterial wall to changes of internal pressure. J Physiol (London) 28: 220–231
3. Norlen G (1949) Arteriovenous aneurysms of the brain. Report of ten cases of total removal of the lesion. J Neurosurg 6:475–494
4. Nornes H, Grip A (1980) Hemodynamic aspects of cerebral arteriovenous malformations. J Neurosurg 53:456–464
5. Pertuiset B, Posada T, Metzger J (1969) L'exérèse retrograde des malformations artério-veineuses des hémisphères cérébraux sans hématome—Technique, indications et résultats. Ann Chir 22:803–809
6. Pertuiset B, Galal A, Sichez JP, van Effenterre R, Goutorbe J, Dagreou F, Joly-Pottuz G (1976)

Exérèse totale par voie ventriculaire de deux malformations artério-veineuses pallido-caudées sous hypotension profonde. Revue Neurol 132 (11):799–803
7. Pertuiset B, Goutorbe J, Ancri D, Philippon J (1976) L'hypotension profonde préventive par le nitroprussiate de soude dans l'abord direct de 94 malformations vasculaires sus tentorielles. Revue Brésilienne de neuro-chirurgie, Seara Med Neuro (Sao Paulo) anov. 1,2,3,4, pp 51–54
8. Pertuiset B, Sichez JP, Philippon J, Fohanno D, Horn Y (1979) Mortalité et morbidité après exérèse chirurgicale totale de 162 malformations artério-veineuses intracraniennes (1958–1978) Revue Neurol 135 (4):319–327
9. Pertuiset B, Ancri D, Lienhard A (1981) Profound arterial hypotension (MAP ⩽ 50 mmHg) induced with neuroleptanalgesia and sodium nitroprusside (series of 531 cases): Reference to vascular autoregulation mechanism and surgery of vascular malformations of the brain. In: Advances and technical standard in neurosurgery, vol. 8. Springer, Berlin, pp 75–122
10. Pertuiset B, Ancri D, Clergue F (1982) Preoperative evaluation of hemodynamic factors in cerebral arteriovenous malformations for selection of a radical surgery tactic with special reference to vascular autoregulation disorders. Neurol Res 4:209–233
11. Pertuiset B, Ancri D, Sichez JP, Chauvin M, Guilly E, Metzger J, Gardeur D, Basset JY (1983) Radical surgery in cerebral AVM: Tactical procedures based upon hemodynamic factors. In: Advances and technical standard in neurosurgery, vol. 10, pp 81–143
12. Pertuiset B, Ancri D, Arthuis F, Basset JY, Fusciardi J, Nakano H (1985) Shunt-induced hemodynamic disturbances in supratentorial arterio-venous malformations. J Neuroradiol 12:165–178
13. Spetzler RF, Wilson CB, Weinstein P, Nehdorn M, Townsend J, Telles D (1978) Normal perfusion pressure breakthrough theory. Clin Neurosurg 25:651–672

Operative Selection of Patients with Arteriovenous Malformations

Robert F. Spetzler and Joseph M. Zabramski[1]

Surgical treatment of arteriovenous malformations (AVMs) of the brain is intended to eliminate the continued risk of intracranial hemorrhage and neurologic deterioration. The decision of whether to recommend surgery should rest on an objective comparison of the long-term risks presented by the untreated AVM with the more immediate risk of operative treatment. To facilitate the surgical decision making process, we have developed a grading system for AVMs that estimates the risk of resection.

The important factors in assessing the risk of resecting an AVM include size, location, number of feeding arteries, rate of flow through the lesion, degree of steal from adjacent brain, and the pattern of venous drainage. A grading system that accounted for all these variables, however, would be too cumbersome for routine clinical use. Experience with the management of AVMs has established that many of these factors are interdependent. Thus, it is possible to reduce the number of variables considered for the grading process to three without ignoring critical factors. The factors found most important in predicting the risk of surgical resection of an AVM are its size, its pattern of venous drainage, and the eloquence of the surrounding brain.

Size of the AVM

The size of an AVM is responsible for much of the technical difficulty encountered in its surgical removal. The larger an AVM, the greater the amount of surrounding normal neural tissue that is exposed to injury during resection. In addition, the size of an AVM determines, or is closely related to, the number of feeding arteries, the amount of flow, and the degree of vascular steal from the adjacent normal brain. We have cate-

gorized these lesions into three sizes. An AVM is considered small if it is less than 3 cm, medium if it is between 3 and 6 cm, and large if it is greater than 6 cm.

Pattern of Venous Drainage

The pattern of venous drainage is also closely related to the technical difficulty associated with surgical removal of an AVM. Deep venous drainage, no matter how small, always complicates the removal of an AVM. Often, most of an AVM has to be separated from the surrounding brain before this deep component can be approached. These deep arterialized veins are friable, resist bipolar coagulation, and have the dangerous propensity of retracting and bleeding into the parenchyma or ventricle when disrupted. Angiographically, the pattern of venous drainage is considered superficial if all drainage from the AVM is through the cortical venous system. The venous pattern is considered deep if any or all of the drainage is through deep veins such as the internal cerebral veins, basal veins, or precentral cerebral vein.

Eloquence of Adjacent Brain

Eloquent brain can be defined as those areas with readily identifiable neurological function that result in a permanent disabling neurological deficit when injured. In this grading system, we consider the following areas of the brain as eloquent: the sensorimotor, language, and visual cortex, the hypothalamus and thalamus, the internal capsule, the brain stem, the cerebellar peduncles, and the deep cerebellar nuclei. The removal of AVMs adjacent to or surrounded by eloquent areas of brain obviously carries a greater risk of neurologic morbidity than does excision of these same lesions from less critical areas.

[1] Barrow Neurological Institute, Phoenix, Arizona, USA

Determination of AVM Grade

To assign a grade to an AVM, the size, venous drainage, and eloquence of the adjacent brain are determined from angiography, computerized tomography (CT), and/or magnetic resonance imaging (MRI). A numerical value is then assigned for each of these variables (Table 1). The grade of the lesion is then derived by summing the points for each category.

All operable AVMs fall into one of five grades (Fig. 1). The lowest grade possible is grade I: such a lesion would be smaller than 3 cm (1 point), located in a noneloquent region such as the anterior frontal lobe (0 points), and have exclusively superficial drainage (0 points). The complete excision of such an AVM would present relatively minor technical difficulties with little associated risk of morbidity or mortality. The highest grade of an AVM is grade V (Fig. 1). A grade V AVM is larger than 6 cm (3 points), located in or adjacent to eloquent brain (1 point), and would have some portion of its drainage in the deep venous system (1 point). The resection of such lesions is associated with a significant risk of postoperative deficits. Extensive dissection in close proximity to important brain regions is required to remove these large malformations, and removal is further complicated by the difficulties associated with controlling the fragile, deep draining veins. Various combinations of lesion size, location, and drainage patterns result in intermediate grades of AVM from II to IV with an associated increasing degree of technical difficulty for resection (Fig. 1).

Finally, there are lesions not currently considered for surgery. This group contains AVMs dispersed diffusely through critical areas of brain, such as the hypothalamus or brain stem.

Clinical Application of Grading System

To establish the predictive value of this grading system, a retrospective evaluation was carried out in 100 patients undergoing complete resection of their AVM at the authors' institution. Results of this analysis are presented in Table 2. Morbidity has been divided into major and minor deficits: temporary neurologic deficits lasting less than 3 days were not included. There were no deaths in this series.

The results demonstrate a good correlation between AVM grade and the incidence of postoperative neurologic complications. Grade I

Table 1. AVM grading scale

Graded feature	Points assigned
Size of AVM	
Small (<3 cm)	1
Medium (3–6 cm)	2
Large (>6 cm)	3
Eloquence of adjacent brain	
Noneloquent	0
Eloquent	1
Pattern of venous drainage	
Superficial	0
Deep	1

Grade = [size] + [eloquence] + [venous drainage]; for example, grade V = [3] + [1] + [1]

lesions were resected without neurologic complication, while surgery for grades II, III, IV, and V lesions was associated with an increasing incidence of postoperative neurologic deficits (Table 2).

Natural History of AVMs

It is generally accepted that AVMs are congenital lesions resulting from a local aberrant connection between the primitive arterial and venous plexus of the developing brain. Initially, the AVM involves only the arteries destined for the zone of abnormal shunting, and the surrounding cerebral vasculature develops normally. Because of the reduced resistance offered by the AVM, there is a gradual increase in flow through the malformation with a resulting increase in the size of the feeding arteries and the veins draining the lesion. As this shunt increases still further, blood flow to other areas in the hemisphere is deviated through enlarging collaterals to the AVM, producing growth in the size of the malformation and a variety of symptoms that include hemorrhage, headache, seizures, and local ischemic deficits. These vascular changes evolve at different rates and to different degrees depending on the original embryonic characteristics of the AVM. Rarely, diffuse lesions with markedly enlarged feeding and draining vessels will become symptomatic in childhood, or a small lesion with slow flow will persist into adulthood.

At diagnosis, about 50% of AVMs are less than 3 cm, 40% are between 3 and 6 cm, and 10% are greater than 6 cm in maximum diameter. Most AVMs do not become symptomatic until the third decade of life; fewer than 10% become

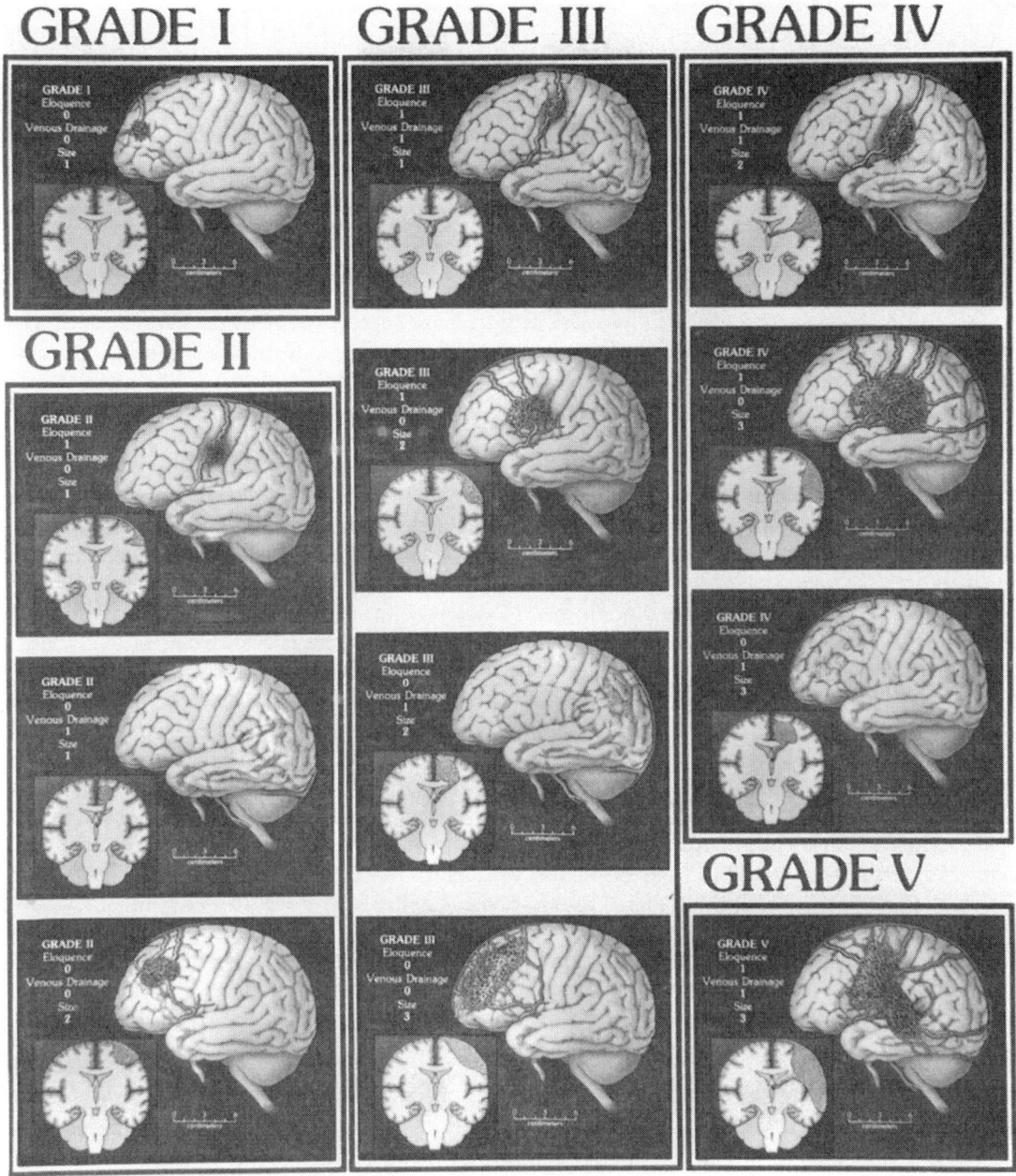

Fig. 1. AVM grading scale. After Spetzler and Martin [11]; reprinted with permission of Journal of Neurosurgery

symptomatic before the end of the first decade [5]. In terms of the general incidence among all patients with AVMs, spontaneous bleeding is the most common presentation in nearly all clinical series, and it is the most serious complication facing the patient. Indeed, as data have accumulated, it has become apparent that the long-term prognosis for the patient with an AVM is grim.

The ongoing risk of first hemorrhage from an AVM has been reported between 1% and 3% per year, and the risk of recurrent hemorrhage is as high as 6% for the first year after a bleeding episode, and 2%–3.8% thereafter [2–4]. The age range for the maximum incidence of bleeding appears to be between the ages of 11 and 35 years, and smaller AVMs appear to have a somewhat greater propensity to bleed than do larger malformations [4]. The risk of death associated with initial AVM rupture is approximately 10%, and the mortality appears to rise with each bleed-

Table 2. AVM grade versus surgical results

Grade	No. of cases	Minor[a] deficit		Major deficit		Deaths	
		No.	Percent	No.	Percent	No.	Percent
I	23	0	0	0	0	0	0
II	21	1	5	0	0	0	0
III	25	3	12	1	4	0	0
IV	15	3	20	1	7	0	0
V	16	3	19	2	12	0	0
Total	100	10	10	4	4	0	0

[a] Minor deficits included temporary neurologic changes that resolved completely or left the patient with only minimal residual

ing episode [4, 8]. The incidence of neurologic deficits is reported at approximately 50% for each bleeding episode [12]. In addition to the complications of intracranial hemorrhage, patients with AVM's face the lesser risks of seizures, hydrocephalus, and the development of flow-related symptoms, such as ischemic deficits due to vascular steal.

Patient Selection

Whether to recommend surgery for the individual patient with an AVM requires considering the specific characteristics of both the vascular malformation and the particular patient harboring the lesion. Obviously, the individual patient benefits from surgery only if resection can be accomplished without mortality or disabling morbidity.

We use the grading system described above to assist in the surgical decision-making process. Applying this grading system preoperatively allows the surgeon to objectively assess the risks of complete surgical resection of an AVM in individual cases.

Assuming no contraindications to surgery, we recommend operative excision of nearly all grade I and grade II AVMs, regardless of presentation: exceptions might include the elderly patient or the intact patient with a lesion seated directly within an eloquent area of brain. We think this aggressive approach is justified considering the low risk of surgery for grade I and grade II lesions (Table 2) and the rather grim long-term prognosis associated with AVMs, as outlined above.

Because of the increasing risks associated with the operative excision of AVMs in patients with

grade III and grade IV lesions, the decision for surgery is more individualized: the patient's age and clinical presentation are major factors that must be considered. In general, we recommend surgery for the patient if the AVM is not seated in eloquent brain, or, if the AVM is seated in eloquent brain but there is evidence of hemorrhage, and/or the patient has a fluctuating or fixed neurologic deficit secondary to the lesion.

The excision of grade V AVMs is associated with a significant risk of postoperative neurologic deficits. By definition, these lesions are large (greater than 6 cm), always located in eloquent brain, and have a component of deep venous drainage that further complicates their excision. Clearly, the decision of whether to recommend surgery for patients with such lesions will depend on the surgeon's previous operative experience. Using a combination of staged embolization and surgical excision, we have completely excised 16 grade V AVM's without mortality: three patients in our series had mild postoperative deficits (19%), and two had major neurological deficits (12%). Patients selected for surgery comprise only about 25% of the total of grade V AVM's. Currently, we recommend surgery in patients with grade V AVM's only when the patient has a fluctuating or fixed neurologic deficit in the distribution of the lesion, and/ or there is documented evidence of recurrent hemorrhage.

Technical Considerations

The surgical excision of large AVMs (those greater than 6 cm in maximum diameter) presents special problems. Nearly all of these lesions will have angiographic evidence of vascular steal, and, in the more dramatic cases, there is often a virtual absence of normal hemispheric filling until a portion of the AVM is obliterated. Vascular steal by the AVM can produce a region of chronically ischemic brain surrounding the lesion: the blood vessels in these areas of ischemia are chronically dilated, and, when exposed to sudden changes in the blood flow produced by complete excision of the AVM, they may be unable to respond. As a result there can be local swelling and hemorrhage in a pattern nearly identical to that seen in the patient with malignant hypertension, despite normal or even slightly reduced intravascular pressures. This clinical picture has been labeled normal perfusion pressure breakthrough (NPPB) [10]. We have found that stepwise reductions in blood flow through the AVM produced by the use of staged pre- and intraoperative embolizations reduce the risk of this complication [9].

The initial treatment in large AVMs usually consists of transfemoral embolization. Ivalon sponge particles, ranging in size from 150 to 290 μm, are the material of choice for all embolization procedures. These particles are small enough to pass through the feeding artery and to lodge preferentially in the nidus of the AVM, thereby reducing the possibility of collateral vessels resupplying the lesion. Bucrylate embolization of AVMs is not recommended when surgery is being considered. Bucrylate produces a brittle, noncompressible mass that makes operative dissection of the embolized AVM difficult.

Intraoperative embolization of vessels feeding the AVM is combined with ligation at or near the site of cannulation. Ligation prevents the elevation of proximal pressure, which attends AVM embolization, from being transmitted to residual nonoccluded segments of the nidus supplied by the feeding artery. Permanent occlusion of the feeding vessel is an important factor in avoiding postembolization hemorrhage [7] and a major advantage of intraoperative embolization over transfemoral embolization. Usually, one major group of feeding vessels is embolized during each operative stage of treatment. Thus, the typical large AVM would require two or three separate surgical procedures to embolize and obliterate the major feeding vessels, followed by the operative excision of the AVM.

All surgical procedures are performed under barbiturate anesthesia. Barbiturates reduce cerebral metabolism and blood flow, and may help the brain to adjust to the changes in hemodynamics induced by the embolization and excision of an AVM. In fact, several patients who developed NPPB after removal of large AVMs have been successfully treated by the prompt induction of barbiturate coma [1, 6].

Summary

The decision of whether to recommend operative excision of an AVM should be based on an objective assessment of the long-term prognosis of the untreated lesion and the risks of surgery. We have developed a relatively uncomplicated, preoperative grading system for AVMs. Applying this grading system allows the surgeon to estimate the risk of completely excising a particular AVM. The estimates presented are based on our experience with a series of 100 patients who underwent complete AVM excision.

In our series, staged management was used to reduce the risk of excising large AVMs. These lesions were managed by preoperative transfemoral embolization, intraoperative selective embolization combined with feeding artery ligation and, finally, surgical excision. The stepwise throttling of large AVMs appears to minimize the risks of NPPB. The extensive AVM embolization and feeding vessel ligation integral to this staged approach serve another, equally important purpose; the control of intraoperative bleeding—a factor previously limiting the surgical excision of many large AVMs.

References

1. Day AL, Friedman WA, Sypert GW, et al. (1982) Successful treatment of the normal perfusion pressure breakthrough phenomenon. Neurosurgery 11:625–630
2. Drake CG (1979) Cerebral arteriovenous malformations: Considerations for and experience with surgical treatment in 166 cases. Clin Neurosurg 26:145–208
3. Fults D, Kelly DL Jr (1984) Natural history of arteriovenous malformations of the brain: A clinical study. Neurosurgery 15:658–662
4. Graf CJ, Perret GE, Torner JC (1983) Bleeding from cerebral arteriovenous malformations as part of their natural history. J Neurosurg 58:331–337
5. Luessenhop AJ (1984) Natural history of cerebral arteriovenous malformations. In: Wilson CB, Stein BM (eds) Intracranial arteriovenous malformations. Williams and Wilkins, Baltimore pp 12–23
6. Marshall LF, U HS (1983) Treatment of massive

intraoperative brain swelling. Neurosurgery 13:412–414

7. Mullan S, Kawanaga H, Patronas NJ (1979) Microvascular embolization of cerebral arteriovenous malformations. A technical variation. J Neurosurg 51:621–627

8. Perret G, Nishioka H (1966) Report on the Cooperative Study of Intracranial Aneurysms and Subarachnoid Hemorrhage, section VI. Arteriovenous malformations: An analysis of 545 cases of cranio-cerebral arteriovenous malformations and fistulae reported to the Cooperative Study. J Neurosurg 25:467–490

9. Spetzler RF, Martin NA, Carter LP, et al (1987) Surgical management of large AVMs by staged embolization and operative excision. J Neurosurg 67:17–28

10. Spetzler RF, Wilson CB, Weinstein P, et al. (1978) Normal perfusion pressure breakthrough theory. Clin Neurosurg 25:651–672

11. Spetzler RF, Martin NA (1986) A proposed grading system for arteriovenous malformations. J Neurosurg 65:476–483

12. Wilkins RH (1985) Natural history of intracranial vascular malformations: A review. Neurosurgery 16:421–430

Discussion on Intracranial Arteriovenous Malformations

Yu-Quan Shi[1]

Although there are various kinds of modern treatment for intracranial arteriovenous malformations (AVMs), surgical excision has remained the most efficient and reasonable form of curative treatment, and should be of first choice whenever possible. Since the development of microsurgical techniques, both the operability and the sucess rates of complete excision of AVM have improved remarkably. In my series of 132 cases of AVM upon which I have operated directly, the rate of complete excision is 93% and the overall operative mortality is 0.8%. It is my policy now to advise excision of AVM for every case, provided the predicted surgical outcome is not poorer than the expected natural consequence of the AVM.

With regard to individual cases of AVM, the decision of surgical excision is not so easy to make, because the technical difficulties, as well as the risk of operation, vary a great deal according to grade. We have proposed a scheme to categorize the AVM into four grades. The criteria of each grade have been given in the Journal of Neurosurgery (October issue, volume 65, 1986). It is my experience that, with grades I and II AVMs, excision could be done almost without operation mortality and with very little operative morbidity (excluding the preoperative natural morbidity). For cases above grade II, both the operative mortality and morbidity rates increase as the grading gets higher.

The AVM is designated as a giant one if the maximal dimension of the vascular nidus shown in an ordinary angiogram exceeds 7.5 cm, and is designated as a large one if its maximal diamension lies in the range of 5.0–7.5 cm. Both the giant and the large AVMs are not suitable to be excised radically if they lie in the midst of eloquent brain, such as the Rolandic or Sylvian areas, or in the vital part of the brain, such as the diencephalon or brain stem. As an alternative, intravascular procedures by means of catheterization, and various kinds of intraluminal thromboembolic processes could be recommended. One might also be satisfied by mere ligation of its main feeding arteries, leaving the vascular nidus alone for future trial.

The amount of blood shunting of any AVM is another important factor to be concerned with, particularly for the security of its surgical excision. The greater the amount of blood shunting, the more the risk of excision. By careful examination of the size and number of feeding arteries and draining veins, we can roughly estimate the amount of blood shunting of a given AVM. Excision of a highly perfused AVM will cause a sudden diversion of the voluminous blood stream to the surrounding brain, which is poorly autoregulated. This will result in sudden swelling, edema, disruption, and even diffuse hemorrhage in the surrounding brain substance. This catastrophic event, occurring during operation, has been fully described by various authors in the literatures, and its pathogenesis has been well elucidated by Spetzler and Pertuiset: the name "cerebral perfusion pressure breakthrough phenomenon" has been attached to it. We call this dreadful event "cerebral hyperfusion phenomenon," which results when the perfusion pressure exceeds the upper limit of the autoregulation mechanism of the cerebral vessels. The same phenomenon can sometimes happen in cases of acute intracranial hypertension, when there is suddenly decompression, as in the case of acute traumatic subdural hematoma. To struggle against such a disastrous event during operation, we usually urge enhancement of the hypotension measure in order to lower the perfusion pressure, and the starting of hyperventilation in order to induce vasoconstriction of the cerebral vessels. At the same time, we excise more of the surrounding brain tissue which contains the bleeding spots, instead of attempting to check the bleeders

[1] Department of Neurosurgery, Hua Shan Hospital, Shanghai Medical University, Shanghai, People's Republic of China

individually. We have twice encountered such awkward situations during AVM excision and were able to control both of them. The patients survived at follow-up of 5 and 4 years after the operation, respectively, one in slight morbidity and the other in severe morbidity.

AVMs which lie deep in the cerebral parenchyma usually will not be visible on the surface of the brain during craniotomy. These consist of AVMs which are hidden in the inter-hemispheral fissure (the medial hemispheric AVMs), AVMs of the corpus callosum, AVMs of the striatothalamocapsular region, AVMs of the medial temporal lobe, AVMs of the base of the brain, AVMs in the depth of the cerebellum, AVMs of the C-P angle, and AVMs of the brain stem. With the exception of the last one mentioned, we operated on most of these deep AVMs selectively. Suffice it to say that the operative results of these deep AVMs are poorer than those of the superficial group. If the vascular nidus shown in angiogram is well circumscribed, and its feeding arteries are easy to approach, or if there is a localized area of cerebral softening in CT scannings as a result of previous hemorrhage or infarction, the operation is expected to be less troublesome. Small and deeply seated AVMs are sometimes even more difficult to tackle than medium or large sized ones, because it is difficult to locate the lesion accurately. In that case, the lesion must be approached tactically, either by following its feeding arteries or its draining veins, or by going through the ventricle in the nearest possible route by the least destructive techniques.

Excision of the deep-seated AVMs and AVMs of eloquent brain sites will usually result in some neurological deficits, such as deterioration of sensori-motor paralysis, aphasia, hemianopsia, and sometimes seizure attacks. Most of these deleterious effects of surgery are transient and will last for a couple of weeks to a few months. Since the effect of "cerebral steal" of the AVM has been corrected by the excision, there will be improvement of the blood supply to the surrounding tissue, and the neurological function of the patient will usually be compensated.

Surgical Treatment for Deep-Seated or Large AVM

Takehide Onuma[1] and Jiro Suzuki[2]

Introduction

The best treatment for arteriovenous malformations (AVMs) is their total removal. However, in deeply seated or large AVMs, total resection is not only difficult but also hazardous. Moreover, the surgical results of deep or large AVMs are not always satisfactory and vary depending on the surgical indication, methods, and surgeon's technical experiences.

We discuss the therapy of deep or large AVM, especially the surgical technique, and introduce our new trial method which utilizes a balloon catheter to temporary occlude the feeding arteries under the administration of a new brain protective substance for the prolongation of the temporary occlusion time.

Surgical Technique for Total Removal of AVM

Our characteristic principle for resection of AVM is to temporarily occlude the feeders prior to the dissection of AVM with the aid of brain protective substance, Sendai Cocktail, which prolongs the permissible occlusion time [3, 4]. The surgical procedure, in brief, is as follows: we perform a craniotomy large enough to allow extirpation of the AVM and to expose the feeding arteries or the main feeding trunk arteries at the cerebral base. After the craniotomy, cerebrospinal fluid is aspirated from the subarachnoid space at the chiasmal portion to make the surgical manipulation easy. Then, the feeding arteries of the AVM, or the main artery at the base of the brain which supply the feeders, are disclosed and secured. Meanwhile, a brain protec-

tive substance, Sendai Cocktail (20% mannitol 10 ml/kg vitamin E 10 mg/kg, phenytoin 10 mg/kg), is administered for about 30 min.

Next, temporary clips are applied on these feeders to temporarily interrupt blood flow for the extirpation of the AVM. By this method, since the volume of the AVM and the vascular pressure of feeders and drainers are decreased, hazardous bleeding can be avoided and damage to the brain itself can be minimized.

When the main feeding artery is the middle cerebral (MCA) or the posterior cerebral artery (PCA), we first approach the base of the brain and disclose these feeders before dissection of the AVM. When the anterior cerebral artery is a feeding artery, it is approached interhemispherically (Fig. 1). The feeding artery is then transiently occluded and the AVM is resected. In the dissection of the AVM, relatively large afferent arteries should be cut after applying hemostatic clips, because hemostasis only with a bipolar coagulator is insufficient and often postoperative bleeding occurs. Care also must be taken to prevent postoperative hemorrhage from the small abnormal vessels, the so-called premature vessels, connected to the nidus. Draining veins should be cut last. Using this method, the entire operation can be performed in a dry field, and extirpation is possible in a relatively short time without unnecessary injury to the cerebral parechyma. Therefore, this method is especially useful and effective in cases of deep or large AVMs.

New Technique for Resection of Deep or Large AVMs

In the cases of deep or large AVMs, sometimes we not only encounter difficulties in directly applying the temporary clips on the feeders, but also find it impossible at times to even approach the feeding arteries. In such cases, we have recently tried temporary occlusion of the feeders by intravascular balloon catheter under the admini-

[1] Department of Neurosurgery, Sendai City Hospital, Sendai, Japan
[2] Division of Neurosurgery, Institute of Brain Diseases, Tohoku University School of Medicine, Sendai, Japan

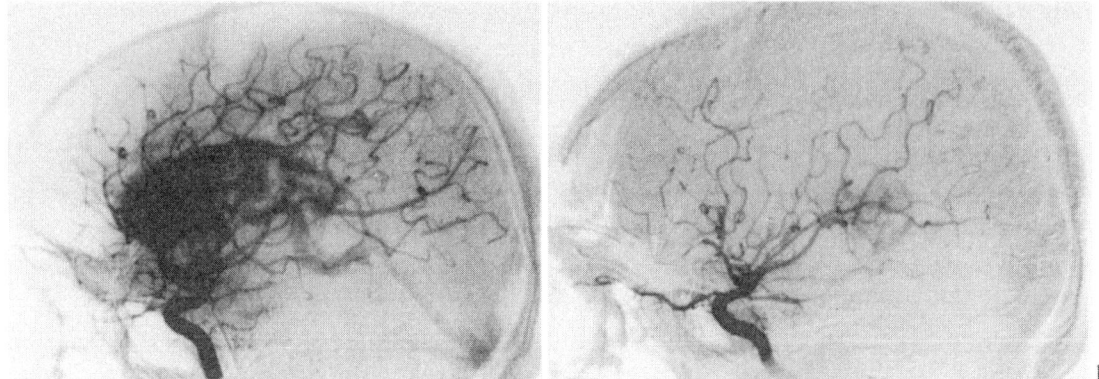

a   b

Fig. 1a, b. A large deep AVM is located on the corpus callosum and in the third ventricle. A bifrontal craniotomy was followed by the temporary clipping of the proximal portion of the bilateral A_2 arteries and the AVM was removed by the interhemispheric approach. **a** Preoperative angiogram. **b** Postoperative angiogram

stration of the Sendai Cocktail [5, 10]. By this new method, surgical excision of the AVMs can be adopted based on the location and the extent of the nidus regardless of the difficulty of access to the feeding arteries. One of the ten cases treated by this method is presented.

Case 1

A 46-year-old male was admitted for headache and vomiting. Carotid angiography disclosed a large AVM in the left temporal region which was fed by the MCA and was associated with an aneurysm of the left internal carotid (IC) bifurcation (Fig. 2). Vertebral angiography showed that the AVM was also fed by the posterior temporal branch of the left PCA (Fig. 3). Since it was impossible to simultaneously clip both feeders, the MCA and the PCA, we first temporary occluded the PCA by balloon cathter under administration of Sendai Cocktail (Fig. 4). Craniotomy was followed by the temporary clipping of the left MCA, total removal of the AVM, and the clipping of the aneurysm neck at the IC bifurcation (Fig. 5).

Materials and Results

A total of 274 cases of cerebral AVM had been treated in Tohoku University from 1961 to October 1986. Total removal was performed in 195 cases, partial removal in nine, feeder clipping in 15, embolization in ten, and conservative treatment was done in 45 cases. The results on discharge are shown in Table 1.

Results of Large AVM

Among 274 cases, there were 41 cases in which the diameter of the nidus of the AVM was greater than 5 cm. Of these, 14 were treated by total removal, one by partial removal, seven by feeder clipping, and four by embolization. Twelve of the 14 cases undergoing total removal showed good results and there were no deaths. We have not experienced "normal perfusion pressure breakthrough," the sudden swelling or hemorrhage of the surrounding cerebral tissue immediately after the total extirpation of the large AVM.

On the other hand, feeder clipping was performed on almost all deep-seated AVMs, and the results were unsatisfactory. One case, in which the AVM extended from thalmus to basal ganglia, died (Table 2).

Results of Deep-Seated AVM

There were 83 cases in which AVM was located in the deep portion. Forty-one cases received total removal and the results were good in 22 cases, fair in 14, poor in one case, and fatal in four. The results of other treatments are shown in Table 3.

Discussion

The greatest obstacles in the surgery of large or deep AVMs are how to safely and totally resect the AVMs and how to reduce or eliminate neurological deficits.

Drake listed the main surgical problems as-

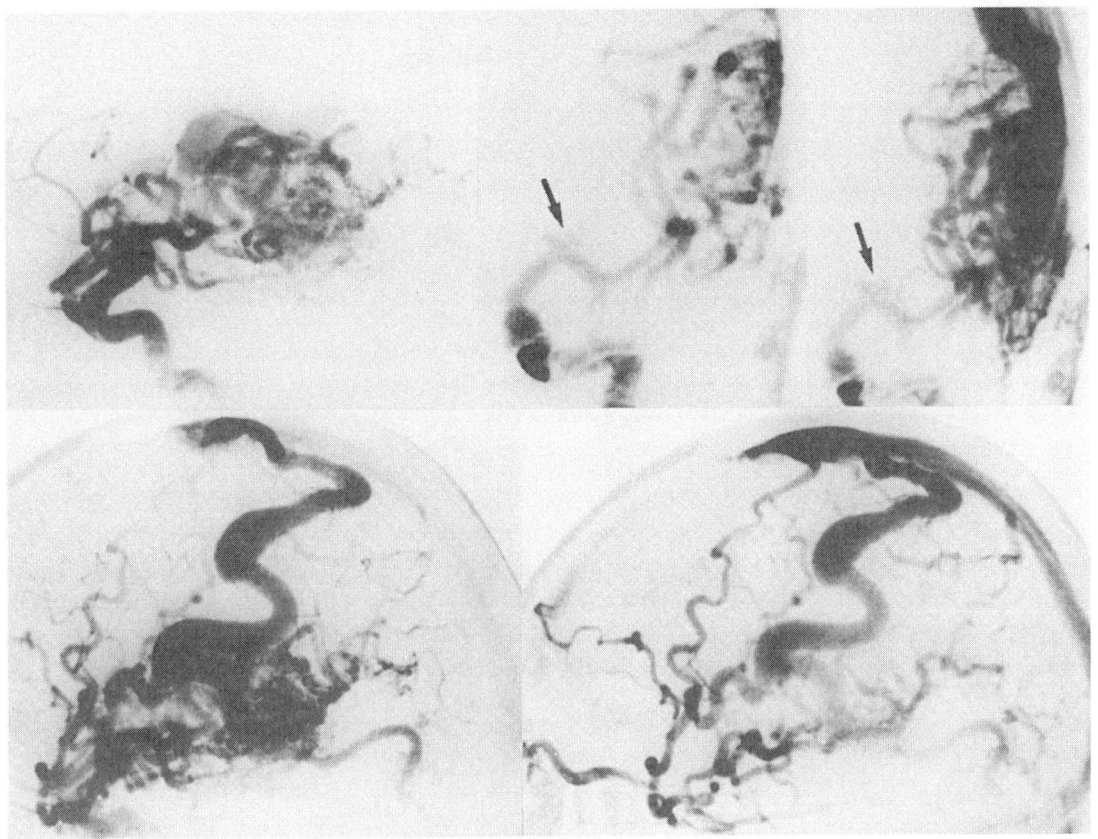

Fig. 2. Case 1. A large AVM in the left temporal region, which was fed by the MCA, and association with an aneurysm of the left IC bifurcation (*arrow*)

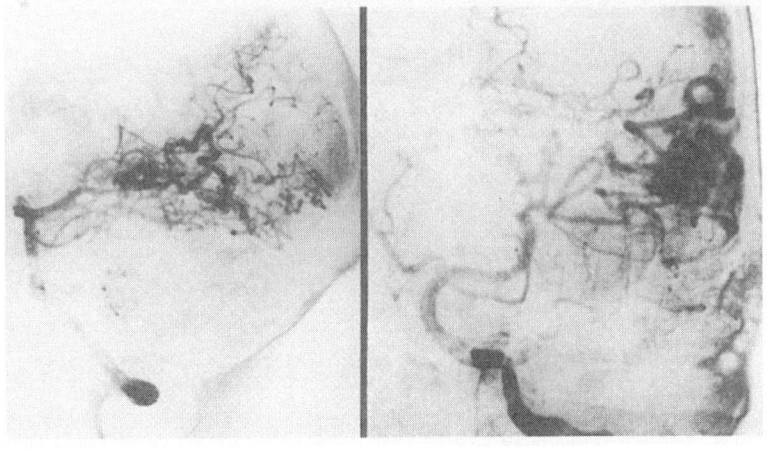

Fig. 3. Case 1. A vertebral angiography shows that the AVM was also fed by the posterior temporal branch of the left PCA

sociated with large AVMs as multiple feeders, difficulties in discriminating arteries and veins, premature rupture, and danger of the sudden elimination of huge sump effects [1]. But our surgical technique to temporarily occlude the feeders under the administration of the brain protective substance, Sendai Cocktail, enabled us to excise large AVMs safely. By occluding feeders temporarily, red veins turn dark and the volume of the nidus is reduced, making dissection of the AVM easy. Even if premature rupture occurs, disastrous bleeding can be avoided.

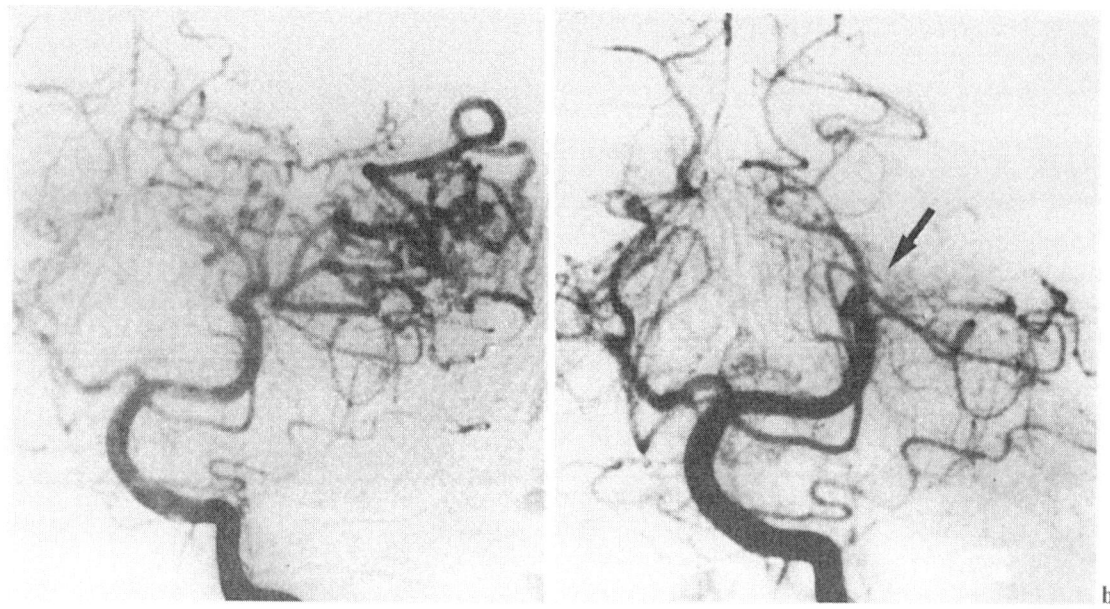

Fig. 4a, b. Case 1. A feeding artery of the posterior temporal branch of the left PCA is well occluded by balloon catheter (*arrow* shows tip of the balloon). **a** before balloon occlusion, **b** after balloon occlusion

Before temporary occlusion, our newly developed Sendai Cocktail, consisting of mannitol, vitamin E and phenytoin, is used as a brain protective substance to prolong the occlusion time of feeders [6–9]. Our results were good in 86% of the cases of large AVMs treated by total removal. We experienced no fatality, nor any normal perfusion pressure breakthrough phenomenon [2], by our present method. In the excision of deep AVMs, problems such as brain damage by direct approach and difficulty in reaching the feeders or AVM itself contributed greatly to the unsatisfactory results in comparison with our overall results. The cases determined as inappropriate for total excision were treated by feeder clipping.

Deep AVMs present much greater operative risks than superficial ones, but surgical treatments are necessitated by frequent episodes of bleeding. In such case, difficulties are sometimes encountered in applying the temporary clips on feeders because of its deep location. For these instances, we have tried our new technique utilizing a balloon catheter for the temporary occlusion of feeders, and it has proved to be useful as described in the case presentation [5, 10].

In conclusion, although our clinical experience with the balloon catheter is still insufficient, we believe that temporary occlusions of the feeders

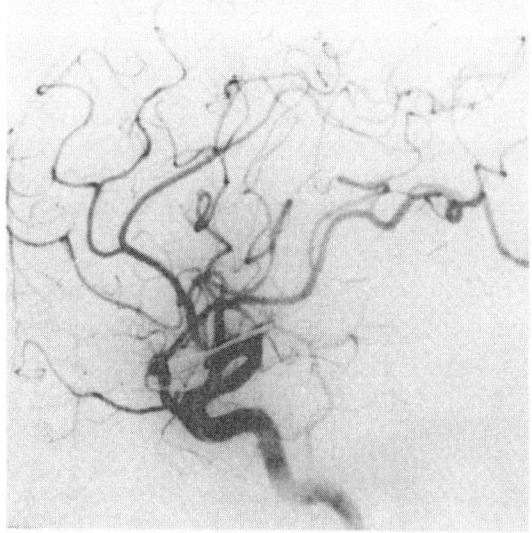

Fig. 5. Case 1. A postoperative angiogram shows the complete removal of the AVM and the clipping of the aneurysm

by intravascular balloon catheter under the administration of the Sendai Cocktail is valuable, especially for the resection of deep-seated or large AVMs. Accordingly, surgical treatments can be expanded to AVMs which are inoperable by conventional methods.

Table 1. Results of AVM on discharge

	No. of cases	Good	Fair	Poor	Dead
Total removal	195	149 (76.4%)	36 (18.5%)	3 (1.5%)	7 (3.6%)
Partial removal	9	6 (66.7%)	1 (11.1%)	1 (11.1%)	1 (11.1%)
Feeder clipping	15	8 (53.3%)	4 (26.7%)	2 (13.3%)	1 (6.6%)
Embolization	10	10 (100%)	0	0	0
Conservative	45	36 (80%)	3 (6.6%)	2 (4.4%)	4 (8.9%)
Total	274	209 (76.3%)	44 (16.0%)	8 (2.9%)	13 (4.7%)

Table 2. Results of large AVM (41 cases > 5 cm)

	No. of cases	Good	Fair	Poor	Dead
Total removal	14	12	1	1	0
Partial removal	1	0	0	1	0
Feeder clipping	7	3	2	1	1
Embolization	4	4	0	0	0
Conservative	15	13	0	0	2
Total	41	32	3	3	3

Table 3. Results of deep AVM (83 cases)

	No. of cases	Good	Fair	Poor	Dead
Total removal	41	22	14	1	4 (9.7%)
Partial removal	3	3	0	0	0
Feeder clipping	13	6	4	2	1
Embolization	6	6	0	0	0
Conservative	20	17	2	0	1
Total	83	54	20	3	6

References

1. Drake CG (1979) Cerebral arteriovenous malformations: Considerations for and experience with surgical treatment in 166 cases. Clin Neurosurg 26:145–208
2. Spetzler RF, Wilson CB, Weinstein P, et al. (1978) Normal perfusion pressure breakthrough theory. Clin Neurosurg 25:651–672
3. Suzuki J, Iwabuchi T, Onuma T (1972) Surgery for the total removal of arteriovenous malformations. Operation 26:1169–1179 (in Japanese)
4. Suzuki J, Onuma T, Kayama T (1982) Surgical treatment of intracranial arteriovenous malformation. Neurol Res 4:191–207
5. Suzuki J, Takahashi A, Yoshimoto T, et al. (1985) Use of balloon occlusion and substances to protect ischemic brain during resection of posterior fossa AVM. J Neurosurg 63:626–629
6. Suzuki J, Yoshimoto T (1979) The effect of mannitol in prolongation of permissible occlusion time of cerebral artery–clinical data of aneurysm surgery. Neurosurg Rev 1:13–19
7. Suzuki J, Yoshimoto T, Kodama N, et al. (1982) A new therapeutic method for acute brain infarction: Revascularization following the administration of mannitol and perfluorochemicals–a preliminary report. Surg Neurol 17:325–332
8. Suzuki J, Fujimoto S, Mizoi K, et al. (1984) The protective effect of combined administration of anti-oxidants and perfluorochemicals on cerebral ischemia. Stroke 15:672–679
9. Suzuki J, Imaizumi S, Kayama T, et al. (1985) Chemiluminescence in hypoxic brain. The second report: Cerebral protective effect of mannitol, vitamin E and glucocorticoid. Stroke 16:695–700
10. Takahashi A, Suzuki J, Sugawara T, et al. (1986) Surgical treatment of AVMs occluding these feeders during the removal: Utilizing intraoperative balloon catheter and the brain protective substances (Sendai cocktail). Neurological Surg 14:179–187 (in Japanese)

Discussion

Hegde (Bangalore): I would like to ask Dr. Spetzler how he makes the diagnosis of a normal perfusion pressure breakthrough when there is brain swelling and hemorrhage during surgery; is it by exclusion of other causes or by the use of particular criteria?

Spetzler (Phoenix): This occurs very infrequently; at the time of surgery this danger should be borne in mind when there is general swelling of the brain: At this point the surgeon should stop. Usually, the normal perfusion pressure breakthrough is a delayed phenomenon; it is exactly the same kind of occurrence as a hypertensive breakthrough except that it is limited to the area surrounding the arteriovenous malformation (AVM). I think the risk of it occurring can be assessed from the angiogram when only the AVM is primarily being filled and particularly from the presenting symptoms—if the patient has a fluctuating or progressive ischemic deficit as opposed to hemorrhage.

Samii (Hannover): I personally belong to the group of Prof. Yaşargil who has never experienced this phenomenon. However, I would like to ask the panelists for their opinion.

Luessenhop (Washington): This brain swelling perhaps occurs frequently to a mild degree. With the kind described by Dr. Spetzer about 1–2 h into the procedure the surgeon suddenly notices that the brain has become massively swollen. Petechial hemorrhages occur in the cortex at some distance from the AVM. When this happens it is a complete disaster and it is difficult to save the patient. My feeling is that this can be controlled and it should not happen.

Pertuiset (Paris): I have observed this phenomenon four times. It is for this reason that I use the multiple stages of operation; the condition arises, as Dr. Spetzler said, following removal of the AVM because all the blood enters the brain, which is unable to deal with the influx due to problems with the autoregualtion capacity. In addition to multiple stages of operation I also reduce the caliber of the internal carotid artery by means of a temporary clamp. In spite of these precautions a brain swelling occurred during surgery at the beginning of this year, but it was stopped by the continuous injection of pentothal. If such swelling occurs pentothal must be administered immediately—as soon as the cavity containing the AVM begins to be reduced.

Suzuki (Sendai): Theoretically, it may happen, however in over 200 cases, I have never experienced such a phenomenon.

Samii: Do you not think it may be residual AVM which bleeds?

Spetzler: Many complications occur with AVM, though the cause of the complication is not evident. It is not infrequent upon removal of an AVM for increasing edema surrounding the AVM to be evident on the postoperative CT scan for a number of days. It is simply a leaking of plasma, which is part of the normal perfusion pressure breakthrough; if it is sufficiently severe, breakdown or hemorrhage will occur. The most common source of postoperative hemorrhage is residual AVM. The evidence obtained clinically, from CBF study, and laboratory findings shows the existence of normal perfusion pressure breakthrough.

Brock (Berlin): We have not observed a breakthrough phenomenon in a large series of AVMs. This is because we operate on them using barbiturate anesthesia. It is known that barbiturates are the most potent agents reducing blood flow, intracranial pressure, and perfusion pressure. There is no evidence that autoregulation is disturbed around a malformation, but if this did occur hypotension would be the most natural way of combating it and the best way of achieving this and providing brain protection at the same time would be with barbiturate administration as described by Prof. Pertuiset.

Spetzler: All the AVMs I operated on were done under barbiturate anesthesia. Of the series of 175, there was only one normal perfusion pressure breakthrough, which occurred very early in my series before the use of barbiturates.

Byrnes (Belfast): Could Dr. Spetzler comment on the timing of the stages of contributary vessel embolization?

Spetzler: Our stages are normally 1 week apart. I feel that it is much better to take out a very large AVM in stages, based on the source of the blood supply. I think that the results are satisfactory considering that the patients had previously been thought inoperable.

Pertuiset: In our staging, the interval is never less than 1 week and never more than 3 weeks. This is based on the record of the flow velocity in the neck, which is a good indication of the blood flow into the malformation. My opinion is that a new equilibrium must be obtained before going on to the next stage. With respect to breakthrough, an interesting observation was made by Dr. Mullan in the Journal of Neurosurgery in 1979; he described vascular brain swelling, which is probably related to breakthrough. At that time, he did not clip the artery but made a ligature. He found it difficult at first to remove the ligature, but 20 min after removal the brain returned to normal.

Pitts (San Francisco): Yesterday, Prof. Yaşargil showed three kinds of vessels entering AVMs: one directly into the AVM, another bypassing it giving feeders, and a third normal type of vessel near an AVM that is very difficult to distinguish angiographically and sometimes also during surgery. I would like to ask the panel how they would deal with this problem.

Samii: I believe that we are unable preoperatively to distinguish precisely between those vessels that are feeding the AVM and those that belong to the normal blood supply of the surrounding area. I think that we will need more help from neuroradiologists in future to perform functional and very selective angiography in order to characterize the hemodynamics of individual vessels. With such preoperative assis-

tance, we will then be in a position to coagulate stepwise the different vessels and thereby reduce the possibility of complications.

Luessonhop: If a vessel is identified contributing to an AVM and which is going on to distal areas it should not be sacrificed: It should be identified, followed, and saved. A major problem for us with very small cortical AVMs has been saving the bypassing artery, particularly in the speech area.

Spetzler: With respect to the grading of AVMs, we feel this should be as objective as possible, which is why we devised our grading system based on volume; flow is also an important factor here and should be assessed with respect to the hemodynamics of an AVM.

Sugita (Matsumoto): In the literature, large AVMs are variously defined as being over 4 cm or over 6 cm, but I feel that measuring the volume gives a more accurate impression of the size. Flow should also be taken into account. High shunt and low shunt are difficult to assess in normal angiograms. Perhaps more recent technologies should be utilized, such as PET or current three-dimensional methods.

Spetzler: The problem of course is that AVMs are not of a shape that readily permits three-dimensional measurement. Drainers should be excluded from the measurement; it is the size of the nidus that is critical.

Sano (Nagoya): We measure large AVMs before, during, and after operation by means of CBF and observe a delayed high CBF in the surrounding area. I would like to ask the panel if they carry out CBF monitoring during operation.

Sugita: Measurement of CBF in large AVMs with respect to breakthrough was discussed yesterday. The number of cases studied by individuals is not very high only 5–20, but 50–100 cases would be required for the results to be meaningful.

Hosobuchi (San Francisco): I think that Prof. Pertuiset is the only presenter to discuss the patient selection criteria. I would like to ask the panel what they think the real indications are for resection of AVMs, bearing in mind the patient morbidity and mortality.

Luessenhop: The current feeling in neurology in

the United States is that if a particular form of surgery offers a mortality of 1% or more it should not be carried out. Recent technical innovations may appear extremely attractive and lead us to think in terms of 5% or 6% mortality, but this is not acceptable. The natural history of AVMs has now been better worked out. We should concentrate on the cases where there is almost zero mortality and be extremely selective with the other cases.

Spetzler: The grade V patients that I operate on have either multiple hemorrhages, progressive neurological deficit, or fluctuating neurological deficit. We do not use seizures or headaches as indications. I was very interested to hear that in Prof. Pertuiset's series 80% of all the AVM cases he operates on present only with seizures.

Luessenhop: I agree with Dr. Spetzler to a certain extent, but I feel that predictability of bleeding is poor in any one patient: A patient who bled 2 or 5 years ago is no different from a patient who has never bled. If a patient bled five times 10 years ago and has not bled subsequently is he any different from a patient who has never bled? There is no clear answer here. If we assume that a person who bled once a long time ago or a person who had a seizure at one time is different from someone who has never had a symptom then Dr. Spetzler may be correct, but we have no evidence that this is so.

Samii: The most important question I feel concerns the limits of surgical indications for AVM. This depends on the experience of the surgeon and different surgeons have different limitations. The decision as to whether surgery should be attempted in any particular case should rest solely with the surgeon based on his own experience. There appear to be two types of AVM: benign ones which are easy to remove and malignant ones which tend to bleed from the beginning to the end of the operation. As I said before I think we need more preoperative angiographic information to indicate which cases are likely to be problematic.

Pertuiset: We have been studying the hemodynamics of AVMs since 1977. It is absolutely essential before carrying out surgery on an AVM to know the hemodynamic factors involved. These factors involve, first, the flow into the AVM from the monitoring of the flow velocity in the arteries of the neck and, second, the capacity for autoregulation of the brain arteries.

Commentator *Handa* (Hamamatsu): I would like to restrict my comments to the practical scoring system of AVMs in connection with Dr. Hosobuchi's question. As many speakers indicated, large and deep-seated AVMs once considered inoperable can now be treated directly and successfully. However, it is also true that in approximately one-third of patients with large and deep-seated AVMs there is still no established treatment available despite recent advances in microsurgery and various kinds of supplementary treatment. Another matter of concern among neurosurgeons is the operability of different regions. I think the indication for surgery of AVMs should be assessed both in terms of accessibility to the region and from the aspect of natural versus surgical risk. At least six factors are of major importance in assessing AVMs from a therapeutic point of view: (a) age of the patient, (b) mode of clinical presentations, i.e., symptoms, (c) size, (d) location, (e) number of feeding arteries, (f) hemodynamics. The first two factors are thus natural, and the latter four surgical. I think that a simple and effective scoring system can be devised based on an objective assessment of the above factors, and from the results of such scoring the operability or inoperability in a particular patient can be judged. Such a scoring system could be established internationally.

RTD 12. Giant Aneurysm

Surgical Management of Giant Intracranial Aneurysms

Lindsay Symon[1]

Giant aneurysms are commonly defined as those with a diameter larger than 2.5 cm. In the past, it was customary to assess this by angiography, but much more accurate assessment of aneurysmal size is now available by the use of computerised tomography or magnetic resonance imaging. These two techniques further present the advantage that the proportion of the aneurysmal sac filled by fluid blood and the proportion filled by clot are more easily assessed, and a true appreciation of the difficulties of approach, therefore, made available. Giant aneurysms present considerable problems because of their bulk, their compression of neighouring structures, and their adhesion both to the parent vessel, a considerable proportion of whose wall they may, at least apparently, take up, and to the important perforating vessels in the region of the base. Overall, aneurysms arise from the bifurcation or trifurcation of major vessels; giant aneurysms are no exception. Therefore, the complexity of their adhesion to the branches of their parent artery may be considerable, and the problems which they present in management may be considerably greater than those presented by a smaller lesion of similar origin. The age distribution of cases of giant aneurysm shows that these patients are generally older than the average age of patients presenting with aneurysmal rupture and subarachnoid hemorrhage. This consorts well with the observation that the majority of these lesions present with space-occupying and compressive effects, though a certain number of them have caused subarachnoid hemorrhage in the recent or remote past. Indeed, in a number of circumstances, false aneurysms or organizing clots without the true aneurysmal wall may increase the apparent size of such aneurysms.

The author's present experience extends to approximately 50 giant aneurysms treated over a 10-year period, with a 7% mortality rate and a 6% unsatisfactory result.

Control of the Afferent Circulation

Adequate dissection of a massive sac tense is substantially impossible, either because of the blood pressure within it or because of the contained clot. Therefore, the first step in the management of these lesions should be control of the afferent and efferent circulation. It is in these circumstances that temporary clips have their main application. Giant aneurysms almost always encourage the collateral circulation, particularly those which have become attached to and have considerably stretched major cerebral vessels. As a result, the as yet ill-defined parameters of safety of temporary vascular occlusion are lengthened in the management of giant aneurysms. The author has found the use of somatosensory- or other-evoked responses of value in assessment of the integrity of perfusion of peripheral circulation, particularly in the middle cerebral and carotid distributions. However, even without this safeguard, it is probable that periods of occlusion of the circulation of up to half an hour may be tolerable in most giant aneurysms without subsequent neurological defect. In the management of the circulation it is important to remember that the integrity of the collateral circulation depends upon the pressure within the collateral vessels. Where intra-aneurysmal pressure is to be lowered by opening the aneurysm, as in the second step of management, it is essential to prevent the collateral circulation bleeding out via the distal vessels into the aneurysm. Therefore, proximal control must be parallelled by distal control. For example, in a middle cerebral aneurysm, not only must the main trunk of the middle cerebral be occluded, but the distal trunks also. Here the situation of the perforating vessels must be very care-

[1] Gough-Cooper Department of Neurological Surgery, Institute of Neurology, Queen Square, London, England

fully borne in mind. While it is true that the leptomeningeal collateral circulation is highly competent, particularly when encouraged by partial proximal vessel obstruction in association with the bulk of the aneurysm in question, the collateral circulation to the perforating vessels is poor. Indeed, these are functionally the end arteries described by Cohnheim. No extended period of vascular occlusion is safe beyond about 10 min where the circulation to the perforating segments is shut off. After this, irreversible damage in the distribution of the perforating circulation is likely to produce dense and unacceptable neurological defects. Therefore, if the opportunity arises to include the perforating segments in continued perfusion without an occluded segment, it should be seized. For example, it may be necessary to dissect a trifurcation aneurysm of the middle cerebral so that the proximal segment of the middle cerebral may be occluded distal to the perforating segment. In the same way, efforts should be made to exclude their recurrent artery of Heubner from an occluded segment if proximal anterior cerebral occlusion is contemplated, although this may be difficult or impossible where the origin of Heubner, proximally from the AC2, is extensively taken up in the aneurysm. Effort should likewise be made to make sure that the anterior choroidal artery remains perfused if proximal and distal terminal carotid occlusion is used in the management of giant terminal carotid aneurysms. These caveats represent a counsel of perfection and, where they cannot be satisfied, the surgeon must be aware that the length of time available to him in which the circulation can be controlled is limited to around 10 min under normothermic and normotensive circumstances.

The question of profound circulatory arrest and hypothermia will not be addressed as this surgeon has no experience in its use, but it is possible, under the circumstances of an otherwise inoperable giant aneurysm, that combined surgery with a thoracic team will present its main advantages.

During temporary vascular occlusion, which the author sometimes refers to as profound local hypotension, the remainder of the circulation may be protected by the maintenance of a normal perfusion pressure. Exactly what this should be will depend on the preoperative blood pressure. An intelligent assessment of the likely threshold of failure of autoregulation may be obtained from the characteristics of the preoperative blood pressure. Thus, a severely hypoten-

sive patient with a blood pressure of 180/110 is likely to show autoregulatory failure below a mean pressure of around 100, whereas a normotensive patient with a blood pressure of 120/70 will show a well-preserved autoregulatory profile down to a mean pressure of 50–60. While moderate hypotension may be employed in the approach to the aneurysm and is of course surgically valuable, due consideration must be made of the likely affects of vascular occlusion in the presence of diminished pressure head. It might be thought advisable to raise the blood pressure during proximal vascular occlusion: greater experience with intraoperative monitoring will confirm or deny this. From somatosensory-evoked response monitoring in the author's hands, it has emerged that dense ischemia distal to proximal occlusion is signalled by a rapid failure of the evoked response within 2 min. This applies only to carotid, middle cerebral, and basilar occlusions, where the somatosensory pathway is affected by the vascular occlusion. Provided the evoked response fails slowly over a period of longer than 4 min, then it is likely that the ischemic lesion is of a less dense character and that the greater part of the area falls into the functional "penumbra," reperfusion of which may restore function provided it occurs within an hour. Thus, middle cerebral occlusion has been tolerated for 45 min maximum in one of the author's cases although, where the perforating segment has been included in the occluded segment, rapid failure of the evoked response has occurred and appreciable though transient neurological disturbance, rectifying over a period of 12-24 h, has signalled a dense ischemia only just recoverable.

Reduction of Sac Bulk

This implies the capacity to expose a sufficient area of aneurysm to open it and evacuate its contents. As a rule, exposure of a portion of the periphery of the aneurysm fundus will have been carried out during the approach. Where the aneurysm is to be opened, it is essential that it be opened far enough away from the neck that the manipulations do not cause a tear of the wall down towards the parent artery, rendering the neck unclipable or incapable of holding a ligature. Therefore, the surgeon must balance the necessity for sufficient exposure of the aneurysm to enable its evacuation prior to the application of temporary clips, with the risks of rupture before control of the circulation has been achieved. As a rule, this author prefers to isolate the afferent and efferent vessels first, then to sufficiently expose the aneurysm to enable it to be collapsed, to apply temporary clips, and finally to open the aneurysm and evacuate its bulk. Most of these aneurysms contain partly fluid blood and partly clot. Sometimes they are almost entirely occupied by laminated thrombus. In previous days, this constituted a considerable difficulty in dissection, the thrombus having to be broken up by blunt hooks and rongeurs, but the availability of the ultrasonic dissecting apparatus has entirely changed the picture. The ultrasonic dissector is without parallel in the management of laminated clot or neuroma tissue. It can be relied upon to handle everything except calcified clot, and it is possible, therefore, to dissect round within the wall of the aneurysm, to remove any calcifying material with rongeurs, and to leave a very thin and malleable wall. Finally, the area of the neck can be cautiously approached from within the aneurysm, the proximal and distal circulation being controlled by clips, and, with the aneurysm wall being pliable and relaxed, fashioning of a neck is much more simple.

Occlusion of the Aneurysm Neck

The ingenuity of colleagues in the design and manufacture of clips of various descriptions has greatly simplified the management of the neck of a giant aneurysm. Thus, it is no longer necessary to reduce the neck to 5 or 6 mm in length. Considerable lengths of neck may now be included in long clips with, if necessary, the addition of a booster clip as described by Sundt to make sure that distal clip closure is adequate. This considerably reduces the risk of disruption of the neck where dissection of the neck from a vessel wedded to it by prolonged contact and fibrosis places both the neck and the parent vessel at risk. The variety of ingenious clips devised by Sugita should be on hand although the author, who is much indebted to his Japanese colleague for a whole variety of clever instruments,

has scarcely ever found it necessary to use these particularly ingenious clips. One maneuver which can occasionally be of help is to apply a straight artery forcep to the neck of the aneurysm once one is certain that the neck contains no material which can be squeezed into the parent vessel. The gentle crushing of the neck will often enable clips to occlude it where they are incapable of doing so in the presence of the grossly thickened fibrous neck originally present. Pásztor has made the point, with which the author concurs, that, following the final preparation of the neck, it is wise to release the distal circulatory occlusion clamps and let the lumen of the vessel clear to make sure that nothing has been squeezed into the vessel lumen by preparation of the neck and evacuation of the clot within the aneurysm.

On the whole, it is the author's preference to use clips for vascular occlusion now rather than ligatures. However, there are still circumstances where a ligature may prove invaluable. Under these circumstances, particular attention must be paid to two major factors: The first is that the ligature does not irreversibly kink the vessel concerned. In this respect, adequate preparation of the neck is essential and it may even be thought desirable to place a temporary clip between the ligature and the neck of the vessel, although if this is feasible it is usually possible to use a permanent clip rather than a ligature. Although the author has occasionally ligated a neck previously crushed by artery forceps, this is fraught with hazard and is not recommended. The second major danger is that, particularly close to the base of skull, as in carotid ophthalmic aneurysms, the neck of the aneurysm may have taken up dura. This must be appreciated during the dissection of the neck, for if a ligature is attempted with dural inclusion, the neck of the aneurysm will undoubtedly tear, leaving a major rupture in the carotid itself. The complete origin of the aneurysm from the parent artery must be in view before ligature can be considered safe. There is little doubt that, with the continued development of clip design, the use of ligatures will progressively decline.

Giant Aneurysms

Sydney J. Peerless and Charles G. Drake[1]

Giant Aneurysms

Our experience with more than 600 giant intracranial aneurysms operated upon in our unit since 1958 includes 55 carotid cavernous aneurysms, 99 posterior communicating aneurysms, 98 carotid ophthalmic aneurysms, 96 carotid bifurcation aneurysms, 47 middle cerebral artery aneurysms, and 17 anterior cerebral artery aneurysms. Of those giant sacs arising from the posterior circulation, 125 have arisen at the basilar bifurcation, 46 from the basilar artery at the superior cerebellar artery origin, 49 on the basilar artery below the superior cerebellar artery, 30 at the vertebral-basilar junction, 27 vertebral, 29 P1 aneurysms, and 22 arising from the second portion of the posterior cerebral artery.

We have recently followed-up on 500 patients in this series. Generally, the more proximal the aneurysm has been on the cerebral vascular tree, the more favorable have been the results and those arising from the anterior circulation have done significantly better than those arising from the posterior circulation. Excellent or good results have been achieved in 94% of the carotid cavernous aneurysms, 89% of the carotid posterior communicating artery (PCoA) aneurysms, 87% of the carotid ophthalmic aneurysms, 84% of the carotid bifurcation aneurysms, and 75% of the middle cerebral artery aneurysms. In the posterior circulation, 74% of the vertebral aneurysms have achieved excellent or good results. Only 66% of the vertebral junction, 67% of the giant aneurysms of the basilar below the superior cerebellar artery, 63% of the basilar superior cerebellar artery aneurysms, and 62% of the giant basilar bifurcation aneurysms have achieved excellent or good results. Of those aneurysms arising from the posterior cerebral artery, 78% of the P1 aneurysms and 100% of the P2 aneurysms

achieved excellent or good results. Excellent results are those patients who, on follow-up, are neurologically normal, without detectable deficit. A good result is achieved when the patient has demonstrable neurologic findings, but whose neurologic dysfunction does not interfere with their activities of daily living or their ability to return to their previous work.

Tables 1 and 2 summarize our operative experience with giant aneurysms by site and by method used in the repair of the aneurysm. Although all giant aneurysms represent a significant surgical challenge, those at the basilar bifurcation have proved to be, for us, the most difficult to achieve consistently good results.

Giant Basilar Bifurcation Aneurysms

Method of Treatment and Results

Direct clipping of the neck of an aneurysm, whether small or giant, is the best treatment method to prevent further enlargement, rupture, or thromboembolic complications arising from clot forming in the aneurysm and migrating out into distal branches. Of the 122 patients with giant aneurysms arising from the basilar bifurcation in our series, 57 were, at the time, thought suitable for direct clipping of the neck: in only 40 (70%) did we ultimately achieve an excellent or good result. Significant permanent neurologic disability occurred in 12 patients and five died.

As an aneurysm grows at the basilar bifurcation, it tends to balloon out the terminal basilar artery and incorporate the origins of both posterior cerebral arteries, the superior cerebellar arteries, and the perforators that arise off the terminal basilar artery and off the original segments of the posterior aspects of the P1 arteries. As well, the necks tend to become thick, atherosclerotic, and even calcified, making compression and obliteration with a clip blade frequently impossible. Because these aneurysms can reach a huge size

---

[1] Division of Neurosurgery, The University of Western Ontario, London, Ontario, Canada

Table 1. Giant anterior circulation aneurysms: methods and results

	No.	Excellent	Good	Poor	Dead
Carotid cavernous ICA ligation					
2 bypass—Silk	1	17		1	1
—Selv	18				
Siphon balloon	28	27		1	
Trapped	4	4			
Total	51	48		2	1
		94%		4%	2%
Carotid posterior communicating					
Packed	1	1			
Carotid occlusion					
Selv	2	4			
Balloon	2				
Neck occlusion	22	13	6	2	1
Total	27	18	6	2	1
		67%	22%		
			89%		
Carotid-ophthalmic					
Explored only	2	1	1		
Trapped (3 EC-IC)	6	4	1	1	
Carotid occlusion					
Silk	1	9	1	1	1
Selv	11				
(3 EC-IC)					
Balloon (3 EC-IC)	4	3	1		
Neck occlusion	70	57	5	4	4
Total	94	74	9	6	5
		78%	10%		
			88%		
Carotid bifurcation					
Explored only	2		1		1
Neck occlusion	6	3	2	1	
Carotid occlusion	16	13	2	1	
Bypass only (carotid not occluded)	1				1
Total	25	16	5	2	2
		64%	20%	8%	8%
			84%		
Middle cerebral					
Explored only	3	2	1		
Excised	2	2			
Wrapped	6	3		2	1
Neck occlusion	19	10	5	3	1
M1 occlusion	14	10		4	
Total	44	27	6	9	2
		61%	14%	20%	5%
			75%		
Anterior cerebral					
Explored only	2		1		1
Wrapped	1		1		
Neck clipped	6	4	1		1
A1 occlusion	4	2	2		
A2 occlusion	3	1		1	1
Total	16	7	5	1	3
		44%	31%	6%	19%
			75%		

Selv Selverstone's clamp

in the interpeduncular and prepontine cistern, often bulging up to invaginate the third ventricle, their shear bulk prevents adequate exposure from any approach, making identification and separation of vital structures from the neck impossible. Under these circumstances, an attempt to clip the neck without regard for the difficulties of exposure and protection of major branches and even tiny perforators has proved to be disasterous. The majority of our poor results and deaths, when we have attempted neck clipping, have been caused by occlusion of the terminal basilar artery, one or both of the P1 segments, or the superior cerebellar arteries, when the clip migrated proximally on to the more normal and soft portion of the vessel, resulting in occlusion of these critical branches and secondary major infarction of the midbrain and diencephalon.

Under these circumstances, we have attempted alternate methods of treatment. One has been to thrombose the aneurysm with the injection of foreign material. Intraluminal thrombosis has been attempted on four occasions. One excellent result was achieved in a patient in whom the basilar artery had already been clipped, but the aneurysm continued to fill through the collateral circulation afforded by the PCoA. Injection of wire brought about complete thrombosis. This patient is counted in the clip occlusion group. Of the three remaining patients where intraluminal thrombosis alone was used, there was one good result, one poor result, and one death. The two patients with unfavourable outcomes both rebled within days or months of their original operation despite more than 90% thrombosis of the sac. In both instances, there was some portion of the neck still filling, which was the site of the recurrent hemorrhage.

If the neck of the aneurysm cannot be clipped, we have come to rely increasingly upon proximal basilar artery occlusion as a method, decreasing the chances of further rupture or enlargement of these giant sacs. The basilar artery has been clipped directly in 20 patients and occluded gradually in 30 patients, using a tourniquet with the patient awake. Excellent or good results were obtained in 30 patients (60%) following basilar artery occlusion, with 14 patients left with neurologic disability and six patients dead. As bad as these results are, they need to be compared to our experience with 12 patients in whom the aneurysm was only explored at a time when no other option or definitive treatment of the aneurysm was thought to be possible. An attempt was made to pack gauze and muscle around the aneurysm in two of these patients, and, in the remaining ten patients, the aneurysm was simply inspected and nothing more done. The results in this explored-only group, including the two in which an attempt was made to wrap the sac, have been dismal. Only four achieved excellent or good results, seven were poor and one died in the immediate postoperative period. Follow-up of this group has shown that these aneurysms characteristically run a progressive and malignant course. All of the patients but two were dead within 22 months and the remaining two became progressively neurologically disabled. The causes of death in this group were progressive aneurysmal enlargement with brain stem compression or rupture of the aneurysm. With 80% of the patients being dead and the remaining being disabled within 5 years of the their first symptoms, a 60% good or excellent result must be considered a therapeutic advance in those managed with hunterian ligation.

The decision to occlude the basilar artery is based primarily upon two considerations: the adequacy of alternate collateral circulation to the terminal basilar artery in the face of basilar occlusion and the lack of any other suitable therapeutic strategy. The adequacy of the collateral circulation is determined by four-vessel angiography. One needs to determine if there are carotid-basilar connections via the PCoA and the P1 segments. If these vessels cannot be seen in the original injections of the carotid or vertebral arteries, then we rely on Allcock's test. In this test, the carotid-basilar communication is assessed by compressing each of the carotid arteries in turn and, with the pressure reduced in the carotid circulation, contrast injected into the vertebral-basilar system will flow from the high-pressure posterior cerebral artery into the carotid circulation, giving the surgeon the opportunity to assess the presence and size of each PCoA. From our experience, we have determined that a single PCoA, 1 mm in diameter or greater, is capable of supplying sufficient flow to the terminal basilar circulation. PCoAs of 1 mm in diameter or greater, particularly if they are of equal size, produce the most satisfactory result; there is no pressure drop between the two P1 segments producing stagnation of blood in the aneurysmal sac and thrombosis. If the PCoAs are 1 mm in diameter or greater and bilaterally present, we are usually confident to directly clip the basilar artery under anesthesia at the time of the original operation. If the PCOAs are smaller than 1 mm in diameter, or if only one is present,

Table 2. Giant posterior circulation aneurysms

	No.	Excellent	Good	Poor	Dead
Basilar bifurcation					
Explored only	12	2	2	7	1
Intraluminal thrombus	3	(1)	1	1	1
One vertebral ligated					
Basilar a. clip	20	11	3	5	1
Tourniquet occlusion Basilar a.	30	10	6	9	5
Neck clipping	57	22	18	12	5
Total	122	46	30	34	14
		38%	25%	28%	11%
			63%		
Basilar—SCA					
Explored only	4		3	1	
Coated	1		1		
SCA ligation	2	1			1
trap	3		2	1	
Basilar clip	5	4		1	
Tourniquet applied only	2	(1)		1	(1)
Neck clip	28	5	12	5	6
Total	45	11	18	9	8
		24%	39%	20%	17%
			63%		
Basilar below SCA					
Explored only	3		1		2
Coated	1	1			
Neck occlusion	5	2		3	
Basilar occlusion					
Clip	17	12	2	2	1
Tourniquet	7	2	2	1	2
Bilateral vertebral occlusion clip	11	4	4	2	1
Trapping	5	2	1	1	1
Total	49	23	10	9	7
		47%	20%	18%	14%
			67%		
V-B junction					
Explored only	2			2	
Neck clipping	5	2		3	
Trapped	2	1			1
Vertebral occlusion					
Single	11	4	3	2	2
Bilateral	10	7	2	1	
Total	30	14	5	8	3
		47%	17%	27%	10%
			64%		
Vertebral					
Explored	1				1
Neck occlusion	3	2	1		
Trapped	4	2	1	1	
Vertebral occlusion	19	11	3	3	2
Total	27	15	5	4	3
		56%	19%	15%	11%
			75%		

(*Table 2 continued on following page*)

Table 2 (*continued*)

	No.	Excellent	Good	Poor	Dead
P1 Aneurysms					
P1 Clip	13	10	2	1	
Trapped	8	5	1	1	1
Neck clipped	6	4		2	
Explored glued	1				1
Total	28	19	3	4	2
		68%	11%	14%	7%
			79%		
P2 Aneurysms					
Neck clipped	6	4	2		
P2 clip	11	10	1		
P2 trapped	5	2	3		
Total	22	16	6		
		73%	27%		
			100%		

SCA superior cerebellar artery

we are more inclined to place a tourniquet around the basilar artery and bring it out through the scalp incision so that the vessel may be progressively stenosed and occluded with the patient awake and under angiographic control. On several occasions, where the aneurysm has continued to fill and enlarge, despite basilar artery occlusion, by flow coming through a large and usually asymmetric PCoA, we have resorted to further stenosis or occlusion of these inflow vessels to finally bring about thrombosis of the aneurysm. As noted above, the use of intraluminal thrombosis techniques would appear to have an enhanced value in those situations when the high jet of pressure and flow has been removed from the sac.

Causes of Poor Results and Deaths

Of the 122 patients with giant basilar bifurcation aneurysms operated on in our unit, we have had 34 poor results and 14 deaths. This 39% combined mortality and morbidity is sobering and deserves further consideration. The single death in the explored-only group and the death in the patient who had horse-hair and wire injected into the aneurysm were both due to rebleeding and occurred within days after the surgical procedure from aneurysms not secured. One patient who died after his basilar artery had been clipped also expired as a result of rebleeding 12 h after

complete occlusion of the basilar artery. This patient had had a small basilar bifurcation aneurysm clipped 8 years previously and was well until a second hemorrhage brought him to hospital and reinvestigation, which demonstrated that the original clip had slipped and the aneurysm had grown to giant size and had rebled in a portion of the present aneurysm, in continuity with the arterial circulation. The neck of the aneurysm could not be clipped at reoperation but, because of the presence of two large posterior communicating arteries, the basilar artery was clipped and he tolerated this well. His recurrent hemorrhage was presumably due to continued high pressure and flow through the posterior communicating vessels. Of the five patients who died following attempted tourniquet occlusion of the basilar artery, four of them rebled before the tourniquet could be actually closed and, in one of these, the fatal hemorrhage was the first bleed from an intact aneurysm at the time of the original operation. The fifth patient developed a progressive deterioration of consciousness, complete with ophthalmoplegia and progressive coma, beginning 14 h after the tourniquet had been closed, and expired from a cardiopulmonary complication 3 months after the original operation. There had been gradual and progressive thrombosis from the aneurysm into the terminal basilar artery, presumably due to insufficient collateral flow after the basilar artery had been occluded. Of the five patients who died following attempts to clip the neck of the aneurysm, two died from temporal lobe hematomas, one after the aneurysm was explored and clipped under deep hypothermia and cardiopulmonary bypass, and one, a grade IV patient at operation, died from continued swelling of a huge temporal lobe clot caused by the original rupture of the aneurysm. The remaining three patients died from midbrain and diencephalic infarction from imperfectly placed or slipped clips that occluded one or both P1s, the superior cerebellar artery, and their associated perforators. In each instance, the surgeon at operation was content that the clip was in a perfect position. However, the patients deteriorated in the postoperative period and postoperative angiography and autopsy demonstrated that the clip had migrated proximally, obliterating the branches of the terminal basilar artery. Recognition of this tendency of a clip to migrate off the hard atherosclerotic base of an aneurysm onto the critical vessels has, in recent years, caused us to attempt to clip this type of neck less often and to rarely use a single clip, but more often rely on multiple tandem clips to progressively narrow the neck from above, with the shorter blades having a higher closing pressure while preserving the critical lumen of adjacent vessels within the aperture. It is also important to collapse the distal sac where possible and be quite certain there is no further filling, however small, which may gradually increase the volume and pressure in the sac and add to the forces that will displace the clip proximally.

Of the poor results, six of the seven patients who were only explored went into the operating room in poor neurologic condition and, understandably, were no better postoperatively. Three had a complete Weber's syndrome, one had a syndrome of four-limb ataxia and pathologic laughter, and one was blind and demented from the massive compressive effect of a giant sac. One patient who was only explored had three further hemorrhages in the postoperative period, each worsening his neurologic condition. The last patient grade II at the time of operation, awoke from the anesthetic dysarthric and confused. Four days postoperatively, a subdural hematoma was recognized and evacuated, but he has remained disabled with dysarthria and a mild right hemiparesis. Of the five patients with poor results following deliberate clipping of the basilar artery, two were grade IV and one was grade V at the time of operation and, although all three patients survived, there has been no significant

recovery of their neurologic deficit caused by massive compression of the midbrain and the effects of their hemorrhage. Two patients who were grade I at the time of operation were initially well upon recovering from the anesthetic, but the clip occlusion of their basilar artery gradually deteriorated 2–12 h following the procedure with signs of mesencephalic ischemia. One patient slowly' improved over several months, but has been left with a troublesome upper extremity ataxia and ophthalmoplegia: the other deteriorated into deep coma with fixed pupils and a persistent vegatative state. This latter tragic result was due to thrombus extending from the aneurysm and occluding P1 on the side of the dominant PCoA.

Of the nine patients who had poor results following tourniquet occlusion of the basilar artery, three patients were grade III, three were grade IV, and one was grade V at the time of operation. All have had complete occlusion of their aneurysm and all have shown some improvement of neurologic deficit, but have been left significantly disabled with hemiplegia, internuclear ophthalmoplegia, and ataxia. One patient, who presented with a rubral tremor, worsened following tourniquet closure and remains unable to work. In the remaining patient, tourniquet occlusion of the basilar artery produced incomplete thrombosis of the aneurysm. All patients deteriorated postoperatively; one from extension of the thrombus out into branch vessels, and two because of rebleeding.

There have been 12 poor results in those aneurysms whose necks were clipped at operation. Three patients were poor-grade (grades III or IV) going into the operation and, although the aneurysm was completely obliterated, they have not significantly improved and remain dependent on their families for their daily care. One patient came through the operation well, but developed postoperative hydrocephalus which was treated initially with a ventriculostomy which became infected and led to the development of a subdural empyema. This avoidable complication has left the patient with a hemiparesis. All of the remaining patients were injured by the operation by the clip slipping or being imperfectly placed, resulting in occlusion of one or both P1s, the superior cerebellar artery, or adjacent perforators, with resulting midbrain and/or thalamic infarction. Today, we would probably not attempt to clip the necks of some of these aneurysms, having a greater appreciation of the necessity of having a perfectly placed clip, with no possibility of slippage or deformity of the terminal basilar artery.

There is considerable room for improvement in the operative results of giant aneurysms in general and in those arising from the basilar bifurcation in particular. Undoubtedly, early recognition of these lesions before they reach giant size will have the most important effect on improving results. By the time the patient presents from a compressed midbrain and diencephalon from these huge sacs, even complete obliteration of the aneurysm often does not permit substantial recovery of the injured brain. Temporary basilar artery occlusion and the use of the new aperture clips, particularly when applied in tandem, will make neck clipping more frequently feasible and safe. The recognition of aneurysms which cannot have the neck clipped with a certain margin of safety is critical. In these situations, one must fall back to proximal vessel occlusion or, perhaps in the future, intravascular balloon occlusion of the neck as a safer alternative.

The early attempts to deal with these giant aneurysms of the posterior circulation, by Cushing, Dandy, Olivecrona, Tonnis, Poppen, Schwartz, Jamieson, and Drake, resulted in very few alive, neurologically intact patients. Today, with the dramatic improvement in radiologic imaging, neuroanesthesia, and modern neurosurgical technology, the outlook for these patients is very much better. Overall, we have achieved 68% good or excellent results by operating on patients harbouring giant aneurysms arising from the posterior circulation. In that 86% good and excellent results have been possible in our unit in anterior circulation giant aneurysms, there remains a need for further innovation and effort.

Giant Aneurysms of the Carotid and Middle Cerebral Arteries

Eugene S. Flamm[1]

This paper will focus on the operative management of patients with giant aneurysms of the carotid and middle cerebral arteries. These comprise approximately 70% of the giant intracranial aneurysms upon which the author has operated. The carotid sites include ophthalmic (Ophth), posterior communicating (PCA), and anterior choroidal (ACh) arteries, and the internal carotid artery bifurcation (ICAB). These cases occurred in the author's personal experience with over 700 aneurysms. This data and the location of the operated aneurysms is summarized in Tables 1 and 2. Although there are many similarities in the management of all patients with subarachnoid hemorrhage (SAH) from aneurysms, specific details of these locations will be stressed.

Surgical Technique

Aids to Exposure

To maximize the exposure of the circle of Willis and reduce the amount of retraction required, several adjuncts are utilized. An infusion of 20% mannitol (0.5–1.0 g/kg) is begun at the time of the skin incision. Patients also receive furosemide (40 mg) on call to the operating room. Another important adjunct is spinal drainage. A catheter introduced through a Touhey needle is inserted into the lumbar subarachnoid space after induction of anesthesia. The drainage is not opened at this time. When the dura has been exposed and tented, the spinal drainage is begun. This delay prevents stripping away of the dura which may cause epidural bleeding that is difficult to control. Furthermore, it is easier to open the leaves of the

arachnoid in the sylvian fissure if there is some CSF present. In addition to the relaxation of the brain and reduction of the need for retraction that this method provides, it facilitates the microdissection, since the surgeon can work in a drier field and does not constantly have to remove CSF while working on the aneurysm. The final step to achieve a slack brain is to maintain a PCO_2 in the range of 25–30 torr before the dura is opened; thereafter, PCO_2 is kept between 30 and 35 torr.

Clip Application

The selection of the appropriate clip should begin early in the course of the dissection so that the surgeon has a good idea which clips and clip appliers will be best suited for the particular aneurysm. It is important to remember that the neck of an aneurysm becomes wider than the initial diameter when it is clipped. It is important to have a clip long enough to account for this increase.

Although smaller carotid aneurysms usually can be safely clipped by placing the clip at right angles with the parent vessel, it is often better to apply the clip so that the blades are parallel to the parent vessel. This is particularly important when dealing with larger, thick-walled aneurysms. Failure to do this increases the chances of compromising the lumen of the vessel or producing a kink in the parent vessel. With aneurysms of 2 cm or larger, a segment of the parent artery and the aneurysm itself often share a portion of the same arterial wall. It often becomes necessary to reconstruct the parent vessel to preserve flow and obliterate the aneurysm. The introduction of the Sugita fenestrated clips has greatly improved our ability to do this. With the different blade lengths and angles, a patent vessel can be formed out of the base of the aneurysm with one or more of these clips.

An addition problem encountered with carotid aneurysms, especially larger ones, is the

[1] Division of Neurosurgery, University of Pennsylvania School of Medicine, Philadelphia, Pennsylvania, USA

Table 1. Distribution of aneurysms (1970–1986)

	No.	Percent
Ophthalmic	65	8.7
PCA	190	25.6
Ant. choroidal	40	5.4
ICAB	30	4.0
ACA	151	20.3
DACA	28	3.8
MCA	162	21.8
V-B	77	10.4
Total	743	100.0

PCA posterior communicating artery, *ICAB* internal carotid artery bifurcation, *ACA* anterior communicating artery, *DACA* distal anterior cerebral artery, *MCA* middle cerebral artery *V-B* vertebro-basilar

Table 2. Giant cerebral aneurysms (2–5 cm, mean 2.5 cm

Location	Total	Giant	Percent
Ophthalmic	65	32	49.2
PCA	190	13	6.8
Ant. choroidal	40	5	12.5
ICAB	30	7	23.3
ACA	151	17	11.3
Distal ACA	28	0	0
MCA	162	28	17.3
V-B	77	19	24.7
	743	121	16.3

PCA posterior communicating artery, *ICAB* internal carotid artery bifurcation, *ACA* anterior communicating artery, *DACA* distal anterior cerebral artery, *MCA* middle cerebral artery, *V-B* vertebro-basilar

tension within the aneurysm. This often prevents the clip from closing completely. There is also an increased chance of rupture if the clip does not completely obliterate the aneurysm when it is applied. Several techniques are available to reduce the tension within the aneurysm. Temporary occlusion of the internal carotid artery in the neck dramatically reduces the pressure in the supraclinoid carotid artery and within the aneurysm. Although temporary clips can be applied directly to the supraclinoid carotid artery, this often reduces the working space necessary to clip the aneurysm and carries the risk of endothelial damage.

Another technique that has been helpful with large, thick-walled aneurysms is suction decompression. A 21-gauge scalp vein needle, with the phlanges removed, is connected to the operating room suction. By puncturing the dome of the aneurysm where it is thick, blood can be suctioned through the aneurysm and the intraluminal tension reduced. Although this may not cause the thick-walled aneurysms to collapse, the aneurysms will become softer and more pliable. The clip can then be closed down easily and more safely. Blood loss has not been more that 150 ml when this technique has been employed.

One further method for dealing with aneurysms with broad necks is to fashion one that is more suitable for clip application. Bipolar coagulation has been used for this. I prefer to use a larger clip or create a neck with a ligature around the base of the aneurysm. This can be done with a 0 silk: the purpose is not to obliterate the aneurysm with the silk but to fashion a neck onto which a clip can be placed.

In almost all cases, the aneurysm should be punctured and opened after it has been clipped. Only in this way can the surgeon be certain that he has achieved his goal of obliterating the aneurysm. It is surprising how often an aneurysm may bleed when this is done after a seemingly perfect clip application. The only exception to this is when no further adjustment of the clip is safe or possible. This occurs with some of the larger, ophthalmic region aneurysms. In these cases, a postoperative angiogram is used to ensure complete closure of the aneurysm.

It is difficult to describe all the nuances of the dissection techniques used in the surgery for giant aneurysms. However, for giant aneurysms of the carotid and middle cerebral arteries, certain general maneuvers can be outlined.

Carotid Ophthalmic Artery Aneurysms

Aneurysms arising from the proximal supraclinoid carotid artery can often be the most challenging of the anterior circulation because of their size, inaccessibility, and relation to the cavernous sinus. Although they represent only 10% of most series, they often reach sizes of 2 cm or more. In the present series, one half of the aneurysms in the region of the ophthalmic artery were 2 cm or greater. Furthermore, it is often difficult, from the preoperative angiographic studies, to determine whether the aneurysm can be selectively clipped. This decision must often be made at the time of surgery.

Aneurysms in this location can present as nonspecific SAH. More often they present with visual complaints due to optic nerve or chiasmal compression. Occasionally, they may present as pituitary tumors because of their projection into the midline suprasellar or even intrasellar location.

Preparation for surgery of these aneurysms must include the availability of a high-speed microdrill with an angled hand piece and a variety of diamond burrs. In cases with aneurysms of 2 cm or greater, or in which there is no chance of obtaining proximal control of the intracranial carotid artery, serious consideration should be given to isolating the carotid artery in the neck. This is particularly useful with the larger aneurysms: temporary occlusion of the common or internal carotid artery at the time of clip application is extremely useful in reducing the tension within the aneurysm as the clip is applied. This reduces the likelihood of rupture and the need for systemic hypotension. In conjunction with suction decompression, this technique is very helpful in achieving accurate clip placement. With aneurysms bigger than 2 cm, it is often necessary to reconstruct the carotid artery, which may share a common wall with the aneurysm itself. This can often be achieved with one or more fenestrated clips that encircle the carotid artery. Accurate placement of this type of clip is greatly enhanced by having the artery and the aneurysm quite slack.

Posterior Communicating Artery (PCA) Aneurysms

The most characteristic presentation of this aneurysm is the sudden appearance of a partial third nerve palsy at the time of the SAH. This almost always manifests itself with some pupillary abnormality. This is probably the only pathognomonic sign associated with SAH, although it is occasionally found with aneurysms of the upper basilar artery.

About 10% of PCA aneurysms do not produce any third nerve deficit. When this occurs, special attention should be given to the angiogram since this often indicates that the aneurysm is projecting laterally onto the medial edge of the temporal lobe rather than in the more common downward position. This is of great importance in planning the surgical approach since care must be taken not to retract the temporal lobe before the aneurysm can be controlled. Aneurysms at this location do not frequently achieve giant size because they produce

compression of the third nerve and are diagnosed before they can enlarge. Those that do reach 2 cm can be particularly difficult because of the involvement of the wall of the carotid artery itself in the makeup of the aneurysm wall.

Although every attempt should be made to preserve the posterior communicating artery itself, this is sometimes not possible with the larger aneurysms at this location. A small PCA may be incorporated into the aneurysm wall or be completely hidden from view by the large sac. If this vessel is small it poses little risk. If the PCA is larger, or if there is a direct carotid artery origin of the PCA, great care must be taken to isolate the normal vessels and preserve them.

Anterior Choroidal Artery Aneurysms

There is no specific clinical presentation of aneurysms arising from the region of the anterior choroidal artery. They are relatively uncommon, comprising only 5.4% of the present series. They presented with SAH in 29 of 40 cases, temporal lobe seizures in two, and a partial third nerve palsy in two. They were found in association with another aneurysm in 12 cases, the most common association being with an adjacent PCA aneurysm. Because of the important territory of the brain supplied by the anterior choroidal artery, every effort should be made to identify the origin of the artery itself. Failure to do this will frequently cause the vessel to be included in the clip. This is poorly tolerated and results in an infarction in the internal capsule which produces a severe hemiparesis from which recovery is incomplete at best.

The dissection and clipping of aneurysms in this location is quite similar to that of PCA aneurysms. The major difference is the need to identify the anterior choroidal artery with certainty. An important aid in visualizing the anterior choroidal artery is to obtain adequate room to work at the distal end of the carotid artery. This is facilitated by widely opening the sylvian fissure. Although this is generally done as part of the initial approach to carotid aneurysms, and certainly for aneurysms of the carotid bifurcation, an extra effort should be made in cases of anterior choroidal aneurysms because there is often a tendency to regard them as PCA aneurysms, which do not require the same amount of exposure. The anterior choroidal artery may course medially to the aneurysm; it becomes necessary to separate it from the aneurysm neck to prevent its inclusion in the clip. Often this can be done by working from the medial side of the carotid artery, between the vessel and the optic nerve.

Internal Carotid Bifurcation (ICAB) Aneurysms

Aneurysms at the distal end of the internal carotid artery are among the less frequent aneurysms of the anterior circulation. Nevertheless, they can be a most challenging problem because of the size that they may attain, the increased likelihood of intraoperative rupture, and the involvement of several major vessels, namely the anterior and middle cerebral arteries, the anterior choroidal artery, and the internal carotid artery itself.

In most reported series and in the author's experience, aneurysms at the ICAB comprise about 5% of intracranial aneurysms. They may present as mass lesions or with SAH. There is no specific clinical presentation that increases the probability of finding an aneurysm in this location. The special considerations for this aneurysm revolve around the local anatomy, particularly the arrangement of the perforating arteries near the bifurcation of the carotid artery and the path of the anterior choroidal artery in relation to the aneurysm.

Even before these planes are well established, the surgeon should develop a mental picture of the location of the neck. Should rupture occur before the dissection has been completed, it is helpful to have a good idea of where the neck is so that a rapid and accurate dissection and application of the clip can be carried out while bleeding is controlled by suction. A point to remember is that the anterior choroidal artery passes behind the carotid artery as seen in this approach. The artery should be located before the clip is applied so that it is not included in the clip as it passes deep to the aneurysm. This is a small detail of the location of this aneurysm which should be stressed.

Middle Cerebral Artery Aneurysms

Aneurysms of the middle cerebral artery (MCA) comprise 20%–25% of intracranial aneurysms in recently reported series. They pose several particular problems. We have operated upon 162 MCA aneurysms in 147 patients, representing 22.8% of 743 aneurysms operated upon in this series. Of the 147 patients, 28 had giant MCA aneurysms that required the use of one or more of the ancillary techniques discussed above. Although the incidence of bilateral MCA aneurysms was only 16.8%, the overall occurrence of multiple aneurysms including the MCA was 43.5% (64/147). This figure is considerably greater than the expected rate for multiple aneurysms.

Three approaches to aneurysms of the middle cerebral artery can be used. The classical approach, and the one that is the most logical from an anatomical standpoint, is to work from proximal to distal along the MCA. This approach begins with the usual exposure of the carotid artery and progresses up the sylvian fissure. Because this often necessitates considerably more dissection and retraction than other approaches, I reserve it for those cases with very proximal MCA aneurysms or cases with other aneurysms, such as internal carotid aneurysms, when the fissure has already been opened.

In most cases of large MCA aneurysms, I prefer to begin the dissection in the distal portion of the sylvian fissure at the level of the pterion. After the arachnoid plane is established, a distal branch can be followed to the aneurysm. Good exposure is obtained and one can easily obtain proximal control of the MCA with this method.

One other approach that has been recommended is through the superior temporal gyrus. Since the dissection must eventually return to the subarachnoid space, I use this approach only when an intracerebral hematoma is present. One is more likely to cause bleeding from the aneurysm by approaching it where it is adherent to brain than through the subarachnoid space.

Because of the number of vessels in the region and the variability of their course, giant aneurysms of the MCA can be among the most difficult. It is important to be sure that all major branches of the MCA have been identified before applying any clip to the aneurysm. This usually requires an extensive and careful delineation of the bifurcation of the MCA. Aneurysms in this location are often well suited for the use of some of the ancillary techniques discussed above. Rather than use systemic hypotension, I now prefer to use temporary clips of the proximal MCA, or combine this with suction decompression of the larger aneurysms. When temporary clips are used, it is advisable to raise the blood pressure to improve the collateral circulation once the aneurysm is protected by the temporary clip.

Aneurysms of the MCA require special care in clip application. Great effort must be made to preserve the bifurcation of the vessel and not compromise the branches by narrowing them or kinking them with the clip. The reduction in tension within the aneurysm by these special methods can be a great aid to the accurate placement of the final clip. Even with this approach, it is sometimes better to leave a portion of the base of the aneurysm unclipped rather than compromise the flow through the bifurcation. The base of these aneurysms is often thick or atherosclerotic; it is not likely to be the site of a future SAH, but it could be the source of compromised flow or emboli if the clip is not carefully applied.

It is often necessary to adopt some compromises with all large aneurysms at these locations. Unlike smaller aneurysms that can be totally obliterated, giant aneurysms may have thickened walls or branches that prevent complete occlusion of the aneurysm. Since the thick part of the wall is an unlikely site of SAH, it may be necessary to leave this portion of the aneurysm unclipped rather than compromise cerebral blood flow. I do not use any wrapping or coating technique when this is done. There is insufficient evidence to suggest that the use of plastic or tissue adhesives do anything to alter the natural history of these aneurysms. The use of intravascular approaches to large aneurysms is beyond the scope of this paper, but it is certainly one additional technique to be considered in the future.

Surgical Management of Giant Intracranial Aneurysms

W. Richard Marsh and Thoralf M. Sundt, Jr.[1]

Giant intracranial aneurysms represent one of the most problematic lesions of vascular neurosurgery because of their complex anatomy and the variety of treatment modalities often required. Since 1969, a total of 263 aneurysms measuring at least 25 mm have been operated upon by our department. These represent nearly 20% of our total group of 1418 aneurysms treated. Of these, 193 were unruptured and presented with symptoms of mass effect; 70 of the aneurysms presented with subarachnoid hemorrhage. Forty aneurysms were in the posterior circulation and 223 were in the anterior circulation. A variety of surgical techniques were required: proximal ligation in 26 patients, simple trapping in 15 patients, direct clipping in 92 patients, direct clipping and thrombectomy in 16 patients, superficial temporal to middle cerebral artery bypass and proximal ligation in 33 patients, superficial to middle cerebral artery and saphenous vein bypass graft in four patients, saphenous vein bypass graft and clipping in six patients, saphenous vein bypass graft and trapping in nine patients, saphenous vein bypass graft and proximal ligation in 12 patients, and direct repair with vessel reconstruction in 13 patients. The results show excellent or good outcome in 198 patients, poor outcome in 15 patients and death in 50 patients. The results will be analysed with respect to aneurysm location and patient preoperative grade.

Giant intracranial aneurysms are, by definition, aneurysms measuring more than 25 mm in diameter. We distinguish these from the smaller saccular aneurysms (<15 mm) and an intermediate size group called globular aneurysms (15–25 mm). This is a useful categorization, as outcome and surgical management is somewhat different for each group. Certainly, giant aneurysms pose special problems related to their

size because of frequent lack of identifiable neck, difficulty with placement and effectiveness of the usual aneurysm clips, and compression of adjacent neural structures by the aneurysm.

Giant aneurysms produce their symptomatology from mass effect, thromboembolic complications, subarachnoid hemorrhage (SAH), or a combination of all three. Any patient harboring such an aneurysm with any suggestion of SAH, including warning leaks, is considered for operation. The natural history of unruptured giant intracranial aneurysms has been the topic of some discussion in the literature. Some have hypothesized that the thick aneurysmal wall and the often present luminal laminated thrombus protect against rupture. Many anecdotal reports have documented cases where such aneurysms have remained static, diminished, or decreased in size over time. Our own experience has been less encouraging: it is our belief that once these lesions become symptomatic with compressive or embolic phenomena, the aneurysm is probably in a dynamic state and has a higher probability of rupture. A recent review from our institution reporting the long-term follow-up of 130 patients with 161 unruptured intracranial aneurysms suggested that aneurysms of less than 10 mm in size had a very low probability of subsequent rupture and that the mean diameter of aneurysms which subsequently ruptured was 21.3 mm [5]. The problem of the incidentally discovered giant aneurysm remains, though the same study suggests strong consideration for operation be given. As these lesions are technically more difficult, decision must be individualized based on the anatomy of aneurysm, the patient's general medical condition, informed consent, and the experience of the operating surgeon.

For purposes of our analysis, five locations are recognized: internal carotid artery (ICA), middle cerebral artery (MCA), anterior communicating artery (ACA), caput of the basilar artery (BAC), and vertebrobasilar trunk (VB). Aneurysms of

---

[1] Department of Neurological Surgery, Mayo Clinic, Rochester, Minnesota, USA

the ICA can be further divided into cavernous sinus, clinoidal, and bifurcation aneurysms. Four categories were used for judging the results of surgery: excellent (normal employment, with normal mentative and little or no neurological deficit), good (neurological deficit but with normal mentation and employment), poor (anything less than full activity), and death. Any death within 6 months is reflected in the mortality figures.

In planning the operative approach to giant aneurysms, it must be remembered that the giant aneurysm base is always thick-walled and the parent vessel may be incorporated within the wall. Small, important, perforating vessels may arise from the aneurysm fundus. These factors often make direct clipping difficult or impossible. Consequently, the operative approach should include contingency plans for establishing a bypass if patency of the parent vessel becomes a problem. In addition, many giant aneurysms contain laminated thrombi within portions of the fundi. We have found this in nearly all giant MCA aneurysms and most giant ICA aneurysms occurring at the fiburcation and projecting ventrally from the supraclinoid carotid artery [3]. This clot can usually be identified on preoperative CT scans. It is often necessary to remove the intraluminal clot to make the aneurysm wall pliable enough to accommodate a clip. The ultrasonic aspirator has proved particularly useful in this task.

All giant aneurysms of the ICA are approached directly at this time. The cervical ICA is exposed for temporary ligation and to measure cerebral blood flow (CBF) before and during temporary occlusion. Most ICA aneurysms can be exposed with the usual pterional craniotomy in the manner of Yaşargil [6]. In past years, the anterior clinoid was removed from an intradural approach using the high-speed air drill [2]: it is our custom now to expose the contents of the cavernous space using the approach developed by Dolenc [1]. If the CBF studies suggest a poor or marginal tolerance of the neural tissue to temporary occlusion, then a bypass is first constructed using either the temporal artery or a saphenous graft. If, after dissection of the aneurysm, it is judged imprudent to attempt clipping of the aneurysm, then either the ICA is ligated or a Selverstone clamp is applied, depending upon the results of CBF studies. If occlusion CBF is above 30 ml/100 g per minute, one can predict with confidence that acute carotid ligation will be tolerated. Flows of 20–30

ml/100 g per minute indicate caution, as ICA ligation should be performed gradually with a Selverstone clamp. Ligation of the common carotid artery or construction of a saphenous vein graft, capable of carrying substantially greater flow, should be strongly considered for any flow less than 20 ml/100 g per minute.

In cases of MCA giant aneurysm, it is usually necessary to open the aneurysm and complete a thrombectomy. If reconstitution of an endothelialized channel is not possible, then resection and reconstruction of the middle cerebral artery is undertaken or some form of bypass is constructed prior to proximal ligation past the distal-most perforating vessel on the M-1 segment of the MCA. During the time of MCA occlusion (a period of 8–10 min), the mean arterial blood pressure is raised 30–40 torr and the patients are given 250 mg pentobarbital. We have had no complications related to temporary MCA occlusion for this period of time.

Giant aneurysms of the posterior circulation remain the greatest challenge in surgery for giant aneurysms. In general, if the aneurysm was not able to be directly repaired, some form of proximal ligation and distal bypass procedure has been performed. In recent years, a saphenous vein graft to the posterior cerebral artery has been used with modest success. Fusiform aneurysms of the basilar artery have been the most resistant to successful treatment.

Of the 263 cases of giant aneurysm surgically treated, 209 aneurysms were in the anterior circulation: 142 ICA aneurysms, 54 MCA aneurysms, and 13 ACA aneurysms. Forty aneurysms were in the posterior circulation: 18 in the region of the BAC and 22 VB aneurysms. Fourteen aneurysms were seen at other sites.

The overall results of treatment (Table 1) show 164 (62%) excellent results, 34 (13%) good results, and 65 (25%) poor results or death. If we look at results for aneurysms of the anterior and posterior circulation, we find 66% excellent, 12% good, 22% poor or death, and 37% excellent, 23% good, and 40% poor or death, respectively.

Most of the aneurysms were unruptured, presenting with symptoms of mass effect or cerebral embolism. This group faired best with 70% excellent results, 10% good results, and 20% poor results or death (Table 2). Seventy patients presented with subarachnoid hemorrhage as their indication for treatment. Patients in better condition prior to surgery did better overall. However, there is an increased risk from operation as

Table 1. Giant aneurysms: Results and locations (263 cases)

Location	Results				
	Excellent	Good	Poor	Death	Total
ACA	7	0	2	4	13
MCA	31	9	3	11	54
ICA	101	15	4	22	142
BAC	6	5	2	5	18
Vertebral	9	4	4	5	22
Other	10	1	0	3	14
Total	164	34	15	50	263

ACA anterior communicating artery, *MCA* middle cerebral artery, *ICA* internal carotid artery, *BAC* caput of the basilar artery

Table 2. Giant aneurysms: Results and preoperative grades (263 cases)

Botterell preop grade	Results				
	Excellent	Good	Poor	Death	Total
0	134	19	10	30	193
I	17	6	1	6	30
II	11	4	2	6	23
III	2	4	0	4	10
IV	0	1	2	4	7
Total	164	34	15	50	263

Table 3. Giant aneurysms: Results and treatment in 227 of the 263 cases

Treatment	Results				
	Excellent	Good	Poor	Death	Total
Proximal ligation	18	2	0	6	26
Simple trapping	6	5	3	1	15
Direct clipping	57	16	6	13	92
Direct clipping and thrombectomy	11	1	1	3	16
STA-MCA and proximal ligation	24	3	1	5	33
STA-MCA and SVG bypass	3	0	0	1	4
SVG and clipping	4	1	0	1	6
SVG and trapping	4	2	1	2	9
SVG and proximal ligation	5	1	1	5	12
Direct repair with vessel reconstruction	9	0	1	3	13
Other	1	0	0	0	1
Total	142	31	14	40	227

SVG saphenous vein graft

compared to a comparable group of saccular aneurysms.

Of 227 of the 263 cases, direct clipping was possible in 92 patients (40%), and in an additional 22 patients (10%) in conjunction with some type of bypass to protect during the period of temporary occlusion (Table 3). Excision of the aneurysm and microvascular reconstriction of the parent artery was accomplished in 13 patients (6%). One hundred patients (44%) required indirect methods of treatment with the sacrifice of the parent artery either by proximal ligation or trapping, with or without construction of a bypass.

Booster clips have become indispensable tools in the management of giant aneurysms (Table 4) [4].

We believe the following points should be adhered to for maximum safety in repairing giant aneurysms:
a) Temporarily occlude major vessels for aneurysm repair
b) Open the aneurysm prior to placing the clips, in order to relieve the tension of the sac, and remove thrombotic material from the base of the aneurysm that might be displaced into the lumen of the parent artery
c) Leave a small cuff of aneurysmal base between the proximal clip and the parent artery
d) Use as strong and heavy a primary clip as is available
e) Use clips in tandem where necessary
f) Check the adequacy of aneurysm repair by elevating blood pressure above normal levels

Table 4. Summary of aneurysm cases repaired using booster clips

Case no.	Age(yrs)	Sex	Date of surgery	Location of aneurysm	Indication for surgery[a]	Result
1	48	F	4-8-82	ICA	Mass effect	Excellent[b]
2	67	M	4-9-82	ACA	Mass effect	Excellent
3	36	F	6-2-82	ICA	Mass effect	Excellent
4	61	F	6-18-82	ICA	Mass effect	Good[c]
5	48	F	7-2-82	ICA	Mass effect	Excellent
6	78	F	7-21-82	ICA	Mass effect	Excellent
7	63	F	7-21-82	ICA	Mass effect	Excellent
8	53	F	8-10-82	ICA	Mass effect	Good
9	40	F	8-20-82	Basilar	Mass effect	Death
10	67	F	9-14-82	MCA	SAH, grade III	Good
11	52	M	10-12-82	MCA	Mass effect	Excellent
12	44	M	1-11-83	ACA	SAH, grade II	Excellent
13	60	F	2-8-83	ICA	Mass effect	Excellent
14	61	F	4-18-83	ICA	Mass effect	Excellent
15	51	F	2-14-83	ICA	SAH, grade I	Excellent
16	73	M	4-7-83	ICA	SAH, grade III	Death
17	37	M	4-13-83	ICA	Mass effect	Excellent
18	56	M	5-6-83	Basilar	SAH, grade II	Excellent
19	59	F	5-27-83	ICA	Mass effect	Excellent
20	50	F	5-24-83	ICA	Mass effect	Excellent

[a] Neurological grade is according to Botterell's classification
[b] No deficit
[c] Patient able to work, mild neurological deficit
ICA internal carotid artery, *ACA* anterior cerebral artery, *MCA* middle cerebral artery, *SAH* subarachnoid hemorrhage

g) Reinforce and clips that appear to be leaking or are precariously perched with one or more booster clips

h) Perform immediate postoperative angiography to verify patency of major and perforating vessels if any doubt about patency exists concerning clip placement.

References

1. Dolenc V (1983) Direct microsurgical repair of intracavernous vascular lesions. J Neurosurg 58:824–832

2. Sundt TM, Piepgras DG (1979) Surgical approach to giant intracranial aneurysms: Operative experience with 80 cases. J Neurosurg 51:731–742

3. Sundt TM (1982) Surgical technique for giant intracranial aneurysms. Neurosurg Rev 5:161–168

4. Sundt TM, et al. (1984) Booster clips for giant and thick-based aneurysms. J Neurosurg 60:751–762

5. Wiebers DO, et al. (1987) The significance of unruptured intracranial saccular aneurysms. J Neurosurg 66:23–30

6. Yaşargil MG, Fox JL (1975) The microsurgical approach to intracranial aneurysms. Surg Neurol 3:7–14

Surgical Treatment for Giant Intracranial Aneurysms

Satoru Fujiwara and Jiro Suzuki[1]

Introduction

Even today, amid significant developments in microsurgical techniques, the surgical results in cases of giant intracranial aneurysms are not satisfactory and there are many cases for which nothing but conservative therapy can be used. Over a period of 25 years, we have actively pursued a policy of surgical treatment for giant aneurysms whenever possible. In the present paper, we report the results of surgical treatment in our giant aneurysm cases and the surgical techniques which we currently use for such aneurysms at various sites in the cerebrum.

Materials and Results

Materials and Therapeutic Techniques

Between 1961 and 1986, we experienced a total of 82 cases of cerebral aneurysm in which the largest diameter of the aneurysm exceeded 2.5 cm. The location of these aneurysms were as follows: 42 (51.2%) on the internal carotid artery (ICA), 15 (18.3%) on the vertebrobasilar artery (VBA), 14 (17.1%) on the anterior communicating artery (AComA), nine (11.0%) on the middle cerebral artery (MCA), and two (2.4%) on the anterior cerebral artery (ACA; Table 1).

Surgical treatment was carried out in 63 of these cases, among which 38 were direct operations, 25 were carotid ligation and/or EC-IC bypass operations, and two were intravascular surgery. The remaining 17 cases were treated conservatively for various reasons (Table 2).

The surgical procedure for the direct operations included excision and neck ligation and/or clipping in 21 cases (12 AComA and ACA, five MCA, three VBA, and one ICA case), neck liga-

tion and/or clipping in 14 cases (eight ICA, three AComA, two VBA, and one MCA case). Unavoidably, trapping was done in three cases (one AComA, one MCA, and one VBA case; Table 3). On the other hand, among the ICA cases, there were 25 located at the infraclinoid or intracavernous portion of the ICA, excluding those on the intracranial bifurcation of the ICA or the internal carotid-posterior communicating (IC-PC) portion, which could not be reached for direct surgical therapy. In such cases we had previously performed ligation of the common carotid (CCA) and external carotid (ECA) arteries, but more recently we ligate the cervical

Table 1. Site distribution of giant aneurysm cases

Site	No. of cases
ICA	42 (51.2%)
AComA	14 (17.1%)
VBA	15 (18.3%)
MCA	9 (11.0%)
ACA	2 (2.4%)
Total	82

(Tohoku University, Sendai 1961–1986)
ICA internal carotid artery, *AComA* anterior communicating artery, *VBA* vertebrobasilar artery, *MCA* middle cerebral artery, *ACA* anterior cerebral artery

Table 2. Treatment for giant aneurysm

Treatment	No. of cases
Surgical	63
Direct operation	38
Carotid ligation and/or EC-IC bypass	25
Intravascular surgery	2
Nonsurgical	17
Total	82

EC-IC extracranial-intracranial

[1] Division of Neurosurgery, Institute of Brain Diseases, Tohoku University School of Medicine, Sendai, Japan

Table 3. Aneurysm site and operative procedure of directly operated cases

Site	Excision and neck ligation and/or clipping	Neck ligation and/or clipping	Trapping	Total
AComA, ACA	12	3	1	16
ICA	1	8	0	9
MCA	5	1	1	7
VBA	3	2	1	6
Total	21	14	3	38

AComA anterior communicating artery, *ACA* anterior cerebral artery, *ICA* internal carotid artery, *MCA* middle cerebral artery, *VBA* vertebrobasilar artery

Table 4. Indirectly operated cases of intracranial internal carotid giant aneurysms

Operative procedures	No. of cases	Results				
		Excellent	Good	Fair	Poor	Dead
CC & ECA ligation	13	8	1	0	0	4
ICA lig. & EC-IC bypass	12	5	4	1	0	2
Total	25	13 (52.0%)	5 (20.0%)	1 (4.0%)	0	6 (24.0%)

CC common carotid, *ECA* external carotid, *ICA* cervical internal carotid artery, *EC-IC* extracranial-intracranial

portion of the ICA and perform an EC-IC bypass operation. These techniques have been used in 13 and 12 cases, respectively (Table 4).

Therapeutic Results

For evaluation of the therapeutic results, a five-group classification was used. Patients who recovered to a normal state were classified as "excellent"; those with mild neurological deficits, but still fit for employment were "good"; those unsuitable for employment due to gait disturbances, psychiatric abnormalities, and/or aphasia, but capable of everyday living without assistance were "fair"; those in a bedridden state were "poor"; and "dead".

The results of directly operated cases at the time of discharge from hospital, grouped according to the operative procedures, are shown in Table 5. Overall, there were nine excellent, 12 good, four fair, and seven poor cases, as well as six deaths (the mortality was 15.8%). The results following aneurysm excision were superior to those following neck clipping only. In comparison with the results in AComA and ICA cases, those in MCA and particularly VBA cases were unfavorable (Table 6). Among the 25 inaccessible ICA giant aneurysms, the follow-up results after 2-12 years from surgery were 13

excellent, five good, one fair, and six dead (Table 4).

Case Presentations

Case 1. The patient was a 54-year-old male. Onset was due to subarachnoid hemorrhage from a giant aneurysm of the AComA. On admission, a round mass was seen at the optic chiasm in CT scans. Bifrontal craniotomy and a subfrontal and interhemishperic approach were used for aneurysm treatment. Under the administration of the Sendai Cocktail, temporary clips were applied to the bilateral A1 and A2 portions of the ACA (Fig. 1) and the aneurysm was excised without bleeding (Fig. 2). The aneurysmal neck was well-formed, so that it could be clipped and then wrapped with muscle pieces and Aron Alpha.

The patient was discharged in a good, rather than an excellent, condition due to the visual field disturbances which had been present preoperatively.

Case 2. The patient was a 62-year-old male. Onset was due to subarachnoid hemorrhage from a giant aneurysm of the AComA. Left carotid angiogram and CT scans showed a giant mass centering on the optic chiasm (Figs. 3, 4). As in case 1, a bifrontal interhemispheric approach was used. Under the administration of the Sendai

Table 5. Operative procedures and results at discharge

Procedures	No. of cases	Results				
		Excellent	Good	Fair	Poor	Dead
Excision and neck ligation and/or clipping	21	7	7	1	3	2
Neck ligation and/or clipping only	14	2	4	3	4	2
Trapping	3	0	1	0	0	2
Total	38	9 (23.7%)	12 (31.6%)	4 (10.5%)	7 (18.4%)	6 (15.8%)

Table 6. Sites and results of direct operation at discharge

Site	No. of cases	Results				
		Excellent	Good	Fair	Poor	Dead
AComA, ACA	16	4	7	3	0	2
ICA	9	5	1	1	0	2
MCA	7	0	3	0	3	1
VBA	6	0	1	0	4	1
Total	38	9 (23.7%)	12 (31.6%)	4 (10.5%)	7 (18.4%)	6 (15.8%)

AComA anterior communicating artery, *ACA* anterior cerebral artery, *ICA* internal carotid artery, *MCA* middle cerebral artery, *VBA* vertebrobasilar artery

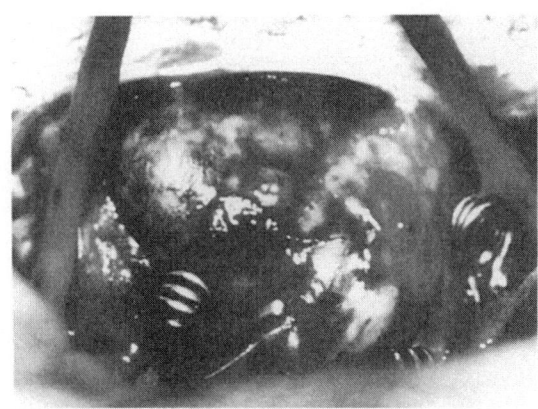

Fig. 1. Operative view of giant aneurysm at the anterior communicating artery of case 1. Four temporary clips were placed at bilateral A1 and A2 under administration of the Sendai Cocktail

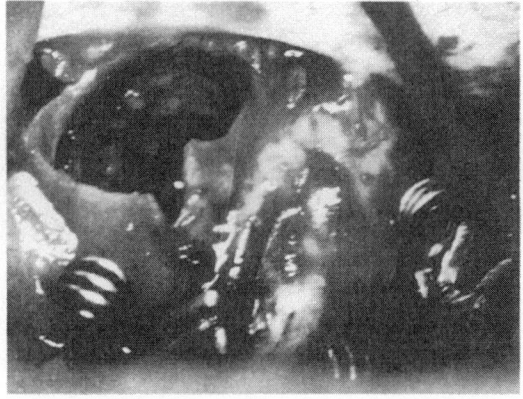

Fig. 2. The same case as Fig. 1. Aneurysm was excised in an entirely dry field

Cocktail, the aneurysm was excised, but the neck of the aneurysm was not able to be preserved. Since the left A1-A2 junction was severed, the Sendai Cocktail was again administered and A1-A2 anastomosis was immediately performed.

The patient had no notable neurological deficits after surgery and, in postoperative angiograms, the blood flow around the affected region was found to be good (Fig. 5). He was discharged in excellent condition.

Case 3. The patient was a 55-year-old female who had a giant aneurysm with a maximal diameter of 2.5 cm on the left MCA. Using a left frontal craniotomy, the Sylvian fissure was dissected enough and, under the administration of the Sendai cocktail, temporary clips were applied to the left M1 and M2 regions. The dome of the aneurysm, which was hidden beneath the sphenoid ridge, was dissected and exposed (Fig. 6). Since the walls of the parent artery and the

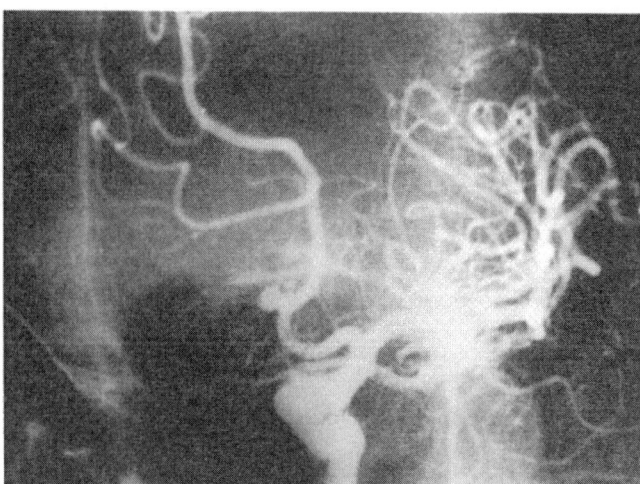

Fig. 3. Left carotid angiogram of case 2. The anterior cerebral artery was curved by a giant mass at the chiasmal region

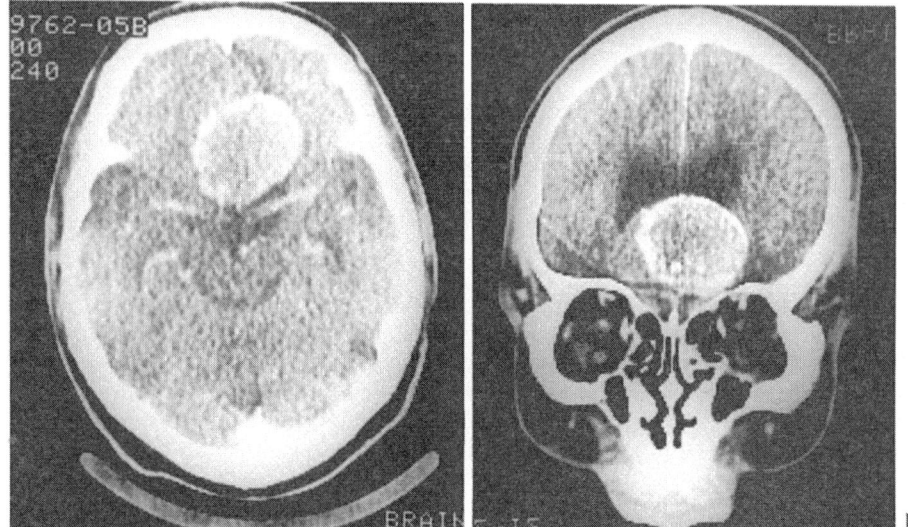

Fig. 4. a Enhanced axial and **b** coronal CT of case 2

aneurysmal neck were nonsclerotic and soft, it was possible to ligate and place a clip on the aneurysmal neck (Fig. 7). Due to mild paresis present preoperatively, she was discharged in good condition.

Case 4. Onset of the disease in this 32-year-old female was convulsive attacks due to a giant aneurysm of the right MCA. CT scans on admission showed a huge bilobular mass which was calcified and occupied the right middle fossa (Fig. 8). Angiograms revealed a cerebral aneurysm with distinct lumen (Fig. 9a). We decided that detachable balloon technique rather than the direct operation was indicated for the following reasons: (a) the aneurysm was large enough to fill the middle fossa; (b) there was

severe calcification of the aneurysmal. wall; (c) massive thrombi were present within the lumens of the aneurysm; and (d) the patient was neurologically intact. In a two-phase operation, occlusion of the lumen was achieved using a balloon (Fig. 9b). The patient was discharged in excellent condition.

Case 5. The patient was a 59-year-old female. Onset was due to subarachnoid hemorrhage from a giant aneurysm of the basilar artery. In CT scans, a 2.5 cm in diameter mass compressing the midbrain was seen (Fig. 10). It was considered that, at surgery, first a huge dome would appear in the operative field and hinder the identification of the parent artery: as a consequence, excision of the aneurysm and treatment of the

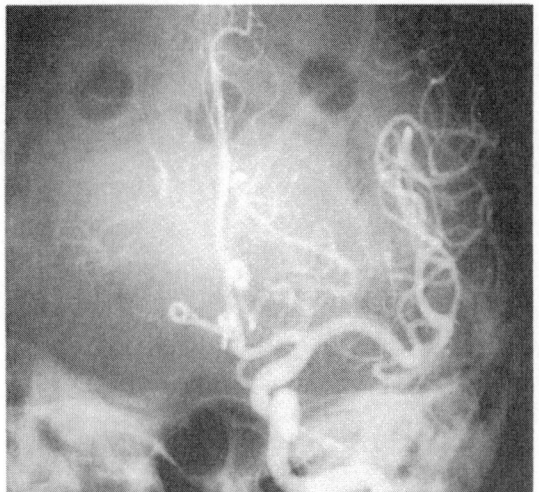

Fig. 5. Postoperative left carotid angiogram of case 2. Blood flow of the A2 of the left anterior cerebral artery was preserved after A1–A2 anastomosis

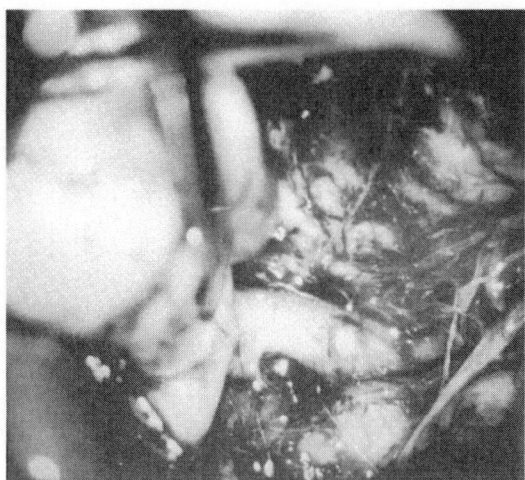

Fig. 6. Operative view of case 3. The dome of the aneurysm, which hid beneath the sphenoid ridge, was dissected and exposed safely by means of temporary clips placed on left M1 and M2

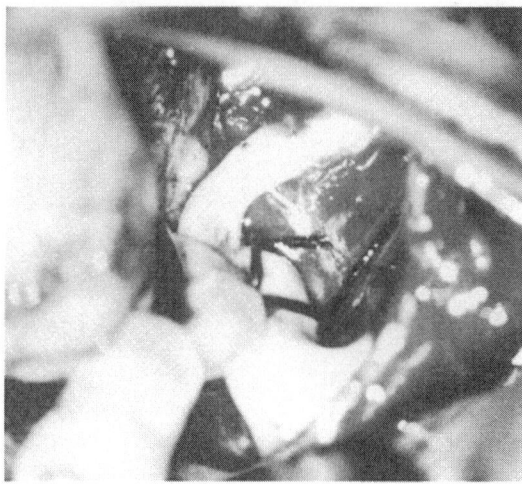

Fig. 7. The same case as Fig. 6. Ligation and clipping of the neck of MCA giant aneurysm

neck would be deemed impossible and treatment with a detachable balloon should be selected. Using the balloon Matas' test under the administration of the Sendai Cocktail, it was possible to occlude temporarily the basilar top region without producing any symptoms. The radical operation was then completed with the balloon in place. As anticipated, identification of the parent artery at surgery was difficult due to the aneurysm itself (Fig. 11a), but, by means of temporary occlusion of the basilar artery due to balloon inflation, excision of the aneurysm and neck clipping were completed in an entirely dry operative field (Fig. 11b). The patient was discharged in excellent condition.

Discussion

It is often necessary to abandon the possibility of performing direct surgery on giant intracranial aneurysms, not only because of their unusual size, but also due to their locations, the difficulty of neck treatment, the frequency of calcification of the aneurysmal walls, and other characteristic features. When direct operation is not possible, the second choice therapy (carotid ligation) or conservative therapy must be employed.

As demonstrated from our results, the mortality rate of direct operations on giant aneurysms was 15.8%, which is at the same level as the average rate (15.5%–20.0%) of major series reported by various institutes [1–8]. It should be noted, however, that, in comparison with a mortality rate of only 5% in the 2000 cases of usual-sized aneurysms in which we have performed direct surgery, the mortality rate in cases of direct surgery on giant aneurysms is high and indicates the extreme difficulty of their treatment. In contrast, the results were surprisingly good for cases in which carotid ligation has been performed for ICA aneurysms at infraclinoid or intracavernous sites which cannot be approached. The mortality rate was particularly low for cases in which superficial temporal artery-middle cerebral artery (STA-MCA) anastomosis was also done.

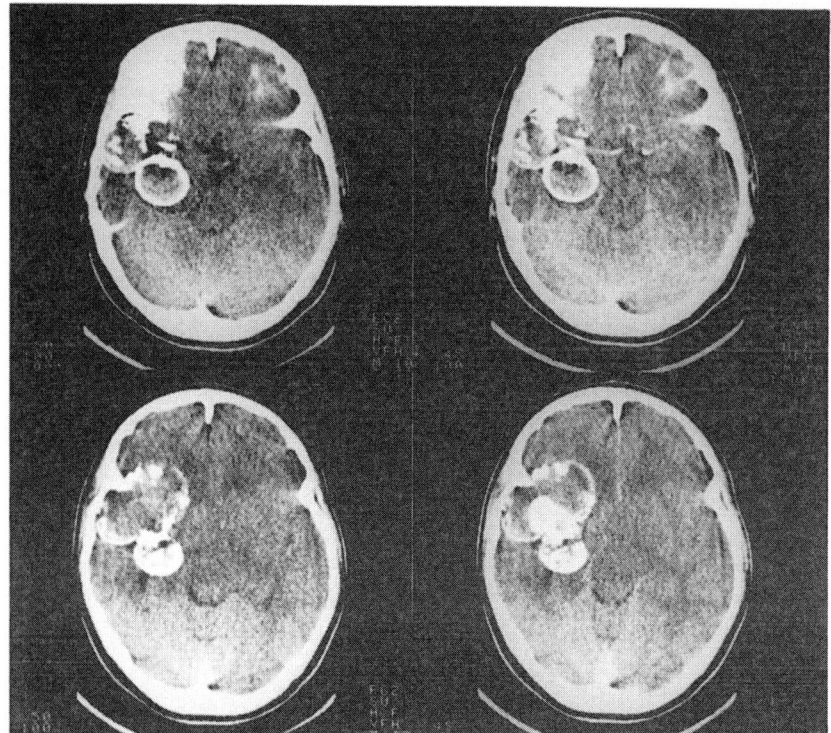

Fig. 8. Enhanced serial axial CT of case 4. A huge bilobular mass with enhanced lumens occupied the left middle fossa were depicted

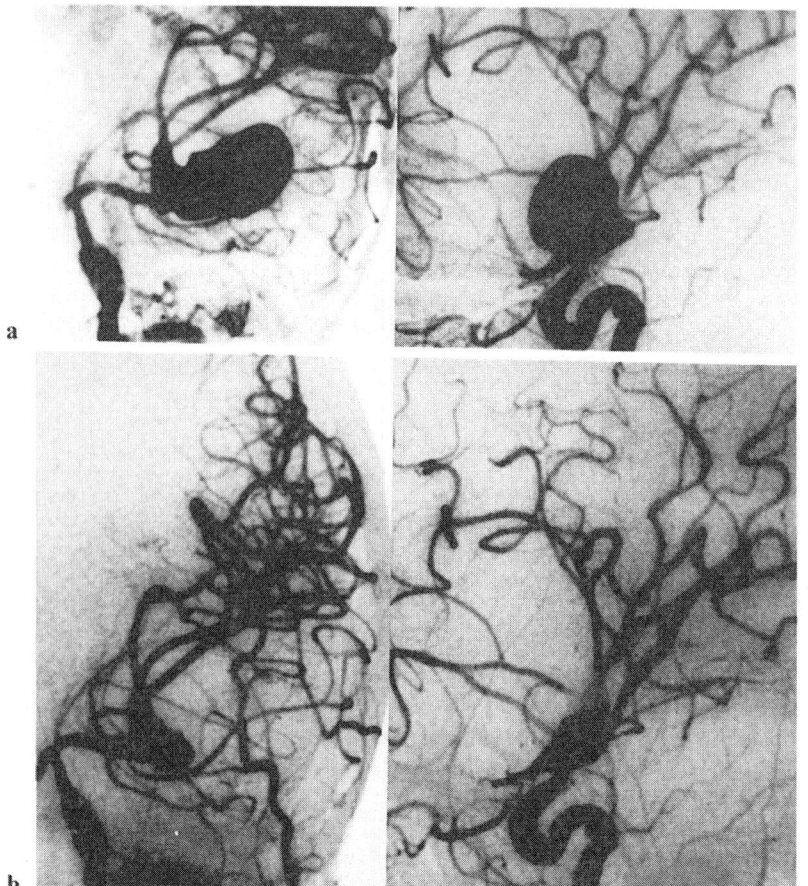

a

b

Fig. 9a, b. Left carotid angiogram of case 4 **a** before and **b** after detachable balloon techniques

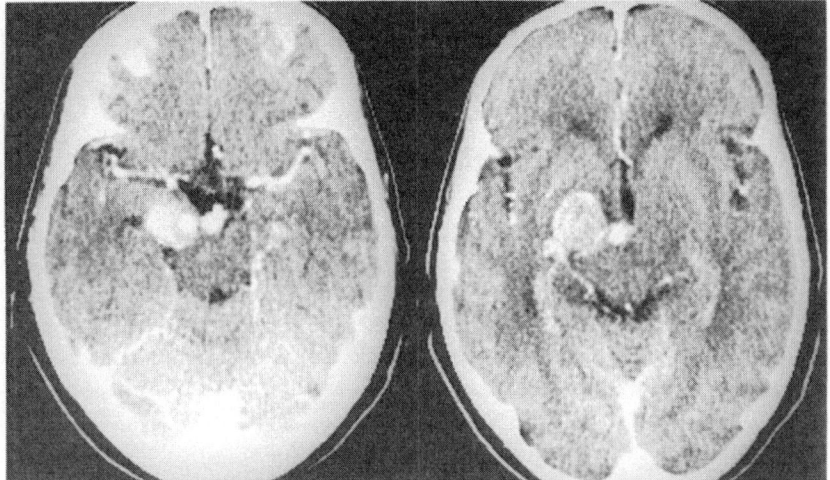

Fig. 10. Enhanced serial axial CT of case 5

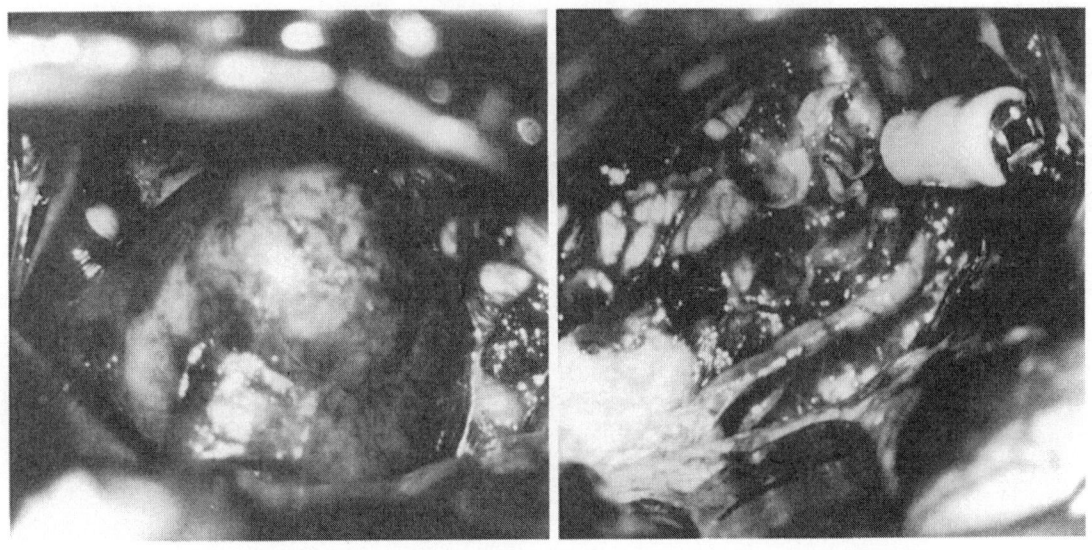

a

b

Fig. 11a, b. Operative view of case 5. **a** Just after retraction of the temporal base. The parent artery and the neck could not be identified because of a big dome of the basilar top giant aneurysm. **b** Excision of the aneurysm and clipping of the neck were successful

As introduced in the presentation of the five cases above, we have adopted the following fundamental guidelines of the treatment for giant aneurysms.

For giant aneurysms of the ICA, direct operation should be done if the parent artery can be identified and the aneurysm neck is distinct, as in cases where the aneurysm is located on the internal carotid bifurcation (ICB) portion or for some aneurysms on the IC-PC or IC-ophthalmic portions. For aneurysms located at inaccessible sites on the infraclinoid and intracavernous portions, gradual occlusion of the cervical ICA and

STA-MCA double anastomosis should be done under the administration of the Sendai Cocktail. Using this technique, satisfactory results can normally be obtained. It should be noted, however, that although the improvement of symptoms due to the aneurysm mass can be achieved in this way, it is rare that all symptoms disappear and it is necessary to do follow-up CT studies to determine whether or not the lumen of the aneurysm has been occluded. From now, the detachable balloon technique will be adapted for treatment of aneurysms at these sites.

For giant aneurysms of the AComA, the

aneurysmal mass should be completely dissected from the optic chiasm and then excised. For this purpose a bifrontal, interhemisperic approach should be used and, under the administration of the Sendai Cocktail, temporary clips must then be applied to the bilateral A1 and A2 portions. By this way, direct surgery can be carried out in almost all cases.

In most giant aneurysms of the MCA, where the aneurysm is nonsclerotic and of a "medium" size (2.5–3.0 cm in diameter), it is normally possible to put temporary clips on the M1 and M2 portions, dissect the aneurysm from surrounding tissues, and then treat the neck region. In such cases, direct operation is recommended. When, however, the aneurysm is "huge" (greater than 4.0 cm in diameter) and fills the middle fossa, or shows a massive thrombus within the aneurysmal lumen, such as serpentine aneurysm, severe calcification of the aneurysmal walls, or sclerosis of the neck, there is a danger of neck occlusion or the inability to treat the aneurysmal neck region, even if direct operation were done and the mass successfully excised. Postoperatively, severe paresis and morbidity may therefore be present. In such cases, direct operation should not be pursued, but rather treatment with a detachable balloon should be performed.

Finally, in the case of VBA giant aneurysms, it is not possible to excise safely the aneurysm since the first big dome of aneurysm occupies the operative field and the parent artery and aneurysmal neck cannot be identified or treated. There occasionally occurs a fortunate case of VBA giant aneurysm, such as in our case 5 above, but the mortality rate of our own cases of giant VBA aneurysms which have undergone direct operations has been 16.7% and, in the literature [1, 7, 8], mortality rates around 20% have been reported. As a consequence, we believe that the detachable balloon technique is indicated in such cases.

Conclusion

We have discussed the operative results which we have obtained in the treatment of our 82 cases of giant intracranial aneurysm. We have found that different therapeutic methods and surgical techniques should be used for giant aneurysms at various cerebral sites and with various characteristics.

References

1. Drake CG (1979) Giant intracranial aneurysms: Experience with surgical treatment in 174 patients. Clin Neurosurg 26:12–95
2. Heros RC, Nelson PB, Ojemann RG, et al. (1983) Large and paraclinoid aneurysms: Surgical techniques, complications, and results. Neurosurgery 12:153–163
3. Hosobuchi Y (1979) Direct surgical treatment of giant intracranial aneurysms. J Neurosurg 51:743–756
4. Kodama N, Suzuki J (1982) Surgical treatment of giant aneurysms. Neurosurg Rev 5:155–160
5. Onuma T, Suzuki J (1979) Surgical treatment of giant intracranial aneurysms. J Neurosurg 51:33–36
6. Sundt TM Jr, Piepgras DG (1979) Surgical approach to giant intracranial aneurysms. Operative experience with 80 cases. J Neurosurg 51:731–742
7. Symon L, Vajda J (1984) Surgical experiences with giant intracranial aneurysms. J Neurosurg 61:1009–1028
8. Whittle IR, Dorsch NW, Besser M (1984) Giant intracranial aneurysms: Diagnosis, management, and outcome. Surg Neurol 21:218–230

Discussion

Symon (London): What is the best form of bypass to use if during an operation a difficult circumstance arises, such as an aneurysm that cannot be clipped or controlled directly?

Flamm (New York): I have never had to perform a bypass on an emergency basis after a major problem has occurred, either because of good fortune or planning to do it ahead of time. If one is at all concerned that the need for it may arise during the course of an operation, it probably should be done before dealing with the aneurysm.

Peerless (Ontario): We have met with this circumstance, but we usually have the patient worked up sufficiently to know that a bypass may become necessary. But in every case, the flap and the superficial temporal artery at the edge of the flap are prepared. The right leg is also prepared and draped so that the saphenous vein can be taken out when an emergency occur. I cannot recall how many times we have had to do this, but most often the circumstance was that the aneurysm was exposed and it was decided that a proximal ligation was the only possibility, particularly in the case of a middle cerebral artery aneurysm or distal carotid aneurysm. The bypass was then put into place and a tourniquet or similar proximal occluding device prepared for eventual occlusion after we were sure that the bypass was open. I think that every time one of these aneurysms is managed in the anterior circulation, this eventuality should be reckoned with; it is the one time when a bypass can save the situation. In the posterior circulation, we have considerable doubt that a bypass is often necessary, although again we preserve the posterior branch of the superficial temporal artery for such an eventuality.

Symon: What you have just said avoids a circumstance where the artery has to be acutely occluded: You would say that you apply the tourniquet and then let the bypass open. However, if a high-flow bypass is required would you use a middle cerebral superficial temporal anastamosis or would you use a high-flow vein bypass?

Peerless: I think this depends on the particular situation. With middle cerebral artery aneurysms, it is very often one major branch of the artery that is at greatest risk and so we would bypass on it and as proximal to it as possible. If, however, the aneurysm is more proximal and all the branches of the middle cerebral artery are at risk we would be more likely to use a vein bypass to a more proximal vessel. I think that the more proximal the aneurysm, the greater the area that needs to be irrigated and so a high-flow shunt is more likely to be necessary.

Flamm: My largest experience with bypass for middle cerebral artery aneurysms was in a group of patient with mycotic aneurysms. In these cases, we went on the distal branch from which the aneurysm arose, performed the bypass, and then resected the aneurysm and the parent vessel. This worked well but only because it was distal and we were only supplying a particular branch beyond the bifurcation of the middle cerebral artery.

Symon: There is a good deal of evidence now which could suggest that the cortical branches of the middle cerebral artery, particularly in giant aneurysms, are not seriously at risk because of the adequacy of the leptomeningeal collaterals. It seems to be more the deep circulation of the middle cerebral artery that is a cause of concern. A point I would like to make concerns the safety of temporary occlusion of major arteries. How long would the panelists be prepared to do this? Some of us may be rather less convinced than the evidence from the multiple vascular occlusion model in the dog would suggest.

Peerless: Temporary proximal occlusion has been carried out in Toronto for about 35 years with the protection of mannitol only. I have always felt that it is a useful procedure. Dr. Drake and I have used it quite frequently over the past 4 or 5 years with mannitol. There is no doubt that it is an important part of the technology and for some aneurysms it is the only way they can be dealt with. Unfortunately, if basilar bifurcation or superior cerebellar artery aneurysms are of giant size there usually is not enough room to get a proximal clip into place. Under those circumstances, we have always fallen back on deep hypotension.

Flamm: I certainly use this procedure, increasingly so in recent years. I use low-pressure closing clips intermittently, putting them on for a couple of minutes and then removing them. The patient's blood pressure is usually raised when the clip is on and I make no attempt to lower it, so that we can make use of whatever collateral we can get. A word of caution is calld for here with regard to large aneurysms: If the aneurysm is opened when the temporary clips are on it is advisable to back-bleed through the parent vessel before opening the circulation, because otherwise an air embolus may be created distally in the arterial circulation.

Symon: Yes, this is an important which should be clearly stated: The distal clip should always be removed first. Dr. Marsh and Dr. Sundt use temporary clips quite a lot, how do you feel about them at the Mayo Clinic?

Marsh (Rochester): Yes, I believe that with middle cerebral aneurysms for example with no bypass in place, he will leave them on for no more than 8–10 min. With more proximal aneurysms on the internal carotid, intraoperative blood flow measurements are carried out in almost every case. If the measured blood flow at surgery is low and there is concern after inspection of the aneurysm that a more prolonged period of temporary occlusion is likely, or that there is a higher probability that this will not be a clippable aneurysm, then a bypass is put in place, either with the temporal artery if it is of good caliber or with a leg vein. The procedure is then carried out: If the aneurysm does in fact turn out to be clippable, fine; if not, the surgeon is well prepared for the other eventuality.

Giombini (Milan): I would like to know something more about the natural history of giant aneurysms. Dr. Peerless has told us that basilar bifurcation giant aneurysms have a very bad prognosis. I would be interested to hear, however,

about giant aneurysms at other sites because we often receive patients with little complaints concerning their aneurysm. If we consider that poor results are about 20%–25% and the natural history of normal aneurysms has a 1%–2% mortality per year, a big gap is seen between the two figures.

My second question concerns the fact that there are many different policies with respect to handling giant aneurysms. Should a decision about the best technique be made case by case or would it be possible to establish a standard or adjustable protocol? Should every case first be embolized, treated with a detachable balloon, or first explored?

Symon: I think that with the natural history question we will acquire more information on this as more and more patients are CT scanned for incidental data. Most of us are dealing with patients who present with neurological symptoms, otherwise they would not have come to us. The patients we receive at the National Hospital, Queen's Square have advanced neurological symptoms since the neurologists have a habit of protecting patients from surgery until they are quite certain that the situation is deteriorating. So we are in no doubt that with the aneurysms we operate on surgery is in fact indicated unless the morbidity and mortality would strongly appear to militate against this. There are a number of cases with giant top basilar aneurysms that have been discovered incidentally. I can think of two cases in which this occurred and I had to leave them alone because I did not feel that I could attack them safely.

With regard to your second question, several of our panelists did address this. It is clear that where you have a service where all the capacity for dealing with aneurysms is available, including intravascular methods, then the proper thing to do is to tailor the therapy to each individual aneurysm.

Marsh: In a recent paper from the Mayo Clinic in the Journal of Neurosurgery, the natural history of unruptured aneurysms is discussed in 130 patients. In those patients, 151 aneurysms were identified, 21 of which were symptomatic only by virtue of mass effect; six of those were 15–25 mm but the majority were over 25 mm and classified as giant. None of those patients underwent surgery, but nine eventually went on to develop hemorrhage, the mean time to hemorrhage being of the order of 4 years. The mean size at rupture in that group was almost 22 mm. Though not exactly clear, the inference was that the likelihood of rupture increased with size; particularly for the large aneurysms this becomes symptomatic by virtue of mass and operation should be strongly considered. The question of how to deal with a truly incidentally discovered giant aneurysm is rather more problematic. The decision there would rest I feel on an honest assessment of the anatomy and the capabilities of the surgeon.

Peerless: We are at present following up a group of patients who either refused operation or because the aneurysm was discovered entirely incidentally we did not push to operate. I have shown you the data from the patients with aneurysms of the basilar bifurcation and these were explored only; the patients were symptomatic and did very poorly. It may well be that there is a quiescent stage of giant aneurysms where the patients do well for a long period of time. We have almost 200 of these patients on our files and hope to have these data published by the end of the year.

The site of the aneurysm plays a major role here. In the past year for example two of our patients have died as a result of giant aneurysm, having refused operation the previous year. One of these was a nondominant middle cerebral artery aneurysm that had quadrupled in size from just over 2.5 cm to over 5 cm in diameter; the patient died of the mass effect without ever having bled.

With respect to standard therapy, there certainly is no standard therapy for giant aneurysms: It would be wrong for the surgeon to approach these aneurysms with only one or two methods at his disposal. At some sites where we could earlier have used the clip, we would now tend to use other methods.

Auer (Graz): In the recent literature, it has become clear that large and giant aneurysms rupture more than we had previously thought. Does this knowledge influence your decision in cases like Dr. Peerless has just described?

Symon: I suppose it must do really; it indicates that we should not leave such aneurysms untreated.

Flamm: I think this has already been answered by Drs. Marsh and Peerless. I would only add that here with aneurysms we are not dealing with cancer; the outcome is not inevitable. As Dr. Marsh said, the surgeon has to consider seriously what the chances are in his hands of a good result as against the natural history. I do not think that every aneurysm should be operated on.

Symon: Yes, I think here that the decision for and against operation depends upon a balanced assessment upon the experience and technology available and on one's balanced assessment of the risks the patient faces.

Commentator, *Steiner* (Stockholm): This session has convincingly demonstrated that the management of giant aneurysms is one of the highlights in the ongoing renaissance in neurosurgery today. The prognosis in untreated partially thrombosed giant aneurysms is poor due to hemorrhage, mass effect, and thromboembolism. This justifies all efforts to achieve a definite cure; therefore, closure of the neck of the aneurysm by surgical or nonsurgical methods should always be tried. Nevertheless, surgery is carried out in 30%–70% of cases with a mortality of 15%–50%. The parameters of the aneurysm, patient, and surgeon limit the use of surgery. The surgeon should use the safest method for the patient, which may not necessarily be the most prestigious technique. The steady improvement in microsurgery and the development of surgical and nonsurgical techniques makes any forecast for the future management of giant aneurysms a little risky. However, it is not wishful thinking I believe to say that the present limitations of the scope and achievement of the surgeon in giant aneurysms will be overcome.

RTD 13. Revascularization in Acute Stage of Cerebral Infarction

Revascularization in the Acute Stage of Cerebral Ischemia

Past Experience, Present Attitude

P. Schmiedek[1]

Soon after extra-intracranial bypass surgery was introduced into clinical practice, its potential usefulness in the situation of acute ischemia was suggested. Over the following years, however, the main indication for cerebral revascularization then became chronic brain ischemia, whereas emergency cerebral revascularization remained a matter of controversy. In fact, in contrast to the many thousand patients who underwent extra-intracranial bypass surgery in order to prevent the development of future ischemic events, only a few series have been published on acute cerebral revascularization, with the total number of cases being in the range of little over 100 operated patients. Most of these underwent extraintracranial bypass surgery: some also had acute middle cerebral artery embolectomy [1, 3, 6, 8]. Among the various reasons to explain this obvious discrepancy is the fact that acute brain ischemia is only rarely being seen immediately following its onset. This is necessary to consider any form of surgical intervention. Furthermore, even in those patients who could be operated on within a reasonable time period (6–8 h after the onset of ischemia), the postoperative results which have been reported over the years were not good enough to recommend it as a standard treatment. While overall good results were obtained in two-thirds of the patients, the remaining ones did poorly or died following surgery. With the introduction of new diagnostic possibilities for brain imaging, and also with the use of potentially beneficial treatment modalities to extend the reversibility of brain ischemia, it seems to be justified and also necessary to continue the consideration of emergency cerebral revascularization in the treatment of acute brain ischemia [9]. In this report, summary of our own experience with extra-intracranial bypass surgery in acute brain ischemia will be presented and more recent illustrative case reports will be given to outline the various problems which may arise when emergency revascularization is considered in clinical practice.

Previous Experience With Acute Bypass Surgery

Our first series of acute bypass surgery included seven patients who interwent surgery within 4–24 h following the onset of ischemia [4]. All patients presented with either spontaneous occlusion of cerebral vessels or, subsequent to complicated neurosurgical procedures, with intraoperative arterial occlusion. Five of the seven patients died postoperatively and the remaining two had severe neurologic deficits. Based on these poor results, it was concluded at that time that patients with acute brain ischemia were no candidates for cerebral revascularization. Autopsy findings in two of these patients showing considerable brain swelling were thought to indicate that the ischemic process might have even been aggravated by the anastomotic blood flow to the brain. This series of acute bypass surgery was not only the first one to be reported in the literature; it was also, when compared with subsequent series by others, the one with the highest mortality by far. Retrospectively, however, it should be noted that all of these patients were operated on when CT scanning of the brain was not yet available. Moreover, these patients underwent surgery at a time when this procedure had just been introduced in clinical practice. It still was a time consuming operation, and was not yet the standard procedure which it later on became with the experience gained from numerous operated cases of chronic cerebrovascular disease.

In 1980, another series was started, which included seven patients [7]. All of these patients had spontaneous occlusion of cerebral vessels and underwent extra-intracranial bypass surgery

---

[1] Department of Neurosurgery, Klinikum Grosshadern, University of Munich, Munich, Federal Republic of Germany

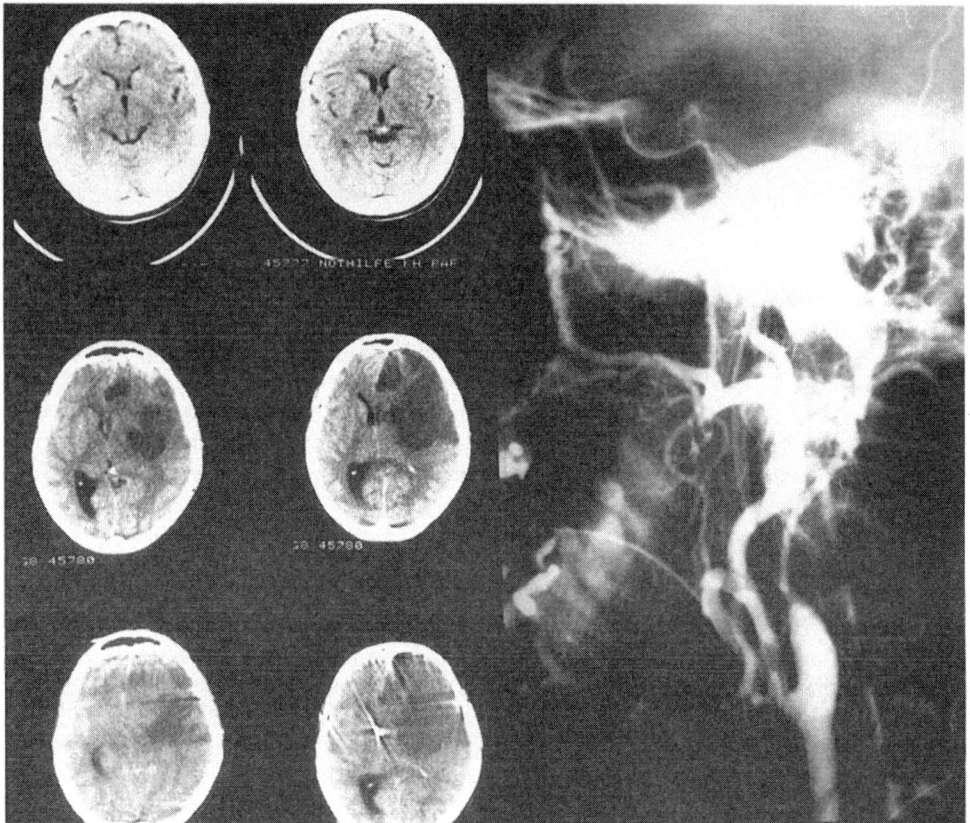

Fig. 1. Acute cerebral ischemia. Case example of suspected traumatic occlusion of internal carotid artery

within 7–24 h following the initial development of ischemic deficits. The postoperative results in this series were considerably better. Three patients had a delayed good improvement of preoperative neurologic deficits, three patients improved postoperatively to some extent, although this could not be definitly attributed to the bypass operation, and only one patient died. However, even with this experience, it was thought that the problems related to acute cerebral revascularization were still too many to encourage its use. The main argument against acute cerebral revascularization is our still incomplete knowledge with regard to the underlying pathophysiological process causing cerebral ischemia and, moreover, our as yet unsatisfactory ability to predict the individual prognosis in a patient with acute brain ischemia. In contrast to a patient where a large cerbral artery has to be occluded intraoperatively, and where, if untreated, a definite and permanent neurologic deficit has to be expected postoperatively, the situation is different in those cases with spontaneous thrombotic or embolic cerebrovascular

occlusion [6]. In these patients, the natural prognosis of the disease includes a large spectrum, ranging from complete recovery without any treatment to death despite all medical or surgical attempts to protect the brain. Following this experience, we have not operated on any further cases with acute brain ischemia, not because we think that it is contraindicated but rather because we feel unable to determine with sufficient accuracy the appropriate candidate for this treatment.

The following three cases reports illustrate our still ambigous attitude toward acute brain revascularization.

Case 1

This was a 43-year-old female who had a car accident, suffered a whiplash injury, and was admitted to another hospital. She was discharged in good condition 24 h later. One week later, she gradually developed a left-sided weakness. A CT scan was done and was found to be normal. Over the next 24 h her neurologic deficits progressed to left hemiplegia and she became stuporous. Another CT scan was done which now showed definite signs of brain ischemia in her right hemisphere. Right carotid angiography was done which demonstrated an occlusion of her internal carotid artery. In view of her history, it was thought to be related to the injury which she had suffered one week earlier. Brain revascularization at this stage seemed to be not indicated and, despite medical treatment, she died after only 24 h from severely elevated intracranial pressure (Fig. 1).

Case 2

This 52-year-old patient underwent cardiac catheterization for suspected heart disease. At the end of the procedure, sudden onset of a left-sided hemisparesis was noted. Three hours later, a CT scan was done, showing only a suspicious area of beginning hypodensity on the right side. With her neurologic deficits still unchanged, a right carotid angiography was performed 6 h after the onset of brain ischemia. However, angiographic findings were negative and this was interpreted as due to spontaneous revascularization of embolic cerebrovascular occlusion. The CT scan was repeated 2 h later and showed a small hemorrhegic lesion in her right hemisphere. Subsequently, her neurologic deficits did not show any significant improvement and on a CT scan 3 weeks later, brain infarction was found (Fig. 2).

Case 3

This 43-year-old patient was admitted following acute subarachnoid hemorrhage in a Hunt-Hess grade II condition. Angiography revealed an anterior communicating aneurysm, which was uneventfully clipped the next day. His postoperative course was good until 13 days following his hemorrhage, when he developed a left-sided hemiparesis. At this time, his transcranial Doppler flow values were rising, suggesting the occurence of postoperative vasospasm. His neurologic condition worsened and right carotid angiography was done, revealing extreme arterial narrowing with almost no intracranial vascular filling. He was immediately brought to the intensive care unit and hypertensive hypervolemic treatment was initiated and continued for the next 10 days. The patient recovered well and was discharged in good condition 4 weeks later. On control angiography his cerebral vasculature appeared to be normal (Fig. 3).

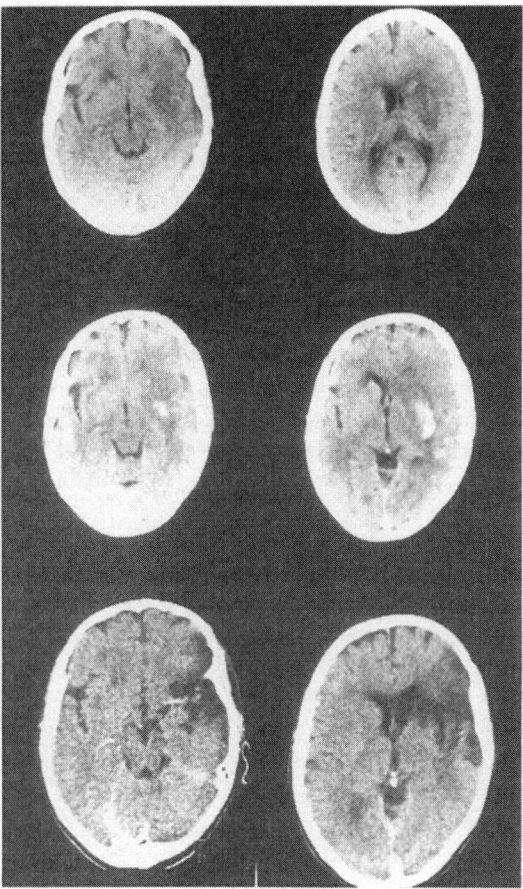

Fig. 2. Acute cerebral ischemia. Case example of spontaneous revascularization following embolic cerebrovascular occlusive disease

Comments

All of these three patients would have qualified as candidates for emergency revascularization.

In the case of the first patient, the diagnosis was made too late. Although it remains speculative, extra-intracranial bypass surgery might have prevented her fatal outcome had the diagnosis been made 24 h earlier. This then illustrates the necessity to obtain immediate diagnostic studies in patients with suspected cerebrovasculr occlusive disease. It also shows that it is necessary to train our colleagues to be aware that emergency revascularization is another therapeutic possibility which certainly does have an alternative value when compared to other forms of treatment.

The second case is an example of the real dilemma of emergency revascularization. This patient, with suspected embolic cerebrovascular occlusion, had cerebral angiography within the 6 h time period following onset of ischemic symptoms. Emergency embolectomy was already planned. However, she had a normal angiogram, and it was thought that spontaneous revascularization had taken place in the meantime. She nevertheless had a permanent neurologic deficit. Moreover, she also developed a hemorrhagic brain lesion. In this case, we have an example of natural emergency revascularization and it is hard to imagine that the result of a surgical revascularization procedure would have been considerably better. From the last case, the lesson to be learned is that, in cerebral vasospasm, emergency revascularization is possibly not the treatment of choice, although this had been suggested recently [2]. Cerebral vasospasm is, by its nature, a transient phenomenon, and all measures should be used before taking surgery, which is a permanent therapeutic measure, into consideration.

In conclusion, in spite of the progress which had been made with regard to new diagnostic possibilities, and despite the introduction of agents to extend the reversibility of brain ischemia, the role of emergency revascularization remains controversial. Since it is difficult to imagine arriving at a definite solution of this problem in the near future, it can only be hoped that, from continuing experience with its use in carefully selected cases, more evidence will acummulate to improve this present state of uncertainty.

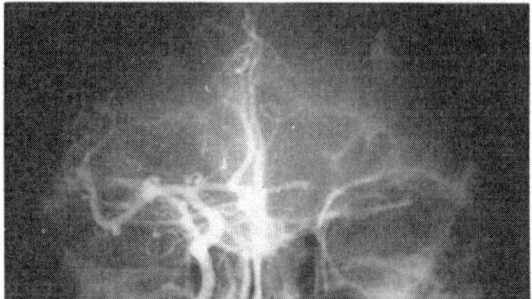
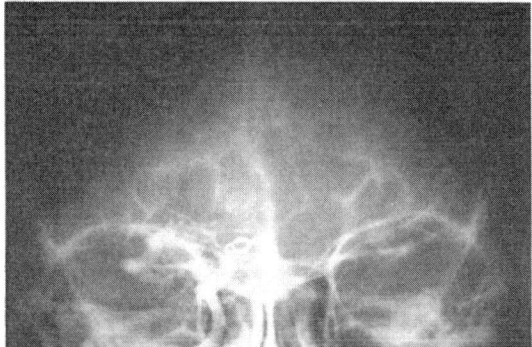
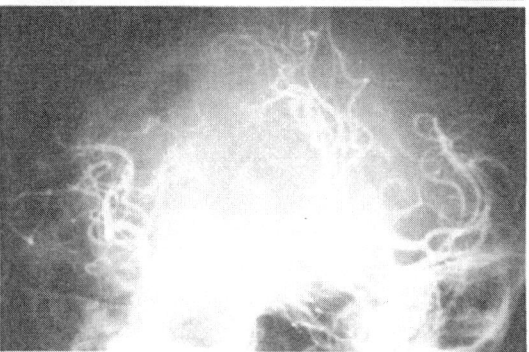

Fig. 3. Acute cerebral ischemia due to severe vasospasm following subarachnoid hemorrhage

References

1. Batjer H, Mickey B, Samson D (1986) Potential roles for early revascularization in patients with acute cerebral ischemia. Neurosurgery 18(3):283–291
2. Batjer H, Samson D (1986) Use of extra-intracranial bypass in the management of symptomatic vasospasm. Neurosurgery 19(2):235–245
3. Diaz FG, Ausman JI, Mehta B, et al. (1985) Acute cerebral revascularization. J Neurosurg 63:200–209
4. Gratzl O, Schmiedek P, Spetzler R, Steinhoff H, Marguth F (1976) Clinical experience with extra-intracranial arterial anastomosis in 65 cases. J Neurosurg 44:313–324
5. Lawner PM, Simeone FA (1979) Treatment of intraoperative cerebral artery occlusion with pentobarbital and extra-intracranial bypass: Case report. J Neurosurg 51:710–712
6. Meyer FB, Piepgras DG, Sundt T, Yanaqihara T (1985) Emergency embolectomy for acute occlusion of the middle cerebral artery. J Neurosurg 62:639–647
7. Schmiedek P, Gratzl O, Olteanu-Nerbe V, Marguth F (1985) Clinical experience with EC-IC arterial bypass surgery in acute cerebral ischemia. In: Handa CR, Kikuchi H, Yonekawa Y (eds) Microsurgical anastomoses for cerebral ischemia. Igaku-Shoin, New York, pp 36–40
8. Suzuki J, Yoshimoto T, Kodama N, Sakurai Y, Ogawa A (1982) A new therapeutic method for acute brain infarction: Revascularization following the administration of mannitol and perfluorochemicals–A preliminary report. Surg Neurol 17:325–332
9. Suzuki, J (1987) Treatment of cerebral infarction: Experimental and clinical study. Springer, Vienna

Revascularization in the Acute State of Cerebral Ischemia

Fernando G. Diaz, James I. Ausman, and Manuel Dujovny[1]

Large numbers of people are affected throughout the world by the development of cerebral ischemic infarcts every year. Seventy percent of these events are caused by occlusive lesions, most of which are not directly accessible by surgical means. It has been suggested by Astrup [1] that a period of grace exists during which the presence of cerebral ischemia is not followed by the development of cell death, as long as the perfusion to the ischemic tissue is reestablished. The major concern voiced by most physicians regarding the possibility of reperfusing the acutely ischemic brain has been the potential for the development of a hemorrhagic infarction in the area of ischemia [4, 5, 20].

Cerebral revascularization has been tried experimentally on several occasions [3, 4, 6, 20], mostly with favorable results. In most early animal experiments, when the ischemic brain was reperfused without any medical pretreatment, it was observed that the animals were able to tolerate regional cerebral ischemia for as long as 4–6 h [4, 6, 20]. In most of these reports, the reestablishment of cerebral perfusion was followed by the recovery of neurological function. We believe this is possible since the ischemic brain can tolerate a profound drop in cerebral perfusion down to 15 ml of blood per 100 g of tissue per minute without losing cellular integrity [1, 9, 13, 24]. There is a total or partial cessation of electrical function, but the cell retains the capacity to return to a normal level of activity as long as it is reperfused [13, 24].

A major problem in the clinical setting is that most patients cannot come to the doctor for treatment before 4 or 6 h have passed since the onset of their deficit [4, 5, 22]. Furthermore, it is necessary to perform several diagnostic tests to determine the exact nature and extent of the cerebral ischemic problem, including a computerized tomographic scan, a four-vessel cerebral angiogram, and, in most cases, a cerebral blood flow study [26]. In the optimum of all cases, it is likely that all these tests and evaluations of the patient would not be completed before 6–10 h have elapsed from the onset of the ischemic deficit. If this is the case, what can we do to prolong the period of grace during which the ischemic brain may tolerate having poor perfusion?

Experimental studies in animals have also revealed that some pharmacological substances may be used to prolong the interval of ischemia which may be tolerated by the brain. Lawner [10] and Spetzler [19] reported on prolonged periods of regional cerebral ischemia tolerated prior to the performance of a cerebral revascularization when the animals were treated with barbiturates and maintained in coma. Suzuki has shown also that the addition of mannitol, phenytoin, and vitamin E also help to prolong the period of ischemia tolerated by the brain prior to the reinstitution of perfusion [23, 27].

The indications for acute cerebral revascularization have not been totally established, and a great deal of controversy still exists regarding its applicability in the treatment of cerebral ischemia [5, 7, 22]. In our opinion, cerebral revascularization is applicable in the treatment of patients who present with an acute cerebral hemispheric deficit, within the first 6–8 h of its occurrence. The clinical picture would include patients with a fixed neurological deficit present for less than 10 h, patients with crescendo transient ischemic attacks (TIAs), and patients with progressing neurological deficits. We have shown that these patients can be operated on safely without the development of any additional neurological deficit in most, and without the development of a hemorrhagic infarction [5].

These patients should have a CT scan which is either negative or shows a small area of decreased density in the region corresponding to the deficit. A patient with a large area of decreased density

[1] Department of Neurosurgery, Henry Ford Hospital, 2799 West Grand Boulevard, Detroit, Michigan, USA

on CT scanning, in our opinion, should not be operated on because we would fear the development of a hemorrhagic infarction, as we observed in some of our experimental animals. Furthermore, these patients should have a selective four-vessel cerebral angiogram which reveals an area of either occlusion or stenosis in the territory corresponding to the ischemic deficit. This area of stenosis or occlusion should also be otherwise inaccessible by any other surgical means. These vascular lesions would include a unilateral internal carotid artery occlusion, a carotid siphon stenosis, a middle cerebral artery stenosis, or occlusion. Those patients with stenotic lesions should have an area of stenosis which is hemodynamically significant, i.e., greater than 85% of the cross-sectional diameter of the vessel confirmed on biplane angiography. In addition, these patients should have a cerebral blood flow study which reveals a perfusion deficit in the area of the brain corresponding to the neurological picture.

The use of positron emission tomography [16] with regional metabolic studies would be ideal in the evaluation of these patients who would be candidates for acute cerebral revascularization, but the cost and availability, even to highly specialized centers, limits its wider application at the present time.

We would not consider candidates for surgery those patients who have a fixed neurological deficit which has been present for longer than 10–12 h. We support this because patients in whom we operated on after this period of time from the onset of their deficit usually did have any meaningful recovery [4]. Other patients who would not be candidates for cerebral revascularization include patients with a large area of decreased density on the CT scan or with evidence of a hemorrhagic infarction. Patients with a history of a recent myocardial infarction, or with advanced neoplastic disease, would not be operated on either. Relative contraindications include patients with serious medical problems including chronic obstructive pulmonary disease, diabetes mellitus, renal failure, or advanced liver disease. The decision to operate on these patients would depend on the relative risk presented by the evaluating internist.

Our current management of patients considered for acute cerebral revascularization is the following: we proceed initially by immediately placing them in barbiturate coma [12, 18], which requires their immediate intubation and mechanical ventilation. Their oxygenation is optimized and they are kept slightly hypocarbic (PCO2 approximately 30–35 torr). A Swan-Ganz catheter is inserted, and their cardiac output and cardiac index are optimized. Those who can tolerate increased cardiac demand are given volume in the form of salt poor albumin, to produce a state of slight hypervolemia and hemodilution [25]. Those who have marginal cardiac function are kept normovolemic, but their hematocrit is reduced to 30% by phlebotomy and salt-poor albumin infusion. A foley catheter and an indwelling arterial line are placed to facilitate their continued monitoring.

The moment the decision is made to transport the patients to surgery, they are given a bolus dose of lidocaine (1 mg/kg) [21], and an intravenous infusion of phenytoin (15 mg/kg) [23] is given over the course of the operation while monitoring their cardiac parameters. Once in the operating room, the patients receive a single injection of furosemide (40 mg/kg) and two doses of mannitol (0.5 g/kg) [11, 27] are given at 1-h intervals from the furosemide. The operative procedure is conducted under barbiturate anesthesia with sodium pentothal (3 mg/kg) given at regular intervals until recirculation to the ischemic area has been reestablished through the bypass procedure [10, 14, 17, 18]. The barbiturates are not continued postoperatively.

The future of cerebral revascularization in the acute state remains, in our opinion, one of the most likely, potentially beneficial forms of treatment for patients with a cerebral deficit secondary to a perfusion deficit caused by an arterial lesion not surgically accessible by any other means [4, 21]. There has been, to date, no scientifically proven benefit from any form of medical treament given in the acute state which prevents the establishment of a fixed neurological deficit in patients with a severe perfusion deficit [4]. Several nonsurgical means have shown promise regarding the possibility of increasing the period of ischemia which may be tolerated by the brain. Medications such as barbiturates [14, 17], phenytoin [23], mannitol [11, 27], and vitamin E [23] have been reported to be of use. Lowering the viscosity of the blood by hemodilution, in combination with moderate systemic hypertension, serves to increase the amount of blood that passes to the area with low perfusion via the collateral circulation [25]. Substances, such as fluorocarbons, administered parenterally or in the subarachnoid space would increase the amount of oxygen delivered to the ischemic tissue by increasing the oxygen carrying capacity of the blood or CSF

[8, 15, 23]. Finally, hyperbaric oxygenation to 2.5 atmospheres would also increase the amount of oxygen delivered to the brain by increasing the amount of oxygen in solution in the serum.

However effective or promising any of the previously mentioned nonsurgical methods may seem in the short run, none are capable of resolving the primary problem of decreased cerebral perfusion faced by these patients. One could argue that some, or a combination of all, of these measures could be used to allow the brain to develop the collaterals needed to reperfuse the brain spontaneously. This would certainly obviate the need for surgery. However, in the practical setting, none of these methods singly or in combination can be maintained long enough for the brain to establish its own collateral supply. Therefore, it is, in our opinion, the patient with acute cerebral ischemia secondary to a perfusion deficit who is most likely to benefit from a rapid intervention which combines some nonsurgical maneuvers with a cerebral revascularization procedure [4]. This will require the establishment of teams of neurologists, neurosurgeons, and neuroradiologists who are willing to work in cooperation and who can establish protocols that can be instituted rapidly and efficiently. Areas of concentration could be developed throughout the world in centers with recognized expertise and support from these teams of physicians. When these centers are established, one could consider a randomized study of best medical and best surgical therapy including all patients with acute cerebral ischemia which fit the description given above.

The International Cooperative Study [7] attempted to evaluate the potential usefulness of cerebral revascularization, but limitations in total numbers and in individual groups of patients with acute ischemic symptoms make their observations not statistically valid [2].

In our opinion, cerebral revascularization remains a viable option in the management of patients with acute cerebral ischemia secondary to hypoperfusion, produced by an arterial lesion not surgically accessible by any other means. We are still evaluating all patients who present with this syndrome in a very aggressive manner, and proceed with an acute cerebral revascularization in those select cases who fit the criteria we have outlined. We believe that these patients have the greatest potential to benefit from the rapid reinstitution of cerebral blood flow to their acutely ischemic brain, and should therefore be given the opportunity of acute cerebral revascularization.

References

1. Astrup J, Siesjo BK, Symon L (1981) Thresholds in cerebral ischemia: The ischemic penumbra. Stroke 12:723–725 (editorial)
2. Ausman JI, Diaz FG (1986) Critique of the Extracranial–Intracranial Bypass Study. Surg Neurol 26:218–221
3. Crowell RM, Olsson Y, Klatzo I, Ommaya A (1970) Temporary occlusion of the middle cerebral artery in the monkey: Clinical and pathological observations. Stroke 1:439–448
4. Diaz FG, Ausman JI, Mehta B, Dujovny M, de los Reyes RA, Pearce J, Patel S (1985) Acute cerebral revascularization. J Neurosurg 63:200–209
5. Diaz FG, Mastri AR, Ausman JI, Chou SN (1979) Acute cerebral revascularization after regional cerebral ischemia in the dog: II. Clinicopathological correlation. J Neurosurg 51:644–653
6. Dujovny M, Osgood CP, Barrionuevo PJ, Hellstrom R, Laha RK (1976) Middle cerebral artery microneurosurgical embolectomy. Surgery 80:336–339
7. The EC/IC Bypass Study Group (1985) Failure of extracranial-intracranial arterial bypass to reduce the risk of ischemic stroke: Results of an international randomized trial. N Engl J Med 313:1191–1200
8. Handa H (1982) Effect of Fluosol–DA on cerebral circulation in humans. In: Frey R, Beisbarth H, Stosseck K (eds) Oxygen–carrying colloidal blood substitutes. Zuckschwendt, Munich, pp 204–207
9. Jones TH, Morawetz RB, Crowell RM, Marcoux FW, FitzGibbon SJ, DeGirolami U, Ojemann RG (1981) Thresholds of focal cerebral ischemia in awake monkeys. J Neurosurg 54:773–782
10. Lawner PM, Laurent JP, Simeone FA, Fink EA (1982) Effect of extracranial–intracranial bypass and pentobarbital on acute stroke in dogs. J Neurosurg 56:92–96
11. Little JR (1978) Modification of acute focal ischemia by treatment with mannitol. Stroke 9:4–9
12. Michenfelder JD, Milde JH (1975) Influence of anesthetics on metabolic, functional and pathological responses to regional cerebral ischemia. Stroke 6:405–410
13. Morawetz RB, Crowell RH, DeGirolami U, Marcoux FW, Jones TH, Halsey JH (1979) Regional cerebral blood flow thresholds during cerebral ischemia. Fed Proc 38:2493–2494
14. Moseley JI, Laurent JP, Molinari GF (1975) Barbiturate attenuation of the clinical course and pathologic lesions in a primate stroke model. Neurology (Minneap) 25:870–874
15. Peerless SJ, Ishikawa R, Hunter IG, Peerless MJ (1981) Protective effect of Fluosol-DA in acute cerebral ischemia. Stroke 12:558–563
16. Powers WJ, Raichle ME (1985) Positron emission tomography and its application to the study of cerebrovascular disease in man. Stroke 16:361–

376

17. Selman WR, Spetzler RF, Roski RA, Roessmann U, Crumrine R, Macko R (1982) Barbiturate coma in focal cerebral ischemia: Relationship of protection to timing of therapy. J Neurosurg 56:685–690
18. Smith AL, Hoff JT, Nielsen SL, Larson CP (1974) Barbiturate protection in acute focal cerebral ischemia. Stroke 5:1–7
19. Spetzler RF, Selman WR, Roski RA, Bonstelle C (1982) Cerebral revascularization during barbiturate coma in primates and humans. Surg Neurol 17:111–115
20. Sundt TM Jr, Grant WC, Garcia JH (1969) Restoration of middle cerebral artery flow in experimental infarction. J Neurosurg 31:311–322
21. Sundt TM Jr, Onofrio BM, Merideth J (1973) Treatment of cerebral vasospasm from subarachnoid hemorrhage with isoproterenol and lidocaine hydrochloride. J Neurosurg 38:557–560
22. Sundt TM Jr, Whisnant JP, Fode NC, Piepgras DG, Houser OW (1985) Results, complications, and follow-up of 415 bypass operations for occlusive disease of the carotid system. Mayo Clin Proc 60:230–240
23. Suzuki J, Fujimoto S, Mizoi K, Oba M (1984) The protective effect of combined administration of anti-oxidants and perfluorochemicals on cerebral ischemia. Stroke 15:672–679
24. Symon L, Branston NM, Strong AJ, Hope TD (1977) The concept of thresholds of ischaemia in relation to brain structure and function. J Clin Pathol 30 (Suppl 11):149–154
25. Wood JH, Fleischer AS (1982) Observations during hypervolemic hemodilution of patients with acute focal cerebral ischemia. JAMA 248:2999–3004
26. Yanagihara T, Wahner HW (1984) Cerebral blood flow measurement in cerebrovascular occlusive diseases. Stroke 15:816–822
27. Yoshimoto T, Sakamoto T, Watanabe T, Tanaka S, Suzuki J (1978) Experimental cerebral infarction. Part 3: Protective effect of mannitol in thalamic infarction in dogs. Stroke 9:217–218

Acute Cerebral Revascularization: Indications and Limits

Rolando Gagliardi and Lucia Benvenuti[1]

Introduction

Many reports dealing with experimental and clinical experiences with acute focal cerebral ischemia have been published in the past years. Nevertheless, no widely accepted protocols of treatment have been established and the published results have been variable, when analyzed in terms of survival and functional recovery.

The lack of proven beneficial therapeutic measures, together with the question of the applicability of experimental models to actual clinical situations, have suggested a treatment chiefly consisting of prevention, supportive measures, and rehabilitation. This conservative approach has been widely accepted up to date.

The purpose of this paper is to present our clinical experience with acute focal cerebral ischemia and discuss the rationale for treatment on the basis of the present knowledge of the pathophysiology of this clinical entity.

Materials, Methods, and Results

Twelve patients with symptoms of acute focal cerebral ischemia have been admitted to our department from September 1976 to March 1987. Seven of them were males and their ages ranged from 24 to 70 years (mean age, 44.1 years). All of them reached us within 2 h of the acute episode. Eight of them had a middle cerebral artery (MCA) occlusion, and the remaining four had an internal carotid artery (ICA) occlusion.

Eight patients received an emergency extracranial–intracranial arterial bypass (EIAB), and the remaining four underwent an MCA embolectomy. All procedures but two were accomplished within $6\frac{1}{2}$ from the onset of neurological symp-

[1] Department of Neurosurgery, USL 10/D, Careggi Hospital, Florence, Italy

toms: in the first patient submitted to EIAB, we were not able to respect the scheduled time because we had been trying to perform at first an embolectomy, and, in the seventh patient of the EIAB–treated series, there was a clinical picture of "stroke in evolution." Surgical data and clinical courses of our patients are reported in Table 1.

Discussion

The neurological appearance of an acute occlusion is the clinical expression of an anatomopathological damage due to progressive cerebral ischemia which begins soon after the stroke and reaches its maximum (becomes irreversible) in a few hours. It was thought that persistence of ischemia for more than a few minutes lead to irreversible brain damage. This opinion was challenged in recent years since experimental and clinical results suggested that brain tissue can tolerate ischemia for a considerable time. This observation stimulated more accurate studies in the pathophysiology of focal cerebral ischemia.

On the basis of current knowledge, the pathophysiology of focal cerebral ischemia can be analyzed in terms of thresholds of ischemia, metabolic derangements, and morphological changes of ischemic brain tissue.

Several teams of investigators proved that the threshold for brain electrical failure is at 15–18 ml/100 g per minute, and the threshold of ionic failure is at approximately 10 ml/100 g per minute Between these two thresholds of electrical and ionic failure exists a small range of flow at which, in spite of functional loss, membrane homeostasis and structural integrity of the tissue are maintained. This restricted range of flow has been defined "ischemic penumbra" [5]. The ischemic penumbra explains the potential for recovery in patients with acute focal cerebral ischemia when a collateral flow, able to satisfy the basic energy requirements, exists. Although the tolerance of

Table 1. Surgical data and clinical course in 12 patients

Case number	Sex	Age (yrs)	Neurol. status on admission	Preoper. angiography	Clip removal (h)	Postop angiography	Surgical outcome	Follow-up
Embolectomy								
1	F	70	Rt. hemiplegia, aphasia	Lt. MCA occl.	6.5	Patent	Moderate hemiparesis speech impair.	Good
2	F	24	Rt. hemiplegia, aphasia	Lt. MCA occl.	5.5	—	Death (2nd day)	—
3	M	32	Rt. hemiplegia, aphasia	Lt. MCA occl.	6	Patent vasospasm	Moderate hemiparesis	Good
4	M	56	Rt. hemiplegia, aphasia	Lt. MCA occl.	5	—	No improv.	Poor
EIAB								
1	M	39	Rt hemiplegia, aphasia	Lt. MCA occl.	8	EIAB Patent MCA recanal.	Rt. hemipar., speech impair.	Good
2	M	45	Rt. hemiplegia, aphasia	Lt. ICA occl.	5	EIAB patent	Slight speech impairment.	Excellent
3	F	33	Rt. hemiplegia, aphasia	Lt. MCA occl.	6.5	EIAB poorly visualized	Rt. hemipar., speech impair.	Good
4	F	29	Lt. hemiplegia	Rt. ICA occl. in siphon	6	EIAB patent	Moderate upper monoparesis	Good
5	M	47	Rt. hemiplegia, aphasia	Lt. MCA occl.	5.5	EIAB patent MCA recanal.	Moderate hemip. speech impair.	Good
6	M	55	Lt. hemiplegia	Rt. ICA occl.	5	EIAB patent	Slight upper monoparesis	Excellent
7	F	65	Lt. hemiplegia	Rt. ICA occl.	10	EIAB patent	Moderate upper monoparesis	Good
8	M	40	Rt. hemiplegia, aphasia	Lt. MCA occl.	5.5	EIAB patent	Slight speech impair.	[a]

EIAB extracranial-intracranial arterial bypass, *MCA* middle cerebral artery
[a] Follow-up restricted to 2 months with excellent result

the nervous tissue for a reduced flow is unknown, experimental reports suggest that after 3–6 h cellular death is unavoidable. Therefore, the ischemic penumbra is a dynamic condition that will deteriorate over time.

At a cerebral blood flow (CBF) of approximately 10 ml/100 g per minute, metabolic derangements occur. These metabolic disorders are multifactorial and reflect both the rapid depletion of energy stores and the lactacidosis due to the anaerobic metabolism [2, 7]. The impairment of the sodium pump (ATP-dependent), and the resultant increase of extracellular potassium and intracellular sodium will depolarize the neuronal membrane. This occurence is responsible for the opening of voltage-sensitive calcium channels and the resulting increase in intracellular free calcium. An increase in intracellular calcium concentration seems to play a crucial role in inducing ischemic cell injury by favoring breakdown of membrane phospholipids with the production of free fatty acids. The intracellular acidosis is responsible for the denaturation of proteins with consequent loss of enzimatic func-

tion, an increase of glial edema that compromises potential collateral flow, and a possible increased production of free radicals. Therefore, after acute occlusion of a vessel, a foregoing cascade of metabolic derangements takes place.

The structural integrity of the tissue is impaired simultaneously with the appearance of metabolic derangements. For the determination of the reversibility of cerebral ischemia, morphological assessment of ischemic damage is important [2, 3]. Morphological damage soon after the onset of ischemia, however, has not been well elucidated because of the relative insensitivity of conventional histologic methods. Further investigations on this subject are expected.

Coming from the abovementioned known pathophysiological aspects, it is possible to affirm that the potential for recovery in acute focal cerebral ischemia can be helped, on the one hand, by slowing down or contrasting the metabolic derangements in order to extend the survival time of the brain tissue and, on the other hand, by the reperfusion of the ischemic area before damage of neurons becomes irreversible.

The definition of adequate pharmacological measures to protect the brain from the development of cerebral infarction has been extensively investigated in recent years [8–10]. Medical therapies can act by decreasing neuronal energy requirements, by improving the CBF, by stabilizing membrane pumps, and by protecting the brain from neurotransmitter release. Of course, drugs can be used in various combinations, some of which are particularly effective in protecting the brain from the development of an extensive damage [9].

The rationale for emergency surgical revascularization is the reestablishment of the flow in the ischemic area which is mandatory, because the abovementioned therapeutic measures are temporary and of limited duration. The flow can be reestablished through lysis of the clot or through the natural development of collateral circulation. However, we do not know in advance whether and when spontaneous recanalization will occur, or the rate of the development of collateral vessels. Therefore, in selected patients, it is justified to consider the possibility of a treatment consisting of surgical revascularization in combination with medical supportive treatment able to stabilize jeopardized neurons until the restoration of flow is accomplished.

According to the literature [1, 4, 6, 10], our surgical results seem to offer a better outcome than natural history to patients with acute occlusion. Our experience cannot be considered conclusive; nevertheless, it allows us to draw some conclusions.

The crucial factor in acute focal cerebral ischemia is the time during which surgery would be helpful. The reestablishement of the flow has to be accomplished during the penumbral state of the neurons.

The 4- to 6-h limit suggested by experimental reports seemed, to us, too long to allow survival and functional recovery of human ischemic tissue. In our series, in fact, surgical procedure did not always bring excellent results, even when accomplished within 6 h after the stroke. Therefore, the identification of the time limit for the survival of human brain tissue after an acute occlusion would be of paramount importance for a conclusive evaluation of the potential for emergency revascularization

Further developments are expected in the identification of brain protective substances. Medical therapies to improve collateral flow and decrease neuronal energy requirements may lengthen the penumbral time and may, thereby, maximize the effects of surgery. Cases 6 and 8 in the EIAB-treated series received mannitol infusion and barbiturate protection, and presented a quicker recovery from neurological deficit.

The angiographic picture of intracranial vessels is the most important prognostic factor, as it permits a qualitative assessment of collateral flow [2]. When the occluded artery is beyond the main anastomotic systems, such as the circle of Willis, the cortical anastomotic network is usually only slightly effective, as the infarct often involves the whole region supplied by the occluded vessel and develops quickly. When the occluded artery is located upstream of the circle of Willis, anastomoses are more often efficient, at least partially. In our series, we observed a better outcome in patients who were affected by an ICA occlusion in comparison with patients suffering from an MCA occlusion.

Obviously, the evaluation of general physical conditions of the patient will be of paramount importance in making any surgical decision, and the lack of preexisting vascular damages will maximize the possibility of success. We believe that our good results can be explained, at least partially, by our rigorous protocol of selection: young age, good health, and the absence of known preexisting vascular diseases.

Although a small area of infarcted tissue may never be prevented, a wider area of infarction can be avoided by allowing the reperfusion of tissue that may be marginally compromised during the early period. In our series, we observed a small infarcted area on CT-scan pictures even when the the patient had an excellent functional recovery.

Embolectomy of the MCA offers the possibility of an immediate reperfusion of the entire arterial tree. However, this surgical procedure is laborious and, therefore, indicated only in very selected cases. In our experience, EIAB has definitely given more encouraging results that thromboembolectomy. EIAB is, of course, a less traumatic procedure and fairly quick in expert hands; nevertheless, it ensures only an initial and limited flow.

Conclusions

The pathophysiological mechanisms responsible for acute focal cerebral ischemia allow for the recognition of the rationale for acute surgical revascularization combined with adequate pharmacological therapies.

The value of this combined treatment could be

clarified only by means of further clinical trials based on standardized criteria of selection for patients who can benefit from the treatment itself, rigorous therapeutical schedule, and universally accepted criteria for evaluating the results.

References

1. Diaz FG, Ausman JI, Metha B, et al. (1985) Acute cerebral revascularization. J Neurosurg 63:200–209
2. Duyckaerts C, Hauw JJ (1985) Pathology and pathophysiology of brain ischemia. In: Bories J (ed) Cerebral ischemia. Springer, Berlin, pp 10–17
3. Heiss WD (1983) Flow thresholds of functional and morphological damage of brain tissue. Stroke 14:329–331
4. Kayama T, Kanako M, Muraki M, et al. (1985) Surgical results of emergent revascularization for the acute major stroke: Hemodynamic observation and clinical course. In: Spetzler RF, Carter LP, Selman WR, Martin NA (eds) Cerebral revascularization for stroke. Thieme-Stratton, New York, pp 555–563
5. Lassen NA, Symon L, Baron JC (1986) Pénombre et ischémie cérébrale. Libbey, London
6. Meyer FB, Sundt TM, Yanagihara T, Anderson RE (1987) Focal cerebral ischemia: Pathophysiologic mechanisms and rationale for future avenues of treatment. Mayo Clin Proc 62:35–55
7. Michenfelder JD, Sundt TM Jr (1971) Cerebral ATP and lactate levels in the squirrel monkey following occlusion of the middle cerebral artery. Stroke 2:319–326
8. Spetzler RF, Selman WR, Roski RA, et al. (1982) Cerebral revascularization during barbiturate coma in primates and humans. Surg Neurol 17:111–115
9. Suzuki J (1987) The development of new brain protective agents. In: Suzuki J (ed) Treatment of cerebral infarction: Experimental and clinical study. Springer, Vienna, pp 158–202
10. Suzuki J (1987) Revascularization in acute stage. In: Suzuki J (ed) Treatment of cerebral infarction: Experimental and clinical study. Springer, Vienna, pp 270–279

Cerebral Revascularization

Robert F. Spetzler and Fred Williams[1]

Carotid and cerebral vascular surgeons have generally opposed early intervention in acute stroke because the nonfunctioning brain tissue was presumed necrosed, and revascularization risked hemorrhagic infarction with little potential benefit. Recently, however, the theory of the ischemic penumbra has described acute stroke as a centrifugal distribution of cell states ranging from death at the center of the lesion through irreversible and reversible intermediate pathologic states to a peripheral region of normal brain tissue. The proportion of cells in each state is a function of collateral blood supply and the duration of ischemia. This theory suggests that early treatment may help in acute stroke. Medical methods have sought to improve the microcirculation by hemodynamic and hematologic manipulation and by cerebral cellular protection with pharmacologic agents. This review, however, focuses on surgical approaches.

Experimental Basis

The survival of neurons depends on their receiving adequate amounts of substrates, most importantly, glucose and oxygen. Although less discussed, cerebral blood flow (CBF) also removes toxic by-products of metabolism. Normal average CBF is 50 $cm^3/min/100$ g of brain tissue and is regionally coupled to the metabolic requirements of the surrounding cells by changes in the resistance to flow of local arterioles. When perfusion pressure is decreased, as occurs in severe arterial stenosis or occlusion, this coupling process is decompensated, and CBF decreases below cellular needs. CBF between 15 and 20 $cm^3/min/100$ g is considered the neuronal threshold of electrical failure. Clinically, neurologic deficits occur in this range. A sudden rise in the extracellular potassium level occurs with a CBF between 6 and 8 $cm^3/min/100$ g and may indicate that the cells no longer have the energy to maintain the integrity of their membranes. This threshold may be near the initiation of the spiraling, irreversible, downhill cascade that precedes cellular equilibrium. The accumulation of intracellular calcium, the liberation of arachidonic acid, and increasing intracellular acidosis are important contributors to cell death. The theory of the ischemic penumbra postulates that neurons subjected to an ischemic insult are positioned along a dynamic spectrum, with reversible and irreversible groups of cells indistinctly delineated. Over time, at a rate inversely proportional to the residual CBF, a continuous downward shift in cell states occurs: an increasing number of cells reach the point of no return and die. Cells in the penumbra are in a temporarily reversible state of dysfunction, and acute revascularization procedures aim to preserve these neurons.

The presence of the ischemic penumbra can be inferred from experiments in animals, where temporary acute cerebrovascular obstructions causing neurologic deficits have been reversed by either bypassing or removing the obstruction [12]. Strong et al., studied an artificial area of ischemia in the monkey and found that CBF values and EEG recordings vary within this region consistent with the penumbra theory [10]. As will be described, clinical evidence supporting this theory also exists.

Natural History

The natural history for stroke secondary to an acute carotid or cerebral vascular occlusion remains obscure. The ideal study has not been performed, and early studies lack angiographic documentation. Many recent studies have been retrospective or have had small numbers of patients. Patients have often been uncategorized with respect to the severity of their deficits. Fol-

---

[1] Barrow Neurological Institute, Phoenix, Arizona, USA

low-up has also been variable. As a result, evaluating surgical series has been difficult.

Comparing the results obtained from operative series with those reported in studies of the natural history of the disease has several problems. For example, the two sets of patients may be unmatched for age or for distribution in the severity of strokes. Computed tomography (CT) scans have generally been ignored in most studies of natural history, even though they have been a crucial factor in the selection of surgical candidates. Basic hospital care for the stroke patient changes from year to year and from region to region. For instance, the outcome of a control group may be quite different if hemodilution-hypervolemic therapy is used. These limitations must be considered when the efficacy of a procedure is compared to natural history.

Finally, one of the most obvious difficulties in evaluating a procedure for the early treatment of acute stroke is differentiating the stroke from a transient ischemic attrack (TIA), given its current definition. The optimal time for surgical treatment in the face of an acute occlusive vascular process has been said to be within the first 6 h after ictus. If revascularization is not performed within this time limit, the ischemic penumbra potentially could be lost. The definition of TIA, however, is an ischemic deficit that resolves within 24 h. In practice, the transience of the TIA usually manifests itself before 24 h. Therefore, the diagnosis of stroke is likely to be accurate, and a spontaneously recovering patient is unlikely to be selected for revascularization surgery. However, this problem with nomenclature questions the generalizability of information from various studies, and interpreting the results of small, uncontrolled, surgical series becomes more difficult.

Grillo and Patterson retrospectively reviewed 44 patients with acute, angiographically-proven arteriosclerotic occlusion of the internal carotid artery [6]. Of these, 26 patients had a stroke related to the event, and 15 patients presented with TIAs. Of these 41 patients with acute neurologic deficits related to carotid occlusion, seven patients died within the first 2 weeks from effects related to the infarction, and nine patients eventually died from the consequences of generalized arteriosclerosis (e.g., myocardial infarction or stroke in the contralateral hemisphere). Therefore, the overall mortality rate in this population was 41%; almost half of the deaths were unattributable to the presenting stroke. Of the 24 patients surviving with mild to moderate deficits,

Table 1. Natural history

	ICA occlusion	MCA occlusion
Total	41	24
Stroke	26	19
TIA	15	5
Mortality	16 (41%)	10 (42%)
Stroke (acute)	7	5
Atherosclerotic degree	9	2
Other	—	3

ICA internal carotid artery, *MCA* middle carotid artery, *TIA* transient ischemic attack

19 had no further progression of their deficits. The strokes that eventually occurred in the others were contralateral to the original occlusion. The authors did not report the grading of the initial stroke, or the nature and time course of the TIAs.

Moulin, et al., reviewed the clinical course of angiographic middle cerebral artery occlusion in 24 patients [7]. This process was hearly always embolic. Five patients presented with TIAs, and the remainder presented with stroke (eight were major). Of the ten deaths, five were secondary to the initial stroke, and four died later: two patients from ipsilateral stroke and two from myocardial infarction. Of the remaining 14 patients, 12 (63%) remained completely functional, although five had further ischemic events. Only one patient had a second stroke. Again, information about the course or grading of the individual strokes, and the number of patients with progressive deficits was not given.

These studies (Table 1) indicate that the prognosis for patients with occlusion of the internal carotid artery or the middle cerebral artery (MCA) without major stroke is fair but limited by the presence of generalized arteriosclerotic disease. Overall, the mortality directly attributable to acute stroke is 20%. However, neither these results, nor most of the reports on the natural history of this disease, are generally applicable to the subset of patients for whom revascularization surgery might be considered.

Clinical Considerations for Revascularization

Situations in which early revascularization surgery might be considered are acute stroke related to occlusion of the internal carotid artery and/or acute stroke related to MCA occlusion. Early revascularization remains controversial, and many neurovascular surgeons claim that surgery is strictly contraindicated. Even among those who perform surgery on patients with an acute stroke, the process of selection is painstaking. In 1969, Blaisdell et al. reported the findings of the Joint Study of Extracranial Arterial Occlusion, which found a mortality of almost 50% in 50 patients operated upon for profound stroke and depressed level of consciousness within two weeks of the initial stroke [1]. Many studies since have also shown high mortality and poor results, even when the patients have been operated upon emergently.

Patients with mild to moderate, progressive, or fluctuating deficits appear to constitute a different category. Ojemann and Crowell reported on 21 patients who underwent emergency endarterectomy for carotid occlusion [8]. Of the 15 patients in whom the patency of the internal carotid could be reestablished, 12 had documented neurologic improvement. This implies that 20% of the patients either did not improve or worsened. Only one of the six patients, in whom the reopening attempt failed, improved postoperatively. The distribution of deficits in each group is not disclosed. It was stated, however, that only the patients with profound neurologic impairment fared poorly in the postoperative period.

In a more recent and uncommonly optimistic report, Meyer described 34 patients with acute carotid occlusions [11]. In contrast to the above studies, these patients all presented with either profound deficits or with neurologic impairment that relentlessly progressed to a profound level. Several of these patients had altered sensorium. More than half of these patients were diagnosed on the basis of clinical findings alone. Of these patients, 70% improved postoperatively; the mortality rate was 20%. Even more striking, 13 patients had good to excellent results, and nine patients were normal. In the two cases in which patency could not be restored, death occurred. Only two patients had hemorrhagic infarctions. Good outcome correlated well with the presence of collateral flow on the preoperative angiogram; correlation with the total time of oligemia was less clear. When an MCA occlusion was associated with the carotid occlusion, the prognosis was poor.

MCA embolectomy has been performed with mixed success. Gagliardi, et al., described four cases of embolectomy all performed within 6 h of an MCA occlusion [4]. Two of these patients died. One patient died as a result of cerebral infarction, but the other patient had a good surgical result and then subsequently died of myocardial infarction. Another patient had restoration of blood flow within 5 h of his occlusion, but remained neurologically impaired postoperatively, and later died as a result of his neurologic state.

MCA embolectomy was performed emergently in 20 patients by Meyer et al. [11]. All these patients presented with severe neurologic impairment, including hemiplegia, reduced level of consciousness, and aphasia if the dominant hemisphere was involved. Seven patients made good to excellent recoveries, and two patients were neurologically normal postoperatively. Of the three patients in whom operation did not restore patency, all died or did poorly. Patients with associated ipsilateral carotid occlusion generally had worse results. Two patients had hemorrhagic infarctions. Collateral flow, tested by the presence of backflow at the time of surgery, was correlated with better prognosis, whereas duration of occlusion was again a poor predictor of outcome. The overall mortality was 10%, with a mortality rate of 6% for patients whose MCA could be reopened, compared to 33% when the MCA could not be reopened.

The superficial temporal to middle cerebral artery (STA-MCA) bypass, designed mainly to treat occlusion or severely stenotic cerebral vascular lesions inaccessible to direct approach, such as lesions of the internal carotid syphon, has been criticized as having no benefit over medical treatment in stroke. A few authors, however, have described this treatment with favorable results, even in acute ischemic deficits. Diaz et al. reported 15 patients operated upon within 12 h after the initiation of ischemic symptoms: eight patients had crescendo TIAs, three had progressive stroke, and four had fixed neurologic deficits [3]. The presenting clinical signs and symptoms resolved in ten patients postoperatively, and no deaths were related to the procedure.

In a series of 65 STA-MCA bypass patients, Gratzl et al., however, had three patients with acute cerebral ischemia die postoperatively from severe brain edema; the operations were performed between 4 and 16 h after the initial event [5]. In four patients with stroke in evolution, the neurologic condition worsened postoperatively.

In summary, surgical results in the early treatment of the various lesions associated with acute

Table 2. Surgical outcome

	No.	Mortality
ICA occlusion		
Blaisdell 1969	50	42%
Ojemann 1975	21	3 (14%)
Successful reopening	15 (12 improved)	1
Unsuccessful reopening	6 (1 improved)	2
Meyer 1987	34	7 (20%)
Successful reopening	32 (23 improved)	5
Unsuccessful reopening	2	2
MCA occlusion		
Gagliardi 1983	4	2 (50%)
Meyer 1987	20	2 (10%)
Successful	16 (7 improved)	0
Unsuccessful	3	1
Unknown	1	1

ICA internal carotid artery, *MCA* middle carotid artery, *TIA* transient ischemic attack

ischemic deficit vary widely (Table 2). Four-vessel carotid angiograms and the state of collateral flow have rarely been reported. CT scanning has not been correlated with preoperative status nor with surgical outcome. The perioperative medical care is rarely described. Because these studies are retrospective, perioperative care has not been strictly controlled. The complications of hemorrhagic infarction, cerebral edema, and failed operation have been encountered. Although the immediate surgical mortality rates have generally been similar to those of the medically treated patients, long-term follow-up has not been available for all series. The available information, then, on cerebral revascularization in the acute phase of stroke should be cautiously interpreted.

Discussion

The ischemic penumbra has been demonstrated experimentally. Its existence and practical uses in the clinical setting have been questioned. It can be inferred from the clinical information presented, however, that the penumbra exists and can be salvaged by revascularization in some cases. In which subgroup of patients can the natural history be improved by operation? The difficulty in using existing studies to determine the natural history of cerebrovascular occlusion in patients that might also be considered as surgical candidates is clear. Patients chosen for neurosurgical consultation are usually a select subset of all patients with the particular disease. Rarely

are they patients with minimal or transient complaints. More commonly, they have moderate, severe, or even profound deficits. Frequently, the neurosurgeon is consulted as a last resort for patients undergoing a progressive deterioration unresponsive to other treatments.

Our experience and the limited information contained in past archives have indicated a careful process of selection based on examination, complete angiography, CT scan results, duration of ischemic deficits, and hospital course is required in patients presenting with acute ischemic deficits (Fig. 1). Although the time factor has been minimized by Meyer [11], we would still consider duration of ischemia one of the more crucial factors determining outcome. The 6-h value given by some is probably more artificial than real. It is more likely that the time limit for the penumbra is determined, in some fashion, by the amount of collateral flow. Patients presenting with acute ischemic deficits undergo CT scanning to rule out a mass lesion secondary to infarction, or the presence of another type of lesion masking itself as an ischemic process. Patients with mass lesions are generally not considered surgical candidates. Patients with altered sensorium are considered poor surgical candidates as well.

Those patients manifesting mild to moderate deficits with normal CT scans are considered for surgery, particularly those with fluctuating deficits. Complete carotid and cerebral angiograms are obtained. Evidence for collateral flow, such as retrograde filling of the carotid syphon in

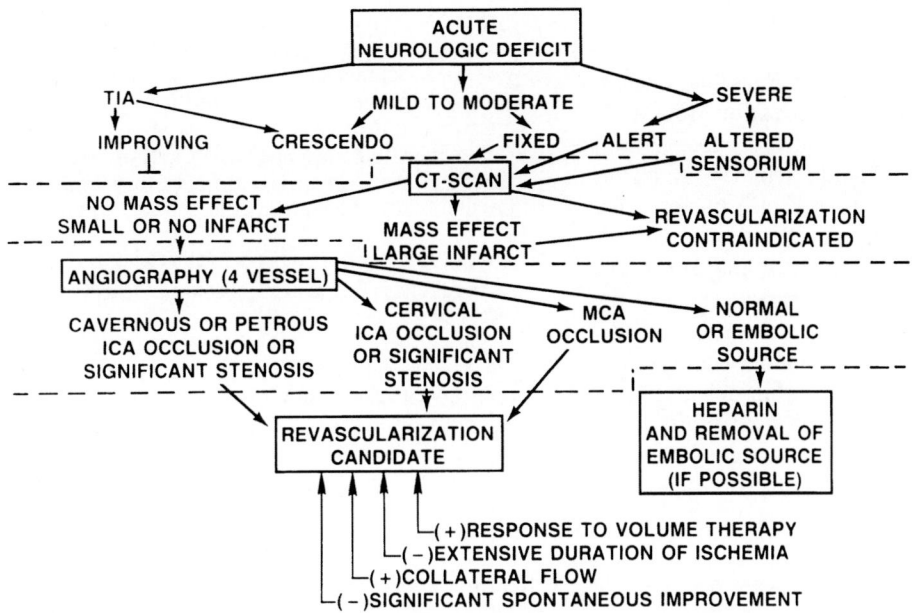

Fig. 1. Decision tree for acute ischemic deficit. Abbreviations as in Table 1

internal carotid occlusion, or the presence of retrograde filling by way of leptomeningeal collaterals in MCA occlusion, argues for revascularization, while a prolonged duration of ischemia argues against it.

Patients with stroke in evolution constitute a distinct group. This phenomenon, occurring in up to 40% of patients presenting with stroke, carries an ominous prognosis [2]. The differential diagnosis in a patient with an acute stroke who becomes worse includes enlarging infarction, worsening edema, intracerebral hemorrhage, embolism, increasing stenosis, hypotension, or hypovolemia. Metabolic abnormalities, such as hypoxia, should also be ruled out. The CT scan may need to be repeated, depending upon the severity of the neurologic change. In such patients, initial bedside therapy usually includes a bolus of colloidal fluid. Patients responding to hemodynamic augmentation should, in theory, be good surgical candidates, because their neurologic function appears to be coupled to their hemodynamic state. Actually, the full nature of progressive deterioration in stroke is poorly understood and in need of further study.

Some question the definition of TIA; however, in our experience, with no improvement of significant deficits after 2 h or with a progressive decline in neurologic function, the likelihood of frank stroke is large. For TIAs in the presence of carotid occlusion, adequate collateral flow is a prerequisite to carotid endarterectomy.

Important points in performing a carotid endarterectomy in the case of an acute carotid occlusion include intraoperative intravenous heparinization as well as continuous heparin irrigation once the vessel is open. The surgical microscope facilitates removal of small fragments and, as with heparin, protects against intraoperative embolic complications. Neurologic status is continuously monitored by EEG. The occluded internal carotid is opened distal to the plaque and inspected for thrombus before clamping the common carotid or the external carotid arteries. After the thrombus is removed, standard endarterectomy is performed. If the thrombus cannot be removed, a small balloon catheter can be carefully inserted to make another attempt at removal. If no significant backflow is obtained, internal carotid ligation and stumpectomy are performed.

MCA embolectomy is performed as described by Meyer et al. [11]. After clipping distal to the embolus, a distal branch of the MCA is incised and the thrombus is removed. Bypass has rarely been used for acute stroke at this institution.

Important adjuncts to the perioperative care of these patients include: speed and efficiency; experienced intensive care staff; tight, continuous control of the blood pressure; hemodilution/hypervolemic therapy; and barbiturates. Barbiturates have been shown to be therapeutic within a short therapeutic window of 2–3 h after the ischemic insult [9].

Summary

Although the ischemic penumbra is an appealing model, emergent revascularization for acute stroke should still be considered experimental. The natural history of acute stroke secondary to cerebral vascular occlusion is still unclear. The qualities that determine the ideal surgical candidate are not completely defined, and our ability to evaluate the efficacy of the surgical procedures awaits better knowledge of the natural history. It may be that, with the adjunctive therapies of cerebral protection with barbiturates and hemodynamic augmentation, the time limit of the penumbra can be lengthened, and early revascularization will become more consistently successful.

References

1. Blaisdell WF, Clauss RH, Galbraith JG, et al. (1969) Joint study of extracranial arterial occlusion. JAMA 209:1889–1895
2. Britton M, Roden A (1985) Progression of stroke after arrival at hospital. Stroke 16:629–632
3. Diaz FG, Ausman JI, Mehta B, et al. (1985) Acute cerebral revascularization. J Neurosurg 63:200–209
4. Gagliardi R, Benvenuti L, Guizzardi G (1983) Acute operation in cases of middle cerebral artery occlusion. Neurosurgery 12:636–639
5. Gratzl O, Schmiedek P, Spetzler R, et al. (1976) Clinical experience with extra-intracranial arterial anastomosis in 65 cases. J Neurosurg 44:313–324
6. Grillo P, Patterson RH (1975) Occlusion of the carotid artery: Prognosis (natural history) and the possibility of surgical revascularization. Stroke 6:17–20
7. Moulin DE, Lo R, Chiang J, et al. (1985) Prognosis in middle cerebral artery occlusion. Stroke 16:282–284
8. Ojemann RG, Crowell RM, Roberson GH, et al. (1975) Surgical treatment of extracranial carotid occlusive disease. Clin Neurosurg 22:214–263
9. Selman WR, Spetzler RF, Roski RA, et al. (1982) Barbiturate coma in focal cerebral ischemia: Relationship of protection to timing of therapy. J Neurosurg 56:685–690
10. Strong AJ, Venables GS, Gibson G (1983) The cortical ischaemic penumbra associated with occlusion of the middle cerebral artery in the cat: 1. Topography of changes in blood flow, potassium ion activity, and EEG. J Cereb Blood Flow Metabol 3:86–96
11. Sundt TM Jr (1987) Occlusive cerebrovascular disease. Saunders, Philadelphia, pp 269–279, 467–476
12. Weinstein PR, Anderson GG, Telles DA (1986) Neurological deficit and cerebral infarction after temporary middle cerebral artery occlusion in unanesthetized cats. Stroke 17:318–324

Peracute Revascularization for the Cases of Major Trunk Occlusion of Major Stroke Type

Mitsuo Kaneko and Keisei Tanaka[1]

For the past 7 years, we have accumulated experience of peracute revascularization for the cases of major trunk occlusion of major stroke type. Since we adopted the dynamic CT scan 5 years ago, it became far easier and clearer to decide the indication for surgery in a short period of time.

Our patients were admitted as early as possible after the onset of stroke, and the emergency revascularization was performed after documenting the site of occlusion in a major trunk of the carotid artery system and then measuring the hemodynamic pattern, by means of dynamic CT scan (DCT), routinely. Preoperative administration of mannitol and barbiturates was initiated earlier, even immediately after the dyanmic CT scan.

In this report, we will discuss how to differentiate the reversible cases by using DCT, what happens in those cases of peracute revascularization (43 cases), and then what ensued on those cases not indicated for peracute revascularization (19 cases).

Vascular reconstruction (EC-IC bypass or direct embolectomy) was performed within 6 h after the onset of stroke in most cases; this could be the approximate maximal time limit for the reversibility of cerebral ischemia of this type in those experiences.

Material and Method

Since 1980, 43 cases of peracute revascularization have been performed for major stroke in our hospital (Table 1). When the patient was admitted within 2–3 h after the onset of stroke, an urgent series of examination were initiated immediately.

Plain CT scan. Most cases, of course, do not show any low-density area in such early stage.

Dynamic CT scan. After administration of 60 cm^3 65% angiografin by bolus injection in a cubital vein, a time-density curve on each ROI (region of interest) is drawn on the selected tomographic scan. The general hemodynamic pattern can be observed by comparison with the opposite side of healthy hemisphere.

Cerebral angiography. The definite site of occlusion or stenosis of the cerebral artery can be pointed out.

Routine preoperative clinical examination. Plain chest X-ray, EKG, several blood examinations, etc.

The patient was sent to the operating room mostly within 1 or 2 h after admission to the hospital. Then, the emergency revascularization was completed mostly within 6 h after the onset of stroke.

A total 28 other cases were not indicated for the peracute revascularization and their clinical courses were analyzed compared to the operated cases.

Hemodynamic patterns on DCT

Hemodynamic patterns were classified into three types from the level of the residual blood flow (Fig. 1).

In type 1, there is considerable residual blood flow in the area of arterial occlusion, with a peak value of more than 50% of the healthy side. In type 2, there is less collateral blood supply in the occluded area, with a peak value of one-third to one-half of the healthy side. In type 3 patterns, there is minimal collateral flow with a peak value of less than one-third of that of the healthy side. The time-density curve is almost flat.

In our experience, those cases showing the time density curve of type 1 responded well for acute revascularization if it was completed within 6 h after onset with enough blood supply.

[1] Department of Neurosurgery, Hamamatsu Medical Center, Hospital, Shizuoka, Japan

Table 1. Clinical summary of the emergency revascularization

Case no.	Age (yrs)	Sex	Clinical manifest.	Occluded vessel	Preop. DCT	Method of revasculn.	Time to Op. (h)	LDA on CT	ADL
1	66	F	Rt-hemi. aphasia	Lt-Ex.IC		EC-IC	4	None	1
2	51	M	Rt-hemi., aphasia	Lt-Ex.IC		EC-IC	5.5	None	1
3	37	M	Rt-hemi., aphasia	Lt-M1		Embolectomy	5	Small cort.	1
4	56	M	Lt-hemi.	Rt-M1		Embolectomy	6	Small cort.	1
5	56	M	Rt-hemi., aphasia	Lt-Ex.IC	Type 1	EC-IC	6	None	1
6	56	M	Rt-hemi., aphasia	Lt-Ex.IC	Type 1	EC-IC	6.5	None	1
7	50	M	Lt-hemi.	Rt-Ex.IC	Type 1	EC-IC	3	Small cort.	1
8	59	M	Lt-hemi.	Rt-M1	Type 1	Embolectomy	4.5	Small cort.	1
9	72	F	Rt-hemi., aphasia	Lt-M1	Type 1	EC-IC	5.5	Small cort.	1
10	61	M	Lt-hemi.	Rt-M1	Type 1	Embolectomy	6	Small cort.	1
11	58	M	Lt-hemi.	Rt-M1	Type 1	EC-IC	6	Lacuna	1
12	59	M	Lt-hemi.	Rt-M1	Type 1	EC-IC	6	Small cort.	1
13	71	M	Lt-hemi.	Rt-M1	Type 1	Embolectomy	6	Lacuna	1
14	64	M	Rt-hemi., aphasia	Lt-M1	Type 1	Embolectomy	5	None	1
15	63	M	Rt-hemi., aphasia	Lt-M1	Type 1	EC-IC	5	Small cort.	1
16	60	M	Rt-hemi., aphasia	Lt-M1		EC-IC	6	Lacuna	1
17	66	M	Rt-hemi., aphasia	Lt-M1	Type 1	EC-IC	13	Small cort.	2
18	57	M	Rt-hemi., aphasia	Lt-Ex.IC	Type 1	EC-IC	14	Small cort.	2
19	68	M	Lt-hemi.	Rt-Ex.IC	Type 1	EC-IC	6	Small cort.	2
20	62	F	Lt-hemi.	Rt-M1	Type 1	EC-IC	5.5	Small cort.	2
21	74	M	Rt-hemi., aphasia	Lt-Ex.IC	Type 1	EC-IC	6.5	Moderate cort.	2
22	69	M	Lt-hemi.	Rt-M1		EC-IC	11	Small cort.	2
23	56	M	Rt-hemi., aphasia	Lt-Ex.IC	Type 1	EC-IC	3	Border	2
24	59	M	Lt-hemi.	Rt-M1	Type 2	EC-IC	7	Border	2
25	58	F	Rt-hemi., aphasia	Lt-Ex.IC		EC-IC	7	Border	3
26	66	M	Lt-hemi.	Rt-M1	Type 1	EC-IC	8	Border	3
27	71	M	Lt-hemi.	Rt-M1	Type 2	EC-IC	4	None	3
28	61	F	Rt-hemi., aphasia	Lt-Ex.IC	Type 2	EC-IC	4.5	Small cort.	3
29	65	M	Lt-hemi.	Rt-Ex.IC	Type 1	EC-IC	6	Small cort.	3
30	76	F	Rt-hemi., aphasia	Lt-M1		EC-IC	4	Small cort.	3
31	76	M	Rt-hemi., aphasia	Lt-M1	Type 1	Embolectomy	4	Lacuna	3
32	69	M	Lt-hemi.	Rt-M1		EC-IC	6	Small cort.	3
33	61	M	Rt-hemi., aphasia	Lt-M1	Type 2	EC-IC	5	Moderate cort.	3
34	70	F	Lt-hemi.	Rt-In.IC		Embolectomy	6	Moderate cort.	3
35	72	M	Rt-hemi., aphasia	Lt-M1	Type 1	EC-IC	12	Large cort.	3
36	75	M	Lt-hemi.	Rt-In.IC	Type 2	Embolectomy	4	Moderate cort.	3
37	70	F	Lt-hemi., aphasia	Rt-M1	Type 2	EC-IC	6	Moderate cort.	3
38	57	F	Rt-hemi., aphasia	Lt-M1	Type 3	EC-IC	5	Moderate cort.	3
39	77	F	Rt-hemi., aphasia	Lt-Ex.IC		EC-IC	6	None	4
40	57	M	Rt-hemi., aphasia	Lt-In.IC	Type 1	EC-IC	6	Moderate cort.	4
41	78	M	Rt-hemi., aphasia	Lt-M1		Embolectomy	5	Large cort.	5
42	58	M	Rt-hemi., aphasia	Lt-In.IC		EC-IC	7.5	Massive	Died
43	73	M	Lt-hemi.	Rt-Ex.IC	Type 3	EC-IC	4	Massive	Died

Hemi hemiplegia, *EC-IC* extracranial-intracranial bypass, *Ex.IC* extracranial internal carotid, *In.IC* intracranial internal carotid, *M1* M-1 portion of the middle cerebral artery, *cort* cortical

Summary of Operated Cases

We have performed 43 cases of peracute revascularization during the past 7 years: 32 men and ten women, ranging from 37 to 78 years old (average, 63.7 years old; Table 1). In 13 cases, there was a previous history of some cardiac disease, mostly atrial fibrillation.

On admission, all patients had severe hemiplegia: on the right side in 25 patients, and on the left in 18 patients. All 25 right hemiplegic patients and one left hemiplegic had associated aphasia.

The site of occlusion, as indicated by emergency cerebral angiography, was in the extracranial segment of an internal carotid artery in 14 patients, in the intracranial segment of an internal carotid artery in five patients, and in a middle cerebral artery in 24 patients.

The time interval from the onset of stroke to the completion of revascularization ranged from 3 to 14 h; 35 patients were completed within 6 h after the onset (Table 1).

Superficial temporal artery to middle cerebral artery (STA-MCA) anastomosis or EC-IC bypass was performed in 34 patients and embolectomy was done in nine patients.

Postoperative prognosis was classified in activity of daily life (ADL) according to standards set by the Japan Neurosurgical Society for Stroke. Fifteen patients recovered to ADL 1 (full recovery to daily activity). Nine patients returned to ADL 2, or partial recovery, with remarkable relief of hemiplegia. Thirteen patients remained in ADL 3 (required assistance in daily life). These might correspond to the natural course of cerebral infarction: in other words, revascularization may have played no part in the lack of improvement in these patients. Another four patients worsened to ADL 4 (restricted to bed). In an early series, two patients died of hemorrhagic infarction, in which the residual blood flow must have been very poor or the time-density curve was flat. Such a case is contraindicated for revascularization these days, due to those experiences.

On retrospective review, preoperative hemodynamic patterns on DCT could predict well the functional recovery of patients after revascularization. Of 23 cases of type 1 on preoperative DCT, 18 cases returned to ADL 1 or 2, and four cases resulted in ADL 3. Of six cases of type 2, one case returned to ADL 2, and five cases remained in ADL 3. Of two cases of type 3, which were operated upon in our early series, one remained in ADL 3 and another died of hemorrhagic infarction.

On postoperative CT scan, eight cases showed almost normal findings, 22 cases had small low-density areas in the subcortex, basal ganglia, or borderzone area, and 13 cases showed moderate or large areas of low density.

Summary of Unoperated Cases

Two unoperated cases of type 1 on early DCT became ADL 3 or 4, each showing moderate size of low-density areas on late CT scans. Of seven unoperated cases of type 2, all became ADL 3 or 4, showing large low-density areas on late CT scan.

Of 19 unoperated cases of type 3, eight cases became ADL 4, one became ADL 5 (vegetative), and ten cases died. All showed hemispheric low-

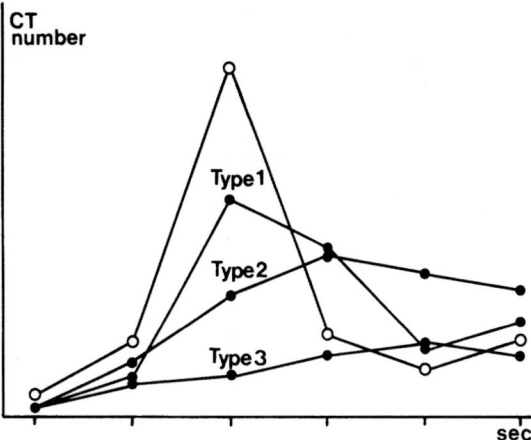

Fig. 1. Hemodynamic patterns in the acute stage of stroke on dynamic CT scan

density areas associated with remarkable cerebral swelling.

Conclusion

In those cases of major trunk occlusion of major stroke type, peracute revascularization is effective if it is done for cases of type 1 on DCT and within 6 h after the onset of stroke with the securing of an adequate route to give enough blood supply.

References

1. Kobayashi S, Oka H, et al. (1984) Hemodynamic study in cerebral infarction using dynamic CT scan. Neuro Surg (Tokyo) 12(13):1477–1484
2. Shimada T, Kaneko M, et al. (1983) Clinical study on dynamic CT scan in cases of acute revascularization performed within 6 hours after onset. CT research (Japan) 5(1):295–296
3. Shimada T, Kaneko M, et al. (1986) A Clinical study of major stroke cases of a low perfusion pattern on a dynamic CT scan. CT research (Japan) 8(5):529–535
4. Kaneko M (1984) Peracute revascularization for cerebral arterial occlusion of major stroke type. Japan J Stroke 6(1):150–152

Acute Stage Revascularization Under the Administration of a New Cerebral Protective Agent, "Sendai Cocktail"

Takashi Yoshimoto, Akira Ogawa, and Jiro Suzuki[1]

Introduction

Following Suzuki's discovery in 1969 that mannitol is capable of protecting the brain against the effects of ischemia [2], numerous experimental and clinical studies have been carried out in our department on substances which might have similar protective effects [3, 5, 6, 10]. Since 1980 we have been able to apply the results of that research to the treatment of ischemic vascular disorders, which had previously been treated conservatively for want of an effective therapeutic technique [4, 7]. Specifically, we currently use a new technique which entails the administration of brain protective substances at an early stage following onset. While such drugs are acting to suppress the development of pathology due to the brain ischemia, acute stage vascular reconstruction is performed. In 1982, we reported on our first series of successful cases in a preliminary study [4]. In the present paper, we discuss the results in the 52 cases experienced thus far, details of the therapeutic technique, and our current thoughts on acute stage vasculr reconstruction under the administration of cerebral protective agents.

Therapeutic Methods and Indications

Therapeutic Methods

On the arrival of a patient with an ischemic cerebrovascular disorder, we administer, by intravenous drip over 60 min, the following drugs: 10 ml/kg 20% mannitol, 10 mg/kg vitamin E, and 10 mg/kg phenytoin (the so-called Sendai Cock tail) [9]. Over the next 2 h, we intravenously administer drugs which are known to be efficient oxygen carriers and which have a molecular diameter less than 1/80th that of erythrocytes, namely, the perfluorochemicals (1000 ml of Fluosol-DA) [1]. During this period, we perform cerebral angiography, CT scanning, etc. For those patients deemed suitable for surgery, vascular reconstruction is performed immediately. As a rule, the vascular reconstruction is bypass surgery for thrombosis cases and embolectomy for embolism cases (Fig. 1).

Indications

Cases in which the responsible lesion has been identified in cerebral angiograms and, moreover, in which distinct low-density areas have not yet developed in CT scans, are suitable for surgical correction. Neurologically, cases in which deficits, such as motor paresis, are severe or deteriorating are also considered suitable for vascular reconstruction, provided that the level of consciousness has not yet fallen to that of a semicomatose state. However, when a notable improvement in the neurological symptoms is observed during the administration of the Sendai cocktail, surgery is not performed and the course of the disease is closely observed.

Materials and Methods

Between November 1980 and December 1985, acute stage vascular reconstruction using this technique was performed in 52 cases. The patients ranged in age from 20 to 71 years. The therapeutic results were evaluated 2 months postoperatively, using a five grade classification as follows: excellent, where the patient was entirely normal; good, in which mild neurological deficits remained but a return to a normal social life was possible; fair, in which independent domestic life was still possible; poor, in which the patient was dependent upon others in daily life; and dead.

[1] Division of Neurosurgery, Institute of Brain, Diseases, Tohoku University School of Medicine, Sendai, Japan

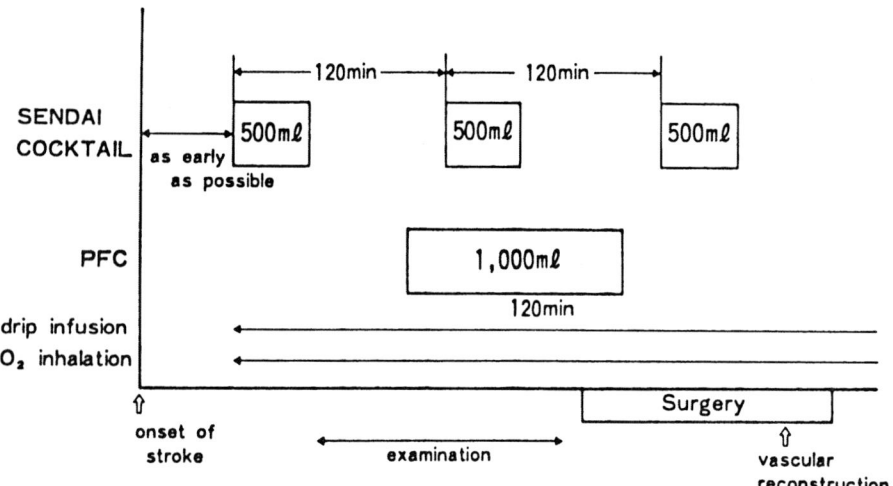

Fig. 1. Therapeutic methods. *PFC* perfluorochemicals

Results

Overall Results

The outcome of the 52 cases included 21 in excellent condition (40%), 11 in good condition (21%), nine in fair condition (17%), three in poor condition (6%), and eight dead (15%).

Major Stroke and Progressing Stroke

For the major stroke cases, the Sendai Cocktail was administered and vascular reconstruction begun as soon as possible. The time from onset until recirculation ranged from 6 to 24 h, with a mean of 12 h. For the progressive stroke cases, however, the Sendai Cocktail was administered soon after admission and, depending upon the case, hypertensive therapy begun; however, the course of the disease was observed before surgery was undertaken. In cases where symptoms persisted or deteriorated, vascular reconstruction was performed. The time until surgery varied from 1 to 8 days, with a mean of 4 days. The results were as follows: among the major stroke cases, 14 were excellent (41%), four good (12%), six fair (17%), three poor (9%), and seven dead (21%). Among the progressing stroke cases, there were seven excellent (39%), seven good (39%), three fair (17%), none poor, and one dead (6%). The outcome was favorable in the majority of the progressing stroke cases, with most of the patients returning to useful social lives. The one fatality had an occlusion of the internal carotid artery and contracted pneumonia postoperatively (Table 1).

Thrombosis and Embolism Cases

There were 27 thrombosis cases, including 18 cases of progressing stroke. The outcomes were excellent in 15 cases (56%), good in seven (26%), fair in four (13%), and there was one death (4%). More than 80% of these patients returned to useful social lives. In contrast, among the 25 embolism cases, six had excellent outcomes (24%), four were good (16%), five were fair (20%), three were poor (12%), and there were seven deaths (28%). In other words, the number of favorable outcomes (excellent and good) was similar to the number of unfavorable outcomes (poor and death), at about 40% each. The cause of death in four of the seven fatalities was deterioration of the postoperative systemic condition (renal failure in two cases, myocardial infarction in one case, and pneumonia in one case). The remaining three deaths were due to brain infarction, that is, hemorrhagic infarction or marked brain edema (Table 2).

Site of the Occluded Vessel

The vascular occlusion was in the internal carotid artery (ICA) in 16 cases and in the middle cerebral artery (MCA) in 36 cases. The outcomes in the ICA cases were excellent in five (31%), good in two (13%), fair in three (19%), poor in two (13%), and dead in four (25%). Among the MCA cases, excellent outcomes were found in 16 cases (44%), good in nine (25%), fair in six (17%), poor in one (3%), and there were four deaths (11%). Three of the four ICA deaths were due to cerebral infarction, whereas all of the

Table 1. Results of major stroke and progressing stroke

	Major stroke	Progressing stroke
Excellent	14 (41%)	7 (39%)
Good	4 (12%)	7 (39%)
Fair	6 (17%)	3 (17%)
Poor	3 (9%)	0
Dead	7 (21%)	1 (6%)
Total	34 cases	18 cases

Table 2. Results of thrombosis and embolism cases

	Thrombosis	Embolism
Excellent	15 (56%)	6 (24%)
Good	7 (26%)	4 (16%)
Fair	4 (15%)	5 (20%)
Poor	0	3 (12%)
Dead	1 (4%)	7 (28%)
Total	27 cases	25 cases

MCA deaths were due to systemic complications (Table 3).

Table 3. Results and site of the occluded vessels

	ICA	MCA
Excellent	5 (31%)	16 (44%)
Good	2 (13%)	9 (25%)
Fair	3 (19%)	6 (17%)
Poor	2 (13%)	1 (3%)
Dead	4 (25%)	4 (11%)
Total	16 cases	36 cases

ICA internal carotid artery, *MCA* middle cerebral artery

Summary

Therapeutic Results

Although there is no appropriate control study for comparison with the present results, it is noteworthy that, among the 1000 cases [8] of similar disorders brought to the hospital within 24 h of onset, 44% had excellent or good results after two months of conservative therapy. Moreover, among the 292 cases which had distinct vascular lesions, only 17% had excellent or good results. These clinical findings strongly indicate the superiority of our new technique for acute stage vascular reconstruction, in which 61% were found to have excellent or good outcomes. This new therapeutic method, involving acute stage vascular reconstruction under the administration of brain protective substances (the Sendai Cocktail), has been found to be effective in cases of ischemic cerebrovascular disorder.

Indications

We have discussed our results in cases of major stroke, progressing stroke, thrombosis, embolism, and ICA and MCA lesions. The worst results were for occlusion of the ICA in major strokes due to embolism. This type of occlusion is severe because occlusion at the terminal portion also results in occlusion of the MCA and anterior cerebral artery. Currently, we consider such cases unsuitable for acute stage reconstruction. Among other cases, many will show marked improvements in neurological symptoms due to the therapy, but there have also been some fatalities due to systemic complications—a fact which indicates the importance of postoperative care when treating patients with cerebral infarction.

Surgical Technique

Bypass surgery is normally done in thrombosis cases, and embolectomy in embolism cases. Furthermore, together with recent developments in microballoon catheters, it is becoming possible to use thrombolytic agents, such as urokinase and tissue plasmin activator in localized cerebral regions. These developments suggest that a new intravascular surgical technique for such lesions, in which the surgical invasion is minimal and the entire operation can be completed in a shorter period of time, may become possible.

References

1. Mizoi K, Yoshimoto T, Suzuki J (1981) Experimental study of new cerebral protective substances, functional recovery of severe incomplete ischemic brain lesion, pretreated with mannitol and perfluorocarbon emulsion. Acta Neurochir 56:157–161
2. Suzuki J (1974) A method of prolongation of temporary stopping of the cerebral blood flow. Presidential Address, 33rd Annual Meeting JPN Neurol Surg 1974
3. Suzuki J, Yoshimoto T (1979) The effect of mannitol in prolongation of permissible occlusion time of cerebral artery—clinical data of aneurysm surgery. Neurosurg Rev 1:13–19

4. Suzuki J, Yoshimoto T, Kodama N, et al. (1982) A new therapeutic method for acute brain infarction: Revascularization following the administration of mannitol and perfluorochemicals—A preliminary report. Surg Neurol 17:325–332

5. Suzuki J, Fujimoto S, Mizoi K, et al. (1984) The protective effect of combined administration of antioxidants and perfluorochemicals on cerebral ischemia. Stroke 15:672–679

6. Suzuki J, Imaizumi S, Kayama T, et al. (1985) Chemiluminescence in hypoxic brain. The second report: Cerebral protective effect of mannitol, vitamin E and glucocorticoid. Stroke 16:695–700

7. Suzuki J, Ogawa A, Yoshimoto T, et al. (1985) Indication for surgery in the acute stage of cerebral infarction. The role of new cerebral protective drugs "Sendai cocktail" and perfluorochemicals. In: Spetzler RF, et al (eds) Cerebral revascularization for stroke. Thieme-Stratton, New York, pp 392–396

8. Suzuki J (1987) Clinical course of acute cerebral infarction—analysis from 1,000 cases. Nishimura, Niigata, pp 22–184

9. Suzuki J (1987) Treatment of cerebral infarction—experimental and clinical study. Springer, Vienna, pp 158–202

10. Yoshimoto T, Sakamoto, T, Watanabe T, et al. (1978) Experimental cerebral infarction: III. Protective effect of mannitol in thalamic infarction in dogs. Stroke 9:217–218

Discussion

Schmiedek (Munich): Which patients should be considered for acute revascularization?

Kaneko (Hamamatsu): We have examined more than a thousand cases of cerebral infarction within 2 or 3 h after the onset over the past 7 years. In our series, there have been more than 50 cases of minor (lacunar) stroke. Even with major stroke, the patients are often older and have complications. Cases with definite indications are quite rare. We operated on 50 of 1000 cases. We did hemodynamic studies in most of the patients.

Yoshimoto (Sendai): We studied the natural course of 1000 patients with cerebral infarction. Particularly in cases of middle cerebral artery occlusion with good recovery, there was improvement in the acute stage in 2–3 h, but after that almost all showed deterioration. The indication should be based on a CBF study or some other modern means of diagnosis. However, in those patients who show improvement in the acute stage; acute revascularization may be appropriate.

Tsubokawa (Tokyo): Does this mean that acute revascularization may be indicated if the patients do not improve with 3 h?

Yoshimoto: When we carry out revascularization, we use the Sendai Cocktail to protect the brain. When the patient comes in, we diminish the amount of the Sendai Cocktail and an examination is carried out. If the patient improves, surgery is not indicated. I agree with Dr. Ausman that barbiturate therapy, which induces a comatose state may be misleading in selecting the candidates for acute revascularization. In very severe cases where the consciousness is disturbed we cannot do anything.

Kaneko: It has to be decided whether the stroke type is major or minor at the onset. With a minor stroke type there is minor weakness from the beginning. But 20%–25% of cases of major stroke begin as minor strokes and then progress. So we can usually tell from the onset whether to operate or not. In the case of major stroke we will not be in time if we wait.

Ausman (Detroit): What would you do if, say, a patient arrived in the emergency room and presented with acute right hemiplegia, the history indicating that the duration has been 1 h?

Kaneko: Most of our patients are admitted within 2–3 h of onset and we immediately examine the patient. We receive patients with complete hemiplegia—major stroke type. We take a CT scan, of course, and then do a dynamic CT scan. At this point, we can tell which area is becoming infarcted or how severe the ischemic grade is. We carry out angiography immediately.

Ausman: Let us say the angiogram showes a carotid occlusion; obviously, there is other information that you derive from the CT scan which helps you make a decision. What is this information that makes you decide whether to operate or not?

Kaneko: The portion of occlusion is apparent. On dynamic CT scan if the patient has sufficient collateral of 50% or so we are in time and the patient will recover. We will operate immediately. The CT is the critical test.

Spetzler (Phoenix): I have great trouble with acute bypass surgery and have only experience of one case, a 23-year-old woman. Perhaps the surgery was too late or the protective agents were insufficient, but the patient developed severe edema and died. It seems to me that this will always be a problem unless we have stronger protective agents or can get to the patients sooner so that blood can be resupplied in severe ischemia. With less severe ischemia we do not know what the natural history would be.

Suzuki (Osaka): Two hours from the onset to the start of operation is difficult to believe. How do you manage to take the history, do the urinary catheter, electrocardiogram, DSA, or angiogram and discuss the situation with the patient's family in this time?

Kaneko: We start operating within an hour or hour and a half of the patients arriving at the hospital, but this is nothing difficult. Dynamic CT scan and plain CT scan usually take 30 min; angiography takes 30 min. For anastamosis, we train hard to reduce the time; STA-MCA takes us now about 1–1 1/2 h.

Yoshimoto: With regard to time, all the panelists today gave the figure of 6 h for operation, but I find it difficult to complete revascularization within this time. I did not present my experimental data, but if there is a decrease of 60%– 70% in cerebral blood flow even though revascularization is done in 1–2 h the brain function does not return to normal. However, if the brain protective agents were employed, the time threshold was prolonged. In our clinical series, although the mean time until revascularization after onset was 12 h, we still obtained favorable results. This again shows the importance of the brain protective agents.

Weinstein (San Francisco) There is no doubt about the contraindication for any attempted revascularization or even hypertensive and hypervolemic therapy in patients who have an acute onset of severe deficit with impaired levels of consciousness. But in other patients with mild to moderate deficits we need some method of quantitatively assessing the functional metabolic state of the brain. We have some hope for MRI scanning and ultimately magnetic resonance spectrascopy in this regard, but that technology is certainly not presently available for studies in emergency patients. Have any of the panel found a method of blood flow study in the acute situation that has proven to be reliable for patient selection, because without it I think it would be difficult to rationalize a protocol for future study of the problem.

Schmiedek: I personally believe that CBF studies in this group of patients are probably not very useful. We do not need CBF studies because we can actually see the visible manifestations of cerebral ischemia. Another point is that CBF studies are much too time consuming. There has been very little information on CBF in acute ischemia so I think that these findings would be difficult to interpret.

Kaneko: I agree with Dr. Schmiedek. We do not have the time to perform CBF studies in acute patients. We recommend dynamic CT scans.

Cruz (Sao Paulo): The use of stable xenon CT studies as a standard is the same as using any CBF technique. CBF provides no information whatsever about the metabolism itself. So what is the value of your "critical CBF level" Dr. Kaneko to decide whether to operate or not when you just consider the partition coefficient? If you do not deal with O_2 extraction measurements of $CMRO_2$, which would give a more accurate picture of the condition of the patient, how can you make the decision about surgery?

Kaneko: We cannot tell definitely what the critical CBF level is from the dynamic CT scan, but we are able to arrive at a rough evaluation of the hemodynamic situation. After having dealt with 300 cases in the very acute stage, we feel we can decide whether the condition of the patient is above or below the critical level. Perhaps about 30%–40% of healthy signs is about the critical level.

Commentator, *Auer* (Graz): I think at the moment, emergency surgery for acute cerebral ischemia cannot be recommended as a general procedure; it has to be limited to a very few circumstances which, however, are ill-defined. The problems as clearly defined by the speakers are twofold. The first is time: It is a fight against minutes in emergency surgical procedures for patients with cerebrovascular occlusive disease. The second problem is diagnosis: The earlier a patient is admitted to hospital, the greater the problem as to what the patient actually has. Does the patient have transient ischemic attack or will definite ischemia develop? What we do have available at present is adequate surgical techniques, i.e., EC-IC bypass, embolectomy, and thromboendarterectomy. According to the literature, there is about a 50%–70% improvement rate after emergency procedures, but of course no one really knows what could have been the natural history in these patients. What is lacking right now I feel is adequate organization of patient management for a timely admission to hospital provided that we can give these patients adequate diagnosis on a pathophysiological and pathomorphological basis; we must know if we are dealing with a patient who has a reversible or irreversible ischemic deficit.

So, to summarize, I think that at this time none of the procedures can be generally recommended, with perhaps one exception that has not really been discussed in this session—rethromboendarterectomy following thromboendarterectomy. If a patient who has undergone carotid thromboendarterectomy deteriorates neurologically very few hours after surgery, immediate emergency rethromboendarterectomy to my knowledge from the literature has the best rate of recovery among all procedures of emergency surgery in this context.

RTD 14. Intravascular Surgery and Treatment for Dural AVM and CCF

Operative Thrombosis of Aneurysms and Fistulae

Sean Mullan[1]

Aneurysms

Our experience in treatment includes internal carotid occlusion and thrombosis by wire, needles, and balloon.

Internal Carotid Occlusion

This is a perfectly safe procedure for any patient who can tolerate manual carotid compression. The key to safety is to carry out the occlusion under full heparinization as taught by Rasmussen in the early 1950s.

Step 1. The Selverstone clamp is applied (open) under local or general anesthesia.

Step 2. When the patient is fully awake, the clamp is totally closed to verify ischemic tolerance. If the patient tolerates occlusion for one minute, the clamp is set with five-eighths of one turn open, i.e., almost totally closed. If not tolerated for a full minute, we have, on two occasions successfully, slowly occluded the clamp over a period of 2–3 weeks. We have not had any others in which this slow attempt failed. If the total occlusion produces ischemic symptoms very rapidly, we have not attempted a slow occlusion.

Step 3. Over a 2-day period, subtotal occlusion is continued for the patient who tolerates the initial trial occlusion. This interval permits the distal carotid to shrink in proportion to the new volume it transmits, so that, eventually, when a clot is allowed to develop within it, there will be no further elasticity and, therefore, no force to extrude the clot intracerebrally. The clamp is adjusted each day since it sometimes opens slightly under the continued pulsation.

Step 4. The patient is totally heparinized. Heparinization is not started earlier because of the risk of wound hematoma immediately after surgery. The clamp is fully occluded. Heparinization is maintained for 2 days. If symptoms occur, the clamp is opened.

Step 5. The stem of the clamp is removed.

We have twice observed hemispheric signs and symptoms. One patient developed these suddenly, associated with a slight fall in systemic blood pressure. The clip was opened, and he made an immediate recovery. The internal carotid artery was then successfully occluded over a 2-week period. It was never certain whether the problem was ischemic or embolic. Another patient had a slow decrease in higher intellectual function, beginning about 3 h after total occlusion, noted by his family but not observable by the medical and nursing staff, over a period of a few hours. It was finally recognized as dysphasia appeared. All symptoms and signs completely reversed over a few hours upon opening the clamp. It was not reapplied.

A limitation to the carotid occlusion method is that giant aneurysms are frequently bilateral.

Thrombosis of Carotid Cavernous Aneurysms

We have attempted to occlude the aneurysms while preserving carotid flow by three methods.

Wire thrombosis. This has been described in detail in the literature [1]. It is suitable for small aneurysms of about 1 cm in diameter with small necks. It is not suitable for giant aneurysms, most of which have broad necks which permit the thrombus to extend into the carotid. In one patient with a very small aneurysm, the wire itself, finding inadequate room within the aneurysm, extended into the carotid and thrombosed it asymptomatically.

Needle thrombosis. This method is suitable for relatively small aneurysms with a well-defined neck. Copper clad steel needles of 0.2-mm diam-

---

[1] Department of Neurosurgery, University of Chicago Medical Center, Chicago, USA

eter inserted transdurally across the neck will effectively thrombose them. These are so small that they have not injured the extraocular nerves in any instance.

Ballon thrombosis. This is our current area of interest. It is indicated for patients with giant symptomatic aneurysms who may not tolerate carotid occlusion, in whom carotid occlusion is inadvisable because of bilateral aneurysms, or in whom there is contralateral atherosclerosis. Our experience has been with the use of DeBrun balloons and Fogerty balloon catheters (no. 4). Neither is ideal. The DeBrun balloon catheter is too flexible and cannot be forced against the neck. It floats freely within the blood stream. The Fogerty catheter, cut off short, can be pushed against the neck, but the volume of each balloon (0.75–1.0 ml) is too small. Three to six such balloons must be used. It is, however, preferable to the DeBrun. One balloon is positioned against the neck and held there by subsequently positioned balloons.

The balloon catheters are inserted by craniotomy with exposure of the cavernous dura. They are inserted through separate needles which are withdrawn, leaving the balloon catheter in place. Hemorrhage from the needle tract is stopped by Surgicel and slight pressure. The balloons are inflated with saline, one at a time, and occlusion is monitored by serial angiography (usually performed through a retrograde superficial temporal artery catheter). When the exact degree of occlusion has been achieved, the balloons are deflated and then filled sequentially with silastic. The end point should be close to the volume of saline previously used, but may not be identical and must again be arrived at by serial angiography. We have used continous corticography to monitor cerebral function during occlusion [3].

Thrombosis of Supraclinoid Aneurysms

These have smaller necks than cavernous aneurysms; therefore, there is not the same risk of intraarterial spread of thrombosis. Quite larger aneurysms may be safely occluded by wire on the supraclinoid carotid and on the anterior and middle cerebral arteries. We have also occluded very thick-walled giant middle cerebral arteries by the balloon insertion method. This method employs a large needle through which the no. 4 Fogerty catheter is inserted, which

could rupture a very thin wall. Wire insertion, on the other hand, using a 31-gauge needle, can be carried out safely through the most delicate wall.

Carotid Cavernous Fistulae

The technique employed has varied somewhat since that previously described [2]. We had previously advocated the insertion of thrombogenic material in a retrograde manner through the ophthalmic vein and the superior petrosal sinus. We also used wire inserted into any cavernous areas not radiographically filled by artery, and needles into the fistulous communication.

As our experience progressed, we continued to utilize the ophthalmic vein and the superior petrosal sinus as the approaches of choice, but have become more familiar with direct incision and packing into the sinus immediately above the foramen rotundum and into the posterior superior bulge lateral to the third and fourth nerves (Parkinson's triangle). We have used wire infrequently, not because it is not effective, but because its insertion is somewhat tedious.

The major problems have resulted from delay in initiating treatment, in four patients due to delay in referral (one), delay in the patient's consent (two), and delay in our judgement (one). These resulted in two instances of blindness and in two deaths. There were, in addition, two technical errors. In one patient, we caused a massive intracerebral hemorrhage when we inserted a preoperative lumbar drain. In another, following the report of the use of a direct cyanoacrylate occlusion of the sinus [4], we placed a small catheter (craniotomy) in the sinus. Two injections of contrast showed no reflux into the carotid, but subsequent to the injection of the thrombogenic liquid, the patient sustained a carotid occlusion and died.

These experiences have taught us that delay in treatment, whether caused by the patient or by those in charge of his management, can have serious consequences. We have also learned that fatal spontaneous subarachnoid hemorrhages can occur, subdural drainage can precipitate a fatal subdural hemorrhage, and a liquid thrombogenic agent should not be used in the cavernous sinus.

There have been no ischemic complications and no permanent extraocular or motor palsies. One patient completely recovered from a sixth nerve palsy at the end of a year.

Balloon Occlusion of Fistulae

This is now the method of choice for the acute traumatic fistula if the patient can tolerate unilateral manual carotic compression. It is recognized that, in a large number of cases, occlusion is effected by occluding the carotid rather than the fistula itself. For all patients who cannot tolerate manual occlusion, for those with contralateral cavernous fistulae or aneurysms, and for those with evidence of atherosclerosis, we prefer to maximize the possibility of saving the carotid by using the craniotomy and direct packing method. For those in whom balloon embolization has failed or for those in whom symptoms recur despite a previous trapping operation, there seems to be no good alternative to direct occlusion in most instances. A very occasional recurrence after direct trapping might be subject to arterial embolization if only one external arterial branch was involved.

Cavernous Dural Fistulae

They are mostly unilateral, low flow fistulae producing unilateral visual symptoms. A few shunt to both sides but are unilateral in origin. A very few are independently bilateral: They are distinguished from traumatic- and aneurysm-derived fistulae in that the blood supply is primarily from the external carotid and secondarily from the dural branches of the internal carotid. These smaller fistulae may be embolized by percutaneous catheterization of the external carotid through the femoral. For the larger fistulae with multiple feeders, operative thrombosis of the cavernous sinus is simpler for both the patient and the surgeon.

Lateral Sinus and Other Dural Fistulae

These are commonly found in relation to the cavernous sinus, or, less frequently, in association with the lateral sinus. They can also be found in relation to the superior or inferior petrosal sinus, to the sagittal sinus, or to the vein of Galen, and sometimes to a cortical vein attached to, but not draining into, a sinus. Except for those obviously congenital malformations relating to the vein of Galen, these are acquired lesions which probably arise from a segment of thrombosed sinus or vein. Apparently, in the process of recanalization, the arterial and venous ingrowing channels join up.

Lateral sinus fistulae usually carry a very high volume of blood and are filled from many external carotid, internal carotid, vertebral, and cervical arterial branches, unilateral or bilateral, even when the fistula is unilateral. They are best dealt with by operative thrombosis of the lateral sinus. This is done by trapping the segment by a proximal and distal balloon and then packing it with thrombogenic material.

Fistulae of veins entering into the sagittal or lateral sinus are usually accompanied by evidence that a sinus thrombosis had once occurred at this site. The sinus has either recanalized separately from its entering vein, or has established an adequate collateral. Surgical excision of the fistulous point is relatively simple. In our experience, the surface area that is fistulous in the lateral sinus has been very large, but in the venous, or the sagittal, and in the petrosal fistula, the exact site of the fistula has been small, though the arterial and venous components have been quite extensive.

Thrombosis of Cerebral Arteriovenous Malformations

It has long been known that clipping of the distal anterior cerebral artery was not necessarily followed by devastating disability and, in fact, the method was once used in the treatment of some anterior communicating aneurysms. Therefore, it appeared possible to consider thrombosing cerebral arteriovenous malformations that were located in the distal anterior cerebral distribution. The pericallosal and calloso-marginal were catheterized above the corpus callosum and the malformations were obliterated by the injection of thrombogenic glue. There were three groups: Those confined to the medial surface of the hemisphere had no postoperative complications. Those that extended over the surface and deep into the hemisphere had a temporary hemiparesis which disappeared within a week or two. The third group had an established preoperative hemiparesis either due to a hemorrhage or due to a steal. They developed an increased hemiparesis which took up to 3 months to return to preoperative levels. Since no patient suffered a permanent disability, we believe that this method has less morbidity than a conventional excision in this AVM.

References

1. Mullan S (1974) Experiences with surgical thrombosis of intracranial berry aneurysms and carotid cavernous fistulas. J Neurosurg 41:657–670
2. Mullan S (1979) Treatment of carotid cavernous fistulas by cavernous sinus occlusion. J Neurosurg 50:131–144
3. Mullan S, Duda EE, Patronas NJ (1980) Some examples of balloon technology in nurosurgery. J Neurosurg 52:321–329
4. Sampson D, Ditmore QM, Beyer CW (1981) Intravascular use of isobutyl 2-cyanoacrylate: II. Treatment of carotid cavernous fistulas. Neurosurg 8:52–55

Intraoperative Metallic Thrombosis of Carotid-Cavernous Fistula

Y. Hosobuchi[1]

It has long been known that red blood cells, white blood cells, and fibrinogen are negatively charged at the normal pH of blood. It is also known that white blood cells and washed platelets migrate to the positive pole in an electrophoretic cell [1, 10]. Thus, the intravascular presence of a metal with a high dissociation constant of positively charged metallic ions, such as Fe^{2+}, Cu^{2+}, and Be^{2+}, should attract these negatively charged intravascular elements to form a thrombus; this reaction should be enhanced by passage of an anodal current through the metal. The earliest attempts to apply this logic to the formation of an intravascular thrombus were made independently by Velpeau in 1831 [11] and Phillips in 1832 [9], who described a method of occluding an artery by introducing needles into the lumen and withdrawing the needles after a thrombus had formed about them. Velpeau [11] and Phillips [9] both suggested that this method might be utilized in the treatment of aneurysms. Moore and Murchison [5] first reported insertion of a permanent wire into an aneurysmal sac to create an intrasaccular thrombus.

Hamby [3] described how Ciniselli, in 1847, was the first to use electrical current to aid in the deposition of fibrin and the formation of a clot, passing it through needles temporarily-inserted into an aneurysmal sac. The feasibility and therapeutic potential of this method were recognized by others. Blackemore and King [2] and Linton and Hardy [4] reported particularly favorable results in the treatment of aortic aneurysms before the development of the artificial aortic bypass.

Electrothrombosis of intracranial aneurysms was introduced by Werner et al. [12] in 1941, but it was not favorably received by neurosurgeons. The technique was reintroduced by Mullan et al. [6] in 1964; Peterson et al. [8] applied this technique to the treatment of a carotid cavernous fistula in 1968. After introducing a copper wire through the dilated superior ophthalmic vein into the carotid-cavernous sinus, Peterson and coworkers [8] applied 2 mA positive current to the wire for 4 h and progressively obliterated the fistula by thrombosis; however, 3 days later, the internal carotid artery thrombosed spontaneously and vision in the patient's ipsilateral eye was lost.

I have used the electrometallic thrombosis technique in the treatment of 80 patients who had a total of 90 fistulas, ten of which were bilateral. This paper describes the technique, its results and complications, and its role in relation to other modes of treatment of carotid-cavernous fistulas.

Methods

Introduction of Copper Wire Through the Superior Ophthalmic Vein

A dilated superior ophthalmic vein receiving arterial blood can easily be identified through simple incisions of the upper eyelid. The vein is cannulated with a polyethylene, barium-impregnated catheter which is advanced to the cavernous sinus under fluoroscopic control. Size 29- to 34-gauge copper wires (10–40 mm in length) are then inserted through the catheter into the cavernous sinus. Direct current from a constant direct-current generator, varying from 0.2 mA to 0.8 mA, is applied for 10–30 min to initiate thrombosis in the cavernous sinus. The cathether is removed, the copper wires are cut flush with the superior ophthalmic vein as it joins the naso-frontalis vein, and the incision in the eyelid is closed. It then takes a few days before thrombosis of the fistula is complete.

After a week following the initial procedure, carotid arteriography is repeated to verify occlusion of the fistula. When occlusion is confirmed,

---

[1] Department of Neurological Surgery, School of Medicine, University of California, San Francisco, California, USA

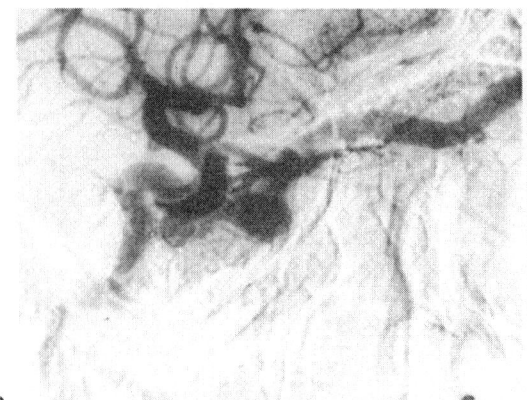

a

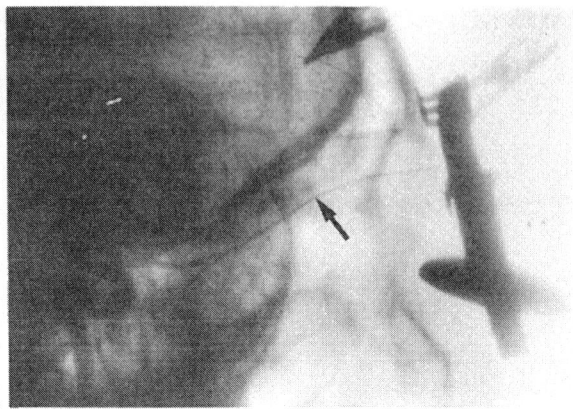

b

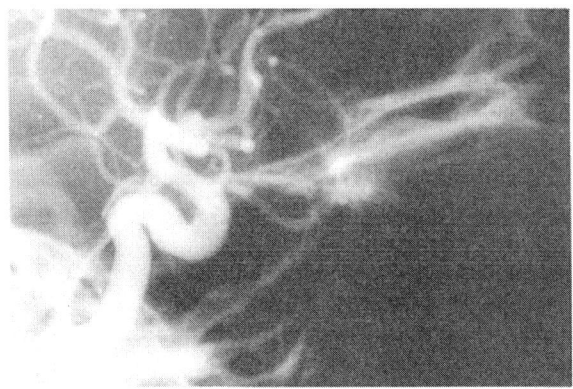

c

Fig. 1. a A spontaneous carotid-cavernous fistula in a 34-year-old woman involved only the anterior segment of the sinus to the superior ophthalmic vein. b An intraoperative X-ray film shows 28-gauge copper wires (*arrow*) inserted to the anterior cavernous sinus through the ophthalmic vein. c Postoperative angiogram shows total obliteration of the fistula

the palpebral incision is reopened under local anesthesia and the copper wire is removed. This technique is simple, although only applicable to a fistula located at the anterior portion of the cavernous sinus, because it is generally difficult to manipulate the catheter or wire beyond the midpoint of the cavernous sinus (Fig. 1). In my series of 90 fistulas, I was able to use this method in only four cases.

Direct Introduction of Copper Wires and Needles into the Cavernous Sinus by Craniotomy

With the patient positioned on his or her side and under general anesthesia, the ipsilateral superficial temporal artery is cannulated for operative angiography. The temporal lobe, approached through a frontotemporal craniotomy, is retracted, and the tentorial incisura and the ipsilateral third nerve are identified. A small metallic clip is applied to the tentorium just posterior to the ingress of the third nerve; angiograms are made to establish the topographical relationship of the metallic clip, carotid artery, and the cavernous sinus. If the fistula drains to the posterior segment of the sinus, and therefore to the superior and inferior petrosal veins, various lengths

of 29- to 34-gauge copper wires (10–40 mm in length) are inserted into the posterior half of the "Parkinson triangle." This area, described by Parkinson [7], contains no neurovascular structures except the meningohypophyseal branch of the internal carotid artery.

A 15-cm length of 22-gauge, thin-walled hypodermic tubing, shaped to a fine, penetrating point, is used as an insertion needle for the copper wires, which range from 30- to 34-gauge. A finer inserting needle is used for wires of smaller gauge (e.g., a 31-gauge needle for 40- to 46-gauge copper, beryllium-copper, or stainless steel wire).

Because the fine metallic wire is soft and may bend where it enters the needle, a "pump" is used to advance the wire. This pump is made with 4 cm of 22-gauge, thin-walled hypodermic tubing passed over the 31-gauge tubing. The wire and the end of the pump are grasped together and pushed forward. When the wire meets resistance, the insertion needle is withdrawn from the sinus, and the wire is cut off 2–3 mm from the wall of the sinus. Direct anodal current (0.2–0.5 mA) may be applied to the cut end of the wire for 60–120 s to initiate thrombosis. When the surgeon can insert the copper or beryllium-copper wire no further into the sinus because of the softness of the wire and the fistulous flow over the portion of the sinus in the operative field, stiffer stainless steel wire may be used for mechanical packing of the remaining space.

Usually, three to four separate copper or beryllium-copper wires are needed to thrombose the posterior segment of Parkinson's triangle [7]. The progression of thrombosis following the insertion of each copper wire or needle is monitored with intraoperative angiograms.

If a fistula still exists, the inferior drainage through the pterygoid plexus is next approached. The engorged pterygoid plexus can be identified easily after the posterior venous drainage is closed, because the major force of shunted arterial blood is now directed inferiorly toward it, the ophthalmic veins, and sometimes toward the circular sinus and the basal vein of Rosenthal. Copper wires (10–12 mm long, 28-gauge to 30-gauge) are inserted parallel to the overlying dura and perpendicular to the course of the pterygoid plexus. Small amounts of direct current can be applied, but usually are not necessary, as thrombosis occurs spontaneously within a few minutes. Usually, after the posterior segment of the fistula has been thrombosed, the venous plexus is so engorged that the surgeon has no difficulty in inserting the copper superficially and avoiding damage to the first and second divisions of the trigeminal nerve.

If the fistula still exists after both the posterior drainage and the inferior drainage have been thrombosed, it must certainly be located at the anterior segment of the cavernous carotid artery or on its medial aspect. At this stage, unless the cavernous carotid artery can be clearly delineated by angiography, blind insertion of the wire or needles into the sinus may be hazardous because of possible damage to cranial nerves and perhaps direct puncture of the very cavernous portion of the carotid artery that the surgeon is attempting to save. One easy access to anterior and medial segments of the cavernous sinus is the orifice from the sphenoparietal sinuses. If the middle cerebral vein drains separately into the anterior segment of the cavernous sinus, it also can be used. The insertion needle is slipped into the cavernous sinus through one of these orifices, and through it 30–40 mm of copper wire can be threaded easily to the anterior and medial segments of the cavernous sinus.

The presence of wires medial to the cavernous carotid artery is pertinent, for this prevents recanalization of the fistula and formation of a contralateral cavernous sinus fistula through the circular sinus. A direct current of 0.2–0.5 mA can again be applied for 2–5 min to each inserted wire.

An angiogram taken at this point should reveal complete occlusion of the fistula.

Results and Complications

I have used the cavernous sinus thrombosis technique in treating 80 patients with a total of 90 fistulas, ten of which were bilateral (Table 1). The fistulas were obliterated in all but three cases. In five patients, the thrombosis extended to the involved carotid artery because of a large tear in the carotid artery that was incurred during the initial trauma. These five patients lost flow through the involved carotid artery; three of them died and two developed hemiparesis as a result of this complication. Among the 77 patients who survived, none suffered further impairment of their vision after treatment; in fact, except in the patients who were blind before

Table 1. Experience with 110 carotid-cavernous fistulas occurring in 99 patients (1969–1986)

Type of fistula	No. of cases
Spontaneous fistulas	
Dural AVM	
External carotid artery supply only	12
Supply from both the external and internal carotid artery	37[a]
Ruptured cavernous carotid aneurysm	7
Total	56
Treatment	
None	3
External carotid embolization only	8
Spontaneous thrombosis	6
Stereotactic heavy particle irradiation	2[b]
Operated by cavernous sinus thrombosis technique	37[c]
Posttraumatic fistulas	
Treatment	
Spontaneous thrombosis	1
Operated by cavernous sinus thrombosis technique	53[d]
Total	54

[a] Includes three bilateral fistulas
[b] One treated by external carotid artery embolization; also includes bilateral fistula
[c] Includes 15 fistulas operated after external carotid artery embolization
[d] Includes seven bilateral fistulas
AVM arteriovenous malformations

the operation, vision usually improved greatly after occlusion of the fistula. Partial or total ophthalmoplegia was observed preoperatively in 36 of 80 patients. After the operation, all but four patients who had third-nerve palsy regained total function. Five patients had postthrombotic ophthalmoplegia, but the problem resolved completely within 3 months in each case. In all cases, proptosis, chemosis, and bruit disappeared after the fistula was totally thrombosed.

Suggested Approach to Carotid Cavernous Fistulas

A carotid-cavernous fistula is rarely a life-threatening condition. As the fistula is likely to disappear spontaneously in 5% of cases, the mere presence of a fistula is not an indication for surgery unless the patient's vision continues to deteriorate, the bruit is intolerably loud, or the cosmetic appearance of the eye is unacceptable. If proptosis and chemosis are minimal and if there is no threat to vision, patients can forego surgical repair of the fistula indefinitely, provided that they are followed carefully by an ophthalmologist. It is not necessary for a surgeon to follow patients who tolerate a fistula with no difficulty. Ocular tension should be monitored carefully, as chronic elevation of the venous pressure may produce glaucoma of a type that does not respond well to medical management. If the visual acuity begins to diminish, an operation to repair the fistula should be performed promptly because changes in vision reflect rapid decompensation of retinal and orbital circulation that may result in massive infarction of the globe and the total orbital contents [3].

Although the entrapment procedure is still a widely used method for treating these fistulas, it involves all the hazards inherent in an open craniotomy and occlusion of a carotid artery. As satisfactory alternative procedures for the treatment of carotid-cavernous fistulas are becoming readily available, it is probable that the entrapment method will become obsolete within a decade. If the patient is young and is able to tolerate cervical carotid occlusion, the balloon-catheter technique is useful. If the fistula has multiple arterial feeders or if the patient cannot tolerate the loss of blood flow in the carotid artery, then carotid sinus thrombosis induced by copper wire is indicated in order to preserve circulation through the involved carotid artery while obliterating all arterial feeders. As the detachable balloon procedure is refined and used more widely, this method may become the preferred technique for treating the posttraumatic fistula which does not have collateral feeders.

References

1. Abramson HA (1924) A possible relationship between the current of injury and the white blood cell in inflammation. Am J Med Sci 167:702–710
2. Blakemore AH, King BG (1938) Electrothermic coagulation of aortic aneurysms. JAMA 111:1821–1827
3. Hamby WB (1966) Carotid-cavernous fistula. Charles C Thomas, Springfield
4. Linton RR, Hardy IB Jr (1952) Treatment of thoracic aortic aneurysms by the "Pack" method of intravascular wiring. N Engl J Med 246:847–855
5. Moore CH, Murchison C (1864) On a new method of procuring the consolidation of fibrin in certain incurable aneurysms: With the report of a case in which an aneurysm of the ascending aorta was treated by the insertion of wire. Proc R Med Chir Soc London 4:327–335
6. Mullan S, Beekman, F, Vailati G, et al. (1964) An experimental approach to the problem of cerebral aneurysm. J Neurosurg 21:838–845
7. Parkinson D (1964) Collateral circulation of cavernous carotid artery: Anatomy. Can J Surg 7:251–268
8. Peterson EW, Valberg J, Whittingham DS (1969) Electrically induced thrombosis of the cavernous sinus in the treatment of carotid cavernous fistula. Excerpta Med Int Congr Series 193:105
9. Phillips B (1832) A series of experiments performed for the pupose of showing that arteries may be obliterated without ligature, compression, or the knife. Logman, London, p 66
10. Sawyer PN, Pate JW (1953) Bio-electric phenomena as an etiologic factor in intravascular thrombosis. Am J Physiol 175:103–107
11. Velpeau A (1831) Memoire sur la piqure ou l'acupuncture des arte'res dans le traitement des aneurismes. Gaz Med Paris 2:1–4
12. Werner SC, Blakemore AH, King BG (1941) Aneurysms of the internal carotid artery within the skull. JAMA 116:578–582

Treatment of Dural Arteriovenous Fistulae

V. Van Halbach, R.T. Higashida, and G.B. Hieshima[1]

Dural arteriovenous fistulae (DAVF) account for 10%–15% of all intracranial arteriovenous malformations. Signs and symptoms can vary from a pulse synchronous tinnitus, bruit, headache, papilledema, hemorrhage, proptosis, visual decline, altered mental status, to transient or permanent neurological deficit. Except for bruit and tinnitus, these signs and symptoms are related to the venous drainage. Over the past 6 years, we have treated 79 patients with dural arteriovenous malformations (DAVMs): forty involved the region of the transverse and sigmoid sinus, 32 involved the region of the cavernous sinus, and seven involved the superior sagittal sinus. Each location presents with different signs and symptoms and requires various treatment modalities.

Cavernous Sinus Dural Fistulae

We treated 32 patients with dural fistula involving the cavernous sinus. The most common presenting symptoms were proptosis in three-fourths of patients; nearly one-half had bruit or diplopia from ophthalmoplegia. Twenty-seven percent had visual decline related to the DAVM.

Treatment Modalities

Carotid Jugular Compression

Patients who were compliant, and had no evidence of cortical venous drainage, were begun on compression therapy. This consisted of the patient compressing his/her own carotid for 10 s per treatment, several times per hour. If tolerated, the length of compression was gradually increased to 30 s. The combination of carotid artery

inflow and jugular vein outflow compression helps promote thrombosis in the involved cavernous sinus. The patient's initial treatments should be monitored by a physician checking for signs of bradycardia, hypotension, or cerebral ischemia. The contralateral hand is used so that, if ischemia develops unknowingly to the patient, the patient's hand will fall away and terminate the compression. Maximal effectiveness is seen within 4–6 weeks. Figure 1 is of a patient with a dural fistula involving the cavernous sinus. Following compression therapy for 4 weeks the fistula resolved. Of 23 patients treated by this modality, there was complete cure in eight and improvement in two. There were no complications with this treatment modality.

Embolization

In patients with cortical venous drainage or visual decline, or who fail compression therapy, embolization is highly effective in treatment of DAVMs. The choice of embolic agents, most commonly polyvinyl-alcohol sponge (PVA) or liquid adhesive agents such as isobutyl-cyanoacrylate (IBCA), depends on many factors and must be individualized to each case. Figure 2 is of a patient with a dural fistula cured with PVA embolization. Of the 22 patients treated by embolization, there was complete cure in 17 and improvement in four.

There was one permanent complication in this series; a mild weakness was suffered when thrombus dislodged from a catheter following direct carotid puncture.

Transverse and Sigmoid Sinus Fistulae

There were 25 females and 15 males with DAVMs involving the posterior fossa. Abnormal venous drainage in 34% was demonstrated and 29% suffered hemorrhage related to their fistula. Figure 3a is a DAVM located at the transverse sigmoid junction supplied by middle

[1] Department of Neurological Surgery and Radiology, U.C.S.F. Hospitals, San Francisco, California, USA

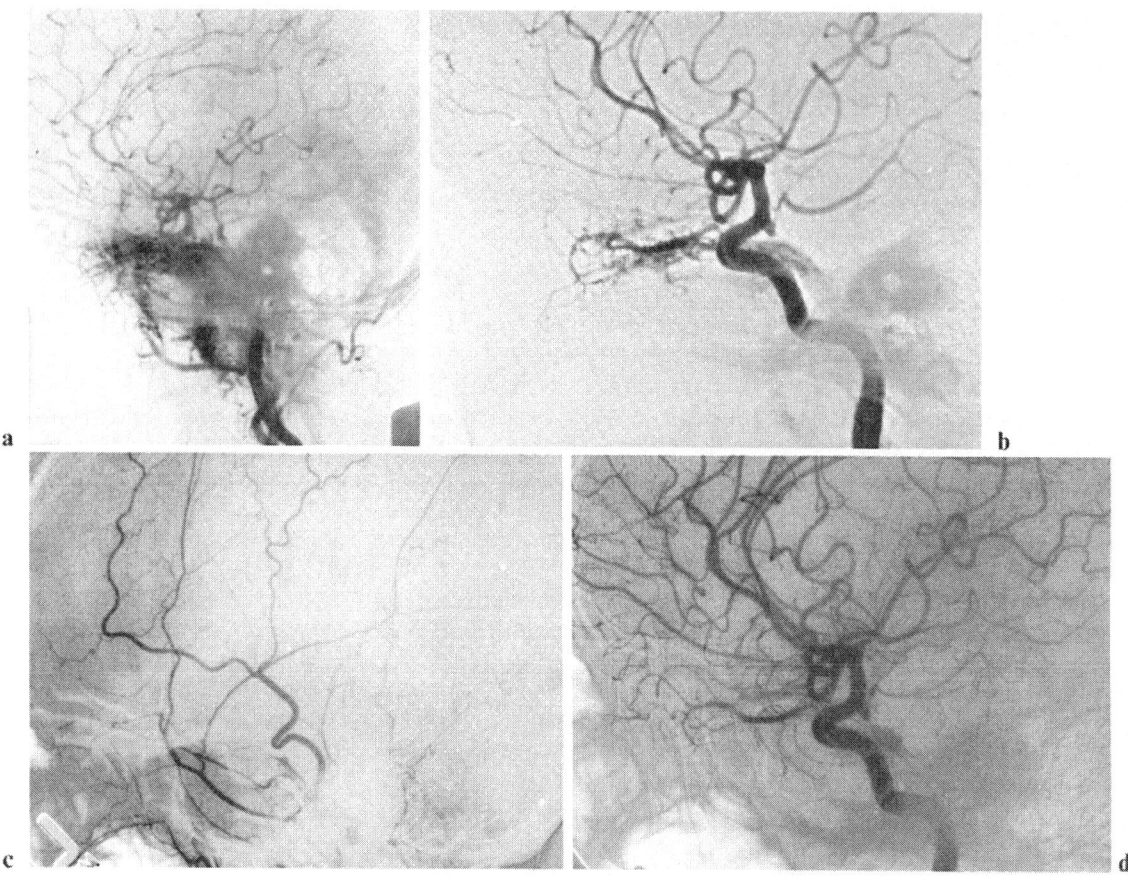

Fig. 1. a Lateral common carotid angiogram showing a dural fistula involving the cavernous sinus. **b** Selective internal carotid angiogram. **c** Selective external and **d** internal show occlusion of the fistula following compression

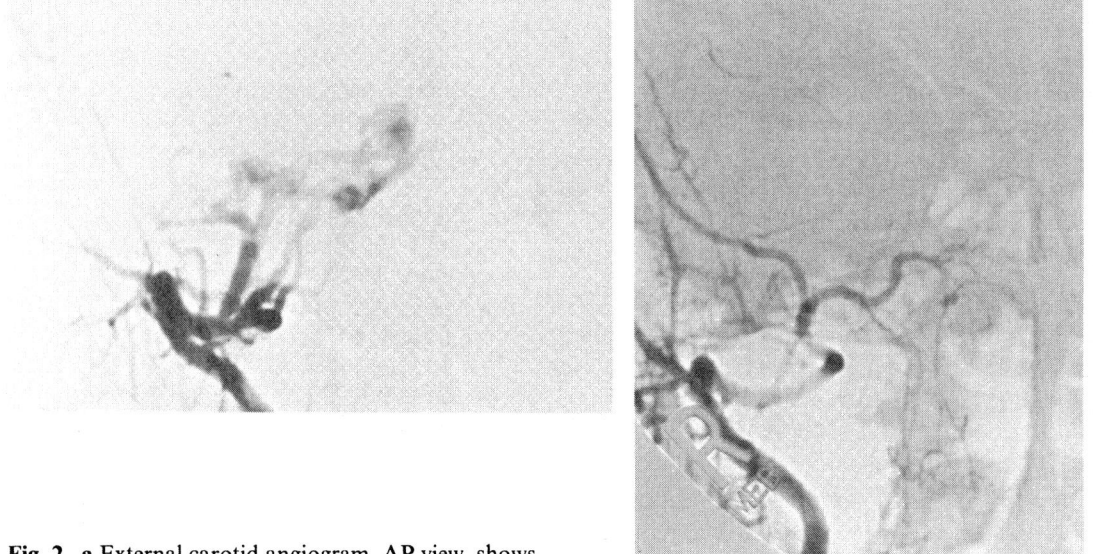

Fig. 2. a External carotid angiogram, AP view, shows fistula supplied by branches of the internal maxillary artery. **b** Postembolization angiogram shows complete cure

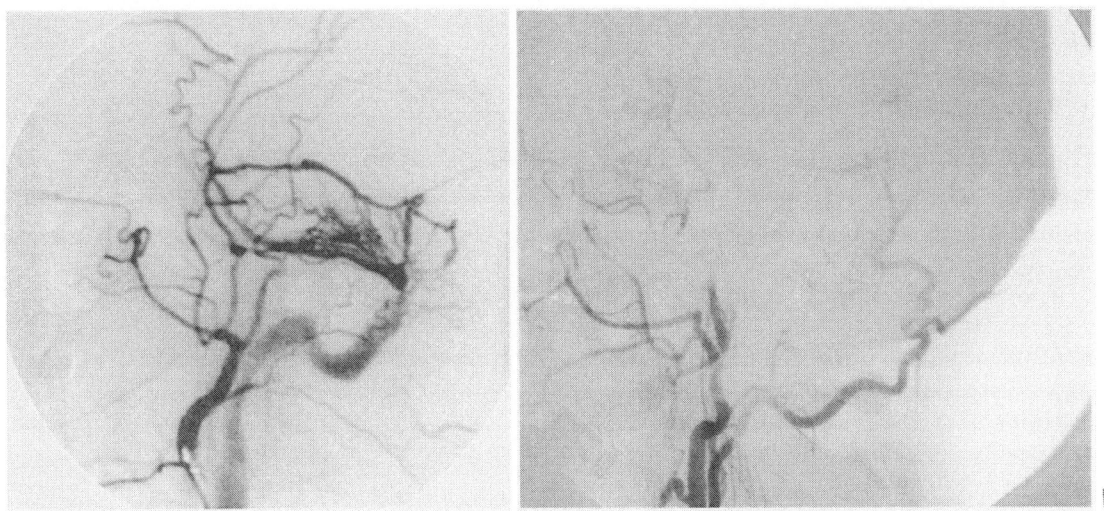

Fig. 3. a External carotid artery angiogram shows fistula at transverse sigmoid junction supplied by middle meningeal, posterior auricular, and occipital arteries. **b** Postembolization angiogram demonstrates complete cure

meningeal, posterior auricular and occipital arteries, treated with liquid adhesive and demonstrates cure of the DAVM (Fig. 3b)

Treatment Modalities

Occipital Artery Compression

Patients with a large, easily palpable occipital artery and angiographic features indicating a low risk of hemorrhage or deficit, were begun on compression therapy. Patients were instructed to compress the feeding occipital artery for up to 30 min. During effective compression, the bruit decreased or was absent. Of the 11 patients treated by this modality, four had complete cure and three improved.

Embolization

Twenty patients underwent embolization treatment with 13 resulting in complete cure and six clinically and angiographically improved. There were two complications related to embolization. The first was a nonsurgical patient who suffered repeated subarachnoid hemorrhages and had prior ligation of the occipital artery. Reflux of embolic material from a C1 collateral arising from the vertebral artery resulted in a posterior fossa stroke. The second patient developed a homonymous hemianopsia secondary to venous occlusion related to liquid adhesive agents.

Embolization and Surgery

Ten patients underwent a combination of embolization and surgery. All had prior embolization, surgery, or unsafe transvascular embolization routes. Operative exposure and embolization of arterial feeders was performed in six, and embolization of the dural sinus or draining vein was performed in four. All were performed with liquid adhesives. Complete cure was achieved in seven, and improvement in three.

Superior Sagittal Sinus Fistulae

Seven patients with fistulae involving the superior sagittal sinus were treated. Three were cured by embolization alone, and four required surgical exposure and embolization. Two patients presented with hemorrhage, both with drainage to a cortical vein.

Discussion

DAVFs are rare lesions and can present with a wide variety of symptoms. While some have advocated surgical excision of the involved dura and dural sinus for definitive cure, this is not without risk of morbidity and mortality. With advances in neuroangiographic techniques and materials, endovascular treatment may emerge as a safe and effective treatment for these lesions. The angiographic and clinical spectrum of

DAVFs is wide. Spontaneous closure as well as closure following diagnostic angiography is well documented. On the opposite end of the spectrum, some DAVFs can present with massive intradural hemorrhage, blindness, or neurological deficits. As discussed by Lasjaunias, Vinuela, and Kuhner, symptoms are often related to the venous drainage, which may change with thrombosis of venous outflow pathways. Recognition of angiographic and clinical features which indicate a poorer prognosis is essential in the decision of treatment modalities. Of the patients in our series with repeated subarachnoid hemorrhage, a narrowing of the venous outflow was present. A combined neurosurgical and neuroradiological approach is often essential in the treatment of more complex fistulae, especially when previous feeding artery ligation has been performed or supply arises entirely from intracranial vessels which are dangerous to embolize.

Compression therapy is a highly effective treatment modality in patients without hazardous clinical or angiographic features. Because the venous compression of the jugular vein increases venous pressure and may theoretically increase the risk of venous hemorrhage or infarction in patients with cortical venous drainage, these patients are excluded from compression therapy. Cortical venous drainage is often accompanied by a fluctuating mental status and is an indication for emergent treatment. Thrombosis of the fistula by either compression therapy or embolization is often accompanied by pain which may last several days or weeks.

The decision to use more hazardous treatments such as embolization and surgery must be individualized. The goal of therapy is clinical improvement, not angiographic resolution.

Often subtotal occlusion of the fistula is adequate for clinical improvement and subsequent thrombosis and cure is common, especially following liquid adhesive agents.

In conclusion, DAVFs can present with a wide spectrum of signs and symptoms. While not all fistulae need treatment, and many may undergo spontaneous cure, the prognosis of some may be quite poor. Recognition of angiographic and clinical features which may signify a more hazardous fistula is important. Compression therapy, in selected patients, may be quite effective in treatment of less hazardous fistulae. Both embolization and surgery in conjunction with embolization are effective modalties for the treatment of more hazardous fistulae.

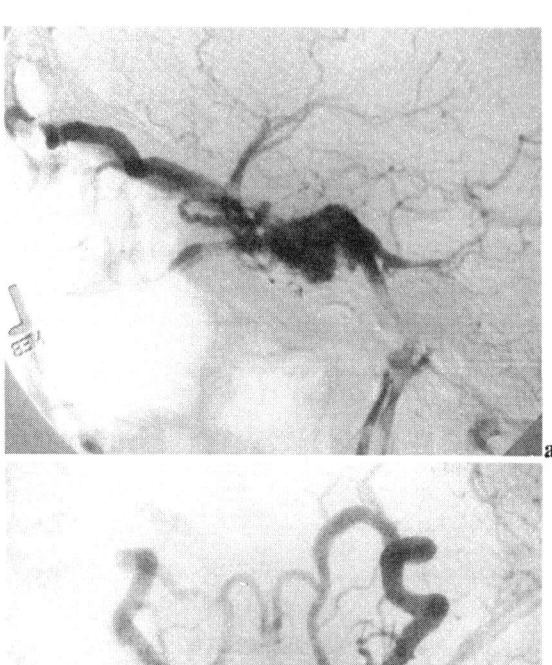

Fig. 4. a Lateral and **b** AP view of cavernous sinus injection during a transvenous treatment of direct cavernous sinus fistula

Treatment of Carotid Cavernous Fistulae

Direct carotid cavernous sinus fistulae (CCFs) are usually secondary to severe head trauma associated with basal skull fracture or ruptured intracavernous aneurysms. The most common presenting symptoms include retroorbital bruit, pulsating exophthalmos, conjunctival edema, and ophthalmoplegia. The indications for emergent treatment include progressive visual loss, rapidly progressive proptosis, intractable orbital pain, and cerebral ischemia. Over the past 14 years we have evaluated 147 patients with direct CCFs. Of these, five closed spontaneously and four died from intracerebral hemorrhage before treatment could be instituted. A total of 138 patients were treated by transvascular embolization techniques. In 116, excellent results were achieved with marked improvement in symptoms. Of the remaining 22 cases, the following complications were noted; 18 patients developed cranial nerve palsy (16 transient, two permanent), three patients with stroke, two patients with transient ischemia, one case of retroorbital hemorrhage and one death. Transarterial balloon occlusion was performed in 83%, transvenous embolization in 10%, and direct surgical exposure and intraoperative embolization was performed in 3%. The remaining 4% were cured by compression therapy (described above). Patients with a small fistula, minimal symptoms, and thrombosis or outflow pathways were often treated effectively with compression therapy alone. Transarterial embolization with silicone balloons was effective in the majority of the cases; only when the orifice of the fistula was too small for the balloon to enter (less than 1.5 mm) was a transvenous route attempted (Fig. 4).

References

1. Berenstein A, Kricheff II, Ransohoff J (1980) Carotid cavernous fistulas: Intraarterial treatment. AJNR 1:449–457

2. Debrun GM, Lacour P, Caron JP, Hurth M, Comoy J, Keravel Y (1978) Detachable balloon techniques in treatment of cerebral vascular lesions. J Neurosurg 49:635–649

3. Debrun GM (1983) Treatment of traumatic carotid-cavernous fistula using detachable balloon catheters. AJNR 4:355–356

4. Hieshima GB, Grinnell VS, Mehringer CM (1981) A detachable balloon for therapeutic transcatheter occlusions. Radiology 138:227–228

5. Higashida RT, Hieshima GB, Halbach VV, Goto KG (in press) Closure of Carotid Cavemus Sinus Fistulae by Extend compression of the carotid artery and jugular vein. Acta Radiologica Supp 369:580–583

6. Norman D, Newton TH, Edwards MS, DeCaprio V (1983) Carotid-cavernous fistula: Closure with detachable silicone balloons. Radiology 149:149–157

7. Sanders MD, Hoyt WF (1969) Hypoxic ocular sequelae of carotid cavernous fistulae. Br J Ophthalmol 53:82–97

8. Serbinenko FA (1974) Balloon catheterization and occlusion of major cerebral vessels. J Neurosurg 41:125–145

9. Taki W, Handa H, Yonekawa Y et al. (1981) Detachable balloon catheter systems for embolization for cerebrovascular lesions. Neurol Med Chir (Tokyo) 21:709–719

Anatomy of the Cavernous Sinus and Dural AVM

Tomio Ohta[1], Shuro Nishimura[1], and Sumiko Magari[2]

Introduction

The cavernous sinus was named by Winslow [6], who described it as being similar in structure to the corpus cavernosum of the penis. Since then, the anatomy of this portion of the dural sinuses has been referred to by many researchers, but their detailed anatomical descriptions on this point are not in agreement. Some anatomists are opposed to the name "cavernous sinus." The histopathological findings of the dural arteriovenous malformation (AVM) in the region of the cavernous sinus, observed in our autopsy case, were completely different from the normal anatomy usually depicted in the standard textbooks of human anatomy. This investigation was undertaken to get some idea of the relationship between the cavernous sinuses of normal adults and fetuses, and those with dural.

Methods

The normal cavernous sinuses (adult and fetus) were removed en bloc with the bone from autopsy cadavers. These materials were fixed with 10% formalin solution and decalcified with 10% formic acid solution. After dehydration with ethanol, they were embedded with celloidin. The blocks were sectioned serially, and stained with H and E, azan stain and Bielschowsky's silver impregnation. The preparations were analyzed both microscopically and three-dimensionally by the Cosmozone 2S computed system. The cavernous sinuses of dural AVM were examined microscopically and were morphologically compared with normal cavernous sinuses.

Department of Neurosurgery[1], Department of Anatomy[2], Osaka Medical School, Takatsuki, Japan

Results

The cavities of cavernous sinuses in normal adults were traversed with a few thin or thick trabeculae (Fig. 1). The thick trabeculae were mostly composed of fatty tissue, but the thin trabeculae rarely had fatty tissue and were composed of fibrous connective tissue. These trabeculae are connected to each other between the inner layer of the dura mater and the adventitia of the internal carotid artery. Some bundles of collagenous and reticular fibers were shown by azan stain and Bielschowsky's silver impregnation. The internal carotid artery runs apart from the wall of the cavernous sinus except at its entrance and exit. The cranial nerves did not always lie in the lateral wall of the cavernous sinus, and, in some portions, they were in the venous cavity, surrounded by connective tissue in their outer layers.

Normal fetal cavernous sinuses almost always had thick trabeculae not composed of fatty tissue (Fig. 2), and their appearance was not venous sinus but, rather, venous plexus like the "primitive cavernous sinus of fetus" described by Paget [4]. Interstitial tissue (trabecula) of the fetal cavernous sinus was composed of mesenchymal connective tissue which consisted of numerous mesenchymal cells, some extracellular fibers, and a fluid ground substance. The mesenchymal cells were stellate or fusiform with long and slender extensions.

The cavernous sinus of dural AVM had thick trabeculae, which were composed of much loose connective tissue and scanty fatty tissue (Fig. 3). These findings resembled the fetal venous plexus. Arteries of the dural AVM ran in a serpentine form in the trabeculae, and these lumina showed stenosis in various degrees. The intimas were partially hypertrophic, and the internal elastic lamina was interrupted in some parts and hypertrophic in others.

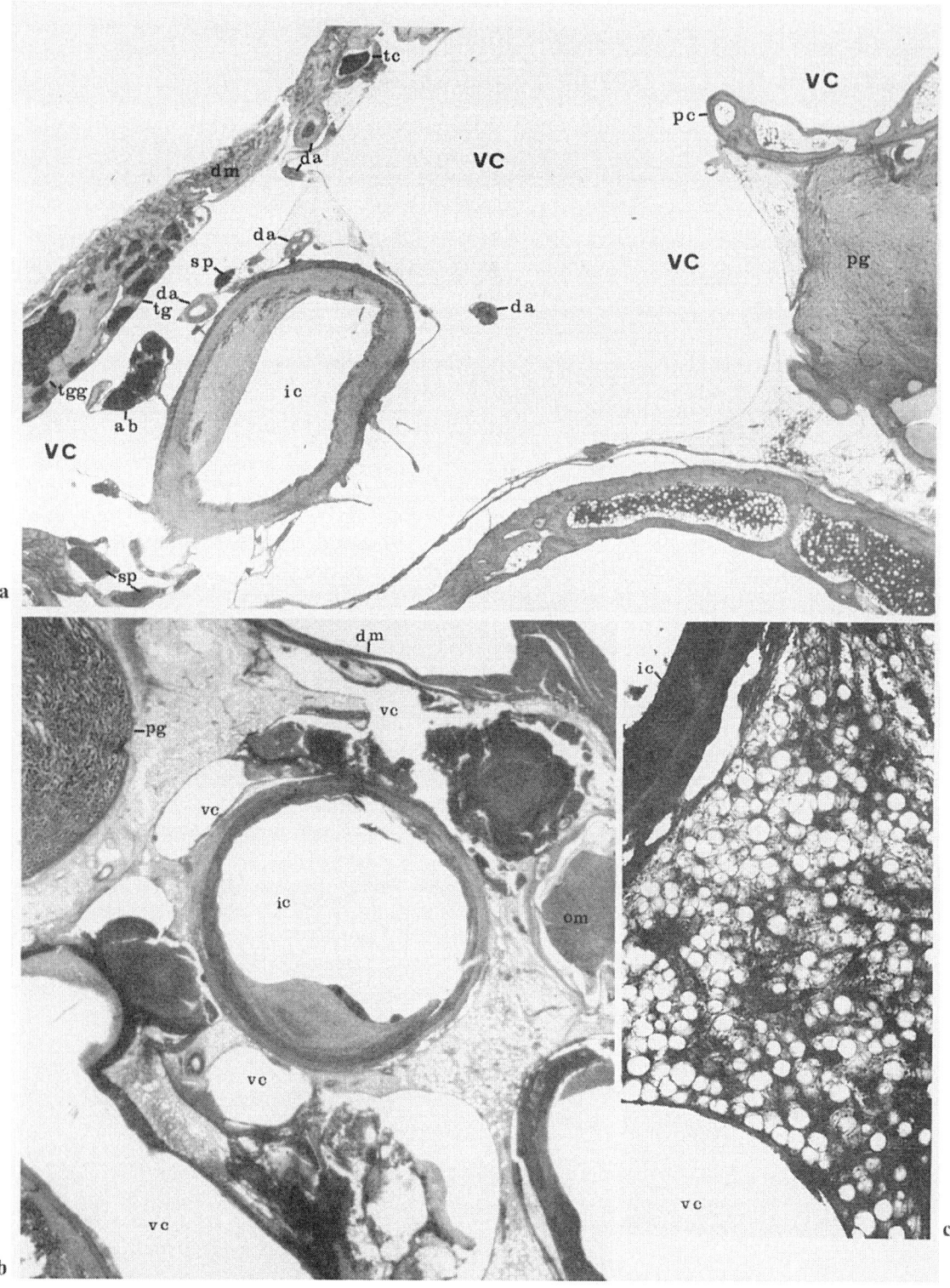

Fig. 1a–c. Normal adult cavernous sinus sectioned coronally. **a** Thin trabecula type in a 51-year-old male. In large venous sinus the internal carotid artery (*ic*) is suspended by trabeculae. The abducens nerve (*ab*), some sympathetic nerve fibers, and dural arteries (*da*) in the venous cavity are surrounded by connective tissue in their outer layers. H and E. **b** Thick trabecula type in a 67-year-old male. Venous cavity (*vc*) is traversed with thick trabeculae, which are largely fatty tissue. H and E. **c** Trabecula is largely composed of fatty tissue. H and E, × 8. *dm* dura mater, *om* oculomotor nerve, *pc* posterior clinoid process, *pg* pituitary gland, *sm* sympathetic nerve, *sp* sympathetic plexus, *tc* trochlear nerve, *tg* trigeminal nerve, *tgg* trigeminal nerve ganglion

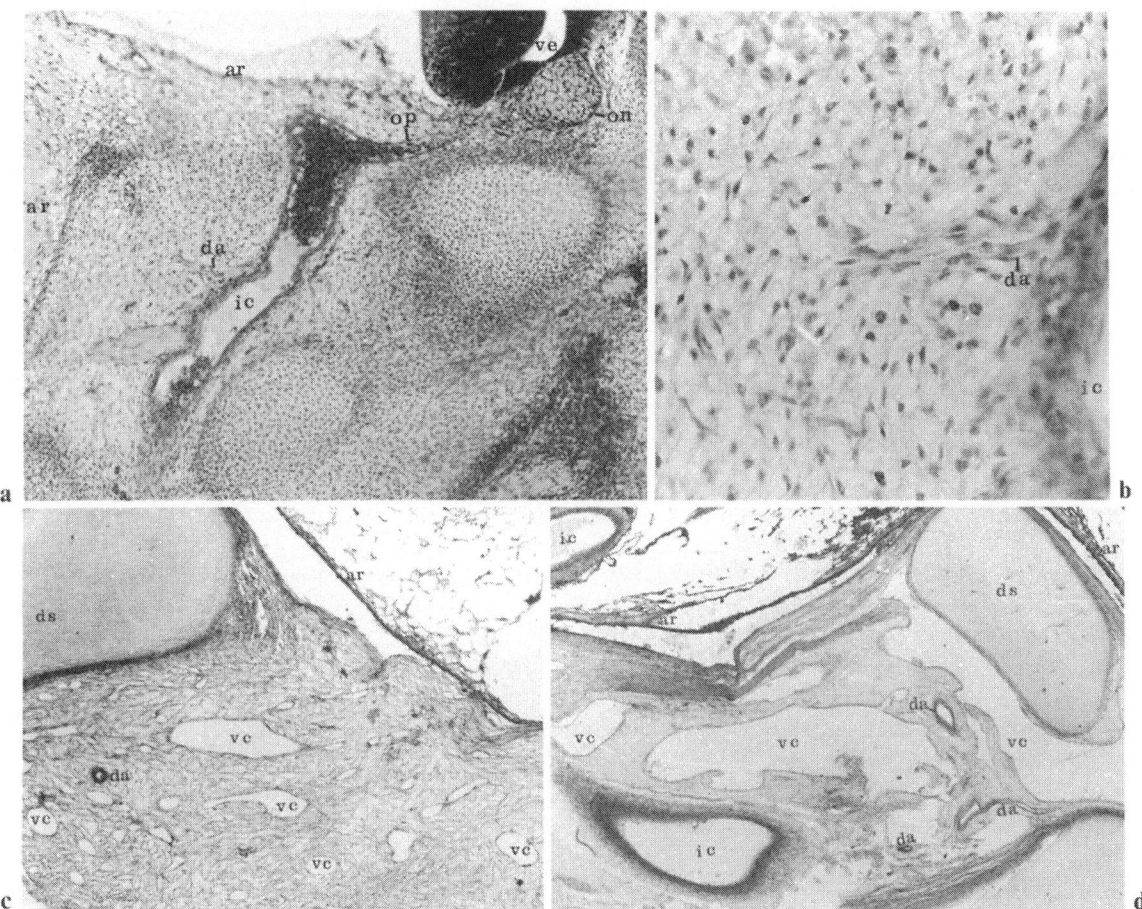

Fig. 2a–d. Fetal cavernous sinus sectioned sagittally. **a** Sixth-week embryo. Area surrounding the internal carotid artery (*ic*) is filled with mesenchymal connective tissue and includes no large veins. The cavernous sinus has not developed. Bielschowsky's silver impregnation, ×20. **b** Sixth-week fetus. The mesenchymal connective tissue of cavernous sinus region consists of numerous mesenchymal cells, some extracellular fibers and a ground substance. The mesenchymal cells are stellate or fusiform with long and slender extension. H and E, ×80. **c** Twentieth-week fetus. Area between the pituitary gland and the internal carotid artery is composed of small veins and loose connective tissue without fatty tissue. This appearance is not that of a venous sinus but rather of the venous plexus (primitive cavernous sinus). Bielschowsky's silver impregnation, ×7. **d** Twenty-fifth-week fetus. Between the internal carotid artery and the dorsum sellae (*ds*), irregular venous cavities (*vc*) are traversed by the interstitial tissue which consists of the mesenchymal connective tissue without fatty tissue. H and E, ×7. *ar* arachnoid, *da* dural artery, *on* optic nerve, *op* opthalmic artery, *vc* venous cavity, *ve* ventricle

Discussion

Whether the cavernous sinus is a venous sinus with a few trabeculae or a venous plexus with many trabeculae is a matter of controversy even at the present time. Why did the previous studies result in different conclusions?

Difficulties of Methods

The cavernous sinus is situated in a complicated structure of the skull base, which is composed of bone, periostium, dura mater, cranial nerves, sympathetic nerves, the pituitary gland, and the internal carotid artery and its branches. Because of different tissues in this area, observations are very difficult to make, not only macroscopically but also microscopically. Observations with a resin cast carry a risk of producing artifacts by the high injection pressure of resin into veins whose pressure should be low in the living case. Histological examination is possible for differentiating arteries, veins, nerves, glands, and connective tissues, but it is difficult to study these

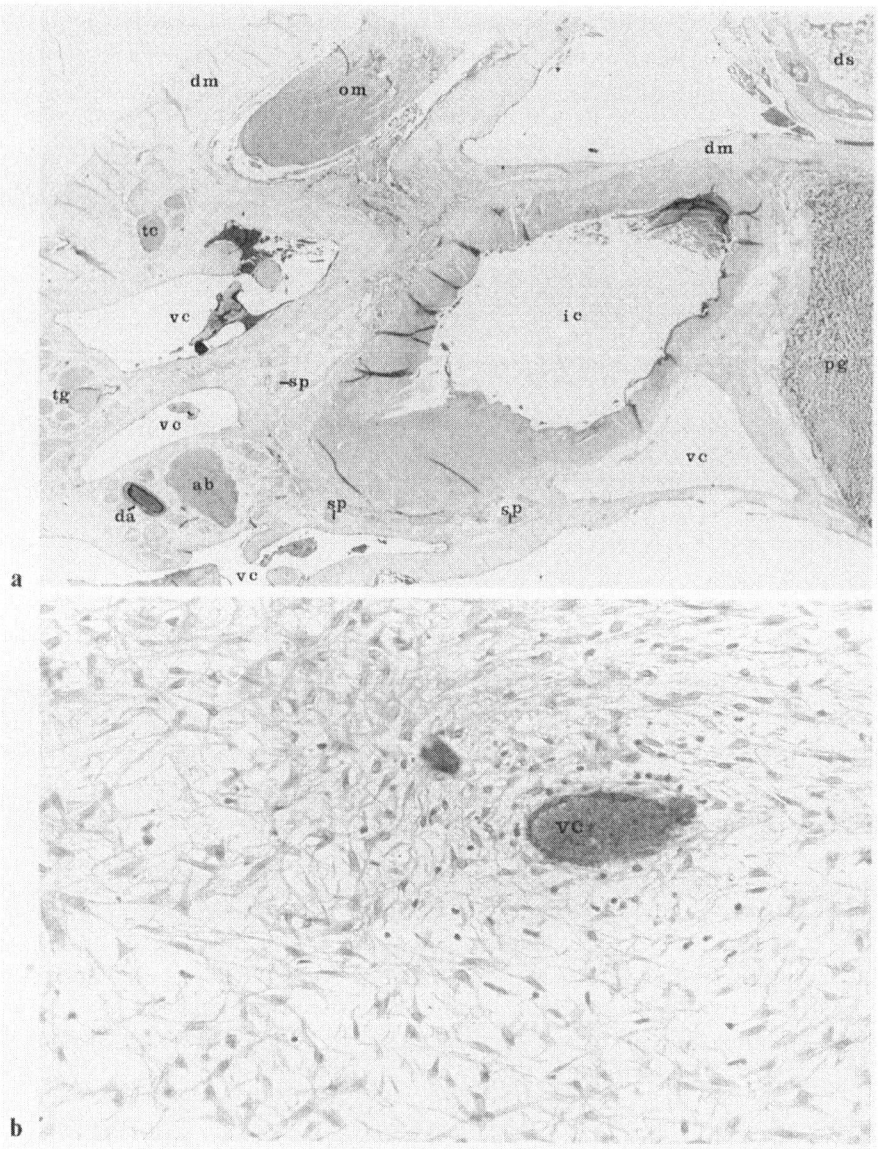

Fig. 3a, b. Cavernous sinus of dural AVM sectioned coronally. **a** The cavernous sinus consists of many small veins like the fetal cavernous sinus, and does not include much fatty tissue as in normal adults. H and E. **b** The trabecula of dural AVM consists of loose connective tissue like the mesenchymal connective tissue of fetus. H and E × 100. *Abbreviations* are the same as those used in Figs. 1 and 2

structures three-dimensionally. We analyzed serial histological preparations by a computed three-dimensional examination.

Development of the Cavernous Sinus and Its Variations

According to a report by Bedford [1], and later by Miyazaki [3], the cavernous sinuses are quite different individually. The fetal cavernous sinus is a venous plexus type (the primitive cav-

ernous sinus) [4]. The fetal plexiform venous cavities develop into venous sinuses, and the interstitial tissue probably would develop and degenerate into fibrous trabeculae or fatty tissue. The interstitial tissue of the fetal cavernous sinus is composed of the mesenchymal connective tissue, which is multipotential and can develop many kinds of connective tissues including vessel walls. The cavernous sinus of dural AVM observed in our autopsy case is plexiform in appearance and resembles a primitive cavernous sinus. The cavernous sinuses of normal adults have merely thin trabeculae or thick trabeculae, which are composed largely of fatty tissue, and there are rarely mesenchymal connective tissues. Normal dural vessels, including those in the cavernous sinus region, have rich collateral nets of arteries and artery-vein bypasses [2, 5]. If the mesenchymal connective tissue in the cavernous sinus leaves without degeneration during the developmental process, dural AVM may possibly be malformed from a physiological artery-vein bypass. Blood flow of dural arteries is definitely poor compared with the cerebral arteries, and, therefore, a small dural AVM must be almost asymptomatic until it ruptures in the cavernous sinus and the surrounding tissue. When dural AVM ruptures for some cause (hypertension, diabetes mellitus, fluctuation and elevation of intracranial pressure, delivery, or trauma), the signs and symptoms usually experienced in a case of dural AVM become apparent. As a result, the arteriovenous shunt flow will be increased and nearby arteries, which have rich collateral nets, will send blood to the dural AVM by a pressure gradient (siphoning effect). The dural AVM, including normal collaterals of the dural arteries, becomes enlarged. Because of the minor leakage from the dural AVM, natural healing or healing after angiography may be possible in some cases. Since other dural sinuses develop from plexiform veins into a single sinus, the same process will occur in the development of dural AVM in other regions of the dural sinuses.

References

1. Bedford MA (1966) The "cavernous" sinus. Br J Opthalmol 50:41–46
2. Kerber CW, Newton TH (1973) The macro- and microvasculature of the dura mater. Neuroradiology 6:175–179
3. Miyazaki H (1981) The "cavernous" sinus. Neurological Surgery 9(10):1131–1138
4. Paget DH (1956) The cranial venous system in man in reference to development, adult configuration, and relation to the arteries. AM J Anat 98:307–355
5. Rowbothan GF, Little E (1965) Circulation of the cerebral hemispheres. Br J Surg 52:8–21
6. Winslow JB (1732) Exposition anatomique de la structure de corps human. 2:31, Prevost, London

Intravascular Neurosurgery and the Treatment of Abnormalities in the Central Nervous System

Akira Takahashi and Jiro Suzuki[1]

Due to the recent development of intravascular surgery, many disorders can be treated by means of a newly developed method known as "interventional neuroradiology" [1], "endovascular surgery," or, recently, "surgical neuroangiography" [4], but better named "intravascular neurosurgery." This term refers to the fundamentally "surgical" property of this technique which should be performed by neurosurgeons or under very close cooperation with them. Since August 1983, we have performed more than 150 balloon catheterizations and, 91 cases of various central nervous system abnormalities were treated intravasculary. In this communication, our experiences are summarized with special reference to the effectiveness of intravascular neurosurgery.

Material and Method

We have adopted the use of mainly three different types of balloon catheters as the tools of treatment; various types of detachable balloons, calibrated leak balloons, and nonleak balloons. Among them, we developed a super-selective leak balloon with a floppy tip (Fig. 1). With the great improvement in selectivity by using this new balloon catheter, we made it possible to use liquid diffuse embolizing materials (estrogen-alcohol followed by polyvinyl acetate).

The cases which were treated by intravascular surgery were assigned to five groups according to the methods used (Table 1). Detachable balloon catheters were used for the patients of group I. Group II consisted of 19 cases arteriovenous malformation (AVM) and 11 cases of meningioma who were managed with chemical embolization using leak balloon catheters. Group III

consisted of super-selective infusion of drugs for acute cerebral infarction and malignant glioma. Group IV consisted of four cases of balloon angioplasty for vasospasm due to subarachnoid hemorrhage. Group V was managed with conventional neurosurgical operations using the intraoperative balloon temporary occlusion. Among these cases, chemical embolization for AVM and intraoperative occlusion are discussed elsewhere in this volume; here, we will briefly describe the other 50 cases.

Results

Group I: Detachable Balloon Occlusion

Six cases of arteriovenous fistula, including traumatic carotid cavernous fistulas (CCFs), were occluded with the preservation of parent artery, with one exception (Fig. 2). Among the aneurysm cases, all cases of vertebral fusiform aneurysm and infraclinoidal internal carotid aneurysm were treated by proximal parent arterial occlusion without complications (Fig. 3). The proximal parent arterial occlusion appeared to be useful, especially in the cases of vertebral fusiform aneurysm, because it could be performed immediately after the diagnostic angiography and the safety could be confirmed by the neurological tolerance test under local anesthesia prior to permanent occlusion. Intraaneurysmal balloon occlusions were performed in two cases of giant aneurysm. Rerupture was observed in a case of basilar top aneurysm which was treated with contrast-filled balloons, while almost all cavities of aneurysms remained occluded in a patient with a middle cerebral artery (MCA) aneurysm who was treated with silicone-filled balloons.

Group II: Chemical Embolization

As the adjunctive preoperative devascularization, 11 cases of meningioma were embolized

---

[1] Division of Neurosurgery, Institute of Brain Diseases, Tohoku University School of Medicine, Sendai, Japan

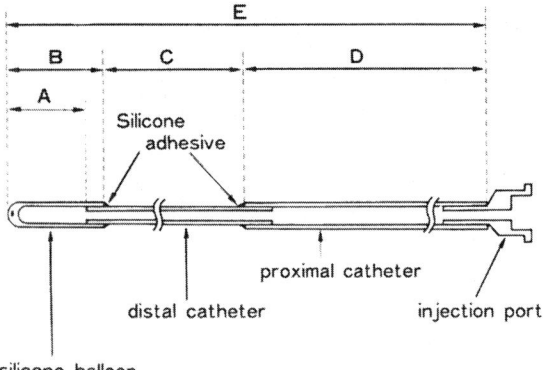

Fig. 1. Specifications of the new balloon catheter. *A* balloon length, 3.0–5.0 mm (O.D. 0.7–0.9 mm); *B* total balloon length, 5.0–7.0 mm; *C* distal catheter length, 100–300 mm (O.D. 0.63 mm, I.D. 0.31 mm); *D* proximal catheter length, 1200–1400 mm (O.D. 0.83 mm, I.D. 0.40 mm); *E* total length of the system, 1500 mm

Table 1. Intravascular neurosurgery of head and neck abnormalities (August 1983–February 1987)

Group of procedure	No. of cases
I. Detachable balloon occlusion	
Arteriovenous fistulas	5
Aneurysms	
Vertebral	6
Carotid	2
Giant	2
Tumor	1
II. Chemical embolization	
Arteriovenous malformations	19
Meningiomas	11
III. Superselective infusion of drugs	
Acute cerebral infarction (fibrinolytic agent)	16
Malignant gliomas (anticancer drugs)	2
IV. Percutaneous transluminal angioplasty	
Angioplasty for vasospasm due to subarachnoid hemorrhage	4
V. Intraoperative temporary occlusion	
Arteriovenous malformations	11
Intracranial aneurysms	8
Vascular rich tumors	4
Total	91

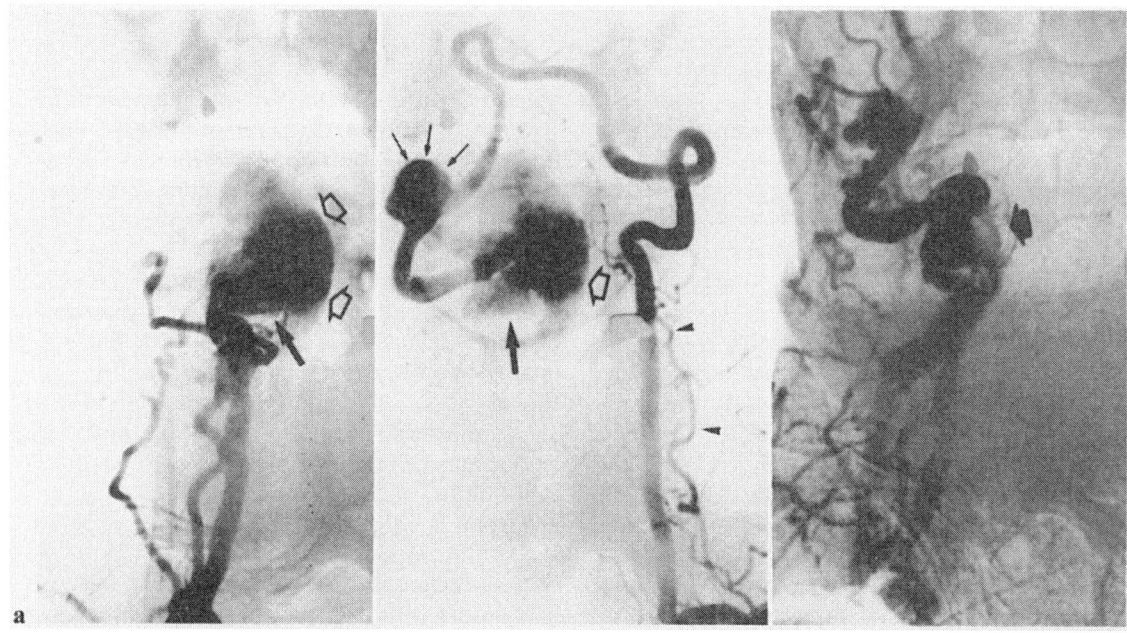

Fig. 2a–c. Detachable balloon occlusion of right vertebral arteriovenous fistula (AVF). **a** This 39-year-old female, who had suffered from von Recklinghausen's disease, complained of progressive tetraparesis due to right vertebral AVF. Preembolization of the right vertebral angiogram (VAG) revealed huge arteriovenous shunt at the level of the right C2 and C3 (*arrow*) drained into the dilated spinal vein (*open arrows*). **b** Preembolization of the left VAG revealed an arterial steal with evidence of a right vertebral aneurysm (*small arrows*). An *arrow* and *open arrows* also indicate the site of the fistula and draining vein respectively. **c** Postembolization of the right VAG indicated complete closure of fistula by balloon (*large arrow*). Right vertebral flow had been preserved. However, it was occluded spontaneously without symptoms, probably due to primary disease

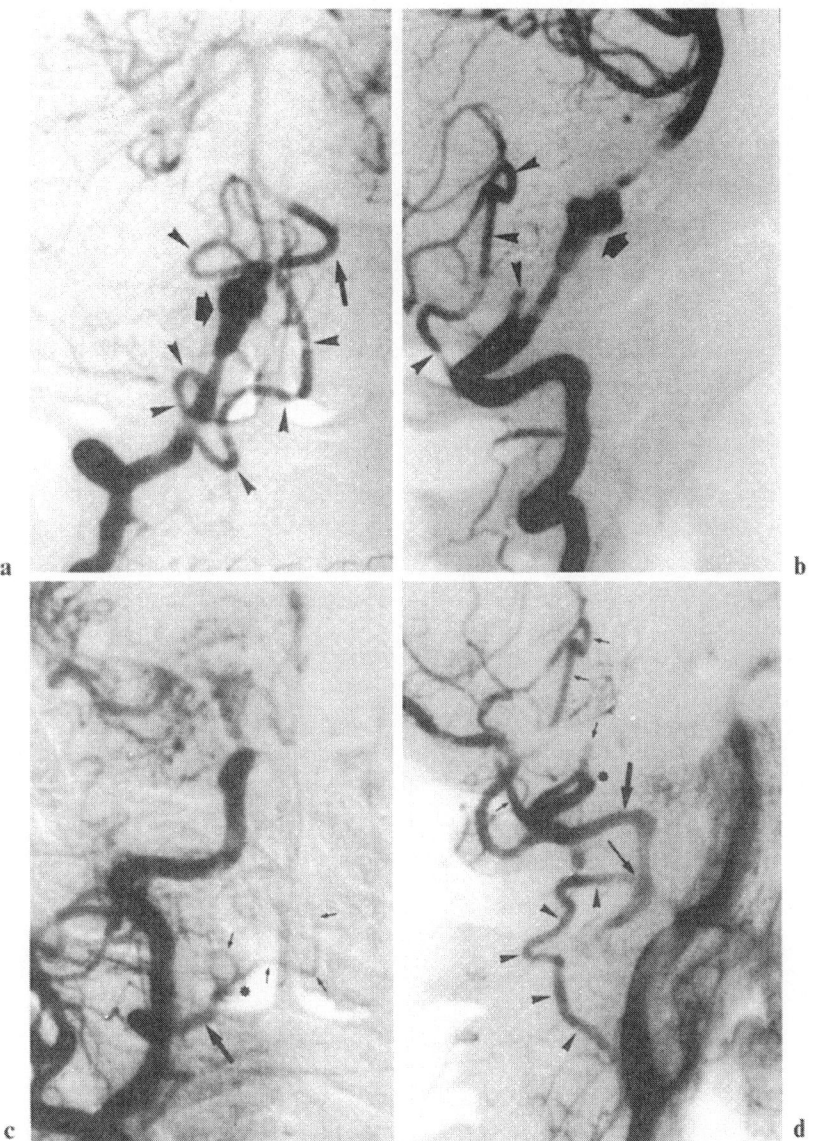

Fig. 3a–d. Vertebral dissecting aneurysm treated in acute stage. **a** This 35-year-old female was admitted on the day of sudden onset of severe headache. Preembolization of the right VAG, straight A-P view, shows a fusiform aneurysm (*thick arrow*) distal to the posterior inferior cerebellar artery (PICA) (*arrow-heads*). The *thin arrow* indicates the junction of the bilateral vertebral arteries. **b** Preembolization of the right VAG, lateral view, shows aneurysm (*thick arrow*) as well as PICA (*arrow-heads*). **c** Right vertebral artery (C_5) was occluded with detachable balloon just after the diagnosis had been made. Postembolization of the right retrograde brachial angiogram, A-P view, shows no filling of the aneurysm. *Arrow, small asterisk,* and *small arrows* indicate right vertebral artery, stump of right vertebral artery (VA), and right PICA, respectively. **d** Postembolization of the right retrograde brachial angiogram, lateral view, shows the right vertebral artery (*thin arrow*) filled through the ascending cervical to the C_1–C_2 collateral (*arrow-heads*). The right PICA (*small arrows*) is well preserved

by the superselective injection of estrogen-alcohol (E-A) or E-A followed by polyvinyl acetate (PVac). Embolized feeding arteries remained obliterated until surgical removal. Postembolization CT scans showed various amount of low-density area within the tumor which might represent the necrosis. In all cases, embolization facilitated the surgical removal. There was some different effect between the two embolization materials. While the cases which were embolized with

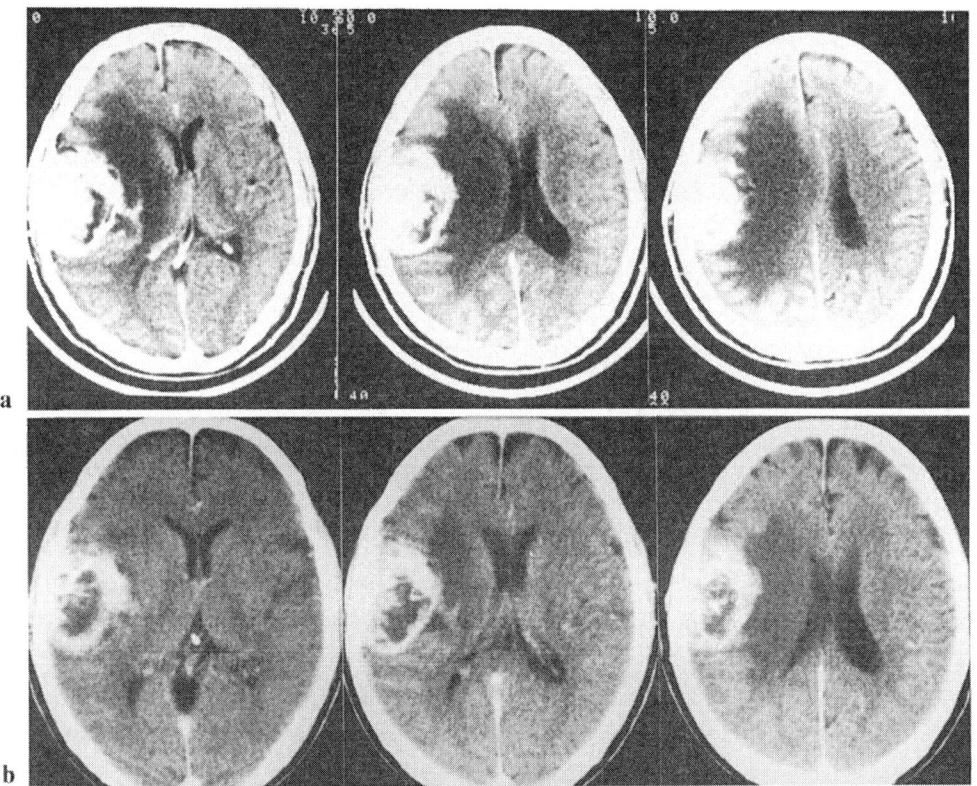

Fig. 4a, b. Embolization of left convexity meningioma. **a** Preembolization enhanced CT scans show enhanced mass at left temporoparietal area with marked peritumoral low-density area. **b** After the embolization of the feeding branch of the left middle meningeal artery with estrogen-alcohol and polyvinyl acetate, enhanced CT scans reveal increased low-density area within the tumor and also a decrease in the size of tumor and perifocal edema

E-A showed some increase of peritumoral edema in the postembolization period, the cases which received combined embolization with E-A and PVac showed clinical improvements with a decreased size of tumor (Fig. 4).

Group III: Superselective Infusion of Drugs

Cerebral infarction in the acute stage has been treated by superficial temporal artery-middle cerebral artery (STA-MCA) anastomosis or surgical embolectomy with the aid of Sendai Cocktail. Recently, it became possible to recanalize the embolic occluded artery with the superselective infusion of urokinase (120 000–1 200 000 IU). Among 16 cases of acute infarction (treated within 12 h after onset), 11 were thought to have embolic occlusion, of which 80% were recanalized (Fig. 5). Hemorrhagic infarction was observed in three cases (M1 in two cases, C1 in one case). In two cases of malignant glioma, superselective infusion of ACNU was carried out with improvement of clinical symptoms.

Group IV: Percutaneous Transluminal Angioplasty

In the cases of vasospasm after aneurysmal subarachnoid hemorrhage (SAH), we have tried to dilate the spastic basal arteries by means of balloon angioplasty. When the patients showed clinical deterioration after the aneurysm surgery, diagnostic angiography was performed to confirm the symptom-related constriction of the basal cerebral arteries. Then nondetachable silicone balloon was introduced into a spastic segment and a 5-s inflation was carried out. In four cases, six basal cerebral arteries were dilated and remained unchanged in the follow-up angiography (Fig. 6). While clinical improvement was observed in two cases, we could not prevent the ischemic consequences in the other two cases who had suffered from the most severe SAH.

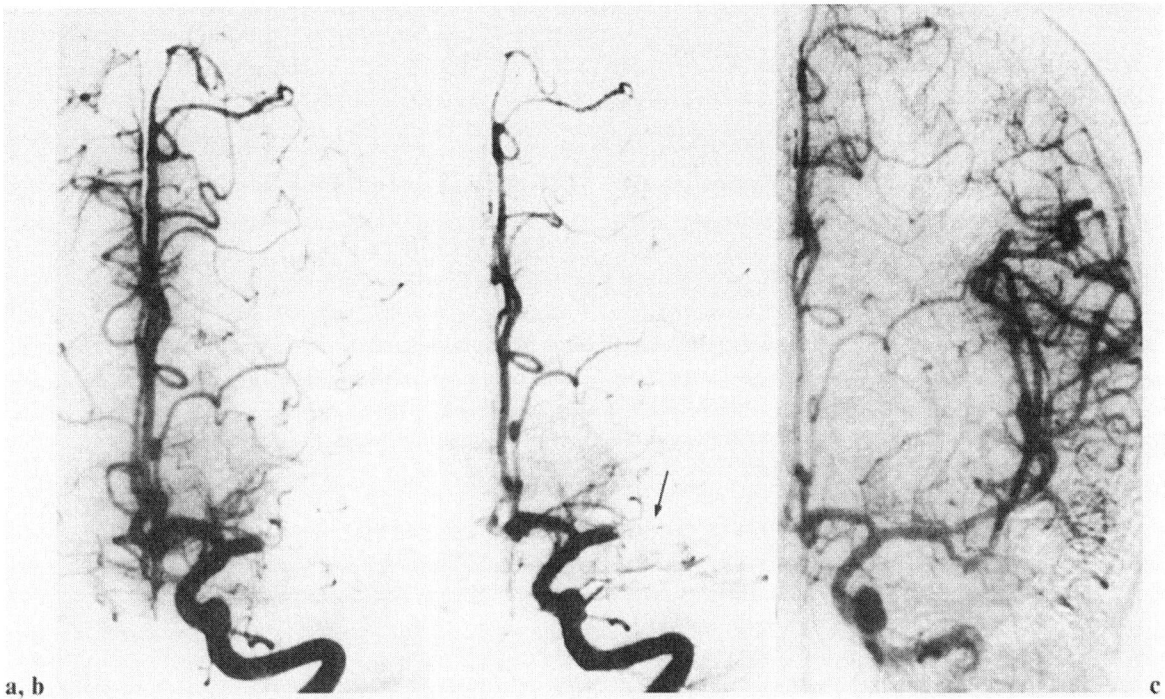

a, b   c

Fig. 5a–c. Acute cerebral embolism recanalized by urokinase infusion. **a** This 37-year-old male was admitted 3 h after onset of right hemiparesis and total aphasia. Left carotid angiogram (CAG), performed during the administration of "Sendai cocktail", discloses abrupt occlusion of left M1. **b** Leak balloon (*arrow*) was easily introduced into embolus, then infusion of urokinase was carried out. **c** Left CAG immediately after the infusion shows recanalization of occluded vessel (5.5 h after the onset). He discharged without neurological deficits

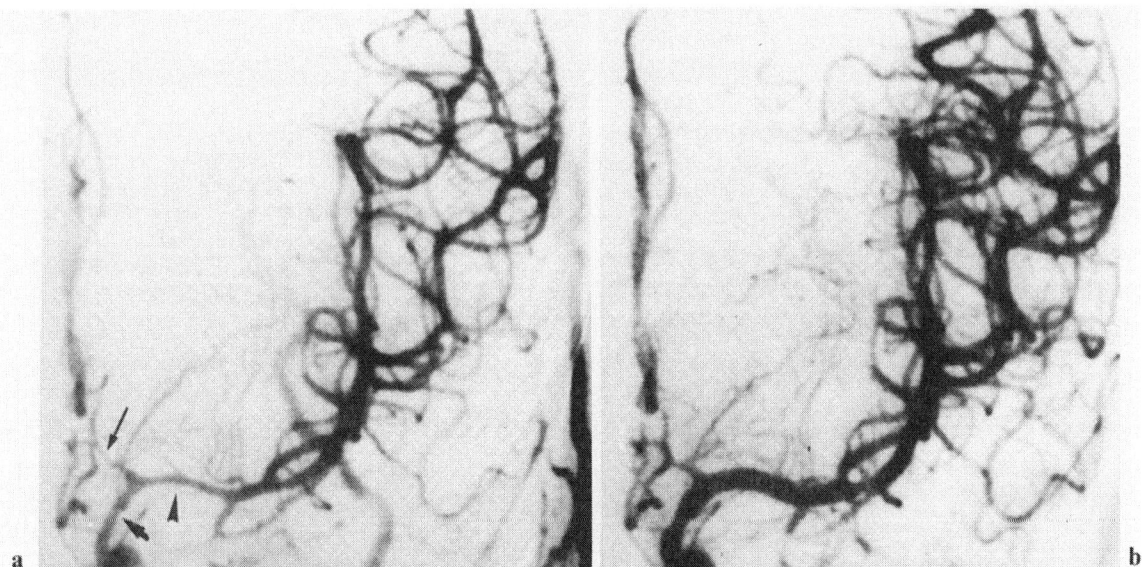

a   b

Fig. 6a, b. Angioplasty for vasospasm due to subarachnoid hemorrhage (SAH). **a** This 38-year-old male had been operated due to an anterior communicating aneurysm on the second day of SAH. On the 10th day of attack, he became stuporous and developed right hemiparesis. Left CAG revealed servere vasospasm in C1 (*arrow*), A1 (*small arrow*), and M1 (*arrow-head*). **b** Postangioplasty left CAG revealed dilatation of vasospastic segments of arteries, and clinical symptoms relieved completely within 12 h

Discussion

In the progress of intravascular neurosurgery, it has become possible to manage more various types of abnormalities of the central nervous system. Concerning our experiences, this technique provides us with the capabilities to handle difficult cases by conventional neurosurgery, and also makes possible less invasiveness and expense. Since we consider this technique is not yet an established one, the key point to improving its effectiveness is thought to be the investigation of catheters and embolic materials.

Interventional neuroradiologists and intravascular neurosurgeons have used various types of balloon catheters as the most important tool. Calibrated leak balloons have proved their effectiveness in the embolization therapy, but they also have problems such as overdistension of balloon and difficult manipulation [2, 3]. The new balloon catheter, the superselective balloon with floppy tip, is characterized by the combination of a silicone flexible distal catheter and a relatively stiff proximal one. This combination allows us to catheterize the fine branches of arterial feeders with less difficult manipulation. The connection between the three different silicone materials (balloon, distal, and proximal catheter) is tight enough that they cannot be detached even when destruction of the balloon or catheter occurs.

Concerning embolic materials, a new method (estrogen alcohol followed by polyvinyl acetate) is reported. Although details are presented in another report in this volume, this method has the possibilities of a cytocidal effect for tumors. Moreover, this material did not harden the lesion after the embolization, so it should have more indications in this field of treatment.

In this paper, we have reported two fields of newly developed treatment; superselective fibrinolytic therapy for acute cerebral infarction and angioplasty for vasospasm. These therapies seem to be too young to accurately assess their potentials yet: however, our preliminary results were encouraging. For the recanalization of embolic occluded arteries, it was suggested that superselective injection of urokinase would be effective [5]. We need to confirm the suitable cases for this procedure with objective indicators. Angioplasty for vasospasm was first reported in 1984 [6] and seems to be very effective in the early stage of symptomatic vasospasm. According to our preliminary results, symptoms cleared quickly after the dilatation therapy. More extensive investigations are also necessary for this treatment.

In conclusion, intravascular neurosurgery is very useful if it is adopted for suitable cases. However, as it is still in its developmental stage, this type of treatment must be performed by the appropriate specialists who are aware of the possible complications and many pitfalls.

References

1. Debrun GM, Vinuela FV, Fox AJ (1982) Aspirin and systemic heparinization in diagnostic and interventional neuroradiology. AJNR 139:139–142
2. Debrun GM, Vinuela FV, Fox AJ, et al. (1982) Two different calibrated leak balloons: Experimental work and application in humans. AJNR 3:407–414
3. Kerber CW (1976) Balloon Catheter with a calibrated leak. Radiology 120:547–550
4. Lasjaunias P, Berenstein A (1987) Surgical neuroangiography, vol. 1. Functional anatomy of craniofacial arteries. Springer, Berlin
5. Zeumer H, Ringelstein EB, Hassel M, Poeck K (1983) Locale fibrinolysetherapie bei subtotaler stenose der a. cerebri media. Dtsch Med Wochenschr 108:1103–1105
6. Zubkov YN, Nikiforov BM, Shustin VA (1984) Balloon catheter technique for dilatation of constricted cerebral arteries after aneurysmal SAH. Acta Neurochir 70:65–79

Discussion

Commentator: *Konovalov* (Moscow): In the past 10 years, many successful methods of treatment of carotid cavernous fistulas and dural arteriovenous malformations have been developed. Practically all these new methods have been discussed today: electrothrombosis, balloon catheterization of arteries, venous catheterization, and the direct approach to carotid cavernous fistulas. Since the cavernous sinus has a different anatomy from other sinuses, carotid cavernous fistulas must be distinguished from dural arteriovenous malformations. From the surgical point of view, this problem is not very far from being solved in my opinion. At most institutes of neurosurgery, fairly extensive experience has now been accumulated—over 1100 cases of carotid cavernous fistulas and dural sinus fistulas of other localizations—using a different kind of vascular surgery. Some very important anatomical work has been presented today on carotid cavernous fistulas. We know the important work of Prof. Parkinson on the surgical approach and the branches which are given off by the carotid artery. The structure of the carotid cavernous sinus is of importance here since ideal surgery is occlusion of those parts of the sinus that are closest to the fistula. This can be done in different ways—the venous route, which seems to me more difficult, and the arterial route. Comparing different methods now, balloon catheterization seems to be the most effective. At the Moscow Institute of Neurosurgery, for example, we have operated on 450 patients with this method; in 98% of cases, or even more, the tissue was completely occluded. The mortality was lower than 1%. The number of complications was also low, usually temporary vascular insufficiency. But of course this problem is not completely solved; there is the problem of how to preserve the artery. We can now preserve the artery in about 75% of cases, but these results can be improved upon. Prof. Romodanov has better results with the patency of the artery.

With respect to arteriovenous communications in the region of cavernous fistulas, this is a different problem. These malformations are more benign and can be spontaneously treated. Prof. Serbinenko, who developed a method of treatment of carotid cavernous fistulas many years ago, saw signs of such a dural communication in the region of the cavernous sinus. Spontaneous cure occurred, but he was strongly motivated to develop methods of treatment of this pathology.

Because this kind of malformation has a lot of communications it is quite difficult to occlude them completely. Now the best method of treatment is superselective catheterization and embolization of the artery; to occlude completely such a malformation is quite a difficult problem. That is why the method of radiosurgery is very important. We have quite a limited experience here—only ten patients with dural malformations with lesions of the carotid cavernous sinus. We irradiated with a proton beam but with good results. I hope that in future this will be one of the important methods of treatment of such malformations. The vasculopathology is more difficult in the dural communications in other parts of the head—in the posterior part, in the region of the transverse, sagittal, and sigmoid sinuses. This communication produces very serious disturbances in the blood circulation. Many aspects of the pathology still remain to be clarified.

I was very much impressed with the presentation of Prof. Mullan. In some cases, we can see thrombosis of the sinus and in several cases we examined postmortem material; it was like a cavernous angioma in the sinus which occluded it. So perhaps the best method of occlusion of this fistula here is dissection of the sinus with all the feeding vessels.

There are many aspects associated wth this problem that are still unclear. For example, we investigated ten patients who died for reasons other than sinus dural communication. In all cases, there was serious calcification of the vessels of the brain and even of the neurons. But perhaps of greater interest is that the calcification was also found in peripheral organs. We cannot explain these findings. This problem needs to be evaluated.

After surgery sometimes, very serious circulatory distubances can occur—the breakthrough phenomenon, hemorrhage into the brain stem. Thus far, we do not know the best way to treat these patients.

Commentator, *Samii* (Hannover): The first question that arises is whether we should treat the patients or not. To decide this we need to have some practical guidelines. The natural history can be summarized as follows. First, there are minor neurological symptoms which may stabilize with time, then progressive neurological deficit, and spontaneous resolution, which appears in approximately 5% of all cases. Based on this, there will be an absolute indication for treatment when progressive neurological symptoms are present; for patients with minor neurological stable symptoms, age, general condition, and quality of life will be determining factors. The diagnostic work-up which follows once the indication for treatment has been made should evaluate the exact location and size as well as the hemodynamics, arterial supply, and venous drainage of the lesion. These hemodynamic evaluations require angiographic study, selective angiographic protocols, and visualization of all possible venous connections. The location and hemodynamic features will influence the choice of approach and the application of different techniques. Treatment can be achieved by endovascular techniques or direct surgical approach.

Since 1964, with the introduction of endovascular techniques by Luessenhop, many authors have developed the methods further. There is no doubt in my mind that the ideal therapy should consist of superselective catheterization and occlusion of the shunt fistula, maintaining the patency of the carotid artery. The method of choice today seems to be the sophisticated detachable balloon technique. Nevertheless, due to the anatomical variations of the vascular network in this area, there are cases in which even a master of endovascular techniques cannot reach the vessels involved using the materials available today. In such cases, a direct surgical approach, as demonstrated by Parkinson in 1973, should be the method of choice. In recent years Dr. Issamad and myself have used pieces of muscle with fibrin glue and achieved satisfactory results. I am sure that in the next few years we will continue to develop the technique of catheterization so that

we will be able to achieve good results in more than 75% of patients.

Negoro (Nagoya): For the embolization of dural AVM, some authors use PVA, others IBCA. There is some controversy here. Did Dr. Halbach report a greater bleeding tendency after IBCA embolization?

Holbach (San Francisco): I think that with an emboic agent the factors involved are very complex; the location of the catheter, the vessel concerned, and the potential for dangerous collaterals are all involved. Each time it has to be individualized. Sometimes, in one vessel we will use IBCA, and in the next vessel PVA. I think that IBCA involves a somewhat greater risk and is rather more permanent. I think each case is individual and that we do not have ideal agent as yet.

Negoro: Could you say something about collagen treatment?

Halbach: We use collagen in a selected number of patients. As the collagen prepared now is too small and often goes through the fistula; we are always concerned about the danger of lung embolization. Investigations are underway into the development of large particles. It may be a useful agent in future.

Ishii (Tokyo): Dr. Steiner observed that there is little place for radiosurgery in CCF and Dr. Hosobuchi thinks that 10 years from now electric current or copper wire techniques will not be used. Can you comment on this Dr. Steiner?

Steiner (Stockholm): I would just like to emphasize that since spontaneous thrombosis is very frequent in spontaneous carotid cavernous fistulas we cannot say that our results are due to the radiation. Traumatic fistulas do not appear to respond to radiosurgery.

Hosobuchi (San Francisco): Where spontaneous thrombosis did not occur in cases of dural AVM of the cavernous sinus region, those patients always showed chornically elevated ocular pressure of above 25 mmHg for 2–3 years; they also had decreased arteriovenous perfusion pressure difference in retinal vessels, which in our experience never disappears. We have treated three such dural AVMs obtaining a supply both from the external and internal and had good results.

These patients were followed up for 4 years and did not show spontaneous thrombosis. However, some patients came to our hospital after making a long plane journey from Europe or the East Coast of the United States and upon landing found that their bruit was gone. We admitted the patients and demonstrated angiographically that the fistula had disappeared.

Mullan (Chicago): I think it is the interval that is important here. Some of my patients after crossing Chicago by automobile lost their fistulas.

Vinuela (Los Angeles): I think it has to be emphasized here that in the treatment of fistulas one has to be aware that one is treating a patient and not an angiogram. I say this because the lesion is difficult to eradicate by any means—surgical or endovascular; its natural history most of the time is benign, and it does sometimes thrombose spontaneously. In endovascular therapy, we have two goals: first, we try to change the local hemodynamics, promoting further thrombosis, second, we try to be very superselective knowing the neuromeningeal branches from the external. The external carotid artery supplies the dura mater but also supplies the cranial nerves going through the foramina. I do not think we can justify a cranial nerve palsy produced by embolization of a lesion whose natural history is benign. I think that in neuroarterial malformations at any localization, our policy should be to change the local hemodynamics, be very patient, and try to protect the arterial supply to cranial nerves through the dura.

Steiner: I found what Prof. Mullan presented today was very interesting. Is there anyone who would care to challenge or comment on what he said?

Vinuela: I do not challenge what Prof. Mullan has said. The superselectivity has taught us exactly the same as what he has seen in his great experience. What I would perhaps find questionable is a radical excision of those lesions which do not present either hemorrhage or increased intracranial pressure.

Mullan: We would never remotely think of radical excision. We simply thrombose the lateral sinus; there is no question of radical excision. It is merely the isolated lesion of the sinuses.

Ishii: Were there any complications?

Mullan: There were with the last case I showed with the sagittal sinus thrombosis and the left lateral sinus thrombosis. When we thrombosed the right one there were no problems until the day after when the patient developed hemianopia. That was the only problem.

Steiner: Could the panel briefly define carotid fistula, arteriovenous dural malformation?

Mullan: I think dural arteriovenous fistulae are entirely different from carotid fistulae which come from trauma or aneurysm. Those carotid fistulae that come from trauma or aneurysm are best suited for balloon embolization. The dural AV fistula into the carotid is an entirely different phenomenon and it can be handled either by arterial embolization or by exposure of the cavernous sinus and packing, whichever one prefers. Of course, here the balloon does not play a role as it does in traumatic and aneurysm fistulae.

Ohta (Osaka): At first, we tried to treat CCF with Hamby's method; however, it turned out to be ineffective in cases of spontaneous CCF. We then examined spontaneous CCF and realized that it was supplied by dural branches of both the internal and external carotid systems. Thus, we think it is a malformation. There may be dural AVM in regions of occlusion or thrombosis of spontaneous CCF.

Holly (West Palm Beach): There has been much talk about the carcinogenicity of the glues we are using. Could the panel comment on this?

Vinuela: We have been using PVA and IBCA since 1978. In neurosurgery, they have been using glues since the early 1960s. More than 3000 patients have been treated over the last 10 years with glues. There is no clinical indication of a malignant degeneration. A study that has been carried out in London, Ontario for many years shows no evidence of malignant degeneration. At our institution, we had a meeting of neuroscientists and we decided to continue using IBCA as in the past, though of course with caution. But there is no clinical or experimental evidence of carcinogenesis in the literature.

Part 3. Selected Papers

Selection of Candidates for EC/IC Bypass and Evaluation of the Benefit of This Surgery Through a SPECT Study

Tsuneyoshi Eguchi, Shigeo Iai, Takahumi Ide, and Motoo Nagane[1]

An ischemic stroke has two causes in its pathogenesis; hemodynamic and microembolic. For the hemodynamic ischemic stroke, in which a misery perfusion plays a major clinical role, a revascularization such as an EC/IC bypass has the benefit of augmenting the cerebral blood flow (CBF).

The phenomenon of misery perfusion has been detected only through PET studies observing the values of regional CBF (rCBF) and cerebral oxygen extraction fraction (OEF). However, there was a recent report [2] in the field of nuclear medicine which stated that the OEF has a good correlation with a cerebral mean transit time (MTT), the value of which can be obtained through a SPECT study. The MTT can be calculated from the values of rCBF and regional cerebral blood volume (rCBV). Thus, the phenomenon of a misery perfusion in cases of hemodynamic ischemic strokes can be assayed through the SPECT study. We are now selecting the candidates for the EC/IC bypass through the study of rCBF, rCBV, and rMTT.

A postoperative examination of these three values with and without digital donor closure (compression) will show how much the bypass flow contributes to the cerebral circulation; the benefit of the EC/IC bypass.

Material and Method

Two cases of the progressing stroke with a sign of hemiparesis due to an occlusion of the proximal middle cerebral artery were examined.

Both of them were operated on (STA-MCA anastomosis) during an acute stage. One of the patients has recovered to a normal neurological status and the other, on the contrary, has shown no neurological improvement. We checked these two cases and tried to find the differences between them in the values of rCBF, rCBV, and rMTT.

Following are the methods used for obtaining the values of the territory of the middle cerebral artery as the region of interest (ROI). The value of rCBF was obtained as a three-dimentional value using a SPECT of TOMOMATIC 64 by the ^{133}Xe inhalation method. The value of rCBV was obtained as a relative one using the same machine with ^{99m}Tc-labelled red blood cells. The value of rMTT was obtained from the value of rCBV divided by the value of rCBF.

If hemodynamic deficiency (rCBF ↓) exists, the cerebral vessels are forced to dilate to compensate for the lowered cerebral perfusion [1]. Therefore, rCBV is increased and rMTT is consequently increased, indicating a correlative increase in OEF, which means the existence of a misery perfusion.

In 11 typical cases with decreased rCBF and increased rCBV and rMTT, the degree of increase in rCBV or rMTT was compared with the degree of decrease in rCBF, in order to detect the correlation between a cerebral ischemia and the compensatory dilatation of the cerebral vessels.

In another 20 cases with neurological signs of ipsilateral hemispheric ischemia, the EC/IC bypass was performed. rCBF, rCBV, and rMTT were examined postoperatively, with not only pre-, but also post-digital donor closure (compression). The changes of these values under this maneuver were evaluated and the benefit of the bypass flow was estimated.

The values of rCBF, rCBV, and rMTT are expressed as a ratio of the value of the affected side divided by that of the nonaffected side.

The changes of rCBF (ΔrCBF) under digital donor closure is obtained through subtraction of its value of post-donor closure from that of pre-donor closure. The changes of rCBV and rMTT (ΔrCBV, ΔrMTT) under digital donor closure are obtained from the ratio of values (affected side/nonaffected side, because these values are

[1] Division of Neurosurgery, Kameda General Hospital, Kamogawa, Chiba, Japan

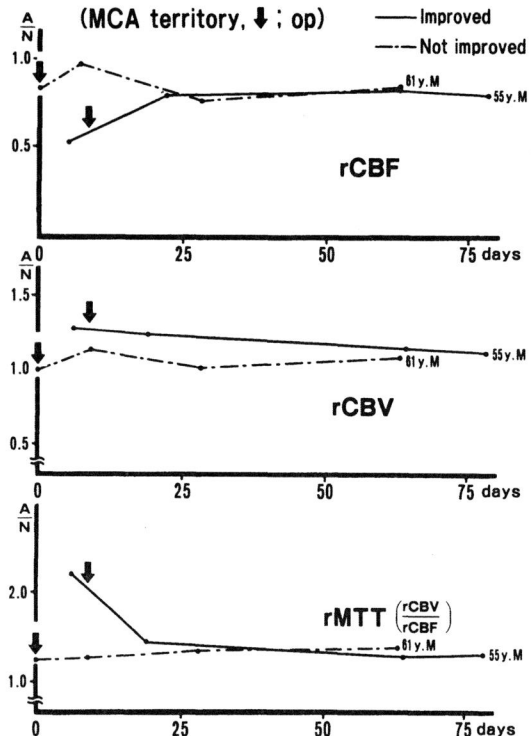

Fig. 1. Pre- and postoperative values of rCBF, rCBV, and rMTT on two cases of progressing stroke. One is improved clinically and the other is not improved

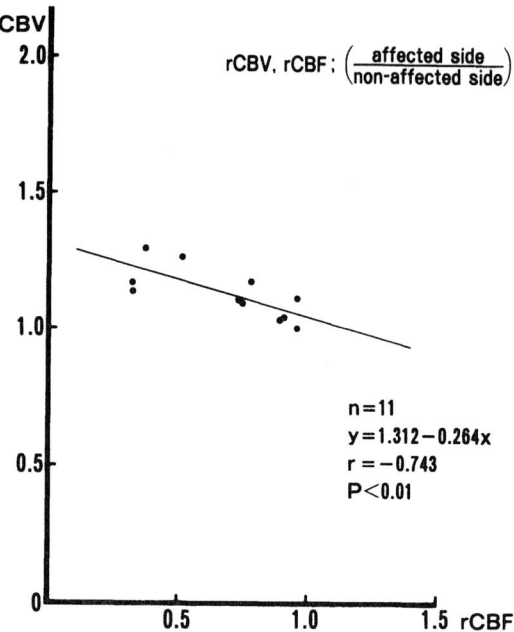

Fig. 2. Correlation between the degree of decrease in rCBF and the degree of compensatory increase in rCBV. Both values are shown as a ratio of that of the affected side to that of the non-affected side

not absolute but relative ones) of post-digital donor closure with the pre-digital donor closure ratio subtracted.

Results

As Fig. 1 shows, in the case of a progressing stroke which has recovered to a normal neurological status (solid line), the preoperative rCBF is decreased, and both rCBV and rMTT are compensatorily increased, indicating the existence of a misery perfusion. These values are improved postoperatively.

To the contrary, in the other case of progressing stroke, which has shown no neurological improvement, the preoperative values of rCBV and rMTT are not increased in spite of decreased rCBF, indicating the existence of a matched perfusion. These values did not essentially change postoperatively.

In this way, we may select the candidates for an EC/IC bypass surgery, if we get the values of not only rCBF, but also rCBV and rMTT, which can be substituted for the value of OEF.

There is a good correlation between the value of decreased rCBF and that of increased rCBV or

rMTT ($n = 11$, r $= -0.7$, $P < 0.01$, and $n = 11$, r $= -0.98$, $P < 0.001$, respectively). This indicates that the severer the cerebral ischemia is, the more the cerebral vessels dilate and, consequently, the more the rCBV (Fig. 2) or rMTT increases.

In 20 cases of EC/IC bypass surgery, rCBF, rCBV, and rMTT were examined postoperatively with both pre- and post-digital donor closure.

After the donor was closed, rCBF in the territory of the middle cerebral artery on the affected side was decreased significantly, and rCBV or rMTT was increased significantly ($n = 20$, $P < 0.001$, respectively).

The rCBV increased when the bypass flow was shut down, indicating that the bypass flow is beneficial for the cerebral circulation (Fig. 3). The shutdown of the bypass flow makes the cerebral vessels dilate to compensate for the hemodynamic deficiency which has been improved postoperatively with this bypass flow. The more the bypass flow contributes to the cerebral circulation, the more rCBV and rMTT are increased, if the bypass flow is shut down ($P < 0.05$ and $P < 0.001$; Fig. 4).

These findings suggest that the shutdown of

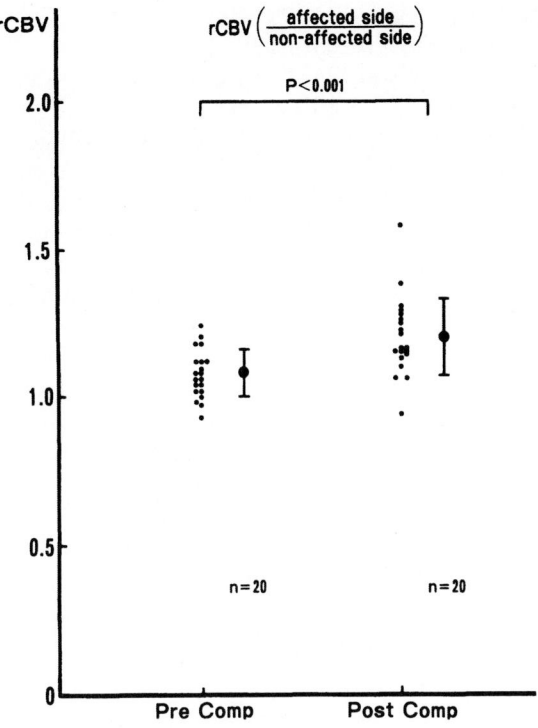

Fig. 3. Postoperative examination of rCBV with and without digital donor closure (compression). rCBV is increased significantly when the bypass flow is shut down, indicating that the bypass flow is beneficial for the cerebral circulation

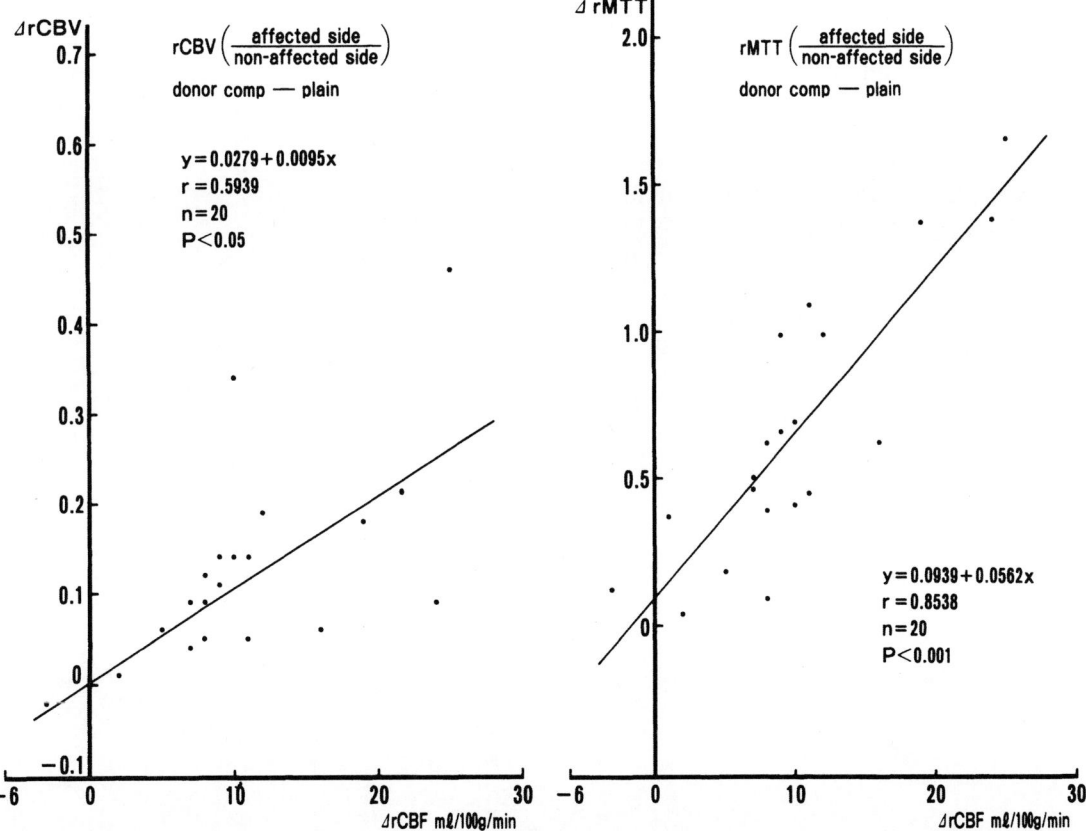

Fig. 4. Correlation between the bypass flow (ΔrCBF; pre-donor closure—post-donor closure) and the compensatory change in rCBV or rMTT (ΔrCBV or ΔrMTT; post-donor closure—pre-donor closure). The more the bypass flow contributes to the cerebral circulation, the more rCBV or rMTT is increased, if the bypass flow is shut down

the bypass flow may expose the brain to a misery perfusion, especially if the bypass flow (ΔrCBF) is large. In other words, the bypass flow contributes well to the cerebral circulation, indicating the benefit of the EC/IC bypass surgery.

Discussion

It was reported in the International Cooperative Study of EC/IC Bypass [3] that this operation had no benefit in preventing strokes on the patients who had suffered from transient ischemic attack, reversable ischemic neurological deficit or minor completed stroke. In this study, however, the values of cerebral circulation or hemodynamic reserve were not examined at all.

Among the patients enrolled in the study, there might be ones with a matched perfusion or ones with a misery perfusion, and there might be ones with an embolic origin or a hemodynamic origin. The sample is not uniform but mixed. The results of the study, therefore, cannot confirm that the EC/IC bypass has no benefit for every kind of cerebral ischemic patient.

The important point is to differentiate the patients with a hemodynamic deficiency from those with an embolism, to differentiate the patients with a misery perfusion from those with a matched perfusion.

The state of a misery perfusion has been evaluated with the aid of a PET scan but this instrument is, at the moment, not popular. We have, therefore, tried to find the state of a misery perfusion with a SPECT scan, examining not only rCBF, but also rCBV and rMTT, which can be obtained through a SPECT study, while OEF,

which is obtained only through a PET study, has a good correlation with MTT [2].

As the cases in Fig. 1 show, we can select the candidates for an EC/IC bypass surgery after we evaluate not only rCBF, but also rCBV and rMTT. If rCBV and rMTT are increased with decreased rCBF, there is a misery perfusion and a revascularization to augment the cerebral blood flow is beneficial. If rCBV and rMTT are not increased in spite of decreased rCBF, there is a matched perfusion and a revascularization is meaningless. In this way, examination of rCBV and rMTT together with rCBF is useful in selecting candidates for EC/IC bypass surgery.

On the other hand, an examination of the post-operative rCBF, rCBV, and rMTT with pre- and post-digital donor closure is useful and helpful to evaluate the efficacy and benefit of the EC/IC bypass surgery for those operated patients.

References

1. Powers W, Martin W, Herscovitch P, Raichle M, Grubb R (1983) The value of regional blood volume measurements in the diagnosis of cerebral ischemia. J Cereb Blood Flow Metab 3(1):S598–599
2. Shishido F, Uemura K, Inugami A, et al. (1986) Cerebral circulation and metabolism in cerebral infarction of middle cerebral artery territory—a positron CT study with HEADTOME III and ^{15}0 labelled gases. J Nucl Med (Tokyo) 23(2):123–134
3. The EC/IC Bypass Study Group (1985) Failure of extracranial-intracranial arterial bypass to reduce the risk of ischemic stroke. Results of an International Randomized Trial. N Eng J Med 313:1191–1200

Single Photon Emission Study of Hemodynamic Reserve in Internal Carotid Occlusions
Value of Combined Measurement of Cerebral Blood Flow and Cerebral Blood Volume

J.M. Derlon, G. Bouvard, M.C. Petit, J.P. Thenint, F. Viader, S. Khoury, B. Dupuy, and J.P. Houtteville[1]

Unlike carotid endarterectomy which can theoretically prevent both hemodynamic and embolic strokes from atherosclerotic plaques, extracranial-intracranial (EC-IC) bypass is advisable only for lesions determining a chronic decrease of brain perfusion pressure potentially responsible for hemodynamic strokes. Nevertheless, these operations have usually been decided on clinical and angiographic data, and have seldom taken into account objective hemodynamic intracranial parameters. Using positron emission tomography (PET), some authors have shown that permanent disturbances of hemodynamic [6, 7] and metabolic [2] data was a relatively infrequent occurrence in patients with carotid obstructive lesions, but that, in some of them, carotid endarterectomy [6] or EC-IC bypass [10] could reverse these disturbances.

Following these studies, we have shown [3–5] that the measurement of resting regional cerebral blood flow (rCBF) alone was not enough to assess the hemodynamic consequences of obstructive (stenotic and occlusive) lesions of the internal carotid artery (ICA). However, the combined study of rCBF and resting regional cerebral blood volume (rCBV) could provide a very accurate assessment of both pre- and postoperative hemodynamic conditions. Similarly, other authors showed that the measurement of the "perfusion reserve" after CO_2 inhalation [9] or i.v. acetazolamide (R) [8] provided a better hemodynamic assessment of ICA occlusions than did resting rCBF measurement alone.

After a thorough analysis of the cooperative study results [1], we decided to reexamine all our cases of ICA uni- and bilateral occlusions in order to determine which percentage of these patients exhibited a permanent decrease of auto-regulation reserve downstream of the lesion.

Patients and Methods

Eighty patients were studied, belonging to three clinical groups: asymptomatic ($n = 8$), transient ischemic attacks (TIAs, $n = 19$), and completed stroke (CS, $n = 53$, with 37 mild strokes and 16 severe strokes). In 66 patients, a CT scan was performed, showing a normal or atrophic brain ($n = 26$), or an ischemic hypodensity relevant to the occlusion side ($n = 40$). All patients underwent an angiographic study of at least both ICA (Table 1).

In all patients, a combined study of resting rCBF (clearance of inhaled ^{133}Xe studied with a 32 probe Novo-Cerebrograph) and resting rCBV (single photon computed emission tomography [SPECT] after autotransfusion of ^{99m}Tc-labeled erythrocytes) was performed. Detailed information about methods and normal and pathologic values were published previously [4, 5]. In 49 patients, a dynamic study of rCBF and rCBV before and after intravenous injection of 1 g acetazolamide was performed. Considering all data together, hemodynamic reserve (HR)

Table 1. Angiography

	Number
Results	
Unilateral ICA occlusion with no or moderate contralateral stenosis	61
Unilateral ICA occlusion with severe contralateral stenosis	11
Bilateral ICA occlusion	8
Etiology	
Atherosclerosis	63
Spontaneous dissection	11
Traumatic dissection	1
Ligation	4
Moyamoya	1

Methods used were bilateral selective carotid arteriography, four axes arteriography, DIVA

[1] CHRU, Avenue de la Côte de Nacre, Caen, France

assessment results were analyzed in unilateral ICA occlusions.

A normal HR was diagnosed if the rCBF, after i.v. acetazolamide, was bilaterally and symmetrically increased, with no asymmetry of rCBV before or after i.v. acetazolamide. A decreased HR was diagnosed when the rCBF, after i.v. acetazolamide, was not increasd on the ICA occlusion side. The rCBV was increased on this side at rest, but the asymmetry disappears after i.v. acetazolamide.

In bilateral ICA occlusion (eight cases), only dynamic rCBF studies were usable, for resting rCBV were symmetric.

Results

Among 80 patients, 36 exhibited a decreased HR at first exploration (which was performed between 6 days and 3 months after the onset of the ischemic attack). A spontaneous normalization was observed within a short delay (1–2 weeks) after the first exploration in seven patients (of whom five had a spontaneous ICA dissection). Therefore, only 32% of all patients had a permanently decreased HR.

In 54 patients with unilateral ICA occlusion, we could study the importance of anterior communicating artery (ACA) patency in the occurence of an HR impairment (Table 2). We confirmed our previous observations that, even if an HR is more likely to occur in the case of a noncross-filling of the intracranial arterial bed via the ACA, the ACA angiographic patency cannot predict this occurence in individual patients.

Among the whole population of 80 patients, 56 were eligible for an EC-IC bypass, according to the clinical and angiographic criteria of the International Cooperative Study. An isotopic HR impairment was demonstrated in 20, which means that EC-IC bypass was justified in only 31% of conventionally eligible patients.

Discussion

The International Cooperative Study [8] began in 1977, at a time where the decisive works on hemodynamic ischemic brain disorders with PET and SPECT were not yet performed or published. Therefore, it was justifiable to set operative indications on clinical and angiographic grounds only, and in a relatively large

Table 2. Coating materials

	Biobond	Aron alpha
Total coating	9	1
	Gelfoam 1	
	Oxycell cotton 1	
Partial coating	11	2
	Gelfoam 1	Gelfoam 2
	Muscle piece 1	

way owing to neurosurgical practice which was very confident in the safety and effectiveness of the procedure. Since that pionneering period, a bulk of data has been gathered, mainly by isotopic methods, on intracranial hemodynamics during ischemic disorders. PET studies [6] showed that true hemodynamic impairment was relatively infrequent at the subacute or chronic stage of ICA obstructive lesions, but that it could be reversed by surgery. Single photon assessment methods [3–5] have more recently concluded in the same way, with the advantage of being routinely available in most centers. In our own study, the fact that 70% of all conventionally eligible patients for EC-IC bypass study had no HR impairment and were not, therefore, truly eligible, indicates a very important bias in the Cooperative Study statistics and conclusions. A new clinical trial would therefore be necessary, in which isotopic HR study should be one of the eligibility criteria.

References

1. Barnett HJM, Peerless SJ, Fox AJ, et al. (1985) Failure of extracranial arterial bypass to reduce the risk of ischemic stroke: Results of an International Randomized Trial. N Engl J Med 313:1191–1200
2. Baron JC, Bousser MG, Laplane D, Comar D, Castaigne P, Kellershorn C (1982) Noninvasive study of cerebral blood flow and oxygen metabolism with positron emission tomography in human cerebral ischemic disorders. In: Rose, FC (ed) Advances in stroke therapy. Raven, New York
3. Derlon JM, Bouvard G, Hubert P, et al. (1987) Etude hémodynamique des lésions obstructives de l'axe carotidien interne: Intérêt de la mesure couplée du débit et du volume sanguins cérébraux. Rev Neurol 143(1):32–39
4. Derlon JM, Bouvard G, Lechevalier B, et al. (1985) Haemodynamic study of internal carotid artery stenosis and occlusion: Value of coupled measurements of regional cerebral blood and regional cerebral blood volume. In: Meyer JS,

Lechner H, Reivich M, Ott E (eds) Cerebral vascular disease, vol. 5, World Federation of Neurology, 12th Salzburg Conference, Excerpta Medica. Elsevier, Amsterdam, pp 170–176

5. Derlon JM, Bouvard G, Lechevalier B, et al. (1986) Haemodynamic study of internal carotid disease: Value of combined measurement of regional cerebral blood flow and blood volume. Ann Vasc. Surg 1:86–97

6. Gibbs JM, Leenders KL, Wise RJS, Jones T (1984) Evaluation of cerebral perfusion reserve in patients with carotid artery occlusion. Lancet 28:182–186

7. Gibbs JM, Wise RJS, Legg MJ (1983) Progress in emission tomography studies in acute stroke and in patients with carotid occlusion: Pathophysiology of cerebral ischemia and diminished perfusion reserve. In: Progress in stroke research, vol. 2. Pitman, London, pp. 214–226

8. Lassen NA (1983) ^{133}Xenon tomography of cerebral blood flow in cerebrovascular disease. In: Greenhalgh RM, Rose FC (eds) Progress in stroke research. Pitman, London, pp 197–204

9. Norrving B, Nilson B, Risberg J (1982) rCBF in patients with carotid occlusion: Resting and hypercapnic flow related to collateral pattern. Stroke 13(2):155–162

10. Samson Y, Baron JC, Bousser MG, Rey A, Derlon JM, David P, Comoy J (1985) Effects of extra-intracranial arterial bypass on cerebral blood flow and oxygen metabolism in human. Stroke 16:4

Preoperative Evaluation and Postoperative Follow-up of Extra-Intracranial Arterial Bypass in Ischemic Cerebrovascular Disease

Functional Neuroimaging with Single Photon Emission Computed Tomography Using ^{99m}Tc-Hexamethyl-Propylene-Amine-Oxime and ^{123}I-Iodoamphetamine, and with Positron Emission Tomography Using ^{18}F-2-Deoxy-2-Fluoro-D-Glucose and 3-O-(^{11}C-Methyl)-D-Glucose

N. Roosen[1], K.-J. Langen[2], H. Wieler[2], E. Rota[3], H. Herzog[3], W.J. Bock[1], L.E. Feinendegen[2,3], and D.D. Patton[3,4]

Introduction

The report of the EC-IC Bypass Study Group, which was published in 1985, seemed to constitute the ultimate disqualification of extra-intracranial arterial bypass (EIAB) in cerebrovascular disease [9]. However, it was not unanimously accepted [1]. Particularly, the importance of functional neuroimaging using emission tomography has received little attention in the selection of patients for inclusion in the EC-IC Bypass Study [10].

At the University of Düsseldorf, and in collaboration with the Nuclear Research Center Jülich GmbH, positron emission tomography (PET), as well as single photon emission computed tomography (SPECT), have been used in both pre- and postoperative examinations of patients undergoing EIAB surgery. We performed a retrospective study of these patients and analyzed their clinical history and computed tomography (CT), PET, and SPECT findings. Early results on SPECT imaging in this condition have been presented elsewhere [7], and we now report an extended review of our series with longer follow-up and with additional patients included.

Case Material and Methods

Patient Characteristics

All patients were operated by one of the authors

Neurosurgical Clinic[1], Department of Nuclear Medicine[2], University Hospital Düsseldorf, Düsseldorf, Federal Republic of Germany[3], Institute of Medicine, Nuclear Research Center Jülich GmbH, Jülich, Federal Republic of Germany[4], Division of Nuclear Medicine, Department of Radiology, College of Medicine, Health Sciences Center of the University of Arizona, Tucson, Arizona, USA

(N.R.) in the period from January 1984 to December 1986. Most of these patients had surgery in 1984 or 1985. We performed 36 operations in 34 patients (25 male and 9 female; Table 1). Usually the superficial temporal artery (STA) was anastomosed end-to-side to the middle cerebral artery (MCA): 17 patients were operated on the left side, 14 on the right side, and two bilaterally. In one patient, an occipital artery (OccA) to posterior inferior cerebellar artery (PICA) anastomosis was done. Follow-up was adequate for 32 of 36 EIAB. Long-term patency rate (>6 months) was determined by Doppler sonography to be 94%. After publication of the negative results of the EC-IC Bypass Study Group [9], very few patients with cerebrovascular disease have been referred to the Neurosurgical Department of the University Hospital Düsseldorf for evaluation of microvascular surgical therapy, and an EIAB was performed in only two of them. Both patients had evidence of a hemodynamic cause for their cerebrovascular symptoms. CT in these cases has been within normal limits.

Table 1 reveals a preponderance of arterial occlusions and of unilateral atherosclerotic disease, involving only one vessel.

SPECT Studies

All 27 SPECT examinations were performed with a Philips GAMMA DIAGNOST tomograph, according to a modification of the technique described by Herzog et al. [4, 7]. In 19 SPECT studies, we used ^{123}I-iodoamphetamine (IMP) as a tracer of regional cerebral blood flow (rCBF) [5]. Recently, a new radiopharmacon, ^{99m}Tc-hexamethyl-propylene-amin-oxime (HMPAO) was developed for rCBF determination [8]. Eight SPECT investigations were obtained with HMPAO.

Table 1. Clinical findings in 34 patients with atherosclerotic cerebrovascular disease treated with EIAB

	Without other pathology	With contralat. ICA stenosis	With contralat. ICA occlusion	n
ICA or siphon stenosis	3	2	—	5
ICA or siphon occlusion	12	7	4	23
MCA stenosis	1	—	—	1
MCA occlusion	5	—	—	5
		9	4	
Total	21	13		34

Operations performed (36)
STA-MCA left 17 patients, right 14 patients, bilateral 2 patients, OccA-PICA left 1 patient
n = 34 patients; 25 ♂ ⟨56 years⟩; 9 ♀ ⟨50 years⟩
follow-up: 32 of 36 EIAB; patency rate [> 6 months]: 30 of 32 EIAB (94%)
ICA internal carotid artery, *MCA* middle cerebral artery, *EIAB* extra-intracranial arterial bypass

PET Studies

An ECAT II tomograph [GG&G, Ortec] was used for PET scanning with ^{18}F-2-deoxy-2-fluoro-D-glucose (FDG) or 3-O-(^{11}C-methyl)-D-glucose (CMG) [11]. Eight PET studies were performed with FDG and five with CMG.

Results

Transient ischemic attacks (TIA) or partially reversible neurological deficits were the reason for performing EIAB in 41% of patients (Fig. 1). In 47% of our cases there were stable neurological deficits, i.e., completed stroke, on preoperative evaluation. In 12% there were TIAs or partially reversible neurological deficits, associated with completed stroke symptomatology: one half of this group had TIAs complicated by stroke, and the other half showed completed stroke with changing severity of neurological symptoms.

In patients with TIAs or partially reversible deficits, there were no further ischemic symptoms after EIAB in a group of 81%. In patients with stable neurological deficits, this was only 62%. However, they showed some postoperative functional improvement in 41% of cases.

Pre- and post-EIAB SPECT was performed in eight patients. Tracer uptake, correlating with rCBF, increased in six of them. Five out of these six concurrently showed a clinical improvement (Fig. 2), i.e., no further occurrence of TIA or an improvement of a previously stable neurological deficit [7]. However, a post-EIAB neurological amelioration could also be seen without increase

in rCBF, as determined with SPECT. As to the extent of the lesions demonstrated with SPECT, this was generally larger than with CT [7].

The results of PET scanning were similar to those reported in the literature on ischemic cerebrovascular disease [11]. There was a fairly good correlation between SPECT and PET findings, especially in the chronic phase of cerebral ischemia. Pre- and post-EIAB PET was performed in one patient with TIA, and in a second patient, who had suffered a cerebral infarction. The TIA patient had a post-EIAB increase in regional cerebral metabolic rate (rCMR) of glucose (rCMRgluc), correlating with the cessation of TIA's. In the stroke patient, we could not show a change in rCMRgluc, although some clinical improvement occurred after EIAB.

Discussion

The report of the EC-IC Bypass Study Group corroborated earlier findings on the extreme variability of the clinical course of atherosclerotic cerebrovascular disease, thus emphasizing the necessity of studying large populations in therapeutic trials [9]. Criteria for patient entry into such randomized trials are very important [1, 10]. Biased criteria may lead to wrong results and conclusions, thus making the whole effort of conducting a large scale study worthless [1]. One of the critiques of the EC-IC Bypass Study Group report concerns the negligence of functional studies in the entry criteria [1, 10]. PET is the gold standard for evaluation of rCBF and rCMR, but it also is a very expensive and com-

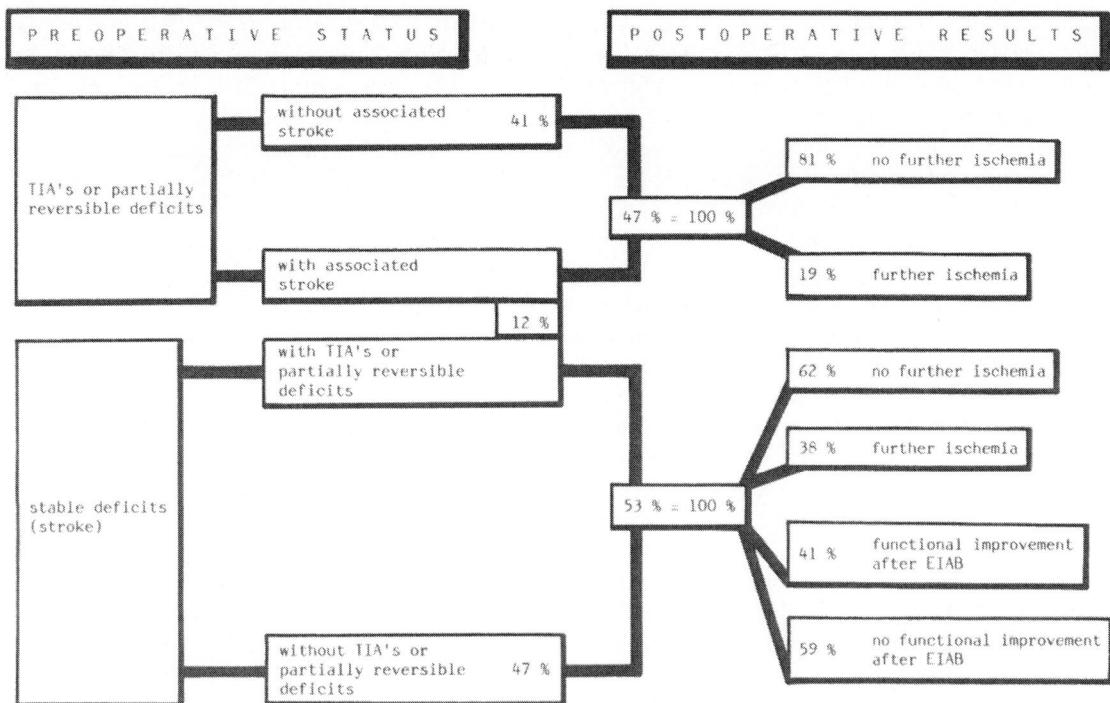

Fig. 1. The preoperative status of 34 patients with 36 EIAB operations is compared with the postoperative results. Preoperatively, patients were divided into two groups, according to the first neurological symptoms with which they presented: either reversible symptoms or primarily completed stroke. In a minority of patients of each group, another type of symptomatology secondarily became superposed on the primary clinical picture. After EIAB, most patients with reversible neurological symptoms had no further ischemic episodes. This was less marked in patients with primarily completed stroke. A significant proportion of them showed some functional improvement after EIAB. *TIA* transient ischemic attack

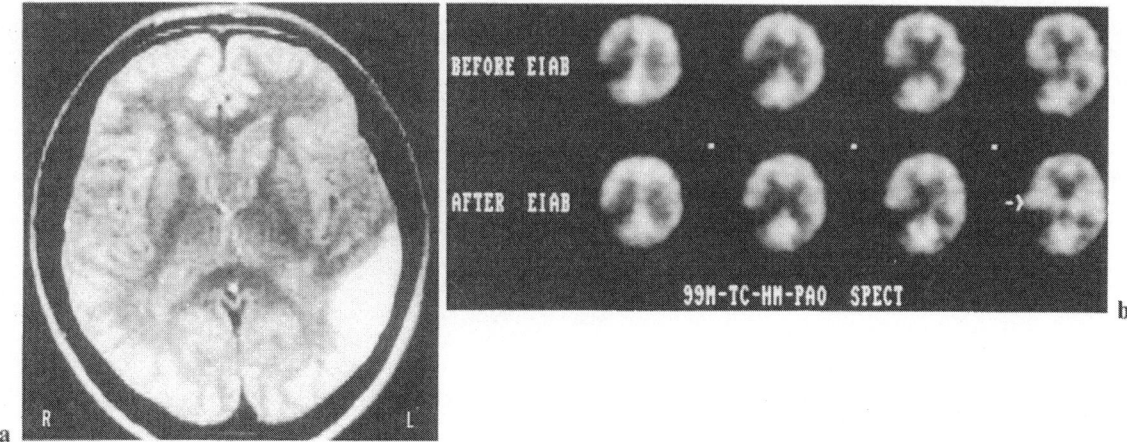

Fig. 2a, b. This patient suffered a stroke in part of the territory of the left MCA. Neurological symptoms included a right hemiparesis and Gerstmann's syndrome. During the ensuing weeks, the severity of the hemiparesis showed marked fluctuations. Angiography demonstrated a left ICA occlusion and delayed left MCA filling from the right ICA and the vertebrobasilar arterial circulation. CT did not show a hypodense lesion, but (**a**) MR (SE 2000/56 scan is depicted) revealed a hyperintense area within the MCA territory on the left side. (**b**) HMPAO SPECT before EIAB revealed a large region of decreased or abolished HMPAO uptake. After EIAB there was a clear increase in HMPAO uptake in part of the hypoperfused area (*arrow*), and, concurrently, the hemiparesis showed a marked amelioration. Also, there were no transient deteriorations in muscle strength seen anymore on the right side. The Gerstmann's syndrome was unchanged, as could be expected from the HMPAO SPECT findings

plex technique not suitable for routine investigation of large numbers of patients [11]. There clearly is a need for easy-to-perform techniques of physiological neuroimaging. With the exception of Xe-CT [3], all such techniques involve SPECT [2], but use different tracers. The (patho)physiological parameter studied is rCBF [2]. The biochemical disturbances in cerebrovascular disease, however, are rather complicated: fairly well established and constant relations between rCBF, rCMR of oxygen (rCMRO$_2$), regional oxygen extraction ratio (rOER), rCMRgluc, etc., are known for chronic, stable cerebrovascular ischemic lesions, but not for the early stages of ischemia [11]. Therefore, rCBF determination with SPECT gives only an incomplete description of cerebrovascular insufficiency. Nevertheless, the clinical value of this technique is not questioned, due to its ready availability, low cost, and low work load [2].

The different radiotracers for determination of rCBF using SPECT, viz., ^{133}Xe, ^{81m}Kr, ^{99m}Tc-labeled microspheres, IMP, and HMPAO have been discussed in the literature [6, 8]. Some of them have to be administered using rather invasive methods. ^{133}Xe SPECT is an inhalation technique, which offers the possibility to study the reactivity of the cerebral vasculature; on the other hand, it requires specially dedicated SPECT systems [6]. IMP and HMPAO can be injected intravenously and rCBF determined with regular SPECT systems [6,8]. Both IMP and HMPAO are simple to use, but IMP, in contrast to HMPAO, is expensive and not readily available [5,6,8]. Furthermore, ^{99m}Tc has a shorter half-life than ^{123}I, thus allowing higher levels of radioactivity to be given, which results in better resolution of SPECT images. For these reasons, HMPAO, and not IMP, is to be preferred as a radiotracer in SPECT studies of rCBF.

Our clinical results compare favorably with those of the literature [1,9], although admittedly our series is not prospective and not randomized. On the basis of our findings and a review of the literature, we believe there are still indications to perform EIAB surgery, despite the results of the EC-IC Bypass Study Group [9]. Hemodynamic ischemia can be treated with EIAB, and HMPAO SPECT offers good possibilities to demonstrate this.

The ultimate result of surgical management of cerebrovascular ischemia depends upon the progression of the underlying multivessel disease. This progression is probably hardly influenced by EIAB surgery. However, EIAB can acutely abolish TIAs and can cause an immediate postoperative amelioration of a previously fixed neurological deficit, as has been described in our clinical series. In general, the correlation of rCBF changes after EIAB with neurological outcome was fair. Therefore, selection of suitable candidates for EIAB surgery by functional neuroimaging is of prime importance, and HMPAO SPECT seems to be very useful in this regard.

Acknowledgments. The authors are indebted to Dr. Ackermann, Amersham Buchler GmbH & Co KG, 3300 Braunschweig, F.R.G., for providing detailed information and data on HMPAO, and for generous support of the presentation of this report during the symposium. The continuous assistance on technical matters of CT and SPECT investigations, as well as the kindly offered support for the preparation of this study, which were given by Dipl.-Ing. Fechner, C.H.F. Müller-Philips Medical Systems, 4000 Düsseldorf, F.R.G., are acknowledged. The help provided by Dr. Ackermann and Dipl-Ing. Fechner is gratefully appreciated.

References

1. Ausman JI, Diaz FG (1986) Critique of the extra-cranial-intracranial bypass study. Surg Neurol 26:218–221

2. Esser PD (1985) Improvements in SPECT technology for cerebral imaging. Semin Nucl Med 15:335–346

3. Hellma RS, Collier BD, Tikofsky RS, Kilgore DP, Daniels DL, Haughton VM, Walsh PR, Cusick JF, Saxena VK, Palmer DW, Isitman AT (1986) Comparison of single-photon emission computed tomography with [^{123}I] iodoamphetamine and xenon-enhancement computed tomography for assessing regional cerebral blood flow. J Cereb Blood Flow Metab 6:747–755

4. Herzog H, Wieler H, Vogt E, Spohr G, Feinendegen LE (1985) Improved brain SPECT using a single head SPECT camera with a conventional LFOV detector. Nucl Med Commun 6:560

5. Holman BL, Hill TC, Lee RGL, Zimmerman RE, Moore SC, Royal HD (1983) Brain imaging with radiolabeled amines. In: Freeman LM, Weissmann HS (eds) Nuclear medicine annual 1983. Raven, New York, pp 131–165

6. Lassen NA, Rommer P (1986) Cerebral blood flow tomography by single photon emission computerized tomography using ^{133}Xe in cerebrovascular disease. In: Ventura A, Crepaldi G, Senin U (eds) Monographs on atherosclerosis, vol 14. Karger, Basel, pp 71–82

7. Roosen N, Wieler H, Herzog H, Patton DD,

Feinendegen LE (1987) Effect of extra-intracranial arterial bypass (EIAB) on regional cerebral blood flow measured by brain-SPECT and ^{123}I-amphetamines (IMP) or ^{99m}Tc-hexamethyl-propylene-amine-oxime (HMPAO) using a single head camera with a 30-degree slant-hole collimator. In: Gagliardi R, Benvenuti L (eds) Controversies in EIAB for cerebral ischemia. Proceedings of the Eighth International Symposium on Microsurgical Anastomoses for Cerebral Ischemia, Florence, 14–17 September, 1986. Monduzzi Editore, Bologna, pp 273–279

8. Sharp PF, Smith FW, Gemmell HG, Lyall D, Evans NTS, Grozdanovic D, Davidson J, Tyrrell DA, Pickett RD, Neirinckx RD (1986) Technetium-99m HM-PAO stereoisomers as potential agents for imaging regional cerebral blood flow: Human volunteer studies. J Nucl Med 27:171–177

9. The EC-IC Bypass Study Group (1985) Failure of extracranial-intracranial arterial bypass to reduce the risk of ischaemic stroke: Results of an international randomized trial. N Engl J Med 313:1191–1200

10. The EC-IC Bypass Study Group (1985) The international cooperative study of extracranial/intracranial arterial anastomosis (EC-IC bypass study): Methodology and entry characteristics. Stroke 16:397–406

11. Wieler H, Herzog H, Patton DD, Schmid A, Rota E, Feinendegen LE (1986) Functional studies in brain and heart with positron emission tomography. Med Prog Technol 11:73–106

Effect of Preexisting STA-MCA Bypass on rCBF and SSEP's Following Acute Stroke in Dogs

CHRISTOPHER M. LOFTUS[1], JULIUS A. SILVIDI[2], and DANIEL D. BERNSTEIN[3]

Hypothesis

This study was predicated on the hypothesis that a preexisting extracranial to intracranial bypass can support hemispheric blood flow even in the face of an acute severe proximal vascular occlusion, and that delayed reopening of a bypass graft may also provide significant restoration of flow to a profoundly ischemic hemisphere. It was also designed to investigate the possible preservation of somatosensory evoked responses (SSEP's) by bypass blood flow and the potential for return, if any, of SSEP function following delayed revascularization.

Materials and Methods

Seven adult mongrel dogs (20 ± 5 kg) were anesthetized with intravenous sodium pentothal 25 mg/kg, intubated, and maintained with 1% halothane, N_2O, and 30% O_2. The $PaCO_2$ was maintained at 40 mmHg, and the PaO_2 at 90 mmHg with a mechanical ventilator. Muscular paralysis was achieved utilizing metocurine iodide in doses of 1 mg every 1-2 h as necessary. The superficial temporal artery was dissected from the scalp, occluded proximally with a Dietrich clamp, transected distally, filled with heparinized saline, and retracted from the field. A unilateral fronto-temporal craniectomy, flush to the floor of the frontal and middle fossae, was performed after resection of the zygomatic arch. After opening the dura, the frontal and temporal lobes were retracted and secured with a self-retaining retractor system, and microdissection of the ipsilateral anterior cerebral (A2), ophthalmic, ethmoidal, middle cerebral (MCA),

posterior communicating, and anterior cerebellar arteries [10] was performed in preparation for later cautery occlusion of these vessels. A standardized 3-mm STA-MCA anastomosis was then performed on a middle cerebral branch just distal to the bifurcation of the MCA. This branch was customarily 0.6–0.8 mm in diameter. Following completion of the anastomosis, and throughout the remainder of the experimental manipulations, patency was confirmed with a microvascular Doppler probe (Titronics Medical Instruments, Iowa City, Iowa, USA) in both the donor and recipient vessels.

Cerebral blood flow (rCBF) was studied in this model with infusion of radiolabeled microspheres at five times. For rCBF measurements via microsphere injection, a 7-F pigtail catheter was introduced into the left ventricle via the right femoral artery. A Swan-Ganz catheter was introduced through the right femoral vein and flow directed into the pulmonary artery for monitoring of pulmonary capillary wedge pressure (PCWP). Catheters were also placed in the left femoral and brachial arteries for withdrawal of reference blood samples, in right brachial artery for monitoring of mean arterial pressure, and in the inferior vena cava via the left femoral vein for injection of drugs. Core temperature and heart rate were continuously monitored. Blood gases and hematocrit were determined and recorded prior to each blood flow measurement. Labeled 15 micron microspheres (Gadolinium[153], Tin[115], Strontium[85], Niobium[95], and Scandium[46]) in sufficient volume to obtain approximately 400 spheres per tissue sample were injected into the left ventricle and flushed with 5 cm³ saline over 5 s for blood flow determination. Blood reference samples were also drawn from the left brachial and femoral arteries at the rate of 2.06 ml/min for a total of 2.5 min starting 30 s prior to microsphere injection.

At the end of the experiment, 4% neutral red was intraarterially injected to define the ischemic zone. The animals were killed with intravenous

The Cerebrovascular Neurosurgical Laboratory[1], Iowa City Veterans Administration Hospital[2], The University of Iowa Hospitals and Clinics[3], Iowa, USA.

pentobarbital 300 mg/kg and the brains removed. The brains were sectioned in the midline and the cortical ischemic zone (as defined morphologically by neutral red) was dissected from the nonischemic tissues. A mirror-image control zone from the nonoperated hemisphere was likewise dissected out. These tissues, together with biopsies from the right and left renal cortices and right and left cardiac ventricles, were divided into uniform samples, weighed, and counted in a 3-in well-type gamma counter for a period of 5 min each. Reference blood samples were likewise counted. Comparison of flow rates from right and left kidneys served as a control on adequate dispersion of microspheres throughout the vascular system. An analysis of variance statistical technique (pairwise comparisons with Duncan's follow-up test) was used to compare all flows in the ipsilateral ischemic zone and to compare left versus right hemispheres for each individual flow.

Somatosensory evoked potentials (SSEP's) were also studied in these animals. An epidural recording electrode was placed through a separate burr hole 1 cm lateral to the midline at the level of the coronal suture, with a midline reference electrode in the snout. The brachial plexus of the right forelimb was stimulated at 3.0 mA for 500 repetitions, and stimulation-recording sequences, using a Nicolet CA-1000 evoked response averager, were performed at four times: (a) bypass open—no lesion created, (b) bypass open—proximal occlusions performed, (c) bypass clipped—occlusions per-

formed (complete ischemia), and (d) 30 min following bypass reopening. Responses were recorded with a 20-ms time analysis and a bandpass of 150–1500 Hz. The SSEPs were stored on magnetic discs for later retrieval and plotting.

Results

The ischemic zone blood flow values for both hemispheres are summarized in Table 1. As we have shown in previous experiments [7], a mild decrease in rCBF on the operated side can be attributed to brain retraction and dissection alone, but this interhemispheric variation was not statistically significant, and does not, in the authors' estimation, contaminate the experimental data.

As shown in Fig. 1, ischemic zone measurements with the bypass first closed (68.9 ± 10 SEM cm^3/100 g/min) and then opened (76.8 ±

Table 1. Ischemic zone flow measurements (cm^3/100 g/min ± SEM)

	Left (operated)	Right (control)
Flow #1	68.9 ± 10.0	85.93 ± 9.39
Flow #2	76.8 ± 8.9	108.06 ± 9.69
Flow #3	60.18 ± 8.95	86.27 ± 11.55
Flow #4	7.95 ± 2.55	84.94 ± 10.79
Flow #5	46.61 ± 6.29	78.54 ± 14.15

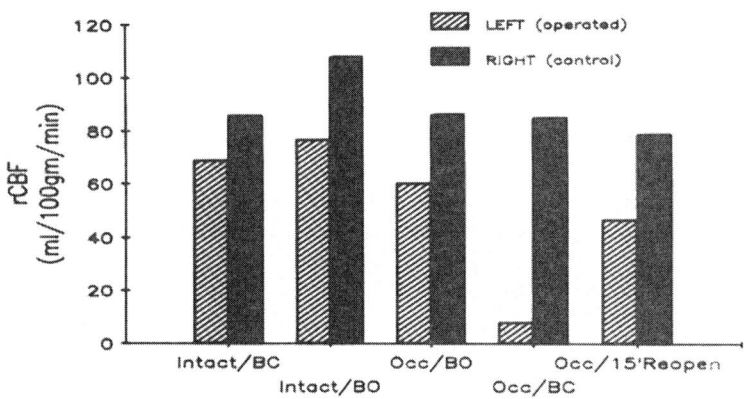

Fig. 1. MCA Ischemic zone rCBF determinations in dogs using radiolabeled microspheres. The bypass had no significant contribution in the intact vascular system. Flow was largely preserved following creation of the arterial lesion but almost completely abolished with subsequent bypass clipping. Reopening of the bypass reestablished significant ipsilateral flow. *MCA* middle cerebral artery, *BO* bypass open, *BC* bypass closed, *Occ* occluded

8.9) showed no significant contribution of bypass flow in the intact vascular system. Following proximal vascular occlusion, rCBF was preserved by bypass flow (60.18 ± 8.95). There was no statistical difference between these flow values and either of the intact system flows.

A significant flow decrease ensued when the bypass was subsequently clipped (7.95 ± 2.55, ANOVA $P < 0.05$). This confirmed both the adequacy of this ischemic model and the protective effect of the preexisting bypass. Reopening of the bypass graft following 15 min of ischemia restored flow to 76% of previous levels (46.61 ± 6.29). This restoration was a significant increase from the global ischemia values ($P < 0.05$), and was not statistically different from preocclusive values. Statistical analysis of flows in left versus right hemispheres showed no significant differences in flows #1, 2, and 3. The global ischemia flow #4 was significantly lower on the ischemic side, as was the revascularization flow #5, indicating that, by this type of left-right comparison, delayed revascularization was statistically inferior to preischemic bypass protection flow #3.

Preocclusion SSEP's showed a consistent biphasic wave at 8–10 ms (Fig. 2). This wave, with some decrease in amplitude, was preserved by bypass flow following the arterial lesion. Bypass clipping (complete ischemia) abolished the ipsilateral SEEP. Variable return SEEP's occurred following reestablishment of bypass flow, but never reached the amplitudes seen prior to bypass clipping.

Discussion

Choice of Ischemic Model

Initial studies in this laboratory began with models of cerebrovascular bypass followed by occlusion of either middle cerebral artery alone or both the middle cerebral and intracranial internal carotid (IC) arteries. Despite the suitability of these models as reported by previous investigators [4, 5], in our pilot studies, these ischemic models were ineffective in producing a reproducible decrease in rCBF. The collateral contribution in the dog brain was felt to be still too rich to provide reproducible results with these occlusions alone. Accordingly, attention was focused on validating with microsphere flows the "cerebral mantle infarction model" described by Suzuki et al. [10], in which six major

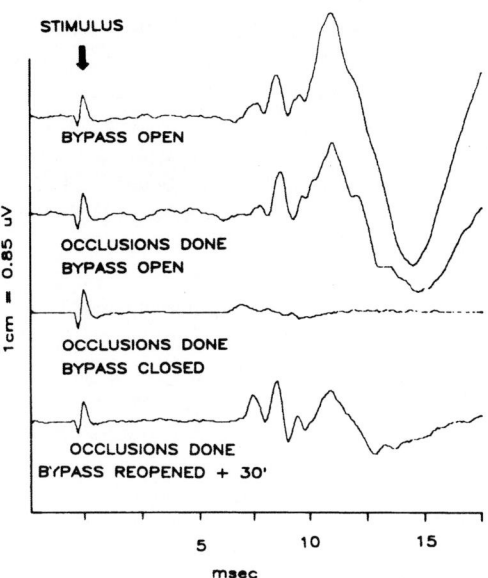

Fig. 2. Somatosensory evoked potentials (SSEP's) from a representative experimental animal. SSEP's were preserved to some degree by bypass blood flow, and universally disappeared following bypass clipping. Although some recovery ensued following reopening of the graft, this was variable, and usually not as extensive as shown here. Stimulus: 30 mA, 10.3/s, 200 μs. Display: 20 ms, ± 50 μV. Fitter bandpass: low 150 Hz, high 1500 Hz. Notch: on, Artifact: on. Repetitions: 500

vessels are occluded at the base of the brain. This model produced consistent and reproducible decreases in rCBF and served for the remainder of the studies. Occlusion of these vessels also clearly abolished the ipsilateral SSEP [7].

Cerebral Blood Flow Studies Following Cerebral Revascularization

The contributions of bypass blood flow to hemispheric blood flow in both intact and ischemic brain have been studied in several ways. Laboratory investigations have employed dog models exclusively. Crowell, in an early study using an electromagnetic flow meter on the STA branch, showed that graft flow was low to unrecordable in an intact system, but increased significantly following proximal MCA clipping, and also increased when collateral flow was abolished by ligation of the contralateral common carotid artery [1]. Fein and Molinari significantly increased hemispheric flow (measured by xenon washout) when a temporal cortical artery was used for anastomosis after MCA occlusion; this augmentation of flow was not found when a parietal branch was employed [4]. Diaz and Meyer showed return of rCBF (measured by hydrogen clearance) to preocclusive levels following an immediate revascularization procedure [2], and Lawner et al. reported a 31.6% increase in rCBF with bypass 3 h post combined MCA-ICA clip occlusion [5].

Aside from Crowell's electromagnetic flow measurements in the STA branch itself [1], no study has established the contribution of bypass blood flow in an intact system. This point has clinical relevance, where revascularization procedures may be performed prophylactically in preparation for operative manipulation and possible occlusion of major intracranial arteries. Two groups have shown that preocclusion bypass in the dog afforded clinical protection against infact during subsequent clip occlusion of intracranial trunk arteries, but neither study measured cerebral blood flow in these animals [3,6]. All other prior investigators have performed the anastomosis and studied bypass flow at some point after proximal occlusion has occurred, without determining the ability of a preexisting STA-MCA bypass to augment flow in a setting of acute arterial occlusion.

The present study thus addresses several issues not previously evaluated experimentally [8]. All data must of course be evaluated in the context of the species employed, although every effort has been made to simulate clinical rCBF parameters and to model as nearly as possible the anatomical bypass procedure. It has been shown that no significant augmentation of hemispheric flow occurs following STA-MCA bypass in the intact system, and this model thus lends support to the concept that there is little or no risk of precipitating intracranial hemorrhage with a prophylactic bypass procedure. Preexisting bypass grafts were able to maintain hemispheric flow well above ischemic thresholds (60.18 cm^3/100 g/min) even following acute severe vascular occlusion, and the adequacy of the experimental lesion in producing severe ischemia (7.95 cm^3/100 g/min) was proven with subsequent bypass occlusion. This data speaks against the need (in this canine model) for bypass "maturation" before adequate flow levels can be delivered. Finally, postischemic bypass reopening, simulating revascularization of an ischemic area with delayed bypass graft placement, restored significant flow to the ischemic zone, but was not as effective in augmenting flow as prophylactic bypass surgery. The data thus lend support to preischemic by-

pass placement, both because of its low risk, and because of its superior ability to maintain flow in the face of acute severe ischemia.

Somatosensory Evoked Potentials

Measurement of both latency and amplitude of somatosensory evoked responses in models of cerebral ischemia has been performed by several groups, although at the present time SSEP amplitude appears to be the more critical and reproducible measurement [9]. The present SSEP studies has several purposes. Abolition of SSEP's with this ischemic model has been previously documented in our laboratory [7], and was used to assess the effectiveness of the ischemic lesion in each individual experiment. This study also showed preservation of both SSEP latency and amplitude by bypass flow alone, and subsequent loss of these responses following bypass occlusion. Although some recovery of the evoked potentials did occur following bypass reopening, the limited and sporadic nature of this recovery again lends support to placement of a preexisting bypass graft rather than delayed postischemic revascularization.

Conclusions

It is clear that acute or subacute cerebral revascularization will be a less common therapeutic option in most cases of cerebrovascular ischemic disease. The role of prophylactic cerebral revascularization, however, remains a current and controversial topic among neurovascular specialists, many of whom continue to propose prophylactic EC-IC bypass prior to pericarotid surgery at the medial sphenoid wing or in preparation for surgical obliteration of difficult carotid aneurysms. These recommendations have been formulated primarily on theoretical considerations or clinically based reports, with no clear laboratory confirmation of the ability of prophylactic revascularization to support hemispheric flow in cases of acute vascular occlusion.

The studies reported here, while limited by interspecies variations, have elucidated the relationship of extracranial-intracranial revascularization to cerebral blood flow in both subcritical (intact system) and critical (ischemic) situations through multiple rCBF determinations with the radiolabeled microsphere technique, and have extended current knowledge of the relationships of cortical SSEP's to cerebral ischemia and revascularization. This data lends experimental support to the placement of a prophylactic STA-MCA bypass graft prior to elective carotid sacrifice, or prior to treacherous surgical procedures where the possibility of acute vascular injury is high.

References

1. Crowell RM (1973) Electromagnetic flow studies of superficial temporal artery to middle cerebral branch artery bypass graft. In: Austin GM (ed) Microneurosurgical anastomoses for cerebral ischemia. Thomas, Springfield, pp 116–124

2. Diaz FG, Meyer M (1981) Acute cerebral revascularization: III. Cerebral blood flow. Surg Neurol 15(6):458–466

3. Eller TW, Cozzens JW, Groothuis DR (1985) Extracranial-intracranial bypass in experimental stroke. Protective effect of bypass prior to acute vascular occlusion. In: Spetzler, Carter, Selman, Martin (eds) Cerebral revascularization for stroke. Thieme-Stratton, New York, pp 261–266

4. Fein JM, Molinari G (1973) Hemodynamic evaluation of superficial temporal cortical artery microanastomosis in the dog. In: Austin GM (ed) Microneurosurgical anastomoses for cerebral ischemia. Thomas, Springfield, pp 5–14

5. Lawner PM, Laurent JP, Simeone FA, Finke EA (1982) Effect of extracranial-intracranial bypass and pentobarbital on acute stroke in dogs. J Neurosurg 56:92–96

6. Levinthal R, Moseley JI, Brown WJ, Stern WE (1979) Effect of STA-MCA anastomosis on the course of experimental acute MCA embolic occlusion. Stroke 10(4):371–375

7. Loftus CM, Bernstein DD, Starr J, Yamada T, Wegrzynowicz E, Kosier T (1987) Measurement of rCBF and somatosensory evoked potentials in a canine model of hemispheric ischemia. Neurosurgery 21:503–508

8. Loftus CM, Silvidi JA, Bernstein DD, Hitchon PW, Kosier T (1987) Effects of preexisting bypass graft on rCBF and SSEP's following acute canine stroke. J Neurosurg 67:421–427

9. Ropper AH (1986) Evoked potentials in cerebral ischemia. Stroke 17:3–4

10. Suzuki J, Yoshimoto T, Tanaka S, Sakamoto T (1980) Production of various models of cerebral infarction in the dog by means of occlusion of intracranial trunk arteries. Stroke 11(4):337–341

The Effect of Mannitol, Nimodipine, and Indomethacin, Singly or in Combination, on Cerebral Ischemia

Garnette Sutherland[1,2], Howard Lesiuk[1,2], Ranjan Bose[1], and Anders A.F. Sima[3]

Summary

The effects of mannitol, nimodipine, and indomethacin on ischemic neuronal injury were examined in 45 rats (divided equally into nine groups) subjected to 10 min of forebrain ischemia. Of two control groups, one received maintenance fluids, while the other, a normal saline bolus. In the remaining seven groups, mannitol, nimodipine, and indomethacin were administered either singly or in combination 5 min prior to forebrain ischemia. Seven days postischemia, the brains were perfusion-fixed, sectioned coronally into 2.8-mm slices, and stained with hematoxylin and eosin. Quantification of dying neurons was performed by direct counting of standardized levels chosen from the serial sections.

Considerable amelioration in ischemic injury was observed with mannitol. The beneficial effect with nimodipine reached significance in only the hippocampal CA3 sector. Indomethacin showed no significant benefit. Pairing of the agents resulted in significantly reduced neuronal injury compared to the control groups, although this was not greater than that achieved with mannitol alone. The degree of ischemic injury was least when all three agents were used in combination, suggesting a synergistic effect between the agents. These data support the concept that successfully blocking the ischemic cascade with a multifaceted single agent or multiple agents will evoke the most beneficial response.

Introduction

Cellular functions are differentially sensitive to increasing cerebral ischemia. Synaptic transmission ceases with a reduction in cerebral blood flow (CBF) to 15–20 ml/100 g cerebral tissue/min [10]. One to two minutes following the onset of severe ischemia (CBF <6–10 ml/100 g/min), membrane depolarization and efflux of potassium occurs, and sodium, water, and calcium enter the cell [4]. These processes represent "membrane failure"; they are correlated with "energy failure" and mark the initiation of a complex sequence of metabolic events that, if not corrected, will lead to irreversible cellular damage [1–3, 7].

Investigators have attempted to modify the cascade of effects induced by ischemia by blocking one or more of the cascading processes resulting therefrom. This may be effected by agents that maintain CBF above ischemic thresholds or agents that alter the metabolic consequences of ischemia [5, 6, 9].

Given the variety of derangements in ischemia, it is not surprising that a number of investigators have hypothesized that combinations of agents may act synergistically to produce a significantly greater beneficial effect than any of the agents used singly. In this study, we further test this hypothesis utilizing the agents mannitol (M), nimodipine (N) and indomethacin (I), administered either singly or in combination in a rat forebrain ischemia model [8]. This model was chosen as it induces an incomplete, short duration ischemic insult that is mild, uniform, and is subject to chronic qualitative and quantitative analysis.

Materials and Methods

Experimental Model

Forty-five male Sprague-Dawley rats weighing 400–600 g were used for the experiments. The animals were divided into nine groups. There were two control groups; one received main-

Departments of Pharmacology[1], Surgery[2], and Pathology[3], The University of Manitoba, Winnipeg, Manitoba, Canada

tenance fluids while the other received an additional normal saline bolus (1.5 cm³). In the remaining seven groups M, N, and I were administered 5 min prior to 10 min of forebrain ischemia as follows: M 0.25 g/kg (over 60 s), I 4 mg/kg (over 60 s) and N at staged intervals, the first 10 μg/kg 5 min prior to ischemia and an additional two injections of 5 μg/kg at 10-min intervals after the first injection.

On day 7 postischemia, the animal was perfusion-fixed with 2.5% glutaraldehyde in cacodylate buffer (pH 7.25). The brains were cut coronally into 2.8-mm-thick slices from which 8 μm thick serial sections were stained with hematoxylin and eosin. All sections were examined to determine the qualitative and topographic extent of ischemic brain damage. For quantification of ischemic neuronal injury, a standard section, including cerebral cortex and hippocampus, was used. Predetermined regions of this section, consisting of frontal cortex, inferior frontal cortex, and hippocampus including the dentate gyrus, were photographed, and ischemic neuronal injury was quantitatively determined by direct visual counting of all neurons.

Results

Physiological Observations

The infusion of normal saline or therapeutic agent(s) resulted in a transient decrease in hematocrit values (Table 1). In keeping with N's pharmacologic action, its infusion (10 μg/kg), either singly or in combination with other agents, resulted in a significant fall in mean blood pressure ($P < 0.05$). This decrease was transient, and the blood pressure returned to the preinfusion value over 2–3 min. As the second N infusion (5 μg/kg) took place during the induction of ischemia, fluctuations in blood pressure were controlled through either the administration or withdrawal of additional blood. The third infusion of N (5 μg/kg) produced a relative fall in blood pressure which was not significantly different from its preinfusion value ($P > 0.05$).

Following the ischemic insult, the mean blood pressure significantly increased in the control, normal saline, I, and N + I groups ($P < 0.05$). In all groups, a mild metabolic acidosis followed the ischemic insult, which was reflected by a small increase in $PaCO_2$ (3.2 ± 0.5 torr), a decrease in HCO_3^- (2.2 ± 0.2 mmol/l), and a negative base excess (− 2.8 ± 0.2 mmol/l). These changes were not significantly different between groups.

Histopathology: Qualitative Findings

The distribution of ischemic changes was similar in all groups, varying only in severity. Neocortical damage was restricted to cortical layers III and VI. Striatal damage was noted in only the most severely affected animals (three of the control, three of the normal saline, and two of the I-treated animals). In the hindbrain, ischemic injury was restricted to the superior vermis and observed in only those animals that had severe ischemic injury. Of all brain regions, ischemic injury was found to be most severe within the hippocampus. Within this area, the CA1/CA2 and CA3 sectors sustained the greatest injury. Ischemic injury to the outer dentate blade and the subiculum was restricted to animals that had sustained extensive injury. In all but three cases, the hippocampal injury was bilateral and of equal severity.

Histopathology: Quantitative Results

Hippocampus. In the CA1/CA2 sector, ischemic neuronal injury exceeded 60% in both the control (64% ± 10%) and normal saline (70% ± 10%) groups (Fig. 1). Only M, when used singly, showed a significant reduction in ischemic neuronal injury when compared with the control ($P < 0.05$), normal saline ($P < 0.01$), and I ($P < 0.05$) groups. When compared to either the control or normal saline groups, pairing of the agents resulted in a significant decrease in neuronal injury in both the M + N and N + I groups ($P < 0.05$). All three agents in combination resulted in significantly less neuronal injury compared to the control ($P < 0.05$) or normal saline ($P < 0.01$) animals.

A similar effect was observed in the CA3 sector (Fig. 2), which differed from the CA1/CA2 sector in that N used as a single agent showed significantly less neuronal injury compared to the control group ($P < 0.05$), as did all paired drug combinations ($P < 0.05$). No significant intergroup differences were obtained in the CA4 sector.

Dentate gyrus. Ischemic injury was mild within the outer dentate blade, and in no group was a significant reduction in ischemic neuronal injury observed. In the inner dentate blade, however, ischemic injury exceeded 50% in the control group (54% ± 11%). Compared to this, ischemic

Table 1. Mean blood pressure and hematocrit results prior to and following drug or ischemic manipulation

Group (n = 5)	Preischemia				Postischemia	
	Prior to agent		Following agent		(20 min)	
	BP	Hct	BP	Hct	BP	HCT
Control	112.0 ± 5.6	45.0 ± 1.1	—	—	135.0 ± 2.2[a]	45.6 ± 1.2
Normal saline	108.8 ± 5.0	45.7 ± 1.1	117.7 ± 5.0	38.7 ± 2.1	126.7 ± 4.6[a]	44.2 ± 1.1
Mannitol	133.0 ± 5.2	48.8 ± 1.2	135.6 ± 5.9	43.4 ± 3.7	142.6 ± 6.0	45.8 ± 2.3
Nimodipine	113.4 ± 3.2	47.3 ± 1.4	69.0 ± 6.9[b]	44.7 ± 3.4	122.0 ± 8.0	44.0 ± 2.0
Indomethacin	112.0 ± 5.8	45.6 ± 1.0	114.0 ± 6.2	42.9 ± 1.0	130.0 ± 4.5[a]	44.7 ± 0.9
Mannitol + nimodipine	116.4 ± 7.2	45.8 ± 1.7	94.6 ± 4.0[b]	43.3 ± 1.3	124.3 ± 3.3	42.4 ± 2.8
Mannitol + indomethacin	116.2 ± 7.1	45.1 ± 2.2	116.2 ± 7.1	42.6 ± 0.04	127.0 ± 6.4	45.0 ± 0.4
Nimodipine + indomethacin	111.8 ± 7.2	48.7 ± 0.6	75.0 ± 8.1[b]	46.7 ± 1.0	130.4 ± 8.5	46.9 ± 1.1
Mannitol + nimodipine + indomethacin	115.0 ± 8.0	47.6 ± 1.2	79.2 ± 9.5[b]	44.7 ± 1.0	117.8 ± 6.0	45.3 ± 1.0

[a] $P < 0.05$ compared with preischemia
[b] $P < 0.05$ compared with prenimodipine blood pressure
BP blood pressure, *Nct* hematocrit

neuronal injury was significantly less in the M-, M + I- and M + N + I-treated animals ($P < 0.05$).

Frontal cortex. In the medial frontal cortex, ischemic neuronal injury was relatively mild. Nevertheless, M- and M + N + I-treated animals demonstrated significantly less neuronal injury ($P < 0.05$) compared to the control group. Similar results were observed in the inferior frontal cortex (Fig. 3), where only the M + N + I-treated animals demonstrated significantly less neuronal injury compared to the control group ($P < 0.05$).

Discussion

Agents Used Singly

This study has demonstrated considerable amelioration of ischemic injury with M. Other reports have attributed similar observations [5] to improvement in local CBF secondary to decreases in blood viscosity and hemoglobin content and direct vasodilatation. In addition, M favorably affects ischemic edema and functions as a hydrophilic free radical scavenger.

The beneficial effect of N on neuronal ischemia was not as pronounced, although it reached significance in the hippocampal CA3 sector. Calcium antagonists have two potentially beneficial effects. Through vasodilatory mechanisms, they may enhance CBF during and following ischemia, although evidence for such remains controversial. They also inhibit calcium fluxes into the ischemic cell, thereby preventing the secondary effects of cytosolic free calcium [2]. Any potential effect observed with N may reflect either of the above mechanisms. The failure of N to equal the beneficial effect of M suggests that calcium may not have a central role in ischemic neuronal injury.

Indomethacin failed to produce a statistically significant beneficial effect. Prostaglandins are known to accumulate during incomplete ischemia and reperfusion is associated with an inbalance between the production of thromboxane A_2 and prostacyclin favoring thromboxane A_2 and, hence, vasoconstriction [6]. The failure of I to prevent ischemic neuronal injury in the present study suggests that ischemic prostaglandin formation and/or postischemic hypoperfusion are not major factors in the initiation or propagation of ischemic neuronal injury.

Combinations of Agents

The combinations of M + N or M + I produced a favorable response; however, this benefit is no

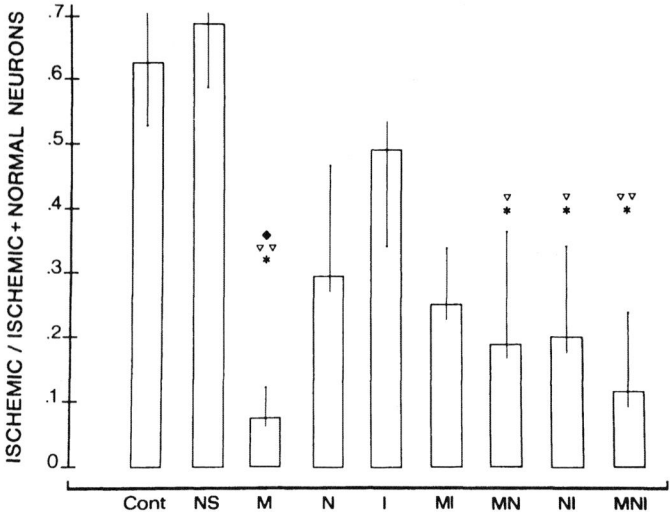

Fig. 1. Quantitative results for the hippocampal CA1/CA2 sector with ischemic neuronal injury expressed as mean ± SEM. Average number of total cells in CA1/CA2 was 730 ± 33. *$P < 0.05$ compared to control; ▽$P < 0.05$, ▽▽$P < 0.01$ compared to normal saline; ◆ $P < 0.05$ compared to indomethacin. Analysis of variance followed by Duncan's test for multiple comparisons (ANOVA/D). *NS* normal saline, *M* mannitol, *N* nimodipine, *I* indomethacin

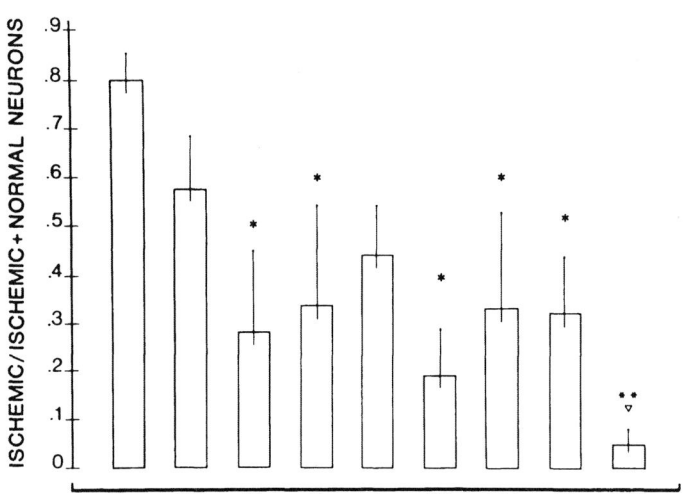

Fig. 2. Quantitative results for the hippocampal CA3 sector expressed as mean ± SEM. Average number of total cells in CA3 was 561 ± 23. *$P < 0.05$, **$P < 0.05$ compared to control; ▽$P < 0.05$ compared to normal saline; ANOVA/D. *Abbreviations* are the same as in Fig. 1

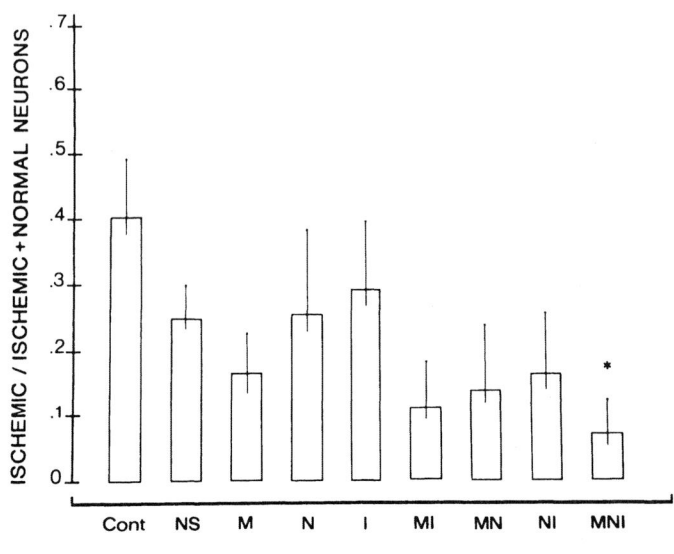

Fig. 3. Quantitative results for the inferior frontal cortex expressed as mean ± SEM. Average number of total cells was 755 ± 53. *$P < 0.05$ compared to control; ANOVA/D. *Abbreviations* are the same as in Fig. 1

greater than that achieved with M alone. These observations are further evidence for the multifaceted effects of M that override further benefit which might be achieved through the addition of N or I. The combination of N + I resulted in qualitatively less ischemic injury than was observed with either agent alone, suggesting synergism between the two agents.

The degree of ischemic injury was least when all three agents were used in combination. In the CA3 sector, this combination resulted in significantly less neuronal injury than in either the control or normal saline groups. Its protective effect appeared greater than that of M, which was significantly different only from the control group. Similarly, for the inferior frontal cortex, only the M + N + I-treated group showed significantly less neuronal damage than the control group.

These data support the concept that successfully blocking the ischemic cascade with a multifaceted single agent or multiple agents (that may not be effective singly) will produce the most beneficial response. Combinations of agents may elevate CBF above ischemic thresholds, thereby preventing energy failure and its resulting dissipative ion fluxes. Mannitol would favorably affect ischemic cerebral edema, thus maintaining the optimal diffusion distance for both oxygen and substrate. Preventing calcium influx into the ischemic cell may inhibit the accumulation of free fatty acids and their metabolites, prostaglandins, leukotrienes, and endoperoxides. In addition, it would prevent the activation of several calcium-dependent enzyme systems, and the uncoupling of oxidative phosphorylation by mitochondrial sequestration of calcium. The addition of indomethacin, which inhibits the ischemic-induced imbalance between thromboxane A_2 and prostacyclin, could favorably affect the postischemic, hypoperfusion state.

Acknowledgments. The authors gratefully acknowledge the grant support of the Canadian Heart Foundation (Manitoba Branch), the Manitoba Research Council, and the Dean's Fund, Faculty of Medicine, The University of Manitoba.

References

1. Ames A, Nesbett FB (1983) Pathophysiology of ischemic cell death. 1. Time of onset of irreversible damage; importance of the different components of the ischemic insult. Stroke 14:219–226
2. Cheung JY, Bonventre JV, Malis CD, Leaf A (1986) Calcium and ischemic injury. N Engl J Med 314:1670–1676
3. Dienel GA, Pulsinelli WA, Duffy TE (1980) Regional protein synthesis in rat brain following acute hemispheric ischemia. J Neurochem 35:1216–1226
4. Harris R, Symon L (1984) Extracellular pH, potassium and calcium activities in progressive ischaemia of rat cortex. J Cereb Blood Flow Metabol 4:178–186
5. Little JR (1979) Treatment of acute focal cerebral ischemia with intermittent boluses of low-dose mannitol. Neurosurgery 5(6):687–691
6. Shigeno S, Fritschka E, Shigeno T, Brock M (1985) Effects of indomethacin on rCBF during and after focal cerebral ischemia in the cat. Stroke 16(2):235–240
7. Siesjo BK (1981) Cell damage in the brain: A speculative synthesis. J Cereb Blood Flow Metabol 1:155–185
8. Smith M-L, Auer RN, Siesjo BK (1984) The density and distribution of ischemic brain injury in the rat following 2–10 min of forebrain ischemia. Acta Neuropathol (Berl.) 64:319–332
9. Steen PA, Newberg La, Milde JH, et al. (1983) Nimodipine improves cerebral blood flow and neurologic recovery after complete cerebral ischemia in the dog. J Cereb Blood Flow Metab 3:38
10. Symon L (1985) Flow thresholds in brain ischemia and the effects of drugs. Br J Anaesth 57:34–43

Recovery of Cortical Evoked Potential and LCGU Following Transient MCA Occlusion in the Rat

Kazuhiro Sako, Akira Hashizume, Shigeki Yura, and Yukichi Yonemasu[1]

Introduction

Recent evidence indicates that the development of infarct is a function of residual blood flow and duration of ischemia [3, 4]. However, it is difficult to predict whether ischemic tissue is viable or not in the early postischemic period. The present investigation was designed to study the relationship of somatosensory evoked potential (SEP), local cerebral glucose utilization (LCGU), and histopathological changes in the transiently MCA-occluded rat.

Materials and Methods

Preparation and Experimental Protocol

Male Wistar rats were used throughout the experiments. A preparatory operation for the autoradiography was performed under 1.5% halothane anesthesia. A burr hole was made on the left coronal suture 5 mm lateral from the midline for the measurement of cortical SEP. Following subtemporal craniectomy, the left MCA was exposed. After preparatory operation, the concentration of halothane was decreased to 0.75%. In each experiment, after a control measurement of SEP, the MCA was occluded with a microclip. The animals were divided into two groups. In the first group ($n = 8$), the clip was removed 1 h after occlusion and four rats were used for the measurement of LCGU. Another four rats were allowed to recover from anesthesia and used for histopathological examination after 72 h. In the second group ($n = 8$), the clip was removed 2 h after occlusion, and the same procedures as the first group were done. Local cerebral blood flow (LCBF) was measured 1 h after MCA occlusion in another group of rats. Body temperature was kept around 37°C with a heating lamp. Blood pressure and gases were checked before and after MCA occlusion.

Recording of SEP

The recording system (Cadwell 5200) was adjusted to a band width of 10–2000 Hz, and averaging was performed over 256 responses. Stimulating electrodes were inserted around the median nerve in the right fore limb, and stimuli were given as 0.1 ms duration square waves at 4/s with voltage adjusted to 1.5 times threshold levels for paw twitch. A silver ball electrode, as a recording electrode, was placed on the epidural space through the burr hole. The small screw electrode was placed in the frontal sinus as a reference.

Measurement of LCGU and LCBF

LCGU was measured by the quantitative autoradiographic technique [7] using 14C-deoxyglucose (DG) at 30 min after reperfusion. LCBF was measured by the quantitative autoradiographic technique [6] using 14C-iodoantipyrine (IAP) at 1 h after MCA occlusion. Details of these methods are described elsewhere [5, 10].

Histological Studies

The rats were killed with saturated potassium chloride and brains were perfused with normal saline and 10% formaldehyde 72 h after reperfusion. The brains were removed and were stored in 10% formaldehyde until they were embedded in paraffin. Coronal sections were taken every 1 mm and were stained with cresyl violet and hematoxylin-eosin.

[1] Department of Neurosurgery, Asahikawa Medical College, Asahikawa, Japan

Results

SEP

Through the experiment we were able to obtain a well defined first positive wave (P1) and a first negative wave (N1) constantly in 5.6 ms and 7.6 ms, respectively, before MCA occlusion (Fig. 1). We used the interpeak latency and amplitude for the evaluation of SEP. At 5 min after MCA occlusion, SEP showed no definite peak. Partial recovery of SEP was noted in 2 of 18 rats at around 20 min after MCA occlusion, and these two rats were excluded from analysis. Following the removal of the clip, nearly complete recovery of the SEP was observed in the first group of rats (Fig. 2a). However, in the second group, recovery of SEP was minimal (Fig. 2b; Table 1.).

LCGU

LCGU in the ischemic side of the first group returned to 78% compared to that of the contralateral homologous area. In the second group, in contrast, the recovery of LCGU after restoration of blood flow was proportional to the depth of ischemia. LCGU in the ischemic core (sensorimotor cortex) with 2 h of ischemia and 30 min reperfusion was 0.29 μmol/g/min, which was 34% of the contralateral homologous area (Fig. 3; Table 2).

LCBF

Mean LCBF in the ischemic core at 1 hour after MCA occlusion was 0.27 ml/g per min. LCBF in the thalamus (ventral posterolateral nucleus) revealed a slight reduction which was statistically insignificant (Table 3).

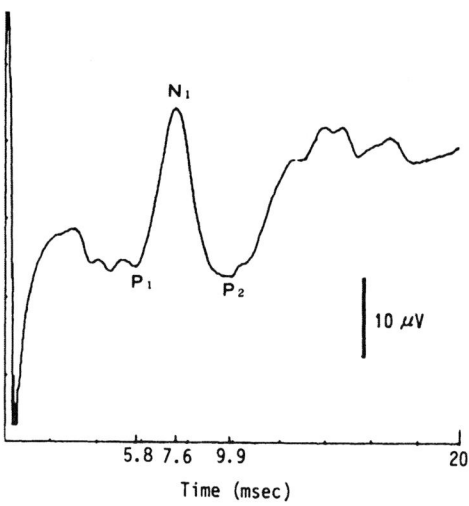

Fig. 1. The representative cortical SEP obtained in our experiment

Histopathology

There was no histological evidence of ischemic brain damage in the first group of rats. On the other hand, cerebral infarct was observed in the sensorimotor cortex in all of the second group of rats.

Discussion

The reversible focal cerebral ischemic model in the rat utilized in this experiment is very useful for the investigation of ischemic stroke. This was developed by Tamura et al. [8], and reproducibility of the ischemia has been well established.

Partial recovery of SEP during MCA occlusion was observed in 2 of 18 rats in this experiment. This was probably due to development of

Table 1. Changes in interpeak latency and amplitude of the SEP recorded before MCA occlusion and after reperfusion

		Latency (ms) P1–N1	Amplitude (μV) P1–N1
Preocclusion	($n = 8$)	1.85 ± 0.27	29.47 ± 8.79
After reperfusion 1st group	($n = 4$)	1.98 ± 0.30	31.93 ± 10.75
2nd group	($n = 4$)	3.62 ± 0.63^{b}	19.42 ± 4.30^{a}

Values are mean $\pm$ SD
a $P < 0.05$
b $P < 0.01$

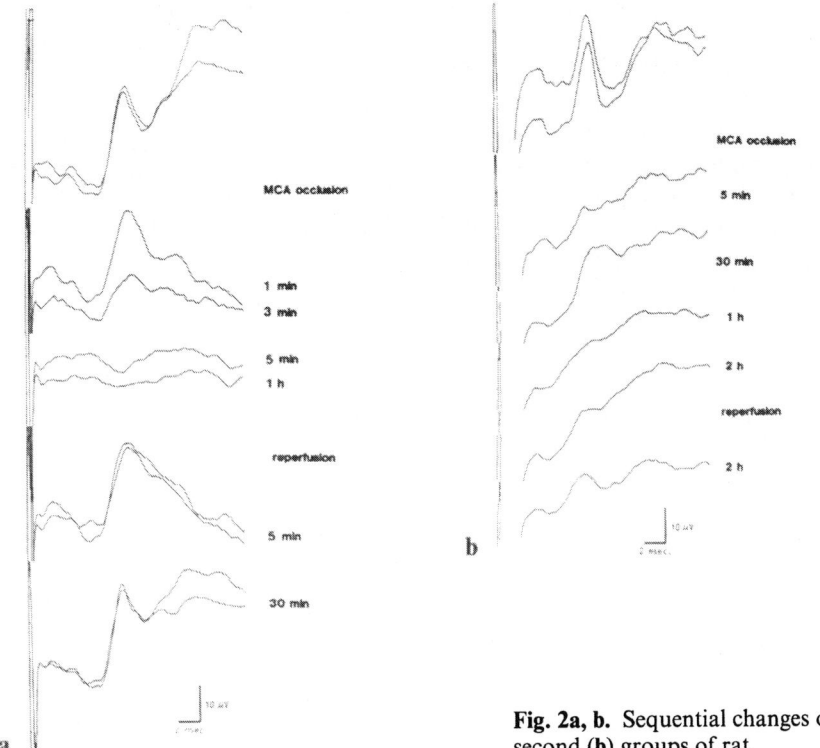

Fig. 2a, b. Sequential changes of SEP in the first (**a**) and the second (**b**) groups of rat

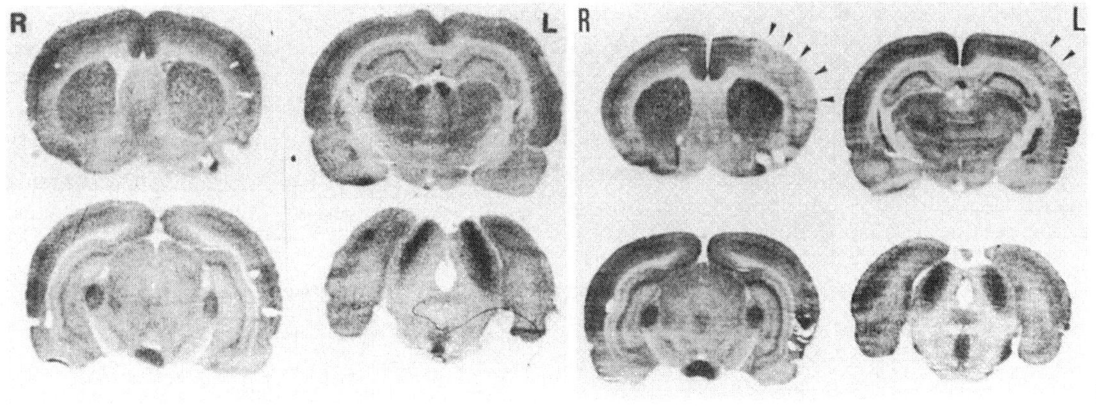

Fig. 3a, b. The representative 14C-DG autoradiograms in the first (**a**) and the second (**b**) groups of rat

Table 2. LCGU measured 30 min after reperfusion in rats subjected to 1-h and 2-h left MCA occlusion

Structure	1st group (n = 4)		2nd group (n = 4)	
	Ischemic side	Nonischemic side	Ischemic side	Nonischemic side
Sensorimotor Cx	0.78 ± .16	1.00 ± .15	0.29 ± .05	0.85 ± .05
Parietal Cx	0.71 ± .08	0.88 ± .08	0.32 ± .06	0.84 ± .04
Auditory Cx	1.06 ± .16	1.36 ± .13	0.54 ± .13	1.11 ± .12
Occipital Cx	0.83 ± .03	0.90 ± .03	0.64 ± .06	0.73 ± .06

All measurements are μmol/g/min

collateral circulation. In these rats, the distal portion of the MCA occluded by clip appeared dark
red, indicating that the clipping was complete. In
the state of critical blood flow level, small increases in flow may be enough for the recovery of
SEP. There have been several reports in which
the CBF threshold for the irreversible ischemic
damage was investigated. The reported CBF
values vary slightly depending on the methods
of CBF measurement or animal species. According to Tamura et al. [8], the CBF values that
were associated with consistent histological
changes in rats using the 14C-IAP method was
0.24 ± 0.03 ml/g/min. The average value for
CBF in the ischemic core obtained in our experiment was 0.27 ± 0.06. These values are very
close and there could be no significant difference
statistically. As already described by Morawetz
et al. [4] and Heiss and Rosner [3], present results
also indicated that ischemic brain damage was
defined by severity and duration of ischemia.

Only a few investigations of SEP in rats have
been reported [1], and there has been no report
investigating the SEP change of ischemic brain in
rats. In the present study, the initial change of
SEP after ischemia was a decrease in amplitude
as previously described. However, 5 min after
MCA occlusion, it seemed to be difficult to define N1 and P1. There are several reports [2]
that have investigated the SEP change during
ischemia, and many of them have analyzed
the relationship between alteration of CBF
and changes of both amplitude and latency. In
our experience, interpretation of SEP during
ischemia is very difficult. There are certainly
some electrical activities after MCA occlusion,
but it seems impossible to define the activities as
N1 and P1. SEP is an integration of each neuronal activity and reflects the neuronal function.
Therefore, disappearance of N1 and P1 does not
mean the stop of each neuronal activity. It is a
result of disintegration of each neuronal activity
and signifies neuronal dysfunction.

After restoration of blood flow, the 1-h occlusion group showed complete recovery of SEP.
On the other hand, the 2-h occlusion group revealed minimal recovery of SEP, increase of
interpeak latency, and decrease of amplitude.
The recovery of SEP was well correlated with the
LCGU in the sensorimotor cortex. In the 1-h
occlusion group, which revealed no histological
change, LCGU in the left sensorimotor cortex
recovered by 78%, compared to the contralateral
homologous area. However, in the 2-h occlusion
group, which showed infarction in the sensori-

Table 3. LCBF in rats 1 h after left MCA occlusion

Structure	Ischemic side ($n = 3$)	Nonischemic side ($n = 3$)
Sensorimotor Cx	$0.27 \pm .06$	$1.80 \pm .11$
Parietal Cx	$0.31 \pm .12$	$1.67 \pm .17$
Auditory Cx	$0.42 \pm .14$	$2.02 \pm .10$
Occipital Cx	$0.72 \pm .23$	$1.47 \pm .18$
Thalamus (VPL)	$1.18 \pm .18$	$1.36 \pm .15$

All measurements are ml/g/min

motor cortex, the LCGU recovered by only 34%
of the contralateral homologous area. This observation is comparable to the previous study
reported by Tanaka et al. [9], which showed
the relationship between LCGU recovery and
histological change in cats with transient MCA
occlusion model. According to their report, the
LCGU in the regions with severe histological
damage was below 44.2% of the sham level.

The present investigation suggests that LCGU
and SEP are well coupled with the consequent
histological damage. In other words, LCGU and
SEP in the early recovery period of ischemia are
able to predict the reversibility of ischemic brain.
However, in order to determine the threshold for
the irreversible damage during ischemia, further
studies that correlate the metabolic alterations
and SEP changes are required. This correlation
is relevant to the interpretation of glucose metabolism and SEP as a predicting tool for therapeutic interventions in the acute phase of strokes.

References

1. Allison T, Hume AL (1981) A comparative analysis of short-latency somatosensory evoked potential in man, monkey, and rat. Exp Neurol
   72:592–611
2. Branston NM, Symon L, Crockard HA, Pasztor
   E (1974) Relationship between the cortical evoked
   potential and local cortical blood flow following
   acute middle cerebral occlusion in the baboon.
   Exp Neurol 45:195–208
3. Heiss WD, Rosner G (1983) Functional recovery
   of cortical neurons as related to degree and duration of ischemia. Ann Neurol 14:294–301
4. Morawetz RB, DeGirolami U, Ojemann RG,
   Marcoux FW, Crowell RM (1978) Cerebral blood
   flow determined by hydrogen clearance during
   middle cerebral artery occlusion in unanesthetized
   monkey. Stroke 9:143–149
5. Sako K, Kobatake K, Yamamoto YL, Diksic M
   (1985) Correlation of local cerebral blood flow,

glucose utilization, and tissue pH following a middle cerebral artery occlusion in the rat. Stroke 16:828–834

6. Sakurada O, Kennedy C, Jehle J, Brown JD, Carbin GL, Sokoloff L (1978) Measurement of local cerebral blood flow with iodo (14C) antipyrine. Am J Physiol 234:H59–H66

7. Sokoloff L, Reivich M, Kennedy C, Rosiers MH, Patlak CS, Pettigrew KD, Sakurada O, Shinohara M (1979) The 14C deoxyglucose method for the measurement of local cerebral glucose utilization: Theory, procedure, and normal values in the conscious and anesthetized rat. J Neurochem 28:897–916

8. Tamura A, Graham DI, McCulloch J, Teasdale GM (1981) Focal cerebral ischemia in the rat: II. Regional cerebral blood flow determined by (14C) iodoantipyrine autoradiography following middle cerebral artery occlusion. J Cereb Blood Flow Metabol 1:61–69

9. Tanaka K, Greenberg JH, Gonatas NK, Reivich M (1985) Regional flow-metabolism couple following middle cerebral artery occlusion in cats. J Cereb Blood Flow Metabol 5:241–252

10. Yura S, Sako K, Aizawa S, Suzuki N, Yonemasu Y, Kojima M (1986) The effect of hyperglycemia on ischemic brain damage: Relevance to the local cerebral blood flow. Brain Nerve (Tokyo). 38:1117–1125

Sequential Changes of Brain Metabolism During Temporary Global Ischemia in the Rat Detected by Simultaneous 1H and 31P MRS

Reizo Shirane[1], Lee-Hong Chang[1,2], Philip R. Weinstein[1], and Thomas L. James[2]

Introduction

In vivo magnetic resonance spectroscopy (MRS) provides a noninvasive method for evaluating brain metabolism. Previous studies with 31P MRS have developed techniques for continuous monitoring of phosphate metabolites and intracellular pH (pHi) during ischemia and reperfusion [1]. Furthermore, recent progress has made it possible to monitor brain lactate content quantitatively with 1H MRS [2]. In this study, we utilized a double-tuned surface coil for 1H and 31P MRS. With this recently described method, in vivo 1H and 31P spectroscopy can be carried out simultaneously without retuning or replacement of the coil [3].

The present study explores the dynamic changes of inorganic phosphate (Pi), phosphocreatine (PCr), and ATP levels as well as pHi and lactate alterations during 15-min global ischemia and 60-min reperfusion. A seven-vessel occlusion model in the rat was used in this study. During occlusion, no uptake of isotope in the forebrain is observed by C-14-IAP autoradiography.

Animal Preparation

Male Sprague-Dawley (SD) rats, weighing 300-400 g, were initially anesthetized with 3% isoflurane, orotracheally intubated with a plastic 16-gauge angiocatheter, and connected to a rodent respirator (Harvard 683). Muscle paralysis was achieved by an intraperitoneal injection of pancuronium (1 mg/kg). Anesthesia was maintained with 1.5% isoflurane during surgery and 1% during experimental observation, together with administration of a 70% N_2O and 30% O_2

mixture. A ventral cervical skin incision was made and the subsequent dissection was performed using a surgical microscope. The omohyoid muscles were transected bilaterally. The external carotid and pterygopalatine arteries were occluded with bipolar cauterization. The basilar artery was then occluded as described by Kameyama et al. [6]. Next, silastic tubing (0.047 cm in diameter, Dow Corning) was looped around each common carotid artery and sternomastoid muscle, and the ends were brought out though small separate stab incisions to form a snare for remote controlled arterial occlusion with the rat positioned in the spectrometer. A PE-50 catheter was inserted into the left femoral artery. Blood pressure and arterial blood gases were monitored during the experiment. Scalp, periosteum, and temporal muscles were reflected. A small cranial window was made over the temporal region bilaterally, and epidural electrodes were placed to monitor electroencephalograph (EEG) with a Neurotrac monitor (Interspec). Blood glucose was measured (YSI 27) before induction of ischemia.

During the experimental period, the arterial PCO_2 was adjusted to 35–40 mmHg, PO_2 to 100–140 mmHg, and body temperature was maintained at 37°–38°C with a temperature-regulated water jacket in the animal cradle. Global ischemia was induced by applying tension to the silastic snares until flattening of the EEG was observed. Tension was maintained for 15-min intervals. Reperfusion was accomplished by release of tension on the carotid snares and verified by inspection under the surgical microscope at the end of the experiment.

MRS Methods

In vivo nuclear magnetic resonance (NMR) spectroscopy was performed on our 5.6T horizontal bore spectrometer (1H at 236.8 MHz and 31P at 95.8 MHz, 10-cm diameter). A two-turn

Department of Neurosurgery[1], Department of Pharmaceutical Chemistry[2], University of California, San Francisco, California, USA

Table 1. Physiological values in experimental animals

	Control	5 min after occlusion	30 min after reperfusion
Body temperature (°C)	37.3 ± 0.2	37.4 ± 0.2	37.6 ± 0.1
MABP (mmHg)	87 ± 3	117 ± 8	93 ± 3
$PaCO_2$ (mmHg)	35.5 ± 0.6	37.0 ± 0.2	37.3 ± 0.1
PaO_2 (mmHg)	124.4 ± 8.0	119.0 ± 4.8	114.6 ± 5.5
Arterial pH	7.47 ± 0.01	7.46 ± 0.02	7.45 ± 0.02

Values are means ± SEM
MABP mean arterial blood pressure

elliptical surface coil (8 × 12 mm), which was double-tuned to 1H and 31P frequencies, was placed over the calvarium. The homogeneity of the magnetic field was optimized by shimming on the water proton signal to a line width of 0.2 ppm. Both 1H and 31P spectra were acquired simultaneously in 5-min blocks. 1H spectra were obtained by using a presaturation-Hahn spin echo pulse sequence [3]. For 31P spectroscopy, a selective saturation pulse sequence was employed [4]. The 1H and 31P pulse sequences were interleaved and applied repetitively for 5 min until a satisfactory signal-to-noise ratio was obtained. Two hundred free induction decays were collected each for 1H and 31P spectrum with a spectral width of ± 3000 Hz and 4K deta points. Chemical shifts were referenced to the N-acetyl aspartate (NAA) resonance at 2.02 ppm or to the PCr resonance at 0 ppm for 1H and 31P, respectively. Absolute lactate concentrations were calculated as described previously [2], i.e., a 1:1 ratio of lactate peak area to NAA peak area corresponding to 19.6 μmol/g lactate in the brain. pH was determined from the chemical shift of the Pi peak relative to the PCr according to the equation described by Seo et al. [9]. After control spectra were obtained, the carotid arteries were occluded for 15 min and released for one hour reperfusion.

Results

Five rats were subjected to the experimental protocol described. Each animal demonstrated a flat EEG tracing within 30 s after applying tension to the snares. EEG activity recovered partially at 36 ± 3 min (mean ± SE) after onset of reperfusion when it was characterised by a low-amplitude slow-wave pattern. The physiological parameters recorded are presented in

Table 1. Blood pressure was elevated during arterial occlusion and returned towards control levels after reperfusion. There was no significant change in blood gases during the experiment. Blood glucose values, measured before induction of ischemia, were 10.1 ± 0.3 μmol/ml.

Both 1H and 31P spectra obtained from one animal are shown in Fig. 1. The percent changes of phosphorus NMR peak areas for ATP, PCr, and Pi are shown in Fig. 2a–c. The sequential changes of pHi and lactate concentration are presented in Fig. 2d,e. Each value at a time point represents the mean observed within a 5-min block. After the induction of ischemia, complete depletion of PCr and ATP was observed, while Pi increased remarkably. Reduction of pHi to 6.25 ± 0.07 (control level, 7.11 ± 0.03) and accumulation of lactate to levels as high as 21.3 ± 2.2 μmol/g (control level, 2.8 ± 0.7 μmol/g) were also observed. These changes occurred rapidly and were demonstrated on the 5- and 10-min spectra. Thefor, the 31P spectra stabilized, although lactate increased continuously during ischemia. After reperfusion, energy metabolites returned towards control level rapidly during the first 15 min, and more gradually over the next 45 min. Lactate and pHi levels recovered more slowly.

At the end of 60-min reperfusion, metabolites returned almost to control levels, except that the PCr was elevated at a slightly higher level (120% ± 6% of control). An alkaline shift of pHi during reperfusion was not evident in this study.

Discussion

Changes in high-energy phosphates, pHi, and lactate during ischemia and recirculation have been studied extensively with in vitro methods in order to define compensatory mechanisms, as

15 min occlusion

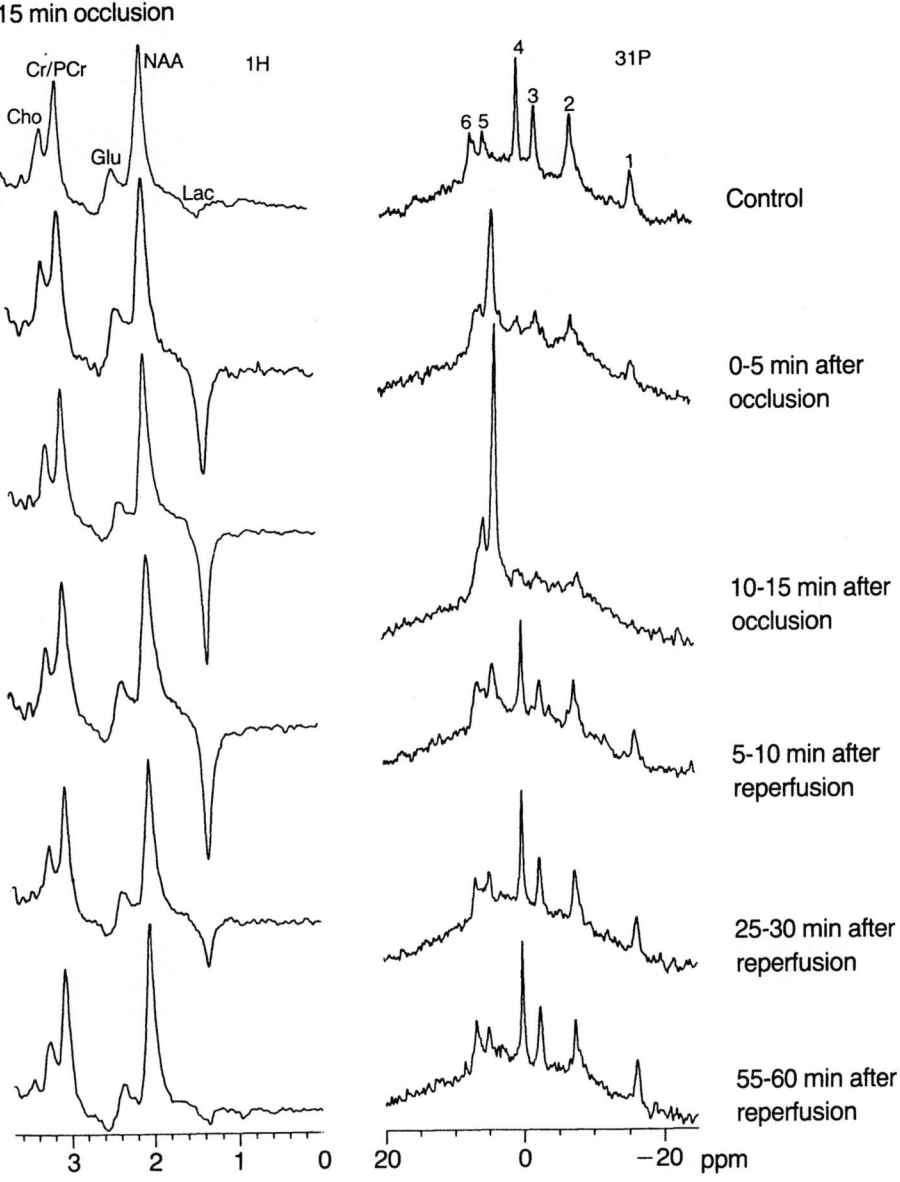

Fig. 1. Sequential change of 1H and 31P spectra during ischemia and reperfusion. *Cho* choline; *Cr/PCr* creatine/creatine phosphate, *Glu* glutamate, *NAA* N-acetylaspartate, *Lac* lactate, *1, 2, 3 β- α- γ*-phosphates of adenosine triphosphate, *4* creatine phosphate, *5* inorganic phosphate, *6* phosphomonoesters

well as to describe metabolic parameters of irreversible cell injury upon which to base investigation of protective therapies. Profound depletion of high-energy phosphates that recovered within 60 min was observed in vivo in our experiment after induction of ischemia. This is in agreement with previous reports describing in vitro results in complete or nearly complete ischemia models [10].

Serial recordings indicate that lactate values progressively increased during the 15-min ischemia and the early phase of recirculation to levels exceeding 20 μmol/g. In complete normoglycemic ischemia, the amount of lactate accumulated is determined by preischemic stores of glucose and glycogen and does not exceed 15 μmol/g [7]. This observation indicates that the experimental model used in the present study produced less than complete ischemia. Since our separate C-14-iodoantipyrine (IAP) CBF studies showed no uptake of radioisotope in the forebrain and cerebellum, and the NMR signal was

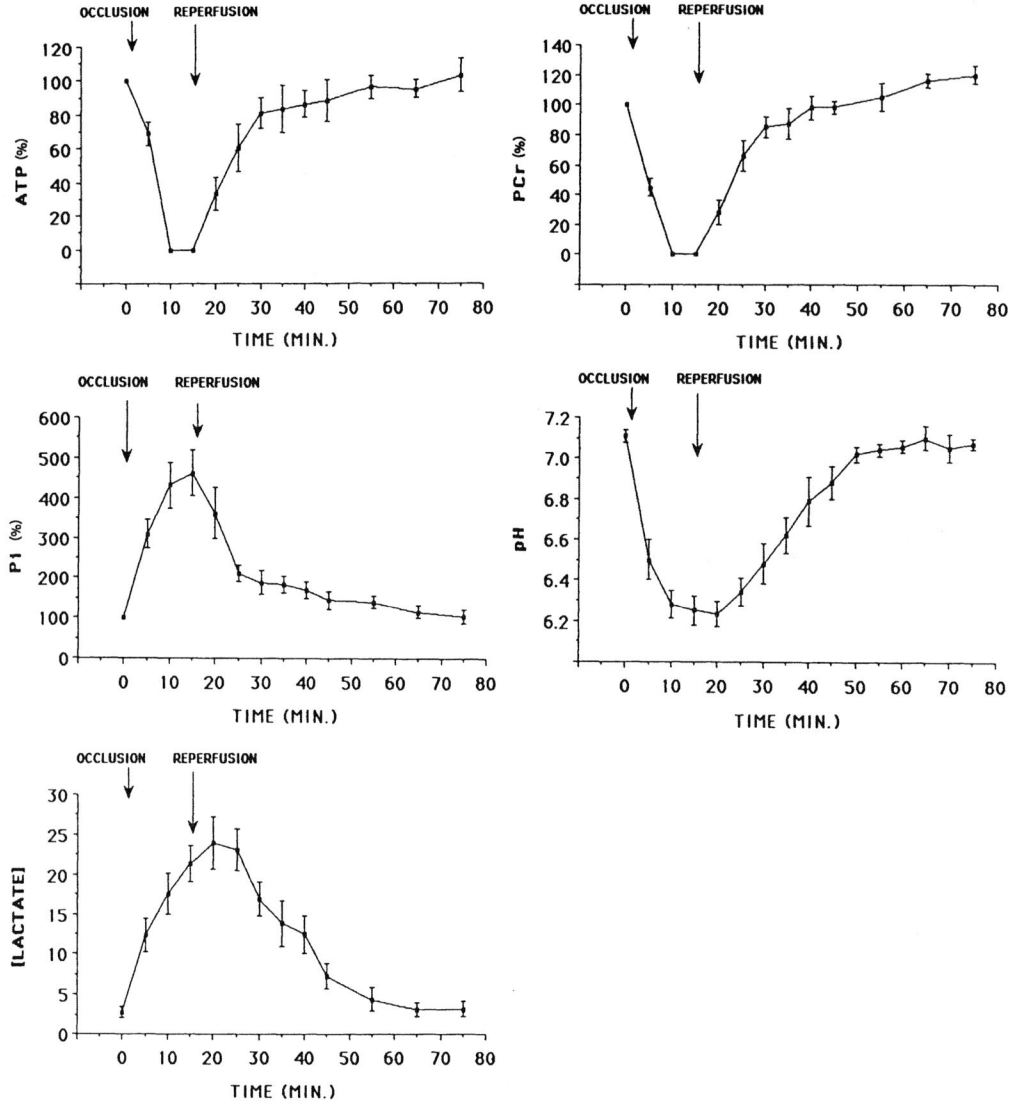

Fig. 2. Plots of changes of ATP, PCr, Pi, pHi, and lactate against time. *Time 0 min* indicates control level of each metabolite, *Time 5–15 min* ischemia, *Time 20–80 min* reperfusion. ATP, PCr, and Pi are shown in percent changes of control level; Lactate is presented as calculated concentrations in μmol/g; All values are means $\pm$ SEM; all time is in minutes

obtained from these areas, the authors explain lactate levels higher than 20 μmol/g as follows. When ischemia was induced in the magnet, the silastic snares were carefully and gradually stretched until a flattened EEG was observed. Some flow may have been possible with this technique. Induction of ischemia caused a rise of the mean arterial pressure (control level +30 mmHg) which might have potentiated minimal extracranial collateral flow.

The control pHi obtained in this study was consistant with the results of previous NMR studies [8]. The changes in pHi and lactate during ischemia and recirculation were similar to the in vitro and microelectrode measurements reported by von Hanwehr et al. [5]. The determination of pHi from Pi chemical shifts is based on the fact that these signals arise predominantly from the intracellular space. Data points below pH 6.0 are not reliable because of the influence of PCr titration [8]. In the present study, pHi levels less than 6.0 were not considered accurate.

Total depletion of PCr and ATP with pHi below 6.5 and lactate levels over 20 μmol/g for 15 min does not indicate immediate and irreversible mitochondrial damage since metabolic recovery occurred. However, since separate studies with a three-vessel occlusion model [6] indicate that a 10% mortality was observed at 7 days after 15 min of nearly complete ischemia, mechanisms of delayed injury may be initiated by this insult.

The results of this study suggest the possibility of using this model for study of treatments that modify cerebral metabolic reaction to global ischemia. Since a uniform response to the ischemic insult was observed in each rat, it should be possible to observe significant protective effects that delay or attenuate changes in energy metabolites, pHi, or lactate levels. Further studies during longer ischemia and reperfusion periods should delineate delayed effects of ischemic acidosis and reperfusion upon recovery from transient global ischemia. Comparison with results of our previous studies of incomplete ischemia produced by the four-vessel occlusion model [1] may define effects of differences in substrate availability and CBF upon metabolic response to ischemia and reperfusion.

References

1. Andrews BT, Keniry MA, Richards TR, et al. (1987) 31-phosphorus nuclear magnetic resonance spectroscopy in global cerebral ischemia and reperfusion in the rat. Neurosurgery 5:699–708
2. Chang LH, Pereira BM, Keniry MA, et al. (1987) Comparison of lactate concentration determinations in ischemic and hypoxic rat brains by in vivo and in vitro 1H NMR spectroscopy. Magn Reson Med 4:575–581
3. Chang LH, Chew WM, Weinstein PR, et al. (1987) A balanced-matched double-tuned probe for in vivo 1H and 31P NMR. J Magn Reson 72:168–172
4. Gonzalez-Mendez R, Litt L, Koretsky AP, et al. (1984) Comparison of 31P NMR spectra of in vivo rat brain using convolution difference and saturation with a surface coil: Source of the broad component in the brain spectrum. J Magn Reson 57:526–533
5. von Hanwehr R, Smith ML, Siesjo BK (1986) Extra- and intracellular pH during near-complete forebrain ischemia in the rat. J Neurochem 46:331–339
6. Kameyama M, Suzuki J, Shirane R, et al. (1985) A new model of bilateral hemispheric ischemia in the rat: Three-vessel occlusion model. Stroke 16:489–493
7. Ljunggren B, Norberg K, Siesjo BK (1974) Influence of tissue acidosis upon restitution of brain energy metabolism following total ischemia. Brain Res 77:173–186
8. Petroff OAC, Prichard JW, Behar KL, et al. (1985) Cerebral intracellular pH by 31P nuclear magnetic resonance spectroscopy. Neurology 35:781–788
9. Seo Y, Murakami M, Watari H, et al. (1983) Intracellular pH determination by a 31P NMR technique: The second dissociation constant of phosphoric acid in a biological system. J Biochem 94:729–734
10. Yoshida S, Busto R, Martinez, et al. (1985) Regional brain energy metabolism after complete versus incomplete ischemia in the rat in the absence of severe lactic acidosis. J Cereb Blood Flow Metabol 5:490–501

Microsurgical Anatomy of the Posterior Clinoid Region

Operative Approach to the Posterior part of the Cavernous Sinus

Lucia J. Zamorano, Manuel Dujovny, James I. Ausman, Fernando G. Diaz, S. Kim Berman, and Haresh G. Mirchandani[1]

Introduction

The posterior clinoid region (PCR) is related to many important structures, such as the cavernous sinus (CS), internal carotid artery (ICA), extraocular nerves, pituary gland, and clivus. The aim of our study was to characterize the microsurgical anatomy of the posterior clinoid region (PCR), including the posterior clinoid process (PCP) and its relationships to surrounding neurovascular structures.

Material and Methods

Forty-three tissue blocks, containing 86 cavernous sinus, were removed from the cranial base of adult unfixed cadavers with the help of an electric saw. Each block contained the sphenoid bone, part of the petrous temporal bone, anterior and posterior clinoid, pituitary gland, both cavernous sinus, carotid artery and cranial nerves II, III, IV, V, and VI. The petrous carotid arteries were cannulated and injected with colored silicone rubber (MICROFIL, Canton Bio-Medical Products, Inc., Boulder, Colorado). Microdissection under an operating microscope was performed. The microsurgical anatomy of the PCR was studied with reference to the PCP and its arterial and neural relationships. Simulated surgical procedures were also carried out in 20 specimens. A superoposterior surgical approach to the posterior part of the cavernous sinus, including the removal of the PCP, was investigated.

Results

Microsurgical Anatomy of PCR

The PCR includes the PCP and related structures: the posterior part of the CS, the CC1 and CC2 portions of the cavernous carotid artery and its branches, and the IIIrd, IVth, Vth, and VIth cranial nerves.

Posterior clinoid process. The posterior clinoid processes (PCPs) are the lateral and superior extensions of the dorsum sellae. The tips of the PCP varied considerably in size and shape. We found six different types, the most common being the symmetrical and rounded type, projecting forward and slightly lateral. The diameters of the PCP at its base on the dorsum sellae, and the distance from the tip of the PCP to the midpoint of the base in coronal and sagital planes, are shown in Table 1.

The distance between both anterior clinoid processes was 30.1 +/− 5.5 mm (range = 22–43 mm), and between both posterior clinoid processes it was 15.4 +/− 2.6 mm (range 11–20 mm). The distance between the tips of the anterior and PCPs was 12.32 +/− 5.1 mm (range 2–20 mm) on the right and 11.95 +/− 4.5 mm (range 3–20 mm) on the left.

Arterial relationships. We found three main courses of the carotid artery at this level. The most common was a right angled curvature at the junction of CC1 and CC2 (52%). In 30% a pronounced convexity was found, with the artery ascending as far as the top of the PCP. In 18%, the artery ran in a straight course from the carotid canal to the junction of CC2 and CC3.

The more common branches of the intracavernous carotid artery were the meningohypophyseal trunk (present in all cases), the inferior cavernous sinus (present in 95%), and capsular artery (present in 20% of the cases). Less frequent branches were the clival and ophthalmic arteries (present in 15% of the cases). Related to and partially covered by the PCP is the junction of the ascendent (CC1) and horizontal (CC2) portions of the intracavernous carotid artery, with an outer diameter of 5.8 +/− 0.62 mm (range 4.5–8 mm).

[1] Department of Neurological Surgery, Henry Ford Hospital, Detroit, Michigan, USA

Table 1. Posterior clinoid process (PCP) diameter (mm)

	Right		Left	
	diameter +/− SD	Range	diameter +/− SD	Range
Coronal	7.45 +/− 1.9	5–9	5.9 +/− 1.1	4–8
Vertical	3.05 +/− 1.2	1.5–5	2.4 +/− 1.4	1–7
Saggital	3.7 +/− 2.0	0–55	3.7 +/− 0.9	2.5–5

In spite of marked variations in curvature of the carotid artery and its branching pattern, a constant fact was the relationship to the PCP of the meningohypophyseal artery and its branches, the clival artery and the posterior division of the inferior cavernous sinus artery. The meningohypophyseal trunk arose at the level of the dorsum sellae at the union of CC1 and CC2, from the posterior, lateral, or superior surface of the carotid. Although different branching patterns were found, the trunk gave rise to three branches: the tentorial artery (present in all cases), which coursed laterally to the tentorium, giving branches to the IIIrd and IVth cranial nerves and anastomosing with the meningeal branches of the ophthalmic artery; the inferior hypophyseal artery (present in 97% of the cases) which coursed medially to supply the posterior pituitary capsule, often with one or two branches proximal to entering the sella, with one of these branches supplying the dura around the PCP; and the dorsal meningeal artery (present in 97% of the cases), which perforated the dura of the posterior cavernous sinus wall to supply the clival area and the VIth cranial nerve. It accompanied the VIth cranial nerve into the cavernous sinus and past Dorello's canal toward the clivus.

The inferior cavernous sinus artery (present in 95% of the cases) arose from the lateral CC2 and gave rise to two branches, the anterior and posterior division, the last one being related to the PCP. The clival artery (present in 15% of the cases) was the most proximal branch of the intracavernous carotid artery and arose from the dorsal surface of the CC1 segment.

Neural relationships. Cranial nerves were located in relationship to the lateral wall of the cavernous sinus. This wall was formed by two layers: a smooth superficial layer formed by the dura mater, and a deep layer where the IIIrd, IVth, and VIth nerves were embedded. The two layers were loosely attached to each other and could be easily separated. After the superficial layer of dura was removed, the course of the cranial nerves and their relationship to each other and the PCP were studied from their dural entry points to the superior orbital fissure. The distance between the anterior borders of "entry pores" and the posterior clinoid process is discussed in Table 2.

The IIIrd cranial nerve pore was situated rostrally (20 cases on the left, 19 on the right), at the same level (13 cases on the left, nine on the right), and dorsally (ten cases on the left, 15 cases on the right). The trochlear nerve pore was situated on the lower surface of the tentorial notch in 22 cases, in the basin region in 28, and in the apical region of the basin in 36 cases. The VIth cranial nerve was split into two rootlets in ten cases, and into three rootlets in one case.

Microsurgical Approach to the Posterior Cavernous Sinus

A semicircular incision of the roof of the posterior cavernous sinus was done, 3 mm medial to the oculomotor nerve pore extending posteriorly on the dura, covering the PCP up to a distance about 10 mm above the abducens nerve pore. The dura was reflected laterally to protect against the cranial nerves. The PCP was drilled off to its base, as was the superolateral border of the clivus. This approach allowed a wide exposure of the CC1 and CC2 portions of the intracavernous carotid artery and its branches (Fig. 1). In 70% of the cases, there was a wide space between CC1, CC2, and the PCP; in 30% of the cases, where a pronounced loop was found, the artery was protected from injury during drilling. The artery is mobile and easy to reach at that level, especially on its medial aspect where no branches were found. More laterally, the meningohypophyseal artery (with its branches), the posterior division of the inferior cavernous sinus, and the clival artery need to be protected. The lateral wall of the cavernous

Table 2. Distance between "entry pore" of cranial nerve and PCP

	Right	Left
IIIrd cranial nerve	5.4 +/− 1.9 mm	5.9 +/− 1.9 mm
IVth cranial nerve	12.6 +/− 5.49 mm	12.5 +/− 3.4 mm
Vth cranial nerve	13.7 +/− 4.38 mm	13.8 +/− 2.75 mm
VIth cranial nerve	22.6 +/− 0.32 mm	21.5 +/− 2.94 mm

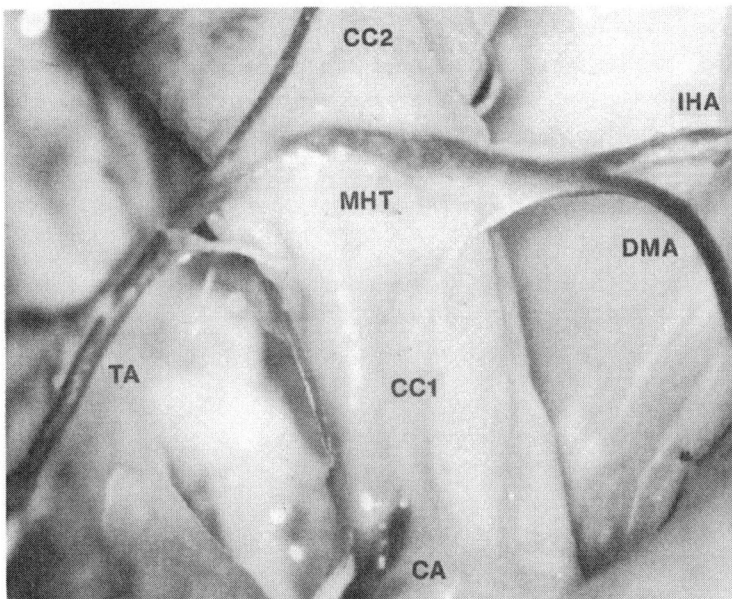

Fig. 1. Superior-posterior view of the intracavernous carotid artery after removal of the PCP (Posterior clinoid process). *CC1* and *CC2* are widely exposed as is the MHT (meningohypophyseal trunk), with its branches IHA (inferior hypophyseal artery), *DMA* (dorsal meningeal artery), and *TA* (tentorial artery). The *CA* (clival artery) is also visible

Discussion

Many authors have described different approaches to the cavernous sinus since Parkinson described his lateral approach to the cavernous portion of the carotid artery [5]. The operative approaches that have been used include the "lateral" (through the lateral wall between the trochlear and ophthalmic nerves or between the ophthalmic and maxillary nerves), the "inferior" approach (from the infratemporal fossa following the petrous internal carotid artery), the "anterior," including the removal of the anterior clinoid process, the "superior" (through the superior wall), and the "medial" approach (through the sphenoid sinus) [1, 4]. Our study suggests that the exposure of the posterior region of the cavernous sinus can be achieved through an incision of the roof of the cavernous sinus medial to the pore of the oculomotor nerve, with resection of the PCP and the superolateral aspect of the clivus. Drilling off the PCP has also been described as a useful technique for the clipping of basilar tip aneurysms [2].

Two major problems are involved in direct surgery in the cavernous sinus: vascular morbidity (due to hemorrhage), and cranial nerve damage. Hemorrhage from the cavernous sinus has often been successfully controlled with packing [1]. Hemorrhage, due to injury of the intracavernous carotid artery, is a real cause of morbidity and mortality, and can be reduced significantly if the petrous ICA and the supraclinoid carotid artery are exposed [3]. The wide space between the carotid artery and PCP in the superoposterior approach, the mobility of the intracavernous carotid at this level, and the absence of branches on the medial side make this approach safer. Cranial nerve morbidity can be reduced by intraoperative monitoring [6], and in the proposed superposterior approach, the cranial nerve remains intact in the lateral wall.

sinus, with the included cranial nerves, remained intact.

The wide exposure of the CC1 and CC2 portions of the intracavernous carotid artery and some of its branches (achieved through this superoposterior approach), suggests that this would be a feasible approach for vascular surgery at that level. Endarterectomy, reconstructive procedures of the carotid artery, and bypass surgery to the meningohypophyseal trunk (or some of its branches), as well as direct treatment of aneurysms, fistulas of the posterior portions of the intracavernous carotid artery, or dural arteriovenous fistulas could all be treated using this approach.

References

1. Dolenc V (1983) Direct microsurgical repair of intracavernous vascular lesions. J Neurosurg 58:824–831

2. Dolenc V, Skrbec M, Skrap M, Morina A (1986) Transcavernous approach to carotid-ophthalmic artery and basilar tip aneurysms. Proc. International Symposium on Cavernous Sinus, Ljubljana, Yugoslavia, pp 226–234

3. Glasscock M (1969) Exposure of the intrapetrous portion of the carotid artery. In: Hamberger C, Wersall J (eds) Disorders of the skull base region. Proc. of the Tenth Nobel Symposium, Stockholm, 1968, Almqvist and Wiksell, Stockholm, pp 135–143

4. Hakuba A, Suzuki T, Komiyama M (1986) Surgical approaches to the cavernous sinus: Report on 52 cases. Proc. International Symposium on Cavernous Sinus, Ljubljana, pp 226–234

5. Parkinson D (1965) A surgical approach to the cavernous portion of the carotid artery: Anatomical studies and case report. J Neurosurg 25:474–483

6. Sehkar L, Moller M (1986) Operative management of tumors involving the cavernous sinus. J Neurosurg, 64:879–889

Acute Surgery for Ruptured Posterior Circulation Aneurysms

Shigeru Nemoto, Charles G. Drake, Sydney J. Peerless, and Gary G. Ferguson[1]

Posterior circulation aneurysms are less commonly encountered and surgical access is less straightforward. The timing of surgery for these uncommon lesions has not been discussed. This report concerns our recent experience with early management of ruptured posterior circulation aneurysms.

Clinical Material

Eighty-six patients with ruptured posterior circulation aneurysms have been operated on at our unit within seven days following their last subarachnoid hemorrhage (SAH) since 1970. Twenty-two patients were male and 64 were female, aged 8–68 years (mean age 47 years).

The basilar bifurcation was the most common site (Table 1). Of 86 ruptured aneurysms, 59 were small (<12 mm), 22 large (12–25 mm), and five giant (>25 mm).

At the time of surgery, 46 patients were Botterell grade I, 27 grade II, 10 grade III, and 3 grade IV.

Surgical Management, Postoperative Course, and Results

Basilar Bifurcation Aneurysms

Of 50 patients with ruptured basilar bifurcation aneurysms, 28 were grade I, 15 grade II, and seven grade III. Forty-seven patients had their aneurysms clipped, and three were treated with upper basilar artery occlusion.

Seventeen patients developed major neurological deficits immediately after surgery from various causes; intraoperative rupture, temporal lobe swelling, extradural hematoma, rupture of

the aneurysm following tourniquet closure, and probably perforator injury. Of these 17 patients, however, 13 recovered completely within several weeks, three remained disabled, and one died.

Ten patients developed delayed neurological deficit between days 7 and 13, caused by ischemia with vasospasm. Three of them responded to hypervolemic-hypertensive therapy. Five patients remained disabled and two died.

Of 26 patients operated on within 96 h of the last SAH, and 24 patients operated on between days 5 and 7, good results were obtained in 22 (85%) and 18 (75%), respectively. Operative mortality was 6% in both groups.

SCA Aneurysms

Fourteen patients had ruptured superior cerebellar artery (SCA) aneurysms; six grade I, five grade II, two grade III, and one grade IV, All underwent direct clipping of the aneurysms. Five patients were operated on within 96 h of SAH, and nine patients between days 5 and 7.

Postoperatively, five patients became drowsy, probably due to perforator manipulation, but all recovered completely within a week. One patient (grade I) developed hemiparesis, resulting from major intraoperative bleeding and incomplete clip placement. Another grade III patient de-

Table 1. Location of the ruptured aneurysms on the posterior circulation (treated within 7 days of SAH)

Location	Number
Basilar	66
Bifurcation	50
SCA	14
V-B Junction	2
Vertebral	15
Posterior cerebral	5
Total	86

[1] Division of Neurosurgery, University Hospital, London, Ontario, Canada

Table 2. Results of surgery for the posterior circulation aneurysms (treated within 7 days of SAH)

Grade[a]	No.	Excellent	Good	Poor	Dead
I	46	30	9	5	2
II	27	12	12	3	0
III	10	4	3	2	1
IV	3	0	0	0	3
Total	86	46	24	10	6
		(81%)			(7%)

[a] Botterell grading

veloped hemiparesis which was caused by vasospasm, and showed satisfactory recovery in 3 months.

Results were excellent or good in 11 patients (79%), poor in two, and fatal in one (mortality 7%).

Vertebrobasilar Junction Aneurysms

Two patients with ruptured vertebrobasilar junction aneurysms underwent clipping. One patient (grade I) was operated on day 5 and suffered 6th, 7th, and 8th cranial nerve palsies postoperatively. The other patient (grade IV after four hemorrhages), who was operated on day 1 of the last SAH, developed severe vasospasm of the basilar artery on day 3 (18 days after the first SAH) and died.

Vertebral Aneurysms

Of 15 patients with ruptured vertebral aneurysms, eight were grade I, six grade II, and one grade IV. Fourteen patients underwent direct clipping of the aneurysm and one patient was treated with proximal occlusion of the vertebral artery. Seven patients were operated on within 96 h of SAH, and the remainder between days 5 and 7.

Eight patients developed postoperative neurological deficit. Four had transient lower cranial nerve palsies. Three became confused or more drowsy, due to vasospasm, or, probably, retraction of the brainstem. A grade IV patient was complicated by postoperative subdural hematoma and died. Of 15 patients with ruptured vertebral aneurysm, 14 had satisfactory outcome.

Posterior Cerebral Aneurysms

Of five patients with ruptured posterior cerebral aneurysm (three P-1 and two P-2 aneurysms),

Table 3. Results of surgery for the posterior circulation aneurysms

Grade	Timing	No.	Excellent/good	Dead
I, II	<96 h	30	28 (93%)	0
	Days 5–7	43	35 (81%)	2
III, IV	<96 h	11	5	4
	Days 5–7	2	2	0

Table 4. Results of surgery for the ruptured posterior circulation aneurysms

Grade	Timing of surgery	No.	Excellent or good (%)	Dead (%)
I, II	<7 days	73	86	3
	Elective	888	90	3
III, IV	<7 days	13	54	31
	Elective	132	57	15

three were grade I, one grade II, and one grade III. Aneurysms were clipped within 4 days of SAH in two patients, and between days 5 and 7 in three patients. Postoperatively, two patients with P-1 aneurysm developed hemiparesis from undetermined etiology. One of them recovered useful function but the other remained disabled. One patient with a grade I P-2 aneurysm developed aphasia and hemiparesis on day 12 and recovered completely. Finally, four out of five patients had good results.

Grade, Timing, and Results

The overall results are shown in Table 2. In grades I and II patients, surgery within four days of SAH and between days 5 and 7 resulted in a 93% and an 81% good outcome, respectively (Table 3). Elective surgery (later than day 7) in 888 patients of grades I and II showed a 90% satisfactory outcome. Operative mortality in the surgery within 7 days was 3%, which is the same as in elective surgery.

In patients of grades III and IV, surgery within seven days resulted in a 54% good outcome and a 31% mortality, while a 57% good outcome and a 15% mortality occurred in elective surgery (Table 4). In this series, grade IV patients all died. In elective surgery of ten grade IV patients, only two had good outcome, five remained disabled, and three died (morbidity 50% and mortality 30%).

In good risk patients with posterior circulation aneurysm, early surgery can be performed with satisfactory results.

Size of Aneurysms and Results

Early surgery of small and large aneurysms resulted in an 83% and an 82% good outcome, respectively. In elective surgery, good outcome was obtained in 91% of small aneurysms and 82% of large aneurysms. Small and large aneurysms were treated with the same risk.

Of five patients with giant aneurysm, results were excellent or good in three (60%), which is similar to elective surgery.

Age and Results

Sixty-eight patients aged under 60 years and 18 patients over 60 years had similar operative results.

Rebleeding and Results

Forty-six patients who suffered only one SAH had an 82% good outcome and a 7% mortality, while 40 patients with multiple bleeds showed similar results.

Intraoperative Rupture

Intraoperative rupture occured in ten patients; four with basilar bifurcation aneurysm, five with SCA aneurysm and one with vertebral posterior inferior cerebellar artery -(PICA) aneurysm.

Minor leak from the aneurysm sac was seen in five patients and all had good results. Five patients sustained major intraopertative bleeding and all developed major neurological deficits. Two of them showed good recovery, one remained disabled, and two died.

Incomplete Obliteration of the Aneurysms

Of 82 patients who underwent clipping of the aneurysm, neck occlusion was incomplete in three (two with a large basilar bifurcation aneurysm and one with a large SCA aneurysm). Reclipping was performed in two patients, one of whom had good results and the other (grade IV) died. An-

other patient with a large basilar bifurcation aneurysm became disabled and no further surgical treatment was carried out.

Proximal vessel occlusion was performed in four patients resulting in complete thrombosis of the aneurysm in three. One patient with a giant basilar bifurcation aneurysm suffered from major rebleeding following tourniquet closure and became disabled.

Operative Complication

Of 64 patients with basilar bifurcation or SCA aneurysm, the brain was slack for subtemporal approach in 60 patients, and only one of them suffered temporal lobe swelling causing hemiplegia. In four patients, a swollen hemorrhagic brain made retraction of the temporal lobe difficult, but ultimately a satisfactory exposure was obtained and three of them had no operative damage to the brain, although one grade IV patient died shortly after surgery. With the subtemporal approach, most patients developed some degree of oculomotor nerve paresis which usually recovered satisfactorily within 6 months. Aside from temporary third nerve palsy, 31 patients deteriorated postoperatively, resulting from intraoperative rupture in five patients, subdural or extradural hematoma in two, temporal lobe swelling in one, manipulation of the lower cranial nerves in five, and probably perforator injury in 18.

Vasospasm

Fourteen patients developed delayed neurological deficit (16%) between days 3 and 14. Five responded to treatment with satisfactory results. Two patients recovered from their deficit over a year, although hypervolemic-hypertensive therapy was not successful. Four patients remained disabled and three died.

Of 73 grades I and II patients, 11 suffered from ischemia with vasospasm (15%), as did three of 13 grades III and IV patients (23%).

CT scan was performed shortly after SAH in 60 patients. Of 30 patients with CT scan grading (+)-(++), two developed delayed neurological deficit secondary to vasospasm (7%). Both responded to the therapy and showed complete recovery. Of 30 patients with CT scan grading (+++)-(++++), nine developed delayed neurological deficit (30%). Five were permanently

Table 5. Delayed neurological deficit following rupture of the posterior circulation aneurysms

CT Grade	Neurological deficit		Total
	Transient	Permanent or dead	
+, + + (n = 30)	2	0	2 (7%)
+ + +, + + + + (n = 30)	4	5	9 (30%)
Total	6	5	11 (18%)

+ no subarachnoid blood visualized
+ + diffuse or thin sheet
+ + + clot or thick layer
+ + + + diffuse or none with intracerebral or intraventricular clots

Table 6. Results of surgery for the posterior circulation aneurysms (within 7 days of SAH) by CT grade

CT Grade	No.	Excellent	Good	Poor	Dead
+, + +	30	17	11	2	0
		(93%)			
+ + +, + + + +	30	16	7	4	3
		(77%)			(10%)

Table 7. Results of early surgery for ruptured aneurysms (within 96 h of SAH)

Grade (Botterell)	Location of aneurysms	No.	Excellent or good (%)	Dead (%)
I, II	Anterior circulation	41	93	2
	Posterior circulation	30	93	0
III, IV	Anteiror circulation	8	50	25
	Posterior circulation	11	45	31

disabled or died (Table 5). Of the patients with CT grading (+)-(+ +), 93% had good outcome and no mortality, whereas with CT grading (+ + +)-(+ + + +), there was a 77% good outcome and a 10% mortality (Table 6). CT scan finding seems to correlate with vasospasm and surgical outcome [3].

Early Surgery in Aneurysms on the Anterior and Posterior Circulation

The results of early surgery of ruptured aneurysms on the anterior and the posterior circulation are shown in Table 7. In this small series, there seems no significant difference in outcome between these two groups of patients.

Discussion

The incidence of vasospasm associated with ruptured posterior circulation aneurysms is not well known. In the present series, 14 patients developed delayed neurological deficit (16%), which seems as common as in the aneurysms on the anterior circulation. In retrospect, the CT scan findings are correlated with the incidence of vasospasm and surgical outcome. Obliteration of the aneurysmal neck is the goal of surgical treatment to prevent rebleeding. Proximal vessel occlusion may be a method of treatment to giant or fusiform aneurysms, which are not uncommon in the posterior circulation [2]. In this series, four patients underwent proximal vessel occlusion and two of them benefited from this treatment. Although occlusion of the basilar or vertebral artery may be feasible in an acute SAH patient of good risk, it is not yet known how a freshly hemorrhagic brain will tolerate this procedure.

Ruptured posterior circulation aneurysms have a high natural mortality due to recurrent bleeding (48%–83%) [4, 7, 10]. Of 1300 posterior circulation aneurysms treated by the senior authors, 1020 were ruptured; 86% of them had good results and operative mortality was 5% [8]. In this series, acute surgery was performed with the same outcome as elective surgery.

Surgical mortality in the early operation of ruptured aneurysms on the anterior circulation has been reported at 7%–15% [1, 5, 6, 9], to which the results in this series are comparable.

Experience in this series suggests that, with appropriate microsurgical techniques, patients with freshly ruptured aneurysms arising from the vessels of the posterior circulation probably can be treated as early as those with anterior circulation aneurysms.

References

1. Auer LM (1983) Acute surgery of cerebral aneurysms and prevention of symptomatic vasospasm. Acta Neurochirur (Wien) 69:273–281
2. Drake CG (1979) The treatment of aneurysms of the posterior circulation. Clin Neurosurg 26:96–144
3. Fisher CM, Kistler JP, Davis JM (1980) Relation of cerebral vasospasm to subarachnoid hemorrhage visualized by computerized tomographic scanning. Neurosurgery 6:1–9
4. Hook O, Norlen G, Guzman J (1963) Saccular aneurysms of the vertebrobasilar arterial system. A report of 28 cases. Acta Neurol Scand 39:271–304
5. Hori S, Suzuki J (1979) Early intracranial operations for ruptured aneurysms. Acta Neurochirur (Wien) 46:93–104
6. Kassell NF, Boarini DJ, Adams HP, et al. (1981) Overall management of ruptured aneurysms: Comparison of early and late operations. Neurosurgery 9:120–128
7. Locksley HB (1969) Natural history of subarachnoid hemorrhage. In: Sah AL, Perret GE, Locksley HB, et al. (eds) Intracranial aneurysms and subarachnoid hemorrhage. Lippincott, Philadelphia, pp. 37–108
8. Peerless SJ, Drake CG (in press) Management of aneurysms of posterior circulation. In: Youmans JR (ed) Neurological surgery, 3rd edn. Saunders, Philadelphia
9. Sano K, Saito I (1978) Timing and indication of surgery for ruptured intracranial aneurysms with regard to cerebral vasospasm. Acta Neurochirur (Wien) 41:49–60
10. Troupp H (1971) The natural history of aneurysms of the basilar bifurcation. Acta Neurol Scand 47:350–356

Long-Term Operative Results in a Series of 450 Consecutive Anterior Circulation Aneurysms
Relationships Among Operative Timing, Clinical Outcome, and Angiographic Vasospasm

Sergio Giombini, Carlo L. Solero, Antonio Melcarne, Stefano Ferraresi, and Franco Pluchino[1]

Introduction

Focal ischemic deficits are frequently associated with ruptured intracranial aneurysms. They may present as a reversible phenomenon or may be seen as a complete cerebral infarction. The former usually is a consequence of temporary disfunction in the distribution of the vessel harbouring an aneurysm; the latter may vary from a single infarct appropriate to a given vessel to a picture of diffuse patchy areas of infarction covering one or both cerebral hemispheres.

As several authors have stated [6–8], these findings are the result of a large range of pathological conditions which contribute to severely reduce cerebral blood flow after subarachnoid hemorrhage (SAH). These include atherosclerosis of the cerebral arteries, poor collateral circulation through the circle of Willis, subarachnoid hematoma, systemic hypertension, raised intracranial pressure, and the presence of vasospasm.

The narrowing of the conducting vessels may be the final step of many coincidental factors after SAH. Presently, the most widely accepted cause of vasospasm after rupture of cerebral aneurysm is the response of the arterial wall to substances liberated from blood, but it is still unclear why no vasospasm is found in angiograms of patients presenting with SAH from ruptured arteriovenous malformations, and the strikingly lower percentage of vasospasm in cases of SAH of unknown etiology.

Many other issues about vasospasm are still under debate, one of them being the correlation between clinical and angiographic features. Angiograhic diagnosis of vasospasm is not always associated with neurological ischemic symptomatology; this finding is not shared by other investigators [2] who instead believe that a definite correlation, within limits, does exist.

It is still uncertain if angiographic arterial narrowing after SAH is, per se, of prognostic value, and if it represents a conditioning factor for operative timing.

The purpose of this paper is to add our experience in aneurysmal pathology to this debated issue.

Material and Methods

Among the 420 consecutive cases of ruptured cerebral aneurysms of the anterior circulation admitted to the Istituto Neurologico of Milan, Italy, during the period January 1972 to December 1985, 164 patients (39%) demonstrated vasospasm on angiographic examination. Angiography included both carotid trees and, in most cases, also posterior circulation.

We divided angiographic vasospasm into three types, according to Saito et al. [8]. Type 1 (extensive and diffuse) involves all conducting vessels of the circle of Willis which show thread-like diffuse narrowing. In type 2 (multisegmental), extensive parts of cerebral arteries show segmental narrowing or tapering. Type 3 (local) is restricted to the parent vessel or to its branches near the ruptured aneurysms.

Of our series, 104 patients presented features of type 1 or type 2 vasospasm. They represent 25% of the whole series of SAH and 63% of all types of vasospasm. Patients with type 3 vasospasm were not considered because of the well known good prognosis of this angiographic pattern.

The ruptured aneurysms, in our series, were more frequently at the level of the anterior communicating artery (37 cases, 35.5%): the carotid siphon and middle cerebral artery were involved in 29 cases each (27.8%). In six cases, the aneurysms were on the anterior cerebral artery and on the carotid bifurcation in three other cases. These figures fit with the data reported by some authors [1], and are in contrast with others. We

---

[1] Department of Neurosurgery, Istituto Neurologico C. Besta, Milan, Italy

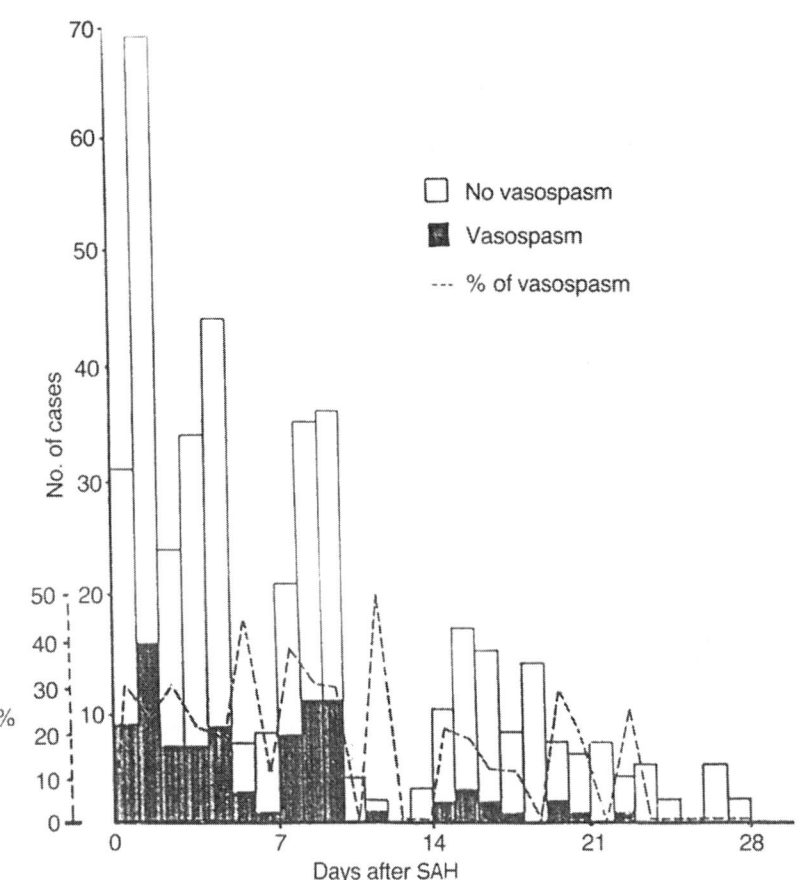

Fig. 1. Daily incidence of angiographic vasospasm after aneurysmal rupture

agree with the view that no single aneurysm site is significantly predisposed to the onset of vasospasm, although it tends to begin and become most severe on the artery harboring the aneurysm or on the artery enveloped in the greatest amount of blood, which often are one and the same.

Our institution being a "second referral" hospital, patients are admitted at varying time intervals from the onset of SAH. It follows that angiography, performed as soon as possible after admission, is obtained over a broad range of time after SAH, and our data may represent a real and valuable standard sample of the onset and evolution of vasospasm.

Angiographic vasospasm was seen both soon after SAH and later on—as far as the 3rd week after bleeding—with higher incidence on day 5 and day 8 (Fig. 1). For the purpose of this study, we have considered the clinical grade (according to Hunt and Hess) noticed just before direct operation on the ruptured aneurysm, which did not necessarily coincide with the grade reported at admission.

The patients and their preoperative grading

were divided into two groups, according to the interval from SAH (Table 1). Day 14 was chosen as a watershed because it represents the average duration of vasospasm [8–10]: the patients operated on before day 14 are considered the "early" surgery group (57 cases), while the patients operated on after day 14 were assigned to the "delayed" surgery group. When symptoms of vasospasm were present, the first being a disturbance of alertness, operations were performed soon after their improvement. The patients of the early surgery group belonging to grades IV and V were operated upon because of intracerebral hematoma (five cases) or after rebleeding; the grades IV and V patients of the delayed surgery group were operated on still in bad conditions due to severe late rebleeding, while their clinical picture was stable or in slight improvement.

The survivors were controlled as outpatients or were requested to fill up a questionnaire together with their family physician. Follow-up ranged from 1 to 9 years (mean 5.8 years). Long-term operative results were classified as "good" if the patients had resumed their previous occu-

Table 1. Aneurysms of the anterior circulation with angiographic vasospasm: results of early ($n = 57$) and delayed ($n = 47$) surgery

	Preop grade	No. of cases	Op. death	Follow up results			
				Good (%)	Fair (%)	Poor (%)	Lost (%)
Operation before day 14	I–II	26	0	20 (76.8)	2 (4.1)	1 (3.8)	3 (11.5)
	III	18	3 (16.6)	10 (55.5)	4 (22.2)	0	1 (5.5)
	IV–V	13	5 (38.5)	2 (15.4)	3 (23.0)	0	3 (23.0)
Operation after day 14	I–II	21	0	17 (80.9)	2 (9.5)	2 (9.5)	0
	III	18	0	11 (61.1)	5 (27.7)	0	2 (11.1)
	IV–V	8	2 (2.5)	1 (12.5)	5 (62.5)	0	0

pations, with no or minimal nerve deficit; "fair" when neurological and/or psychological impairment was only partially incapacitating and patients were still able to work; "poor" if patients, even if self-caring, were invalid. Nine patients were lost at follow-up.

Results and Discussion

All patients underwent direct operations using microsurgical techniques, in most cases without administration of hypotensive drugs.

As shown in Table 1, operative mortality was nil in grades I and II patients, and good results were achieved both in early and delayed surgery groups. In these cases, the absence of consciousness impairment and of nerve symptoms are of greater prognostic value than angiograhic vasospasm.

The same number of grade III patients were operated on before and after day 14. Mortality in the former group was rather high (16%), while no patient of the latter died. One may conclude that delayed surgery seems advisable when grade III is associated with radiological vasospasm, but the tendency for rebleeding must be taken into account: In fact, Nibbelink et al. [5] found an increased incidence of aneurysm rebleed in the presence of vasospasm (21%) as opposed to no vasospasm (11%). The best policy seems to be a compromise between opposite demands: operating early or waiting. We are convinced that as soon as alertness begins to improve, clipping of the aneurysm should be attempted. Then, when the rebleeding risk is none, therapeutic steps, like emodilution, hypervolemia, or induced sistemic hypertension can be adopted to fight arterial narrowing.

The worst prognosis was seen in grades IV and V patients with angiographic severe vasospasm.

The contemporary presence of an intracranial hematoma urged us to perform emergency operation, which was fatal in every case. In two patients of the early surgery group, the long-term result was surprisingly good, and two more fared fairly well: these four patients were in grade IV at admission, and rebled while slightly improving. They underwent emergency operations with satisfying final outcomes. Eight patients in grades IV and V received delayed surgery: all of them had a massive rebleeding which probably occurred when vasospasm was subsiding. This coincidence, together with timely operation, probably offers the explanation of relatively low mortality and fair late results.

The unclear relationship between vasospasm and clinical picture already underlined by several authors [4–9] is suggestive of two different anatomopathological mechanisms. Angiograms give very imprecise information about the actual state of conducting vessels and, most of all, about the reversibility of the phenomenon called arterial narrowing, compared to what cerebral blood flow (CBF) studies may instead offer. It can be assumed that when a discrepancy exists between the neurological picture and angiography (grades I and II patients), vasospasm is the result of a true smooth muscle constriction of the vessel wall, rapid in onset, transient in duration, and easily counteracted by collateral circulation. On the contrary, there is mounting evidence that delayed vasospasm is not muscular spasm at all, but rather a morphological change in the arterial wall [11]. This vascular injury reaction is also referred to as an acute proliferative vasculopathy, which consists of the initial loss of portions of the endothelial lining, accompanied by necrosis of the smooth muscle in the tunica media, and followed by intimal thickening [7]. These features justify fair correlation between angiographic vasospasm and bad neurological conditions, like we have observed in high-grade patients. When clinically significant, the vasospasm causes a reduced CBF and defective metabolism (CMRO2), while cerebral blood volume is increased [3]. This picture represents narrowing of angiographically visible arteries and massive dilatation of intraparenchymal vessels, as a consequence of the loss of autoregulation caused by ischemia. The next step will be cerebral edema. When this stage is reached, the clinical condition will undoubtedly deteriorate, and a clearer relationship with vasospasm and its prognostic significance will be evident. Our efforts should be directed toward the possibility of avoiding the onset or arresting the evolution of vasospasm: the combination of acute surgical repair of ruptured cerebral aneurysms, washout of major subarachnoid cisternal clots, and preventive treatment with new compounds, like calcium antagonistic nimodipine, seems to provide the best treatment and progonsis for these patients.

Summary

This work deals with the problem of the prognostic value of angiographic vasospasm after SAH.

It is based on our series of 420 ruptured aneurysms of the anterior circulation; out of these, 160 (39%) showed arterial narrowing on angiograms. Vasospasm was diffuse or multisegmental in 104 cases. These patients are divided into two groups, according to the interval between SAH and operation: group 1 ("early" surgery) consists of 57 patients who have been operated upon before day 14 from bleeding; group 2 ("delayed" surgery) consists of 47 patients operated on after this date. When comparing the early and long-term operative results of the two groups, we have noticed that clinical picture, especially impairment of consciousness, is a more reliable prognostic factor than angiographic vasospasm. We concluded that the scanty relationship between vasospasm and clinical status may be explained by a different mechanism of the arterial narrowing seen on angiograms: in low-grade patients,
vasospasm rapid in onset but transient in duration, due to a real smooth muscle constriction of the vessel wall, can be hypothized; in high grade cases, vasospasm sustained by long-lasting proliferative vasculopathy may be suspected.

References

1. Dickmann GH, Zamboni O, Driollet Laspiur R (1972) Aneurysms and vasospasm: Clinico-radiological correlation. In: Fusek I, Kunc Z (eds) Proceedings of the Fourth European Congress of Neurosurgery. Present Limits of Neurosurgery. Avicenum, Czechoslovak Medical Press, Prague, pp 229–232
2. Fisher CM, Robertson GH, Ojeman RG (1977) Cerebral vasospasm after ruptured aneurysm. Stroke 8:11
3. Grubb RL, Rhichle ME, Eichling JO (1977) Effects of subarachnoid hemorrhage on cerebral blood volume, blood flow, and oxygen utilization in humans. J Neurosurg 46:446–453
4. Millikan CH (1975) Cerebral vasospasm and ruptured intracranial aneurysm. Arch Neurol 32:433–449
5. Nibbelink DW, Torner JC, Henderson WG (1975) Intracranial aneurysms and subarachnoid hemorrhage. A cooperative study. Antifibrinolytic therapy in recent onset subarachnoid hemorrhage. Stroke 6:622–629
6. Peerless SJ (1979) Pre- and postoperative management of cerebral aneurysms. Clin Neurosurg 26:209–231
7. Peerless SJ, Kassell NJ, Komatsu K, Hunter IG (1980) Cerebral vasospasm: Acute proliferative vasculopathy? II Morphology. In: Wilkins RH (ed) Cerebral arterial spasm: Proceedings of the 2nd International Workshop. Williams and Wilkins Baltimore, 88–96
8. Saito I, Veda Y, Sano K (1977) Significance of vasospasm in the treatment of ruptured intracranial aneurysm. J Neurosurg 47:412–429
9. Symon L (1974) Vasospasm. In: Sano K, Ishii S, Le Vay D (eds) Recent progress in neurological surgery. Excerpta Medica, Amsterdam, pp 176–181
10. Weir B, Grace M, Hansen J, Rothberg C (1978) Time course of vasospasm in man. J Neurosurg 48:173–178
11. Wilkins RH (1980) Attempted prevention or treatment of intracranial arterial spasm: A survey. Neurosurgery 6:198–210

"Scavenger Surgery" for Prevention of Vasospasm Following Subarachnoid Hemorrhage

Surgical Results of 109 Cases Compared with Acute Conventional Surgery

Takeshi Kawase[1], Ryuzo Shiobara[1], Shigeo Toya[1], and Yasuyuki Miyahara[2]

Summary

Subarachnoid blood was actively removed in the acute stage of Subarachnoid hemorrhage (SAH; scavenger surgery) after the clipping of aneurysms in 109 patients with ruptured cerebral aneurysms. The effect on prevention of vasospasm was evaluated to compare the results of 89 conventional acute surgeries without removal of the blood. Both the incidence of ischemic complication and mortality were lower in the "scavenger surgery" group than in the "conventional surgery" group in patients with high SAH scores on CT. Two-thirds of those patients with severe SAH were freed from cerebral infarction and half of the patients had no neurological deficits.

It is well known that the presence of a thick blood clot in the subarachnoid space causes vasospasm of the cerebral artery, which leads to ischemic complications after subarachnoid hemorrhage (SAH). The trials to clear the subarachnoid blood have been performed during aneurysm surgery in the acute stage [1, 5, 7], whereas the effect on vasospasm and the surgical indication were not always clear because of lack of control data of acute aneurysm surgery. In this series, the patients were classified by SAH score on CT as well as the clinical grade, and the surgical results were analyzed and compared to the surgery without blood removal.

Clinical Materials and Surgical Methods

During the past 9 years, 789 patients with SAH were admitted to our hospitals, and 246 patients underwent surgery in the acute stage (days 0–4). This series consists of 198 patients whose preoperative SAH scores on CT scan we were able to analyze. Eighty-nine of these patients underwent conventional aneurysm surgery without active blood removal, and 109 received scavenger surgery. The preoperative conditions were graded by the Hunt and Kosnik grading system. The degree of SAH was classified according to Fisher's CT grade [2] in each of eight cisterns, and the SAH score was calculated by integration of CT grade in all cisterns (0–16 points; Fig. 1). The evolution of ischemic symptoms was examined at bed side during the course of vasospasm, and the appearance of cerebral infarction was detected on CT. The clinical conditions of patients are summarized in Table 1. The patients who received scavenger surgery were more handicapped both on the Hunt-Kosnik grade and on SAH score than the patients received conventional surgery, because of the surgeon's temptation to clear the blood in patients with severe

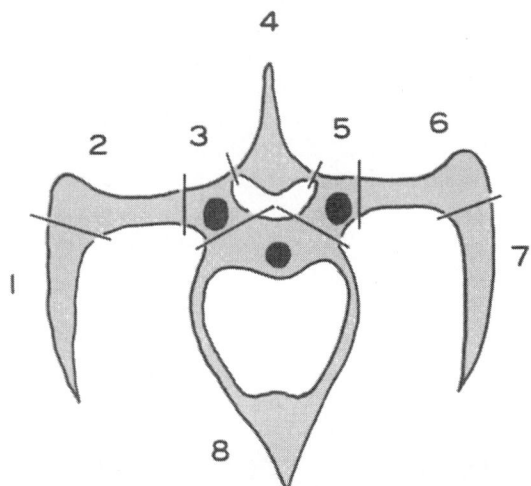

Fig. 1. Calculation of SAH score on CT. *1, 7* insular cistern, *2, 6* sylvian cistern, *3, 5* carotid cistern, *4* interhemispheric fissure and prechiasmatic cistern, *8* cisterns around brainstem. Fisher's SAH grade on CT = 0–2; Total SAH score = $\sum$(grade on each cistern)

[1] Department of Neurosurgery, Keio University, Tokyo, Japan
[2] Ohtawara Red Cross Hospital, Tochigi, Japan

Table 1. Clinical data in series of 198 patients

	Surgery	
	Conventional	Scavenger
Number of cases	89	109
Age (yrs)	51.9	53.0
Sex (% of male)	41.6	56.0
Post. fossa (%)	7.9	1.8
Grade III·IV·V (%)	43.8	59.6
SAH score	5.9	9.3
CT SDH (%)	1.1	3.7
ICH (%)	15.7	18.3
IVH (%)	14.6	9.2
Rebleeding (%)	19.1	18.3

SAH 789 cases, day 0–4 surgery 246 cases, CT performed 198 cases (past 9 years)
Patients with scavenger surgery were mere handicapped in terms of both clinical grade and SAH score
SDH subdural hemorrhage, *IDH* intracranial hemorrhage, *IVH* intraventricular hemorrhage, *SAH* subarachnoid hemorrhage

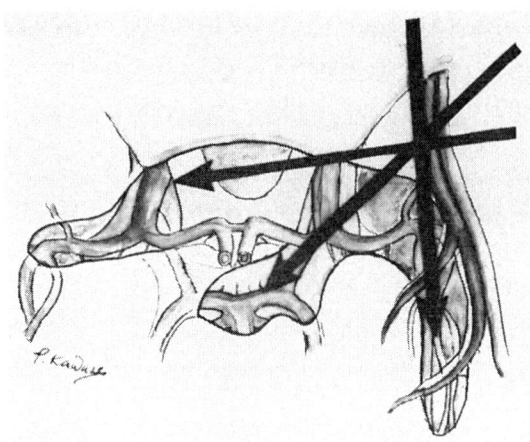

Fig. 2. The cisterns accessed by scavenger surgery. Microscope is turned in three directions

subarachnoid hemorrhage. The number of high-grade patients (III–V) were more in the former group (65 cases, 59.6%) than the latter group (39 cases, 43.8%). The average CT score of SAH was higher on the former group (9.3 points) than the latter group (5.9 points).

An important point of this surgery is how to protect the vulnerable brain and vessels during removal of the blood being packed in the complicated subarachnoid space. The side of craniotomy was selected considering the distribution of SAH, as well as the strategy for aneurysm removal. To access the basal cisterns with minimal brain retraction, the lateral orbital rim was exposed and the eminentia of the sphenoid ridge was drilled out until the superior orbital fissure was opened. The cortical surface was protected with a piece of thin sponge, and the sylvian fissure was widely opened with the preservation of large cortical veins. The microscope axis was turned in three directions to suction the subarachnoid blood (Fig. 2). When the distal sylvian fissure was cleared, the microscope axis was turned posteriorly to allow the basal overview. When the thick blood extended into the contralateral basal cisterns, the microscope was positioned laterally to overlook the contralateral M1 beyond the optic nerves. The liliequist membrane was cut to clear the prepontine cistern and ipsilateral ambient cistern. An appropriately sized suction tube is necessary to avoid damage to the perforating arteries of the posterior communicating artery. When the surgical manipulation caused mechanical vasospasm of the arterial tree, papaverine hydrochloride was topically applied on the arteries. The blood clots in the interhemispheric fissure and in the contralateral distal sylvian fissure were not cleared (Fig. 3).

The postoperative ventriculocisternal drainage was performed in 65% of patients who underwent scavenger surgery and in 41% of those with conventional surgery. The indication for drainage was determined by the severity of hemorrhage, not by the surgical policy. When the postoperative CT showed insufficient reduction of SAH score, ventriculocisternal irrigation was started with an artifical CSF mixed with urokinase (ten cases) [6].

The conventional surgery in this series was categorized as surgery in which surgical blood removal was not done or was limited to the area around the aneurysm.

Results

The results of scavenger surgery and conventional surgery done in the acute stage of SAH were compared in each group and classified according to the preoperative Hunt-Kosnik

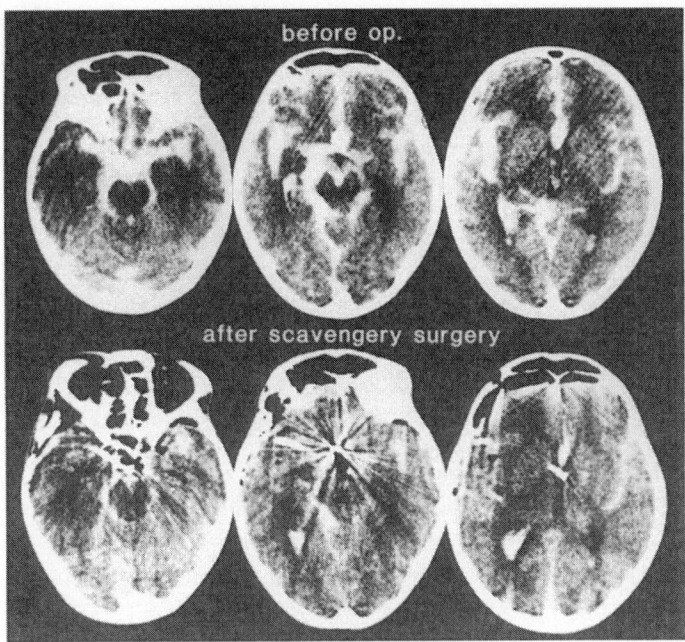

Fig. 3. CT scan of a patient with a high score SAH (16 points). After scavenger surgery, thick blood clots in most cisterns were cleared, except for those in the hemispheric and contralateral insular cisterns. Ventriculocisternal drainage tubes were inserted. The patient was discharged without neurological deficit

grade and the SAH score on CT. The average point decrease of SAH score by the scavenger surgery was double (6.6 points) of that by the conventional surgery (3.4 points).

Preoperative Grade and Infarction Rate

As mentioned above, the decision to perform scavenger surgery was based on the severity of the SAH. Therefore, even if the clinical grade of the patients were judged as II, they received the scavenger surgery when he had a thick SAH as seen in the grade IV patients (Fig. 4).

The infarction rates were smaller in grades II and III patients who underwent scavenger surgery: however, the difference was obscured by the handicap of the severity of SAH.

Preoperative SAH Score, Infarction Rate, and Outcome

Patients were classified into four groups according to the SAH score on CT, with neglect of clinical grades. Throughout all groups, the incidences of cerebral infarction were less in the scavenger surgery group than in the conventional surgery group (Fig. 5). The difference increased in the group with a high SAH score.

Two-thirds of patients were freed from cerebral infarction, even in the most severe SAH group (13–16 points). On the overall outcome,

half of the patients in this group had a excellent outcome although they had severe SAH (Fig. 6). In contrast, the results of conventional surgery for the patients with high SAH scores was disappointing, even if they had a good clinical condition before surgery. The results of patients with a score of less than 12 points showed little or no difference in overall outcome. The cerebral infarction rates in patients with thick SAH (9–16 points) were 30% in scavenger surgery and 41% in conventional surgery. The mortality rates were 18% and 32%, respectively, with a statistical difference of $P < 0.09$ by chi-square test (Fig. 7). The mortality rate of 85 "waiting" patients who did not undergo acute surgery under the same degree of SAH was 55% in our series, and had a more significant difference from those who underwent scavenger surgery ($P < 0.001$). The details of this group will be mentioned elsewhere.

Discussion

It was reported that the degree of vasospasm is closely related to the presence and degree of hematoma in the subarachnoid space. This means the reduction of volume of the hematoma will be effective in preventing vasospasm. However, the surgical technique stated only to clip the aneurysm to prevent rebleeding, and not on the hemorrhage already present. Delayed surgery

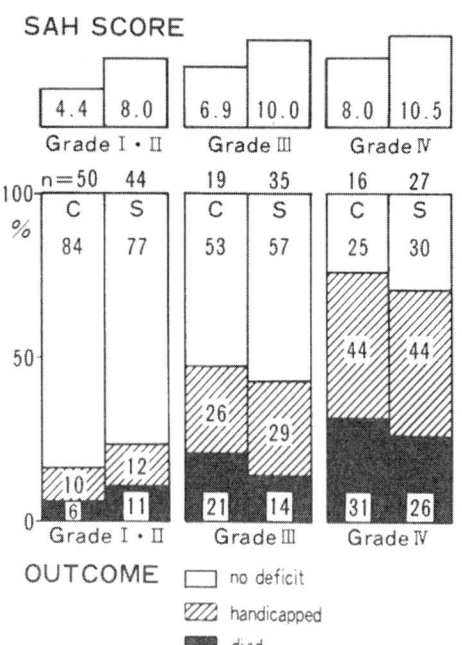

Fig. 4. SAH score and surgical outcomes classified by preoperative Hunt-Kosnik grades. Scavenger surgery patients are more handicapped than conventional surgery patients in SAH score in all clinical grades. The outcomes are a little better in grades III and IV. *C* conventional, *S* scavenger

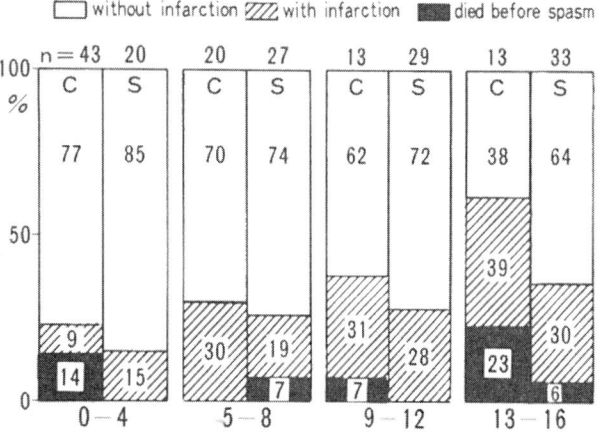

Fig. 5. Incidence of patients with cerebral infarction caused by vasospasm. Note the low rate of infarction in patients who underwent scavenger surgery in the group with the highest SAH score. The infarction rate is decreased to the same levels as the patients with SAH score of 5–12 who underwent conventional surgery. *C* conventional, *S* scavenger

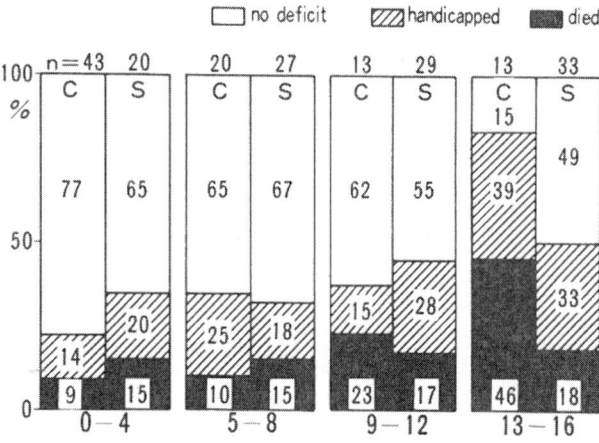

Fig. 6. SAH scores and surgical outcomes. Note the marked difference in mortality and morbidity rates in the group with the highest SAH score. Half of the patients completely recovered, although they had been in a severe condition. There was no remarkable difference in groups with SAH scores of less than 12 points. *C* conventional, *S* scavenger

still has strong support for patients with severe SAH, because of the vulnerability of the brain in the acute stage. The results of delayed surgery are, of course, better than that in the acute stage when discussed only in cases which underwent surgery. However, it must be noted that many patients worsened and died before surgery due to vasospasm or rebleeding. In our data, we lost more than half of the patients with high SAH scores by waiting.

In the recent international cooperative study of aneurysm surgery, the result of surgery in the acute stage was determined beneficial in the prevention of rebleeding but not ishemic complications. This may be because the surgery only concerned the clipping of the aneurysm. In the acute stage of SAH, the blood clots were not yet adhesive to the brain structures, and suction of these masses offered a suitable surgical space. One of the key points of this surgery is to make a basal craniotomy to overview each cistern with minimal brain compression. Preservation of veins buried in the hematoma is also important. We experienced two cases of venous hemorrhage after sacrificing a large cortical vein.

The results of scavenger surgery in this series were superior to those of conventional surgery, and the difference was more clear when the severity of SAH was classified based on CT scores rather than on the clinical grade. Thus, when a patient is in a good clinical condition but has a high CT score in the basal cisterns, the risk of vasospasm may increase. An active treatment to reduce the SAH score should be utilized.

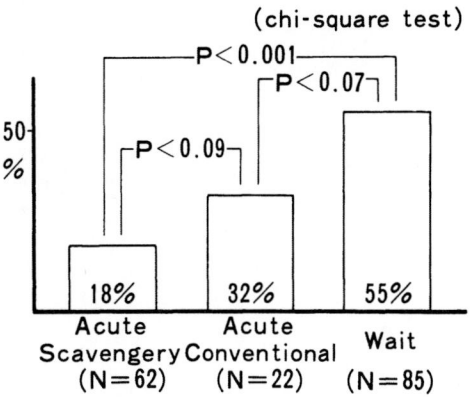

Fig. 7. Mortality rates among three different treatment policies for severe SAH. A large number of patients were lost while waiting for surgery, resulting in a high mortality rate. The mortality is lowest in the scavenger surgery group. SAH score, 9–16; grade on adm. II–IV

References

1. Dolenc M, Fettich M, Korsic R, Pregelj M, Skrap Z, Lamovec M, Cerk M, Kregar T (1982) Blood clot evacuation in aneurysm surgery in the acute stage (Arguments pro and con). Acta Neurochir 63:105–109
2. Fisher CM, Kistlar JP, Davis JM (1980) The correlation of cerebral vasospasm and amount of subarachnoid blood detected by computerized cranial tomography after aneurysm rupture. In: Wilkins RH (ed) Cerebral arterial spasm, Proceedings of Second Intl. Workshop. Williams and Wilkins, Baltimore, pp 397–408
3. Kassell NF, Torner JC (1984) The international cooperative study on timing of aneurysm surgery: An update. Stroke 15:566–570
4. Kawase T, Shiobara R, Toya S, Miyahara Y (1985) "Scavengery surgery" for subarachnoid hemorrhage 1. A surgical technique subarachnoid clot removal. In: Auer LM (ed) Timing of aneurysm surgery. Gruyter, Berlin, pp 357–363
5. Mizukami M, Kawase T, Usami T, Tazawa T (1982) Prevention of vasospasm by early operation with removal of subarachnoid blood. Neurosurgery 10:301–307
6. Shiobara R, Kawase T, Toya S, Ebato K, Miyahara Y (1985) "Scavengery surgery" for subarachnoid hemorrhage 2. Continuous ventriculo-cisternal perfusion using artifical cerebrospinal fluid with urokinase. In: Auer LM (ed) Timing of aneurysm surgery. Walter de Gruyter, Berlin, pp 365–372
7. Taneda M (1982) Effect of early operation for ruptured aneurysms on prevention of delayed ischemic symptoms. J Neurosurg 57:622–628

Treatment of Ruptured Cerebral Aneurysms in the Acute Stage

Correlation Between CT Findings and Vasospasm

Hiroshi Higuchi, Yoshihide Nagamine, Hisashi Abiko, Shinichi Kobayashi, Hideyuki Kamii, and Yoichi Suzuki[1]

Summary

Computed tomography (CT) findings from 320 cases of ruptured intracranial aneurysm, admitted to our department between 1977 and 1986, were graded from I to V as follows: grade I, no abnormality or isodensity in CT findings; grade II, high-density area only in the cistern in which the intracranial aneurysm exists; grade III, high-density areas also in cisterns other than that in which the ruptured intracranial aneurysm exists; grade IV, symmetrical, extremely high-density areas in all cisterns; grade V, presence of massive intracranial or intraventricular hematomas. Comparisons were then made of the morbidity and mortality rates between 156 cases operated on within 3 days of subarachnoid hemorrhage (SAH; group A) and 98 cases operated on four or more days afterwards (group B). It was found that early operations performed within 3 days on patients with CT findings of grades I-III were remarkably successful in preventing cerebral vasospasm and rebleeding. However, in patients with grade IV CT findings, early surgery was not so effective in preventing postoperative vasospasm. The overall mortality rate of 12.1% in group A was better than that of 19.5% in group B.

As a result of the introduction of computed tomography (CT), it has become possible to determine the extent and degree of subarachnoid hemorrhage (SAH) in the early stage of ruptured intracranial aneurysms. We discovered that early surgery, performed within 3 days of the rupture, is useful in preventing not only recurrence of hemorrhage, but also cerebral vasospasm, through the removal of the subarachnoid clot at an early stage [1]. The overall mortality and morbidity in the early operations of our series, the correlation between CT findings and surgical results, and the usefulness of CT grading of SAH are discussed.

[1] Department of Neurosurgery, Neurological Center, Iwate Prefectural Central Hospital, Morioka, Japan

Clinical Materials

Between 1977 and 1986, a total of 320 cases of ruptured intracranial aneurysms were admitted to the Iwate prefectural Central Hospital. A CT scan was performed within 3 days in all cases. Operations were performed within 3 days in 156 cases (group A), and after 3 days in 98 cases (group B). The remaining 66 cases (group C) died before operations could be performed (Table 1).

CT findings on SAH obtained within 3 days of onset were graded from I to V as follows, according to the extent and density of the high-density area (Fig. 1): grade I, no abnormality or isodensity area in CT findings; grade II, high-density area only in the cistern in which the ruptured intracranial aneurysm exists; grade III, high-density areas also in cisterns other than that in which the ruptured intracranial aneurysm exists; grade IV, symmetrical extremely high density areas in all cisterns; grade V, CT findings also suggest the presence of massive intracranial or intraventricular hematomas.

A total of 320 cases of our series were divided into three groups as mentioned above. Comparisons were then made of morbidity and mortality due to cerebral vasospasm between group A and group B. Correlation between CT grading and surgical results, together with the grading of Hunt and Kosnik in group A, were studied.

Table 1. Clinical materials

Group	Number
A Surgery within 3 days	156
B Surgery after 3 days	98
C Nonoperative deaths	66
Total	320

SAH subarachnoid hemorrhage
320 cases 1 October 1977 to 31 December 1986 admitted within 3 days of SAH

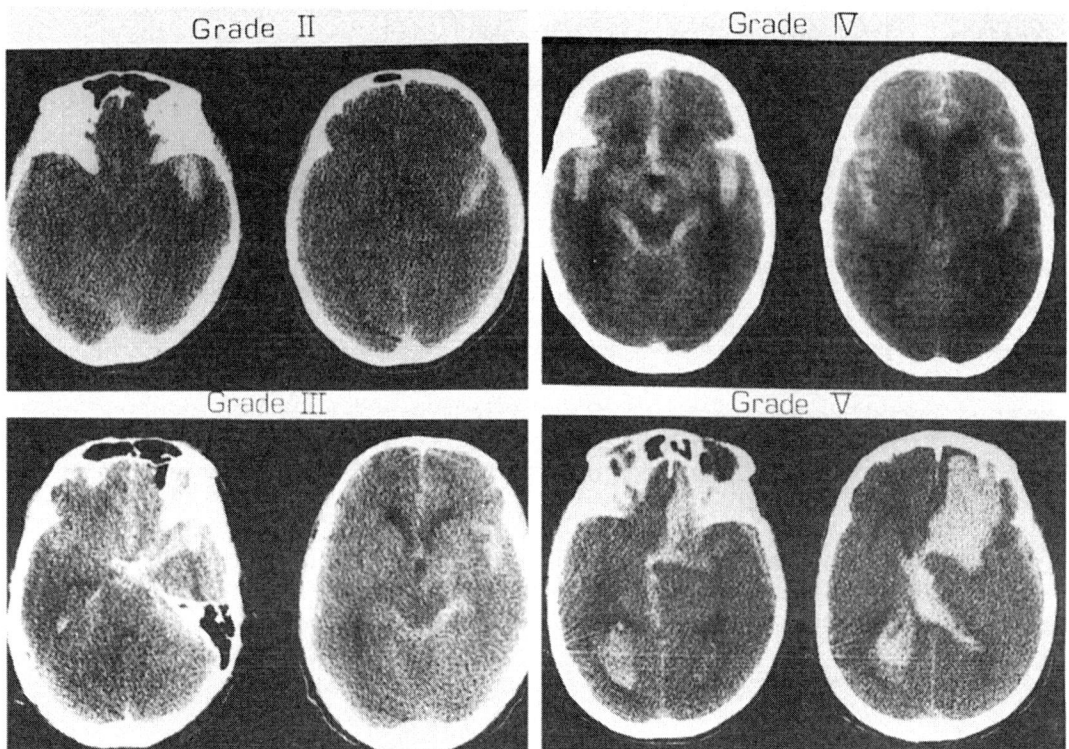

Fig. 1. Criteria for grading of CT findings. In grade II, the HDA is only in the cistern, near the ruptured aneurysm. In grade III, the HDA is also in more distant cisterns. In grade IV, symmetrical extremely HDA is in all cisterns. In grade V, massive intracerebral or intraventricular hematoma is seen

Surgical results were judged after 6 months from admission. In our studies, "good" indicates the ability to return to social activities, "fair" signifies inability to return to social activities but ability to live without the assistance of others, and "poor" indicates confinement to bed or a prolonged vegetative state. Morbidity includes both fair and poor cases. Vasospasm indicates symptomatic vasospasm only.

Results

Comparison of Morbidity and Mortality Between Group A and Group B

In group A, 107 of 156 cases (68.6%) were good, 30 cases were fair or poor (morbidity, 19.2%), and 19 cases died (mortality, 12.1%; Table 2). Almost all of the morbid cases were due to postoperative vasospasm. In group B, 70 of 98 cases (71.4%) were good and 25 cases were fair or poor (morbidity, 25.5%). Almost all of the morbid cases were due to the occurrence of preoperative

vasospasm while awaiting surgery. Three patients died (mortality, 3.0%). In group C, 13 cases died of rebleeding and seven cases died of vasospasm. In these 20 cases, early surgery was possible because their consciousness was good on admission, but they died while awaiting surgery. Forty-six patients died of massive intracerebral or intraventricular hemorrhage. These cases were comatose and without surgical indication. For all cases in group A and group B, mortality was 8.6% and morbidity was 21.6%. The overall mortality of all the cases in our series was 27.5%.

Correlation Between CT Gradings and Surgical Results

In group A, the morbidities of CT grades I–V were 9.5%, 8.0%, 15.7%, 23.0%, and 57.1%, and the mortalities were 0%, 0%, 5.2%, 33.3%, and 21.4%, respectively (Tables 3, 4).

In group B, the morbidities of CT grades I–V were 3.3%, 18.2%, 37.0%, 56.3%, and 33.3%, and the mortalities were 0%, 4.5%, 3.7%, 6.2%, and 0%, respectively.

Table 2. Distribution of ruptured cerebral aneurysms and surgical results

Group		ICA	Sites of ruptured aneurysm MCA	ACOA	ACA	V-BA	Total	Morbidity	Mortality		Total mortality
A (within 3 days)	Good	37	42	22	6		107	30/156 (19.2%)	19/156 (12.1%)		
	Fair	4	9	1			14				
	Poor	4	8	3	1		16				
	Dead	6	6	5	1	1	19ª				
B (after 3 days)	Good	20	24	20	1	5	70	25/98 (25.5%)	3/98 (3.0%)	23/118 (19.5%)	88/320 (27.5%)
	Fair	4	1	10		1	16				
	Poor	5	3	1			9				
	Dead	1		1		1	3ᵇ				
C (nonoperative deaths)	Rebleeding	5	1	2		5	13				
	Vasospasm	1		6			7				
	ICH or IVH	9	10	24	2	1	46				
Total		96	104	95	11	14	320				

ª Seven postoperative vasospasm, eight brain edema or ICH, and four other general complications
ᵇ One vasospasm, one slip out of clip, and one after bleeding
ICA internal carotid artery, *MCA* middle cerebral artery, *ACOA* anterior communicating artery, *ACA* anterior cerebral artery, *V-BA* vertebral-basilar artery, *ICH* intracerebral hemorrhage, *IVH* intraventricular hemorrhage

Correlation Between Surgical Results and the Gradings of Both CT and Hunt-Kosnik in Group A

The morbidities in each group of patients of grades I–IV of Hunt and Kosnik were 5.0%, 8.9%, 32.5%, and 50.0%, and the mortalities were 10.0%, 6.4%, 22.5%, and 11.1%, respectively (Table 4). No patients of Hunt-Kosnik grade V were operated on in our clinic, because they should be without surgical indication.

Discussion

In our series, the mortality of group A, the group with early operation within 3 days, was 12.1%, while that of group B, operated after three days, was 3.0%. The latter was lower than the former. However, if the overall mortality rate of group B is calculated with the inclusion of the 20 non-operated patients who had a good level of consciousness on admission but who died of rebleeding or vasospasm, it would be 19.5%, higher than that of group A (Table 2). Most of the 20 nonoperated cases were high-risk patients, i.e., geriatric cases over 65 years old, patients with general complications, and patients with a giant aneurysm or a vertebro-basilar aneurysm. If early surgery had been performed on these patients, there is no certainty that all the patients would have been saved. Thus, it cannot be said that early surgery is always useful for all SAH patients.

Next, the causes of death in 19 cases of group A were examined. Fifteen patients died of post-operative vasospasm, brain edema, and intra-cerebral hemorrhage, although neck clipping of the aneurysm was successful. The CT grading in these 15 cases was either grade IV or V. The remaining four cases died of accidental general complications (Table 4).

With regard to correlation between CT grading and morbidity, in group B, the higher the CT grading was, the higher was the morbidity due to preoperative vasospasm. In patients with a high CT grade, the frequency of preoperative vasospasm in group B was greater than that of postoperative vasospasm in group A after early removal of subarachnoid clot when possible. In the cases graded CT grade IV, morbidity due to postoperative vasospasm was 23.0% in group A, while morbidity due to preoperative vasospasm in group B was 50.0%. This great difference in morbidity between group A and group B concerning CT grade IV indicates that the greater the extent of the subarachnoid clot, the higher is the risk of occurrence of vasospasm [3], and that the frequency of vasospasm could possibly be reduced by removal of subarachnoid clots in early surgery [3, 4].

Characteristic findings based on correlations between the grading of Hunt and Kosnik [2] and CT grading were that the cases with a high CT grade displayed high mortality and morbidity, in spite of moderate Hunt-Kosnik grades (grade II or III). CT grading is thought to be more sensitive and useful in predicting postoperative vasospasm, cerebral edema, intracerebral hemorrhage, etc. What a surgeon most wants to know when performing an early operation is the extent and degree of SAH. The CT grading of SAH was classified grade I–V, based on how much clot could be removed by minimal invasion, or to what extent what parts of cisterns subarachnoid clot should remain. This grading

Table 3. Correlation between CT grading and surgical results

Group		CT grading I	II	III	IV	V	Total	Morbidity	Mortality		Total mortality
A (within 3 days)	Good	19	23	45	17	3	107 ⎫	30/156 (19.2%)	19/156 (12.1%)	⎫	
	Fair	1	1	6	3	3	14 ⎬ 156				
	Poor	1	1	3	6	5	16 ⎭				
	Dead			3	13	3	19[a]			⎬	
B (after 3 days)	Good	29	17	16	6	2	70 ⎫	25/98 (25.5%)	3/98 (3.0%)	23/118 (19.5%)	88/320 (27.5%)
	Fair		3	6	6	1	16 ⎬ 98				
	Poor	1	1	4	3		9 ⎭				
	Dead			1	1	1	3[b]				
C (nonoperative deaths)	Rebleeding	2	3	2	6		13			⎭	
	Vasospasm				7		7				
	ICH or IVH					46	46				
Total		53	50	86	68	63	320				

[a] Seven postoperative vasospasm, eight brain edema or ICH, four other general complications
[b] One vasospasm, one slip out of clip, and one after bleeding
Abbreviations same as in Table 2

Table 4. Correlation between CT grading and grading of Hunt and Kosnik

Grading of Hunt & Kosnik	Grading of CT I	II	III	IV	V	Morbidity (%)	Mortality (%)
IV		△	△×○	×○×■○○	×○■●△×△○	9/18 (50)	3/18 (11.1)
III	○○	○○○○	○○△△×○	●●×△○■○● ■○×○△○■× △⊗○○○□	×△××■○	13/40 (32.5)	9/40 (22.5)
II	○○○○○×○○ ○○△	○○○○○○○○ ○○×○○○	○○○○○○○○○ ○○○○○○○○○ ○○△○○○△○○ ○○△○○○○○○ ○○○○○○⊗	●○●■●○○ ○○×		7/78 (8.9)	5/78 (6.4)
I	○○○○○○○○	○○○○○○	×⊗⊗○○	○		1/20 (5.0)	2/20 (10.0)
Morbi. (%)	1/21 (9.5)	2/25 (8)	9/57 (15.7)	9/39 (23.0)	8/14 (57.1)	30/156 (19.2)	
Morta. (%)	0/21	0/25	3/57 (5.2)	13/39 (33.3)	3/14 (21.4)		19/156 (12.1)

○ good, △ fair, × poor, dead due to (● vasospasm, ■ brain edema or ICH, ⊗ other complications)

is thought to be practical and suitable for clinical management. In fact, in the case of CT grades I and II, subarachnoid clots can be totally removed by early surgery, postoperative vasospasms are few, and no fatal vasospasms have been encountered. In patients with CT grade III, the incidence of postoperative vasospasm was 21.0%, but fatal vasospasm occurred in less than 3.5% of the cases. A problem, however, arises in grade IV patients. In grade IV, good recovery was 43.6%, but the incidence of fatal vasospasm was 33.3%, and morbidity was 23.0%. This fact means that, in early surgery for grade IV cases, the removal of the subarachnoid clot is limited. Therefore, it is important not to extend damage to the brain while trying to remove the subarachnoid clot in an early operation.

References

1. Higuchi H, Nagamine Y, Satoh H (1982) Direct operation on intracranial aneurysms within 48 hours of subarachnoid hemorrhage: Correlation between CT findings and vasospasm. In: Brock M (ed) Modern neurosurgery. Springer, Berlin, pp 436–441
2. Hunt WE, Kosnik EJ (1974) Timing and preoperative care in intracranial aneurysm surgery. Clin Neurosurg 21:79–89
3. Komatsu S, Sato T, Ogawa A, et al. (1981) Correlation between CT findings and subsequent development of cerebral infarction due to vasospasms in subarachnoid hemorrhage cases. Neurol Med Chir (Tokyo) 21:373–377
4. Suzuki J, Onuma T, Yoshimoto T (1979) Results of early operations on cerebral aneurysms. Surg Neurol 11:407–412

Outcome of Aggressive Aneurysm Treatment with Early Operation and Adjunct Nimodipine in a Strictly Defined Swedish Population Served by a Small Neurosurgical Unit

Jan Hillman and Claes von Essen[1]

Introduction

Recently, much interest has been focused on improvement of the overall outcome in aneurysmal subarachnoid hemorrhage (SAH). Clinical work has demonstrated that surgery performed early after aneurysmal bleeding yields equally good or better results than does delayed surgery on a number of selected survivors from the early disasters characterizing this disease [3]. Furthermore, attempts to treat manifest brain ischemia during the course of SAH by hemodynamic manipulations [4], or to prevent its occurence by use of the calcium entry blocker nimodipine, seem promising [1, 8]. The structure of the medical care system in this country permitted almost every patient in a strictly defined population of 934 000 people, who survived long enough after aneurysm rupture to be transported, to be seen in this center. Furthermore, 86% of all patients were seen within 24 h post-SAH. This provides us with a unique opportunity to roughly evaluate the overall outcome of aneurysm bleeding obtained by the therapeutic principles presently applied, and permits a good understanding of the causes of clinical deterioration in a number of patients.

Treatment Policy

Surgical intervention was planned to be carried out as soon as possible after admission. The surgical procedures were performed by six different members of the team. A right-sided pterional approach was utilized if another approach was not necessitated by aneurysm location or multiplicity. Multiple lesions were treated whenever possible during the first operation. The area immediately surrounding the aneurysm was cleansed of clotted blood, but no attempt was made to remove cisternal clots extensively outside the actual operative field. Postoperatively, all patients were mobilized as early as possible.

The basic management program was uniform throughout this study. Ventricular drainage, assisted ventilation, mannitol infusions, antihypertensives, anticonvulsants, and antipyretics were used as dictated by acute alterations in the patients' clinical condition. In early operated cases, nimodipine infusion (2–3 mg/h) was started either at the time of clipping or at the time of aneurysm diagnosis and was then continued for a minimum of 10 days. At the slightest clinical sign suggestive of developing cerebral ischemia, the nimodipine dose was increased up to three times the previous dose. No hemodynamic manipulations were utilized in this study.

Results and Comments

Each university center in Sweden provides neurosurgical service to a strictly defined population and there is almost no interregional cross flow of patients. Knowledge of the local incidence of aneurysm rupture [7] thus permits us to conclude that nearly every patient still alive directly after aneurysm bleeding in this region of 934 000 people (Fig. 1) has been included in this study of consecutive cases obtained during a 34 month period ($n = 121$). By assuming an immediate mortality rate of 17% [7], the incidence of aneurysmal SAH can be roughly estimated at 6/100 000 per year, which corroborates data from several western populations.

Figure 2 depicts a flow scheme distribution of the patients into various analysis groups. The total patient population is comprised of 146 cases, 121 of whom arrived at this center alive and the remaining 25 of whom were considered as immediate deaths. Eleven cases (7.5%) were admitted late (>72 h post-SAH), in seven of these cases due entirely to patients' own delay.

[1] Neurosurgical Service, Department of Surgery, University Hospital, Linköping, Sweden

The remaining 110 patients were admitted to this center within 72 h after bleeding (see below). Twelve of these early admitted cases were planned for delayed operation, mainly because of old age. Another 12 patients were devastated immediately upon bleeding and most of them perished soon after arrival without ever being candidates for surgical intervention.

Eighty-six patients were planned for acute operation and nimodipine therapy, which corresponds to 58.9% of all patients with assumed aneurysm rupture. In this subgroup, 62.8% were in grades I and II, 23.3% in grade III, and 14% in grades IV and V when classified according to best grade during the first 24 h. Poor-grade cases also include patients requiring emergency evacuation of large intracranial hematomas. The age distribution and the distribution of ruptured aneurysms were not at significant variance from that obtained for the entire material and, further, corroborates data in the previous literature. In this early surgery group, 11.6% of the patients had aneurysms in the vertebro-basilar circulation.

Of all the patients, 37.7% recovered without evidence of incapacitating neurological or mental sequelae and returned to their premorbid activities. Despite this, several of these patients still complained of discrete psychological disturbances, mainly involving memory, concentration, and endurance. Another 8.9% had permanent neurological or psychological disturbances severe enough to force the patient to enter a less demanding occupation or to conflict with the patient's social reintegration. In 9.6% there were severe incapacitations, and, in most, cases, these patients were institutionalized. The overall mortality, including immediate death, was 43.8% (Fig. 3).

It appears important to understand and to accept that further improvement in overall outcome after aneurysm bleeding rests on two fundamentally different problem complexes. Analysis of causes for poor outcome revealed, as previously stated by others [7], that by 6 months, 55 patients were dead or suffered severe morbidity related to the initial aneurysm bleeding. This figure is equivalent to 60% of all cases with unfavorable outcome (91 patients; Fig. 3). To influence recovery from such brain injury, new dimensions of therapy must be introduced. The most radical approach would be preventive surgery for all aneurysms, although this seems hardly realistic with the methods available today. Hence, much more important at present is the

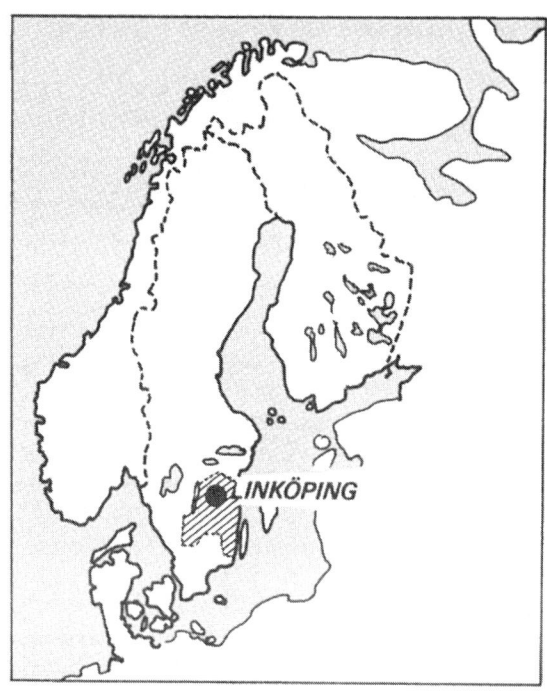

Fig. 1. Map of Scandinavia demonstrating area for which neurosurgical service is provided by the University Hospital Clinic in Linköping

task of optimizing treatment for those patients not devastated by the original bleeding (Hunt-Hess grades I–III; 64.4%, $n = 146$) by striving to eliminate morbidity and mortality from rebleeds, late ischemia, and complications. This group of patients constitute at present 40% of all unfavorable cases and corresponds to 25% of all aneurysm victims in our population.

In the nimodipine group ($n = 86$), delayed brain ischemia with permanent neurological sequelae occurred in 9.3% of the patients when including three cases in which the cause for deterioration could not be definitely ascertained. In grades I–III patients ($n = 75$), four cases (5.3%) suffered from severe ischemia resulting in permanent neurological sequele (three patients) or death (one patient). Several patients with progressive ischemic symptoms responded promptly to increased doses of nimodipine. In our opinion, these observations indicate a true anti-ischemic effect of nimodipine in SAH, although this complication has not been entirely abolished. It may well be that this result can still be further improved through the addition of hypervolemic therapy once ischemia begins despite calcium antagonist medication.

Medical and surgical complications occurred in 10.5% of all surgical cases.

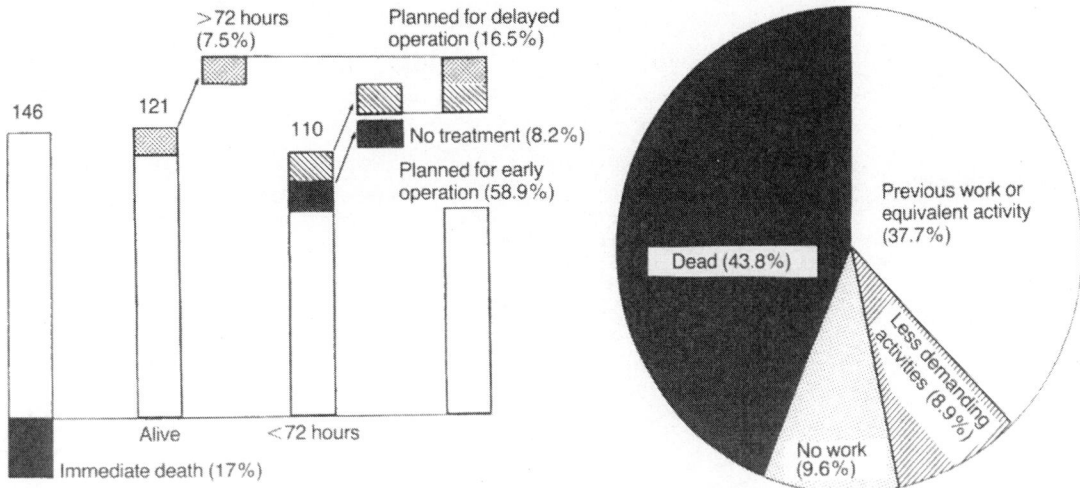

Fig. 2. Flow scheme distribution of 146 consecutive aneurysm bleedings into various analysis groups

Fig. 3. Late overall outcome in a consecutive series of 146 aneurysm victims collected in a defined population of 934 000 people ($n = 146$)

Despite the fact that early operation was undertaken an average of 30.6 ± 1.8 (SEM) hours post SAH, and that nearly 50% of the procedures were started within 24 h and 76% within 48 h after bleeding, no less than 11 patients (10%) suffered severe, proven or strongly suspected rebleedings prior to operation (Fig. 4). The fact that these very early rebleedings were found seems linked to the extreme efficacy of our regional referral system, with 94.5% of all cases admitted in the early stage being seen in this center within 24 h and 50% within 6 h post SAH (Fig. 4).

In six of these 11 cases, clinical deterioration occurred before any diagnostic steps had been undertaken. However, their medical history is strongly suggestive of "ultra-early" rebleedings, since no other reasonable cause for deterioration was revealed either by clinical or radiological examination, and since the final CT findings hardly seemed compatible with the initial condition of the patients. Five rebleedings occurred within 6 h after aneurysm rupture and ten within the first 24 h. "Ultra-early" rebleedings caused death in 7.4% of all patients seen ($n = 121$), which is to be compared with the combined mortality from late cerebral ischemia and surgical-medical complications of 9.1%. This important contribution of "ultra-early" rebleedings to potentially avoidable causes of mortality constitutes the most conspicuous finding of this study [5]. It strongly emphasizes the importance of expeditious transfer of all SAH patients to specialized centers and of minimizing the time used for investigation and preparation for operation. As stated by Ausman et al, the time factor is actually just as important as in the analogous case of a ruptured aortic aneurysm [2]. However, data also clearly show that there is no possibility of completely abolishing rebleedings by only increasing the efficacy of the referral system. It appears necessary to find complementary pharmacological tools to prevent disastrous rebleedings from occurring prior to surgery, and to introduce immediate control of the systemic blood pressure when needed.

It is commonly argued that surgical intervention in the early phase following SAH, especially in patients not being truly grade I, may severely jeopardize outcome by provoking an increased risk for late ischemic complications. However, in our nimodipine-treated cases, all surgical procedures were commenced within three days, 75% within 48 h, and 50% within 24 hours post SAH. With this treatment, 5.3% of grades I–III patients suffered severe late ischemia, which is less than has been observed in recent studies of aneurysm treatment not utilizing calcium antagonists [6, 9], and which corroborates the findings of other authors working with this substance [1, 8].

In a previous series of grades I and II (24 hours) patients operated in this clinic either by delayed approach or early surgery without concomitant nimodipine administration, ischemic symptoms ranging in severity from mild transient deficits to lethal brain infarction occurred in 25%–30% in both groups. Based on these

Rebleedings

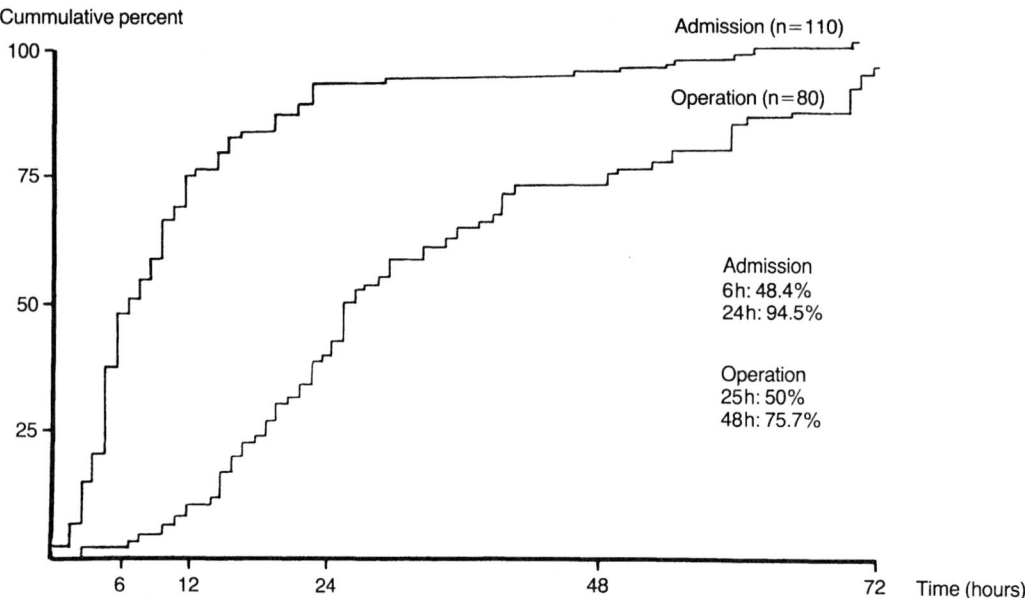

Fig. 4. Time distribution of early rebleeds and cumulative precent as related to admission time and time for surgical intervention of all cases seen within 72 h

data, we cannot agree with authors advocating delayed operation, because of a proposed increased risk for brain infarction with early operation. On the contrary, in our material, "ultra-early" rebleeds have proven fatal with few exceptions, and every effort to prevent this eruptive termination of the patient's life should be undertaken. Obviously, the complex of management problems in SAH is much more multifaceted than a sole requirement for master surgical performance. It appears that, in many countries, restructuring of the regional referral pattern of aneurysmal victims to neurosurgical centers would easily become one of the most rewarding efforts to combat potentially avoidable causes for poor outcome in this serious disease. Active search for yet unruptured aneurysms on a broad scale and their preventive occlusion largely rests in the future neurosurgery.

References

1. Auer LM (1984) Acute operation and preventive nimodipine improve outcome in patients with ruptured cerebral aneurysms. Neurosurgery 15:57–66

2. Ausman JI, Diaz FG, Malik GM, Fielding AS, Son CS (1985) Current management of cerebral aneurysms: Is it based on facts or myths? Surg Neurol 24:625–35

3. Flamm E (1986) Timing of aneurysm surgery 1985. Clin Neurosurg 33:145–158

4. Kassell NF, Peerless SJ, Durward QJ, Beck DW, Drake CG, Adams HP (1982) Treatment of ischemic deficits from vasospasm with intravascular volume expansion and induced arterial hypertension. Neurosurgery 11:337–343

5. Kassell NF, Torner JC (1983) Aneurysmal rebleeding: A preliminary report from the cooperative aneurysm study. Neurosurgery 13:479–481

6. Ljunggren B, Brandt L, Kågström E, Sundbärg G (1981) Results of early operations for ruptured aneurysms. J Neurosurg 54:473–479

7. Ljunggren B, Säveland H, Brandt L, Uski T (1984) Aneurysmal subarachnoid hemorrhage: Total annual outcome in a 1.46 million population. Surg Neurol 22:435–8

8. Ljunggren B, Brandt L, Säveland H, Nilsson P-E, Cronqvist S, Andersson K-E, Vinge E (1984) Outcome in 60 consecutive patients treated with early aneurysm operation and intravenous nimodipine. J Neurosurg 61:864–873

9. Ropper AH, Zervas NT (1984) Outcome 1 year after SAH from cerebral aneurysm. J Neurosurg 60:909–915

Clinical Examination of the Somatosensory Evoked Potential, Auditory Brainstem Response, and Electroencephalography with Ruptured Cerebral Aneurysm in the Acute Stage

Yoji Node and Shozo Nakazawa[1]

Introduction

There are many reports concerned with the monitoring of the multimodality evoked potentials (MEPs) of the hypertensive intracerebral hemorrhage and cerebral infarction [1–3]. However, there exists little information on the MEPs about the ruptured cerebral aneurysm in the acute stage. So, we studied somatosensory evoked potential (SEP), auditory brainstem response (ABR), and electroencephalography (EEG) in patients with ruptured cerebral aneurysms in the acute stage.

Materials and Methods

Forty-six patients were subjected to this study (Table 1). Eighteen were male and 28 were female. The mean age of these patients was 54 years, with a range of 32–79 years. The position of aneurysms were as follows: 22 were anterior communicating artery, 12 were internal carotid

[1] Department of Neurosurgery, Nippon Medical School, Tokyo, Japan

artery, and 12 were middle cerebral artery. We divided these patients into two groups. "Mild" group means the patients of grade III or IV according to Hunt and Kosnik; the number of the patients in this group was 33. "Severe" group means the patients of grade V by Hunt and Kosnik; the number was 13.

SEP, ABR, and EEG was classified into grades I–V (Table 2). The prognosis of the patients was assessed by the Glasgow Outcome scale at 3 months after onset.

Results and Conclusion

The prognosis of the patients was as follows: in the mild group, 14 had a good recovery or moderate disability, seven had severe disability or persistent vegetative state, and 12 were dead. On the other hand, in the severe group, the prognosis of all patients was dead. Figures 1 and 2 show the serial SEP, ABR, and EEG in the patients with ruptured cerebral aneurysm in the mild and severe group. In the mild group, the initial SEP showed that three were grade I, 14 were grade II, ten were grade III, four were grade IV, and two were grade V. In the severe group,

Table 1. Summary of 46 patients with ruptured cerebral aneurysms

Position of aneurysm	Hunt-Kosnik	No. of patients	Prognosis			Total
			GR/MD	SD/PVS	Dead	
Anterior communicating artery	III, IV	16	5	6	5	22
	V	6	0	0	6	
Internal carotid artery	III, IV	9	6	0	3	12
	V	3	0	0	3	
Middle cerebral artery	III, IV	8	3	1	4	12
	V	4	0	0	4	
Total	III, IV	33	14	7	12	46
	V	13	0	0	13	

GR good recovery, *MD* moderate disability, *SD* severe disability, *PVS* persistent vegetative state

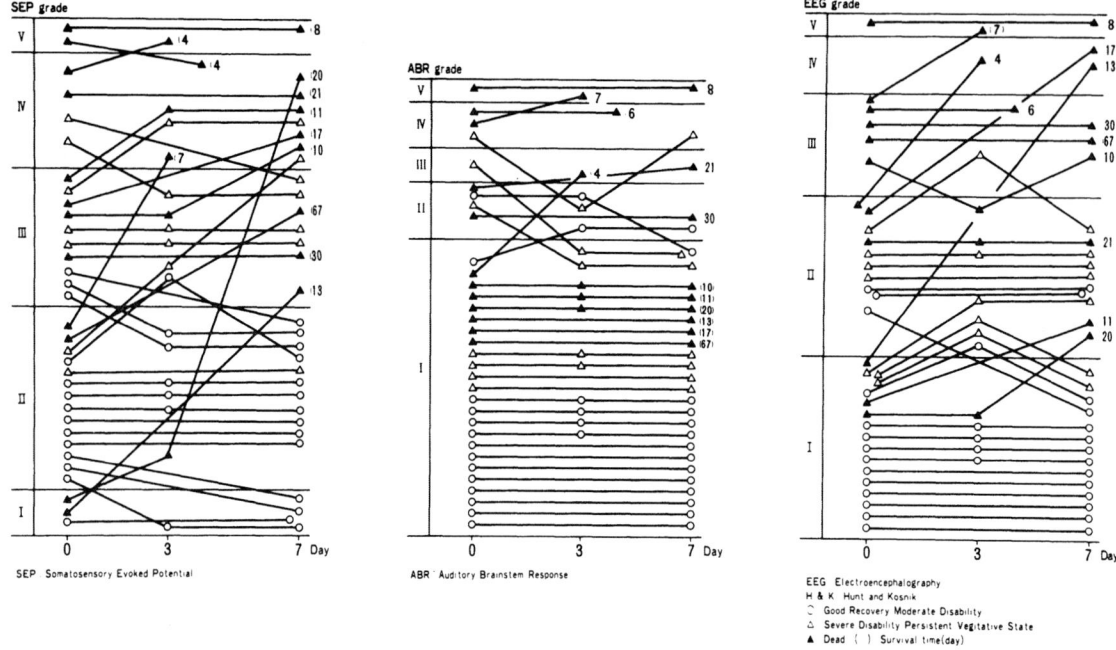

Fig. 1. Serial SEP, ABR, and EEG in the patients with ruptured cerebral aneurysms (Hunt-Kosnik grade III, IV)

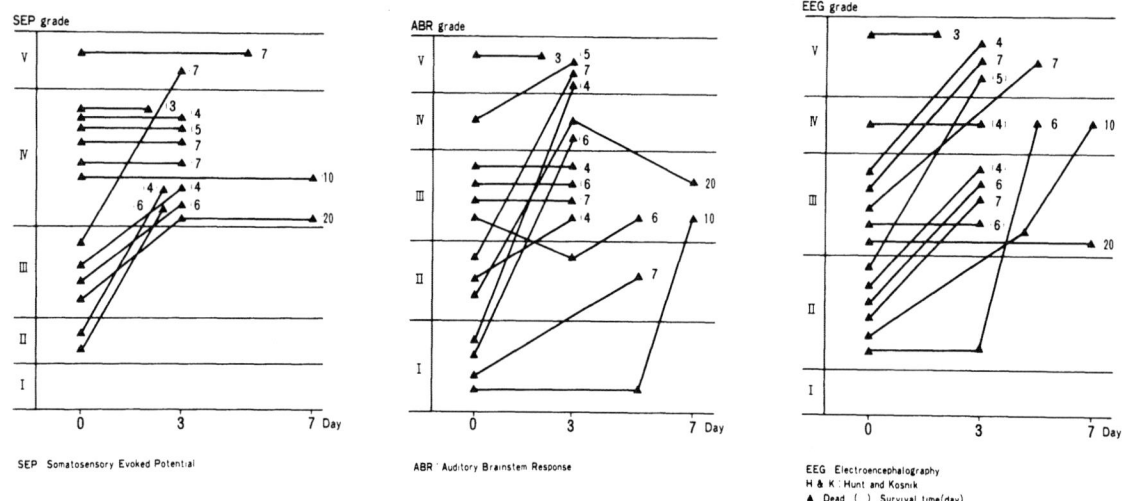

Fig. 2. Serial SEP, ABR, and EEG in the patients with ruptured cerebral aneurysms (Hunt-Kosnik grade V)

two were grade II, four were grade III, six were grade IV, and one was grade V. In the good outcome group, the SEP showed grade II or I within 7 days, even if the initial SEP showed grade III. In the poor outcome group, SEP remained at least grade III, except in one case in which no improvement in SEP was shown. In the dead outcome group, 76% of the patients showed over grade III, and, in the patients presenting grade II or I, SEP became worse from the early stage.

In the mild group, 24 cases (73%) showed grade I in the initial ABR. Meanwhile, in the severe group, four cases (31%) showed grade I in the initial SEP, and another nine patients showed from mild to severe abnormality. In the mild group, 17 cases (52%) showed grade I in the initial EEG, and three dead cases showed grade I, but soon after showed more than grade II. In the severe group, no patient presented grade I upon

Table 2. Classification of SEP, ABR, and EEP

	Grade	Signs
SEP	I	Normal
	II	Remarkable delays in the latency or remarkable decrease in the amplitude of waves over P-3
	III	Disappearance of waves over P-3
	IV	Remarkable delays in the latency or remarkable decrease in the amplitude of waves from P-1 to N-2
	V	Only wave P-1 or flat wave
ABR	I	Normal (I–V latency $\leq$ 2SD)
	II	2SD < I–V latency $\leq$ 4SD
	III	4SD < I–V latency $\leq$ 6SD
	IV	6SD < I–V latency
	V	Only wave I or nearly flat record
EEG	I	Predominant alpha with or without rare theta
	II	Predominant theta
	III	Predominant theta with some delta
	IV	Predominant delta
	V	A nearly flat record or EEG at all

SD standard deviation, *SEP* somatosensory evoked potential, *ABR* aiditory brainstem response, *ABR* aiditory brainstem response, *EEG* electroencephalography

initial EEG, and, in the mildly abnormal group, EEG showed grade III or IV gradually. From these results, initial SEP, ABR, and EEG presented mild to severe abnormality from the early stage. On the contrary, in the mild group, there was a tendency for the SEP to show abnormality earlier than the ABR or EEG.

References

1. Kuchiwaki H, Kageyama N, Furuse M, Nakaya T, Tohyama K (1984) A study of somatosensory-evoked potential and intracranial pressure in a lateral type of experimentally induced hematoma in the internal capsule of dogs. Jpn J Stroke 6:398–404
2. Shigemori M, Yuge T, Kawasaki K, Watanabe M, Kuramoto S (1984) Significance of multimodality-evoked potentials (SEPs) in hypertensive intracerebral (basal ganglionic) hemorrhage. Jpn J Stroke 6:398–404
3. Shigemori M, Yuge T, Kawasaki K, Nakashima H, Kuramoto S (1986) Extension of hematoma and brain dysfunction in hypertensive ganglionic hemorrhage: II. Analysis by multimodality-evoked potentials (MEPs). Jpn J Stroke 8:219–223

Somatosensory Evoked Potential Monitoring in Aneurysm Surgery

J.J.A. Mooij[1], A. Buchthal[2], and M. Belopavlovic[2]

Introduction

The only adequate treatment for cerebral saccular aneurysms is careful dissection by microsurgical techniques and clipping of the existing or surgically created neck. Dissection can be done more safely in difficult aneurysms when the intraluminal pressure has been lowered, thus avoiding inadvertent rupture of the aneurysm. Elective temporary occlusion of parent arteries is now being increasingly used for this purpose as an alternative to pharmacologically induced systemic arterial hypotension [2, 4, 9]. After subarachnoid hemorrhage (SAH), systemic hypotension can result in cerebral hypoperfusion due to failure of blood flow autoregulation in affected areas. Moreover, aneurysm rupture can occur in spite of systemic hypotension; this can have devastating consequences.

Temporary occlusion of a parent artery reduces the risk of aneurysmal rupture to a minimum and creates the best circumstances for an ideal dissection. Occlusion of a cerebral artery, although allowing most of the brain to be perfused normally, carries the risk of ischemic damage in a circumscribed area of the artery's territory. Somatosensory evoked potential (SEP) monitoring has been shown to be promising as an intraoperative technique for indicating the time for which occlusion can be allowed without the risk of permanent ischemic neuronal damage [3, 5, 6]. This is due to the fact that when cerebral blood flow is reduced, synaptic transmission—and thus neuronal function—starts to fail when the flow falls to below 20 ml/100 g/min. At flow values of 8–10 ml/100 g/min, membrane failure occurs, with a massive release of intracellular potassium, resulting in permanent damage. Between these two flow thresholds there is a range of cerebral blood flow where neurons no longer function but retain a capacity for full functional recovery. This capacity becomes time limited, with more severe degrees of ischemia being tolerated for progressively shorter periods of time. Cerebral tissue perfused by flows in this range is known as the ischemic penumbra, and implies that the SEP might serve as an early warning of a critical degree of ischemia during temporary occlusion of a cerebral artery. In the case of the middle cerebral artery (MCA), SEPs by contralateral median nerve stimulation at the wrist monitor part of the MCA territory, being the cortex representing the palm of the hand.

The value of this type of SEP monitoring in elective temporary occlusion of the MCA during surgery on large MCA bifurcation aneurysms was assessed in a preliminary series of patients.

Material and Methods

In 15 cases with aneurysms at the middle cerebral artery (MCA) bifurcation, SEP monitoring was employed during temporary occlusion of the M_1 segment. All cases except one were in Hunt and Hess's grade I or II preoperatively. Two cases underwent early surgery. Two patients were operated upon for unruptured aneurysms.

Surgery

Surgery was carried out under dexamethasone cover via a pterional transsylvian approach using microsurgical techniques. In 13 of the 15 cases, the M_1 segment of the MCA was occluded distally, about 5 mm proximal to its termination and distal to the proximal lateral striate arteries. A proximal occlusion was employed in two cases.

Anesthesia

Anesthesia was induced with sodium thiopentone and suxamethonium chloride and maintained with pethidine, pancuronium, and ventilation

---

Departments of Neurosurgery[1] and Anaesthesia[2], University Hospital, Groningen, The Netherlands

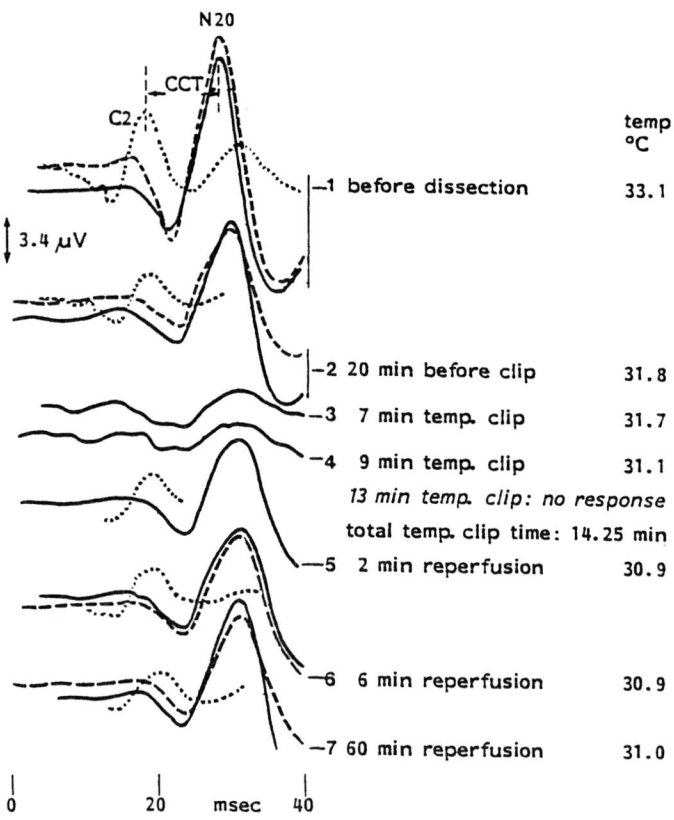

Fig. 1. Intraoperative SEP monitoring during dissection and definite clipping of a large MCA bifuraction aneurysm, using temporary occlusion of M1 for 14.25 minutes. (...) recording over cervical spine (C2), (---) recording N_{20} peak over cortex, nonoperated side, (—) recording N_{20} peak over cortex, operated side, CCT central conduction time. SEPs are recorded negative upward; temperatures are nasopharyngeal throughout

with a nitrous oxide oxygen mixture. Moderate hypothermia was induced by surface cooling following premedication with a lytic cocktail. Sodium nitroprusside was used as needed to control the arterial blood pressure (SABP). During the arterial occlusion the SABP was raised to a high normal level. Arterial carbon dioxide tension (PCO_2) was kept constant at 4.0 to 4.5 kPa. Volatile anesthetic agents other than nitrous oxide were not used.

One case was ventilated with 100% oxygen starting a short time before the arterial occlusion, and given barbiturates to ensure an adequate depth of anesthesia during that time. One case with two MCA aneurysms was loaded prophylactically with 44 mg/kg pentobarbitone.

SEP Monitoring

SEPs in response to median nerve stimulation at the wrist were monitored using recording electrodes at C_3 and C_4 (American EEG Society), and over the cervical spine with a frontal reference. Square waves of 200 μs were delivered via skin contact electrodes over the median nerve at the wrist at a rate of five–seven per second and

with an intensity of 12–15 mA. Nicolet CA 1000 equipment was used and 500 responses averaged whenever possible; during the occlusion period, however, a smaller number usually had to be accepted. Evaluation of the recordings was based on the technique of Hume and Cant [1], using the central conduction time (CCT) to compare responses in the two hemispheres. The CCT is the time interval between the peak recorded over the cervical spine and the N_{20} peak recorded over the cortex, and eliminates the contribution of variations in peripheral conduction time.

Results

An example of SEP monitoring is presented in Fig. 1. The SEP has disappeared after 13 min. MCA occlusion and full recovery of the response is seen after 2 min of reperfusion.

Occlusion times ranged between 6.3 and 52 min at nasopharyngeal temperatures of 28.6°–31.1°C.

Table 1 summarizes the data of the seven patients in whom the SEP was lost during temporary clipping of the M_1. Three of these cases lost

Table 1. Loss of SEP in MCA occlusion

Case	SEP lost (min)	Comments
1	5	Early surgery
2	6, 5	Severe vasospasm, prox. M_1 occlusion
3	6	Early surgery, deficit at SAH
4	9	H & H III, extensive deficit at SAH, no backflow
5	11	Deficit at SAH
6	13	Slight deficit at SAH, prox. M_1 occlusion
7	17	None

SAH subarachnoid hemmorhage

Table 2. Loss of SEP in MCA occlusion and outcome

Case	SEP lost (min)	SEP absent (min)	Complications
1[a]	5	4	Transient new deficit 2 weeks
2	6	4	Transient new
	5	11	deficit <24 h
4[b]	9	7	Increased deficit
3[a], 5–7	6–17	2	None

[a] Early surgery
[b] Hunt-Hess III + infarct

Table 3. SEP preserved in MCA occlusion

Case	Occlusion time (min)	CCT prolong	Comments
9	18	2 ms	Some backflow
10	19.1	0.9	None
11	9	1.2	Unruptured
	11.8	0.6	
	3	None	
12	18.4	0.52	Unruptured
8	13	None	None
14	6.3	None	100% O_2
15	28, 29	None	44 mg/kg PB
13	16, 52	None	Good backflow

CCT central conduction time, *PB* pentobarbitone

the SEP within 6 min; two of these had early surgery, one had intraoperative vasospasm. A further three lost the SEP between 9 and 13 min. All of these had a deficit at the time of SAH, and in one of these the deficit persisted to the time of operation.

In Table 2, the relation is shown between the time for which MCA occlusion was continued in these cases after the evoked potential was lost and the clinical results. Only one patient showed a permanently increased deficit, after a loss of the SEP within 9 min of occlusion, and a total occlusion time of 15.8 min. The transient deficit in case 1 resolved after 2 weeks, and that in case 2 within 24 h. Two minutes of occlusion after the SEP was lost was tolerated well by four cases.

The SEP was preserved in the other eight cases (Table 3). In half of these cases, the CCT was prolonged during temporary M_1 occlusion. No prolongation of the CCT was seen in the other four cases. These include the two cases given a pentobarbitone load and ventilated with pure oxygen. The length of occlusion time in case 13 without any change in SEP is perhaps remarkable. Neurological outcome was excellent in all eight cases.

Discussion

The use of the SEP as a monitor of brain ischemia during the occlusion of a cerebral artery presupposes that the cortical area or pathway being monitored will be maximally affected by the ischemia resulting from the occlusion. The modality or modalities to be monitored must, therefore, be carefully chosen in order to achieve this. In the case of the MCA, the sensory cortex representing the palm of the hand can conveniently be monitored by means of the SEP in response to stimulation of the contralateral median nerve at the wrist, together with the intervening pathway. It must nevertheless be borne in mind that any one SEP modality provides information pertaining exclusively to that specific pathway, from stimulus and sense organ to cortex, while the state of other sensory pathways and cortical areas, the motor cortex and subcortical structures supplied by perforating vessels, can only be inferred. Inhomogeneities of perfusion within the territory of a cerebral artery cannot be ruled out and may be accentuated during occlusion of that artery in the presence of vascular pathology, such as a spastic or stenotic segment. Even severe local ischemia cannot be detected if the monitored pathway is not significantly affected. This must be regarded as a limitation of the technique.

The wide variation in MCA occlusion time before the SEP was lost or affected in the cases presented here must be related at least in part to correspondingly large variations in backflow or collateral perfusion. Some specific risk factors, however, seem to appear from the present data. These are early surgery and neurological deficit immediately preoperative or transiently manifest at the time of the SAH. From experimental work it is known that repeated episodes of cerebral ischemia render the brain more susceptible to further episodes [8]. Since SAH must be regarded as an ischemic insult whose severity is indicated by any neurological deficit at that time, a temporary vascular occlusion during early surgery, or in the presence of a neurological deficit, being a second period of ischemia, entails a higher risk than in healthy brain.

The factors associated with poor tolerance of temporary occlusion seen in the cases discussed here are factors recognized to carry an increased risk in aneurysm surgery in general. Appropriate SEP monitoring during temporary clipping in aneurysm surgery provides a means for early detection of imminent dangers, and this offers the possibility of taking appropriate measures in time. These include a period of reperfusion before reapplying the temporary clip, completing the dissection, and clipping the aneurysmal neck. Raising the arterial blood pressure during the occlusion period maximizes collateral flow [10]. Oxygen demand can be reduced by the use of hypothermia, which was used in all our cases. It is striking that under these circumstances, long occlusion times could be used with a relatively low morbidity compared with those reported at normothermia [2–5,9]. Tolerance to ischemia can also be increased by the use of high doses of barbiturates [7], as we did in one of the cases presented. SEP monitoring remained possible under those circumstances. Ventilation with 100% oxygen, infusion of hypertonic mannitol, and the use of perfluorocarbons may provide further means of increasing tolerance to temporary vascular occlusion.

The data presented here on 15 MCA aneurysm cases suggest that SEP monitoring has the capacity to make a major contribution to the avoidance of neurological damage in cerebral aneurysm surgery. Criteria about critical values of CCT prolongation and times for which absence of the SEP can be tolerated in the prevailing circumstances have to be established in larger series [3, 5].

References

1. Hume AL, Cant BR (1978) Conduction time in central somatosensory pathways in man. Electroenceph Clin Neurophysiol 45:361–375
2. Jabre A, Symon L (1987) Temporary vascular occlusion during aneurysm surgery. Surg Neurol 27:47–63
3. Kidooka M, Nakasu Y, Watanabe K, Matsuda M, Hauda J (1987) Monitoring of somatosensory evoked potentials during aneurysm surgery. Surg Neurol 27:69–76
4. Ljunggren B, Säveland H, Brandt L, Kagström E, Rehncrona S, Nilsson PE (1983) Temporary clipping during early operation for ruptured aneurysm: Preliminary report. Neurosurgery 12:525–530
5. Momma F, Wang AD, Symon L (1987) Effects of temporary arterial occlusion on somatosensory evoked responses in aneurysm surgery. Surg Neurol 27:343–352
6. Mooij JJA, Buchthal A, Belopavlovic M (1987) Somatosensory evoked potential monitoring in temporary middle cerebral artery occlusion during aneurysm surgery. Neurosurgery 21:492-496
7. Selman WR, Spetzler RF, Roessmann UR, Rosenblatt JI, Crumrine R (1981) Barbiturate-induced coma for focal cerebral ischemia: Effect after temporary and permanent middle cerebral artery occlusion. J Neurosurg 55:220–226
8. Spetzler RF, Selman WR, Weinstein P, Townsend J, Mehdorn M, Tellos D, Crumrine RC, Macko R (1980) Chronic reversible cerebral ischemia: Evaluation of a new baboon model. Neurosurgery 7:257–261
9. Suzuki J, Yoshimomto T, Kayama T (1984) Surgical treatment of middle cerebral artery aneurysms. J Neurosurg 61:17–23
10. Symon L (1978) Disordered cerebrovascular physiology in aneurysmal subarachnoid hemorrhage. Acta Neurochirurg 41:7–22

The Role of Intraoperative Monitoring of Sensory Evoked Potentials During Cerebrovascular Surgery

Fred Gentili, William M. Lougheed, Hemant Ghate, and Fumio Shichijo[1]

Despite advances in instrumentation and the use of microsurgical techniques, major neurovascular procedures still carry significant risk for neurological deficit. This is, in part, related to our inability to properly monitor brain function in the anesthetized patient and, thus, interpret the effects, beneficial or otherwise, of our various intraoperative manipulations. Raw electroencephalogram (EEG) activity, compressed spectral array, and cerebral blood flow have all been used to monitor the central nervous system during surgery, but these techniques are cumbersome, the results obtained not uniform, and their reliability inconsistent.

More recently, there has been an increasing interest in the use of evoked potentials to monitor brain function intraoperatively in a more direct and reliable manner [1]. The technique appears to satisfy a number of criteria required for a good central nervous system (CNS) monitoring system. It allows monitoring of patients under anesthesia, independant of their level of consciousness, and recordings can be made continuously and safely from surface or needle electrodes. As direct electrophysiological responses of the nervous system to specific external sensory stimuli, sensory evoked potentials (SEPs), unlike spontaneous EEG activity, reflect the functional capabilities of specific neuronal pathways. SEP parameters also provide objective measurements that can be quantitatively and statistically analyzed. This report summarizes our experience with intraoperative monitoring of SEPs and details our findings in a group of patients undergoing neurovascular procedures.

Methods and Materials

From September 1982 to December 1986, SEPs were monitored intraoperatively in 223 patients undergoing a variety of neurovascular procedures (Table 1). While in the majority of patients, somatosensory evoked potentials (SSEP) alone were monitored, patients with vascular lesions in the posterior fossa usually had both SSEP and brain stem auditory evoked potentials (BAEP) recorded.

The technique for intraoperative recording of SSEP was modified from that of Symon et al. [3]. SSEPs are generated by stimulation of the median nerve at the wrist or posterior tibial nerve at the ankle. Square wave pulses of 0.15 ms duration were delivered at a rate of 4.1 per second using a constant current stimulator (Nicolet 1003). Stimulus intensity was sufficient to sustain a thumb twitch. Recording electrodes were placed on the scalp over the areas of the right and left somatosensory cortex (C3 and C4 positions on the International 10/20 EEG system), over the surface of the C2 vertebra, and over Erb's point. With lower limb stimulation, recording was from a vertex electrode placed 2 cm behind Cz. The reference electrode was placed in the midforehead (FPz). Usually 128 or 512 responses were averaged and short latency (less than 50 msec) responses recorded simultaneously over Erb's point (N 9, brachial plexus wave), C2 (N 14, dorsal column wave), and from the ipsilateral and contralateral cortex (N 20 wave).

BAEPs were recorded using standard parameters [2]. In addition to the standard analysis of

Table 1. Intraoperative monitoring of sensory evoked potentials

Cerebrovascular procedures	No. of cases
Carotid endarterectomy	125
Cerebral aneurysm	67
EC-IC/long vein bypass	20
AVM	11
Total	223

EC-IC extracranial-intracranial, AVM arteriovenous malformations

[1] Division of Neurosurgery, Toronto General Hospital, University of Toronto, Toronto, Canada

amplitude, wave form, and latency of the various waves, derived variables such as central conduction time (CCT), interpeak latencies, and interhemispheric difference (IHD) were also measured. All recordings were carried out using a Nicolet CA 1000 system and data stored on floppy disks.

Patients to be monitored intraoperatively had preoperative recordings to obtain preanesthetic values and to document any preexisting central or peripheral nervous system abnormality. A standardized anesthetic protocol was followed whenever possible to minimize anesthetic and other drug variables. Once anesthetic baseline values were obtained, each patient acted as his own control by comparing one cerebral hemisphere to the other. Recordings were carried out almost continuously throughout the operative procedure. With experience, we have been able to record SEPs intraoperatively in a reliable and reproducible manner in over 90% of patients. The most frequent cause of failure remains electrical interference. With experience, SEP monitoring should rarely prolong the average surgical procedure by more than 10–15 min.

Results

Minor alterations in intraoperative SEP parameters were noted in the majority of patients monitored, and were most often related to changes in anesthetic concentration, drug administration, and alteration in cardiovascular and respiratory parameters. More significant changes in amplitude and latencies were most commonly seen with temporary vessel occlusion and the use of induced hypotension.

Based on our initial experience in 50 patients, a grading system for SEP changes was developed in an attempt to better analyze the data and assess the reliability and prognostic value of the technique [3]. The grading system for SSEP, based on central conduction time (CCT), amplitude of the major cortical wave (N 20), and IHD is shown in Table 2. Note that all grades refer to anesthetic baseline values and not preoperative parameters.

SSEP during Carotid Endarterectomy

Monitoring of SSEPs was used in 125 patients undergoing carotid endarterectomy as a means

Table 2. Grading of intraoperative somatosensory evoked potential changes

Grade	Criterion (changes from anesthetic baseline)
I	No change from anesthetic baseline
II	↑In CCT < 1.0 ms IHD < 0.5 ms
	↓In amplitude < 50% (N_{20} wave)
III	↑In CCT ≥ 1.0 ms IHD ≥ 1.0 ms
	↓In amplitude ≥ 50% (N_{20} wave)
IV	Loss of N_{20} wave

CCT central conduction time, *IHD* interhemispheric difference

of assessing the adequacy of cerebral perfusion and, thus, the need for placement of a temporary bypass shunt. Fifty-five percent of the patients showed only minor changes in SSEP parameters (grades I and II) at the time of carotid clamping. Only one patient in this group developed an immediate postoperative deficit. A major change in SEP parameters (grades III and IV) was noted following carotid clamping in 45% of patients. Nine of these patients developed immediate postoperative neurological deficits which were permanent in two. In patients with grades I and II changes, the occurrence of immediate or delayed postoperative deficit was independent of the use of a bypass shunt. Of the patients showing grades III and IV changes at the time of carotid clamping, the changes reverted back to grades I and II with placement of a temporary bypass shunt in 55%. None of these patients developed an immediate postoperative neurological deficit. Of the 20 patients showing persistent grades III and IV changes despite shunting, the changes had reverted to grades I and II in two-thirds by the time of closure, with no patient showing an immediate postoperative deficit. By contrast, of seven patients showing grades III and IV changes which persisted until the time of closure, five developed immediate postoperative deficit. Of patients with grades III and IV changes at carotid clamping who did not have placement of a temporary bypass shunt, a full 50% showed immediate postoperative deficit. By contrast, of patients with grades III and IV changes at clamping who had shunt placement, 11% showed immediate postoperative deficit.

Of the parameters utilized to grade SEP changes, alteration in amplitude of the major cortical wave (N 20) appeared to be more sensitive in predicting postoperative deficit than either changes in central conduction time or in IHD.

SSEP Monitoring in Aneurysm Surgery

Sixty-six patients undergoing clipping of intracranial aneurysms were monitored. There were 39 females and 27 males, aged 15–78 years. SSEPs were monitored in all patients. In addition, patients with vertebrobasilar aneurysms had BAEP recorded. While minor changes in BAEP and SSEP parameters from anesthetic baseline values were seen in all patients, significant alterations (grades III and IV) were noted in only 17 (25%). Of the 49 patients showing only grades I and II changes, only one patient developed a postoperative sensorimotor deficit. Of 17 patients with grades III and IV changes intraoperatively, seven experienced postoperative sensorimotor deficits. A grades III and IV change, which was reversible, was seen in 13 patients and was associated with an immediate postoperative sensorimotor deficit in three. All patients who developed permanent grade III or IV changes intraoperatively, developed a postoperative deficit. A three month follow-up of the patients with immediate postoperative sensorimotor deficits revealed that the one patient with the grades I and II changes, and the three patients with the temporary and reversible grades III and IV alterations, all had complete or significant improvement in their neurological deficits. By contrast, of the four patients with permanent grades III and IV change, three remained with persistent hemiplegia and one patient died.

Grades III and IV changes were related in the majority of patients either to temporary clipping of parent vessels during aneurysm dissection or to the use of induced hypotension. The level of blood pressure at which grades III and IV changes occurred varied considerably from one patient to another. While dural opening and turning of the bone flap did not significantly alter SEP parameters from anesthetic baseline, brain retraction alone was associated with grades III and IV changes in three patients. Complete loss of the major cortical wave was seen in five patients; in four related to temporary clipping of a major parent vessel and in one to profound hypotension. The cortical wave was lost for periods ranging from 3 to 35 min. Removal of temporary clips or blood pressure elevation resulted in progressive recovery of conduction velocity and amplitude over a 5- to 10-min period in all but one patient.

Discussion

There is a need to monitor neurological function during major neurovascular procedures which are known to carry risk for neurological deficit. The ideal method of intraoperative monitoring of brain function would be applicable to the anesthetized patient, easy to use, accurate, and directly reflect the functional status of neural structures. None of the methods currently available have proven successful. The use of SEP monitoring would appear to offer promise in this regard. Our results suggest that intraoperative monitoring of SEPs may provide a reliable and objective assessment of brain function and accurately predict the development of postoperative neurological deficits. The development of a grading system for SEP changes has been important in determining quantitative tolerance limits for intraoperative SEP alterations. Presently, we use changes in SSEP parameters as the only criteria for tolerance to carotid clamping and the need for temporary shunting during carotid endarterectomy. Sensitivity and specificity of the technique in predicting postoperative deficit has been 90% and 82%, respectively. In our last 50 patients, using the criteria of shunting with the development of grades III and IV changes, we have had only one postoperative deficit which occurred 1 week postoperatively, and only 15% have required shunt placement.

In aneurysm surgery, SEP monitoring has been useful in determining the degree of hypotension, the duration of temporary clipping, and in helping perfect the position of the permanent clip. There has been a high correlation between grades III and IV changes and the development of immediate postoperative sensorimotor deficits. The sensitivity and specificity of the technique has been 87.5% and 82.8%, respectively. In addition, there has been a very high correlation with long-term prognosis in patients with postoperative sensorimotor deficit. The important question—whether surgical intervention based on SEP changes can actually prevent such deficits—remains to be answered. Only with further experience and proper data analysis will the ultimate role of this technique be defined.

References

1. Gentili F, Lougheed WM, Yamashiro K, Corrado C (1985) Monitoring of sensory evoked potentials during surgery of skull base tumors. Can J Neurol Sci 12:336–340

2. Grundy BL (1983) Intraoperative monitoring of sensory-evoked potentials. Anaesthesiology 58: 72–87

3. Symon L, Wong AD, Costa E, Silva I, Gentili F (1984) Perioperative use of somatosensory evoked responses in aneurysm surgery. J Neurosurg 60:269–275

Increase in Cerebral Blood Flow Produced by a Serotonin Antagonist Following Experimental Carotid Arteriotomy

B.A. Bell, B.K. Misra, and J.D. Miller[1]

Introduction

The value of carotid endarterectomy in the management of carotid stenosis remains controversial. The chances of a patient subjected to carotid endarterectomy sustaining a major stroke or dying varies widely, but can be as high as 21% [3]. The variation in surgical results and the plethora of operative techniques, show that the ideal technique has yet to be defined. There is clearly room for the evaluation of measures that would make the operation safer in the hands of all surgeons.

The patients are elderly, and many have hypertension and are long-term smokers with chronic obstructive airways disease [4]. They are therefore prone to systemic insults like arterial hypotension, hypoxia, hypovolemia, pneumonia, and pulmonary emboli. The brain is normally cushioned from insults of this sort by the physiological mechanisms producing cerebral vasodilatation. Impairment of these protective cerebrovascular responses occurs after concussive head injury [8] after cerebral ischemia [10] and after subarachnoid hemorrhage [5]. Impairment after common carotid artery surgery has been detected in baboons [9] and in rats [2]. Impaired cerebrovascular reactivity following carotid endarterectomy may be a major contributor to the morbidity and mortality in man, bearing in mind the possibility of hypoxia and hypercapnia in the postoperative phase, due to underlying lung disease. Measures that restore cerebrovascular reactivity where it is impaired by surgery would therefore be a valuable therapeutic maneuver. These experiments aim to explore the effect of a serotonin S_2 receptor antagonist on cerebral blood flow (CBF) and CO_2 reactivity, after common carotid arteriotomy in a rat model of carotid endarterectomy [2].

---

[1] University Department of Clinical Neurosciences, Western General Hospital, Edinburgh, Scotland

Methods

Rats weighing between 300 and 450 g were anesthetised with intraperitoneal urethane (1.2 g/kg), and a tracheostomy was performed. The femoral artery and vein were cannulated and blood pressure was measured from the femoral arterial catheter. Femoral arterial samples of 50 μl were taken for blood gas analysis. Naftidrofuryl was given via a microprocessor controlled pediatric infusion pump at 2 mg/kg/h via the femoral vein, and an equivalent volume of normal saline was given to untreated animals via the femoral vein.

A silver/silver chloride reference electrode was placed in a subcutaneous pouch on the abdominal wall, and two parasagittal burr holes were made with a high speed drill, leaving the dura mater intact. Gallamine triethiodide (4 mg/kg) was given to paralyse the rat, and intermittent positive pressure ventilation was applied to the tracheostomy with a Harvard 680 rodent ventilator. Micromanipulators were used to pass 90% platinum/10% iridium electrodes through the dura tangentially into the cortex. The burr holes were sealed and the electrodes were anchored with cold setting dental acrylic. Two blood flow measurement electrodes were used in each cerebral hemisphere and regional cerebral blood flow was measured by hydrogen clearance [1, 7]. Up to ten CBF measurements were made in each rat by mixing hydrogen gas in a concentration of 5% into the ventilation circuit. Blood pressure and arterial oxygen tension were kept stable, but ventilation rate and volume were altered to vary arterial carbon dioxide tension within the range of 20–60 mmHg, to allow flow measurements at differing levels of pCO_2 within this range. A control series of 15 rats determined the normal response of CBF in this particular rat model to variations in arterial pCO_2. A second control group of 15 rats had the measurements repeated during treatment with naftidrofuryl.

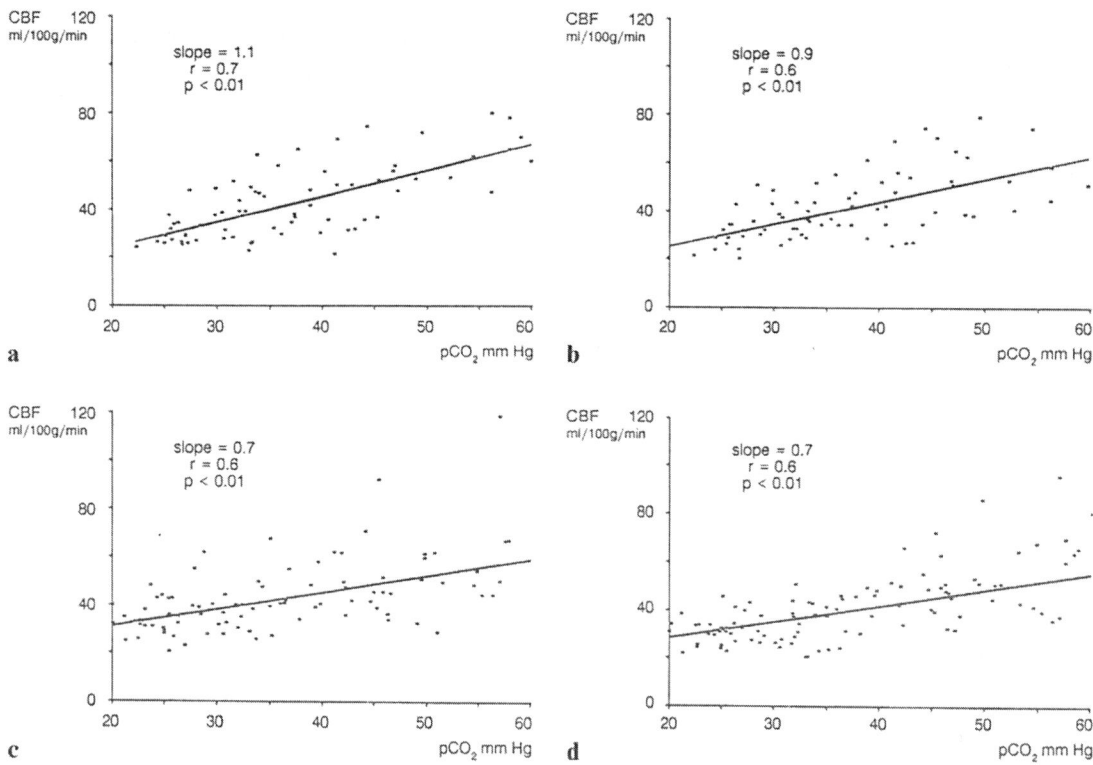

Fig. 1a–d. Cerebral blood flow (*CBF*) in 15 control rats. **a** Left hemisphere. **b** Right hemisphere; CBF in 15 control rats given naftidrofuryl. **c** Left hemisphere. **d** Right hemisphere

The third series of 15 rats had the measurements repeated after dissection and ligation of the common carotid artery, and the effect of permanent carotid ligation was determined. In a fourth series of 15 rats, measurements were repeated after a 5-mm linear arteriotomy between temporary clamps using the operating microscope, and microvascular closure with 10/0 prolene. A fifth series of 15 rats had the measurements repeated following arteriotomy, with an infusion of naftidrofuryl running throughout the experiment.

The sixth series of 15 rats had measurements made after sham arteriotomy, where one common carotid artery was temporarily isolated between microvascular clamps for 30 min, but no arteriotomy incison was made. A final series of 15 rats had an identical sham arteriotomy, but were treated with naftidrofuryl infusion. Rats undergoing arteriotomy and sham arteriotomy were heparinized with 100 units/kg intravenously before application of the temporary clamps.

Results

In the control group, mean CBF at normocapnia (pCO_2 of 40 mmHg) was 44.7 ml/100 g/min and mean CO_2 reactivity was 1 ml/100 g/min/torr (Fig. 1a, b). In the second group of 15 control rats given a naftidrofuryl infusion, normocapnic CBF was 43.5 ml/100 g/min and CO_2 reactivity was 0.7 ml/100 g/min/torr (Fig. 1c, d). In the third group of rats subjected to permanent carotid ligation, normocapnic CBF was 41.5 ml/100 g/min and reactivity 0.8 ml/100 g/min/torr (Fig. 2a, b). In the fourth group of 15 rats subjected to carotid arteriotomy, normocapnic CBF fell to 32.3 ml/100 g/min, and CO_2 reactivity to 0.4 ml/100 g/min/torr (Fig. 2c, d). In the fifth group of 15 rats subjected to arteriotomy with a naftidrofuryl infusion, normocapnic CBF improved to 39.2 ml/100 g/min, and CO_2 reactivity to 0.9 ml/100 g/min/torr (Fig. 3a, b). In the sixth group of 15 rats subjected to sham arteriotomy, normocapnic CBF was 28.1 ml/100 g/min, and CO_2 reactivity was 0.3 ml/100 g/min/torr (Fig. 3c, d). In the seventh group of 15 rats, where a

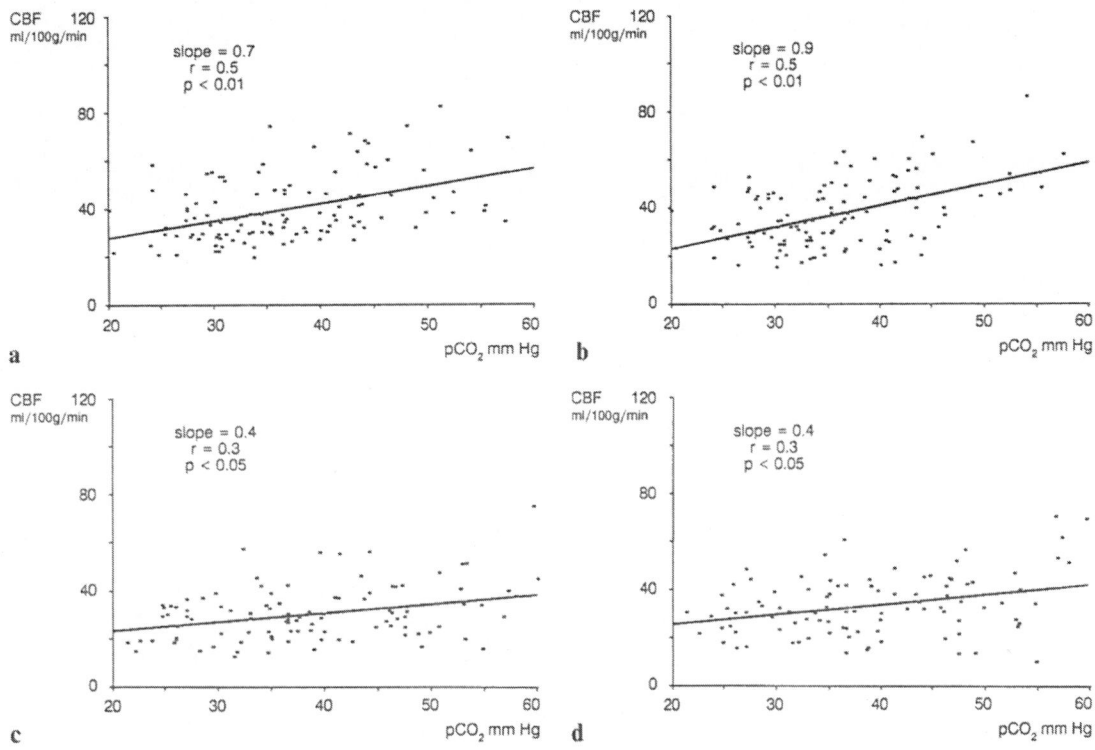

Fig. 2a–d. Cerebral blood flow (*CBF*) in 15 rats subjected to carotid ligation. **a** Contralateral hemisphere. **b** Ipsilateral hemisphere; CBF in 15 rats subjected to carotid arteriotomy. **c** Contralateral hemisphere. **d** Ipsilateral hemisphere

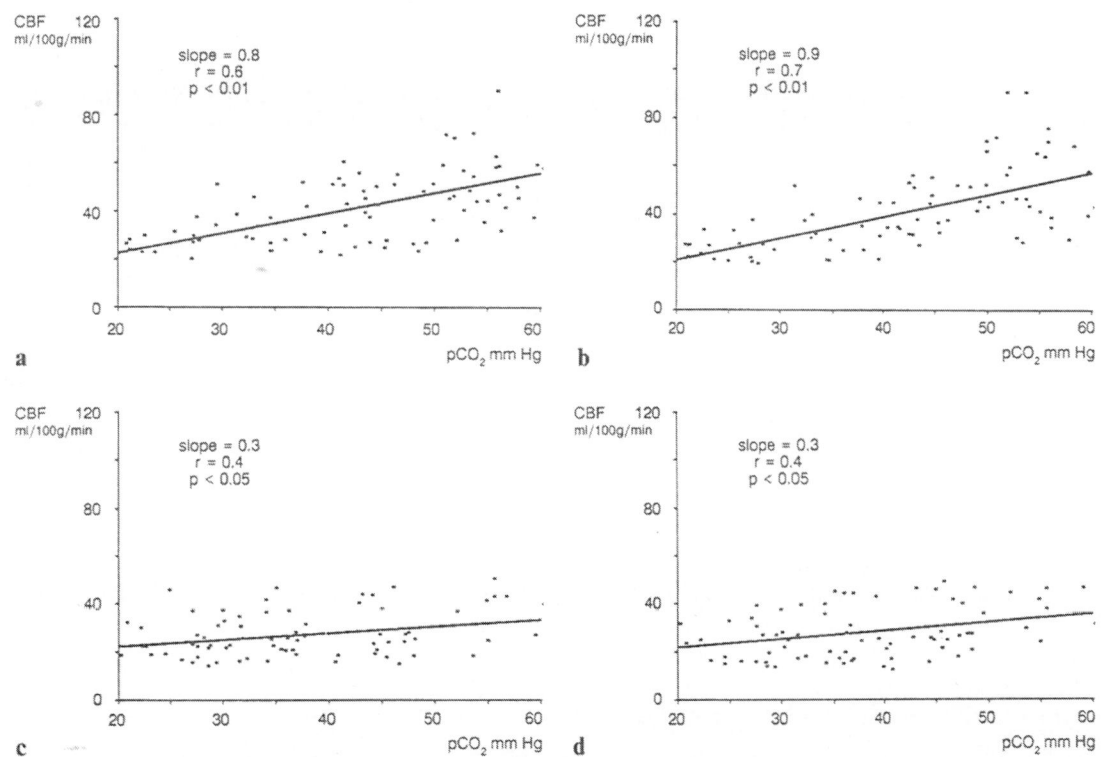

Fig. 3a–d. Cerebral blood flow (*CBF*) in 15 rats given naftidrofuryl and subjected to arteriotomy. **a** Contralateral hemisphere. **b** Ipsilateral hemisphere; CBF in 15 rats subjected to sham arteriotomy. **c** Contralateral hemisphere. **d** Ipsilateral hemisphere

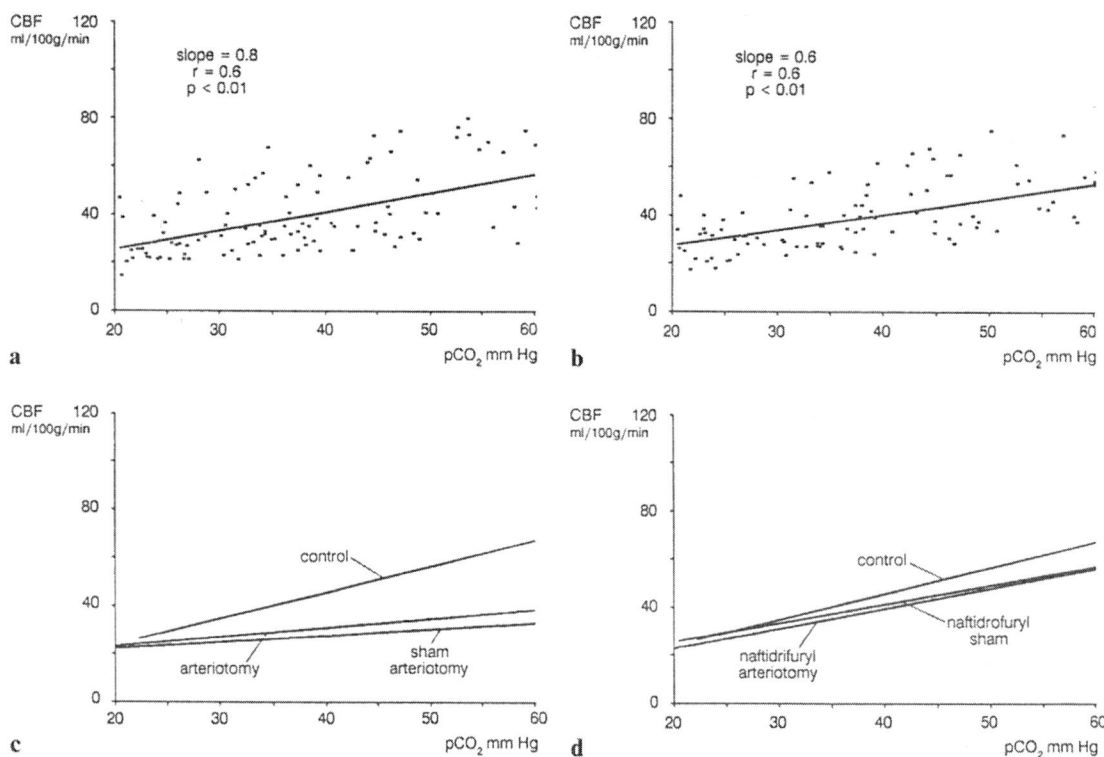

Fig. 4a–d. Cerebral blood flow (*CBF*) in 15 rats given naftidrofuryl and subjected to sham arteriotomy. **a** Contralateral hemisphere. **b** Ipsilateral hemisphere; CO_2 reactivity in control group compared with **c** Arteriotomy and sham arteriotomy groups. **d** Naftidrofuryl-treated arteriotomy and sham arteriotomy groups

sham arteriotomy was performed with a naftidrofuryl infusion, normocapnic CBF improved to 40.5 ml/100 g/min, and CO_2 reactivity to 0.7 ml/100 g/min/torr (Fig. 4a, b).

Discussion

The CBF and CO_2 reactivity results in the first group of control rats are very close to the values found in man [6]. The naftidrofuryl infusion did not produce a significant change in mean normocapnic CBF or CO_2 reactivity in the control rats, and neither did permanent unilateral carotid ligation in the third group of rats. Rats withstand unilateral permanent common carotid ligation well, which is the usual finding in man. The similarity between findings from the first and third experimental groups and observations in man allow the results from these experiments to be extrapolated to man with a reasonable degree of confidence.

Unlike permanent carotid ligation, carotid arteriotomy produced a significant fall of 28% in

normocapnic CBF and a 50% fall in reactivity: the results for sham arteriotomy were similar, with a 37% fall in flow and a 70% fall in reactivity (Fig. 4c). Because these reductions were not seen with permanent carotid ligation, the release of an arteriolar vasoconstricting substance from the clamped vessel during reperfusion through it is postulated. If these findings apply to man, the cerebral circulation in patients with any degree of respiratory embarrassment may be precarious following carotid endarterectomy because CBF will be reduced below the preoperative level and will not increase when pCO_2 rises.

If serotonin is one of the vasoconstricting agents released during reperfusion through the isolated carotid segment, a serotonin antagonist would improve CBF and CO_2 reactivity. This has indeed been found to be the case in the experiments where naftidrofuryl was given following arteriotomy and sham arteriotomy. A flow improvement of 30% occured in both these groups, and CO_2 reactivity improved by over 100%, when compared to the untreated rats (Fig. 4d).

These findings support the hypothesis that serotonin is released after carotid surgery where reperfusion occurs through a segment of vessel isolated during surgery. If the improvement in CBF and CO_2 reactivity produced by naftidrofuryl in these experiments is mirrored after carotid endarterectomy in man, therapy with this agent carries the potential to considerably reduce postoperative morbidity and mortality from cerebral ischemia.

References

1. Aukland K, Bower BF, Berliner RW (1964) Measurement of local blood flow with hydrogen gas. Circ Res 14:164–187
2. Bell BA, Foubister GC, Neto NGF, Miller JD (1985) Effect of experimental common carotid ateriotomy on cerebral blood flow in rats. Neurosurgery 16:322–326
3. Fode NC, Sundt TM, Robertson JT, Peerless SJ, Sheilds CB (1986) Multicentre retrospective review of results and complications of carotid endarterectomy in 1981. Stroke 17:370–376
4. Geevarghese KP, Patel TC (1977) Anaesthesia and surgical treatment of cerebrovascular insufficiency. Int Anesthesiol Clin 15:57–110
5. Jakubowski J, Bell BA, Symon L, Zawirski MB, Francis DM (1982) A primate model of subarachnoid haemorrhage: Change in regional cerebral blood flow, autoregulation, carbon dioxide reactivity, and central conduction times. Stroke 13:601–611
6. Kety SS, Schmidt CF (1948) The effects of altered arterial tension of carbon dioxide and oxygen on cerebral blood flow and cerebral oxygen consumption of normal young men. J Clin Invest 27:484–492
7. Pasztor E, Symon, L, Dorsch NWC, Branston NM (1973) The hydrogen clearance method in assessment of blood flow in cortex, white matter and deep nuclei of baboons. Stroke 4:556–567
8. Saunders ML, Miller JD, Stablein D, Allen G (1979) The effects of graded experimental trauma on cerebral blood flow and responsiveness to CO_2. J Neurosurg 51:18–26
9. Sengupta D, Harper M, Jennett B (1973) Effect of carotid ligation on cerebral blood flow in baboons 2: Response to altered arterial pCO_2. J Neurol Neurosurg Psychiat 36:736–741
10. Symon L (1970) Regional cerebrovascular responses to acute ischaemia in normocapnia and hypercapnia: An experimental study in baboons. J Neurol Neurosurg Psychiat 33:756–762

Cerebral Blood Flow Monitoring in Early Stage of Subarachnoid Hemorrhage

Sen Yamagata[2], Haruhiko Kikuchi[2], Ikuo Ihara[1], Izumi Nagata[2], Yoshito Morooka[1], Yoshito Naruo[1], Takayuki Koizumi[1], Kenji Hashimoto[2], Jun Minamikawa[2], Susumu Miyamoto[2], Kameyoshi Mitsuno[1], Masato Matsumoto[1], Naohiro Yamazoe[2], and Yoshinori Akiyama[2]

Because of the high risk in the development of cerebral ischemia, it is of great importance to know the change of cerebral blood flow (CBF) in the acute stage of subarachnoid hemorrhage (SAH). Especially in cases with diffuse and thick clot in the subarachnoid space, symptomatic cerebral vasospasm is strongly expected and intensive care of these patients is required to prevent the decrease of CBF. However, because of the difficulty of repeated measurement of CBF in these patients, it seems impossible to know the sequential changes of CBF.

We have recently developed a monitoring system for the measurement of local cortical blood flow using a thermal diffusion flow probe with a Peltier stack, and reported its feasibility in clinical use [5, 6]. In this study, we tried to monitor the CBF continuously in patients with diffuse thick subarachnoid clot on CT, using this thermal diffusion method.

Materials and Methods

The local cortical CBF was monitored in 14 patients who were operated within 2 days after SAH (Table 1). The neurological grade was I and II in two, III in seven, and IV in five patients. In all patients, SAH on CT was diffuse and thick, and cerebral vasospasm was strongly expected. The CBF monitoring was performed by thermal diffusion using a small flow probe with a Peltier stack. This probe was left on the brain surface during surgery. The details of this CBF monitoring system has already been described elsewhere. The intracranial pressure (ICP) was also monitored in all patients. Because of the necessity of good contact between flow probe and

---

[1] Department of Neurological Surgery, National Cardiovascular Center, Osaka, Japan

[2] Department of Neurological Surgery, Kyoto University, Kyoto, Japan

brain surface to obtain the correct CBF values, the record of CBF values was started when the ICP was substantially increased. In most cases, it took several hours after surgery. Cerebral angiography was carried out in all patients, except in two who died, to comfirm the presence of cerebral vasospasm.

Results

Local CBF monitoring could be continued for 7–19 days after surgery without any trouble in all except one patient. In this case, a flow probe could not be removed at bedside, so it was done in the operating room. In the initial measurements after surgery, definite low values of CBF were obtained in grade IV patients (mean CBF, 25 ml/100 g/min). On the other hand, a variety of CBF values were found in grade III patients compared to the only minimal decrease of CBF in grades I or II patients (mean CBF, 40 ml/100 g/min). The sequential changes of CBF monitored were well correlated with outcomes. In two patients of grades I and II, no definite decrease of CBF was observed, resulting in excellent outcomes (Fig. 1a). In five of seven grade III patients, CBF was maintained with only a slight decrease, resulting in a good or excellent outcome. However, marked decrease of CBF was found 3–5 days after SAH in another two patients with poor outcomes; one of them died (Fig. 1b). A good recovery of CBF was observed in one of five grade IV patients, and an excellent postoperative outcome was obtained. In another four patients, moderate or marked decrease of CBF was found, resulting in poor outcomes; two of these patients died (Fig. 1c).

A practical chart of CBF and ICP observed in the grade III patient with poor outcome is shown in Fig. 2. This 55-year-old female patient with a ruptured anterior communicating aneurysm was operated on the next day (day 1) after SAH. On the 2nd day, the CBF value was measured above

Table 1. A summary of 14 patients with subarachnoid hemorrhage due to ruptured cerebral aneurysm subjected to local CBF monitoring

No.	Name	Age	Sex	Grade	Location	(op)	CT	CBF Follow-up	Spasm Angiogram	(day)	Symptom	Result
1.	S.T.	50	F	I	Lt IC, A com	(1d)	III	11 d	+	(10)	−	Excellent
2.	N.M.	49	F	II	Lt MC	(1d)	III	8 d	−	(18)	−	Excellent
3.	K.M.	51	F	III	A com, Rt IC	(1d)	III	14 d	+	(14)	−	Excellent
4.	A.Y.	53	F	III	Rt MC	(1d)	III	8 d	−	(10)	−	Excellent
5.	I.C.	62	F	III	A com	(0d)	III	11 d	+ +	(10)	+	Good
6.	N.S.	72	F	III	Rt MC, Lt VA	(2d)	III	8 d	−	(21)	−	Good
7.	H.K.	68	M	III	Rt PC, Anast.	(1d)	III	7 d	+ + +	(10)	+ + +	Death
8.	S.A.	72	F	III	Rt IC	(0d)	III	7 d	+	(12)	+	Good
9.	I.S.	50	F	III	A. com	(1d)	III	8 d	+ +	(11)	+ +	Poor
10.	I.K.	50	F	IV	Lt IC	(1d)	III	8 d	+	(10)	−	Excellent
11.	T.G.	54	M	IV	Rt IC ×2	(0d)	III	19 d	n.d.		+ + +	Death
12.	O.M.	63	M	IV	A com	(0d)	III	16 d	+	(30)	unknown	Fair
13.	I.H.	65	F	IV	Lt IC	(0d)	III	11 d	−	(21)	−	Fair
14.	F.H.	52	M	IV	Lt MC	(0d)	III	7 d	n.d.		+ + +	Death

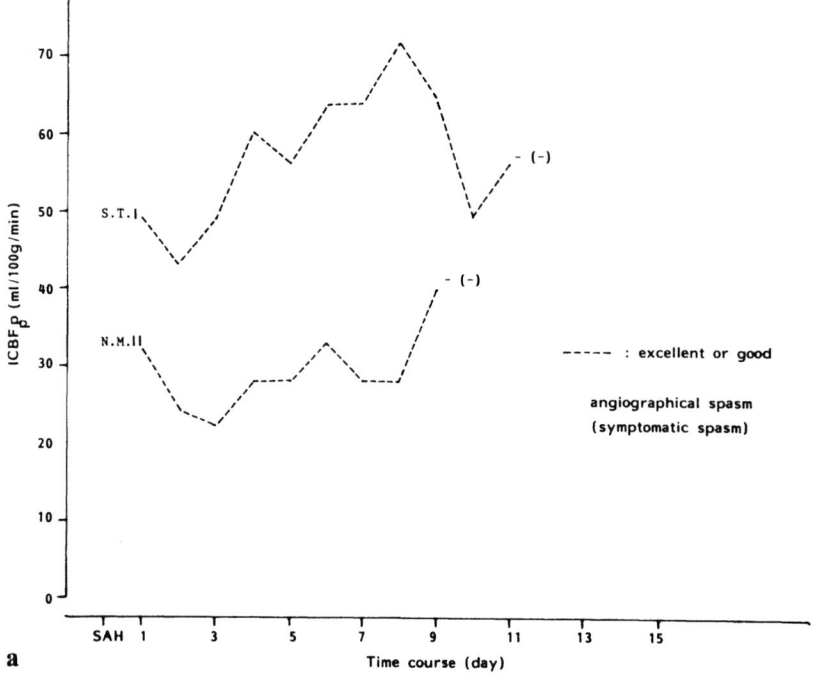

Fig. 1a–c. Sequential changes of local cerebral blood flow (*CBF*) monitored by a thermal diffusion flow probe **a** in two grades I and II patients, **b** seven grade III patients, and **c** five grade IV patients

30 ml/100 g/min and the ICP was about 7 mmHg. In spite of an increase in blood pressure with the infusion of dopamine, an increase of CBF as well as ICP was not observed at this time (Fig. 2a). However, the CBF fluctuated, depending on the change in blood pressure, and gradually decreased on the 3rd day. Thereafter, the CBF value began to be strongly influenced by increases in the ICP. Finally, a barbiturate was administered to protect the brain from the fur-ther decrease in CBF, induced by an uncontrollable increase in the ICP (Fig. 2b, c).

In comparison to the values of CBF and the degree of vasospasm, it was observed that there was no definite correlation between these two, and, in patients with good outcomes, the CBF was preserved in spite of the presence of moderate vasospasm. However, the patients with poor outcomes had a low CBF even if the degree of vasospasm was similar.

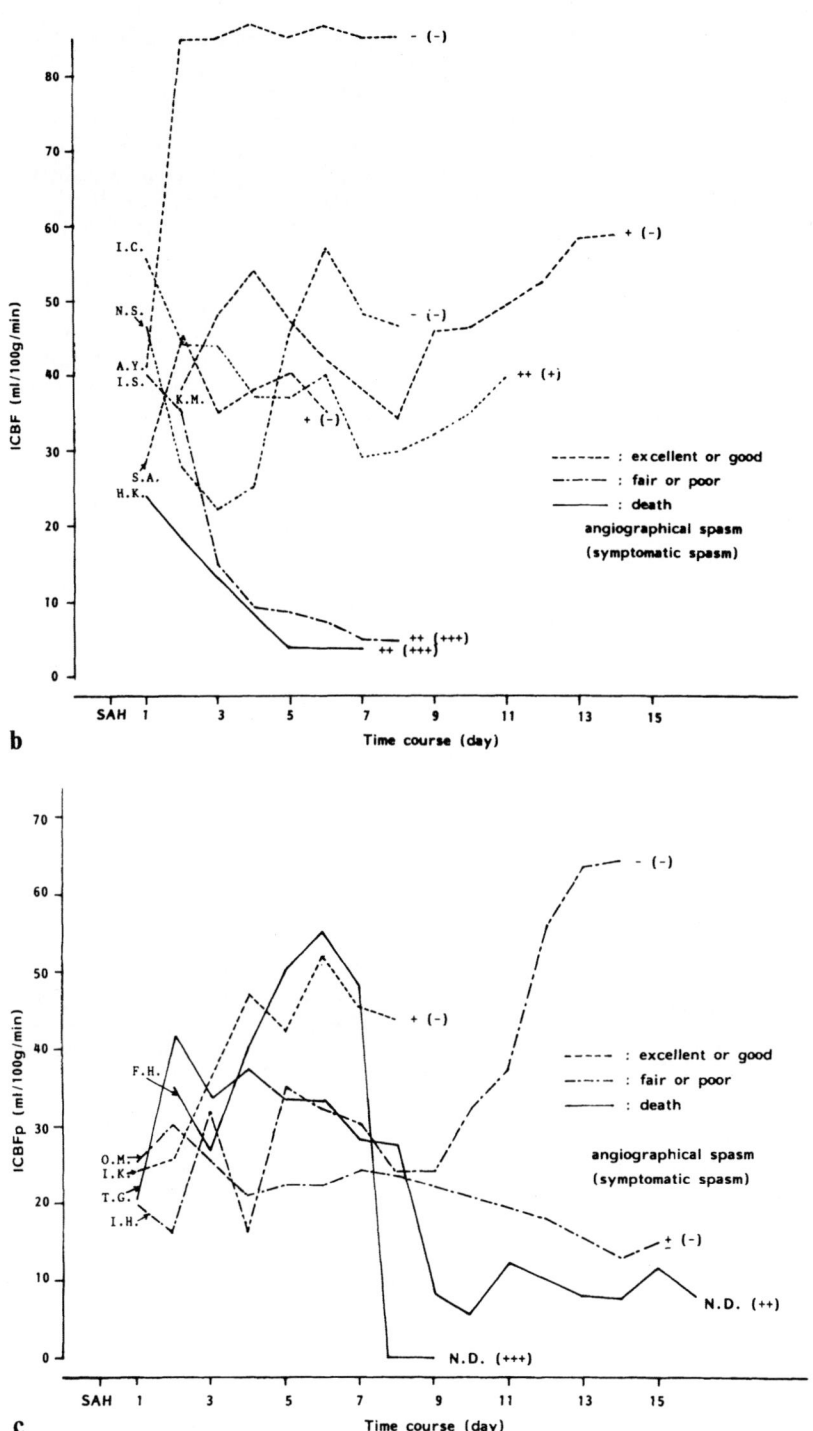

Fig. 1b, c

Discussion

The results of the present study indicate that, with this CBF monitoring, it was possible to know the initiation in the decrease in CBF induced by cerebral vasospasm and other causes. Moreover, from the monitoring of sequential changes in CBF, it may be possible to predict the prognosis of patients with SAH, due to the high correlation between the changes in CBF in most patients and their outcomes.

On the other hand, the decrease of CBF in patients with SAH seems to be caused by three steps of ischemic insults (Fig. 3). The first insult

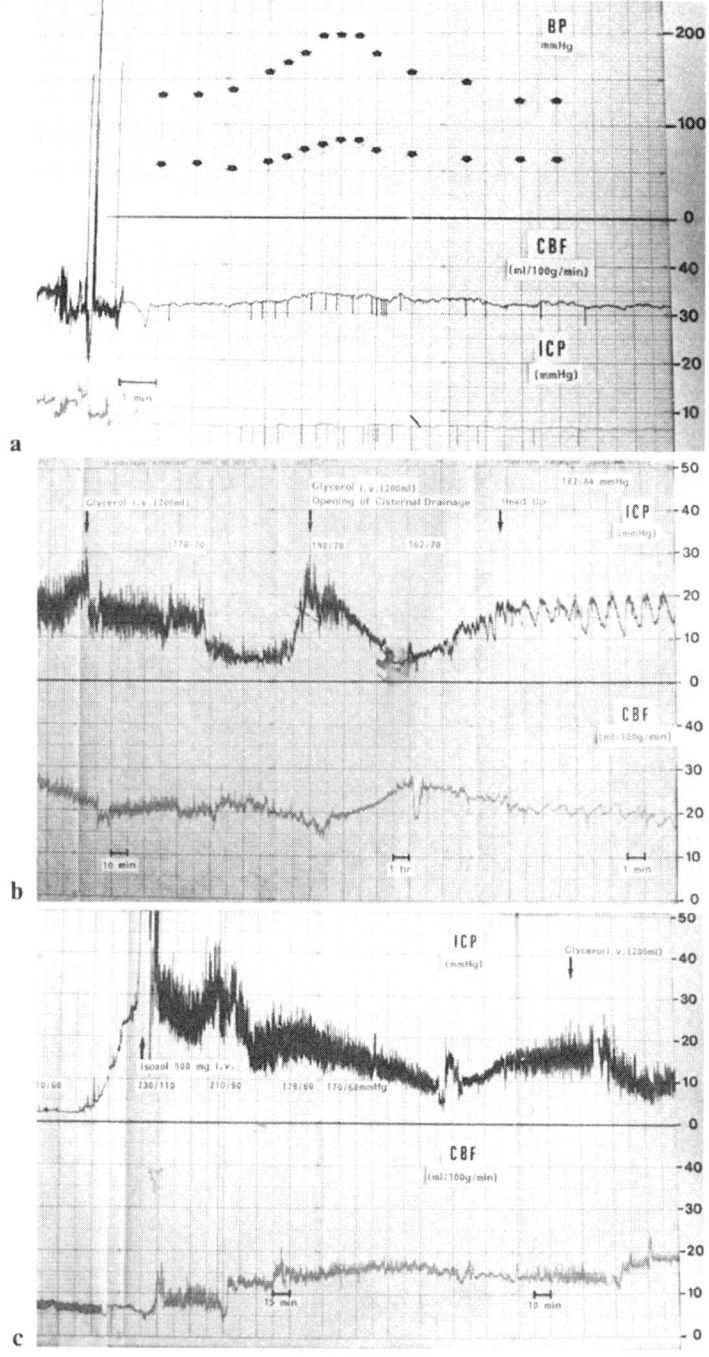

Fig. 2a–c. Case no.9. I.S. charts showing the sequential changes of cerebral blood flow (*CBF*) and intracranial pressure (*ICP*). The record runs from right to left. **a** The CBF was above 30 ml/100g/min and there was no increase of CBF and ICP by the increased blood pressure with the infusion of dopamine on the 2nd day after subarachnoid hemorrhage (SAH). **b** Although decreased CBF and elevated ICP were already observed on the 3rd day after SAH, the CBF was recovered by the reduction of increased ICP with head-up, infusion of Glycerol, or opening of cisternal drainage. **c** However, the ICP was gradually elevated and CBF continued to decrease thereafter in spite of these measurements. Finally, barbiturate was administrated, resulting in immediate reduction both of ICP and CBF

may be induced by the SAH itself [2–4], and cerebral ischemia may be caused by the increased intracranial pressure due to the obstruction of the cerebrospinal fluid pathway, or intracerebral hematoma and the disturbance of microcirculation. The second ischemic insult is caused by cerebral vasospasm, and the third insult is induced by the elevation of the ICP, due to the

ischemic edema or disturbance of cerebrospinal fluid absorption. These ischemic insults are imposed on the brain which has already been damaged by preceding insults. These indicate that similar ischemic events have different effects on the brain, depending on the presence of preceding insults. That is, in cases with low CBF due to the first ischemic insult, the second insult—the

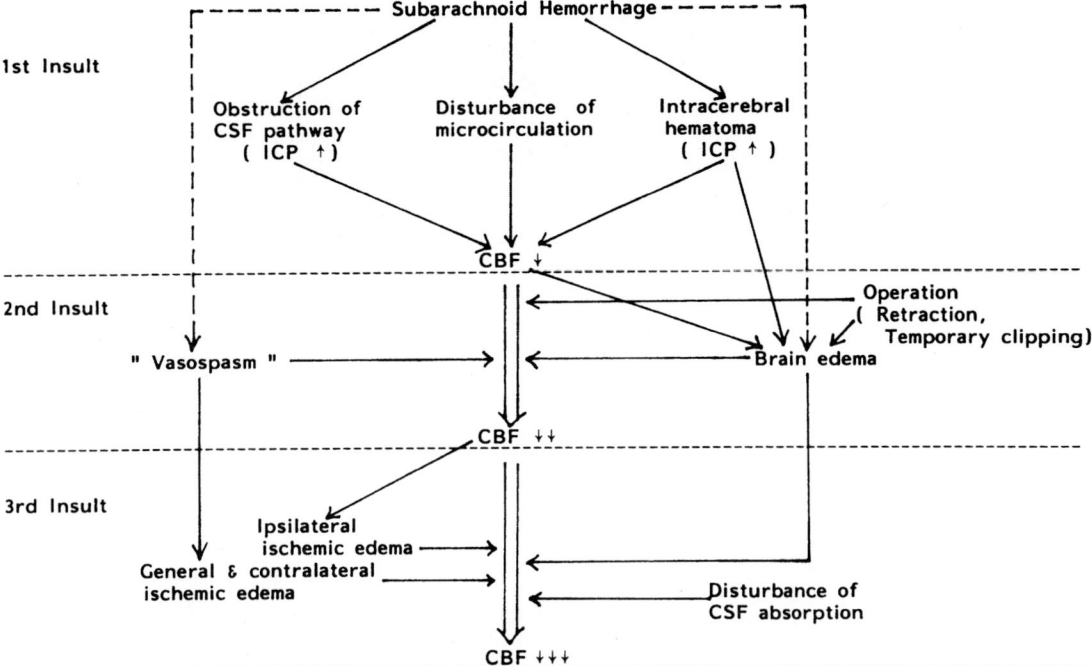

Fig. 3. A schema showing the three steps of ischemic insults after SAH. *ICP* intracranial pressure, *CBF* cerebral blood flow

presence of vasospasm—becomes more severe than in cases with normal CBF, even if the degree of vasospasm is similar. This explains the results of the present study which indicates that there is not a definite correlation between the degree of vasospasm on angiograms and the value of CBF: these facts were also reported in studies by other investigators [1, 4]. The same things occurs upon a third insult. Even a slight increase in the ICP may have a serious influence on the prognosis of patients with a low CBF. In addition to these insults, operative manipulations, such as brain retraction and temporary clipping of major cerebral arteries, may become insults.

Although it is clear that the cerebral vasospasm is the most responsible factor inducing the decrease in the CBF and determining the prognosis in patients with SAH, other factors must be taken into consideration. One of the reasons why the results of cerebral aneurysm surgery have recently improved seems to be the variety of proper treatments for these factors, of which the monitoring of the CBF should be used for more successful management.

References

1. Ishii R (1979) Regional cerebral blood flow in patients with ruptured intracranial aneurysms. J Neurosurg 50:578–594
2. Martin WRW, Baker RP, Grubb RL, et al. (1984) Cerebral blood volume, blood flow and oxygen metabolism in cerebral ischemia and subarachnoid hemorrhage: An in vivo study using positron emission tomograhy. Acta Neurochir 70:3–9
3. Meyer CHA, Lowe D, Meyer M, et al. (1983) Progressive change in cerebral blood flow during the first three weeks after subarachnoid hemorrhage. Neurosurgery 12:58–76
4. Weir B, Menon D, Overton T (1978) Regional cerebral blood flow in patients with aneurysms: Estimation by xenon 133 inhalation. Can J Neurol Sci 5:301–305
5. Yamagata S, Kikuchi H, Karasawa J, et al. (1986) Monitor system for cerebral blood flow: Experimental study of CBF measurement by thermal diffusion using a flow probe with a Peltier stack. Neurol Med Chir 26:195–200
6. Yamagata S, Kikuchi H, Hashimoto K, et al. (1987) Measurement of cerebral blood flow by thermal diffusion using a flow probe with a Peltier stack. Brain Nerve 39:479–484

Clinical and Experimental Studies of Leukotrienes in Subarachnoid Hemorrhage

Yasuaki Nishimura[1], Tatsuaki Hattori[1], Takashi Ando[1], Noboru Sakai[1], Hiromu Yamada[1], and Yoshinori Nozawa[2]

Based on the free radical theory in biological systems, which was proposed in 1973 [3], actions of lipid peroxides relating to the mechanism of cerebral vasospasm after subarachnoid hemorrhage (SAH) have been investigated [1]. Since leukotrienes (LTs) produced from arachidonic acid are suggested to be involved in the cerebral vasospasm, we studied their sequential changes in CSF and also fatty acid composition of the canine basilar artery in SAH.

Materials and Methods

Cases

We examined 19 patients with ruptured cerebral aneurysms who had received surgery within 36 h after SAH, had cranial computerized tomography (CT) before surgery, and had angiography several times during the period when cerebral vasospasm was likely to occur. They were divided into three groups based on the subarachnoid clot on CT according to a modification of Fisher's classification [4, 8]. In group 2a, the Hounsfield number of the highest density area of the clot was less than 55 in Fisher's group 2, and in 2b, over 55 in group 2. Cerebral vasospasm on angiogram (AVS) was assessed and graded by means of angiography based on the rate of reduction in the caliber of the major arteries. In these cases, 6 ml of the cisternal CSF was aspirated from the prepared reservoir on day 1 (the day after the ictus), day 3 and day 7, for the measurements of LTs and lipid peroxides.

Experimental SAH

A canine model of SAH was made as follows. Adult mongrel dogs weighing 8–11 kg were anes-thetized with 30 mg/kg of pentobarbital intravenously. After endotracheal intubation, the animal was left to breathe spontaneously. The cisterna magna was punctured with a No. 22 needle and autologous blood (0.7 ml/kg) was slowly injected following removal of the CSF (0.35 ml/kg).

Then, without SAH, 6 h after SAH, on day 1, day 3, and day 7, 6 ml of CSF was aspirated from the cistern and 10 ml of blood was aspirated from the jugular vein, for measurements of LTs and lipid peroxides. Thirty animals of SAH model and 16 animals without SAH were killed. Their brains were perfused with saline and the basilar arteries were prepared microscopically for the analyses of fatty acid composition.

The Measurement of LTs and Lipid Peroxides

LTs were extracted from 5 ml of the CSF and blood with prostaglandin B_2 (PGB_2) internal standard, according to the method of Powell [9]. Each sample was added to 20 ml ethanol (4 volumes) and 2 ng PGB_2. The mixtures were kept at 4°C for 30 min and centrifuged at $11\,000 \times g$ for 20 min. The supernatants were concentrated on a rotary evaporater at 25°C and the concentrated solutions were then diluted with distilled water, acidified to a pH of 5.6, and passed through an ODS silica cartridge using a syringe. The cartridges were washed with 20% aqueous ethanol, and LTs with PGB_2 were washed from the ODS silica with 60% aqueous ethanol. The eluates were concentrated to 100 μl under reduced pressure and were applied to high performance liquid chromatography (HPLC). The overall recovery of PGB_2 was from 64% to 75%, but the peaks of LTs were undetectable. Thus, each eluate was collected and LTs were determined by radioimmunoassay (Fig. 1). The amounts of lipid peroxides were estimated by measuring the amount of thiobarbituric acid-reactive substance (TRS), according to a modification of Yagi's method.

Department of Neurosurgery[1], Department of Biochemistry[2], Gifu University School of Medicine, Gifu, Japan

Fatty Acid Composition

The canine basilar artery segments were weighed and homogenized in an ice-cold bath with double volume of a 0.1 M Tris-HCL/0.25 M sucrose buffer (pH 7.2). Total lipids were extracted from the homogenates according to a modification of the method of Bligh and Dyer. The neutral lipids were separated by the thin-layer chromatography, and identified by comigration with authentic standards. The analyses of fatty acid composition of neutral lipids and phospholipids were carried out by gas-liquid chromatography after being transmethylated with 10% BF/ CH_3OH. Nonadecanoic acid (C19:0) was added as an internal standard to determine the content of the neutral lipids. Protein content was determined by the method of Lowry et al., using bovine serum albumin as a standard.

Results

Relationship Between AVS and Subarachnoid Clot

As the total subarachnoid blood is considered as a mass (volume × density), we added a factor of density (Hounsfield number) to Fisher's classification [4, 8]. Consequently, it was thought that the subarachnoid clot and AVS were correlated with each other (Table 1).

Changes of TRS and LTs in Patients' CSF

Subarachnoid clot on CT. The mean values of TRS were higher in group 3 than those in group 2a. As to LTB_4, when examined on the 1st day, its levels were significantly higher in group 3 than in group 2a. After 1 week, LTC_4 was higher in group 3. The level of LTD_4 was higher in group 3 on days 3 and 7, while the rate of disappearance of LTD_4 was slower in group 3 than in group 2a (Fig. 2).

AVS. As the cases were the more severe grade of AVS, the more LTs and TRS were accumulated in the CSF after SAH. On days 3 and 7, the levels of LTB_4 were significantly higher in group 3 than in group 2a. On day 3, LTD_4 was higher in group 3 than group 2a.

Delayed ischemic neurological deficits. As for the levels of LTC_4 and LTD_4, and also the rate of disappearance, remarkable significances were found between the cases with and without delayed

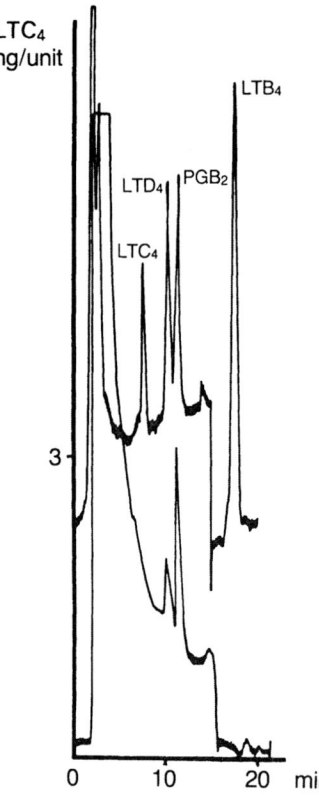

Fig. 1. Upper curve shows a high performance liquid chromatography (HPLC) chromatoaram of an injected mixture of LTC_4, LTD_4, PGB_2, and LTB_4. Lower curve shows a HPLC chromatogram after injection of the pretreated samples. Despite the ca.70% overall recovery of PGB_2, the peaks of LTs could not be detected, so each eluate was collected and leukotrienes were determined by radioimmunoassay. Conditions of HPLC: Shimadzu LC-6A system; Column, TSK ODS-80TM; Solvent, acetonitrile/methanol/ water/acetic acid (40:15:44:1), pH 5.6, flow rate 1.0 ml/min; temp. 35°C. *LT* leukotriene, *PG* prostaglandin

ischemic neurological deficits (Fig. 3). These results indicate that the amounts of LTs and TRS in the CSF produced during the early stage after SAH and the severity of cerebral vasospasm on angiogram may be dependent on the amount of subarachnoid clot, and that delayed ischemic neurological deficits develop in patients with a high amount of LTC_4 and/or LTD_4.

Changes of LTB_4, LTC_4, and TRS in Canine CSF and Plasma

The levels of LTs and TRS in the CSF without SAH were less than 5 pg/ml and 0.05 nmol/ml,

Table 1. Relationship between angiographic vasospasm (AVS) and subarachnoid clot on CT

AVS Classification	None/Slight	Moderate	Severe	Total
Group 2a	○○○	○○ ●●		7
Group 2b	○ ●	○○ ●		6
Group 3		●●●	●●●	6
Total	5	10	4	19

○ no neurological deficit, ● delayed ischemic neurological deficits

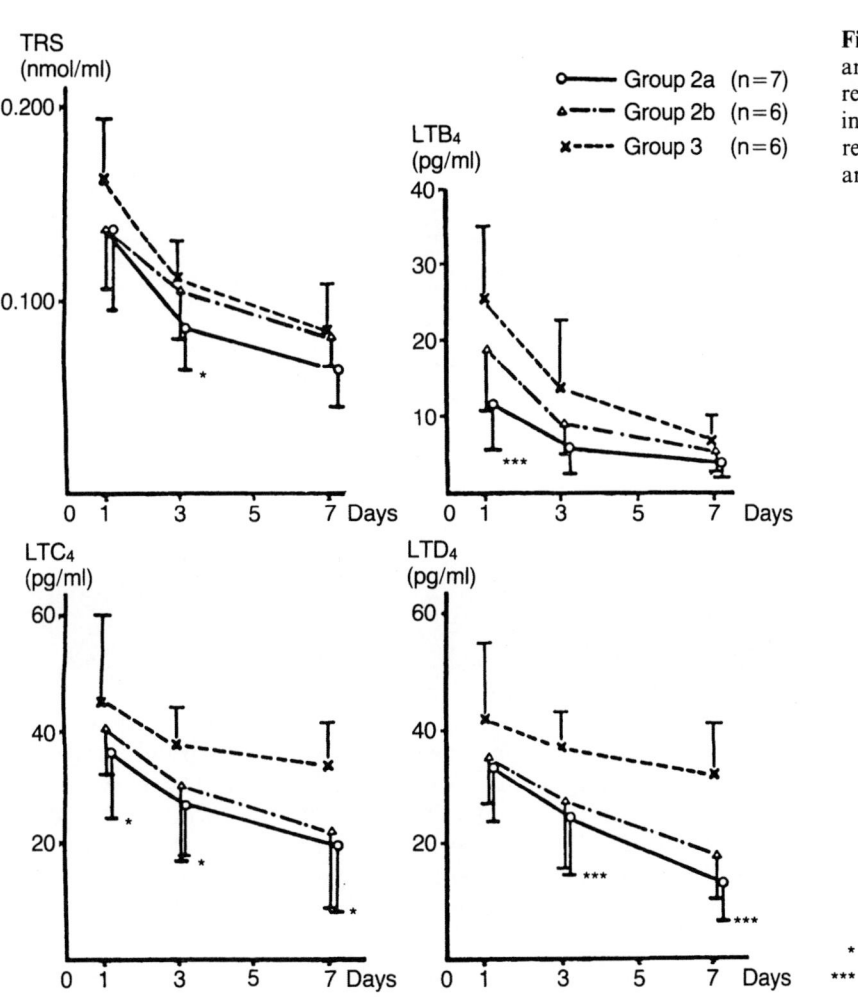

Fig. 2. Changes of LTs and thiobarbituric acid-reactive substance (TRS) in patients' CSF with reference to the subarachnoid clot on CT

respectively. The levels of LTB_4, LTC_4 and TRS 6 h after SAH were elevated 21.7 ± 5.1 pg/ml, 34.1 ± 3.6 pg/ml, and 0.201 ± 0.034 nmol/ml, respectively, and then reduced slowly. The levels of plasma LTC_4 and LTB_4 were than 20 pg/ml, and the plasma TRS was 2.100 ± 0.018 nmol/ml without SAH. These changes were not time-sequential.

Fatty Acid Composition of the Canine Basilar Artery

The concentrations of phospholipid, monoglyceride, free fatty acid, diglyceride, and triglyceride were 222.3 ± 19.8, 6.3 ± 0.8, 13.5 ± 1.1, 3.4 ± 0.3, and 2.2 ± 0.3 nmol/mg protein, respectively. The concentrations of arachidonic

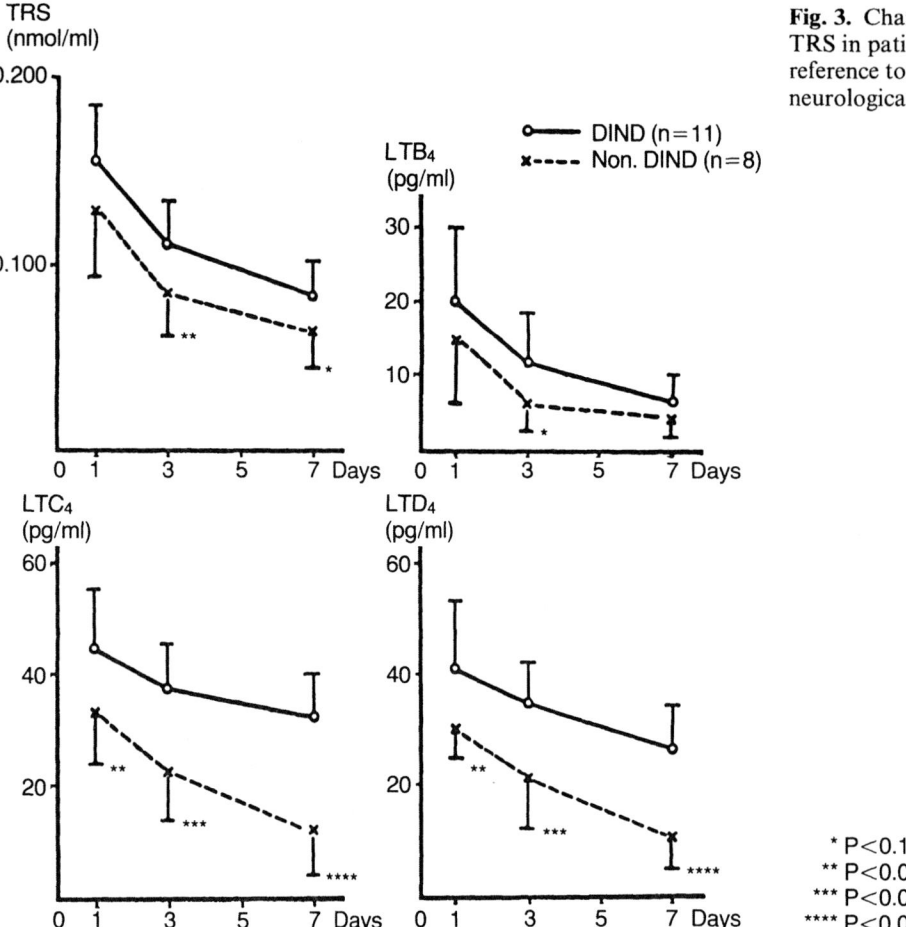

Fig. 3. Changes of LTs and TRS in patients' CSF with reference to delayed ischemic neurological deficits

DIND (n=11)
Non. DIND (n=8)

* P<0.1
** P<0.05
*** P<0.01
**** P<0.001

acid in phospholipid, monoglyceride, and free fatty acid were 21.8 ± 3.9, 0.3 ± 0.1, and 0.01 nmol/mg protein, respectively. Total concentrations of arachidonic acid without SAH, when measured on the 3rd day and 1 week were 22.1 ± 3.9, 15.4 ± 1.8, and 13.2 ± 1.4 nmol/mg protein, respectively. Arachidonic acid as well as other fatty acids gradually attenuated after SAH. It is thus suggested that reacylation is suppressed and deacylation is accentuated in SAH, which leads to accumulation of arachidonic acid during the early stage after SAH (Fig. 4).

Discussion

Since cerebral vasospasm following SAH was observed attentively on angiogram in 1951, massive researches have been rendered for clarifying the mechanism of vasospasm. The roles of LTs in biological systems have been studied from various points of view [2]. LTC_4, LTD_4, and LTE_4 are potent mediators of allergic and inflammatory responses. They all cause major constriction of the small peripheral air ways, increase vascular permeability in postcapillary venules, and produce prompt and dose-dependent constriction of arterioles. LTB_4 is known to be a potent stimulator of both chemotactic and chemokinetic movement of polymorphonuclear leukocytes, which induces degranulation and release of lysosomeal enzymes. Besides, it was reported that it may play a role like Ca^{2+} ionophore, either via thromboxane A_2 or directly. Therefore, several researchers have investigated the roles of these LTs in the pathophysiology of cerebral vasospasm after SAH.

Kiwak et al. reported LTs production in gerbil brain after SAH by the measurement of leukotriene-like immunoreactivity [7], and Rosenblum showed the constricting effect of LTs on cerebral arterioles [10]. Conversely, Holst et al. showed no effect of LTC_4 and LTD_4 on isolated, superfused human cerebral arteries [5], and

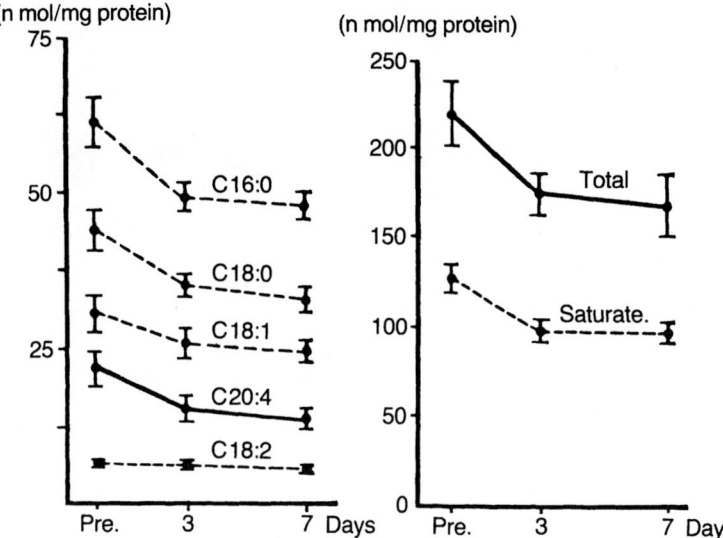

Fig. 4. Changes of fatty acid composition of phospholipids of canine basilar artery

Kamitani et al. reported no roles for LTs in the modulation of arteriolar tone in the normal cerebral circulation, refering to the probability of affects of lipoxygenase compounds on cerebrovascular permeability [6]. At any rate, it is still unclear whether LTs are accumulated in the brain after SAH.

In the present study, we examined the sequential changes of lipid peroxides in CSF following SAH. Furthermore, we detected the LTs or LT-like compounds in CSF during the early stage after SAH. We would suggest that concentration of LTs may be correlated to the amount of subarachnoid clot on CT, the extention of cerebral vasospasm on angiogram, and the severity of development of delayed ischemic neurological deficits. Besides, judging from the sequential changes of LTs, their biological effects, and arachidonate metabolism, it can be speculated that LTs take a part in the initiation of cerebral vasospasm, and that LTC_4 and LTD_4 cause delayed ischemic neurological deficits. Further work will be required to clarify the mechanism of production of LTs in blood vessels and/or brain after SAH.

References

1. Asano T, Tanishima T, Sasaki T, et al. (1981) Possible participation of free radical reactions initiated by clot lysis in the pathogenesis of vasospasm after subarachnoid hemorrhage. In: Wilkins RH (ed) Cerebral Arterial Spasm. Williams and Wilkins, Baltimore, pp 190–201
2. Borgeat P, Samuelsson B (1979) Metabolism of arachidonic acid in polyphonuclear leukocytes: Structural analysis of novel hydroxylated compounds. J Biol Chem 254:7865–7869
3. Demopoulos HB (1973) Control of free radicals in biologic systems. Fed Proc 32:1903
4. Fisher CM, Kistler JP, Davis JM (1980) Relation of cerebral vasospasm to subarachnoid hemorrhage visualized by computerized tomographic scanning. Neurosurgery 6:1–9
5. Holst H, Granstrom E, Hammastrom S, et al. (1982) Effect of leukotrienes C_4, D_4, prostacyclin and thromboxane A_2 on isolated human cerebral arteries. Acta Neurochir 62:177–185
6. Kamitani T, Little MH, Ellis EF (1985) Effect of leukotrienes, 12-HETE, histamine, bradykinin and 5-hydroxytryptamine on in vivo rabbit cerebral arteriolar diameter. J Cerebral Blood Flow Metabol 5:554–559
7. Kiwak KJ, Moskowitz MA, Levine L (1985) Leukotriene production in gerbil brain after ischemic insult, subarachnoid hemorrhage, and concussive injury. J Neurosurg 62:865–869
8. Nishimura Y, Iwama T, Yokoyama K, et al. (1985) Clinical studies of cerebral vasospasm, especially related to the amount of subarachnoid blood found on a CT scan. Prog Comp Tomog 7:285–293
9. Powell WS (1982) Rapid extraction of arachidonic acid metabolites from biological samples using octadecylsilyl silica. Meth Enzymol 86:467–477
10. Rosenblum WI (1985) Constricting effect of leukotrienes on cerebral arterioles of mice, Stroke 16:262–263

Catecholaminergic and Peptidergic Pathways Involved in the Development of Cerebral Vasospasm Following an Experimental SAH in the Rat

Niels-Åa. Svendgaard, Tia J. Delgado, and Mahammed A.-R. Arbab[1]

An experimental subarachnoid hemorrhage (SAH) was produced in the rat by the intracisternal injection of blood. The animals were examined with bilateral vertebral angiography. A biphasic vasospasm was seen with a maximal acute spasm at 10 min and a maximal late spasm at 2 days post SAH.

Systematic selective lesions of the catecholamine pathway and nuclei in the brain stem indicate that A_2, A_1, and one of their projection sites, the median eminence, are involved in the spasm development.

An afferent innervation of the cerebral arteries is demonstrated and a functional role in spasm development is suggested by the prevention of spasm with capsaicin or treatment with a substance P antagonist. The effector mechanism for acute spasm seems to be vasopressin liberated from the median eminence, while the late spasm is probably due to an unknown peptide released from the median eminence in combination with activation of the sympathetic system.

Introduction

Cerebral vasospasm in the major complication of a subarachnoid hemorrhage (SAH) following an aneurysm rupture [6]. The lack of knowledge about the mechanism behind vasospasm has been a stumbling block in the development of a therapy. The diversity in the treatments suggested for vasospasm reflects this lack and stresses the importance of further investigation into the basic mechanism.

In order to study the mechanism behind vasospasm, we developed a spasm model in the rat. Cisternal blood injection induced a biphasic spasm that could be visualized with bilateral vertebral angiography [2]. The effect of the cisternal blood was also evaluated with an autoradiographic, double-isotope technique for simultaneous measurement of cerebral blood flow (CBF) and cerebral metabolic rate of glucose (CMRgl) [3].

The model was used to investigate the central monoamine systems' involvement in the development of spasm. This investigation was carried out via systematic, stereotaxic lesioning of these systems in the brain stem prior to inducing the SAH. Furthermore, the possible existence of a sensory nerve supply to the cerebral arteries was studied with a tracing technique, and a presumed role of the vascular sensory nerves in the spasm development was examined.

Material and Methods

The experiments were performed on male Sprague-Dawley and Brattleboro rats weighing between 200 and 320 g.

Animal Preparation

Stage I. The animals were anesthetized with Brietal (Lilly, Indianapolis, USA). A catheter was permanently implanted with one end connected to the cisterna magna and the other end sutured subcutaneously to the musculature on the vertex [2].

Stage II. Three to seven days after insertion of the cisternal catheter, the animals were prepared for bilateral vertebral angiography. The anesthesia was initiated with halothane. The animals were intubated and artificially ventilated with a nitrous oxide/oxygen mixture. Catheters were inserted into a femoral artery and vein for continuous blood pressure monitoring and for infusion of drugs, respectively. Radiopaque polyethylene catheters were inserted into the axillary arteries for angiography. During the insertion of catheters, 0.75% halothane was added to the gas mixture. Heparin was given

[1] Neurosurgical Research Department, University Hospital, Lund, Sweden

intravenously. After the surgery, the halothane was switched off and suxamethonium chloride was given. Half an hour was allowed to pass before the angiography. Blood samples were drawn periodically for measurements of pH, PaO$_2$ and PaCO$_2$.

Angiography. Metrizamide (Amipaque, Nyegaard and Co, Oslo, Norway) was simultaneously injected into both axillary catheters over two to three seconds (Fig. 1). Measurements of the vertebral and basilar arterial diameters were made using a technique similar to that described by Gabrielsen and Greitz [4]. A vascular index representing the mean value of the diameters at four preselected points within the vertebrobasilar system was calculated.

SAH. Following a control angiography, 0.07 or 0.3 ml homologous blood was injected via the cisternal catheter after aspiration of about 0.03 ml CSF. During the blood injection, the head was lowered by tilting the animal 20°. Ten minutes after the SAH, the angiography was repeated. In a previously published report [2], ten minutes were found to be the point of maximal acute spasm (Fig. 2). After the angiography, the catheters were removed and the axillary arteries were ligated distal to the superficial radial artery to prevent occlusion of the vessel and facilitate perfusion of the limb. The animals were extubated when fully awake.

Stage III. Two days after the SAH, the time for maximal late spasm in normal animals [2], the animals were reanasthetized and intubated. After reinsertion of axillary and femoral catheters, the angiography was repeated. Following the examination, the animals were killed.

Retrograde Tracing of Basilar and Middle Cerebral Arterial Innervation

The basilar artery was exposed through a ventral approach with the animals mounted on a Kopf stereotaxic frame. The middle cerebral artery was exposed through a burr hole in the temporal bone. The dura and the arachnoid overlying the exposed arteries were opened. Wheat germ agglutinin conjugated with horseradish peroxidase (WGA-HRP) was applied over the exposed arteries.

Anterograde Tracing of the Cerebro-Vascular Innervation

The trigeminal ganglion was exposed through

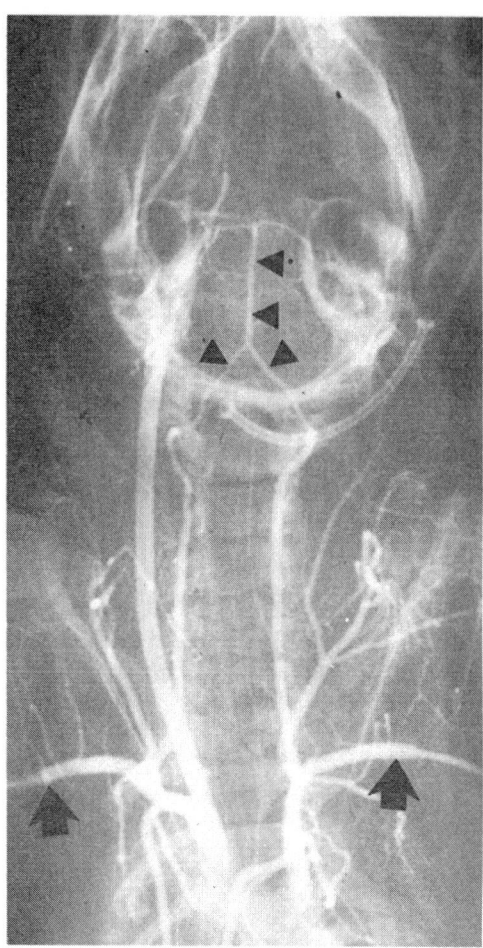

Fig. 1. Bilateral vertebral angiography showing the points (*arrowheads*) at which vertebral and basilar diameters are measured. *Arrows* show axillary catheters

a ventral approach and the upper two spinal ganglia through a hemilaminectomy of the arch of the first cervical vertebra. The exposed ganglia were injected with WGA-HRP.

Transganglionic Tracing of the Basilar and Middle Cerebral Arterial Innervation

WGA-HRP was applied over the exposed proximal basilar and middle cerebral arteries. Unilateral trigeminal and upper two dorsal spinal ganglia rhizotomies were done prior to WGA-HRP application over the arteries in a group of animals. The animals underwent perfusion fixation, and the brain, cervical spinal cord, and the trigeminal, geniculate, nodose, and upper three spinal ganglia were sectioned on a freezing microtome. The sections, including whole mounts of

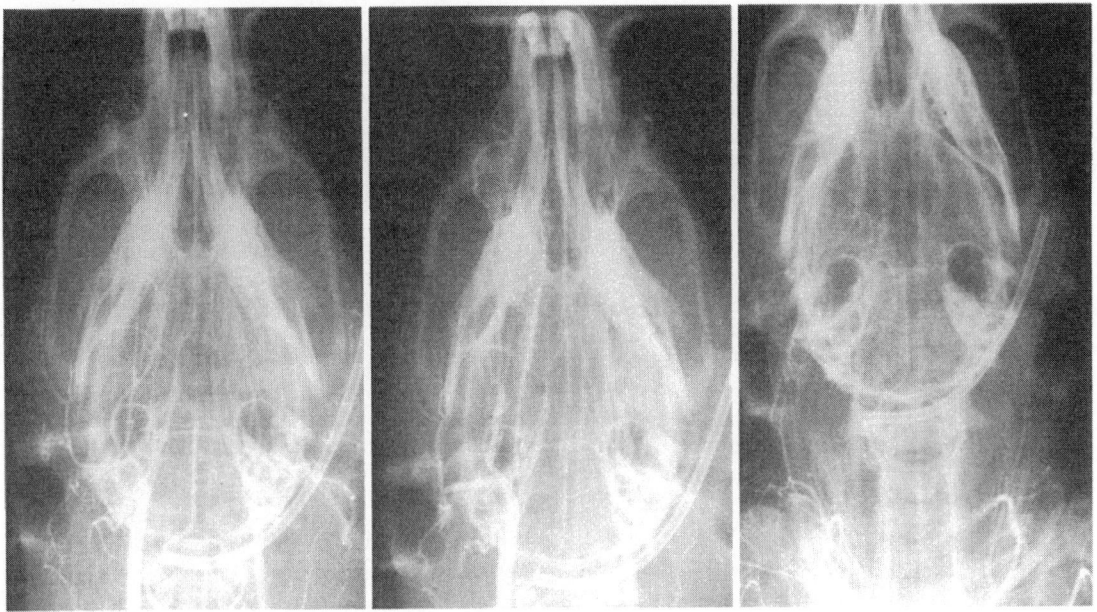

a, b   c

Fig. 2a–c. Vertebro-basilar angiography in a rat. **a** control. **b, c** Ten minutes and 2 days after blood injection. There is spasm at both time points

the cerebral arteries, were reacted according to the tetramethylbenzidine method for demonstration of HRP reactivity according to Mesulam [7] and Gibson et al. [5].

Lesions

Lesions were made chemically, electrothermically, or surgically in Sprague-Dawley rats about 2 weeks prior to angiography. The animals were anesthetized with Brietal or halothane as described previously. Appropriate sham lesions were made in all the experimental groups.

Lesion I. The ascending catecholamine (CA) pathways originating from A_1, A_2, and A_6 (nomenclature according to Dahlström and Fuxe) [1] were lesioned bilaterally in the caudal mesencephalon with 6-hydroxydopamine (6-OHDA). 6-OHDA selectively lesions CA-containing neurons, leaving neurons containing other transmittors intact (Fig. 3a, lesion 1).

Lesion II. The ascending CA pathways from A_2 and A_1 were lesioned bilaterally in the medulla oblongata with 6-OHDA (Fig. 3a, lesion 2).

Lesion III. A_2 in the dorsomedial region of the medulla oblongata was lesioned bilaterally with 6-OHDA (Fig. 3a, lesion 3).

Lesion IV. A_1 in the ventrolateral region of the

medulla oblongata was lesioned bilaterally with 6-OHDA (Fig. 3a, lesion 4).

Lesion V. Since A_1 and A_2 are known to project to the hypothalamus and to the pituitary, selective lesions were made in the hypothalamus-pituitary, region. The caudal part of the pituitary stalk was lesioned surgically from the ventral surface of the brain (Fig. 3b, lesion 5).

Lesion VI. The median eminence was lesioned surgically from the ventral brain surface or electrothermically with a dorsal approach (Fig. 3b, lesion 6).

SAH in Brattleboro Rats and Effect on Spasm of Vasopressin (AVP) Antagonist and AVP Antiserum

Brattleboro rats which congenitally lack the capacity to produce AVP were subjected to an SAH. An AVP antagonist was administered intravenously and the AVP antiserum intracisternally 15 min before the SAH in Sprague-Dawley rats.

Capsaicin Treatment and Effect on Spasm of a Substance-P Antagonist

Newborn and adult Sprague-Dawley rats were injected subcutaneously with capsaicin, a drug that destroys substance P-containing neurons.

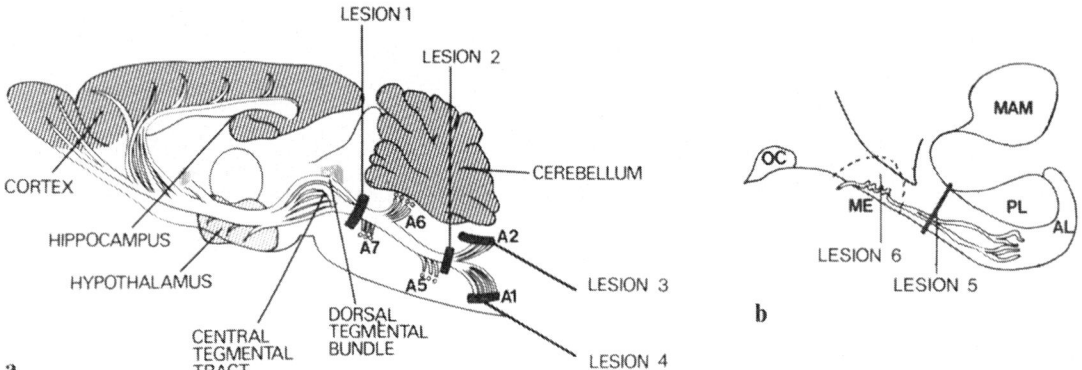

Fig. 3a, b. Schematic illustration of the CA pathways in the rat brain (**a**) and of the hypothalamus (**b**) showing the different lesion sites. *AL* anterior lobe, *MAM* mammilllary body, *ME* median eminence, *OC* optic chiasma, *PL* posterior lobe

An SAH was induced when the neonatally treated animals were 2–3 months old. Adult rats were capsaicin-treated 1–2 weeks prior to the SAH. A substance P antagonist (SP 152) was given intracisternally 2 h prior to the SAH.

Control of Lesions

The lesions of the CA pathways or nuclei were controlled with determination of the noradrenaline content of the frontal cortex and diencephalon-hypothalamus. Microscopy of the lesion sites was performed in some animals in each experimental group 1–6.

Results

Normal Sprague-Dawley animals showed a biphasic spasm pattern after cisternal blood injection. There was a maximal acute spasm of 40% and a maximal late spasm of 27%. The sham-lesioned animals showed the same degree of spasm post SAH. The animals with spasm were noticeably drowsy and passive, but no paralysis was noted.

Lesioning of the ascending CA pathways either in the mesencephalon or in the medulla oblongata prevented the development of both the acute and the late spasm (Fig. 4). Selective lesions of the A_2 nuclei not only prevented the development of acute spasm, but resulted in a significant dilatation of the cerebral arteries at day two post SAH (Fig. 4b). Lesioning of the A_1 nuclei prevented the late, but not the acute spasm phase. The acute spasm in these animals was similar to that seen in normal animals. Transec-

tion of the pituitary stalk did not change the degree of spasm, while lesion of the median eminence prevented the development of both spasm phases.

Brattleboro rats subjected to an SAH did not demonstrate acute spasm, while the late spasm still developed (Fig. 5). Sprague-Dawley rats treated with a vasopressin antagonist intravenously or a vasopressin antiserum intracisternally did not have acute spasm (Fig. 6). The degree of late spasm was not affected.

Innervation of Cerebral Arteries

Following application of the tracer over the middle cerebral artery, retrogradely labelled neurons were identified in the ipsilateral trigeminal ganglion. The geniculate, nodose, and upper three spinal ganglia were devoid of neuronal labelling. Application of tracer over the proximal basilar artery resulted in labelling of neurons in the upper two spinal ganglia bilaterally, while application over the distal basilar artery in addition resulted in cell body labelling within the trigeminal ganglia bilaterally. The third spinal ganglia was devoid of labelling.

Anterograde labelled fibers originating in the trigeminal ganglion projected to the ipsilateral circle of Willis and the distal part of the basilar artery (Fig. 7a). Fibers originating in the upper two spinal ganglia contributed to the innervation of the vertebro-basilar arteries (Fig. 7b).

The central projections of the neurons innervating the middle cerebral arteries were identified above all in the nucleus tractus solitarius, including the A_2, and the nucleus motorius dorsalis nervi vagi (Fig. 7c). Fibers were also identified in the trigeminal brain stem nuclear

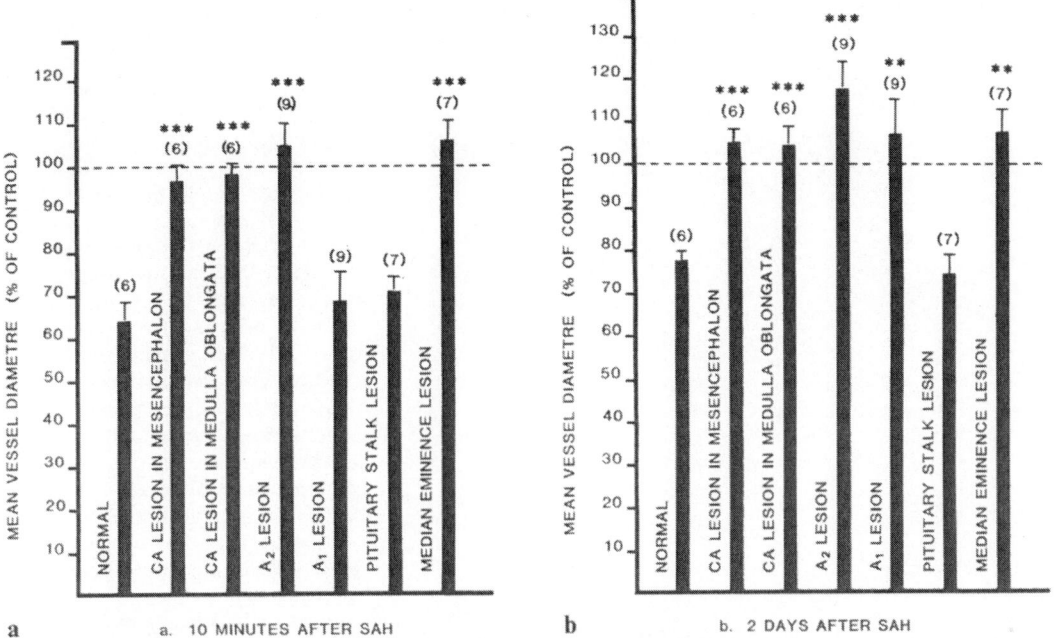

Fig. 4a, b. Angiographical changes in vertebro-basilar diameter post SAH after lesions in the brain stem and the pituitary. Numbers in brackets represent numbers of animals. The values are means ± SEM in percent of control. Student's-*t* test was used for statistical analysis. Each lesion group was compared to the appropriate sham group. *$P < 0.05$, **$P < 0.01$, ***$P < 0.001$

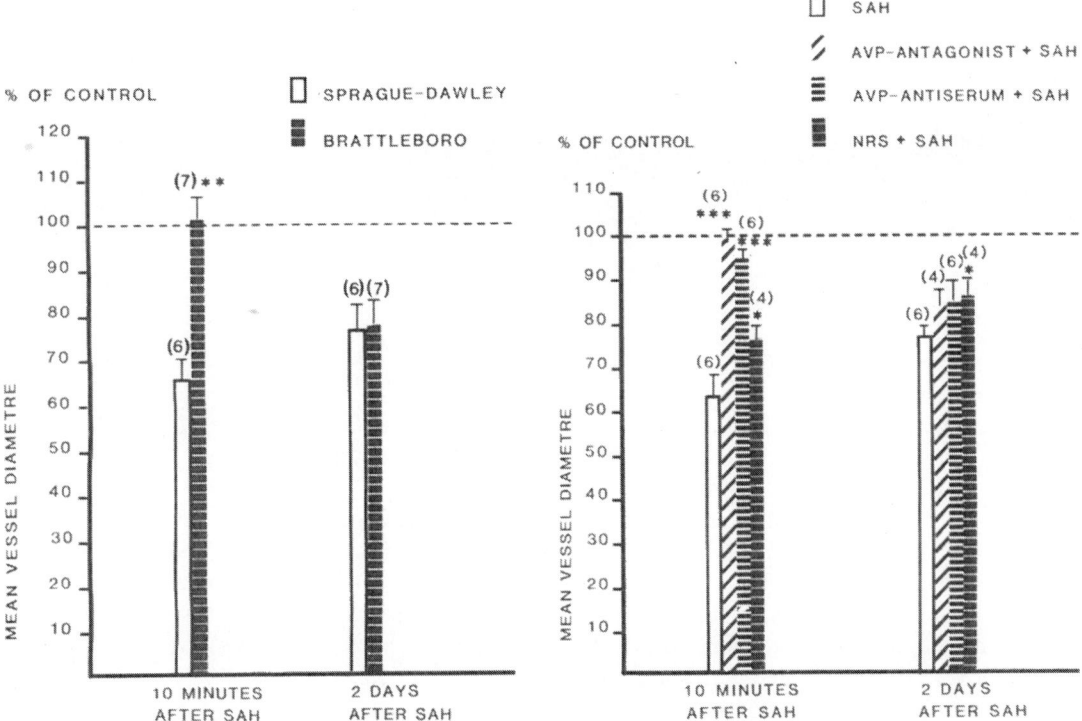

Fig. 5. Angiographical changes in mean vertebro-basilar diameter post SAH in Sprague-Dawley and Brattleboro rats 10 min and 2 days post SAH

Fig. 6. Angiographical changes in mean vertebro-basilar diameter post SAH in Sprague-Dawley rats treated with AVP antagonist or AVP antiserum prior to a SAH

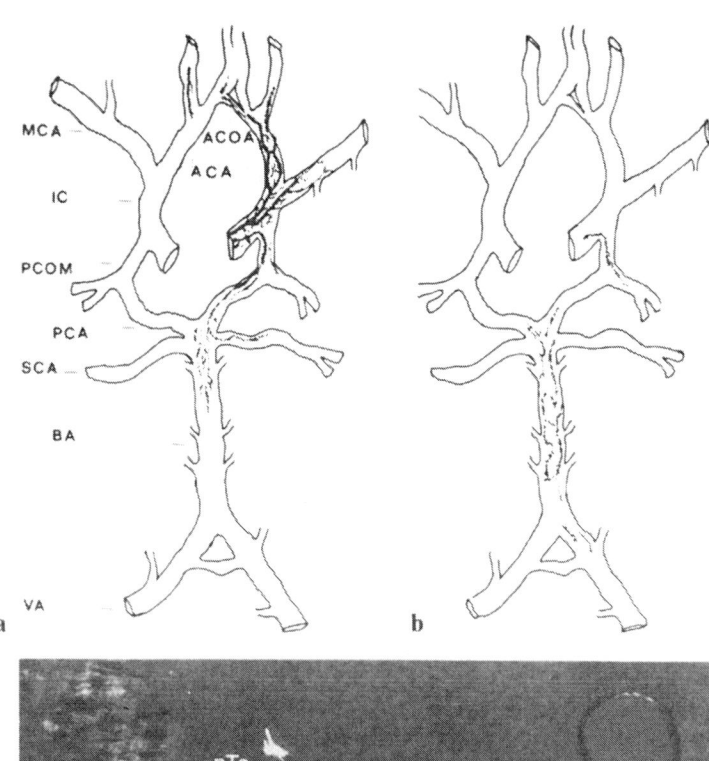

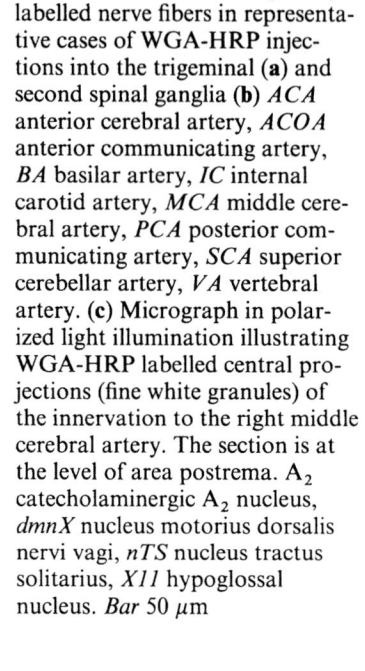

Fig. 7a–c. Schematic drawing of the distribution of anterogradely labelled nerve fibers in representative cases of WGA-HRP injections into the trigeminal (**a**) and second spinal ganglia (**b**) *ACA* anterior cerebral artery, *ACOA* anterior communicating artery, *BA* basilar artery, *IC* internal carotid artery, *MCA* middle cerebral artery, *PCA* posterior communicating artery, *SCA* superior cerebellar artery, *VA* vertebral artery. (**c**) Micrograph in polarized light illumination illustrating WGA-HRP labelled central projections (fine white granules) of the innervation to the right middle cerebral artery. The section is at the level of area postrema. A_2 catecholaminergic A_2 nucleus, *dmnX* nucleus motorius dorsalis nervi vagi, *nTS* nucleus tractus solitarius, *X11* hypoglossal nucleus. *Bar 50 μm*

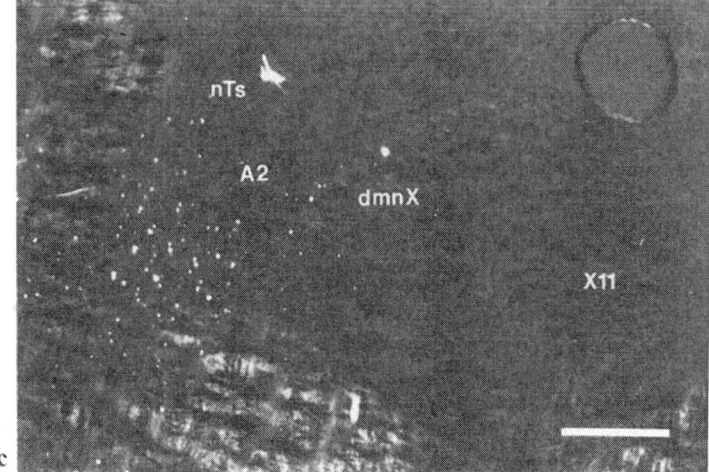

complex, the ventral periaqueductal gray, and the dorsal horns at the level of C_2. Nerve fibers innervating the basilar artery terminated in areas similar to the middle cerebral artery projections with the addition of the cuneate nuclei. The trigeminal brain stem complex, however, was devoid of terminals. Trigeminal and upper spinal ganglia rhizotomies, prior to WGA-HRP application over the middle cerebral and basilar arteries, impeded visualization of labelled terminations in the brain stem and upper spinal cord.

Effect on Cerebral Vasospasm of Capsaicin and Substance-P Antagonist

Treatment with capsaicin of neonatal or adult animals, or intracisternal administration of a substance P antagonist prior to an SAH, prevented the development of both the acute and the late spasm phase (Figs. 8, 9).

Discussion

The present study shows that the intracisternal injection of blood in the rat induces an angio-

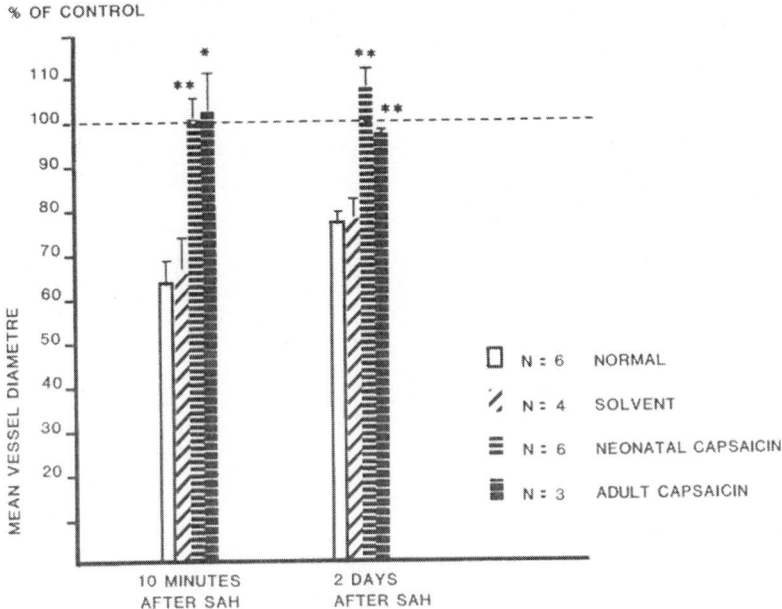

Fig. 8. Angiograhical changes in vertebro-basilar diameter 10 min and 2 days post SAH in Sprague-Dawley rats treated neonatally or as adults with capsaicin prior to the SAH. Values are means $\pm$ SEM. *$P < 0.05$, **$P < 0.01$, ***$P < 0.001$

graphically demonstrable cerebral vasospasm. The spasm has an acute phase maximal at 10 min and late phase maximal at 2 days. The late phase in the rat appears earlier than in other species.

Selective destruction of CA pathways or nuclei in the lower brain stem indicates that the A_2 and A_1 nuclei in the medulla oblongata are involved in the development of vasospasm following an SAH. The findings suggest that blood does not induce spasm via a direct action on the musculature of the cerebral arteries, but that a neural mechanism is involved. Moreover, the different spasm pattern after selective A_1 and A_2 lesions indicates that there is a different mechanism behind acute and late spasm. This is further supported by the finding that cranial sympathectomy reduces the late spasm, but does not affect the acute spasm [8].

Lesions of the median eminence, a projection site of A_1 and A_2 within the hypothalamus-pituitary, prevented the development of both spasm phases. The median eminence is a channel that can liberate hypothalamic peptides into the CSF or blood, or to the pituitary. Investigation of the role of vasopressin using Brattleboro rats, a vasopressin antagonist or antiserum, suggests

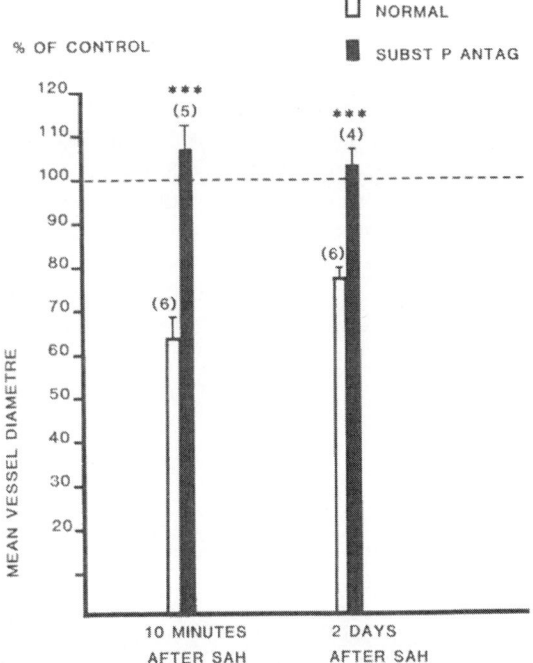

Fig. 9. Angiographical changes in vertebro-basilar diameter 10 min and 2 days post SAH in Sprague-Dawley rats treated with a substance P antagonist intracisternaly prior to the SAH. Values are means $\pm$ SEM. *$P < 0.05$, **$P < 0.01$, ***$P < 0.001$

that vasopressin is involved in the development of acute spasm.

This finding raised the question as to whether a peptide mechanism also could be implicated in the late spasm phase. Investigation of CSF from patients and rats during the late phase with high-performance liquid chromatography revealed the presence of a protein, probably a peptide, in the same position in the chromatogram, suggesting that it could be the same substance (unpublished observations).

Investigations of the cerebrovascular innervation demonstrated that the anterior cerebral circulation is innervated from the trigeminal ganglia and the posterior from the upper two spinal ganglia, and that the neurons innervating the cerebral arteries project monosynaptically to the nucleus tractus solitarius at the level of A_2. The findings indicate that there is an anatomical basis for the transmission of "information" from the cerebral arteries to the A_2. A role for this innervation is indicated by the data from capsaicin and substance P treatment, i.e., that substance P-containing fibers constitute the sensory link in a reflex arc system involved in the development of spasm.

Our findings allow the proposal of the following theory for spasm development: blood in the subarachnoid space gives rise to a signal that is transmitted through capsaicin-sensitive nerve fibers via the trigeminal and upper two spinal ganglia to the nucleus tractus solitarius. From A_2, which is a part of the nucleus tractus solitarius. an impulse is relayed to the paraventricular and supraoptic nuclei, and to the median eminence releasing vasopressin and an unknown spasmogenic compound. Vasopressin seems to underlie the acute spasm, while the late phase

could be induced by the sympathetic system in combination with a spasmogenic factor liberated from the median eminence.

References

1. Dahlström A, Fuxe K (1964) Evidence for the existence of monoamine containing neurons in the central system. 1. Demonstration of monoamines in the cell bodies of brain stem neurons. Acta Physiol Scand 62 (Suppl 232): 1–55
2. Delgado TJ, Brismar J, Svendgaard N-Aa (1985) Subarachnoid hemorrhage in the rat: Angiography and fluorescence microscopy of the major cerebral arteries. Stroke 16: 595–602
3. Delgado TJ, Arbab M A-R, Diemer NH, Svendgaard N-Aa (1986) Subarachnoid hemorrhage in the rat: Cerebral blood flow and glucose metabolism during the late phase of cerebral vasospasm. J Cereb Blood Flow Metab 6: 590–599
4. Gabrielsen TO, Greitz T (1970) Normal size of the internal carotid, middle cerebral and anterior cerebral arteries. Acta Radiol (Diagn) 10: 1–10
5. Gibson AR, Hansma DI, Houk JC, Robinson FR (1984) A sensitive low artifact TMB procedure for the demonstration of WGA-HRP in the CNS. Brain Res 298: 235–241
6. Kassell NF, Sasaki T, Colohan ART, et al. (1985) Cerebral vasospasm following aneurysmal subarachnoid hemorrhage. Stroke 16: 562–572
7. Mesulam M (1978) Tetramethylbenzidine for horseradish peroxidase neurohistochemistry: A non-carcinogenic blue reaction product with superior sensitivity for visualizing neural afferents and efferents. J Histochem Cytochem 26: 106–117
8. Svendgaard N-Aa, Brismar J, Delgado TJ, Diemer NH (1985) The effect on the development of cerebral vasospasm in the rat of lesioning of the peripheral and central catecholamine systems. Neurol Res 7: 30–34

Preventive Action of Cisternal Heparin Injection for Vasoconstriction After Experimental Subarachnoid Hemorrhage

Masahiro Asada[1], Kazuhiko Ishida[1], Norihiko Tamaki[1], Satoshi Matsumoto[1], Kieth Baker[2], John W. Peterson[2], and Nicholas T. Zervas[2]

Summary

We investigated the action of heparin in reducing the degree of vasoconstriction in the experimantal subarachnoid hemorrhage (SAH) models of rabbits. Heparin, injected intrathecally, reduced the degree of constriction significantly. On the other hand, systemic heparin injection or physiological saline cisternal injection did not reveal any preventive effect on constriction. From this experiment, we suppose that heparin might neutralize thrombin which was activated in the CSF after SAH and considered to be one of the constrictive factors producing vasospasm.

Introduction

The etiological factors of vasospasm following subarachnoid hemorrhage (SAH) have been considered to be multiplex. The preventive methods of vasoconstriction and the treatment for symptomatic vasospasm have not been established yet.

Heparin is believed to prevent endothelial injury, thrombin generation, and platelet adhesion to endothelium, and to have inhibitory effects on arterial smooth muscle cell proliferation. The present studies were designed to investigate the action of heparin in reducing the degree of vasoconstriction following experimental SAH in rabbits.

Materials and Methods

Adult rabbits weighing 2.5–3.5 kg were anesthetized with a gas mixture containing oxygen

and 4% halothene. After endotracheal intubation, the halothene was decreased to 2%. The rabbit was placed in a supine position and the right brachial artery was exposed and cannulated with a 19-gauze catheter. The tip of the catheter was placed medial to the brachial plexus and lateral to the origin of the right vertebral artery. The left vertebral artery was coagulated at the point where it enters the foramen transversarium of the sixth vertebra. After the blood gas content was confirmed to be within physiological range, a baseline angiography was performed. Contrast material, 3 cm^3, was injected through the catheter in the right brachial artery. The rabbit was placed in the sphinx position, with the head flexed downward, and the percutaneous puncture into the ciserna magna was done, using a 21-gauge butterfly needle. CSF, 1 cm^3, was removed and unheparinized, autologous, arterial whole blood was injected in the amount of 0.66 cm^3/kg body weight [1]. The rabbit was tilted at 30° in a head down position for 1 h. The catheter in the brachial artery was irrigated and placed subcutaneously for serial angiographies.

The rabbits being injected with blood intrathecally, were divided into four groups. Six rabbits of the first group were followed up without any treatments. Three rabbits of the second group were reinjected with 0.5 cm^3 physiological saline into the cisterna magna at 6 h after the cisternal blood injection. Six rabbits of the third group were similarly reinjected with 0.5 cm^3 (500 units) of heparin (Elkins-Simm, Inc.) into the cisterna magna. Two rabbits of the fourth group were injected with 600 units of heparin intravenously every 8 h from 6 h after the cisterna blood injection. Serial angiographies were performed in all of the groups. The diameters of the basilar arteries were measured at three selected points on the arteries, using a microscope. The most constrictive diameter was adopted for comparison and the percentile to control diameters were calculated. The rabbits which had died immediately due to respiratory failure

[1] Department of Neurosurgery, Kobe University, Kobe, Japan

[2] Service of Neurosurgery, Massachusetts General Hospital, Harvard Medical School, Massachusetts, USA

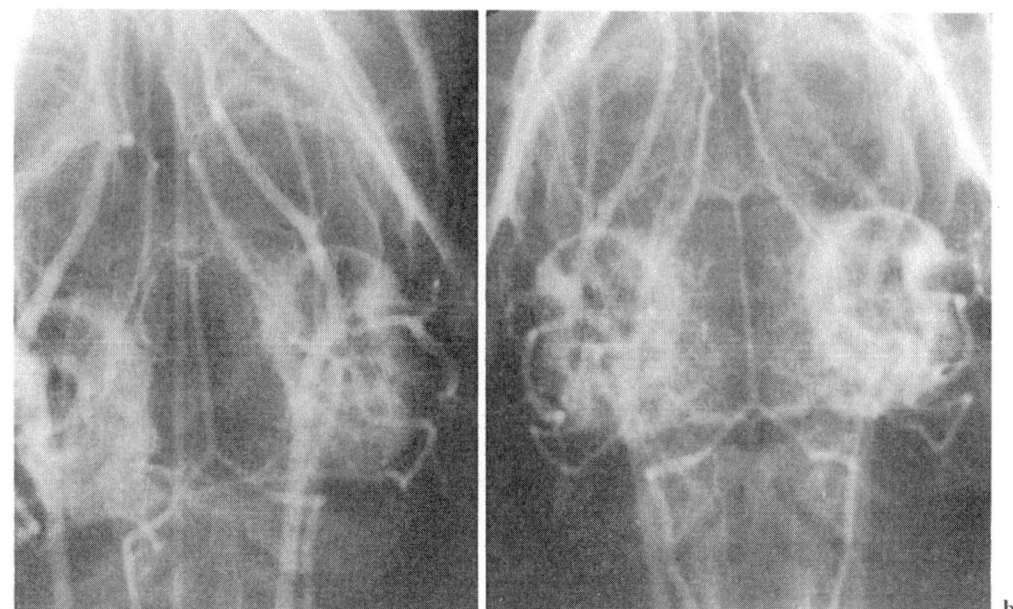

a   b

Fig. 1a, b. Control basilar artery and vertebral artery. **b** Prominent vasoconstriction at the top of the basilar artery 1 day after blood cisternal injection

or brain stem impairment after the cisternal injection, were excluded from this study, and the rabbits without clot around the basilar arteries on the day of killing were also neglected because of the possibility of failure in cisternal injection.

Results

The rabbits which survived after cisternal injection showed inactivity and loss of appetite: however, there were no gross differences in the general conditions between the untreated group and the other three groups. Adverse effects due to the cisternal heparin injection or intravenous heparin injection were not observed. In one rabbit, an electrocorticogram was done at 1 and 2 h after heparin cisternal injection. It revealed no abnormalities. This injection also did not show any significant inhibitory effect on the process of clot formation around the basilar artery and the prepontine cistern.

The prominent vasoconstrictions in the untreated group were observed on days 1 and 2. Typical angiography is shown in Fig. 1. These constrictions subsided on days 5 and 6 (Fig. 2). The physiological saline cisternal injection group showed similar changes in the degree of vasoconstriction (Fig. 3). On the other hand, the cisternal heparin injection group did not reveal

any significant constriction on day 1 and day 2. Only slight constriction was observed on day 3 in this group (Fig. 4). There were statistically significant differences in the degrees of constriction on day 1 ($P < 0.01$) and day 2 ($P < 0.05$) between the untreated group and the heparin cisternal injection group, and on day 1 ($P < 0.05$) and day 2 ($P < 0.05$) between the physiological saline cisternal injection group and the heparin cisternal injection group (Table 1). On days 3 and 4, the average degrees of constrictions were still more severe on the untreated group in comparison with those of heparin cisternal injection group, but there were no satistically significant differences.

One of the two rabbits with heparin intravenous injection was followed up until the 5th day. The change in the degree of constriction was parallel to the one in the untreated group. The other rabbit also showed significant constriction on day 1 and serial angiography was not performed because of thrombosis in the vertebral artery. Therefore, it seemed that intravenous heparin injection had no preventive effect on vasoconstriction (Fig. 5).

Discussion

According to these data, intrathecally injected heparin significantly reduced the degree of vaso-

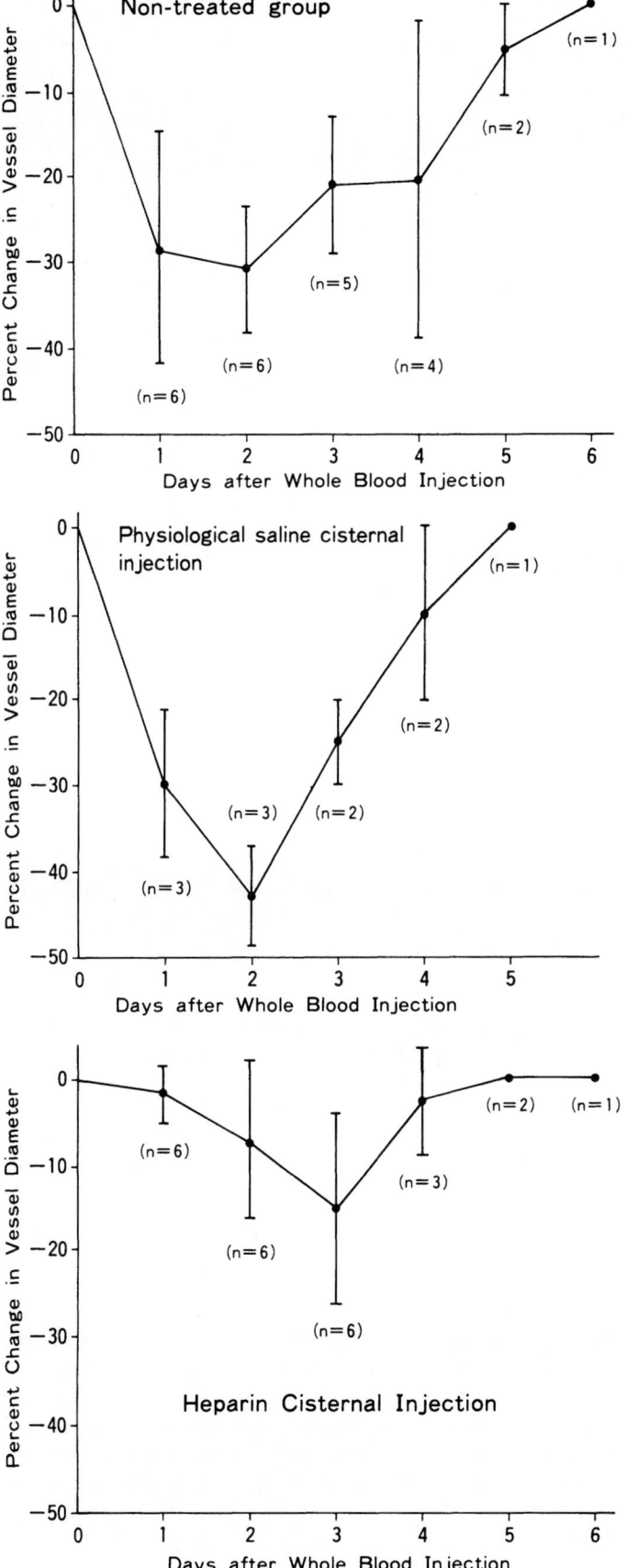

Fig. 2. The percentile change in the diameter of the basilar artery after blood cisternal injection

Fig. 3. The percentile change in the diameter of the basilar artery after physiological saline cisternal injection following cisternal blood injection

Fig. 4. The percentile change in the diameter of the basilar artery after heparin cisternal injection following blood cisternal injection

Table 1. Differences in degrees of constriction among groups. Each figure represents the mean percentile to control diameter of the basilar artery in three groups

	Nontreated group	Heparin cisternal injection	Physiological saline cisternal injection
Day 1	71.8 ± 13.1 ($n = 6$)[a]	98.3 ± 4.1 ($n = 6$)	70.0 ± 8.2 ($n = 3$)[b]
2	69.7 ± 7.4 ($n = 6$)[b]	93.3 ± 10.3 ($n = 6$)	56.7 ± 4.8 ($n = 3$)[b]
3	79.2 ± 7.7 ($n = 5$)	85.0 ± 12.2 ($n = 6$)	75.0 ± 5.0 ($n = 2$)
4	79.3 ± 18.0 ($n = 4$)	96.7 ± 5.8 ($n = 3$)	90.0 ± 10.0 ($n = 2$)
5	95.0 ± 5.0 ($n = 2$)	100 ± 0 ($n = 2$)	100 ($n = 1$)
6	100 ($n = 1$)	100 ($n = 1$)	

[a] $P < 0.01$
[b] $P < 0.05$ in the analysis by U-test

constriction following experimental SAH in rabbits, whereas intermittent intravenous heparin injection or physiological saline cisternal injection had no effects on vasoconstriction. These findings suggest that heparin might decrease the activity of extraluminal vasoconstrictive factors which were released into the CSF following SAH.

It is known that the coagulating system in the subarachnoid space is activated in the early stage of SAH: fibrinopeptide A, as an indicator of thrombin, was measured at extremely high levels in the CSF on the 1st and 2nd day after SAH [5]. Thrombin has been shown to produce vasoconstriction in vivo [7] and in vitro [3], and to be more potent in generating sustained contractions than either serotonin or prostaglandin F2 [8]. The bovine thrombin which had been intrathecally injected for rabbits produced the prolonged vasoconstriction and it continued for 24 h (our unpublished data).

Thrombin also destroys endothelium [6], promotes platelet aggregation, and causes platelets to release vasoconstrictors, such as prostaglandin and thromboxane A2. It also has mitogenic activity. These functions and effects of thrombin might participate in the process of vasospasm.

Heparin is an effector in the inactivation of thrombin by antithrombin III, and promotes the effect of antithrombin III. Therefore, the preventive effect on vasoconstriction by heparin might be derived from the inhibitory action of heparin against thrombin which was activated in the CSF after SAH. White [9] explained that thrombin induced tachyphylaxis in the constrictive response and that thrombin was not likely to be the causative factor in delayed spasm. He stressed the significance of antithrombin III in delayed spasm, which was a nonspecific vasodilator [10].

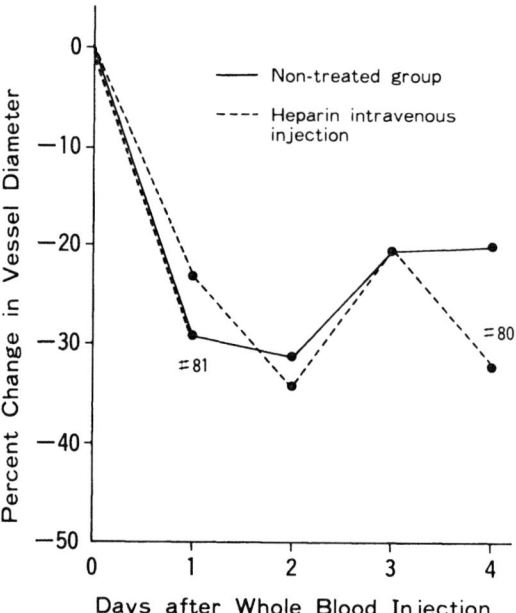

Fig. 5. The percentile changes in the diameter of basilar arteries in the non-treated group and systemic heparin injection group

If this is so, it is worthwhile to investigate the quantitative balance between antithrombin III and thrombin in the CSF after the administration of heparin, heparin plus antithrombin III, or hirudin, a specific inhibitor of thrombin .

Kapp reported that systemic heparin reduced proliferative angiopathy following SAH in cats [4]. This mechanism might result from heparin's inhibitory effect on the platelet derived growth factor (PDGF), which stimulates the proliferation of fibroblast and arterial smooth muscle cells. PDGF also works as a potent vasoconstrictor [2]. It is not clear whether heparin inhibits the vasoconstrictive activity of PDGF or not. However, our experiment of intravenous heparin injection did not prevent vasoconstriction in the early stage of SAH. The preventive action of cisternal heparin injection for vasoconstriction might be explained as follows: heparin neutralized thrombin which was activated in the CSF after SAH and is considered to be one of the constrictive factors producing vasospasm. Studies with another accumulative dosage of heparin or intermittent injections should be done to clarify the action of heparin.

References

1. Baker KF, Zervas NT, Pile-Spellman J, Vacanti FX, Miller D (1987) Angiographic evidence of basilar artery constriction in the rabbits: A new model of vasospasm. Surg Neurol 27:107–112
2. Berk BC, Alexander RW, Brock TA, Gimbrone MA, Webb RC (1986) Vasoconstriction: A new activity for platelet-derived growth factor. Science 232:87–90
3. Haver VM, Namm DH, (1984) Characterization of the thrombin-induced contraction of vascular smooth muscle. Blood Vessels 21:53–63
4. Kapp JP, Clower BR, Azar FM, Yabuno N, Smith RR (1985) Heparin reduces proliferative angiopathy following subarachnoid hemorrhage in cats. J Neurosurg 62:570–575
5. Kasuya H, Shimizu T, Okada T, Takahashi K, Summerville T, Kitamura K (1986) Coagulation and fibrinolytic system and bradykinin in the subarachnoid space after subarachnoid hemorrhage. Blood Vessel (Jpn) 17:233–241
6. Lough J, Moore S (1975) Endothelial injury induced by thrombin or thrombi. Lab Invest 33:130–135
7. White RP, Hagen AA, Morgan H, Dawson WN, Robertoson JT (1975) Experimental study on the genesis of cerebral vasospasm. Stroke 6:52–57
8. White RP, Chapleau CE, Dugdale M, Robertson JT (1980) Cerebral arterial contractions induced by human and bovine thrombin. Stroke 11:363–368
9. White RP. Robertson JT (1985) Role of plasmin, thrombin, and antithrombin III as etiological factors in delayed cerebral vasospasm. Neurosurgery 16:27–35
10. White RP (1987) Comparison of the inhibitory effects of antithrombin III, α_2-macroglobulin, and thrombin in human basilar arteries: Relevance to cerebral vasospasm. J Cereb Blood Flow Metab 7:68–73

Role of Prostacyclin, Thromboxane A_2, and Leukotrienes in Experimental Cerebral Vasospasm

Takashi Ohmoto, Keiko Irie, Junji Yoshioka, and Kozo Iwasa[1]

Introduction

It has been reported that prostacyclin (PGI_2) deficiency with a predominance of thromboxane A_2 (TXA_2) might be involved in the development of cerebral vasospasm following subarachnoid hemorrhage [1]. Recent advances in the research into other forms of arachidonic acid cascades have disclosed the biological properties of leukotrienes (LT), 5-hydroxygenase products of arachidonic acids [7]. Both LTC_4 and LTD_4 have been reported to have a dose-dependent constrictive action on pial arteries in mice [6], suggesting that they might be involved in the development of cerebral vasospasm. The purpose of this study is to clarify the role of eicosanoids, including PGI_2, TXA_2, and 5-lipoxygenase products in experimental cerebral vasospasm.

Materials and Methods

Adult cats weighing 3-4 kg were used in this study. Under general anesthesia (intramuscular injection of 20 mg/kg of ketamin), each cat was immobilized by a stereotaxic instrument. Three milliliters of CSF was withdrawn from the cisterna magna, followed by a cisternal injection of the same volume of autologous arterial blood to induce subarachnoid hemorrhage. Then, a blood and CSF mixture (2:1) was incubated at 37°C for 3 days. Three days after the cisternal injection, the basilar artery was exposed by the transclival approach, using a surgical microscope. It was soaked in the incubated blood-CSF mixture for 10 min, which was then continuously applied by infusion pump at 0.5 ml/h for 2 h.

Photographs of the basilar artery were taken at $2.5 \times$ magnification through a surgical micro-scope at 10 and 120 min after the production of cerebral vasospasm. The inside diameter of the vessel was later measured on a screen. Regional cerebral blood flow (rCBF) measurement was continuously made by the temperature-controlled thermoelectric method, using a tissue flow meter (TF Monitor: UFW-101, Unique Medical Co., Ltd.). rCBF measurement by the hydrogen clearance method (Digital UH-Meter, Unique Medical Co., Ltd.) was also done intermittently to confirm the rCBF values obtained through the temperature-controlled thermoelectric method. Platelet aggregation was monitored by a Platelet Aggregation Profiler (Model PAP-2A, BIO/DATA). Platelet aggregation was induced by the addition of arachidonic acid ($5 \times 10^{-3}M$).

All cats underwent all of the surgical procedures mentioned above. They were then divided into five groups. Group I (ten cats) served as the control, receiving a physiological saline. Cats in groups II, III, IV, and V were treated respectively, with the TXA_2 antagonists ONO-3708 (100 µg/kg/min) and ONO-1270 (100 µg/kg/min); the PGI_2 analogues OP-41483 (75 ng/kg/min) and OP-2507 (100 ng/kg/min); the lipoxygenase inhibitors AA-861 (500 µg/kg/min), ONO-5349 (100 µg/kg/min), and nordihydroguaiaretic acid (NDGA; 300 µg/kg/min); and the LTC_4, D_4 antagonist FPL-55712 (200 µg/kg/min). The intravenous infusion of each drug began 30 min prior to topical application of the incubated blood-CSF mixture onto the basilar artery. Infusion was maintained throughout the experiment.

Results

Changes in Arterial Diameter During Experimental Vasospasm

Topical application of the incubated blood-CSF mixture elicited an initial contraction of not only

---

[1] Department of Neurological Surgery, Kagawa Medical School, Kagawa, Japan

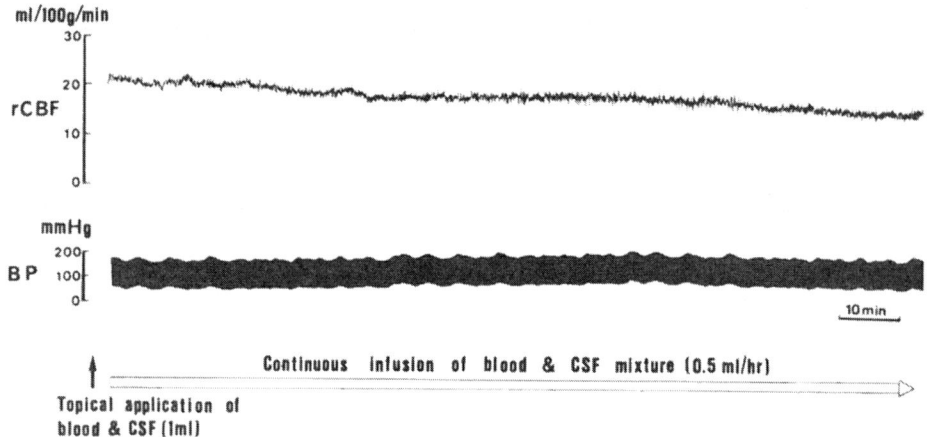

Fig. 1. Time course of rCBF of pontine tegmentum during basilar arterial spasm induced by incubated blood-CSF mixture. Note the gradual decrease of rCBF from 21.2 to 15.2 ml/100 g/min in accordance with elapsed time, while the basilar artery maintains 32% vasospasm

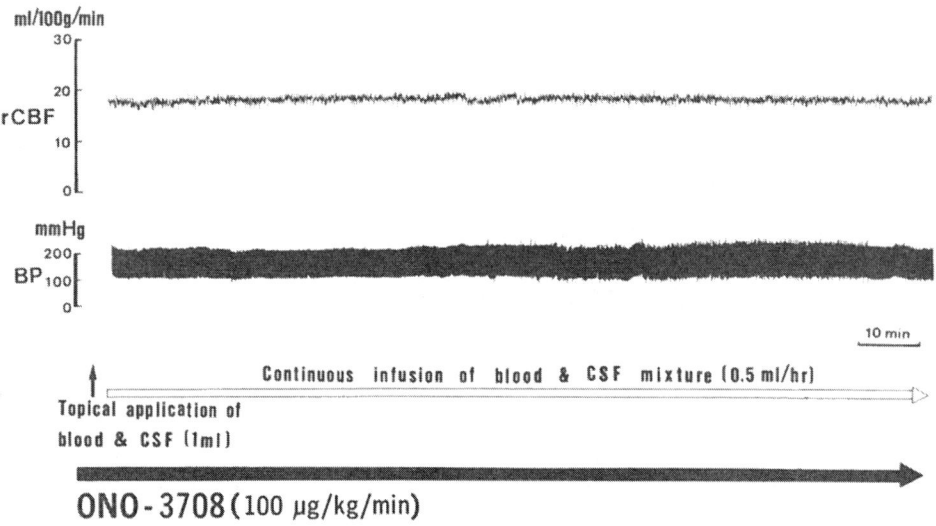

Fig. 2. Time course of rCBF of pontine tegmentum in cats treated with the TXA_2 antagonist (ONO-3708). rCBF of pontine tegmentum remained unchanged

the basilar artery but also its branches. The vasospasm remained unchanged as long as the artery was irrigated with the mixture, although some individual difference of severity was evident.

In group I (ten cats), topical application of the incubated blood-CSF mixture induced vasospasm in 29.4% ± 4.4% (mean ± S.E) and 36.5% ± 4.3% at 10 and 120 min, respectively. None of the PGI_2 analogues (OP-41483, OP-2507), TXA_2 antagonists (ONO-3708, ONO-1270), 5-lipoxygenase inhibitors (NDGA, ONO-5349, AA-861), or LTC_4, D_4 antagonists (FPL-55712) suppressed the constrictor response of feline basilar arteries to the incubated blood-CSF mixture. The degree of vasospasm achieved with these drugs was not significantly different from that of group I.

Changes in rCBF

The measurement of rCBF began 10 min after the onset of cerebral vasospasm induced by topical application of the incubated blood-CSF mixture. The rCBF of the pontine tegmentum in group I was 24.4 ± 1.5 ml/100 g/min at 10

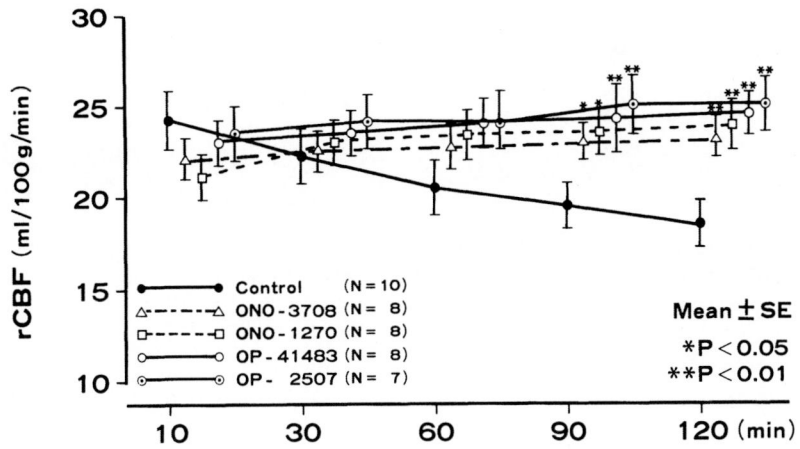

Fig. 3. Effects of TXA$_2$
antagonists and PGI$_2$
analogues on rCBF of
feline pontine tegmentum.
Note the prevention of
gradual decrease of rCBF
in treated cats

min, 76% of rCBF of the normal feline pontine tegmentum (32.0 ± 4.4 ml/100 g/min), as measured in our laboratory. rCBF gradually decreased as more time elapsed, reaching 18.2 ± 1.2 ml/100 g/min at 120 min. However, the caliber of the spastic vessels remained unchanged during this time (Fig. 1).

Treatment with TXA$_2$ antagonist (ONO-3708, 100 μg/kg/min) did prevent the gradual decrease of rCBF of the pontine tegmentum but did not affect mean arterial blood pressure (Fig. 2). Figure 3 shows the effects of TXA$_2$ antagonists and PGI$_2$ analogues on rCBF. Treatment with these agents halted the rCBF decrease of the pontine tegmentum. However, vasospasm did occur to the same degree as in group I.

The effects of 5-lipoxygenase inhibitors (AA-861, ONO-5349, NDGA) and LTC$_4$, D$_4$ antagonist (FPL-55712) on rCBF of the pontine tegmentum are shown in Figs. 4 and 5. With these agents, rCBF did not decrease during vasospasm, but actually increased somewhat in most cats. At 120 min, the rCBF values of those cats were significantly higher than those of the control group.

Platelet Aggregation Studies

In the control cats, 5×10^{-3} M arachidonic acid (AA) induced platelet aggregation before topical application of the incubated blood-CSF mixture. The capacity of platelet aggregation produced by AA remained unchanged at 120 min after topical application. Treatment with PGI$_2$ analogues and TXA$_2$ antagonists inhibited the platelet aggregation induced by AA at 120 min. On the other hand, treatment with 5-lipoxygenase inhibitors

and FPL-55712 did not affect platelet aggregation (Table 1).

Discussion

Morphological studies have disclosed that endothelial cells in spastic arteries are detached from the vessel wall and that platelets adhere and aggregate on the exposed internal elastic lamina [2, 3]. Such platelet adhesion and aggregation could produce a predominant thromboxane pathway inverted from a prostacyclin pathway, which in turn would produce further aggregation and adhesion to the denuded vessel wall, resulting in impaired microcirculation. In this experimental model, treatment with PGI$_2$ analogues or TXA$_2$ antagonists prevented a gradual decrease of rCBF in the territory of the basilar artery, though cerebral vasospasm occurred in the basilar artery even after treatment with those agents.

In these cats, platelet aggregation was inhibited due to the antiplatelet aggregation properties of PGI$_2$ analogues and TXA$_2$ antagonists. These results suggest that TXA$_2$ and PGI$_2$ do not play an important role in the occurrence of vasospasm in major blood vessels, but that treatment with these drugs can affect microcirculation by inhibiting platelet aggregation.

It is known that leukotrienes are generated in various tissues [5]. Rosenblum [6] reported the constriction of cerebral arterioles when mice were given even a low dose (3×10^{-6} M) of LTC$_4$ or D$_4$. It has also been reported that the baseline level of LTC$_4$, D$_4$ in a normal gerbil brain was 0.7 ng/g, and that a subarachnoid injection of blood elevated the LTC$_4$, D$_4$ to 6.82

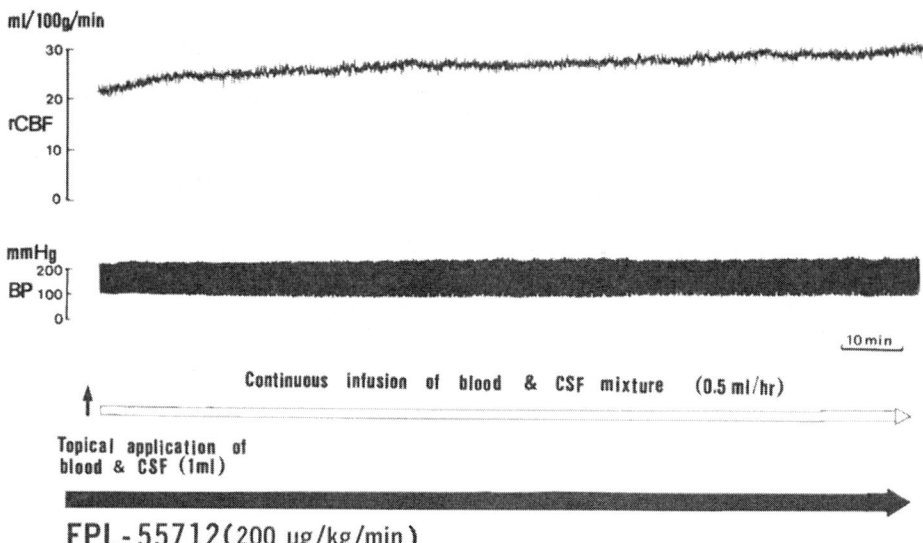

FPL-55712(200 µg/kg/min)

Fig. 4. Effect of LTC$_4$, D$_4$ antagonist (FPL-55712) on rCBF of pontine tegmentum in experimental cerebral vasospasm. The basilar artery demonstrated 26% vasoconstriction upon topical application of blood-CSF mixture, and maintained the same arterial diameter during subsequent continuous infusion of the mixture (0.5 ml/h). rCBF of pontine tegmentum, showing 22.0 ml/100 g/min as its initial value, increased gradually to 29.8 ml/100 g/min

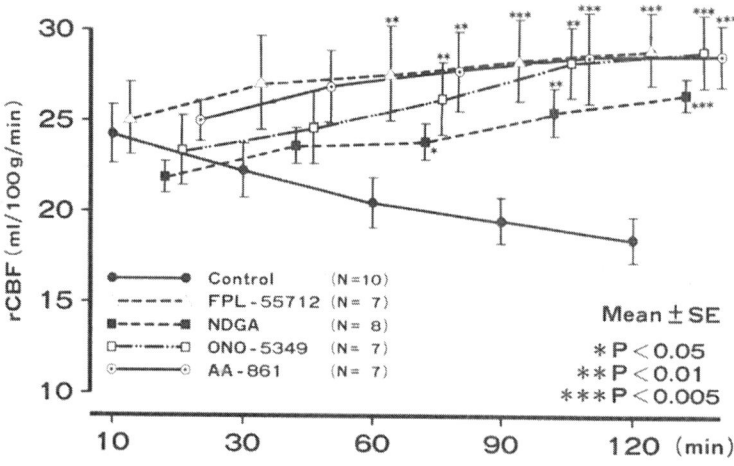

Fig. 5. Effects of LTC$_4$, D$_4$ antagonist and 5-lipoxygenase inhibitors on rCBF of feline pontine tegmentum. The gradual decrease of rCBF is prevented by treatment with LTC$_4$, D$_4$ antagonist and 5-lipoxygenase inhibitors

ng/g [4]. Our recent study revealed that 10^{-6} M LTC$_4$ and D$_4$ constricted the feline basilar artery. Moreover, the contractile activity of LTC$_4$ and D$_4$ was more prominent in small arteries than in large ones. In this study, neither the 5-lipoxygenase inhibitors nor the LTC$_4$, D$_4$ antagonist could prevent cerebral vasospasm in the basilar artery or inhibit platelet aggregation. However, infusion of either the 5-lipoxygenase inhibitors or the LTC$_4$, D$_4$ antagonist did halt

the decrease of the rCBF of the feline pontine tegmentum. If levels of LTC$_4$ and D$_4$ were elevated in the brain as a direct effect of the application of hemolyzed blood or an ischemia caused by vasospasm, rCBF might further decrease as a result of constriction of cerebral arterioles.

From these results, PGI$_2$ analogues, TXA$_2$ antagonists, 5-lipoxygenase inhibitors, and LTC$_4$, D$_4$ antagonist might be useful in pre-

Table 1. Effects of TXA$_2$ antagonists, PGI$_2$ analogues,[a] 5-lipoxygenase inhibitors, and LTC$_4$, D$_4$ antagonist on cat platelet aggregation induced by sodium arachidonate (AA)

Agents	Maximum platelet aggregation rate	
	Before infusion (%)	After 2.5-h infusion (%)
Control ($n = 5$)	86 ± 14	92 ± 10
ONO-3708 ($n = 5$)	90 ± 12	21 ± 7
ONO-1270 ($n = 5$)	94 ± 20	15 ± 10
OP-41483 ($n = 5$)	86 ± 2	30 ± 18
OP-2507 ($n = 5$)	92 + 11	28 ± 13
FPL-55712 ($n = 5$)	82 ± 11	86 ± 4
NDGA ($n = 5$)	92 ± 6	90 ± 10
ONO-5349 ($n = 5$)	80 ± 12	76 ± 10

[a] Treatment with either TXA$_2$ antagonists or PGI$_2$ analogues inhibits platelet aggregation induced by AA (5×10^{-3} M)

venting the progressive decrease of cerebral blood flow due to cerebral vasospasm.

Summary

The role of PGI$_2$, TXA$_2$, and LTC$_4$ and D$_4$ was studied in experimentally induced cerebral vasospasm in cats. PGI$_2$ analogues, TXA$_2$ antagonists, 5-lipoxygenase inhibitors, and LTC$_4$, D$_4$ antagonist had no effect on the development of cerebral vasospasm, but did prevent the gradual decrease of rCBF in the territory of spastic vessels. Platelet aggregation induced by arachidonic acid was inhibited by treatment with PGI$_2$ analogues and TXA$_2$ antagonists, but not by treatment with 5-lipoxygenase inhibitors or with LTC$_4$, D$_4$ antagonist. Eicosanoids may play a key role, not in the occurrence of cerebral vasospasm, but rather in the delayed and progressive decrease of cerebral blood flow that results from cerebral vasospasm.

References

1. Boullin DJ (1980) Cerebral vasospasm. Wiley, Chichester
2. Grady PA, Blaumanis OR, Nelson ER (1980) Morphology and flow dynamics of focal arterial constriction. In: Wilkins, RH (ed) Cerebral arterial spasm. Williams and Wilkins, Baltimore, pp 107–112
3. Kapp JP, Neil WR, Neil CL, et al. (1982) The three phases of vasospasm. Surg Neurol 18:40–45
4. Kiwak KJ, Moskowitz MA, Levin L, et al. (1985) Leukotriene production in gerbil brain after ischemic insult, subarachnoid hemorrhage, and concussive injury. J Neurosurg 62:865–869
5. Piper PJ, Letts LG, Galton SA (1983) Generation of a leukotriene-like substance from porcine vascular and other tissues. Prostaglandins 25:591–599
6. Rosenblum WI (1985) Constricting effect of leukotrienes on cerebral arterioles of mice. Stroke 16:262–263
7. Walker V, Pickard JD (1985) Prostaglandins, thromboxane, leukotrienes and the cerebral circulation in health and disease. In: Symon L, et al. (eds) Advances and technical standards in neurosurgery. Springer, Vienna, vol. 12, pp 3–90

Topographic Peculiarity in Spastic Changes of the Cerebral Artery After Subarachnoid Hemorrhage

Relationship Between Alteration of the Arachidonic Cascades and Electron-Microscopic Findings

Saburo Nakamura, Takashi Tsubokawa, and Kenshi Yoshida[1]

Introduction

Clinical observations have suggested that delayed ischemic neurological deficit caused by cerebral vasospasm is not always correlated with the location of spasm as revealed by angiography. Recent investigations have indicated an important role for arachidonic acid metabolites, especially prostacycline and thromboxane A_2, in the genesis of cerebral vasospasm following subarachnoid hemorrhage [7, 10].

In order to demonstrate the topographic peculiarity of the vascular response to subarachnoid hemorrhage, the concentration of eicosanoids at various levels of arterial segments corresponding to alterations in the electron-microscopic findings was studied.

Methods

Experimental subarachnoid hemorrhage (SAH) was produced by percutaneous administration of 2 ml/kg body weight of fresh autogenous blood into the cisterna magna of adult cats. The animals were killed by exsanguination following transcardiac perfusion of saline solution containing indomethacin and EDTA at various intervals after the production of SAH.

The basilar artery (BA), anterior inferior cerebellar artery (AICA), cerebral pial artery (PA), parietal cortex (PC), and temporal cortex (TC) were obtained and the concentrations of thromboxane B_2 (TXB_2), 6-keto-prostaglandin $F_1\alpha$ (6-keto-PG $F_1\alpha$), and leukotriene (LT) B_4 and C_4 were determined by radioimmunoassay following Murphy's method [9].

The ultrastructural changes in the vessels were examined at various levels of the arterial segments by transmission and scanning electron microscopy.

[1] Department of Neurological Surgery, Nihon University School of Medicine, Tokyo, Japan

Results

The control TXB_2 levels of the arteries ranged from 7.50 pg/mg wet tissue weight (mgWW) to 27.40 pg/mgWW. The mean control TXB_2 concentration was 19.65 pg/mgWW in the BA, 16.90 pg/mgWW in the posterior inferior cerebellar artery (PICA), and 23.26 pg/mgWW in the PA. The control TXB_2 levels of the cortex ranged from 0.62 pg/mgWW to 4.88 pg/mgWW. The mean normal TXB_2 concentration was 2.65 pg/mgWW in the TC and 3.09 pg/mgWW in the PC.

The TXB_2 levels of the SAH group were generally higher than those of the control. In the BA, the mean TXB_2 concentration rose to 26.68 pg/mgWW on the 5th day after the production of SAH, while that of the AICA showed a slight change. The mean concentration of TXB_2 in the PA showed the highest level (33.40 pg/mgWW) on the 7th day after the production of SAH.

The mean levels of TXB_2 in the cerebral cortex rose significantly to 13.35 pg/mgWW in the TC and 9.20 pg/mgWW in the PC, respectively, on the 7th day after the production of SAH (Fig. 1a).

The control 6-keto-PG $F_1\alpha$ levels in the arteries ranged from 6.32 pg/mgWW to 24.60 pg/mgWW. The mean control 6-keto-PG $F_1\alpha$ concentration was 16.53 pg/mgWW in the BA, 14.32 pg/mgWW in the AICA, and 15.21 pg/mgWW in the PA. The control 6-keto-PG $F_1\alpha$ levels of the cortex ranged from 0.44 pg/mgWW to 1.37 pg/mgWW. The mean normal 6-keto-PG $F_1\alpha$ concentration was 0.77 pg/mgWW in the PC and 0.87 pg/mgWW in the TC.

The 6-keto-PG $F_1\alpha$ levels in the SAH group were generally lower than those of the control. The mean 6-keto-PG $F_1\alpha$ concentration in the BA decreased to 6.20 pg/mgWW on the 5th day after the production of SAH, and that of the AICA decreased to 7.79 pg/mgWW on the 3rd day. The mean concentration of 6-keto-PG $F_1\alpha$ in the PA showed unstable changes.

The mean levels of 6-keto-PG $F_1\alpha$ in the cerebral cortex revealed little change in both the PC

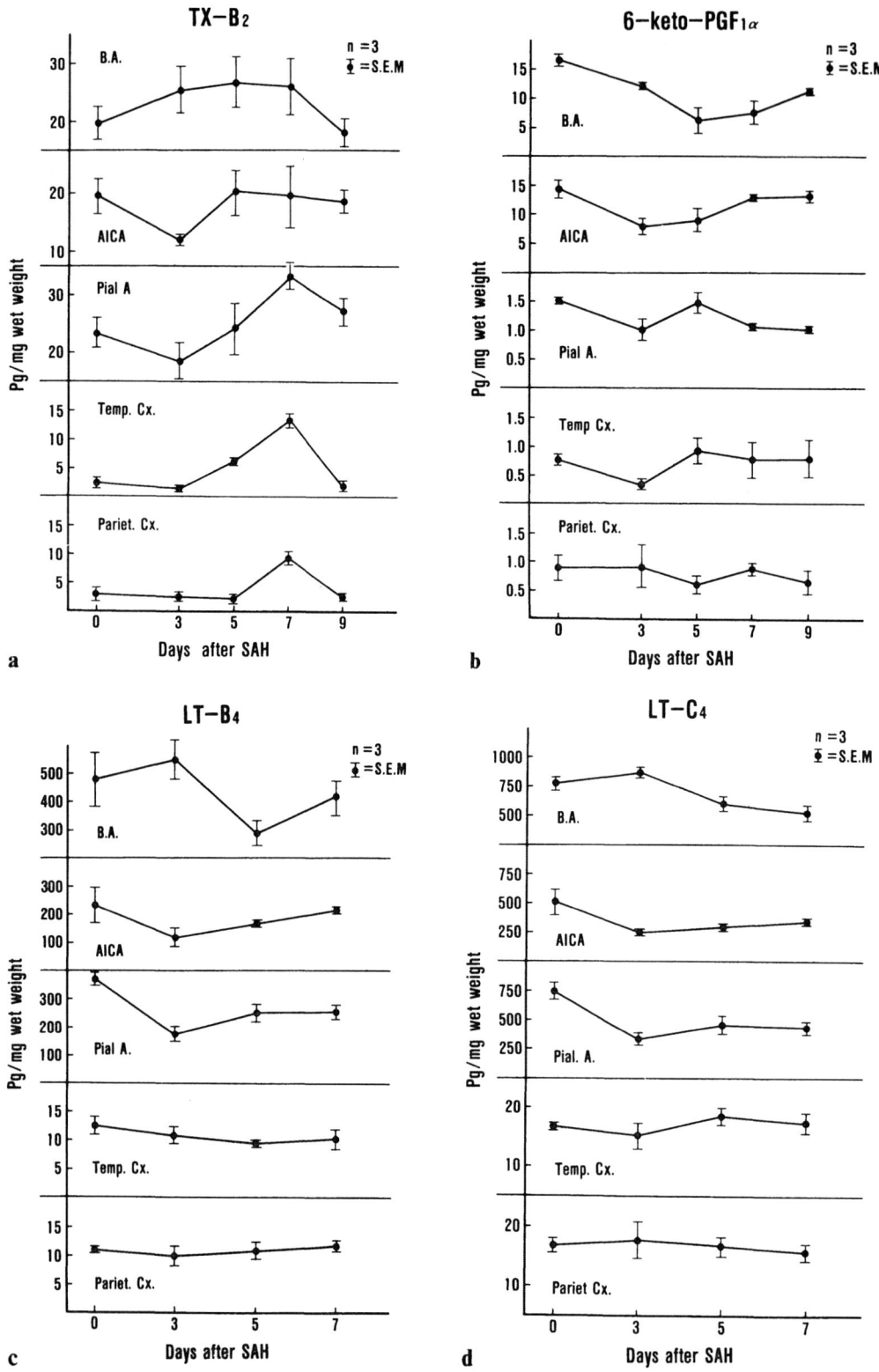

Fig. 1a–d. The eicosanoid levels of the control and the SAH group. **a** Thromboxine B_2 (TXB_2); **b** 6-keto-prostaglandin (*PG*) $F_{1\alpha}$; **c** leukotriene B_4; **d** leukotriene C_4. *BA* basilar artery, *AICA* anterior inferior cerebellar artery

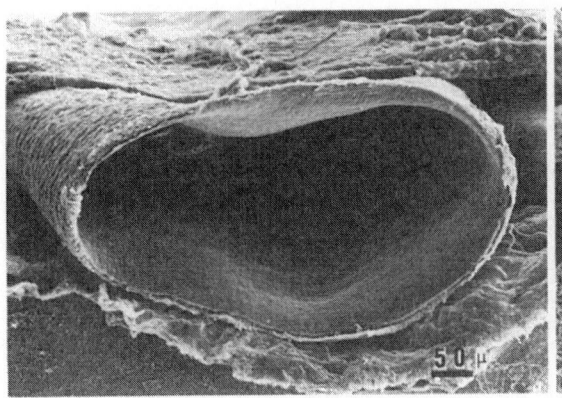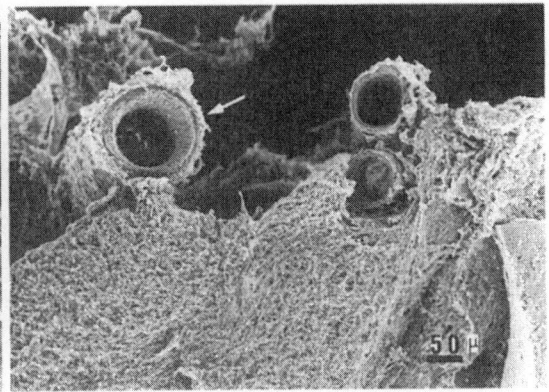

a b

Fig. 2a, b. Scanning electron micrographs. **a** The basilar artery showing little change on the 7th day after the production of SAH. **b** The pial vessels showing the most remarkable change (*arrow*) on the 7th day after the production of SAH. Calibration = 50 μm

and the TC, respectively, after production of SAH (Fig. 1b).

The levels of both LTB_4 and LTC_4 in the arteries and the cerebral cortices showed no steady changes after the production of SAH, and were little changed even on the 7th day when the TXB_2 level increased to the greatest degree (Fig. 1c, d).

Ultrastructural studies revealed extreme deformation of the endothelial cells along the corrugated internal elastic membrane of the spastic arteries. The smooth muscle cells in the tunica media were distorted and the intercellular spaces were irregularly widened. In some areas, adhesion of blood cells and platelets to the intimal surface was observed. Although such findings were recognized in the BA and AICA (Fig. 2a), the most remarkable changes were seen in the pial vessels at the 7th day after SAH production (Fig. 2b), which themselves showed the greatest increase in TXB_2 level.

Discussion

Among the many etiological factors which may be involved in cerebral vasospasm following SAH, arachidonic acid metabolites have attracted the attention of several groups. Experimental studies have revealed an important role for prostacyclin (PGI_2), thromboxane A_2 (TXA_2), and, recently, leukotrienes, in the genesis of cerebral vasospasm [6]. A reciprocal relationship between PGI_2 (a potent vasodilator and inhibitor of platelet aggregation) [8] and TXA_2 (a strong vasoconstrictor and accelerator of platelet aggregation) is considered essential for the maintenance of the cerebrovascular tone [2, 3]. PGI_2 is synthesized in the vascular wall [1], and TXA_2 is generated from aggregating platelets. During the course of SAH, various pathological events give rise to a decreased synthesis of PGI_2 [10]. Thus, the balance between PGI_2 and TXA_2 is shifted to a disproportionate concentration of TXA_2, leading to constriction of the cerebral vessels and platelet aggregation.

One significant finding of our experimental study was that alteration of TXA_2/PGI_2 homeostasis in the vascular wall is demonstrable during the course of SAH. The level of 6-keto-$PG F_1\alpha$, measured as a converted stable product of PGI_2, was decreased in the arterial walls, but changed little in both cortices after the production of SAH.

In contrast, the level of TXB_2, measured as a stable product of TXA_2, was elevated in both the arterial walls and cerebral cortices on the 7th day after SAH production. In particular, the levels of TXB_2 in the pial arteries and both cortices rose significantly (Table 1).

In view of the fact that TXA_2 is generated from aggregating platelets through the activity of the enzyme thromboxane-synthetase, it seems reasonable to suppose that a rise in TXB_2 levels in the cortices indicates pathological events in the vessels rather than in the cerebral parenchyma. Accordingly, arteries of small diameter, such as the pial arteries and intraparenchymal vessels, are affected by increased TXA_2.

Ellis and his coworkers [4] reported that the contraction produced, by TXA_2, in vitro, was as great as that produced by $PG F_2\alpha$ and approximately twice that produced by serotonin.

A falling level of PGI_2, on the other hand,

which is thought to be synthesized in the vascular wall by the action of its specific enzyme prostacyclin-synthetase, indicates a disturbance of its synthesis in the vascular wall. This is thought to be one of the sequelae of the ultrastructural damage [5], which was demonstrated by electron microscope examinations, and the action of specific inhibitors, such as lipid peroxides and free radicals, which are thought to be synthesized through the lysis of subarachnoid blood clots during the course of SAH.

Ultrastructural observations revealed a topographic difference in response to SAH. That is, the vessels of smaller diameter, such as the pial vessels, showed more marked spastic changes than those of larger diameter, such as the BA or AICA. Accordingly, a decline in the 6-keto-PG $F_1\alpha$ level is attributable to pathological events other than vasospasm.

Comparison of the morphological changes with the levels of arachidonic acid metabolites in the arterial walls indicated that vasospasm may be correlated more distinctly with an elevation of the TXA_2 level than a decline in PGI_2 or a change in the levels of leukotrienes.

In conclusion, it is suggested that the ischemic events after SAH may have been induced by vasospasm and increased coagulability, caused by changes in the concentration of arachidonic acid metabolites at the arteries of smaller diameter, such as the pial or cortical arteries.

Table 1. Changes of eicosanoids in the arterial walls and cerebral cortices during the course of SAH

	BA	AICA	PA	Cortex
TXB_2 (TXA_2)	↑	↓↑	↑↑	↑↑↑
6-keto-$PGF_{1\alpha}$ (PGI_2)	↓	↓	↓↑	→
LT-B_4	↓	→	↓	→
LT-C_4	↓	↓	↓↓	→

BA basilar artery, *AICA* anterior interior cerebellar artery, *PA* pial artery, *TXB₂* thromboxane B_2, *PG* prostaglandin, *PGI₂* prostacyclin, *LT* leukotriene

References

1. Abdel-Haim MS, von Holst H, Meyerson B, Sachs C, Änggard E (1980) Prostaglandin profiles in tissue and blood vessels from human brain. J Neurochem 34:1331–1333
2. Bouillin DJ (1980) Potential use of prostacyclin in the treatment of vasospasm. In: Wilkins RH (ed) Cerebral arterial spasm. Williams and Wilkins, Baltimore, pp 533–539
3. Chan RC, Durity FA, Thompson GB, Nugent RA, Kendall M (1984) The role of the prostacyclin-thromboxane system in cerebral vasospasm following induced subarachnoid hemorrhage in the rabbit. J Neurosurg 61:1120–1128
4. Ellis EF, Nies AS, Oates JA (1977) Cerebral arterial smooth muscle contraction by thromboxane A_2. Stroke 8:480–483
5. Fein JM, Flor WJ, Cohan SL, Parkhurst J (1974) Sequential changes of vascular ultrastructure in experimental cerebral vasospasm: Myonectrosis of subarachnoid arteries. J Neurosurg 41:49–58
6. Hagen AA, White RP, Robertson JT (1979) Sythesis of prostaglandins and thromboxane B_2 by cerebral arteries. Stroke 10:306–309
7. Maeda Y, Tani E, Miyamoto T (1981) Prostaglandin metabolism in experimental cerebral vasospasm. J Neurosurg 55:779–785
8. Moncada S, Vane JR (1979) The role of prostacyclin in vascular tissue. Fed Proc 38:66–77
9. Murphy RC, Hammarstrom S, Samuelsson B (1979) Leukotriene C: A slow-reacting substance from murine mastocytoma cells. Proc Natl Acad Sci USA 76:4275–4279
10. Seifert V, Stolke D, Kaever V, Dietz H (1987) Arachidonic acid metabolism following aneurysm rupture. Evaluation of cerebrospinal fluid and serum concentration of 6-keto-prostaglandin F_1 and thromboxane B_2 in patients with subarachnoid hemorrhage. Surg Neurol 27:243–252

Surgical Indication and Approach to Deep-Seated Arteriovenous Malformation

Norio Nakamura, Soji Shinoda, and Koji Akachi[1]

Total extirpation of the nidus is fundamentally the best choice for treatment of intracranial arteriovenous malformations (AVMs). It is never acceptable, however, to allow a persistent postoperative deficit to develop, which would burden the patient after surgery [2]. The only exception is when the patient is in a critical condition.

Materials and Method

At present, we define so-called "deep AVMs" after Pellettieri (Fig. 1) [5]. In the frontal projection, a curved line is drawn from the sagittal sinus through the external capsule to the base of the frontal, temporal and occipital lobes. When the principal portion of the nidus is situated deeper than this line, it is called a deep AVM. Deep cerebellar and brainstem AVMs are included, too.

Forty-seven deep AVMs were encountered in the Tokyo Jikei University Hospital (Table 1). Even though the preponderant positions were the thalamus and paraventricular regions, the deep temporal and interhemispheric and deep cerebellar regions were also frequent. Total extirpation of the nidus was successful in 32 cases, whereas no surgery was undertaken in 15.

Up to the present time, we have taken three risk factors into consideration in judging surgical indication of deep AVMs: the size of the nidus, the position of the nidus, and the pattern of demarcation around the nidus on CT view (Table 2). The profound demarcation of the nidus by previous hemorrhage, cyst, or ventricular wall indicates good risk. We then determine grades of risk on each factors and count a risk score in each case.

The long-term result of our 47 patients was judged by the response to questionnaires, sent recently to all surviving patients. In the case of total extirpation, the preoperative neurological state was compared with the latest activities in daily life (ADL). In the cases without surgery, the neurological state on admission was used.

Results

Of the 15 patients who did not undergo surgery, ten survived without either improvement or aggravation. One became more impaired and four died on account of rebleeding (Table 3).

Of the 32 operated patients, two died immediately after surgery. One was comatose prior to admission because of massive hemorrhage. The other was lost as the result of postoperative hematoma (Table 4).

The neurological condition was aggravated after surgery in 7 of the 30 surviving patients (Fig. 2). Three of the seven complained of hemonymous hemianopsia caused by injured optic radiation. Three suffered hemiparesis after a parietal or sylvian approach. One had mild aphasia after a left temporal approach. Another had hemiparesis caused by accidental subdural hematoma. These neurological deficits of the seven patients still remain, more or less. The risk score of these seven cases prior to surgery was not always very poor.

Discussion

The natural history of cerebral arteriovenous malformation is still a subject of dispute. Graf et al. [1] emphasizes the disaster of rebleeding, recently as high as 6% in the 1st year followed by 2% per year in ruptured AVMs. In the case of deep AVM ruptures, the problem is more serious because the hemorrhage often gives rise to severe disability or death of patients depending on its location [6].

[1] Department of Neurosurgery, Tokyo Jikei University School of Medicine, Tokyo, Japan

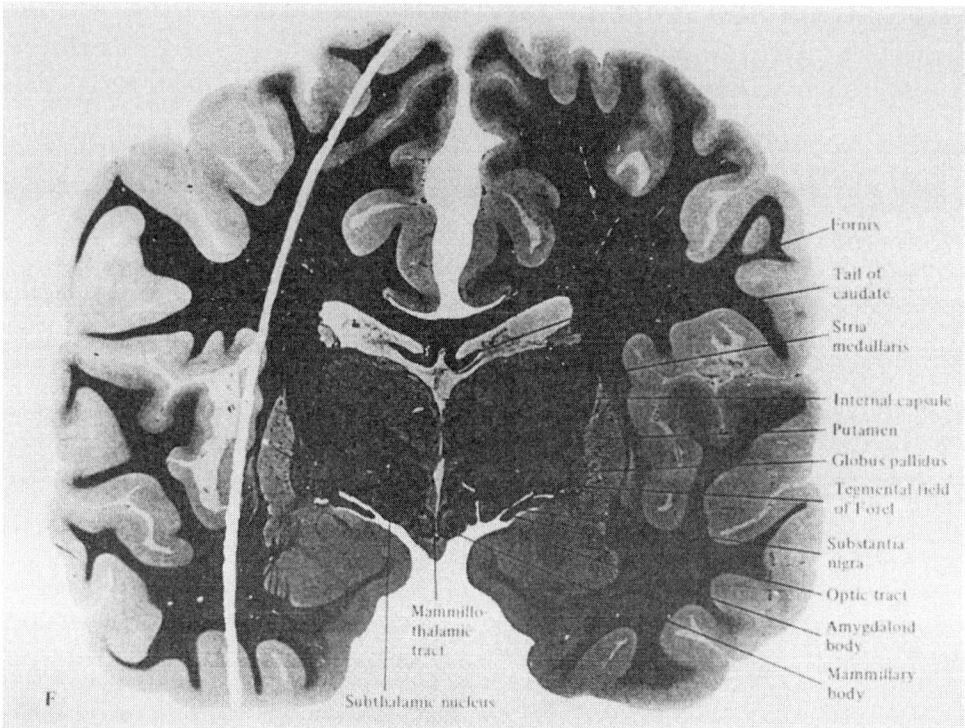

Fig. 1. Definition of deep-seated AVMs

Table 1. Positions of AVMs

Position	Surgery	No surgery	Total
Frontal base	4	1	5
Interhemispheric	3	2	5
Interal occipital	2	1	3
Corpus callosum	1	1	2
Paraventricle	7	2	9
Deep sylvian	2	0	2
Deep temporal	4	2	6
Thalamus	2	5	7
Basal ganglia	2	1	3
Brainstem	0	0	0
Deep cerebellar	5	0	5
Total	32	15	47

Table 2. Risk factors and risk score

Graded feature		Points assigned
A	Size of AVM	
	Small (<3 cm)	1
	Medium (3–6 cm)	2
	Large (>6 cm)	3
B	Eloquence of adjacent brain	
	Noneloquent	1
	Eloquent	2
C	Demarcation of the nidus	
	Demarcated	1
	Not demarcated	2

Spetzler and Martin [4] recently suggested three factors to estimate the risk of surgery for AVM: size of AVM, eloquence of adjacent brain, and pattern of venous drainage. Shi and Chen [3] proposed four factors supplementing arterial supplies.

In the case of deep AVMs, there are serious problems which are different from superficial AVMs. Because the nidus is situated deep in the brain, not only feeding arteries but also draining veins commonly take their course deeply. Moreover, it is frequently necessary to dissect an intact cortex in order to reach the nidus and to compress it with spatulas for a long time while keeping the opening wide.

Taking these peculiarities into consideration, we proposed both the size and position of the nidus as anatomical risk factors. When the nidus is bordered by hemorrhage, cyst, or ventricular wall, dissection of the nidus is facilitated and injury to adjacent brain tissue is minimized. This is the reason why we included profound demarcation around the nidus as the third factor.

In this presentation, the fate of patients who did not undergo surgery seems fairly optimistic; however, this is not true. The lapse of time under observation after discharge from hospital is less than 4 years in the majority of surviving patients. On the other hand it is more than 7 years in the nonsurviving ones; 15 years on the average. Therefore, the longer the patient having deep AVM survives, the more likely the disaster of fatal rebleeding. The basic policy of total extirpation as the best choice for deep AVM also is supported, especially when there is a low-grade risk score to surgery.

Of the 32 patients who underwent surgery, 23 survive in an improved state or without any aggravated neurological deficit, and 22 of these 23 cases have no burden in daily lives at present. However, another seven patients complain of some additional postoperative symptoms as mentioned previously. It might be fair to say that the cause of aggravation after surgery in these seven cases was attributable primarily to the surgical approach to the nidus, in combination with the technical difficulty in accomplishing total extirpation.

In summarizing our cases, the group with a

risk score of 5 is the largest in number and most problematic, when we have to judge the surgical indication as well as the most appropriate approach to the nidus (Table 5).

At first, we discussed ten cases of risk score 5 who did not undergo surgery. Three of ten pa-

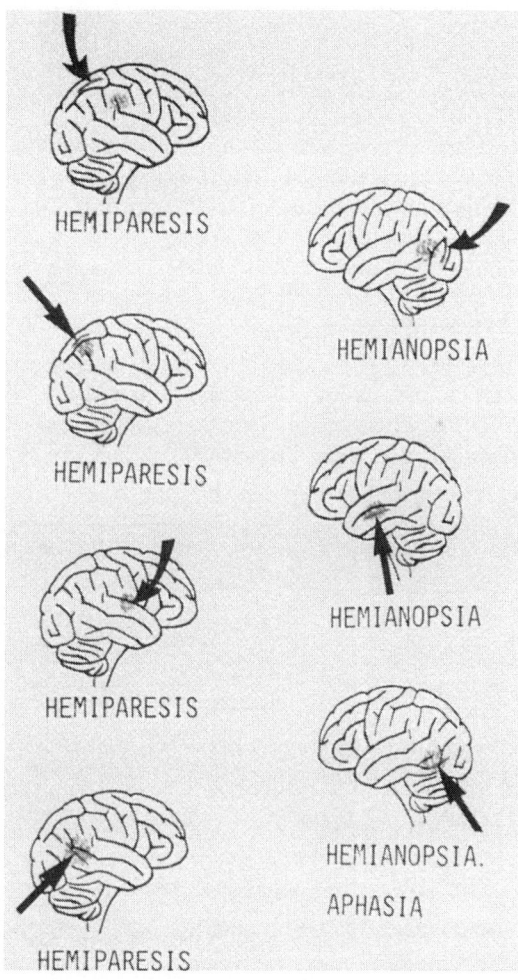

Fig. 2. Postoperative neurological deficits in combination with the approches to the nidus in seven cases

Table 3. Long-term outcome nonoperated group

Score	No change	Aggravated	Dead	Total
3	0	0	0	0
4	1	0	1	2
5	7	0	3	10
6	1	0	0	1
7	1	1	0	2
Total	10	1	4	15

Table 4. Long-term outcome surgery group

Score	Improved			No change			Aggravated			Dead	Total
	EXC	G	F	EXC	G	F	EXC	G	F		
3	1	1	1	0	1	0	0	2	0	0	6
4	2	0	0	3	2	0	0	1	0	2	10
5	0	0	0	5	5	0	0	1	3	0	14
6	0	0	0	1	1	0	0	0	0	0	2
7	0	0	0	0	0	0	0	0	0	0	0
Total	3	1	1	9	9	0	0	4	3	2	32

EXC excellent = ADL 5, *G* Good = ADL 4, *F* fair = ADL 3 (or 2)

Table 5. Cases with risk score 5

	No-surgery group				Surgery group				
Score	Total	Aggravated	Dead	Score	Total	Aggravated			Dead
						EXC	G	F	
3	0	0	0	3	6	0	2	0	0
4	2	0	1	4	10	0	1	0	2
5	10	0	3	5	14	0	1	3	0
6	1	0	0	6	2	0	0	0	0
7	2	1	0	7	0	0	0	0	0
Total	15	1	4		32	0	4	3	2

Combination of risk features in risk score 5

Size	Position	Demarcation
<3 cm	Unlucky	No
3–6 cm	Lucky	No
3–6 cm	Unlucky	Yes
>6 cm	Lucky	Yes

EXC excellent = ADL 5, *G* good = ADL 4, *F* fair = ADL 3 (or 2)

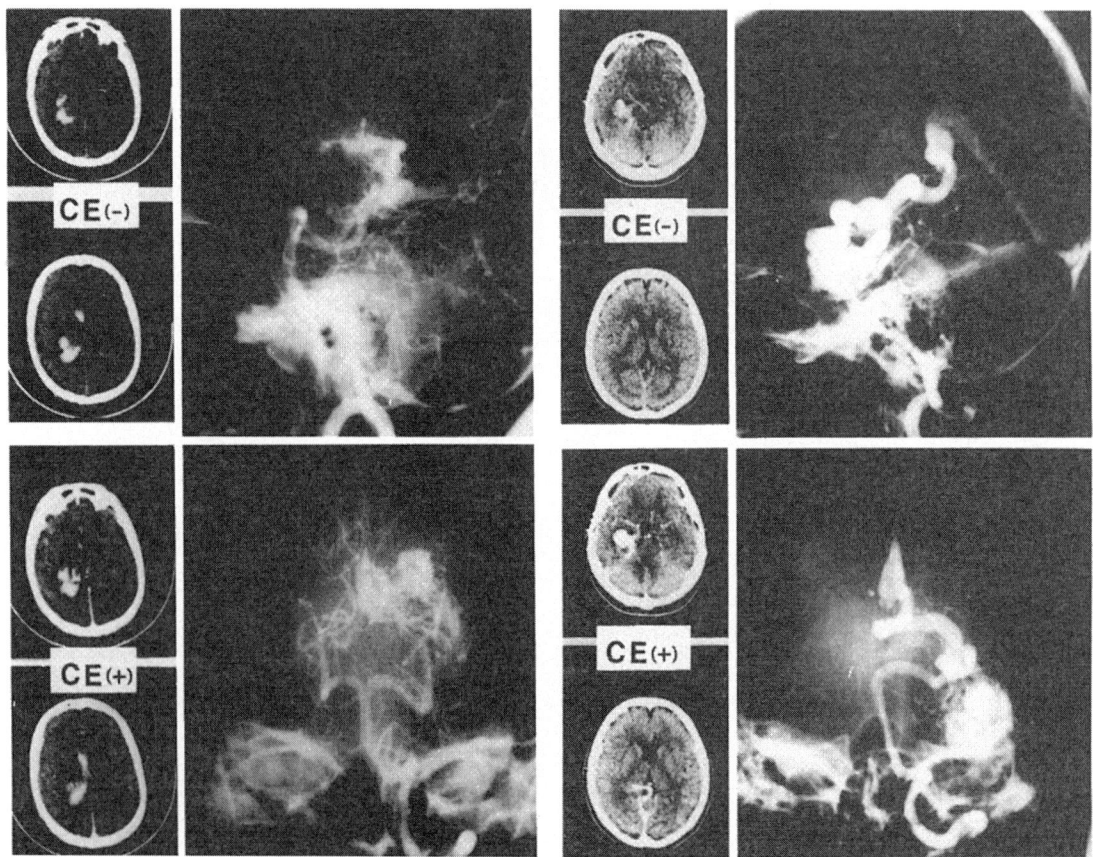

Fig. 3. Case 1. 29-year-old male with left paraventricular AVM of risk score 5   **Fig. 4.** Case 2. 34-year-old female with left paraventricular AVM of risk score 5

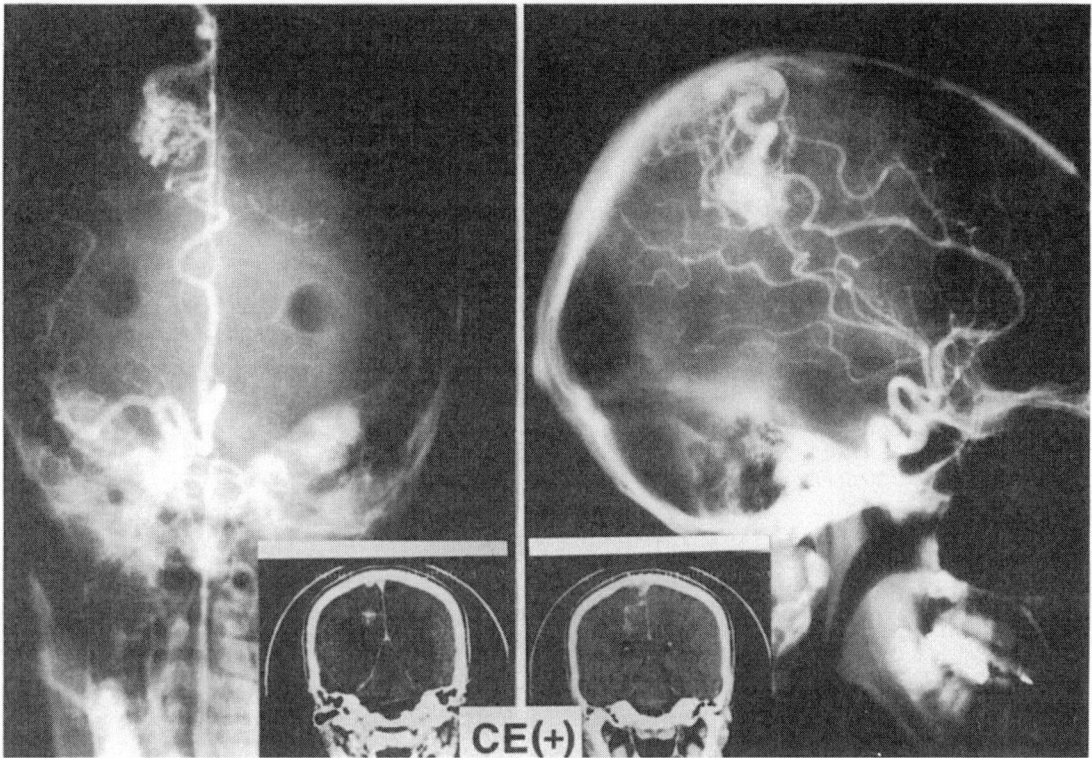

Fig. 5. Case 3. 20-year-old female, now handicapped, who underwent surgery after admission with mild motor weakness

tients died after discharge from the hospital. The following two patients have survived until now.

Case 1. Left paraventicular AVM of risk score 5 was discovered in a 29-year-old male who had suffered from intracranial hemorrhage (Fig. 3). We withheld surgery in fear of postoperative development of both Gerstmann's syndrome and hemiparesis. He has been well for 3 years.

Case 2. Left paraventricular AVM of risk score 5 was found in a 34-year-old female (Fig. 4). She had slight aphasia because of four previous hemorrhages of her AVM. She did not agree to an operation and has survived for 2 years without surgery.

Of 14 cases of risk score 5 who underwent surgery three had mild motor weakness on admission, which was aggravated after surgery; they have spent a handicapped daily life. Case 3 is an example of this group (Fig. 5).

In conclusion, the most deliberate care and the highest technical skill are indispensable requirements for surgery of deep AVMs of risk score 5.

References

1. Graf CJ, Perret GE, Torner JC (1983) Bleeding from cerebral arteriovenous malformations as part of their natural history. J Neurosurg 58:331–337
2. Jomin M, Lesion F, Lozes G (1985) Prognosis for arteriovenous malformation of the brain in adult based on 150 cases. Surg Neurol 23:362–366
3. Shi Y, Chen X (1986) A proposed scheme for grading intracranial arteriovenous malformations. J Neurosurg 65:484–489
4. Spetzler RF, Martin NA (1986) A proposed grading system for arteriovenous malformations. J Neurosurg 65:476–483
5. Pellettieri L (1980) Surgical versus conservative treatment of intracranial arteriovenous malformations. Acta Neurochir Suppl 29:8–9
6. Perria L, Viale GL, Rosa M (1971) Remarks on the pathology and surgery of midline intracranial angiomas. Neurochir 14:71–78

Prediction of Postoperative Perfusion Breakthrough During Removal of High-Flow Arteriovenous Malformation

Kazuo Yamada, Toru Hayakawa, Kazuo Kataoka, Kazutami Nakao, Toshiki Yoshimine, and Heitaro Mogami[1]

Introduction

Surgery of large and high-flow arteriovenous malformations (AVMs) encounters the risk of normal perfusion pressure breakthrough syndrome [6]. The phenomenon might occur after removal of large and high-flow AVM and may relate to the abrupt diversion of intracerebral flow direction. However, the precise changes in hemodynamics after clipping the feeders of the AVM remains uncertain.

We have measured cortical blood flow with a heat clearance method during craniotomy [2, 3, 5] This is safe and reliable method for detection of blood flow changes during cerebrovascular surgery. In the present report, we describe changes in cortical blood flow after clipping the feeder of the AVM. These changes are compared to angiographical findings and postoperative clinical courses.

Case Materials and Methods

Criteria for High-Flow Arteriovenous Malformation

According to the criteria by Wilson et al. [7], we defined high-flow arteriovenous malformation as having a diameter larger than 4 cm, large feeders and high-flow shunts, and with the surrounding vessels being large and dilated for competing sink effect of AVM, or thin due to a steal phenomenon of the AVM. During the last 4 years, we have encountered 20 cases that fulfilled the criteria for high-flow AVM. Of these, surgical removal was attempted in 14 cases. The age of these patients ranged from 14 to 64 years of age, and the median was 29 years old. The initial symptoms of these cases were seizure (six cases),

hemiplegic attack due to steal (four cases), subarachnoid hemorrhage (seven cases), and headache (three cases). Most of the AVM were located in the cerebral convexity, except for four cases situated in the deep temporal lobe, deep frontal lobe, putamen, and corpus callosum. Feeding arteries were derived from the middle cerebral artery in 17 cases, anterior cerebral artery in nine cases, and posterior cerebral artery in 11 cases. Four-vessel cerebral angiogram was performed to delineate all feeding arteries. Interhemispheric and transtentorial steal was also evaluated by those cerebral angiograms.

Blood Flow Measurement by Heat Clearance Method

Intraoperative measurement of cortical surface blood flow was performed in 14 cases. Details of this method were the same as reported previously [2, 3, 5]. Briefly, two to four plate-type probes [Unique-Medical Co. Ltd., Tokyo, Japan] were placed on the cortical surface: one on the nidus of the AVM and the others on the adjacent cortex. Probes were covered with wet cottonoids, with care being taken not to deform the cortex. The probes were connected with a thermocouple flowmeter [UM meter Model 2000, Unique-Medical Co. Ltd., Tokyo, Japan]. The output direct current from the thermocouple probes was amplified and recorded on an X-Y recorder. The heating current for the thermocouple heating circuit was 20 mA, and the sensitivity was adjusted as 10 μV of the output current was equivalent to 3.0 cm on the recording graphs. After the steady-state recording was obtained, feeding arteries of the AVM were clipped one by one, and hemodynamic changes were recorded on the X-Y recorder. Systemic arterial blood pressure was monitored continuously during these procedures. The calibration curve between the output current and blood flow values was obtained from the cat cortical surface using a heat clearance

[1] Department of Neurosurgery, Osaka University Medical School, Osaka, Japan

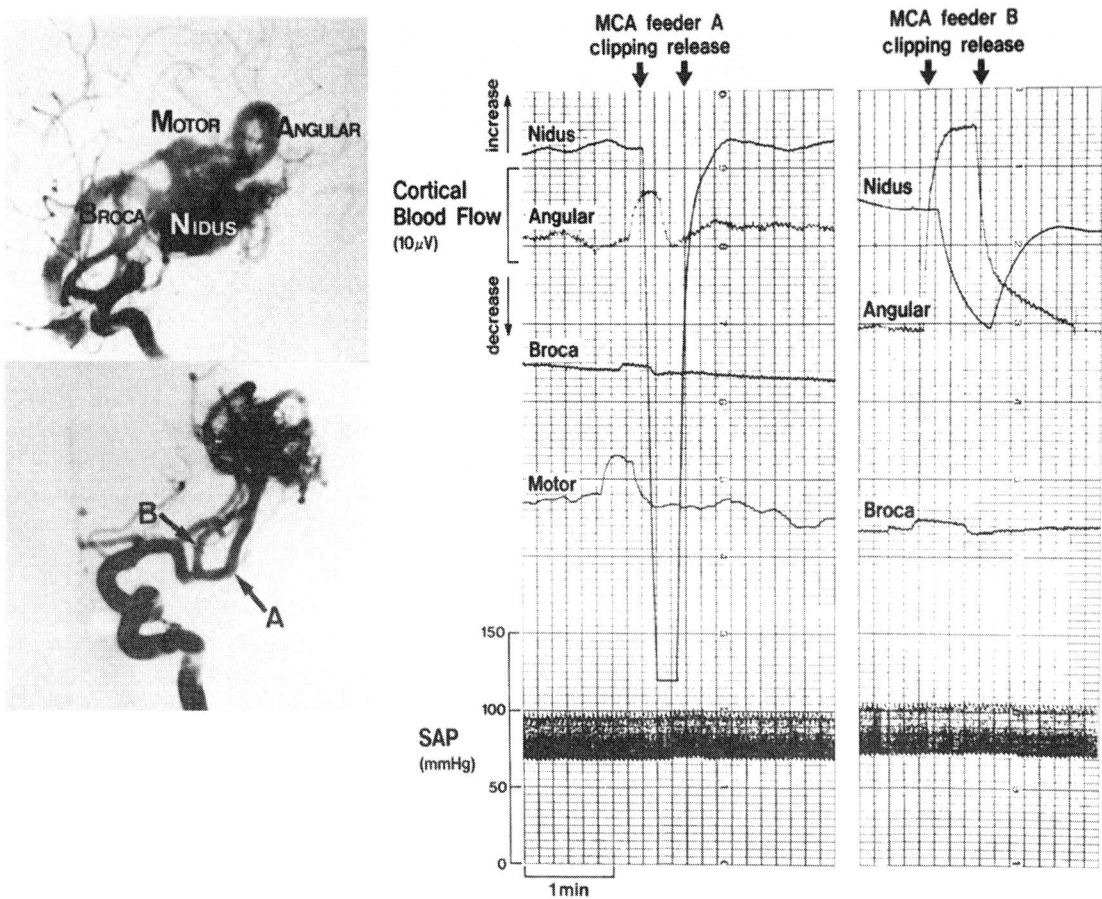

Fig. 1. A case of high-flow AVM showing an increase in adjacent cortical flow due to feeder clipping. *Arrows* indicate feeders A (first) and B (second); *SAP* systemic arterial pressure

method [2]. Ten microvolts of the output current is equivalent to about 8 ml/100 g/min of blood flow changes.

Results

Of 14 cases subjected to blood flow measurements, four cases showed increase in blood flow after clipping the feeders. In a typical case, with a large AVM in the left temporal lobe, the malformation was supplied by two feeders from the left middle cerebral artery (Fig. 1). The thermocouple probes were placed on the surface of the nidus, angular cortex, motor cortex, and Broca area, and the first feeder was clipped. The nidus flow dropped deeply and cortical flow ineased paradoxically. The angular and motor cortices close to the nidus showed more increase in blood flow than the Broca cortex which was

apart from the nidus. After the first feeder was clipped permanently, the second feeder was clipped. The nidus flow dropped further, but the blood flow in the angular cortex increased significantly. The increase in angular cortical flow after the second feeder being clipped was about three times of that after the first feeder was clipped. This suggests that blood flow of the adjacent cortex increased maximally after the final feeding arteries were clipped.

In this case we encountered postoperative hemorrhage at 2 days after the first surgery and removed the clot. Histological observation indicated that the brain tissue adjacent to the AVM showed spotty hemorrhage around the small capillaries. It is possible that the perfusion breakthrough mechanism was responsible for this postoperative hemorrhage, though several alternative possibilities were present. The computed tomography scan taken a week after surgery

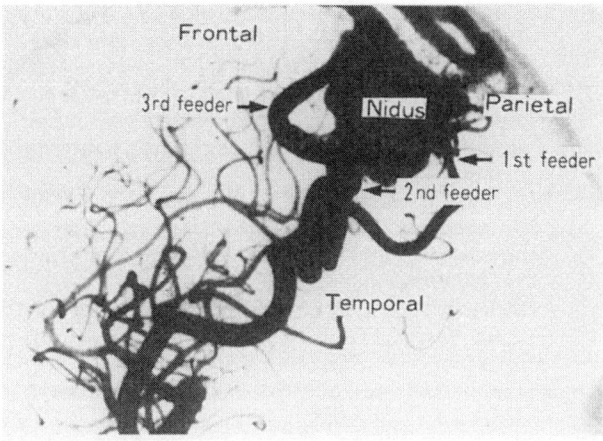

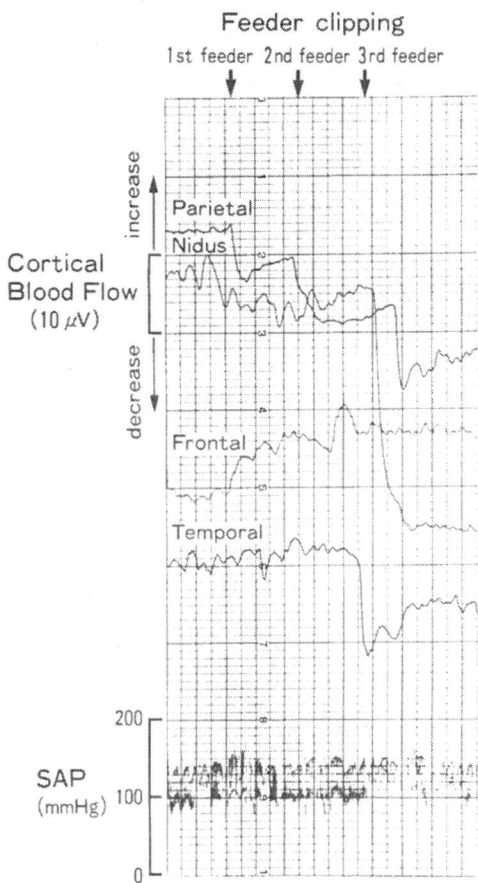

Fig. 2. The right parietal AVM with 3 feeders. Despite feeder clippings, no increase in adjacent cortical flow was noted. *SAP* systemic arterial pressure

showed the area of contrast enhancement in the frontal operculum. This enhancement was disclosed as proximal hyperemia by dynamic computed tomography scan.

Three other cases had similar increases in blood flow in the cortex adjacent to the AVM after feeder clipping. Of these, one case had postoperative hemorrhage and another case had transient confusion and motor aphasia.

Ten cases showed no increase in blood flow at the adjacent cortex when clipping the feeding artery. In one typical case, a parietal AVM had three feeders from the middle cerebral artery (Fig. 2). The thermocouple probes were placed on the nidus and adjacent parietal, temporal, and frontal cortices. When the first and second feeders were clipped, only the parietal flow reduced to some extent. Then the third feeder was clipped, and the nidus flow reduced abruptly. At this time the parietal and temporal flow reduced simultaneously. In these ten cases which showed no increase in cortical flow by the feeder clipping, there were no postoperative complications.

Discussion

During or immediately after the surgery for AVM, formidable hemorrhage occurs occasionally in the brain adjacent to the AVM. This event is explained as normal perfusion pressure breakthrough [6], proximal hyperemia [4], or elimination of sump effect [1]. With this in mind the important point is to predict this syndrome before removal of the AVM. As suggested by Wilson et al. [7], angiographical findings are one of the useful sources of information in predicting this syndrome.

From this aspect, we have undertaken intraoperative measurement of the cortial blood flow during surgery for AVM. We have especially tried to detect blood flow increase after feeder clipping, since this event is caused by an abrupt increase in blood flow after clipping of the feeder and removal of the AVM. As predicted, an increase in blood flow was observed in 4 of 14 cases. Two of those cases had postoperative hemorrhage, and one case had transient confusion and dysphasia. On the other hand, ten cases had no increase in adjacent cortical flow and had no postoperative complications. Therefore, intraoperative blood flow measurement is a useful tool to predict postoperative perfusion breakthrough events. Based on this data, we might plan multistaged surgery, if the cortical blood flow is increased by feeder clipping.

References

1. Drake CG (1979) Cerebral arteriovenous malformations: Considerations for and experience with surgical treatment in 166 cases. Clin Neurosurg 26:145–208
2. Hayakawa T (1984) Intraoperative measurement of cortical blood flow by heat clearance method. In: Kikuchi H (ed) Neurosurgeons, vol 4. The Japanese Congress of Neurological Surgeons, Tokyo, pp 183–190
3. Hayakawa T, Yamada K, Iwata Y, Kato A, Yoshimine T, Ushio Y, Nakatani S, Ikeda T, Mogami H (1985) Usefulness of intraoperative cortical blood flow measurement by heat clearance method for monitoring cerebral ischemia during therapeutic carotid ligation. J Neurol Neurosurg Psychiat 48:819–825
4. Mullan S, Brown FD, Patronas NJ (1979) Hyperemic and ischemic problems of surgical treatment of arteriovenous malformations. J Neurosurg 51:757–764
5. Nakao K, Yamada K, Hayakawa T, Tagawa T, Yoshimine T, Ushio Y, Mogami H (in press) Intraoperative measurement of cortical blood flow and its CO_2 response in childhood moyamoya disease. Neurosurgery
6. Spetzler RF, Wilson CB, Weinstein P, Mehdorn M, Townsend J, Telles D (1978) Normal perfusion pressure breakthrough theory. Clin Neurosurg 25:651–672
7. Wilson CB, U HS, Domingue J (1979) Microsurgical treatment of intracranial vascular malformations. J Neurosurg 51:446–454

Problems in Surgical Management of Giant Intracranial Aneurysms

Minoru Shigemori, Shinken Kuramoto, Jun Miyagi, Yasuo Sugita, and Akihiko Kuratomi[1]

Introduction

The surgical results of cerebral aneurysms have been improved with recent diagnostic and therapeutic advances. However, many problems still remain in the management of giant intracranial aneurysms [1, 2, 6]. In this paper, the problems in the surgical treatment of giant aneurysms of the anterior circulation were studied based on our experiences.

Materials and Methods

The patients included 14 females and two males with ages ranging from 18 to 76 years. The aneurysms, determined on neuroradiological and operative findings, were all larger than 25 mm in the maximum dimension. The aneurysms were located at the internal carotid artery (ICA) in ten patients, including five of infraclinoid, three of paraclinoid, and two of supraclinoid portions. Four patients had aneurysms of the middle cerebral artery (MCA), and two of the anterior cerebral artery (ACA). Five of sixteen patients presented with subarachnoid hemorrhage, and one patient of MCA aneurysm had several attacks of unconsciousness. The other ten patients had manifestations of intracranial space-occupying lesions. Eye signs, including visual disturbance and ocular nerve palsies, were found in nine patients (Table 1).

Of 16 patients, direct operation for the aneurysms was performed in ten patients, and six patients were treated by indirect methods. The surgical results were graded as excellent (with normal neurological function), good (with minimal residual neurological deficits), fair (with moderate neurological deficits), and poor (with severe neurological deficits), at 3 months after operation. Eye signs were classified as the same, better, and worse compared with preoperative conditions.

Results

Of 16 patients, ten had craniotomy, and direct clipping was performed in eight patients in whom the aneurysms were excised or opened (in seven instances). Multiple clipping, including tandem clip placement, was used in three patients of paraclinoid ICA aneurysms. Two giant aneurysms arising from the MCA were treated by excision of the aneurysm and end-to-end anastomosis of the parent artery. Of the other six patients, two had ICA ligation combined with extracranial-intracranial (EC-IC) bypass, and one was treated by ligation of the common carotid artery. Three patients of infraclinoid ICA aneurysms were treated by electrothrombosis using copper wire [3]. The surgical results showed that 10 of 16 patients were excellent or good, but three patients were poor, and one died of pulmonary complication. Eye signs were improved in seven patients, but worsened in two patients (Table 2). The operative complications will be discussed by presenting three illustrative cases.

Case 7. This 40-year-old man was admitted with progressive loss of visual acuity and field on both sides related to a giant aneurysm of the left paraclinoid ICA (Fig. 1a). The aneurysm projecting medially from the left ICA was exposed through the pterional approach. The left optic nerve was markedly stretched over the giant aneurysm and was densely adhered to the dome of the aneurysm. After extensive drilling of the anterior clinoid process, the aneurysm was successfully clipped with Sugita's fenestrated clips, used in tandem, while the cervical ICA was temporarily occluded in the neck. The dome of the aneurysm was then opened. Postoperative re-

[1] Department of Neurosurgery, Kurume University School of Medicine, Kurume, Japan

Table 1. Cases of giant cerebral aneurysms

Case No.	Age (yrs)	Sex	Location of aneurysm	Size of aneurysm (cm)	Clinical presentation
1	57	F	Rt ICA (infraclinoid)	3.5 × 2.5	III, IV, V, VI nervepalsy
2	54	F	Lt ICA (infraclinoid)	3.0 × 2.5	III, IV nerve palsy
3	72	F	Lt ICA (infraclinoid)	3.0 × 2.5	III, V, VI nerve palsy
4	60	F	Rt ICA (infraclinoid)	2.5 × 2.5	III, IV nerve palsy
5	70	F	Lt ICA (infraclinoid)	2.5 × 2.0	IV nerve palsy, loss of v.a.
6	18	F	Lt ICA (paraclinoid)	2.5 × 2.0	Progressive loss of v.a. and field
7	40	M	Lt ICA (paraclinoid)	3.5 × 3.5	Progressive loss of v.a. and field
8	58	F	Rt ICA (paraclinoid)	2.5 × 2.0	Progressive loss of v.a. and field
9	76	F	Lt ICA (supraclinoid)	2.5 × 2.0	SAH (grade III)
10	62	F	Lt ICA (supraclinoid)	2.5 × 1.5	SAH (grade III)
11	66	F	Lt MCA	4.0 × 4.0	SAH, ICH (grade IV)
12	50	M	Lt MCA	3.0 × 2.5	SAH, ICH (grade IV)
13	51	F	Rt MCA	3.5 × 3.0	SAH, ICH (grade III)
14	24	F	Lt MCA	3.0 × 2.5	Unconsciousness fits
15	69	F	Lt ACA (distal)	2.5 × 2.0	Progressive hemiparesis
16	24	F	ACA (A Co A)	2.5 × 2.0	Progressive loss of v.a. and field

ICA internal carotid artery, *SAH* subarachnoid hemorrhage, *MCA* middle cerebral artery, *ICH* intracerebral hematoma, *ACA* anterior cerebral artery, *v.a.* visual acuity, *A Co A* anterior communicating artery

Table 2. Surgical results of giant cerebral aneurysms

Types of treatment	No. of patients	Neurological condition					Eye signs		
		Excellent	Good	Fair	Poor	Dead	Same	Better	Worse
Direct clipping									
Single clip	5	2	0	2	1	0	0	1	0
Multiple clips	3	1	1	0	0	1	0	1	1
Excision of aneurysm and end-to-end anastomosis	2	1	0	0	1	0	0	0	0
CCA ligation	1	0	1	0	0	0	0	1	0
ICA ligation with EC-IC bypass	2	0	2	0	0	0	0	2	0
Electrothrombosis									
with EC-IC bypass	1	0	0	0	1	0	0	0	1
without EC-IC bypass	2	0	2	0	0	0	0	2	0
Total	16	4	6	2	3	1	0	7	2

covery was uneventful. The patency of the parent artery and distal circulation were satisfactory on postoperative angiogram (Fig. 1b). However, he remained blind in the left eye although a visual field defect in the right eye cleared in a few weeks. It is possible that the visual damage in this case resulted from traction and the repeated manipulation of the optic nerve.

Case 13. This 51-year-old woman was referred to us in the diagnosis of subarachnoid hemorrhage and intracerebral hematoma in the right frontal lobe. Angiogram demonstrated a giant MCA aneurysm on the right side (Fig. 2a). On right frontotemporal craniotomy, the sylvian fissure was opened and the aneurysm, as well as the main stem of the MCA, were exposed after evacuating the hematoma. Two clips were placed on the MCA proximal and distal to the aneurysm prior to excision. Following excision of the aneurysms, anastomosis was carried out using 9-0 interrupted black nylon, although the main stem of the MCA was sclerotic and narrow. Postoperatively, the patient continued to be unconscious and severely hemiparetic on the left side.

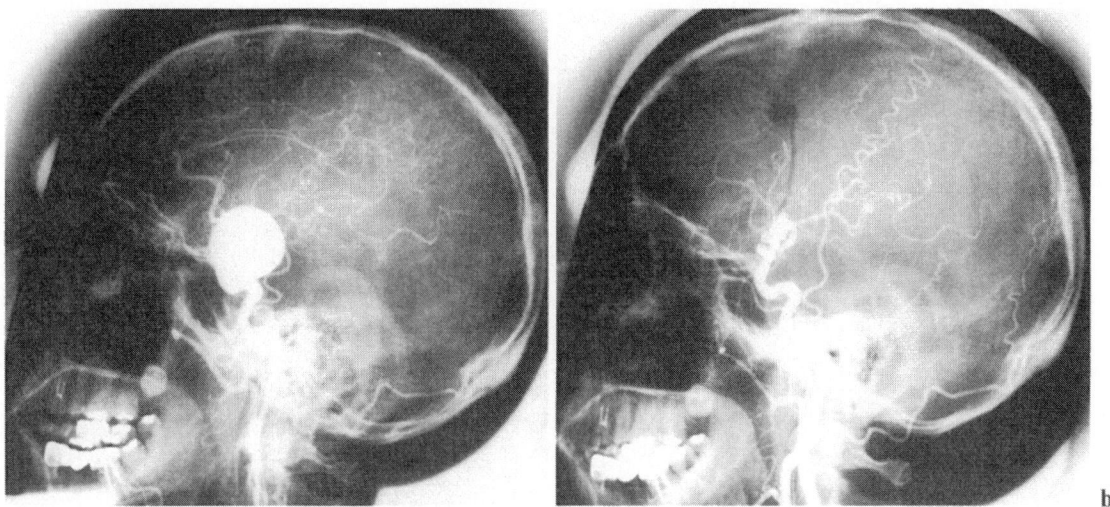

Fig. 1a, b. Case 7. Giant aneurysm of the left paraclinoid ICA **a** before and **b** after surgery

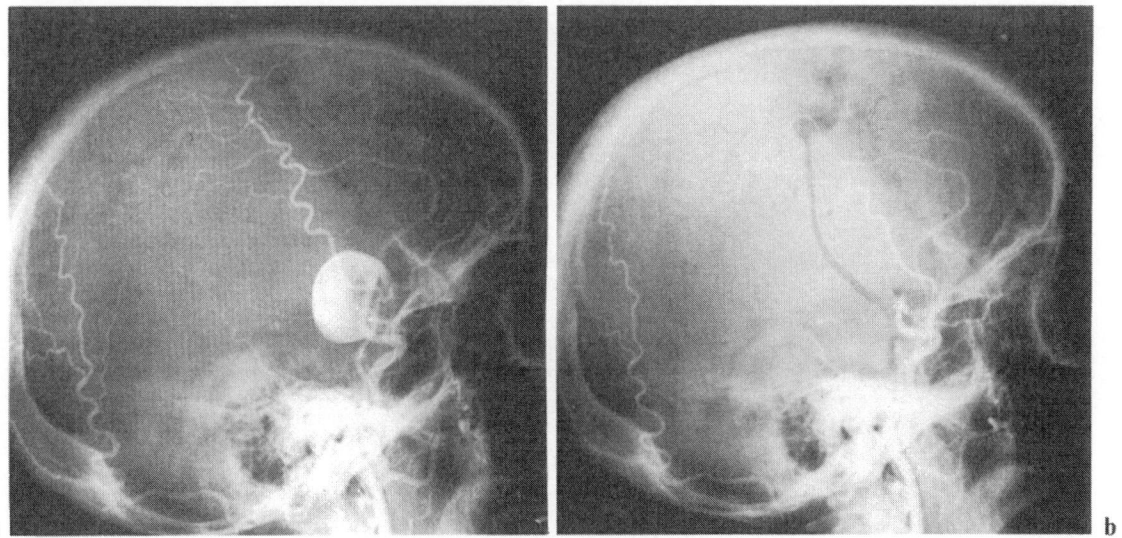

Fig. 2a, b. Case 13. Giant MCA aneurysm on the right side **a** before and **b** after surgery

Postoperative angiogram showed a complete occlusion of the MCA without patency of the anastomosis (Fig. 2b). It is possible that failure of patency of the anastomosis might have enhanced ischemic brain swelling and resulted in poor outcome in this case.

Case 5. This 70-year-old woman was referred for evaluation of progressive loss of vision and ocular nerve palsies in the left eye related to a giant aneurysm of the left infraclinoid ICA (Fig. 3a). For this patient, intramural thrombosis, using copper wire, was employed under monitoring of intraoperative angiogram. A left

frontotemporal craniotomy was performed, exposing the intracranial carotid bifurcation. Intramural thrombosis of the aneurysm was completely achieved, but the parent ICA was also occluded during operation by the progression of the thrombosis. EC-IC bypass was then performed. Postoperatively, she continued to be hemiparetic and eye signs on the left side was worsened. Postoperative angiogram showed complete occlusion of the left ICA (Fig. 3b). More careful control of the amount of wire used for thrombosis might have prevent the occlusion of the parent artery in this case, although an

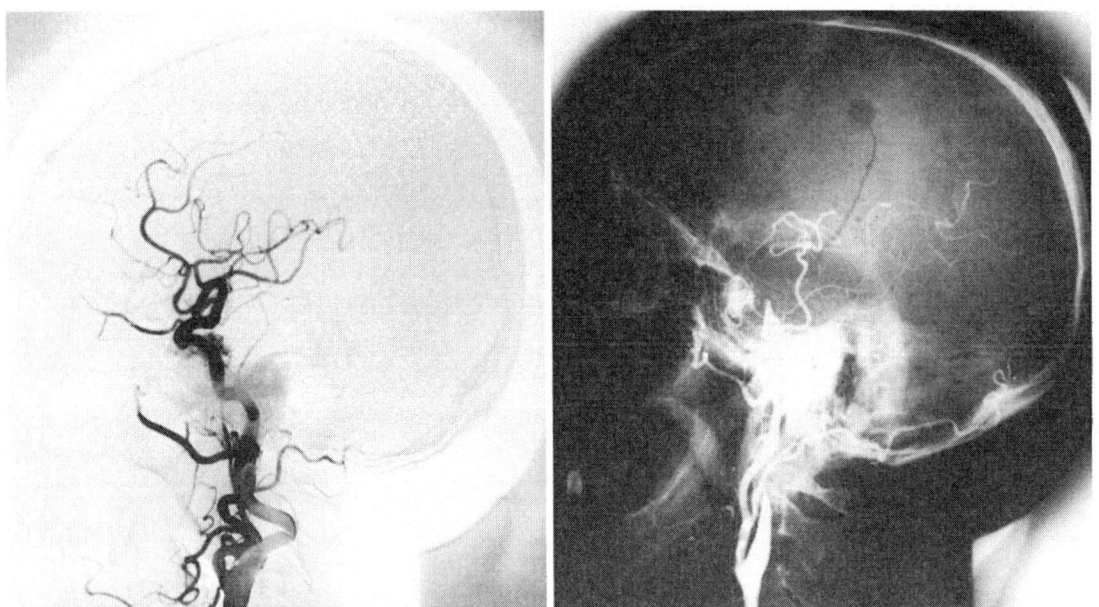

a   b

Fig. 3a, b. Case 5. Giant aneurysm of the left infracliroid ICA **a** before and **b** after surgery

Table 3. Cases of Failed Aneurysm Surgery

Case No.	Age (yrs)	Sex	Location of aneurysm	Types of treatment	Causes of poor result
5	70	F	lt ICA (infraclinoid)	Electrothrombosis	Occlusion of parent artery
9	76	F	lt ICA (supraclinoid)	Multiple clipping	Stenosis of parent artery
12	50	M	lt MCA	Single clipping	Stenosis of parent artery
13	51	F	lt MCA	Excision of aneurysm and end-to-end anastomosis	Failure of patency

intraoperative angiogram was used to evaluate the extent and progression of intramural thrombosis.

The surgical results in this series indicated four patients of poor outcome, including the last two patients. The main cause of poor results were stenosis or occlusion of the parent arteries irrespective of the types of surgical treatment and location of the aneurysms (Table 3).

Discussion and Conclusion

In the surgical management of giant intracranial aneurysms, size, location, and involvement of adjacent structures may be the main determinative factors in deciding the treatment of choice [1, 2, 6]. Many direct or indirect surgical methods

have been reported [1–6]. No matter what method is selected, serious complications sometimes ensue [2]. The present study with a small number of patients indicated that the causes of poor results were ischemic complications and damage to the adjacent structures. Therefore, selection of a suitable clip, its careful application to avoid parent artery stenosis, and careful manipulation to prevent damage of the neighboring structures are mandatory in direct clipping for giant cerebral aneurysms [2, 5, 6]. Even if an indirect method, such as electrothrombosis is employed, patency of the parent artery is most closely related to the postoperative morbidity. Excision of the aneurysm and reconstruction of the parent artery is one of the possible surgical procedures in the selected patients [4].

References

1. Drake CG (1979) Giant intracranial aneurysms: Experience with surgical treatment in 174 patients. Clin Neurosurg 26:12–96
2. Heros RC, Nelson PB, Ojemann RG, Growell RM, Debrun G (1983) Large and giant paraclinoid aneurysms: Surgical techniques, complications, and results. Neurosurgery 12:153–163
3. Hosobuchi Y (1979) Direct surgical treatment of giant intracranial aneurysms. J Neurosurg 51:743–756
4. Smith RR, Parent AD (1982) End-to-end anastomosis of the anterior cerebral artery after excision of a giant aneurysm. J Neurosurg 56:577–580
5. Sugita K, Kobayashi S, Kyoshima K, Nakagawa F (1982) Fenestrated clips for unusual aneurysms of the carotid artery. J Neurosurg 57:240–246
6. Sundt TM, Piepgras DG (1979) Surgical approach to giant intracranial aneurysms: Operative experience with 80 cases. J Neurosurg 51:731–742

Sequential Imaging of Giant IC Aneurysm Following IC Ligation Combined with EC/IC Bypass

Kouzo Moritake[1], Yasuhiro Yonekawa[2], Shiro Nagasawa[1], Hirokazu Ohtsuki[1], Haruhiko Kikuchi[1], Ichiro Fujisawa[1], and Shunsuke Minami[1]

A number of reports have suggested that giant aneurysms of the internal carotid artery can be treated by extracranial-intracranial (EC-IC) bypass and subsequent ligation of the internal carotid artery (IC) with little morbidity [5, 6, 8–11]. Some literature, however, stresses the risk of ischemic complications related to carotid ligation [2, 9]. The purpose of this study is to confirm the effect of this approach and to explore the cause of ischemic complications encountered during or after carotid occlusion by sequential computerized tomography (CT) and magnetic resonance imaging (MRI).

Materials and Method

Fifteen patients were treated for giant aneurysms by IC ligation combined with EC-IC bypass. In all except one patient, who underwent external carotid-middle cerebral artery bypass with the use of a saphenous vein graft, STA-MCA bypass was adopted as an EC-IC bypass. The internal carotid artery was occluded abruptly in eight patients and gradually in seven.

In all of the patients, preoperative and postoperative serial CT studies were performed in order to assess the effect of this combined surgical procedure and to know the fates of the aneurysms after carotid occlusion. In the four most recent cases, MRI was also taken sequentially.

Results

The formation of an intra-aneurysmal thrombus was revealed as a marked increase in density on a plain CT (Fig. 1). This phenomenon could be detected within 2 weeks after IC ligation. A subsequent CT study demonstrated an organization process of intraaneurysmal thrombus, i.e., heterogenous enhancement followed by ring enhancement by contrast material infusion. Further CT study revealed loss of enhancement and a diminution of the size of the aneurysm (Fig. 1).

Figure 2 shows the sequential MRI of a patient treated by this method. On a preoperative MRI, a paraclinoid aneurysm is delineated clearly, as is its relationship to the surrounding structures, such as cavernous sinus, basal cistern, and brain tissue. Most of the aneurysmal lumen was demonstrated as no signal area. Irregular small areas of positive intensity were seen in the thrombosed lumen of the aneurysm, which seemed to reveal turbulence or stasis of blood flow. In an MRI taken 2.5 months after the operation, the aneurysmal lumen was visualized as a low-signal intensity area. The aneurysm shrank remarkably in the 13 months postoperatively.

Figure 3 shows MRIs taken serially in another patient. Two weeks after IC ligation, the aneurysmal lumen was demonstrated as an isointensity mass with peripheral hyperintensity [7]. An MRI taken 5.5 months after IC ligation demonstrated spotty no-signal areas in the thrombus. Sixteen months after occlusion of the IC artery, the aneurysmal lumen became lower and more homogenous in intensity. Spotty areas of no signal intensity disappeared at this stage and the aneurysm shrank remarkably.

Although all patients treated by this method showed excellent or good clinical outcome, 7 of 15 patients developed ischemic complications at early or late postoperative stage. All complications were considered to be related to the brain ischemia caused by carotid ligation; they were all transient. The rate of ischemic complications was much higher in patients who underwent gradual occlusion of the internal carotid artery than in those who underwent abrupt occlusion.

[1] Department of Neurosurgery and Neuroradiology, Kyoto University Medical School Kyoto, Japan
[2] Department of Neurosurgery, National Cardiovascular Center, Suita, Japan

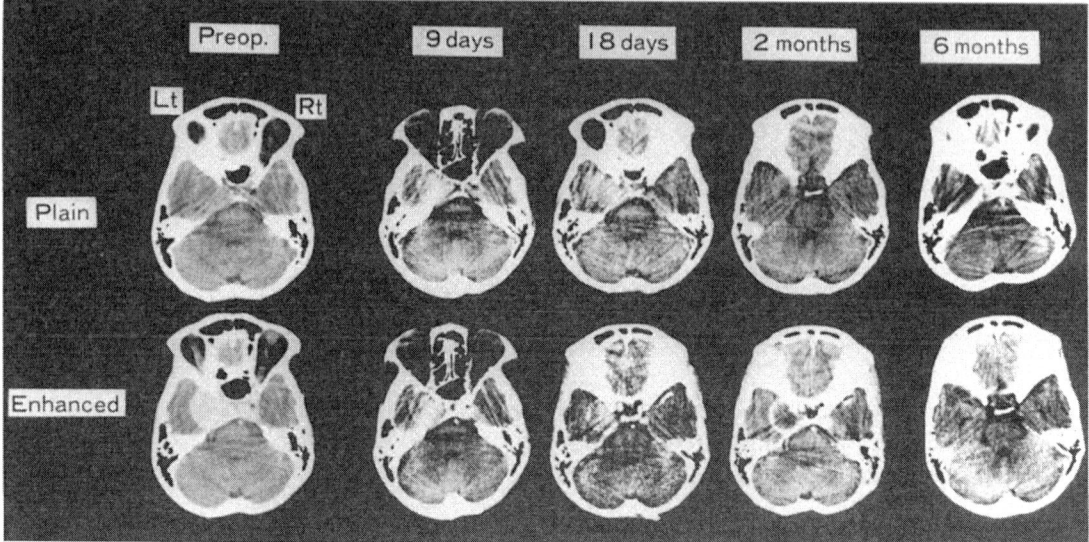

Fig. 1. A 70-year-old female. Giant aneurysm at the cavernous portion of the left internal carotid artery. Preoperative and postoperative serial CT

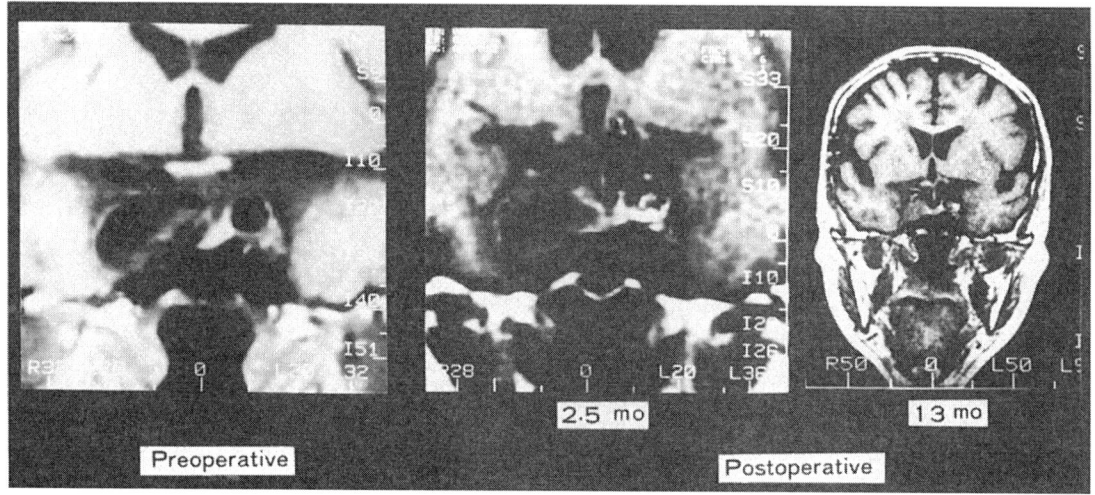

Fig. 2. A 69-year-old female. Giant aneurysm at the cavernous portion of the right internal carotid artery. Preoperative and postoperative serial MRI, T_1-weighted image

Discussion

Sequential CT scans are useful for observing the fate of the giant aneurysm after carotid ligation and for evaluating the effectiveness of therapy [2, 5, 6]. However, a newly developed diagnostic tool, MRI, is able to delineate aneurysms more clearly and depict their relations to the surrounding structures, such as cavernous sinus, basal cistern, and brain tissue, in more detail than the CT [1, 3, 4, 7]. In addition, MRI offers information regarding intravascular and intra-aneurysmal flow states, such as the presence of thrombus or flow pattern, by using flow-related effects as signals [1]. Most aneurysmal lumen were demonstrated as no signal areas by flow-void phenomenon on MRI. Irregular small areas of positive intensity in the aneurysm seem to express turbulent flow or stasis which is demonstrable on angiography and relatively specific to giant aneurysms. Spotty, no signal areas were observed in intraaneurysmal thrombi 2–16 months after internal carotid ligation. They are considered to be the recanalization channels in the thrombi.

It is of great interest that these complica-

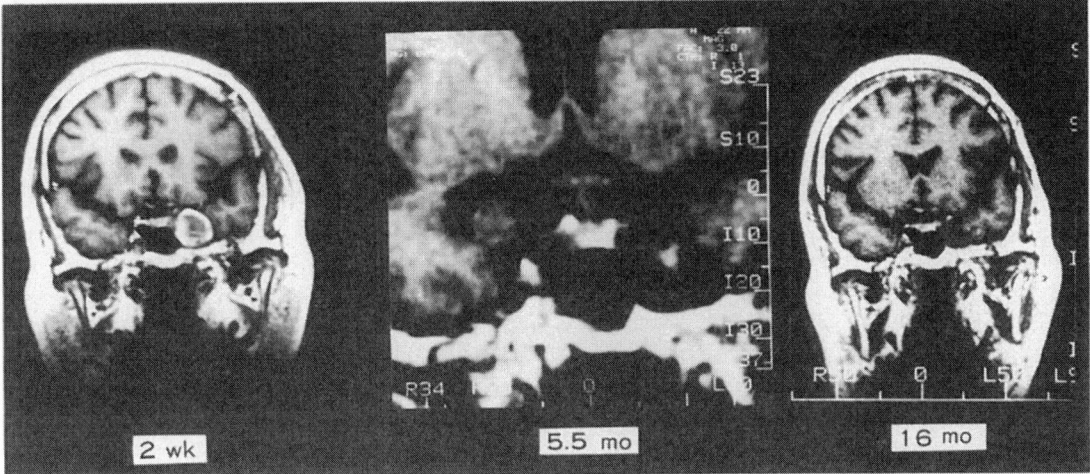

Fig. 3. A 64-year-old female. Giant aneurysm at the cavernous portion of the left internal carotid artery. Postoperative serial MRI, T_1-weighted image

tions occurred either when thrombi formed in aneurysms or when aneurysms shrank. These findings suggest that the ischemic complications after internal carotid ligation are not hemodynamic, but thromboembolic in origin [2, 8]. Namely, ischemic complications after IC ligation are considered to be caused by either primary thrombosis of the aneurysmal lumen or secondary occlusion of recanalized channels in the thrombus. Since both processes are considered to be necessary to cure the aneurysm, postoperative ischemic complications might be inevitable in the treatment of giant aneurysm by this method.

As these complications were transient in any patient, this combined operation seems to be a safe and effective method for the treatment of inaccessible giant aneurysms of the internal carotid artery.

References

1. Crooks LE, Mills CM, Davis PL, Hoenninger J, Arakawa M, Watts J, Kaufman L (1982) Visualization of cerebral and vascular abnormalities by NMR imaging. The effects of imaging parameters on contrast. Radiology 144:843–852
2. Diaz FG, Ausman JI, Pearce JE (1982) Ischemic complications after combined internal carotid artery occlusion and extracranial-intracranial anastomosis. Neurosurgery 10:563–570
3. Edelman RR, Johnson K, Buxton R, Shoukimas G, Rosen BR, Davis KR, Brady TJ (1986) MR of hemorrhage: A new approach. AJNR 7:751–756
4. Eller TW (1986) MRI demonstration of clot in a small unruptured aneurysm causing stroke. J Neurosurg 65:411–412
5. Fujiwara S, Kodama N, Suzuki J (1982) Sequential CT findings on giant aneurysms of the internal carotid artery after carotid ligation. Neurol Med Chir (Tokyo) 22:267–275
6. Gelber BR, Sundt TM (1980) Treatment of intracavernous and giant carotid aneurysms by combined internal carotid ligation and extra- to intra- cranial bypass. J Neurosurg 52:1–10
7. Gomori JM, Grossman RI, Goldberg HI, Zimmerman RA, Bilaniuk LT (1985) Intracranial hematomas: Imaging by high-field MR. Neuroradiology 157:87–93
8. Heros RC, Nelson PB, Ojemann RG, Crowell RM, DeBrun G (1983) Large and giant paraclinoid aneurysms: Surgical techniques, complications, and results. Neurosurgery 12:153–163
9. Mitsugi T, Kikuchi H, Karasawa J, Itoh K, Takahashi N (1982) Surgical treatment of carotid-siphon aneurysms. Neurol Med Chir (Tokyo) 22:513–520
10. Moritake K, Handa H, Yonekawa Y, Taki W, Takebe Y, Konishi T (1985) Clinical and hemodynamic assessments of STA-MCA bypass surgery in 10 patients with giant aneurysm of an internal carotid artery. In: Handa H, Kikuchi H, Yonekawa Y (eds) Microsurgical Anastomoses for Cerebral Ischemia. Igaku-Shoin, Tokyo; pp 127–129
11. Spetzler RF, Carter LP (1985) Revascularization and aneurysm sugery: Current status. Neurosurgery 16:111–116

Clinical Aspects of Endovascular Treatment of Cerebral Aneurysms

Makoto Negoro[1], Keiichi Terashima[1], Tiaming Wang[1], Tsuneo Ishiguchi[2], and Sadayuki Sakuma[2]

Recently, it has been widely accepted that the cerebral aneurysm, ruptured or unruptured, should be treated microsurgically. However, this does not always hold true when treating giant aneurysms. In Drake's series, 62% of giant aneurysm cases couldn't be clipped by usual microsurgical methods [3]. Several attempts had been made to improve these figures, including the direct injection of a thrombotic agent into the aneurysmal sac, or electrothrombosis of the aneurysm. Recent advances in the supercatheterization technique with the detachable balloon makes it possible to cannulate the narrow intracranial arteries [5]. Here we report our current approach toward the cerebral giant aneurysm with the detachable balloon technique.

Clinical Material

Since 1981, at Nagoya University Hospital, 12 patients with giant intracavernous aneurysms have been treated by the detachable balloon technique. All patients presented with cavernous syndromes, such as third or sixth cranial nerve palsies. None of them had any intracranial bleeding episodes.

Therapeutic Measure

A latex detachable balloon catheter (Debrun type) was placed through an introducing sheath in the carotid artery. Under fluoroscopic control, the balloon was navigated into the aneurysmal orifice or within aneurysmal sac. If the balloon occluded the aneurysmal cavity completely, it was detached. If not, the internal carotid artery itself was occluded. In this situation, the patient's tolerance to ischemia had to be determined prior to the permanent occlusion of the internal carotid artery. The test occlusion of the internal carotid artery was carried out with the inflating balloon. The patient was carefully monitored for any neurological signs during 20 min of occlusion. If the occlusion was well tolerated, the balloon was detached and the internal carotid artery was occluded permanently. If not tolerated, the balloon was deflated and the catheter was withdrawn. During these procedures, the patient was kept in systemic heparinization and blood pressure was maintained at the same level.

Postprocedure Follow-Up

All patients were followed by digital subtraction angiography at 6 months and 1 year after the procedure.

Operative Results

The results of the intracavernous aneurysm treatment by balloon are summarized in Table 1. The occlusion of the aneurysmal sac was attempted in three cases and failed in all of them due to technical reasons. The permanent occlusion of the internal carotid artery was accomplished in seven cases, followed by the complete obliteration of aneurysm. After the procedure, two patients developed cerebral complications. One patient demonstrated transient hemiparesis at 24 h after the occlusion, and recovered fully with volume expansion therapy. Another pa-

Table 1. ICA occlusion in cavernous aneurysm

	No. of cases
Permanent	7
Transient	2
Attempted	3
Total	12

Department of Neurosurgery[1], Department of Radiology[2], Nagoya University School of Medicine, Nagoya, Japan

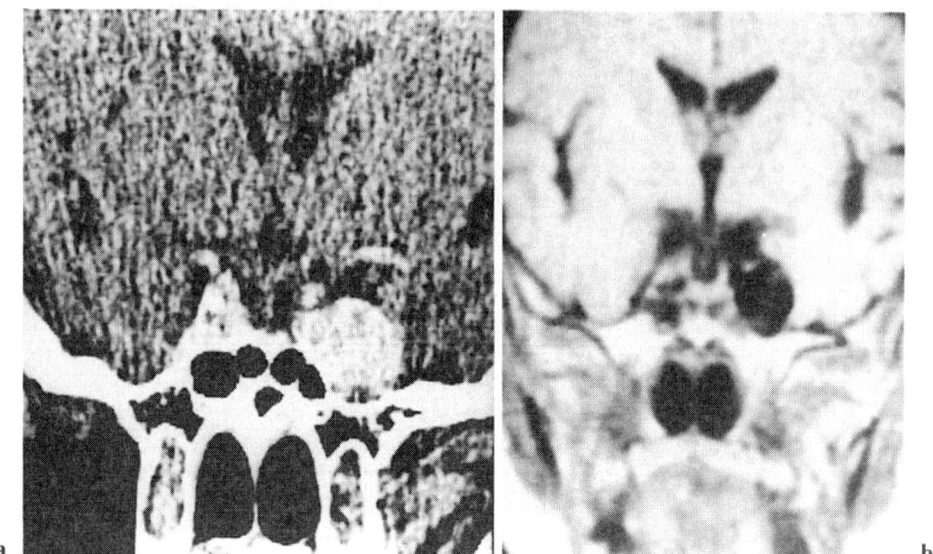

Fig. 1. a CECT scan showing parasellar mass on the left side. **b** MRI-demonstrated low intensity signal within the parasellar mass

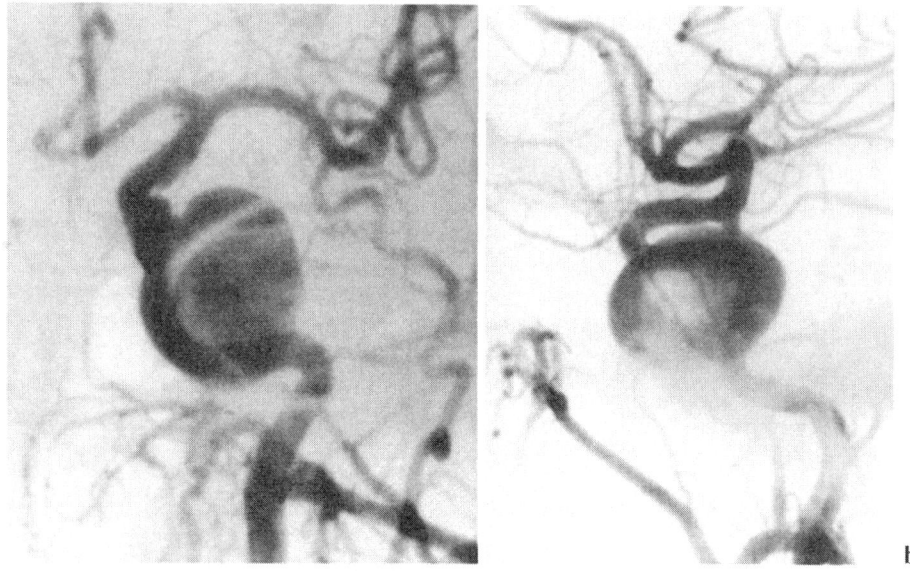

Fig. 2a, b. Cerebral angiogram revealing the giant aneurysm at the cavernous portion of the left internal carotid artery. **a** A-P view. **b** Lateral view

tient, who had EC-IC bypass, developed ischemic symptoms within several hours after the procedure. CT scan showed hemorrhagic infarction at the occluded side. The patient improved slowly, but had significant neurological deficit. Follow-up study revealed aneurysmal occlusions in these treated cases. No change was observed in untreated cases.

Case Presentation

A 51-year-old female developed left abducens nerve palsy several months prior to admission. CT scan demonstrated a parasellar mass (Fig. 1). Cerebral angiography confirmed the presence of a giant intracavernous aneurysm on the left side (Fig. 2). The endovascular occlusion of the left

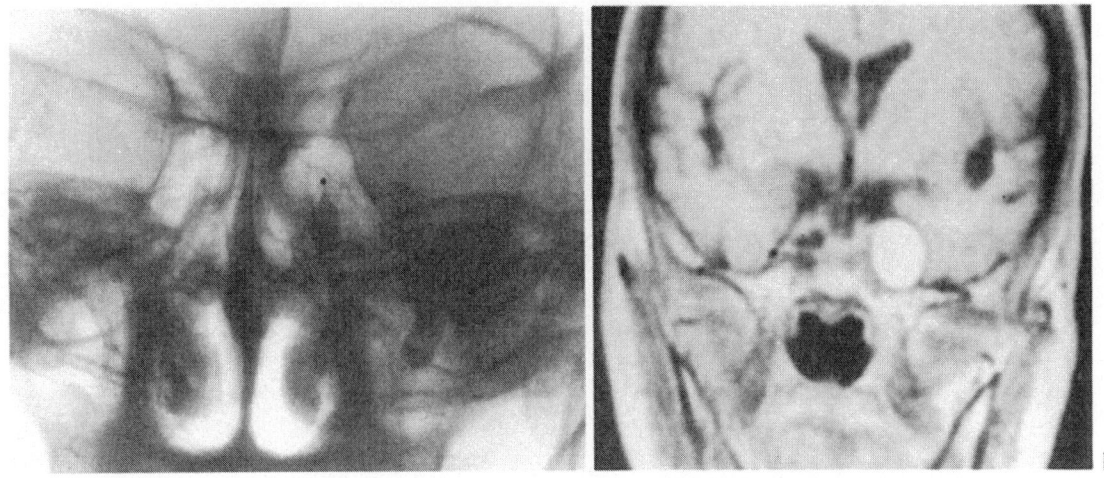

Fig. 3. a Plain craniogram revealing the two detached balloons in the left internal carotid artery. **b** MRI (1 month after the operation) showing the definite change of the signal within the mass, suggesting thrombosis

internal carotid artery was carried out with two, contrast media-filled balloons (Fig. 3a). Magnetic resonance imaging at 1 month after the occlusion revealed the thrombosed aneurysm (Fig. 3b). Her symptoms gradually improved during a 1-year period

Discussion

The endovascular treatment proves to be useful in treating cerebral vascular lesions, but there is still sceptism about the application of this method for cerebral aneurysms. At this point, this treatment is restricted mostly to inoperable cases.

In dealing with those unclippable aneurysms, two methods of endovascular treatment were proposed. One is the proximal occlusion of the parent artery [1, 2, 4, 6, 7], and the other is the aneurysmal sac occlusion [7]. The latter seems to be rational because of the preservation of the parent artery. However, ischemic symptoms occurred more frequently in the saccular occlusion cases [2, 4]. Also, several postoperative bleedings were reported in this method.

Parent artery occlusion is safer and easy to perform. Nevertheless, cerebral ischemia will follow this type of occlusion. According to our experience, 20 min of occlusion is the best way to determine the tolerance to cerebral ischemia. If tolerated well, the parent artery will be occluded without any sequelae. If not, a saccular occlusion or bypass will be required.

Conclusion

The detachable balloon occlusion technique is one of the most important therapeutic measures in dealing with giant unclippable aneurysms. For the moment, the parent artery occlusion is the best method of treatment.

References

1. Berenstein A, Ransohoff J, Kupersmith M (1984) Transvascular treatment of giant aneurysms of cavernous carotid and vertebral arteries. Surg Neurol 21:3–12
2. Debrun G, Fox A, Drake C, et al. (1980) Giant unclippable aneurysms: Treatment with detachable balloons. AJNR 2:167–173
3. Drake C (1979) Giant intracranial aneurysms: Experience with surgical treatment in 174 patients. Clin Neurosurg 26:12–95
4. Fox A, Vinuela F, Pelz D, et al. (1987) Use of detachable balloons for proximal artery occlusion in the treatment of unclippable cerebral aneurysms. J Neurosurg 66:40–46
5. Negoro M, Kageyama N, Ishiguchi T (1983) Cerebrovascular occlusion by catheterization and embolization: Clinical experience. AJNR 4:362–365
6. Raymond J, Theron J (1986) Intracavernous aneurysms: Treatment by proximal balloon occlusion of the internal carotid artery. AJNR 7:587–593
7. Romadanov AP, Scheglov VI (1982) Intravascular occlusion of saccular aneurysms of the cerebral arteries by means of a detachable balloon catheter. In: Krayenbühl H (ed) Advances and technical standards in neurosurgery, vol. 9. Springer, Vienna, pp 25–49

Author Index

Subject Index